Textbook of

Respiratory and Critical Care Infections

Textbook of

Respiratory and Critical Care Infections

Francesco Blasi MD PhD
Professor of Respiratory Medicine
Department of Pathophysiology and Transplantation
University of Milan, Fondazione IRCCS Cà Granda-Ospedale Maggiore Policlinico
Milan, Italy

George Dimopoulos MD PhD FCCP
Associate Professor
Department of Critical Care Medicine, University Hospital Attikon
Medical School Univeristy of Athens
Athens, Greece

JAYPEE *The Health Sciences Publishers*
New Delhi | London | Philadelphia | Panama

Jaypee Brothers Medical Publishers (P) Ltd

Headquarters

Jaypee Brothers Medical Publishers (P) Ltd
4838/24, Ansari Road, Daryaganj
New Delhi 110 002, India
Phone: +91-11-43574357
Fax: +91-11-43574314
Email: jaypee@jaypeebrothers.com

Overseas Offices

J.P. Medical Ltd
83 Victoria Street, London
SW1H 0HW (UK)
Phone: +44 20 3170 8910
Fax: +44 (0)20 3008 6180
Email: info@jpmedpub.com

Jaypee Medical Inc
The Bourse
111 South Independence Mall East
Suite 835, Philadelphia, PA 19106, USA
Phone: +1 267-519-9789
Email: jpmed.us@gmail.com

Jaypee Brothers Medical Publishers (P) Ltd
Bhotahity, Kathmandu, Nepal
Phone: +977-9741283608
Email: kathmandu@jaypeebrothers.com

Jaypee-Highlights Medical Publishers Inc
City of Knowledge, Bld. 237, Clayton
Panama City, Panama
Phone: +1 507-301-0496
Fax: +1 507-301-0499
Email: cservice@jphmedical.com

Jaypee Brothers Medical Publishers (P) Ltd
17/1-B Babar Road, Block-B, Shaymali
Mohammadpur, Dhaka-1207
Bangladesh
Mobile: +08801912003485
Email: jaypeedhaka@gmail.com

Website: www.jaypeebrothers.com
Website: www.jaypeedigital.com

Inquiries for bulk sales may be solicited at: jaypee@jaypeebrothers.com

Textbook of Respiratory and Critical Care Infections

First Edition: **2015**

ISBN: 978-93-5090-298-1

Printed at: Ajanta Offset & Packagings Ltd., New Delhi

Dedications

To my beloved wife Brunella from the bottom of my heart for supporting me each and every day with love and patience

Francesco Blasi

To Deppy and Efi, my family, who endured the many long hours her husband and daddy spent at home uncommunicative, with stoic patience

George Dimopoulos

Contents

Contributors

EDITORS

Francesco Blasi MD PhD
Professor of Respiratory Medicine
Department of Pathophysiology and Transplantation
University of Milan, Fondazione IRCCS Cà Granda-Ospedale Maggiore Policlinico
Milan, Italy

George Dimopoulos MD PhD FCCP
Associate Professor
Department of Critical Care Medicine
University Hospital Attikon
Medical School Univeristy of Athens
Athens, Greece

CONTRIBUTING AUTHORS

Rosanel Amaro MD
Department of Pulmonary and Critical Care Medicine
Hospital Clinic of Barcelona
Barcelona, Spain

Ronald Anderson PhD
Research Professor
Department of Medical Immunology
Faculty of Health Sciences, University of Pretoria
Pretoria, South Africa

Stavros Anevlavis MD PhD
Senior Lecturer of Pneumonology
Democritus University of Thrace
University Hospital of Alexandroupolis
Alexandroupolis, Greece

Apostolos D Armaganidis MD PhD
Professor
Department of Critical Care Medicine
University Hospital Attikon
Medical School Univeristy of Athens
Athens, Greece

Baroukh M Assael MD PhD
Cystic Fibrosis Center
Azienda Ospedaliera-Universitaria di Veron
Verona, Italy

Ilias Athanasiadis MD
Consultant
Mitera Hospital
Athens, Greece

Gianluigi L Bassi MD PhD
Division of Animal Experimentation
Department of Pulmonary and Critical Care Medicine
Hospital Clinic of Barcelona, Barcelona Spain
Centro de Investigación Biomédica en Red de Enfermedades Respiratorias
Mallorca, Spain

Robert P Baughman MD
Professor
Department of Medicine, University of Cincinnati
Cincinnati, Ohio, USA

Stijn I Blot MNSc PhD
Department of Internal Medicine
Faculty of Medicine and Health Sciences, Ghent University Hospital
Ghent, Belgium

Demosthenes Bouros MD PhD FCCP
Professor of Pneumonology
Democritus University of Thrace and
University Hospital of Alexandroupolis
Alexandroupolis, Greece

Ruth Carrico PhD RN FSHEA CIC
Associate Professor of Medicine
Division of Infectious Diseases
University of Louisville
Louisville, Kentucky, USA

Carolina de la Cuesta MD
Attending Physician
Department of Critical Care Medicine
Mount Sinai Medical Center
Miami, Florida, USA

Juan M del Rio MD
Fellow
Division of Pulmonary and Critical Care Medicine
University of Miami Miller School of Medicine
Miami, Florida, USA

Santiago Ewig PhD MD
Head, Deapartmen of Respiratory and Infectious Diseases
Thoraxzentrum Ruhrgebiet
Kliniken für Pneumologie und Infektiologie
Bochum, Germany

Charles Feldman MBBCh DSc PhD FRCP FCP
Professor
Division of Pulmonology
Department of Internal Medicine
Charlotte Maxeke Johannesburg Academic Hospital
University of the Witwatersrand
Johannesburg, South Africa

Miquel Ferrer MD PhD
Department of Pneumology
Thorax Institute, Hospital Clinic of Barcelona
Barcelona, Spain

Mina Gaga MD PhD
Director
7th Respiratory Medicine Department and Asthma Center
Medical Director, Athens Chest Hospital
Athens, Greece

Evangelos J Giamarellos-Bourboulis MD PhD
4th Department of Internal Medicine
University of Athens Medical School, Athens, Greece
Center for Sepsis Control and Care
Jena University Hospital
Jena, Germany

Helen Giamarellou MD PhD
Professor and Head
6th Department of Internal Medicine and
Infectious Diseases Research Lab
Hygeia General Hospital
Athens, Greece

Theoplasti Grigoratou MD
7th Respiratory Medicine Department and Asthma Center
Athens Chest Hospital
Athens, Greece

M Jawad Habib

Lisa A Haglund MD
Associate Professor of Medicine
University of Cincinnati Medical Center
Cincinnati, Ohio, USA

Irene D Karampela MD
Pulmonary and Critical Care Consultant
Department of Critical Care Medicine
University Hospital Attikon
Medical School University of Athens
Athens, Greece

Daniel H Kett MD
Professor of Clinical Medicine
Division of Pulmonary and Critical Care Medicine
University of Miami Miller School of Medicine
Miami, Florida, USA

Benjamin Klapdor MD PhD
Thoraxzentrum Ruhrgebiet
Kliniken für Pneumologie und Infektiologie
Evangelisches Krankenhaus Herne und
Augusta-Kranken-Anstalt Bochum
Bochum, Germany

Petros Kopterides MD
2nd Department of Critical Care Medicine
University Hospital Attikon
Medical School-National and Kapodistrian University of Athens
Athens, Greece

Anastasia Kotanidou MD PhD
Associate Professor
1st Department of Critical Care Medicine and Pulmonary Services
Medical School of Athens University
Evangelismos Hospital
Athens, Greece

Despoina Koulenti MD PhD
Internal Medicine-Intensivist
Department of Critical Care
University Hospital Attikon
Athens, Greece

Georgios Kouliatsis MD
Intensivist, Pulmonologist
Department of Intensive Care Unit
University General Hospital of Alexandroupolis
Alexandroupolis, Greece

Sonia O Labeau MNSc
Faculty of Healthcare Vesalius
University College Ghent
Faculty of Medicine and Health Sciences
Ghent University
Ghent, Belgium

Adamantia Liapikou MD PhD
Consultant
6th Respiratory Medicine
Sotiria Chest Diseases Hospital
Athens, Greece

Alejandra López-Giraldo MD
Department of Pneumology
Thorax Institute
Hospital Clinic of Barcelona
Barcelona, Spain

Nikolaos A Maniatis MD
Assistant Professor
2nd Department of Critical Care Medicine
Medical School of Athens University
Attikon Hospital
Athens, Greece

Ioannis Mastoris
Associate Physician
4th Department of Internal Medicine
University of Athens Medical School
Athens, Greece

Zinka Matkovic MD
Staff Physician
Department for Pulmonary Diseases
Dubrava University Hospital
Zagreb, Croatia

Dimitrios K Matthaiou MD PhD
Internal Medicine-Intensivist
Department of Critical Care
University Hospital Attikon
Athens, Greece

Giovanni B Migliori MD FRCP
WHO Collaborating Centre for TB and Lung Diseases
Fondazione S. Maugeri
Care and Research Institute
Tradate, Italy

Marc Miravitlles MD PhD
Department of Pneumology
Institut d'Investigacions Biomèdiques August Pi i Sunyer
Hospital Clinic of Barcelona
Barcelona, Spain

Gautham Mogilishetty MD
Associate Professor of Medicine
Director of Kidney Transplantation
University of Cincinnati
Cincinnati, Ohio, USA

Muthiah P Muthiah MD FCCP
Division of Pulmonary, Critical Care, and Sleep Medicine
University of Tennessee College of Medicine (MPM and MJH)
Memphis, Tennessee, USA

Nikitas Nikitas MD
2nd Department of Critical Care Medicine
University Hospital Attikon
Medical School-National and Kapodistrian University of Athens
Athens, Greece

Ioanna Nikitopoulou PhD
Research Fellow
1st Department of Critical Care Medicine and Pulmonary Services
GP Livanos and M Simou Laboratories
Medical School of Athens University
Evangelismos Hospital
Athens, Greece

Stylianos E Orfanos MD
Associate Professor
2nd Department of Critical Care
Medical School of Athens University
Attikon Hospital
Athens, Greece

Vasileios Papaioannou MD MSc PhD
Assistant Professor of Intensive Care Medicine
Democritus University of Thrace
Alexandroupolis Hospital
Alexandroupolis, Greece

Maria Pappalettera MD PhD
Fondazione Ospedale Maggiore Cà Granda IRCCS
Dipartimento Fisiopatologia Medico-Chirurgica e dei Trapianti
Università degli Studi di Milano
Padiglione L. Sacco, U.O Broncopneumologia
Milan, Italy

Angelos Pefanis MD PhD
Chief Coordinator
Department of Internal Medicine
"Sotiria" General and Chest Diseases Hospital
Athens, Greece

Tatjana Peroš-Golubičić MD PhD
Professor of Medicine
University Hospital for Lung Disease
University of Zagreb
Zagreb, Croatia

Paula Peyrani MD
Instructor of Medicine
Division of Infectious Diseases
University of Louisville
Louisville, Kentucky, USA

Federico Piffer MD PhD
Fondazione Ospedale Maggiore Cà Granda IRCCS
Dipartimento Fisiopatologia Medico-Chirurgica e dei Trapianti
Università degli Studi di Milano
Padiglione L. Sacco, U.O Broncopneumologia
Milan, Italy

Ioannis Pneumatikos MD PhD FCCP
Professor
Department of Intensive Care Medicine
Democritus University of Thrace
Alexandroupolis Hospital
Alexandroupoli, Greece

Garyphallia Poulakou MD PhD
4th Department of Internal Medicine
University Hospital Attikon
University of Athens Medical School
Athens, Greece

Julio A Ramirez MD FACP
Professor of Medicine
Chief, Division of Infectious Diseases
University of Louisville
Louisville, Kentucky, USA

Gernot GU Rohde MD PhD
Associate Professor
Department of Respiratory Medicine
Maastricht University Medical Center
Maastricht, The Netherlands

Francesco Scaglione MD PhD
Clinical Pharmacologist
Department of Medical Biotechnology and Translational Medicine
University of Milan
Milan, Italy

***Late* Om P Sharma** MD FCCP Master FRCP
Former Professor of Medicine
Division of Pulmonary and Critical Care Medicine
Keck School of Medicine, University of Southern California
Los Angeles, California, USA

Natalie J Slowik MD
Associate Clinical Professor
Department of Medicine
Keck Medical Center - University of Southern California
Los Angeles, California, USA

Ali E Solh

Giovanni Sotgiu MD PhD
Associate Professor of Medical Statistics
Epidemiology and Medical Statistics Unit
Department of Biomedical Sciences, Sassari University
Sassari, Italy

Paolo Tarsia MD PhD
Fondazione Ospedale Maggiore Cà Granda IRCCS
Dipartimento Fisiopatologia Medico-Chirurgica e dei Trapianti
Università degli Studi di Milano
Padiglione L. Sacco, U.O Broncopneumologia
Milan, Italy

Jasna Tekavec-Trkanjec MD PhD
Consultant Pulmonologist
Department for Internal Medicine
Dubrava University Hospital
Zagreb, Croatia

Athanasios Thomopoulos MD
Respiratory Medicine Departmet and Asthma Center
Athens Chest Hospital
Athens, Greece

Antoni Torres PhD MD
Professor
Head of Intensive Care Unit
Department of Pneumology
Clinic Institute of Thorax, Hospital Clinic of Barcelona
Barcelona, Spain

Sotirios Tsiodras MD PhD
Associate Professor of Internal Medicine and Infectious Disease
4th Department of Internal Medicine
University of Athens Medical School
Athens, Greece

Koenraad Vandewoude MD PhD
Faculty of Medicine and Health Sciences
Department of Internal Medicine
Ghent University
Ghent, Belgium

Timothy L Wiemken PhD MPH
Assistant Professor of Medicine
Division of Infectious Diseases
Department of Medicine
University of Louisville School of Medicine
Louisville, Kentucky, USA

Eleftherios Zervas MD
Consultant
7th Respiratory Medicine Department
"Sotiria" Athens Chest Disease Hospital
Athens, Greece

Preface

Respiratory and nosocomial (mainly in the Intensive Care setting) infections and their complications, reflect a major cause of morbitity and mortality. During the last four decades, major advances in the field of infectious diseases have been scored: new pathological entities have been well described (i.e., legionellosis, human immunodeficiency virus infection, Lyme disease, severe acute respiratory syndrome, flu due to H1N1 virus, etc), new drugs were included worldwide in the therapeutic armamentarium, and new mechanisms of resistance to antimicrobials were identified while advances in genomics led to fast and breakthrough therapies. All these efforts targeted the accurate diagnosis and the prevention of infections, the early administration of adequate and appropriate treatment, the infection control and the reduction of antibacterial resistance, and parameters which have been shown to be important of patients' outcome.

The present edition has been planned and designed according to the requirements of the physician who is dealing with respiratory and critical care infections, especially for the critical care practitioners who frequently are the initial providers of care to patients with infections. All the chapter include information from the 2013–2014 literature with table and figures, allowing readers to find help rapidly in the management of their patients. A group of well known international authors has been brought together to address these topics.

The extremely professional work of Jaypee Brothers editions strengthened our efforts and is our hope that this textbook will provide clinicians a reference to help guide the care of their patients.

Francesco Blasi MD PhD
George Dimopoulos MD PhD FCCP

CHAPTER 1

Genetic Predisposition for Respiratory Infections

Natalie J Slowik, Om P Sharma

ABSTRACT

Respiratory disorders are common worldwide. They are a major cause of morbidity and mortality. For many years we have attempted to delineate the exact causes of numerous respiratory pathologies from tuberculosis and sarcoidosis to cystic fibrosis and leprosy. The question has always been why certain individuals exhibit such severe morbidity from illness while others are only mildly affected. In this chapter, we examine the role of genetics and environment in various respiratory pathologies. We attempt to illustrate the various interactions between the human genome and environmental insults. It is clear that much more research is needed on this subject, since it is evident that one pathway is not responsible for all respiratory pathology. It is the interaction between an individual's genetics and the environment that is at the center of most respiratory pathology. When our understanding depends on why certain individuals are more adversely affected than others, we can begin to target therapies more effectively and someday maybe, impact the overall progression and morbidity of the numerous respiratory pathologies.

INTRODUCTION

Respiratory disorders are common worldwide. Many pulmonary infections are genetic in origin, whereas the others are due to environmental factors. Genetic causes of pulmonary infections can be broadly divided into two groups: monogenic (or Mendelian) and complex (or multifactorial). Monogenic diseases are the result of abnormal mutations in single genes. Such mutations are rare and exert a major effect on the gene. An example of a Mendelian single gene disorder is cystic fibrosis, in which the inheritance pattern is clear. In complex and multifactorial genetic disorders, such as tuberculosis and sarcoidosis, the hereditary outlines are blurred. Our understanding of the genetic mechanisms that participate in causing nature-nurture interactions is limited. The conceptual approaches to environmental genomics were established decades ago, but only recently, we have begun to grasp the complex pathways that form the foundation of the interactions between the genes and the environment.

The human genome is made up of 3.2×10^9 DNA base pairs. There are innumerable variations of the DNA sequence within the human genome. many are changes in a single base pair (or nucleotide). Much of the human genome is made up of inconsequential non-functional genetic chains; as a result, small changes or mutations in these areas have little impact on our overall genetic makeup. Our individual genetic makeup is the consequence of small DNA changes, such as single base pair changes that actually happen to occur in close proximity or in the genes that are functional. These minimal changes result in certain persons being affected by some diseases and responsive to some treatments, while others are not. It also explains, why some individuals experience severe side effects, while others are not affected by the treatment at all.

The mechanism by which such minute changes can have a drastic effect is complex. The functional proteins of the body are created by gene sequencing that result in messenger RNAs and lead to protein synthesis. Proteins have multiple functions, including enzyme activity. Because of this close relationship, a single change in the DNA code in a functional area of the genome can impact the amount, type, and function of the protein produced, if it is produced at all. The above discussed single change in the DNA sequence is called single nucleotide polymorphism (SNP). If this SNP occurs in an important functional area of the genome, it is called as functional SNP. As was briefly mentioned above, this change can be minute, or it may be in such an area so as to alter susceptibility to a disease or the efficacy of a drug. There are many functional polymorphisms and are very common.[1] Garantziotis et al., have recently summarized our knowledge of environmental genomics (gene-environment interactions) involved in the pathogenesis of common nonmalignant respiratory diseases.[2] Emerging data indicate that genetic-based disorders are influenced by the environment, and environment-based disorders are modified by personal genetic factors in individual physiologic responses.[3] Many genetic polymorphisms have been shown to be involved in the genetic variance seen amongst individuals when it comes to the susceptibility to acute pulmonary infections, tuberculous as well as nontuberculous. Unfortunately, except for some polymorphisms in mannose-binding lectin, CD14 and the IgG2 receptor, there is no definite theory as to which polymorphisms are important. Waterer et al. have suggested to continue research in this field.[4]

TLR-NF-κB Signaling

Toll-like receptors (TLR) and members of their intracellular signaling pathway play a critical role in the early recognition of invading microorganisms and initiating an inflammatory host response. Despite considerable research, the TLR-nuclear factor-kappa B (TLR-NF-κB) pathway is not completely understood. There are four main components of the TLR-NF-κB pathway:

- TLRs are activating receptors that sense different microbial products
- Protein adaptors [such as myeloid differentiation primary response gene (88) (MyD88) and MyD88 adapter-like/TIR domain containing adapter protein (Mal/TIRAP)]
- Kinases [the interleukin-1 receptor associated kinases (IRAKs) and the IKappa B kinase (IKK) complex]
- Transcription factors (such as NF-κB) that control the expression of proinflammatory genes.

BACTERIAL INFECTIONS

Community-acquired Pneumonia

The chameleon like clinical picture of community-acquired pneumonia (CAP) suggests that something other than the environment and exposure is at play. Genetics must be a factor, in the sense that genes are involved and most likely have some minute changes. It is likely that specific mutations affect the immune response cascade in terms of pattern recognition molecules (PRMs), inflammatory molecules, and the coagulation system. In a current research it is evident that mannose-binding lectin polymorphisms play a more dominant role in CAP than other PRMs, such as the TLRs. There has been extensive research on the possibility of tumor necrosis factor (TNF) and lymphotoxin alpha (LTA) polymorphisms playing a role, but results are not uniform. Also, interleukin (IL)-10 and IL-1 receptor antagonist polymorphisms are important in the anti-inflammatory response. Coagulation gene polymorphisms are also important. The real clinical implications of these genetic studies and variations in CAP and other severe infections in managing such patients remain unclear.[5] A Russian study included 243 patients with acute CAP and 173 healthy subjects. The following candidate loci were used to investigate genetic variability: 3 sites of cytochrome P450, family 1 member A1 (CYP1A1), glutathione S-transferase (GST) M1, GSTT1, GSTP1, angiotensin-1 converting enzyme (ACE) gene of the rennin-angiotensin system, and C-C chemokine receptor type 5 (CCR5). Enhanced predisposition to pneumonia was shown to be characteristic of homozygotes in deletion at the ACE locus [odd ratio (OR) 1.8; $p = 0.013$)], carriers of normal alleles of the GSTM1 locus (OR 1.7; $p = 0.010$), and homozygotes in allele 606T of the CYP1A1 gene (OR 1.6; $p = 0.020$).[6]

One possible mechanism is the genetic variability of the pulmonary surfactant proteins A and D. This change may impact airway clearance of microorganisms and the effect, duration, and severity of the inflammatory response. The genes of these collectins [surfactant protein (SFTP) A1, SFTPA2, and SFTPD)] are located in a cluster at 10q21-24.[6] Garcia-Laorden et al. evaluated the existence of linkage disequilibrium (LD) among these genes. Also, in the same study, there appeared to be a link between the variation in the genes with susceptibility to and eventual sequelae of CAP. Seven non-synonymous polymorphisms of SFTPA1, SFTPA2, and SFTPD were analyzed. For susceptibility, 682 CAP patients and 769 controls were studied in a case-control, prospective study. They showed that missense single nucleotide polymorphisms and haplotypes of SFTPA1,

SFTPA2, and SFTPD were associated with susceptibility and severity of CAP.[7]

TLR signaling and NF-κB activation play a pivotal role in the host immune defense and response to pneumococcal infection. The mutations in the TLR-NF-κB pathway [NEMO (a regulatory subunit in the IKK complex), NFKBIA (which encodes an inhibitor of NF-κB), IRAK4, and MyD88] are involved in predisposition to pneumococcal infections in man and experimental animals. These mutations result in impaired NF-κB activation; NEMO and NFKBIA mutations affect the innate and adaptive pathways, including the TLR pathway that, in turn, affects NF-κB, whereas mutations in IRAK4 and MyD88 appear to disrupt only TLR and IL-1 receptor signaling. The immunodeficiency resulting from hypomorphic NEMO mutations is typically severe and causes a wide range of pathogen susceptibilities. IRAK4 and MyD88 deficiencies, on the other hand, appear to associate with a narrower spectrum of infectious pathogens, primarily pyogenic encapsulated bacteria, particularly *Streptococcus pneumoniae*.[8]

Klebsiella pneumonia

Klebsiella pneumonia is one of the leading causes of nosocomial and community-acquired Gram-negative bacterial pneumonia. Without appropriate treatment, the disease results in severe bacteremia, multiorgan failure, and death. The first line of defense within the primary host is to attempt a quick clearance of the bacteria from the respiratory tract. There are a number of pathways in which this is achieved: direct bacterial phagocytosis by the macrophages, which results in death of bacteria and secretion of cytokines and chemokines, which in turn recruit and activate circulating neutrophils and monocytes into the pulmonary microenvironment. This is in contrast to blood-borne infections, which are primarily cleared through our innate immunity, involving pathways in the liver and spleen. One cell type that plays a role is the Kupffer cell, which phagocytizes bacteria from peripheral blood. Another cell is the neutrophil which is recruited in order to phagocytize and thereby kill the bacteria.

Interferon (IFN)-γ is a vital signal in cell-mediated immunity against a broad array of infectious agents.[9] Its role is very well described when dealing with intracellular pathogens and T-cell mediated immunity. However, when it comes to extracellular pathogens, which most pulmonary pathogens are, its role is not well understood. The complexity of the role of IFN-γ becomes apparent when different bacterial infections are considered. For example, it is of vital importance in successful clearance of pulmonary infections with *S. pneumoniae* and *Pseudomonas aeruginosa*. On the other hand, when models of systemic *Staphylococcus aureus* and *Escherichia coli* infections are evaluated, it has been seen to play a detrimental role. This was further seen when liver specific IFN-γ transgenic mice were examined. Most of these mice Died within 1 year due to infections with mostly Gram-negative bacteria, further suggesting the detrimental role of IFN-γ in these infections.

In order to attempt to illustrate the role of IFN-γ in localized pulmonary infections versus disseminated blood-borne *Klebsiella pneumoniae* infection, IFN-γ knockout mice were used. They were inoculated either intratracheally or intravenously with *K. pneumoniae*. What is seen is that IFN-γ is a critical mediator for the resolution of localized, pulmonary Gram-negative pneumonia. However, the clearance of systemic, blood-borne Gram-negative bacterial infections is independent of IFN-γ secretion.[9] Not only is Gram-negative bacteremia cleared without the use of IFN-γ, its actual production or overproduction may in fact be detrimental.

Another signaling pathway involved in *Klebsiella* pneumonia pathogenesis is Bcl-3. Bcl-3 is an atypical member of the IkB family. Its role is either up- or down-regulation of nuclear NF-κB activity in a context-dependent manner. The role of Bcl-3's is complex. It affects innate immunity and mediates lipopolysaccharides (LPS) tolerance, downregulating cytokine production. Peno et al. studied the role of Bcl-3 in infection with *Klebsiella pneumoniae*. Bcl-3 knockout mice were more likely to be infected with *K. pneumoniae*, vs. their normal counterparts. The mutant mice could not clear bacteria from their lungs, which naturally correlated with increased chances of dissemination. These mice had a profound cytokine imbalance with high IL-10 levels and almost complete absence of IFN-γ, as well as higher production of the neutrophil-attracting chemokines chemokine [C-X-X molif] ligand 1 (CXCL-1) and CXCL-2. Also, the neutrophils found in the Bcl-3 deficient mice were not efficient when it came to intracellular bacterial killing. It becomes evident from this study that the Bcl-3 pathway is vital for clearance of pulmonary infections with Gram-negative bacteria.[10]

Diffuse Panbronchiolitis/Chronic Sinobronchial Inflammation

Diffuse panbronchiolitis (DPB) primarily involves the respiratory bronchioles. It is a persistent bacterial infection that results in the accumulation of lymphocytes and foamy macrophages around the small airways with mucus hypersecretion, so called 'unit lesions of DPB by Professor Kitaichi of Kyoto, Japan. Clinically, DPB resembles idiopathic bronchiectasis. In the past, prognosis of the disease was poor. The use of macrolide therapy, however, has completely changed the dismal outlook of DPB. Because of the occurrence of DPB in Japan, Korea, and South East Asia, a genetic predisposition to the disease was proposed. Immunogenetic studies revealed a strong association with human leukocyte antigen (HLA)-B54 in Japanese and an association with HLA-A11 in Koreans implying that a major susceptibility gene was located between the HLA-A and HLA-B loci on the short arm of human chromosome 6. Keicho and Hijikata have recently cloned mucin-like genes in this candidate region. Although the incidence of DPB has gone down, further analysis of newly identified genes may provide insights into the pathogenesis of other infectious diseases that cause bronchiectasis.[11]

Tuberculosis

Only about 10% of individuals exposed to *Mycobacterium tuberculosis* are actually infected. It appears that complex interactions between environmental and human factors play significant roles in who will and will not develop the disease. Numerous association studies of various candidate genes have been conducted with variable results. The most consistent findings concern certain HLA class II alleles and variants of the natural resistance-associated macrophage protein 1 (NRAMP1) gene.[12] The first major locus identified by genome-wide linkage screening was recently mapped to the chromosome region 8q12-q13. In recent years, a Mendelian predisposition to tuberculosis has been proposed. Tuberculosis was found to be the only phenotypic manifestation in several children with genetic defects of the IL-12/23-IFN-γ circuit and, particularly, those with complete IL-12Rβ-1 deficiency. The human genetics of tuberculosis shows a continuum from Mendelian to complex predisposition with intermediate effects of major genes.[13,14,17]

Clinical studies have suggested the involvement of HLA-DR2 gene and variants of NRAMP1 gene. NRAMP1 is located on chromosome 2q35, and it has been the most studied out of the non-major histocompatibility complex (MHC)-TB susceptibility genes. It is the human version of the same mouse gene that appears to regulate susceptibility to mycobacteria, *Leishmania*, and *Salmonella* with a single amino acid substitution. NRAMP1 is of paramount importance in the early innate response, since it acts on macrophages to activate microbicidal responses.[15] One of the studies of a population in the Western Cape of Africa revealed that two of five polymorphisms of SLC11A1 (NRAMP1) were associated with TB.[16]

Shi et al. examined the polymorphisms of HLA-DRB alleles and the sequences of the HLA-DRB promoter region in 97 unrelated patients with pulmonary tuberculosis and in 62 unrelated normal controls using PCR with sequence-specific primers and PCR direct sequencing. They found that the frequency of HLA-DRB1*15 was significantly higher in the pulmonary tuberculosis group than in the healthy control group (p = 0.001; OR 3.793). The pulmonary tuberculosis group had the same HLA-DRB1 promoter region sequences as the control group. The investigators concluded that the HLA-DRB1*15 allele was associated with pulmonary tuberculosis in the Han nationality from North China.[18]

Takahashi et al. studied the role of SLC11A1 (NRAMP1) polymorphisms affecting the incidence of multidrug-resistant tuberculosis (MDR-TB) amongst other important features of tuberculosis. Using polymerase chain reaction and the restriction fragment-length polymorphism analyses, they investigated four previously reported SLC11A1 polymorphisms, variations in 5'(GT) n, INT4, D543N, and 3'UTR in 95 patients with pulmonary tuberculosis; 10 patients had MDR-TB patients. Clinical information, pertinent to the disease extent and manifestations, was delineated by chart review. Although the number of MDR-TB patients was small, the study showed that the variations of D543N and 3'UTR genes were associated with the incidence of MDR-TB [OR 5.03, 95% confidence interval (CI) 1.24–20.62; p = 0.02], longer time to sputum culture conversion (OR 3.86, 95% CI 1.23–12.23; p = 0.02), and cavity formation (OR 5.04, 95% CI 1.51–23.13; p = 0.02). Also three out of the 10 MDR-TB patients in the study who received appropriate treatment and were compliant, had at least one genetic variation in SLC11A1. The data suggest that genetic variations in SLC11A1 gene play a role in the impact of pulmonary tuberculosis on the host and the likelihood of developing resistant disease.[19] There are instances where obvious environmental risk factors are seen, such as human immunodeficiency virus (HIV) infection, advanced age, diabetes, corticosteroids, or alcohol abuse. However, in the majority of the patients, a complex interaction of genetic and environmental factors drives the course of clinical tuberculosis.[20] Studying ethnic variations and specificity is a major component in understanding the association of genetic variants with outcome of disease susceptibility. SP110, a component of the nuclear body was studied by Abhimanyu et al. They examined SP110 variants in pulmonary (PTB) and lymph node tuberculosis (LNTB) cases in north Indians. They genotyped 24 SP110 variants in 140 north Indian tuberculosis cases and 78 ethnicity-matched controls. Using various techniques, the study demonstrated that SP110 may be a risk factor in LNTB patients.[21]

Mannose-binding Lectin Deficiency

Mannose-binding lectin (MBL) is a protein involved in the innate immune response that combats pathogenic microbes through complement activation. A significant percentage of the human population has an MBL deficiency due to MBL2 polymorphisms. This deficiency may increase the susceptibility to certain infectious diseases, especially respiratory tract infections. A recent meta-analysis illustrated that an MBL deficiency was an independent risk factor for death from pneumococcal infection, even after controlling the comorbidities and bacteremia. There have also been other studies that seem to associate the MBL deficiency with other respiratory infections. However, other bacterial infections, such as tuberculosis, do not appear to be affected by this. Another relevant factor is that the MBL protein is present in small quantities in lung secretions. It is a possibility that these quantities are adequate to activate the complement pathway and combat certain respiratory infections. Therefore, if this protein does play a role in pulmonary immunity, it is presumably prevented by hematogenous dissemination of respiratory pathogens. Given the current literature, MBL is being developed as a new immunotherapeutic agent for prevention of infection in immunocompromised hosts. The available literature suggests that it may also be of benefit in MBL deficient patients with severe pneumonia.[22]

Denholm performed a meta-analysis of 17 trials studying the role of MBL2 genotype and/or MBL levels in tuberculosis. As mentioned previously, no statistically significant relationship was noted between MBL2 genotype and PTB infection. It is noteworthy that MBL levels were measured to be high in patients with tuberculosis. Though it sounds promising, it is relevant to mention that high MBL levels are also consistent with an acute phase reaction. However, it is possible that high MBL levels might somehow, influence tuberculosis infection.[23,24]

Given the possibility of IFN-γ as playing a significant role in the protective immunity against *M. tuberculosis*, Hashemi et al. studied the possible association between single nucleotide polymorphism of IFN-γ +874T/A (rs61923114) and PTB. Their study demonstrated that the AA genotype of +874A/T IFN-γ was a risk factor for PTB (OR 3.333, 95% CI 1.537–7.236, p = 0.002). Also the frequency of the +874A allele was elevated in PTB as compared to normal subjects (OR 1.561, 95% CI 1.134–2.480, p = 0.007).[25]

Mycobacterium Avium Complex

M. avium-complex (MAC) exists freely in nature and is found in water, soil, and dust. MAC infection causes a disseminated disease in immunocompromised hosts and localized lung infiltrate with or without bronchiectasis in immunocompetent hosts, particularly healthy, middle-aged to elderly women. The lesions of MAC often spread, destroy the lungs, impair lung functions and, in some cases, may cause fatal illness. The estimated incidence of MAC is less than 5 cases per 100,000; detailed epidemiological information is not available. A genetic susceptibility paired with an appropriate environmental exposure cause the illness. Genetic defects of INF-γ or IL-12 receptors have been reported to be responsible for disseminating forms of the diseases. Analogy with susceptibility to tuberculosis, HLA and NRMP 1 genes have not produced conclusive results. Shojima et al. investigated genetic loci for MAC. They prepared 3 sets of pooled DNA samples from 300 patients with MAC and 300 controls and genotyped 19,651 microsatellite markers in a case-controlled manner. Although they were able to illustrate certain differences among populations and diseased individuals vs. normal, there were no conclusive data.[26]

Sarcoidosis, a Mycobacterial Infection!

Sarcoidosis is a T cell-driven disease characterized by specific noncaseating granulomas in various organs. There is evidence to suggest that there is a genetic component to the disease, as it appears to cluster among patients who have family members with the disease and the clustering is higher for whites than black families. The majority of family "clusters" involve only parent-child pairs or sibling pairs; more complex pedigrees are rare. This suggests a summation of more than 1 minor genetic influences rather than a single causative gene mutation. In recent years, many of class II MHC alleles have been implicated in certain aspects of the disease. In Japanese patients, HLA-DR5, HLA-DR6, HLA-DR8, and HLA-DR9 seem to be associated with developing sarcoidosis; however, in Scandinavian populations, HLA-DR9 appears to be protective. In German patients, HLA-DR3 is associated with acute versions of disease while HLA-DR5 seems to be seen in chronic forms. Also, in the Scandinavian population, HLA-DR14 and HLA-DR1 are associated with chronic forms of the disease while HLA-DR17 with self-limiting ones.[27] The Acute Candesartan Cilexetil Therapy in Stroke Survivors (ACCESS) study showed a significant link between HLA-DRB1 alleles (specifically HLA-DRB1*1101) and acute sarcoidosis. Two large groups of patients with sarcoidosis were studied and compared to controls. Grutters et al. examined 5 potential functional polymorphisms in the promoter region of the gene for TNF-α. The patients with sarcoidosis displayed an increase in the rare -857T allele. This rare allele, which results from a change of C to T at position 857, was seen in 25.5% of the patients with sarcoidosis vs. 14.1% of controls. With these findings, the investigators summarized that patients with sarcoidosis show higher rates of the rare -857T allele in the promoter region of the gene for TNF-α.[28]

Nevertheless, the genetic aspects of this disease remain poorly understood. One gene that has been studied extensively is the receptor for advanced glycation end-products (RAGE). This gene recognizes multiple tertiary structures like advanced glycation end-products, byproducts of glycation, and oxidation of lipids and proteins. RAGE is seen on biopsies of sarcoid patients. These findings suggest that a genetic link in sarcoidosis may be related to increased RAGE expression or altered function. There are definite pathologic similarities between sarcoidosis and tuberculosis. This raises the possibility that mycobacterial antigen(s) like heat shock proteins (Mtb-hsp) may play a role in both entities. Mtb-hsp, especially Mtb-hsp65, may serve as a connection between infection and autoimmunity through cross-reactivity between the mycobacterial and human hsp. Dubaniewicz believes that in different individuals, the same antigens (Mtb-hsp) may result in a different immune response. As a result, different clinical manifestations ensue and sarcoidosis or tuberculosis develops.[29] This hypothesis is supported by an epidemiological analysis of worldwide sarcoidosis and tuberculosis prevalence. This analysis shows that tuberculosis distribution is opposite to that of sarcoidosis worldwide. About one-third of the Earth's population is infected with *M. tuberculosis*. Also, bacillus Calmette-Guérin (BCG) vaccination has the same heat specific proteins as tuberculosis itself. Therefore, either of these insults, in genetically predisposed individuals, may result in the development of sarcoidosis. Drake et al. investigated this possibility and found Th-1 immune responses to *M. tuberculosis* ESAT-6 and Kat peptides from peripheral blood mononuclear cells in 15 of 26 patients with sarcoidosis.[30]

Acute Exacerbations of Chronic Obstructive Pulmonary Diseases

Chronic obstructive pulmonary disease (COPD) develops in only about 20% of smokers. There is definitely a well-established environmental link between what people inhale and COPD. There is also most likely a genetic component, since not everyone who is exposed is affected. The genetic components are not as well understood. Continued smoking or exposure to second-hand smoke in patients with COPD is a common cause of decline in lung function, and acute respiratory infections become frequent. Many studies have been conducted, investigating the genetic link in COPD. Unfortunately, the results have been inconclusive and animal models have not yielded definite data.[31,32]

Cystic Fibrosis

Cystic fibrosis (CF) is a fatal genetic disease caused by mutations in the cystic fibrosis transmembrane conductance regulator (CFTR) gene. CF is characterized by airway obstruction with recurrent airway inflammation and infection. It is an excellent example of how a thorough understanding of the genetic abnormality of the underlying process can lead to newer treatments leading to improved quality of life and prolonged survival. The CFTR defect was discovered in 1989. There are now more than 1500 mutations of the gene. Pulmonary obstruction in CF is linked to the loss of CFTR function, i.e., regulating chemide channel on the lumen-facing membrane of the epithelium lining the airways. The mutation, F508del-CFTR, caused by deletion of phenylalanine in position 508 (DF508), is found in more than two-thirds of the patients with CF. It causes the protein to misfold and be retained in the endoplasmic reticulum (ER). Recent studies have shown that retention in the ER can be 'corrected' through the application of certain small-molecule modulators. Importantly, 2 such small molecules, a 'corrector' (VX-809) and a 'potentiator' (VX-770) compound are undergoing clinical trial for the treatment of CF. CFTR functions as a regulator of chloride channel in apical membranes. The main defect in CF is one of chloride secretion. CFTR has also been described as a regulator of epithelial sodium channel and bicarbonates transport. This knowledge of CFTR function has resulted in new therapeutic innovations focused on controlling the downstream effects of CFTR dysfunction, e.g., sputum retention, recurrent infections, and associated inflammation.[33] Kim et al. have recently reviewed current knowledge regarding the wild-type CFTR and F508del-CFTR protein and the promise of small-molecule modulators to probe the relationship between structure and function in wild-type protein, the molecular defects caused by the most common mutation, and structural changes required to correct these defects.[34]

Mycobacterium leprae

M. leprae does not cause lung disease but has interesting features that point towards its genetic influences.

M. leprae cannot be cultured in artificial media. Why? Is it possible that this feature was acquired due to genetic loss or mutations during evolution?[35-38] An Indian population showed significantly higher concordance rates in the occurrence of leprosy among monozygotic than in dizygotic twins.[39] Many complex segregation analyses for leprosy phenotypes show that susceptibility to leprosy has a significant genetic component.[40]

Leprosy was the first infectious disease found to have specific HLA variants. Linkage and association studies have shown involvement of class II HLA-DR2 and HLA-DR3 as important genetic risk factors for susceptibility to subtypes of leprosy.[41,42] Other HLA-linked genes involved in innate immune response against leprosy are the TNF-α, NRAMP1 gene, and LTA.[43-45] LTA is a critical effector molecule involved in host defense against intracellular pathogens. A low-expression allele located at position +80 of the LTA gene has been associated with a higher risk of early-onset leprosy in patients from Vietnam and India.[46]

Cytokines play a critical role in the pathogenesis of infectious diseases. Previous studies have established IL-10 as a gene that may play an important role in susceptibility to leprosy infection and disease progression[47] A higher TNF-α/IL-10 ratio was associated with a better prognosis of leprosy in close contacts. Genes such as SLC11A1, Parkinson protein 2 (PARK2), nucleotide binding oligomerization domain containing protein 2 (NOD2) and leucine rich repeat kinase 2 (LRRK2), are associated with leprosy phenotypes.[48-50] NOD2, an intracellular sensing molecule, is expressed by macrophages and epithelial cells that recognize the bacterial cell wall peptidoglycan and the muramyl dipeptides motif. NOD2 gene polymorphism is associated with both types 1 and 2 leprosy reactions. It is assumed that PARK2 participates in NOD2 signaling, whereas LRRK2 regulates PARK2 activity. Variations in TLR1 and TLR2 genes are associated with leprosy reaction. Receptors TLR1, TLR2, and TLR6 are dimmers responsible for antigen recognition, especially mycobacteria, in the innate immune response.[51,52]

FUNGAL INFECTIONS

Aspergillosis

Aspergillus species are solid molds found worldwide. Many members of the *Aspergillus* genus cause lung diseases in human beings, but two species in particular, *A. fumigatus* and *A. flavus*, are common culprits. The spectrum of *Aspergillus*-induced diseases is extensive and depends on the genetic and immunologic make-up of the host (Table 1). Invasive aspergillosis is a rapidly progressive infection that almost exclusively affects severely neutropenic and immunocompromised patients.[53] Bochud et al. studied the involvement of TLR polymorphisms in the development of invasive aspergillosis. The hypothesis of the study was, in recipients of allogeneic hematopoietic stem-cell transplants, there is a link between donor TLR4 haplotype S4 and the risk of invasive aspergillosis. TLRs play a vital role in the innate immune defense system of fruit flies against fungal infection by upregulating the production of the antimicrobial peptide drosomycin.[54] This began the investigation into the possibility of a similar pathway in mammals and led to TLR4. This is a receptor that plays a role in Gram-negative bacterial septic shock through the detection of LPS. Humans have 10 genes that encode TLRs, each with a different role that ranges from detecting microbial glycolipids and lipoproteins to nucleic acids and bacterial flagellin.[55-58]

TABLE 1
Pulmonary Aspergillosis: Clinical Syndromes

Allergic or hypersensitivity reactions
• Allergic asthma
• Allergic bronchopulmonary aspergilllosis
• Extrinsic allergic alveolitis
• Bronchocentric granulomatosis
Invasive (infective) aspergillosis
• Generalized or disseminated
• *Aspergillus* pneumonia
• Lung abscess/cavities
• *Aspergillus* bronchitis
• Infarction
• Pleural effusion/empyema
Chronic necrotizing pneumonitis
• Localized pneumonia
Saprophytic colonization
• Aspergilloma
Mycotoxicosis
• Chemical pneumonitis

Dectin-1 is the major receptor for fungal b-glucans on myeloid cells.[59] Chai et al., studied the association of Dectin-1 Y238X polymorphism with occurrence and clinical course of invasive aspergillosis (IA) in 71 patients who had developed IA after hematopoietic stem cell transplantation (HSCT) and in 21 patients who did not undergo an HSCT but did develop IA. The control group comprised of 108 patients who did have HSCT but not IA. They found some differences. The Y238X allele frequency was increased in non-HSCT patients with IA, and the difference was statistically significant with a p value of <0.05. Also, heterozygosity for Y238X garnered greater likelihood for developing IA post HSCT; however, it did not impact the clinical course of the disease. Furthermore, although there was evidence that mononuclear cells within peripheral blood that were defective in DECTIN-1 function did respond inadequately to infection with *Aspergillus*, the function of macrophages was intact.[60]

A significant proportion of patients with chronic airway obstruction have underlying *A. fumigates* and *A. niger* infections causing a continuum of numerous fungal as well as allergic processes. In order to better illustrate the role of innate immunity in host defense against *A. fumigatus*, Madan studied the function of pulmonary collectins SP-A and SP-D and serum collectin MBL in murine models. There appeared to be an association between the SNPs in SP-A2 and MBL in asthma patients with allergic bronchopulmonary aspergillosis and rhinitis. The mutations of SP-A2 resulting in GCT and AGG alleles as well as the mutation of allele A at position 1011 in MBL resulted in a significantly higher levels of IgE antibodies, eosinophilia, and a lower forced expiratory volume in one second (FEV_1), signifying a greater disease burden than their non-mutated counterparts. As a result, it is possible that these mutations may be used in future to predict susceptibility to allergic aspergillosis.[61]

Coccidioidomycosis

Coccidioidomycosis is a mold that is common to the south-west US, Mexico, and South America. Infection can result after inhalation of spores, which then grow in the pulmonary parenchyma as spherules and are contained by the host immune system forming granulomas. Most people that undergo exposure develop respiratory symptoms without severe sequelae or no symptoms at all. However, less than 1% of infected people may develop a disseminated illness and, sometimes, death. There seems to be a realationship between some ethnic groups and extrathoracic disease. For example, Filipinos and African Americans may be up to 10–175 times more likely to develop dissemination than Caucasians. A look at the genetic constitution of some individuals with dissemination revealed that only particular HLA alleles (e.g., DRB1*1301) and blood type B have been suggested to be associated with dissemination. These molecular phenotypes may simply be surrogate markers for the at-risk ethnic populations.[62-65] Vinh et al. reported an association with IFN-γ receptor 1 deficiency inherited in an autosomal dominant fashion and disseminated coccidioidomycosis. The investigators suggested that the IL-12/IFN-γ axis might play a critical role in controlling autosomal dominant coccidioidomycosis.[66] The clinical implication of this is significant. Therapeutic doses of IFN-γ have been used to treat disseminated disease in patients with this defect as well as in patients who are refractory to current treatments.[67]

Paracoccidioidomycosis

Paracoccidioidomycosis is the result of infection with the dimorphic fungus *Paracoccidioides brasiliensis*. In 2001, there were around 10 million cases throughout South America, 80% of which occurred in Brazil. The organ most often affected by paracoccidioidomycosis is the lung. Infection occurs primarily through inhalation of the pathogen, which primarily affects the lungs and then spreads to other areas of the body causing irreversible physical damage and disability. The clinical spectrum of the disease ranges from a small, localized lesion to severely disseminated systemic infection.[68] Effective defense against *P. brasiliensis* depends mainly upon the ability of the host to mount an efficient, Th1-type of acquired resistance modulated by the interaction of T cells and macrophage-activating cytokines. Resistance or mild type of the disease is related to IFN-γ and TNF-α production, while increased susceptibility to disease is observed with a predominant production of Th2 interleukins IL-4, IL-5, IL-10 and IL-13. Molecular genetic studies have shown evidence of association of paracoccidioidomycosis with specific variants of immune response-related genes. Specific alleles of the TNF-α (-308) polymorphism were associated with paracoccidioidomycosis in a small case-control population sample from Brazil.[69] Variants of Th2 cytokine genes, such as IL10 and IL4 genes, were also found in association with paracoccidioidomycosis. For the IL4 gene, the susceptibility CT genotype was associated with higher production of this cytokine.[70]

Chromoblastomycosis

Chromoblastomycosis is primarily a skin mycosis in man, but in animals, it can cause systemic disease. There are variable presentations of the disease with one being neurological involvement while other exhibiting multifocal dermatitis, the severity of both presentations being broad.[71] A Brazilian study showed that susceptibility to chromoblastomycosis may be influenced by variants of an HLA class I gene located on chromosomal region 6p21, the relative risk for an HLA-A29 carrier to develop chromoblastomycosis was estimated at 10.[72] A recent family-based study performed in a highly consanguineous population from Falcon State, an endemic rural area of northern Venezuela, detected an 11% higher proportion of cases within families, as well as an estimated 65% of heritability for the trait, with the vast majority of cases being caused by *Cladophialophora carrionii*.[73] Interestingly, a previous study had failed to detect association between chromoblastomycosis and polymorphism of the HLA region in a family-based population sample from the same Falcon State.[74]

Histoplasmosis

Histoplasma capsulatum is the most common invasive fungal pulmonary disease worldwide. Histoplasmosis is caused by a small fungus whose natural habitat is soil contaminated by bat or bird excrement. Although considered an endemic mycosis, the fungus has an opportunistic behavior in immunocompromised hosts. The conidial form inhaled in the lungs can cause disease ranging from mild disease in healthy individual to fatal illness in immunocompromised hosts. Protective immunity occurs through the induction of cytokine production by T-cells, particularly IFN-γ and TNF-α, which subsequently activate phagocytes. Mice deficient in IFN-γ have accelerated mortality. Similarly, patients with defective IFN-γ signaling are at risk for severe histoplasmosis.[75]

Inbred mice were used to identify an exceptionally high difference in the levels of fungal burden. A/J mice exhibited less fungal load and morbidity than C57BL/6J mice. This was the opposite than what was observed with bacterial load. The differences were traced to particular locations on chromosomes 1, 6, 15, and 17. Furthermore, the level of fungal load was lowered by a simple substitution of a resistant chromosome 17. These findings lay the foundation for further breakdown and evaluation of the fungal-specific immune program.[76]

The presence of HLA antigens, such as B7 and DRw2 has been associated with the presumed ocular histoplasmosis syndrome (POHs). In a Mexican study, HLA-B22 was found in association with pulmonary histoplasmosis in the state of Guerrero. Allele frequency was highly increased in the Juxtlahuaca and the Olinala populations as compared to controls from the Coyuca population. Importantly, the Juxtlahuaca and Olinala inhabitants are known to live in areas where the disease was considered occupational for peasants, miners, cave tourist guides, anthropologists, archeologists, and others who refer contact with bat guano and/or avian excreta that contain nutrients for fungal growth. In contrast, people from the Coyuca population have no contact with the excreta mentioned above.[77]

PARASITIC INFECTIONS

Hydatid Disease

Azab et al. investigated the immunogenetic predisposition to systemic echinococcosis disease in Egypt. Thirty-five patients with cystic echinococcus (CE) were compared to 100 healthy controls. HLA-DRB1 amplification with PCR and the allele-specific probing technique was used to identify any possible genetic differences in the populations. The study illustrated a positive association between the presence of HLA-DR3 and HLA-DR11 antigens and the development of CE. HLA-DR3 antigen itself correlated with the presence of noncurable disease, larger cysts, multiple cysts, and isolated pulmonary cysts as well as hydatid cyst disease. The presence of the HLA-DR11 antigen on the other hand was associated with smaller cysts.[78]

Filariasis

Lymphatic filariasis is the result of an infection by the the nematode worms *W. bancrofti*, *B. malayi*, and *B. timori*. The infection is transmitted by mosquitoes. The life cycle of these nematodes, discovered by Patrick Manson in 1877, is one of the key factors in infection by these creatures. The mosquito is the key player in this life cycle, as it is the carrier. The larvae get ingested by the mosquito when it feeds, and then they are passed on to the next victim when the mosquito feeds again. A form of infection by these nematodes is elephantiasis, which results in severe swelling of the limbs, breasts, and genitals.

Choi et al. conducted a study to assess if genetic factors influenced susceptibility to human filariasis. A population in South India was studied using common polymorphisms in 6 genes [chitinase-1; chitotriosidase-1 (CHIT1), myeloperoxidase (MPO), NRAMP, cytochrome b-245, α-polypeptide (CYBA), neutrophil cytosolic factor 2 (NCF2), and MBL2]. Two hundred sixteen subjects were studied. The groups included 67 normal controls (N), 63 asymptomatic microfilaria positive (MF+) individuals, 50 patients with chronic lymphatic dysfunction/elephantiasis (CP), and 36 individuals with tropical pulmonary eosinophilia (TPE). The study revealed that the HH variant CHIT1 genotype was associated with decreased activity and levels of chitotriosidase and susceptibility to filarial infection (MF+ and CP; $p = 0.013$). The heterozygosity of CHIT1 gene was over-represented in the normal individuals ($p = 0.034$). The XX genotype of the promoter region in MBL2 was associated with susceptibility to filariasis ($p = 0.0093$). Consequently, they postulated two polymorphisms, CHIT1 and MBL2, predisposing the patients to human filarial infection.[79]

However, in a different study of a different population in Papua New Guniea, Hise et al. examined 906 residents of the area. In this study, they were unable to conclude that there was any association between infection and the CHIT1 genotype.[80]

Leishmaniasis

Leishmaniasis, a vector-borne disease is common in tropical and subtropical countries. Approximately 2 million new cases of leishmaniasis are detected every year. The disease can be divided into visceral leishmaniasis (VL) and American tegumentary leishmaniasis (ATL). ATL can be further subdivided into localized cutaneous leishmaniasis (CL), mucosal leishmaniasis (ML), and disseminated leishmaniasis (DL). ATL is the most common disease form with an estimated 1.5 million cases year. The strong association between *Leishmania* species and different disease forms suggests a prominent role for genetic predisposition. A key step in the immune response against intracellular parasites is the differentiation of IFNγ-secreting CD4 (+) Th 1 cells. Notch receptors have been postulated to play an important role, since they regulate cell differentiation during development. There are 4 Notch receptors; however, only Notch1 (N1) and Notch2 (N2) are seen on activated CD4 (+) T cells. In order to delineate the role of notch receptors further, mice with T cell-specific gene ablation of N1, N2, or both [N1N2 (ΔCD4Cre)] were infected with *Leishmania major*. N1N2 (ΔCD4Cre) mice, on the C57BL/6 L major-resistant genetic background, developed nonhealing lesions and parasitemia. The level of infection was related to impaired secretion of IFN-γ by draining lymph node CD4(+) T cells and increased secretion of the IL-5 and IL-13 Th2 cytokines. However, mice with a single inactivation of N1 or N2 showed immunity to infection and developed a protective Th1 immune response. This signifies that CD4(+) T cell expression of N1 or N2 is redundant in driving Th1 differentiation. Thus, Auderset et al. showed that Notch signaling is required for the secretion of IFN-γ by Th1 cells. However, this effect is not dependent on CSL/RBP-Jκ, the major effector of Notch receptors, since these mice were able to develop IFN-γ-secreting Th1 cells, kill parasites, and heal their lesions.[81]

Most of the genetic studies of host susceptibility factors have been conducted in populations affected by visceral leishmaniasis.[82-85] High circulating level of TNF-α can be observed in plasma of patients with mucocutaneous leishmaniasis (MCL).[86] A subsequent study successfully demonstrated 2 polymorphisms of the TNF-α gene in association with ATL in a case-control Venezuelan population sample, including the (–308) variation of the promoter region of the gene, largely described as a functional regulator of TNF-α plasma levels. Interestingly, the study showed that homozygous females for the susceptibility allele were in higher risk of developing infection, when compared to males with the same genotype.[87] Of note, TNF-α (–308) polymorphism is also associated with other infectious diseases, including leprosy and tuberculosis.[88,89] Also, TNF-α is physically close to the LTA gene, which has also been described in association with leprosy. Both genes are located at chromosomal region 6p21 harboring the MHC/HLA complex, reinforcing the importance of this genome segment in multiple infectious diseases.[90] A study from Sudan detected a haplotype composed of alleles of four polymorphisms of the Interferon Gamma Receptor 1 (INFGR1) gene associated with postkala-azar dermal leishmaniasis, but none of the INFG gene variations were found in association with disease susceptibility.[45] A Brazilian study compared allele frequencies between ATL cases (CL and ML) and healthy controls. It failed to detect association between disease susceptibility/severity and the functional polymorphism INFG (+874). However, INFG (+874) alleles were associated with IFN-γ plasma levels in the same population.[91]

A previously known functional polymorphism (–819) of the IL-10 gene, associated with regulation of IL-10 serum levels, was associated with the development of leishmaniasis skin lesions in a Brazilian population. The same polymorphism is described in association with leprosy. Allele frequencies of a polymorphism in the promoter region of IL-6 gene were differentially distributed among ML patients compared to CL cases. The susceptibility genotype to ML was also correlated with lower IL-6 serum levels leading to higher risk of development of the ML form of the disease. Classical HLA haplotypes are associated with CL and/or MCL and VL type of leishmaniasis.[92-99]

Malaria

Several gene mutations influence severity of malaria. (Table 2).[100] Many of these mutations are linked to erythrocytes, including hemoglobin (Hb) variants, or to proteins, such as haptoglobin and nitric oxide metabolism. There is definitely a spectrum of genetic variation with malaria; for example, heterozygotes, Hbs (sickle cell trait), have protection against severe malaria.[100,101] The major genetic differences occur within the host immunity, HLA genes, cytokine genes, complement regulatory genes, and endothelial receptor genes. Although malaria is a severe public health concern causing significant morbidity and mortality worldwide, especially in developing countries,

TABLE 2

Genetic Mutations Involved in Susceptibility/Resistance to *P. falciparum* Malaria

Gene (Symbol)	Phenotype	Proposed protective mechanisms
Hemoglobin C	↓UM and ↓SM	Reduced cytoadherence of infected erythrocytes
Hemoglobin E	↓SM, ↓parasitemia	Reduced erythrocyte invasion by merozoites, lower intraerythrocytic parasite growth, and enhanced phagocytosis of infected erythrocytes
Hemoglobin S	↓UM and ↓SM	Selective sickling of infected sickle trait erythrocytes leading to enhanced clearance by the spleen. Reduced erythrocyte invasion, early phagocytosis, and inhibited parasite growth under oxygen stress in venous microvessels. Enhancement of innate and acquired immunity
α-thalassemia	↓SM and ↓SMA	Reduced resetting. Increased microerythrocyte count in homozygotes reduces the amount of hemoglobin lost for given parasite density, thus protecting against severe anemia
β-thalassemia	↓SM	—
Glucose-6-phosphate dehydrogenase	↓UM and ↓SM	Increased vulnerability of the glucose-6-phosphatic dehydrogenase deficient erythrocyte to oxidant stress causes its protection against parasitization
Pyruvate kinase	↓Parasitemia	Invasion defect of erythrocytes and preferential macrophage clearance of ring-stage infected erythrocytes
Ovalocytosis	↓SM and ↓CM	Inhibition of merozoite entry into the red cell, impairment of intracellular parasite growth and prevention of the erythrocyte lysis that occurs with parasite maturation, leading to release of merozoites into the bloodstream
Elliptocytosis	↓SM	—
Glycophorins A	↓SM	—
Blood groups	↓SM	Reduced *P. falciparum* rosetting
Haptoglobin	↓SM	Oxidative damage to uninfected cells might be more marked in HP polymorphic individuals since HP proteins bind less efficiently to Hb, increasing premature destruction of erythrocytes and stimulating cytokine release by these circulating cells
Nitric oxide synthase 2	↓SM	Increased NO production induces Th1 cytokines, which activate macrophages and could thus be an antimalarial-resistance mechanism
Heme oxygenase I	↓CM	Release of free heme in the bloodstream

SM, severe malaria; CM, cerebral malaria; UM, uncomplicated malaria; SMA, severe malarial anemia; NO, nitric oxide.

Adapted from Driss A, Hibbert JM, Wilson NO, Iqbal SA, Adamkiewicz TV, Stiles JK. Genetic polymorphisms linked to susceptibility to malaria. *Malar J.* 2011;10:271, *with permission.*

the link between severity of infection and genetics has been rarely studied.

It has been postulated that the macrophage migration inhibitory factor (MIF) may play a protective role against the pathogenesis of malaria.[102] MIF is a cytokine, which regulates immune and inflammatory responses in many diseases, including sepsis, rheumatoid arthritis, cancer, and inflammatory neurological diseases.[103] To investigate its role further, a mouse model was studied that showed MIF levels correlated with malarial anemia.[104] A study of African children illustrated lower levels of MIF in malaria infected children compared with healthy asymptomatic children.[105] Another study, in healthy Eurpoean volunteers, who were exposed to malaria showed a drop in MIF levels.[106] As a result, the role of circulating MIF, other gene polymorphisms, as well as potential interactions with a multitude of other factors needs to be studied further.

A recent review of gene polymorphisms involved in different phenotypes of sickle cell disease showed that multiple genes and pathways mediating sickle cell disease severity are also involved in malaria severity/resistance.[107] Instances and studies, which illustrate genetic similarities across related diseases, are invaluable in identifying important diagnostic biomarkers and for population comparisons.[108-110]

CONCLUSION

The lung plays a critical role in providing the initial defence against respiratory pathogens. Genetic differences modulate responses to pathogens, allergens, and xenobiotics. Many functional gene polymorphisms are associated with gene-environment interactions. Given the complicated aspect of pulmonary infections, it is likely that there is an intricate relationship between our genetics and environmental exposure. However, genetic knowledge related to pulmonary infections is still in its infancy. In this modern world, as our borders become blurred, it is becoming vital that we make every attempt to understand why certain people become very ill, while others never contract the illness. There is an urgent need for well-designed gene association studies to bring therapeutic benefit to the bedside.

REFERENCES

1. Harding D. Impact of common genetic variation on neonatal disease and outcome. *Arch Dis Child Fetal Neonatal Ed.* 2007;92:F 408-13.
2. Garantziotis S, Schwartz DA. Ecogenomics of respiratory diseases of public health significance. *Annual Rev Public Health.* 2010;31:37-51.
3. Workman ML, Winkelman C. Genetic influences in common respiratory disorders. *Crit Care Nurs Clin North Am.* 2008;20:171-89.
4. Waterer GW, Bruns AH. Genetic risk of acute pulmonary infections and sepsis. *Expert Rev Respir Med.* 2010;4:229-38.
5. Wunderink R, Waterer GW. Genetics of community-acquired pneumonia. *Semin Respir Crit Care Med.* 2005;26:553-62.
6. Moroz W, Smelaia TV, Salnikova LE, Golobev AM, Rubanovich AV. Genetic study of predisposition to community-acquired pneumonia. *Vestn Ross Akad Med Nauk.* 2011;(11):12-6
7. García-Laorden MI, Rodríguez de Castro F, Solé-Violán J, Rajas O, Blanquer J, Borderías L, et al. Influence of genetic variability at the surfactant proteins A and D in community-acquired pneumonia: a prospective, observational, genetic study. *Crit Care.* 2011;15:R57.
8. Chapman SJ. Can your genes make you more prone to pneumococcal disease? *Expert Rev Anti Infect Ther.* 2010;8:967-72.
9. Moore TA, Perry ML, Getsoian AG, Newstead MW, Standiford TJ. Divergent role of gamma interferon in a murine model of pulmonary versus systemic Klebsiella pneumoniae infection. *Infect Immun.* 2002;70:6310-18.
10. Pène F, Paun A, Sønder SU, Rikhi N, Wang H, Claudio E, et al. The IkB family member Bcl-3 coordinates the pulmonary defense against Klebsiella pneumoniae infection. *J Immunol.* 2011;186:2412-21.
11. Keicho N, Hijikata M. Genetic predisposition to diffuse panbronchiolitis. *Respirology.* 2011;16:581-8.
12. Cheepsattayakorn A, Cheepsattayakorn R. Human genetic influence on susceptibility of tuberculosis: from infection to disease. *J Med Assoc Thai.* 2009;92:136-41.
13. Bustamante J, Picard C, Boisson-Dupuis S, Abel L, Casanova J. Genetic lessons learned from X-linked Mendelian susceptibility to mycobacterial diseases. *Ann N Y Acad Sci.* 2011;1246:92-101.
14. Abel L, Casanova JL. Human genetics of tuberculosis. *Bull Acad Natl Med.* 2010;194:943-50.
15. Vidal SM, Malo D, Vogan K, Skamene E, Gros P. Natural resistance to infection with intracellular parasites: isolation of a candidate for Bcg. *Cell.* 1993;73:469-85.
16. Hoal EG, Lewis LA, Jamieson SE, Tanzer F, Rossouw M, Victor T, et al. SLC11A1 (NRAMP1) but not SLC11A2 (NRAMP2) polymorphisms are associated with susceptibility to tuberculosis in a high-incidence community in South Africa. *Int J Tuberc Lung Dis.* 2004;8:1464-71.
17. Rezaei N, Aghamohammadi A, Mansouri D, Parvaneh N, Casanova JL. Tuberculosis: a new look at an old disease. *Expert Rev Clin Immunol.* 2011;7:129-31.
18. Shi GL, Hu XL, Yang L, Rong CL, Guo YL, Song CX. Association of HLA-DRB alleles and pulmonary tuberculosis in North Chinese patients. *Genet Mol Res.* 2011;10:1331-6.
19. Takahashi K, Hasegawa Y, Abe T, Yamamoto T, Nakashima K, Imaizumi K, et al. SLC11A1 (formerly NRAMP1) polymorphisms associated with multidrug-resistant tuberculosis. *Tuberculosis (Edinb).* 2008;88:52-7.
20. Milburn H. Key issues in the diagnosis and management of tuberculosis. *J R Soc Med.* 2007;100:134-41.
21. Abhimanyu, Jha P, Jain A, Arora K, Bose M. Genetic association study suggests a role for SP110 variants in lymph node tuberculosis but not pulmonary tuberculosis in north Indians. *Hum Immunol.* 2011;72:576-80.
22. Eisen DP. Mannose-binding lectin deficiency and respiratory tract infection. *J Innate Immun.* 2010;2:114-22.
23. Denholm JT, McBryde ES, Eisen DP. Mannose-binding lectin and susceptibility to tuberculosis: a meta-analysis. *Clin Exp Immunol.* 2010;162:84-90.
24. Affandi J, Price P, Waterer G. Can immunogenetics illuminate the diverse manifestations of respiratory infections? *Ther Adv Respir Dis.* 2010;4:161-76.
25. Hashemi M, Sharifi-Mood B, Nezamdoost M, Moazeni-Roodi A, Naderi M, Kouhpayeh H, Taheri M, et al. Functional polymorphism of interferon-γ (IFN-γ) gene +874T/A polymorphism is associated with pulmonary tuberculosis in Zahedan, Southeast Iran. *Prague Med Rep.* 2011;112:38-43.
26. Shojima J, Tanaka G, Keicho N, Tamiya G, Ando S, Oka A, et al. Identification of MICA as a susceptibility gene for pulmonary Mycobacteriums avium complex infection. *J Infect Dis.* 2009;199:1707-15.
27. Wells AU, Hogaboam CM. Update in diffuse parenchymal lung disease 2007. *Am J Respir Crit Care Med.* 2008;177:580-4.
28. Grutters JC, Sato H, Pantelidis P, Lagan AL, McGrath DS, Lammers JW, et al. Increased frequency of the uncommon tumor necrosis factor-857T allele in British and Dutch patients with sarcoidosis. *Am J Respir Crit Care Med.* 2002;165:1119-24.
29. Dubaniewicz A. Mycobacterium tuberculosis heat shock proteins and autoimmunity in sarcoidosis. *Autommun Rev.* 2010;9:419-24.
30. Drake WP, Dhason MS, Nadaf M, Shepherd BE, Vadivelu S, Hajizadeh R, et al. Cellular recognition of *Mycobacterium*

tuberculosis ESAT-6 and KatG peptides in systemic sarcoidosis. *Infect Immun.* 2007;75: 527-30.
31. Molfino NA. Genetic predisposition to accelerated decline of lung function in COPD. *Int J Chron Obstruct Pulmon Dis.* 2007;2:117-9.
32. Lin CL, Siu LK, Lin JC, Liu CY, Chian CF, Lee CN, et al. Mannose-binding lectin gene polymorphism contributes to recurrence of infective exacerbation in patients with COPD. *Chest.* 2011;139:43-51.
33. Ratjien FA. Cystic Fibrosis: pathogenesis and future treatment strategies. *Resp Care.* 2009;54:595-602.
34. Kim Chiaw P, Eckford PD, Bear CE. Insights into the mechanisms underlying CFTR channel activity, the molecular basis for cystic fibrosis and strategies for therapy. *Essays Biochem.* 2011;50:233-48.
35. Scollard DM, Adams LB, Gillis TP, Krahenbuhl JL, Truman RW, Williams DL. The continuing challenges of leprosy. *Clin Microbiol Rev.* 2006;19:338-81.
36. Cole ST, Eiglmeier K, Parkhill J, James KD, Thomson NR, Wheeler PR, et al. Massive gene decay in the leprosy bacillus. *Nature.* 2001;409:1007-11.
37. Monot M, Honoré N, Garnier T, Araoz R, Coppée JY, Lacroix C, et al. On the origin of leprosy. *Science.* 2005;308: 1040-2.
38. Alter A, Alcais A, Abel L, Schurr E. Leprosy as a genetic model for susceptibility to common infectious diseases. *Hum Genet.* 2008;123:227-35.
39. Prevedello FC, Mira MT. Hanseníase: uma doença genética? *An Bras Dermatol.* 2007;82:483-7.
40. Chakravartti M, Vogel F. A twin study on leprosy. In: Becker PE, Lenz W, Vogel F, Wendt GG, editors. Topics in Human Genetics. Stuttgart:Georg Thieme;1973. p.1-29.
41. Abel L, Demenais F. Detection of major genes for susceptibility to leprosy and its subtypes in a Caribbean island: Desirade Island. *Am J Hum Genet.* 1988;42:256-66.
42. Mira MT. Genetic host resistance and susceptibility to leprosy. *Microbes Infect.* 2006;8:1124-31.
43. Wong SH, Gochhait S, Malhotra D, Pettersson FH, Teo YY, Khor CC, et al. Leprosy and the adaptation of human toll-like receptor 1. *PLoS Pathog.* 2010;6:e1000979.
44. Vanderborght PR, Matos HJ, Salles AM, Vasconcellos SE, Silva-Filho VF, Huizinga TW, et al. Single nucleotide polymorphisms (SNPs) at -238 and -308 positions in the TNF-alpha promoter: clinical and bacteriological evaluation in leprosy. *Int J Lepr Other Mycobact Dis.* 2004; 72:143-8.
45. Abel L, Sánchez FO, Oberti J, Thuc NV, Hoa LV, Lap VD, et al. Susceptibility to leprosy is linked to the human NRAMP1 gene. *J Infect Dis.* 1998;177:133-45.
46. Alcaïs A, Alter A, Antoni G, Orlova M, Nguyen VT, Singh M, et al. Stepwise replication identifies a low-producing lymphotoxin-alpha allele as a major risk factor for early-onset leprosy. *Nat Genet.* 2007;39:517-22.
47. Pereira AC, Brito-de-Souza VN, Cardoso CC, Dias-Baptista IM, Parelli FP, Venturini J, et al. Genetic, epidemiological and biological analysis of interleukin-10 promoter single-nucleotide polymorphisms suggests a definitive role for -819C/T in leprosy susceptibility. *Genes Immun.* 2009; 10:174-80.
48. Mira MT, Alcaïs A, Nguyen VT, Moraes MO, Di Flumeri C, Vu HT, et al. Susceptibility to leprosy is associated with PARK2 and PACRG. *Nature.* 2004;427:636-40.
49. Zhang FR, Huang W, Chen S, Sun L, Liu H, Li Y, et al. Genomewide association study of leprosy. *N Engl J Med.* 2009;361:2609-18.
50. Berrington WR, Macdonald M, Khadge S, Sapkota BR, Janer M, Hagge DA, et al. Common polymorphisms in the NOD2 gene region are associated with leprosy and its reactive states. *J Infect Dis.* 2010;201:1422-35.
51. Misch EA, Macdonald M, Ranjit C, Sapkota BR, Wells RD, Siddiqui MR, et al. Human TLR1 deficiency is associated with impaired mycobacterial signaling and protection from leprosy reversal reaction. *PLoS Negl Trop Dis.* 2008;2:e231.
52. Bochud PY, Hawn TR, Siddiqui MR, Saunderson P, Britton S, Abraham I, et al. Toll-like receptor 2 (TLR2) polymorphisms are associated with reversal reaction in leprosy. *J Infect Dis.* 2008;197:253-61.
53. Sharma OP, Chwogule R. Many Faces of Pulmonary Aspergillosis. *Eur Resp J.* 1998;12:705-15.
54. Bochud PY, Chien JW, Marr KA, Leisenring WM, Upton A, Janer M, et al. Toll-like receptor 4 polymorphisms and aspergillosis in stem-cell transplantation. *N Engl J Med.* 2008;359:1766-77.
55. Lemaitre B, Nicolas E, Michaut L, Reichhart JM, Hoffmann JA. The dorsoventral regulatory gene cassette spatzle/ Toll/cactus controls the potent antifungal response in Drosophila adults. *Cell.* 1996;86:973-83.
56. Medzhitov R, Preston-Hurlburt P, Janeway CA Jr. A human homologue of the Drosophila Toll protein signals activation of adaptive immunity. *Nature.* 1997;388:394-7.
57. Poltorak A, He X, Smirnova I, Liu MY, Van Huffel C, Du X, et al. Defective LPS signaling in C3H/HeJ and C57BL/10ScCr mice: mutations in Tlr4 gene. *Science.* 1998;282:2085-8.
58. Palmer EG. TLR polymorphisms and the risk of invasive fungal infections. *N Engl J Med.* 2008;359:1836-8.
59. Reid DM, Gow NA, Brown GD. Pattern recognition: recent insights from Dectin-1. *Curr Opin Immunol.* 2009;21:30-7.
60. Chai LY, de Boer MG, van der Velden WJ, Plantinga TS, van Spriel AB, Jacobs C, et al. The Y238X stop codon polymorphism in the human b-glucan receptor dectin-1 and susceptibility to invasive aspergillosis. *J Infect Dis.* 2011;203:736-43.
61. MadanT. Potential of lung surfactant proteins, SP-A and SP-D, and mannan binding lectin for therapy and genetic predisposition to allergic and invasive aspergillosis. *Recent Pat Inflamm Allergy Drug Discov.* 2007;1:183-7.
62. Ampel NM. The Complex Immunology of Human coccidioidomycosis. *Ann N Y Acad Sci.* 2007;1111:245-58.
63. Shubitz LF, Dial SM, Perrill R, Casement R, Galgiani JN. Vaccine-induced cellular immune responses differ from innate responses in susceptible and resistant strains of mice infected with Coccidioides posadasii. *Infect Immun.* 2008;76:5553-64.
64. Laniado-Laborin R. expanding understanding of epidemiology of coccidioidomycosis in the western hemisphere. *Ann N Y Acad Sci.* 2007;1111:19-34.

65. Bustamante J, Zhang SY, von Bernuth H, Abel L, Casanova JL. From infectious diseases to primary immunodeficiencies. *Immunol Allergy Clin North Am.* 2008;28:235-58.
66. Vinh DC, Masannat F, Dzioba RB, Galgiani JN, Holland SM. Refractory disseminated coccidioidomycosis and mycobacteriosis in interferon-gamma receptor 1 deficiency. *Clin Infect Dis.* 2009;49:e62-5.
67. Kuberski TT, Servi RJ, Rubin PJ. Successful treatment of a critically ill patient with disseminated coccidioidomycosis, using adjunctive interferon gamma. *Clin Infect Dis.* 2004; 38:910-2.
68. Bozzi A, Reis BS, Pereira PP, Pedroso EP, Goes AM. Interferon-gamma and interleukin-4 single nucleotide gene polymorphisms in Paracoccidioidomycosis. *Cytokine.* 2009;48:212-7.
69. Bozzi A, Pereira PP, Reis BS, Goulart MI, Pereira MC, Pedroso EP, et al. Interleukin10 and tumor necrosis factor-alpha single nucleotide gene polymorphism frequency in paracoccidioidomycosis. *Hum Immunol.* 2006;67:931-9.
70. Sardinha JF, Tarlé RG, Fava VM, Francio AS, Ramos GB, Ferreira LC, et al. Genetic risk factors for human susceptibility to infections of relevance in dermatology. *An Bras Dermatol.* 2011;86:708-15.
71. Bube A, Burkhardt E, Weiss R. Spontaneous chromomycosis in the marine toad (Bufo marinus). *J Comp Pathol.* 1992; 106:73-7.
72. Tsuneto LT, Arce-Gomez B, Petzl-Erler ML, Queiroz-Telles F. HLA-A29 and genetic susceptibility to chromoblastomycosis. *J Med Vet Mycol.* 1989;27:181-5.
73. Richard-Yegres N, Yegres F. Cromomicosis: una endemia rural en la region noroccidental en Venezuela. *Rev Cubana Med Trop.* 2009;61:209-12.
74. Naranjo F, Márquez I, Gendzekhadze K, Zhang S, Fernández-Mestre M, Yegres F, et al. Human leukocyte antigen class I and MICA haplotypes in a multicase family with Cladophialophora carrionii chromoblastomycosis. *Tissue Antigens.* 2006;68:87-92.
75. Ferreira MS, Borges AS. Histoplasmosis. *Rev Soc Bras Med Trop.* 2009;42:192-8.
76. Nosanchuk JD, Gacser A. *Histoplasma capsulatum* at the host-pathogen interface. *Microbes Infect.* 2008;10:973-7.
77. Taylor ML, Perez-Mejia A, Yamamoto-Furusho JK, Granados J. Immunologic, genetic and social human risk factors associated to histoplasmosis: studies in the State of Guerrero, Mexico. *Mycopathologia.* 1997;138:137-42.
78. Azab ME, Bishara SA, Ramzy RM, Oteifa NM, El-Hoseiny LM, Ahmed MA. The evaluation of HLA-DRB1 antigens as susceptibility markers for unilocular cystic echinococcosis in Egyptian patients. *Parasitol Res.* 2004;92:473-7.
79. Choi EH, Zimmerman PA, Foster CB, Zhu S, Kumaraswami V, Nutman TB, et al. Genetic polymorphisms in molecules of innate immunity and susceptibility to infection with *Wuchereria bancrofti* in South India. *Genes Immun.* 2001; 2:248-53.
80. Hise AG, Hazlett FE, Bockarie MJ, Zimmerman PA, Tisch DJ, Kazura JW. Polymorphisms of innate immunity genes and susceptibility to lymphatic filariasis. *Genes Immun.* 2003;4:524-7.
81. Auderset F, Schuster S, Coutaz M, Koch U, Desgranges F, Merck E, et al. Redundant Notch1 and Notch2 signaling are necessary for IFNg secretion by T helper 1 cells during infection with *Leishmania* major. *PLoS Pathog.* 2012; 8:e1002560.
82. Jamieson SE, Miller EN, Peacock CS, Fakiola M, Wilson ME, Bales-Holst A, et al. Genome-wide scan for visceral leishmaniasis susceptibility genes in Brazil. *Genes Immun.* 2007;8:84-90.
83. Jeronimo SM, Holst AK, Jamieson SE, Francis R, Martins DR, Bezerra FL, et al. Genes at human chromosome 5q31.1 regulate delayed-type hypersensitivity responses associated with *Leishmania chagasi* infection. *Genes Immun.* 2007;8:539-51.
84. Mohamed HS, Ibrahim ME, Miller EN, White JK, Cordell HJ, Howson JM, et al. SLC11A1 (formerly NRAMP1) and susceptibility to visceral leishmaniasis in The Sudan. *Eur J Hum Genet.* 2004;12:66-74.
85. Shaw MA, Davies CR, Llanos-Cuentas EA, Collins A. Human genetic susceptibility and infection with Leishmania peruviana. *Am J Hum Genet.* 1995;57:1159-68.
86. Castes M, Trujillo D, Rojas ME, Fernandez CT, Araya L, Cabrera M, et al. Serum levels of tumor necrosis factor in patients with American cutaneous leishmaniasis. *Biol Res.* 1993;26:233-8.
87. Cabrera M, Shaw MA, Sharples C, Williams H, Castes M, Convit J, et al. Polymorphism in tumor necrosis factor genes associated with mucocutaneous leishmaniasis. *J Exp Med.* 1995;182:1259-64.
88. Pacheco AG, Cardoso CC, Moraes MO. IFNG +874T/A, IL10 -1082G/A and TNF 308G/A polymorphisms in association with tuberculosis susceptibility: a meta-analysis study. *Hum Genet.* 2008;123:477-84.
89. Carsin H, Assicot M, Feger F, Roy O, Pennacino I, Le Bever H, et al. Evolution and significance of circulating procalcitonin levels compared with IL-6, TNF alpha and endotoxin levels early after thermal injury. *Burns.* 1997;23:218-24.
90. Salih MA, Ibrahim ME, Blackwell JM, Miller EN, Khalil EA, ElHassan AM, et al. IFNG and IFNGR1 gene polymorphisms and susceptibility to post-kala-azar dermal leishmaniasis in Sudan. *Genes Immun.* 2007;8:75-8.
91. Matos GI, Covas Cde J, Bittar Rde C, Gomes-Silva A, Marques F, Maniero VC, et al. IFNG +874T/A polymorphism is not associated with American tegumentary leishmaniasis susceptibility but can influence *Leishmania* induced IFN-gamma production. *BMC Infect Dis.* 2007;7:33.
92. Blackwell JM, Black GF, Peacock CS, Miller EN, Sibthorpe D, Gnananandha D, et al. Immunogenetics of leishmanial and mycobacterial infections: the Belem Family Study. *Philos Trans R Soc Lond B Biol Sci.* 1997;352:1331-45.
93. Vidal S, Tremblay ML, Govoni G, Gauthier S, Sebastiani G, Malo D, et al. The Ity/Lsh/Bcg locus: natural resistance to infection with intracellular parasites is abrogated by disruption of the Nramp1 gene. *J Exp Med.* 1995;182: 655-66.
94. van Crevel R, Parwati I, Sahiratmadja E, Marzuki S, Ottenhoff TH, Netea MG, et al. Infection with *Mycobacterium tuberculosis* Beijing genotype strains is

associated with polymorphisms in SLC11A1/NRAMP1 in Indonesian patients with tuberculosis. *J Infect Dis.* 2009;200:1671-4.
95. Castellucci L, Jamieson SE, Miller EN, Menezes E, Oliveira J, Magalhães A, et al. CXCR1 and SLC11A1 polymorphisms affect susceptibility to cutaneous leishmaniasis in Brazil: a case-control and family-based study. *BMC Med Genet.* 2010;11:10.
96. Salhi A, Rodrigues V Jr, Santoro F, Dessein H, Romano A, Castellano LR, et al. Immunological and genetic evidence for a crucial role of IL-10 in cutaneous lesions in humans infected with Leishmania braziliensis. *J Immunol.* 2008; 180:6139-48.
97. Castellucci L, Menezes E, Oliveira J, Magalhaes A, Guimaraes LH, Lessa M, et al. IL6 -174 G/C promoter polymorphism influences susceptibility to mucosal but not localized cutaneous leishmaniasis in Brazil. *J Infect Dis.* 2006;194:519-27.
98. Ramasawmy R, Menezes E, Magalhães A, Oliveira J, Castellucci L, Almeida R, et al. The -2518bp promoter polymorphism at CCL2/MCP1 influences susceptibility to mucosal but not localized cutaneous leishmaniasis in Brazil. *Infect Genet Evol.* 2010;10:607-13.
99. Sakthianandeswaren A, Foote S J, Handman E. The role of host genetics in leishmaniasis. *Trends Parasitol.* 2009;25:383-91.
100. Verra F, Mangano VD, Modiano D. Genetics of susceptibility to *Plasmodium falciparum*: from classical malaria resistance genes towards genome-wide association studies. *Parasite Immunol.* 2009;31:234-253.
101. Livingstone FB. Simulation of the diffusion of the beta-globin variants in the Old World. *Hum Biol.* 1989;61:297-309.
102. Jain V, McClintock S, Nagpal AC, Dash AP, Stiles JK, Udhayakumar V, et al. Macrophage migration inhibitory factor is associated with mortality in cerebral malaria patients in India. *BMC Res Notes.* 2009;2:36.
103. Lolis E. Glucocorticoid counter regulation: macrophage migration inhibitory factor as a target for drug discovery. *Curr Opin Pharmacol.* 2001;1:662-8.
104. McDevitt MA, Xie J, Shanmugasundaram G, Griffith J, Liu A, McDonald C, et al. A critical role for the host mediator macrophage migration inhibitory factor in the pathogenesis of malarial anemia. *J Exp Med.* 2006;203: 1185-96.
105. Awandare GA, Hittner JB, Kremsner PG, Ochiel DO, Keller CC, Weinberg JB, et al. Decreased circulating macrophage migration inhibitory factor (MIF) protein and blood mononuclear cell MIF transcripts in children with Plasmodium falciparum malaria. *Clin Immunol.* 2006;119:219-25.
106. De Mast Q, Sweep FC, McCall M, Geurts-Moespot A, Hermsen C, Calandra T, et al. A decrease of plasma macrophage migration inhibitory factor concentration is associated with lower numbers of circulating lymphocytes in experimental Plasmodium falciparum malaria. *Parasite Immunol.* 2008;30:133-8.
107. Mohan A, Sharma SK, Bollineni S. Acute lung injury and acute respiratory distress syndrome in malaria. *J Vector Borne Dis.* 2008;45:179-93.
108. Price RN, Douglas NM, Anstey NM. New developments in *Plasmodium vivax* malaria: severe disease and the rise of chloroquine resistance. *Curr Opin Infect Dis.* 2009; 22:430-5.
109. Sharma VP. Hidden burden of malaria in Indian women. *Malar J.* 2009;8:281.
110. Driss A, Hibbert JM, Wilson NO, Iqbal SA, Adamkiewicz TV, Stiles JK. Genetic polymorphisms linked to susceptibility to malaria. *Malar J.* 2011;10:271.

CHAPTER 2

Upper Respiratory Tract Infections

Tatjana Peroš-Golubičić, Jasna Tekavec-Trkanjec

ABSTRACT

Upper respiratory tract infections are the most common infections in the population. The term "upper respiratory tract" covers several mutually connected anatomical structures: nose, paranasal sinuses, middle ear, pharynx, larynx, and proximal part of trachea. Thus, infection in one part usually attacks the adjacent structures and may spread to the tracheobronchial tree and lungs.

Most of acute upper respiratory tract infections are caused by viruses. Bacterial pathogens can also be the primary causative agents of acute upper respiratory infections, but more frequently, they cause chronic infections.

Although most of the upper respiratory infections are self-limiting, some of them may cause severe complications. These includes intracranial spreading of suppurative infection, sudden airway obstruction due to epiglottitis and diphtheria, rheumatic fever after streptococcal tonsillitis, etc. In this chapter, we will describe clinical settings, diagnostic work-up, and treatment of upper respiratory infections, with special consideration to complications and life-threatening diseases occurring as a result of these infections.

INTRODUCTION

The upper respiratory system includes the nose, nasal cavity, pharynx, and larynx with subglottic area of trachea. In the normal circumstances, air enters the respiratory system through nostrils where it is filtered, humidified, and warmed inside the nasal cavity. Conditioned air passes through pharynx, larynx, and trachea and then enters in lower respiratory system. Dysfunction of any part of upper respiratory tract may change quality of inhaled air and consequently, may impair function of tracheobronchial tree and lung. Upper respiratory tract infections are the most common infections in the population. They are the leading cause for people missing work or school and, thus, have important social implications. They range from mild, self-limiting disease like common cold, syndrome of the nasopharynx to serious, life-threatening illnesses, such as epiglottitis.

Most of these infections are of viral origin, involving more or less all the parts of upper respiratory system and associated structures, such as paranasal sinuses and middle ear. Common upper respiratory tract infections include rhinitis (inflammation of the nasal mucosa), rhinosinusitis or sinusitis (inflammation of the nares and paranasal sinuses, including frontal, ethmoid, maxillary, and sphenoid), nasopharyngitis (rhinopharyngitis or the common cold—inflammation of the nares pharynx, hypopharynx, uvula, and tonsils), pharyngitis (inflammation of the pharynx, hypopharynx, uvula, and tonsils), epiglottitis (inflammation of the superior portion of the larynx and supraglottic area), laryngitis (inflammation of the larynx), laryngotracheitis (inflammation of the larynx, trachea, and subglottic area), and tracheitis (inflammation of the trachea and subglottic area).

In most cases, these diseases are self-limiting and can be managed at home. The more severe cases or those with complications need to seek medical help. In general, symptomatic therapy is sufficient (analgesics, antipyretics, anticholinergic agents, antihistamines, antitussives, adrenergic agonists, corticosteroids, decongestants), in some instances antibiotics, or some traditional way of cure are also used. Rarely, surgical intervention or in most serious cases, care in the intensive care unit (ICU) is necessary.

NATURAL OCCURRENCE OF THE DISEASE

Most upper respiratory tract infections are caused by viruses and bacteria, which invade the mucosa. In most cases, the infection spreads from person-to-person, when touching the secretions by hand or directly by inhaling the respiratory droplets. Bacterial infections could be a prime cause of upper respiratory tract infection, but they may also be due to superinfection of a primarily viral infection.

Risk factors for the development of upper respiratory tract infections are close contact like close contact of small children who attend the kindergarten or school, travellers with exposure to numerous individuals, smoking (second-hand smoke too!), which may alter mucosal resistance, anatomic changes of respiratory tract, and nasal polyposis.

The respiratory tract is very well equipped to combat all kinds of invaders. The defense mechanisms include physical, mechanical, humoral, and cellular immune defenses. Mechanical barrier like hair in nose, which filter and trap some pathogens and mucus coats are very efficient. Ciliated cells with its escalator-like properties help transport all kinds of particles up to the pharynx; from there, they are swallowed into the stomach.

Humoral immunity, by means of locally secreted immunoglobulin A and other immunoglobulins and cellular immunity, acts to reduce the local infections. Inflammatory and immune cells (macrophages, monocytes, neutrophils, and eosinophils) coordinate by means of numerous cytokines and other mediates to engulf and destroy invaders. In case of diminished immune function (inherited or acquired), there is an increased risk for developing the upper respiratory tract infection or prolonged course of disease. Special attention is recommended in those with suboptimal immune defenses like those for instance, without a spleen, those with human immunodeficiency virus (HIV) infection, patients with cancer, patients receiving chemotherapy, dialysis, and those undergoing stem cell or organ transplantation. Adequate antimicrobial treatment and follow-up should be advocated, because a simple upper respiratory tract infection may rapidly progress to a systemic illness in immunocompromised patients.

DIAGNOSIS

The diagnosis of upper respiratory tract infections in most cases rests only upon recognition of the symptoms and physical examination. The classification of those diseases is built upon the clinical manifestations, as already mentioned.

Some of these diseases can be treated at home. If the symptoms are severe, have unexpected prolonged duration, or in some other circumstances like in immunocompromised persons, or during epidemics, medical attention is necessary. The aim is to recognize or detect the causative agent and, thus, enable efficient therapy. In some instances, visualization and imaging techniques help in the management of these patients.

The armamentarium of investigations to reach the final diagnosis is huge.

Microbiology

As most of the upper respiratory tract infections are caused by viruses and as there are no targeted therapies for most viruses, viral testing usually is not indicated, except on several occasions like suspected influenza or in immunocompromised patients.

The search for the type of causative bacterial infection should be performed in some cases. Most frequent is a group A *Streptococcal* infection, especially with pharyngitis, colloquially known as a "strep throat". Group A β-hemolytic streptococcus is the etiologic agent in approximately 10% of adult cases of pharyngitis. The clinical features[1] that can raise a suspicion are:

- Erythema, swelling, or exudates on tonsils or pharynx
- Fever with a temperature of at least 38.3°C for 24 hours
- Tender anterior cervical lymph nodes
- Absence of cough, rhinorrhea, and conjunctivitis (common in viral illness)
- Patient age 5–15 years
- Occurrence in the season with highest prevalence (winter-spring).

If clinical suspicion is high, no further testing is necessary and empirical antibiotic is given. When the diagnosis is inconclusive, further testing is recommended. The rapid antigen test for group A *Streptococcus* is fast, as it gives results in about half an hour, and its specificity is satisfactory. Throat cultures are not recommended for the routine primary evaluation of adults with pharyngitis or for the confirmation of negative rapid antigen tests. Throat cultures may be indicated as part of investigation of outbreaks of group A β-hemolytic streptococcal disease, for monitoring the development and spread of antibiotic resistance, or when pathogens such as *Gonococcus* are being considered.

In most patients with suspected bacterial rhinosinusitis, the search for causative bacteria is not indicated. Sinus puncture aspiration may be performed by trained personnel in rare occasions like in a persistent disease, suppurative spread, and in immunocompromised patients or in nosocomial infections. The search for causative agent in rhinosinusitis may be necessary if the disease has an extended duration, or if influenza, mononucleosis, or herpes simplex is suspected. In rare occasions of laryngitis, the suspicion of diphtheria warrants specific tests.

The materials for microbiology analysis are collected by several procedures: throat swab, nasal wash, swabs, or aspirates for sinus puncture, and aspiration, or by the aid of endoscope.

Diagnostic tests for specific agents are helpful when targeted upper respiratory tract infection therapy follows the isolation of a specific microbe.

Imaging

Radiological studies, plain radiographic films, computed tomography (CT), ultrasound, and endoscopic inspection are not indicated in most cases, for instance, in common cold.[2]

Common plain radiographic findings of sinus include air-fluid levels and mucosal thickening, although all sinusitis patients do not show air-fluid levels (Figure 1).

CT scanning can be helpful in the diagnosis of acute and chronic sinusitis, but it cannot distinguish between acute and chronic paranasal sinusitis. The CT findings have to be interpreted with respect to clinical features.[3]

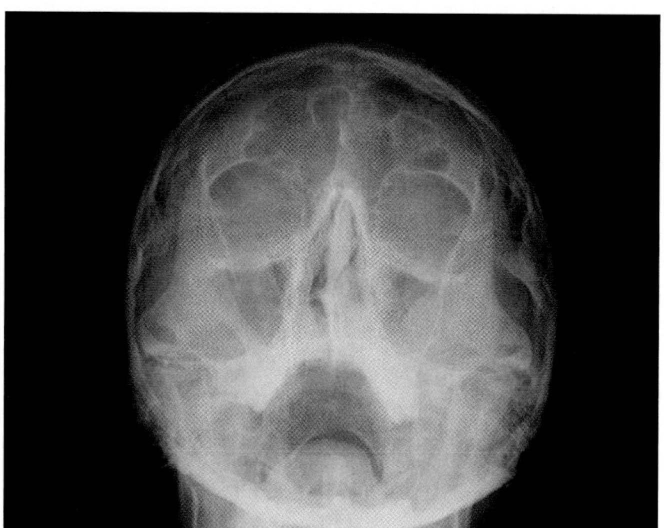

FIGURE 1 Plain radiograph of sinuses shows polypoid edema predominantly on the left maxillary sinus, edema of the nasal conches, and nasal septal deviation.

CT findings of sinus opacification, air-fluid levels, and thickened localized mucosa are all features of acute sinusitis. Many nonspecific CT findings, including thickened turbinates and diffusely thickened sinus mucosa may be detected (Figure 2).

CT findings suggestive of chronic sinusitis include mucosal thickening, opacified air cells, bony remodeling, and bony thickening due to inflammatory osteitis of the sinus cavity walls. Bony erosion can occur in severe cases especially, if associated with massive polyps or mucocele.

If symptoms of rhinosinusitis extend despite therapy or if propagation of disease into adjacent tissue is suspected, sinus imaging is indicated. Signs or symptoms, which warrent intracranial extension of infection, request CT analysis to anfirm the possibility of an intracranial abscess or other suppurative complications. Such symptoms may include proptosis, impaired intraocular movements, decreased vision, papilledema, changes in mental status, or other neurologic findings.

Sinus ultrasonography may also be useful in the intensive care or if radiation exposure is to be avoided. Recently, it has been reported[4] that owing to a very good specificity and negative predictive value, bedside A-mode ultrasound may be a useful first-line examination for intubated and mechanically ventilated patients in intensive care, especially to eliminate suspicion of maxillary sinusitis.

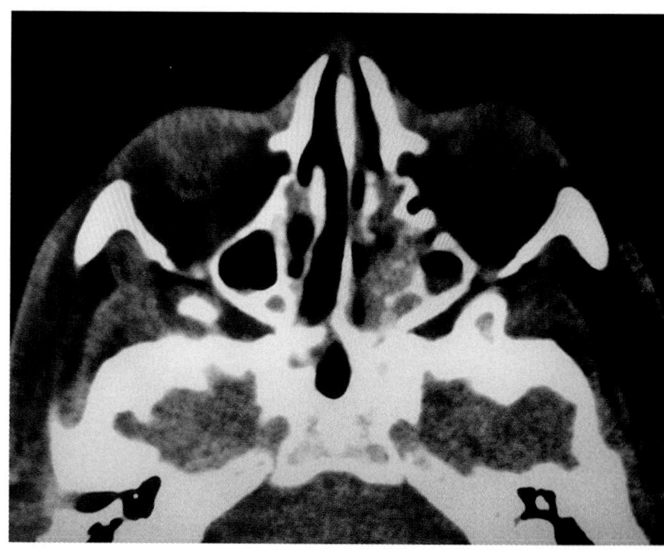

FIGURE 2 Computed tomography scan of paranasal sinuses shows thickening predominantly of the left maxillary sinus, almost diffuse opacification of ethmoid sinuses (especially left sinus) with partially resorbed intracellular septa. Marginal thickening of sphenoidal sinuses and thickening of the nasal passage is also detected.

Nasal Endoscopy and Laryngoscopy

Nasal endoscopy has a definite role in the identification of sinonasal disease. But it has to be underlined that it does not apply to most of the patients with acute diseases who seek medical attention for the first time but only to those with prolonged course, severe symptoms, or when a suspicion of serious complications exists.

The indications for the procedure are the detection of disease in patients experiencing sinonasal symptoms (e.g., mucopurulent drainage, facial pain or pressure, nasal obstruction or congestion, or decreased sense of smell) , evaluation of medical treatment (e.g., resolution of polyps, purulent secretions, convalescence of mucosal edema, and inflammation), evaluation of patients with complications or imminent complications of sinusitis, obtaining a culture of purulent secretions, evaluation of the nasopharynx for lymphoid hyperplasia, Eustachian tube problems, and nasal obstruction.

The laryngoscopy is performed in cases of suspected epiglottitis with great caution, only in well-equipped medical centers where the possible complications could be avoided. The instrumentation can provoke airway spasms and induce respiratory insufficiency.

RHINITIS AND RHINOSINUSITIS

Rhinitis is an inflammation and swelling of the mucous membranes of the nose, characterized by a runny nose, rhinorrhea, sneezing, congestion, obstruction of nasal breathing, and in some cases, pruritus. On the basis of duration of symptoms and changes of nasal mucosa, rhinitis may be acute or chronic. Etiology includes a number of causes, and infectious rhinitis is only one among many (Table 1). Each type of rhinitis may induce associated episode of sinusitis in a predisposed patient because of blockages in intranasal passages.

TABLE 1
Classification and Etiology of Rhinitis

Type of rhinitis	Etiology
Infectious rhinitis	Viruses, bacteria, fungi
Vasomotor rhinitis	Disbalance of the parasympathetic and sympathetic system
Occupational rhinitis	Inhaled irritants
Hormonal rhinitis	Estrogen imbalance
Drug-induced rhinitis	ACEI, β-blockers, methyldopa, aspirin, NSAID, phentolamine, chlorpromazine, penicillamine, inhaled cocaine, estrogen, oral contraceptives
Gustatory rhinitis	Hot and spicy food
Allergic rhinitis	Various allergens
Nonallergic rhinitis with eosinophilia	Abnormal prostaglandin metabolism

ACEI, angiotensin-converting enzyme inhibitors; NSAID, nonsteroidal anti-inflammatory drugs.

Acute Viral Rhinitis (Common Cold)

Acute infectious rhinitis and rhinosinusitis are usually the part of an upper respiratory infection, which involves pharynx known as common cold. Human rhinovirus is responsible for 50–80% of all common colds and the rest are caused by corona virus, adenovirus, parainfluenza virus, respiratory syncytial virus (RSV), or enterovirus.[5]

The incidence of the common cold varies by age. Children younger than 5 years tend to have 3–8 episodes of common cold per year on an average, while adolescents and adults may have approximately 1–4 episodes in an year.[6]

Patients typically present with runny nose, sneezing, congestion, clear-to-mucopurulent nasal discharge, an altered sense of smell, postnasal drip with cough, and a low-grade fever. Facial pain and pressure may also be present. Occasionally, headache, rash (with group A streptococcal infections or enterovirus), gastrointestinal symptoms, myalgia, and fatigue are also present.

Substantial rhinorrhea is a distinctive feature of viral infection. During 2–3 days the nasal discharge turns from clear to mat, greenish and yellow. Fever is unusual in adults. These properties do not differentiate viral from bacterial infection. Due to pharyngeal involvement, the act of swallowing could be transiently disturbed and painful. Nasal blockage may cause mouth breathing and dry mouth.

Viral infections are generally self-limiting and resolve within 7–10 days. Therapy should be directed to symptomatic care, which includes analgesics, antipyretics, and saline irrigation. The use of topical or oral decongestants leads to rebound symptoms and should be avoided. Fluid intake should be encouraged to replace insensible losses and reduced oral intake. If symptoms like fever or cough are present, physical activities should be reduced, because rest is beneficial in the process of recovery.

Because of anatomical predisposition, acute viral rhinitis in young children may be accompanied by congestion of Eustachian tube, reducing air influx in the middle ear space, and resulting in otitis media. Since 1980s, there was controversy regarding antimicrobial therapy versus observation in children with a confirmed diagnosis of acute otitis media due to acute upper respiratory infection, presumably of viral origin. However, recent investigations showed that children recovered more quickly when they were treated with amoxicillin-clavulanate, initiated at the time of diagnosis.[7,8]

Acute Bacterial Rhinosinusitis

Persistent symptoms of acute rhinosinusitis for longer than 10 days or worsening of symptoms after 5–7 days, purulent discharge, and moderate-to-high grade fever suggest a secondary bacterial infection (Figure 3). In children, the most common symptoms of bacterial rhinosinusitis are cough, nasal discharge, fever, and malodorous breath.

In patients with acute bacterial rhinosinusitis, nasal discharge is purulent and minimal, not responding to symptomatic medication and, occasionally, accompanied by sneezing. Hyposmia or anosmia is transitional. Usually, especially in adults, the pain is restricted to diseased sinus. The cough in rhinosinusitis is present all day around, but usually it is most striking in the morning, after waking up, as a reaction to the accumulated secretions in the posterior pharynx during the night.

The inspection reveals mucopurulent secretion, edema and erythema of mucosa, causes of nasal obstruction like polyps or septal deviation, periorbital swelling in ethmoid sinusitis, and facial tenderness in the projection of frontal and maxillary sinus.

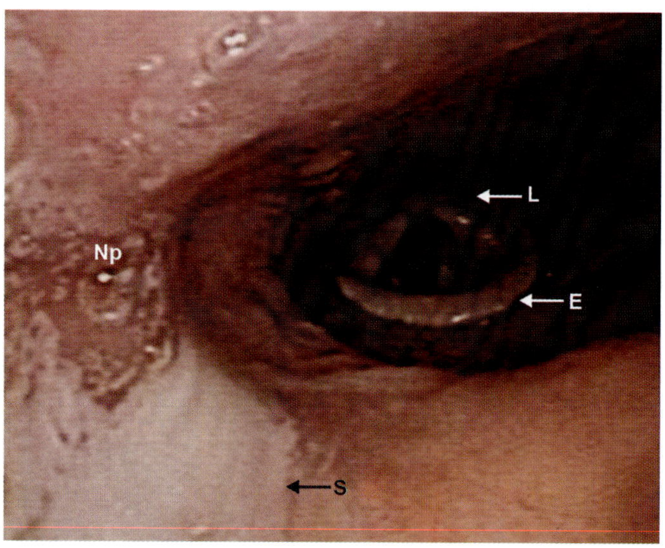

L, larynx; E, epiglottis; Np, nasopharynx; s, secretion.

FIGURE 3 Bacterial rhinosinusitis and nasal drip (endoscopic view). Notice the leakage of purulent secretion from nasopharynx to oropharynx and larynx. Nasal drip induces laryngeal irritation and cough. *Courtesy of Professor Ranko Mladina, MD, PhD. Private Collection.*

Sinusitis is common in persons with viral upper respiratory tract infection, but it refers only to the transitional changes on CT. Yet, it is clinically explicit in only about 2–10% of persons with viral upper respiratory tract infection.[9] The major pathogens of acute bacterial sinusitis are *Streptococcus pneumoniae* and *Hemophilus influenzae*, followed by α-hemolytic and β-hemolytic streptococci, *Staphylococcus aureus*, and anaerobes. In the past decade, *S. anginosus* and methicillin-resistant *S. aureus* (MRSA) has been increasingly recognized as a cause of bacterial sinusitis in children and adolescents.[10] Plain radiograph of the sinuses may reveal complete sinus opacity, air-fluid level, or marked mucosal thickening. CT provides a detailed view of the paranasal sinuses, but this technique is not routinely indicated in evaluation of uncomplicated sinusitis. While nasopharyngeal swab is unreliable, microbiological cultures should be obtained by direct sinus aspiration. Endoscopically guided cultures of the middle meatus may be considered in adults, but their reliability in children has not been established. Due to lack of precision and practicality of current diagnostic methods, the clinical diagnosis of acute bacterial rhinosinusitis is made primarily on the basis of history and symptoms (Table 2).[11] Untreated bacterial rhinosinusitis may cause a number of severe complications: osteitis of the sinus bones, orbital cellulitis, and spread of bacteria to the central nervous system resulting in meningitis, brain abscess, or infection of intracranial cavernous sinus.[12] For this reason empirical antimicrobial therapy should be initiated immediately after the clinical diagnosis of bacterial infection is established. Amoxicillin-clavulanate is the first-choice antimicrobial agent, which is superior to amoxicillin in coverage of increasing β-lactamase-producing pathogens among upper respiratory tract isolates. Doxycycline is an alternative in adults with penicillin allergy. Children

TABLE 2

Viral and Bacterial Rhinosinusitis: Differential Diagnosis

Features	Viral rhinosinusitis	Bacterial rhinosinusitis
Duration of symptoms and signs compatible with acute rhinosinusitis	7–10 days	≥10 days
Fever ≥39°C	No	Yes
Purulent nasal discharge lasting for 3 or more consecutive days	No	Yes
Facial pain lasting for 3 or more consecutive days	No	Yes
New onset of symptoms after initial improvment	No	Yes

with non-type I penicillin allergy may be treated with combination of a third-generation oral cephalosporin and clindamycin. Fluoroquinolones are reserved for patients in whom first-line therapy has failed.[6] Recommended duration of antimicrobial treatment is 5–7 days for uncomplicated bacterial rhinosinusitis in adults, and 10–14 days in children. Intranasal corticosteroids are recommended as an adjunct therapy in individuals with a history of allergic rhinitis. Over-the-counter drugs like decongestants and antihistamines should be avoided.[6] The advantage of probiotics in preventing the antibiotic-associated diarrhea has been reported recently.[13] The pooled evidence suggested that probiotics are associated with a reduction in antibiotic-associated diarrhea, but it was concluded that more research is needed to determine, which probiotics are associated with the greatest efficacy and for which patients should receive which specific antibiotics.

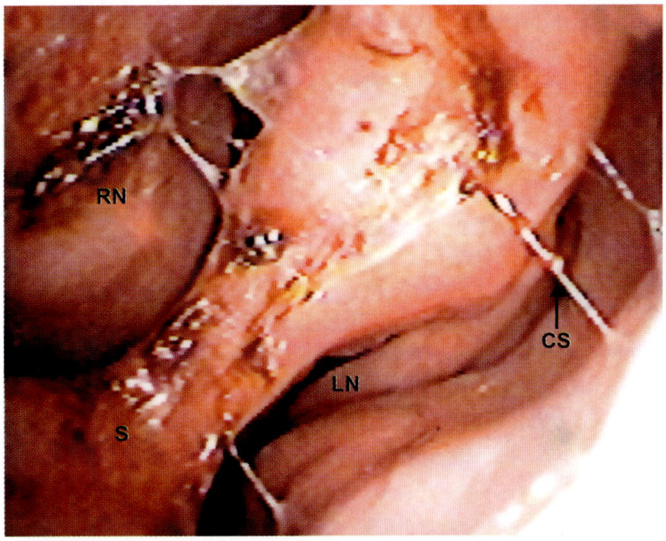

RN, right nostril; LN, left nostril; S, destroyed septum; CS, cobweb pattern of secretion.

FIGURE 4 Chronic "cobweb" rhinitis (endoscopic view from the left nostril). Endoscopy reveals chronic rhinitis with multiple mucosal erosions and almost completely destroyed nasal septum. Cobweb secretion is consistent with colonization and invasion of molds (*Fusarium* spp.).

Chronic Rhinitis

Chronic rhinitis is usually a prolongation of subacute inflammatory or infectious viral rhinitis. Low humidity and airborne irritants may contribute to prolonged inflammation. It may also occur in chronic infective diseases, such as syphilis, tuberculosis, rhinosporidiosis, leishmaniasis, blastomycosis, histoplasmosis, and leprosy. All these diseases are characterized by the formation of granulomas, resulting in destruction of soft tissue, cartilage, and bone (Figure 4). The most common symptoms of chronic rhinitis are nasal obstruction, purulent discharge, and frequent bleeding.

A special form of chronic rhinitis is chronic atrophic rhinitis, which is characterized by progressive atrophy and sclerosis of nasal mucosa and underlying bone. The mucous membrane changes from ciliated pseudostratified columnar epithelium to stratified squamous epithelium, and the lamina propria is reduced in amount and vascularity. Atrophic rhinitis may be primary or secondary due to Wegener's granulomatosis or iatrogenically induced excessive nasal tissue extirpation.[14] Primary atrophic rhinitis (also known as ozena) is a disease of unclear etiology that affects predominantly young and middle-aged adults, especially females, with racial preference amongst Asians, Hispanics, and African-Americans.[15] Most of the patients are from rural or industrial environment with high predisposition to allergic or immunologic disorders.[16] Familial etiology with dominant inheritance has also been described.[17] Patients have prolonged bacterial infection, mainly caused by *Klebsiella* species, especially *K. ozaenae*. The common symptoms in both primary and secondary chronic

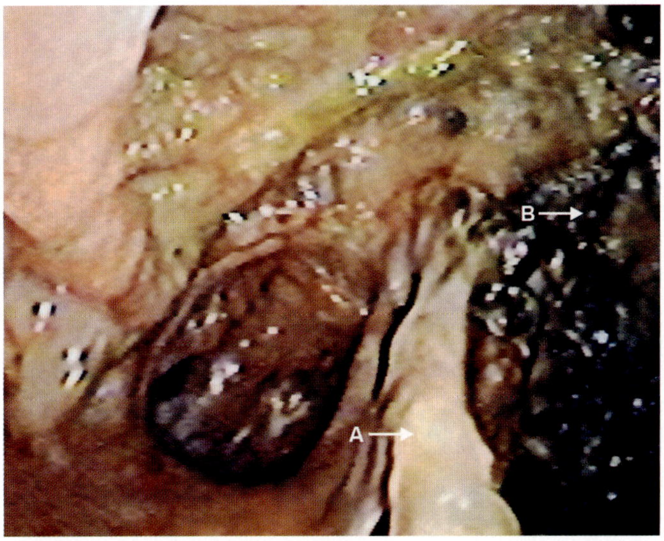

FIGURE 5 Chronic atrophic rhinitis (endoscopic view from the right nostril). Notice the remains of destroyed nasal septum (arrow A) and mucosal crusts in the contralateral nostril (arrow B).

atrophic rhinitis include fetor, crusting, nasal obstruction, epistaxis, anosmia, and sometimes, destruction of soft tissues and cartilages (Figure 5). Different treatment modalities have been described in the literature: nasal irrigation, nose drops (glucose-glycerin, liquid paraffin), topical and systemic antibiotics, vasodilators, estrogens, vitamin A, and D sprayed into the nose or taken through mouth. Surgical treatment aims to decrease the size of the nasal cavities and improves lubrication of dry nasal mucosa. However, there is no evidence from randomized controlled trials concerning the long-term benefits of different treatment modalities for atrophic rhinitis.[9]

PHARYNGITIS

Acute Viral Pharyngitis

Pharyngitis is caused by inflammation and swelling of pharyngeal mucosa. The main symptom of acute pharyngitis is a sore throat. Other symptoms may include fever, headache, joint pain and muscle aches, skin rashes, and swollen lymph nodes in the neck. Inspection discloses pharyngeal erythema, exudates, sometimes mucosal erosions and vesicles, tonsillar hypertrophy, anterior cervical lymphadenopathy, conjunctivitis, and skin rash.

Similar to other upper respiratory infections, the most common cause of acute pharyngitis is a viral infection in settings of common cold or flu. The most common pathogens are rhinovirus, and influenza A and B. Some other viruses can cause specific forms of pharyngitis, such as enteroviruses, Epstein-Barr virus (EBV), and HIV.

Herpangina

Herpangina is a painful pharyngitis caused by various enteroviruses like Coxsackie virus A16, Coxsackie virus B, enterovirus 71, echovirus, parechovirus 1, adenovirus, and herpes simplex virus. Herpangina occurs worldwide, mainly during summer, and most commonly affects infants and young children aged 3–10 years.[18] Clinical manifestation includes high fever, malaise, sore throat, painful swallowing, headache, anorexia, emesis, and sometimes, abdominal pain, which may mimic appendicitis. Enteroviral infections may be accompanied by various type of rash, which depends on viral subtype. In rare cases herpangina may be accompanied by aseptic meningitis and neurological symptoms. Herpangina is characterized by small (less than 5 mm in diameter) vesicular or ulcerative lesions that affect posterior pharyngeal wall, tonsils, soft palate, uvula, and sometimes tongue and buccal mucosa. Enlargement of cervical lymph nodes may also be present. Diagnosis is based upon clinical symptoms, characteristic physical signs, age, epidemiological data, and seasonal appearance. Microbiological standard for diagnosis is based on isolation of enterovirus in cell culture obtained from swabs of the nasopharynx. Other specimens include stool, urine, serum, and cerebrospinal fluid (CSF). However, laboratory analyses are not necessary in most of cases, because herpangina is usually mild and self-limiting illness. Supportive therapy includes hydration, adequate caloric intake, limited activity, antipyretics, and topical analgesics.

Infectious Mononucleosis

EBV causes infectious mononucleosis, which is characterized by fever, tonsillar pharyngitis, lymphadenopathy, lymphocytosis, and atypical mononuclear cells in the blood. EBV spreads by a close contact between susceptible persons and EBV shedders. The majority of primary EBV infections are subclinical and inapparent. Antibodies to EBV have been demonstrated in 90–95% of adults worldwide. The incidence of symptomatic infection begins to rise from adolescence through adult years.[19] Transmission of EBV requires intimate contact with the saliva of an infected person. The incubation period ranges from 4 to 6 weeks. The clinical diagnosis of infectious mononucleosis is suggested in adolescents or young adults with the symptoms of fever, sore throat, and swollen lymph glands. An enlargement of liver and spleen may also be present. Laboratory results include an elevated white blood cell count, an increased percentage of certain atypical white blood cells, and a positive reaction to a "monospot" test. Treatment strategy for infectious mononucleosis is supportive and symptomatic. The use of steroids has also been occasionally reported to decrease the overall prolongation and severity of illness, but there is no available randomized clinical studies to support such therapeutic approach. Persons with infectious mononucleosis may spread the infection for a period of weeks. However, no special precautions or isolation procedures are recommended, since the virus is also found in the saliva of healthy people who carry and spread the virus intermittently for life. These people are usually the primary reservoir of virus, and for this reason the transmission is impossible to prevent.[20]

Acute HIV Infection

Primary or acute HIV infection (also known as acute retroviral syndrome) refers to the interval from initial infection to the time that antibody to HIV is detectable. During this stage of infection, patients are highly infectious due to enormous viral load in blood and genital secretion (>100,000 copies/mL), and negative or indeterminate HIV antibody test results.[21] Approximately, 60% of recently infected persons develop primary acute infection 2–6 weeks after exposure to HIV.[22] Symptoms include fever, fatigue, myalgia, mucocutaneous ulcerations, pharyngitis, anorexia, generalized lymphadenopathy, rash, and sometimes neurologic symptoms. Pharyngitis, usually exudative, is accompanied with cervical lymphadenopathy resembling infectious mononucleosis ("mononucleosis-like" illness).[23] Common laboratory findings include leukopenia, thrombocytopenia, and mild transaminase elevations. Symptoms persist for less than 4 weeks, except lymphadenopathy that may last longer.

Acute Bacterial Pharyngitis

Acute bacterial pharyngitis and tonsillopharyngitis usually occur during the colder months. The most common cause is group A β-hemolytic *Streptococcus* (*S. pyogenes*), which is responsible for 15–30% of all cases of pharyngitis in children and for 10% in adults.[24] Antibiotic therapy is recommended to hasten the resolution of clinical symptoms, and to prevent the occurrence of nonsuppurative complications, such as rheumatic fever. A 10-day course of antibiotic therapy with penicillin is the standard of care for streptococcal tonsillopharyngitis. Alternatives to this "gold" standard are other β-lactams (e.g., amoxicillin, cephalosporins), macrolides, and clindamycin.

EPIGLOTTITIS

Epiglottis is a part of oropharynx, and it forms the back wall of the vallecular space below the base of tongue. During the act of swallowing, it also protects larynx and trachea from aspiration. Infectious epiglottitis is a cellulitis of the epiglottis, aryepiglottic folds, and other adjacent tissues. Infection of epiglottis is a consequence from bacteremia, or direct invasion of the epithelium by microbial pathogens. The primary source of bacteria is posterior wall of nasopharynx. The most frequent causative microorganisms are *H. influenzae*, *S. pneumoniae*, *S. aureus*, and β-hemolytic streptococci. Microscopic epithelial trauma by viral infection or mucosal damage from food during swallowing may predispose to bacterial invasion, inducing inflammation and edema. Swelling of tissue rapidly progresses, and involves aryepiglottic folds and arytenoids.[25] Thus, epiglottitis may cause life-threatening airway obstruction.

In children, symptoms develop abruptly within a few hours of onset. Symptoms and signs include sore throat, dysphagia, loss of voice, inspiratory stridor, fever, anxiety, dyspnea, tachypnea, and cyanosis. Dyspnea often causes the child to sit upright, lean forward, with hyperextended neck, and mouth open for enhancing the exchange of air (tripod position). Treatment of epiglottitis is based on the maintenance of airway. Patients should be monitored continuously in the emergency department or intensive care unit by staff that is able to perform rapid resuscitation, stabilization of airway, and ventilation.[26] Orotracheal intubation or needle cricothyroidotomy should be performed in an emergency situation when respiratory arrest occurs. Antibiotic therapy is necessary but should be initiated after securing the airway. Before culture results, empirically administered antimicrobial therapy should cover the most likely causative pathogens, such as *S. aureus*, group A streptococci,[27] *H. influenzae*, and *Candida albicans* in immunocompromised patients.[28]

Epiglottitis may be fatal due to sudden compromise of airways or complications like meningitis, empyema, or mediastinitis, with a mortality rate of around 1% in adults.

LARYNGITIS

Laryngitis is an acute or chronic inflammation of laryngeal structures. Etiology includes a number of infectious and noninfectious causes listed in table 3. The most common causative agent of acute laryngitis is the rhinovirus. Others include influenza A and B, adenoviruses, parainfluenza viruses, *H. influenzae* type B, β-hemolytic streptococci,

TABLE 3
Classifications and Etiology of Laryngitis

Infectious laryngitis	
Viral	• Rhinovirus • Influenza A, B, C • Adenoviruses • Parainfluenza viruses • RSV • Measles • Varicella-zoster
Bacterial	• *Hemophilus influenzae* type B • β-hemolytic streptococci • *Moraxella catarrhalis* • *Streptococcus pneumoniae* • *Klebsiella pneumoniae* • *Staphylococcus aureus* • Diphtheria (*Corynebacterium diphtheriae, Corynebacterium ulcerans*) • Tuberculosis (*Mycobacterium tuberculosis*) Syphilis (*Treponema pallidum*)
Fungal	• *Candida albicans* • *Blastomyces dermatitidis* • *Histoplasma capsulatum* • *Cryptococcus neoformans*
Noninfectious laryngitis	
Irritant laryngitis due to inhalation of toxic agents, alcoholism, smoking, drugs (crack), allergy, GERD, vocal abuse, laryngeal involvement of rheumatoid arthritis, SLE, hypothyroidism, angioneurotic edema	

RSV, respiratory syncytial virus; GERD, gastroesophageal reflux disease; SLE, systemic lupus erythematosus.

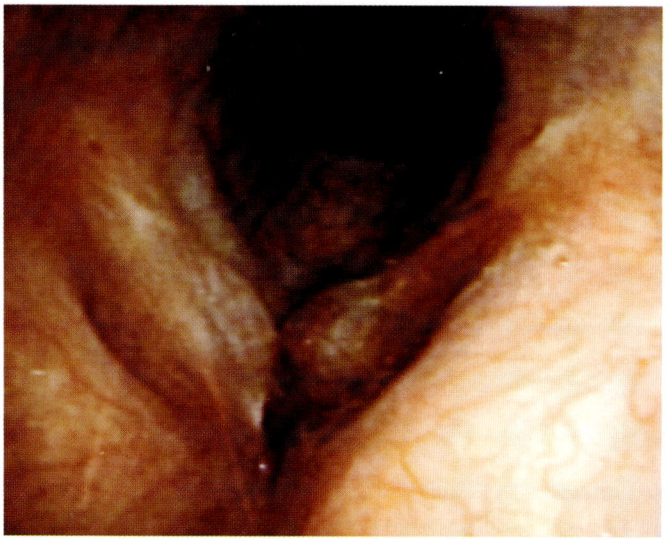

FIGURE 6 Chronic laryngitis (endoscopic view). The laryngeal mucosa appears hyperemic and swollen, forming inflammatory pseudotumors in the anterior part of both vocal folds.

etc. Acute laryngitis may occur as an isolated infection or, more commonly, as a part of a generalized viral or bacterial upper respiratory tract infection. It begins with hoarseness (from mild-to-complete loss of voice), painful swallowing or speaking, dry cough, and laryngeal edema of varying degrees (Figure 6). Fever and malaise are common. Symptoms usually resolve in 7 days. In chronic laryngitis, hoarseness is usually the only symptom that persists for more than three weeks. When the clinical presentation lies between acute and chronic subtype, sometimes it may be of clinical utility to classify as subacute.

Diagnostic procedure begins with comprehensive history of disease that includes chronicity of the condition, epidemiologic data, exposure to environmental fumes and irritants, medication, and smoking habits. In acute laryngitis, indirect laryngoscopy reveals red, inflamed, and occasionally, hemorrhagic vocal cords with round swelling edges and exudates. Physical examination should also include the oropharynx, thyroid, and cervical lymph nodes. Chronic fungal laryngitis caused by *C. albicans* that is a common side effect of inhaled steroids, is characterized by multiple chalk-white mucosal patches spreading on epiglottis, and oropharynx.[29] Laboratory findings (white blood cell count, C-reactive protein) may be an aid in distinguishing viral from bacterial infection. If there is a suspicion on bacterial or fungal cause, laryngeal exudate and oropharyngeal swab should be obtained for cultures. Rapid antigen detection test is also useful in detection of bacterial infection. Diagnosis of diphtheria requires positive culture from respiratory tract secretion, and positive toxin assay. Diagnosis of laryngeal tuberculosis that is usually a complication of extensive pulmonary tuberculosis is based on positive acid fast bacilli in sputum or oropharyngeal swab, and positive cultures for *Mycobacterium tuberculosis*.

Duration of hoarseness is important in differential diagnosis. Acute hoarseness is present in hay fever, acute inhalation of toxic fumes and irritants, aspiration of caustic chemicals, foreign body aspiration, and angioneurotic edema, besides acute infectious laryngitis. Differential diagnosis of chronic hoarseness includes numerous diseases, such as laryngeal cancer, lung cancer with mediastinal involvement, trauma of vocal cords, vocal abuse, gastroesophageal reflux disease (GERD), chronic rhinosinusitis with sinobronchial syndrome, laryngeal involvement in rheumatoid arthritis, systemic lupus erythematosus (SLE), and hypothyroidism.

Diphtheria

Diphtheria is caused by the Gram-positive bacillus *Corynebacterium diphtheriae* and in some cases by *C. ulcerans*. Infected individuals may develop respiratory disease, cutaneous disease, or become asymptomatic carrier. Infection spreads by close contact with infectious respiratory secretions or from skin lesions. The transmission of *C. ulcerans* via cow's milk has been described.[30] Diphtheria occurs throughout the year with peak incidence in winter. At the beginning patients suffer from malaise, sore throat, and low grade fever. Symptoms progress to hoarseness, barking cough, and stridor, also known as croup. Individuals with severe disease develop cervical lymph node enlargement and neck swelling ("bull-neck"). Physical examination reveals hyperemic pharyngeal and laryngeal mucosa with areas of white exudates forming the adherent grey pseudomembrane that bleeds with scraping.[31] Extension of the pseudomembrane into larynx and trachea may lead to airway obstruction with subsequent suffocation and death. Definitive diagnosis requires positive cultures of *C. diphtheriae* from respiratory secretions or cutaneous lesions, and positive toxin assay. Specimens for cultures should be obtained from the throat and nose, including a portion of membrane.

Corynebacterium diphtheriae was first identified in 1880. The first antitoxin against diphtheria was developed in the 1890s, with the first vaccine developed in the 1920s. With the administration of vaccine, the incidence of disease has decreased significantly, although it is still endemic in many parts of the world. Furthermore, while diphtheria primarily affected young children in the prevaccination era, today an increasing proportion of cases occur in unvaccinated or inadequately immunized adolescents and adults.[32]

Croup Illnesses

In prevaccination era the term "croup" was a synonym for diphtheria. Today, the word "croup" refers to a number of respiratory illnesses that are characterized by varying degrees of stridor, barking cough, and hoarseness due to obstruction in the region of the larynx.[33] "That group of illnesses affects infants and children younger than 6 years of age with a peak incidence between 7 and 36 months.[34] Host factors, especially allergic factors, seem to be important in the pathogenesis.[35] Croup illnesses are most commonly caused by parainfluenza viruses, following by influenza virus A, RSV, measles virus, adenovirus, and rhinovirus. In some instances, such as the laryngotracheal bronchopneumonitis and bacterial tracheitis, the croup feature is due to secondary bacterial infection, particularly from *S. aureus*. According to symptoms and signs, croup illnesses are divided in three clinical entities:

1. Spasmodic croup: sudden night time onset of stridor and barking cough, without fever, without inflammation, nontoxic presentation.
2. Acute laryngotracheobronchitis: hoarseness and barking cough, minimal-to-severe stridor, high fever, minimal toxic presentation.
3. Laryngotracheobronchitis, laryngotracheobroncho-pneumonitis, and bacterial tracheitis: hoarseness and barking cough, severe stridor, high fever, typically toxic presentation, and secondary bacterial infection is common.

Treatment of acute laryngitis depends on severity of illness and degree of airway compromise. The most common acute viral laryngitis is usually self-limiting, requiring only supportive treatment, such as analgesics, mucolytics,[36] voice rest, increased hydration, and limited caffeine intake. Antibiotics are needed only when a bacterial infection is suspected.[37] However, sometimes it is a challenge for the physician to recognize when antibiotics are required.

Patients with any degree of airway compromise, especially those suffering from diphtheria and other "croup" illnesses, require particular care. In addition, patients with an underlying risk factor that limits airway, such as subglottic stenosis or vocal cord paralysis, may develop severe airway obstruction even in settings of slight inflammation of laryngeal structures. Corticosteroids should be administered in all patients with possible airway compromise, and airways should be monitored closely to assess the need for tracheotomy.[38]

Patients who are suspected to have diphtheria, need to be hospitalized and should be given diphtheria antitoxin and antibiotic (penicillin or erythromycin). They must be isolated to avoid exposing others to the infection. Diphtheria antitoxin is a crucial step of treatment, and should be administered as early as possible, without waiting for culture results.[39] In severe cases of airway obstruction, when patient cannot breathe on their own, inserting breathing tube and tracheotomy may be necessary.[40]

Treatment of croup illnesses other than diphtheria is based on corticosteroids (intramuscular dexamethasone 0.6 mg/kg). In severe cases, repeated treatments with epinephrine have been used and often decreased the need for intubation.[41] Since the most severe types of croup illnesses are associated with secondary bacterial infection due to *S. aureus*, *S. pneumoniae*, *H. influenzae*, or *Moraxella catarrhalis*, antibiotics should be administered after cultures have been obtained. Most of the children with such severe form of croup require placement of mechanical airway and treatment in an intensive care unit.

Chronic tuberculous laryngitis is almost always a complication of active pulmonary tuberculosis and requires the same antituberculosis drug regimen as pulmonary tuberculosis. Since it is highly contagious, prompt diagnosis and adequate treatment are critical.

Fungal laryngitis commonly appears in immuno-compromised patients, and treatment is based on systemic antifungal drugs. In immunocompetent individuals, fungal laryngitis is often associated with regular usage of inhaled corticosteroids for asthma control. Patients should be advised to rinse mouth before and after inhalation and the dose of corticosteroid should be reduced wherever it is possible.

TRACHEITIS

Tracheitis is an inflammatory process of the larynx, trachea, and bronchi. Most conditions that affect the trachea are bacterial or viral infections; however, irritants and dense smoke can injure the epithelium of the trachea and increase the likelihood of infections. Although infectious tracheitis may affect patients of any age, it presents a special problem in children because of the size and anatomic shape of the airway. The major site of disease is at the subglottic area, which is the narrowest part of the trachea. Airway obstruction may develop secondary to subglottic edema or accumulation of mucopurulent secretion within trachea. The most frequent causes of tracheitis are *S. aureus*' group A β-hemolytic streptococci, *M. catarrhalis*, *H. influenzae* type B, *Klebsiella* species, *Pseudomonas* species, anaerobes, *Mycoplasma pneumoniae*, and influenza A virus (H1N1).[42] Rarely, bacterial tracheitis may develop as a complication of a preceding viral infection or an injury from endotracheal intubation. Bacterial tracheitis is uncommon, with the incidence of approximately 0.1 cases per 100 000 children per year.[43] However, it is the condition of high priority, because the mortality rate has been estimated at 4–20%.[44] Clinical presentation includes high fever, toxic appearance, inspiratory stridor, and bark like cough, hoarseness, dysphonia, and variable degree of respiratory distress. Diagnosis can be confirmed by direct laryngotracheobronchoscopy, which shows inflammation and purulent secretions in the subglottic area or by lateral neck X-ray, which reveals subglottic narrowing. Laryngotracheobronchoscopy enables obtaining specimens for cultures under direct visualization, and may also be therapeutic by performing tracheal toilet. Differential diagnosis includes angioedema, croup, diphtheria, epiglottitis, peritonsillar abscess, retropharyngeal abscess, and tuberculosis. Treatment is based on maintenance of an adequate airway, which implies endotracheal intubation in most of patients, and antibiotics. Initial antibiotics should cover the most common causative bacteria. Empirical antibiotic regimens include a third-generation cephalosporin and a penicillinase-resistant penicillin, or clindamycin administered intravenously. If there is a suspicion of MRSA in the community, vancomycin should be started. Once definitive microbiological diagnosis is made, appropriate antibiotic therapy should continue for more than 10 days. With appropriate airway support and antibiotics, patients improve within 5 days. However, up to 60% of patients may develop one or more complications that include bronchopneumonia, sepsis, toxic shock, adult respiratory distress syndrome (ARDS), post-extubation subglottic stenosis, anoxic encephalopathy, cardiorespiratory arrest, and retropharyngeal abscess or cellulitis.[45] Children with bacterial tracheitis should be admitted in the intensive care unit, with multidisciplinary medical support.

COMPLICATIONS

In most cases, respiratory tract infections resolve entirely but in a minor number of cases, complications may arise.

Otitis media may be a complication in some 5% of colds in children and around 2% in adults. It has recently been shown[46] in adjusted models controlling for the presence of key viruses, bacteria, and acute otitis media risk factors that acute otitis media risk was independently associated with high respiratory syncytial viral load with *S. pneumoniae* and *H. influenzae*. The risk was higher for the presence of bocavirus and *H. influenzae* together. The conclusion was that acute otitis media risk differed with specific viruses and bacteria involved and that the preventive efforts should consider methods for reducing infections caused by RSV, bocavirus, and adenovirus in addition to acute otitis media bacterial pathogens.

The bronchial hyperreactivity may be enhanced or provoked by respiratory tract infections. Symptom-severity of asthma and the frequency of severe exacerbations were associated with previous exacerbations and susceptibility to upper respiratory tract infection, according to novel research on more than 7,000 patients.[47]

Patients with chronic obstructive pulmonary disease may also experience an exacerbation.

Patients who have persistent cough lasting for more than 3 weeks after they have got through acute symptoms of an upper respiratory tract infection, may have a post-infectious cough. In patients who have a cough lasting from 3 to 8 weeks with normal chest radiograph findings, the diagnosis of postinfectious cough has to be taken into consideration. In most patients, a specific etiologic agent will not be identified, and empiric therapy may be helpful. A high degree of suspicion for cough due to *Bordetella pertussis* infection will lead to earlier diagnosis, patient isolation, and antibiotic treatment.[48]

Bacterial superinfection of viral infection may occur occasionally. The propagation of infection into adjacent tissues, or distant organs may ensue but such sequence of events is quite rare.

Possible complications of group A streptococcal pharyngitis are rheumatic fever, acute glomerulonephritis, scarlet fever, and streptococcal toxic shock syndrome.

Complications of influenza are numerous, and include bacterial superinfection, pneumonia, volume depletion, myositis, pericarditis, rhabdomyolysis, encephalitis, meningitis, myelitis, renal failure, and disseminated intravascular coagulation. Influenza also poses a risk of worsening underlying medical conditions, such as heart failure, asthma, or diabetes.

Complications of mononucleosis are splenic rupture, hepatitis, Guillain-Barré syndrome, encephalitis, hemolytic anemia, agranulocytosis, myocarditis, and Burkitt's lymphoma.

The complications of diphtherias may include airway obstruction, myocarditis, polyneuritis, thrombocytopenia, proteinuria, and hearing loss.[49]

CONCLUSION

Upper respiratory tract infections are the most common infections in general population, with important social implications like missed working hours. Most of acute upper respiratory tract infections are caused by viruses, especially rhinovirus, corona virus, adenovirus, parainfluenza virus, RSV, and enterovirus, that are responsible for more than 80% of all common colds. Bacterial pathogens are more commonly causative agents of prolonged and/or chronic infection adhering to primary viral infections.

In most cases of acute infections, diagnostic work-up is based on recognition of symptoms and physical examination. Additional diagnostic procedure should be performed in prolonged and chronic course of infection and special circumstances such as streptococcal pharyngitis, diphtheria and croup disease, epigotittis, and mononucleosis.

Immunocompromised persons have increased risk for developing the prolonged or complicated course of disease. Special attention is recommended in those with HIV infection, splenectomy, cancer, patients receiving chemotherapy, dialysis, and those undergoing stem cell or organ transplantation. Most of the acute upper respiratory infections are self-limiting, requiring no specific treatment. Antimicrobial therapy should be used for streptococcal pharyngitis, bacterial sinusitis and otitis media, pertussis, diphtheria, and chronic bacterial infections.

REFERENCES

1. Choby BA. Diagnosis and treatment of streptococcal pharyngitis *Am Fam Physician*. 2009;79:383-90.
2. Leung RS, Katial R. The diagnosis and management of acute and chronic sinusitis. *Prim Care*. 2008;35:11-24.
3. Tichenor WS. Sinus CT Scans. Available at: http://www.sinuses.com/ctscan.htm. May 2012.
4. Boet S, Guene B, Jusserand D, Veber B, Dacher JN, Dureuil B. A-mode ultrasound in the diagnosis of maxillary sinusitis in ventilated patients. *B-ENT*. 2010;6: 177-82.
5. Macky IM. Human rhinoviruses: the cold wars resume. *J Clin Virol*. 2008;42:297-320.
6. Meneghetti A. Upper respiratory tract infections. Available at http://emedicine.medscape.com/article/302460-overview. April 2012.
7. Hoberman A, Paradise JL, Rockette HE, Shaikh N, Wald ER, Kearney DH, et al. Treatment of acute otitis media in children under 2 years of age. *N Engl J Med*. 2011;364:105-15.
8. Tahtinen PA, Laine MK, Huovinen P,Jalava J, Ruuskanen O, Ruohole A. A placebo-controlled trial of antimicrobial treatment for acute otitis media. *N Engl J Med*. 2011;364: 116-26.
9. Pleis JR, Lucas JW, Ward BW. Summary health statistics for U.S. adults: National Health Interview Survey, 2008. *Vital Health Stat10*. 2009;(242):1-157.
10. Botting AM, McIntosh D, Mahadevan M. Paediatric pre- and post-septal peri-orbital infections are different diseases. A retrospective review of 262 cases. *Int J Pediatr Otorhinolaryngol*. 2008;72:377–83.
11. Chow AW, Benninger MS, Brook I, Brozek JL, Goldstein EJ, Hicks LA, et al. IDSA clinical practice guideline for acute bacterial rhinosinusitis in children and adults. *Clin Infect Dis*. 2012;54:e72-e112.
12. Germiller JA, Monin DL, Sparano AM, Tom LW. Intracranial complications of sinusitis in children and adolescent. *Arch Otolaryngol Head Neck Surg*. 2006;132:969-76.
13. Hempel S, Newberry SJ, Maher AR, Wang Z, Miles JN, Shanman R, et al. Probiotics for the prevention and treatment of antibiotic-associated diarrhea: a systematic review and meta-analysis. *JAMA*. 2012;307:1959-69.
14. Fried MP. Rhinitis. The Merck Manual for Health Care Professionals. Available from: http://www.merckmanuals.com/professional/ear_nose_and_throat_disorders/nose_and_paranasal_sinus_disorders/rhinitis.html
15. Mishra A, Kawatra R, Gola M. Interventions for atrophic rhinitis. *Cochrane Database Syst Rev*. 2012;2:CD008280.
16. Bunnag C, Jareoncharsi P, Tansuriyawong P, Bhothisuwan W, Chantaraku N. Characteristics of atrophic rhinitis in Thai patients at the Siriraj Hospital. *Rhinology*. 1999;37: 125-30.
17. Silbert JR, Barton RP. Dominant inheritance in a family with primary atrophic rhinitis. *J Med Genet*. 1980;17: 39-40.
18. Wang SM, Liu CC. Enterovirus 71: epidemiology, pathogenesis and management. *Expert Rev Anti Infect Ther*. 2009;7:735-42.
19. Heath CW Jr, Brodsky AL, Potolsky AI. Infectious mononucleosis in a general population. *Am J Epidemiol*. 1972; 95:46-42.
20. CDC. Epstein-Barr virus and infectious monnonucleosis. National Center for Infectious Diseases. Available from: http://www.cdc.gov/ncidod/diseases/ebv.htm.
21. Pilcher CD, Joaki G, Hoffman IF, Martinson FE, Mapanje C, Stewart PW, et al. Amplified transmission of HIV-1: comparison of HIV-1 concentrations in semen and blood during acute and chronic infection. *AIDS*. 2007;21:1723-30.
22. Kassutto S, Rosenberg ES. Primary HIV type 1 infection. *Clin Infect Dis*. 2004;38:1447-53.
23. Cooper DA, Gold J, Maclean P, Donovan B, Finlayson R, Barnes TG, et al. Acute AIDS retrovirus infection. Definition of a clinical illness associated with seroconversion. *Lancet*. 1985;1:537-40.
24. Snow V, Mottur-Pilson C, Cooper RJ, Hoffman JR; American Academy of Family Physicians; American College of Physicians-American Society of Internal Medicine; Centers for Disease Control. Principles of appropriate antibiotic use for acute pharyngitis in adults. *Ann Intern Med*. 2001;134:506-8.
25. Fleisher GR. Infectious disease emergencies. In: Fleisher GR, Ludwig S, Henretig FM editors. Textbook of Pediatric Emergency Medicine. Philadelphia:Lippincott Williams & Wilkins;2002. p.783.
26. Sobol SE, Zapata S. Epiglottitis and croup. *Otolaryngol Clin North Am*. 2008;41:551-66.
27. Alcaide ML, Bisno AL. Pharyngitis and epiglottitis. *Infect Dis Clin North Am*. 2007;21:449-69.
28. Chiou CC, Seibel NL, Derito FA, Bulas D, Walsh TJ, Groll AH. Concomitant Candida epiglottitis and disseminated Varicella zoster virus infection associated with acute lymphoblastic leukemia. *J Pediatr Hematol Oncol*. 2006;28: 757-9.
29. Wong KK, Pace-Asciak P, Wu B, Morrison MD. Laryngeal candidiasis in the outpatient setting. *J Otolaryngol Head Neck Surg*. 2009;38:624-7.
30. Bostock AD, Gilbert FR, Lewis D, Smith DC. *Corynobacterium ulcerans* infection associated with untreated milk. *J Infect*. 1984;9:286-8.

31. Farizio KM, Strebel PM, Chen RT, Kimbler A, Cleary TJ, Cochi SL. Fatal respiratory disease due to *Corynebacterium diphtheriae*: case report and review of guidelines for management, investigation, and control. *Clin Infect Dis.* 1993;16:59-68.
32. Galazka AM, Robertson SE. Diphtheria: changing patterns in the developing world and the industrialized world. *Eur J Epidemiol.* 1995;11:107-17.
33. Cherry JD. Croup. *N Engl J Med.* 2008;358:384-91.
34. Segal AO, Crighton EJ, Moineddin R, Mamdani M, Upshur RE. Croup hospitalization in Ontario: a 14-year time-series analysis. *Pediatrics.* 2005;116:51-5.
35. Welliver RC. Croup: continuing controversy. *Semin Pediatr Infect Dis.* 1995;6:90-5.
36. Garett CG, Ossoff RH. Hoarseness. *Med Clin North Am.* 1999;83:115-23.
37. Reveiz L, Cardona AF, Ospina EG. Antibiotics for acute laryngitis in adults. *Cochrane Database Syst Rev.* 2007;(2): CD004783.
38. Fitzgerald DA. The assessment and management of croup. *Pediatr Respir Rev.* 2006;7:73-81.
39. World Health Organization. Diphtheria. Available from: http://www.who.int/immunization/topics/diphtheria/en/index.html. June 2011.
40. BMJ Best practice. Laryngitis. Available from: http://bestpractice.bmj.com/best-practice/monograph/423.html. September 2011.
41. Fogel JM, Berg IJ, Gerbe MA, Sherter CB. Racemic epinephrine in the treatment of croup: nebulization alone versus nebulization with intermittent positive pressure breathing. *J Pediatr.* 1982;101:1028-31.
42. Writing Committee of the WHO Consultation on Clinical Aspects of Pandemic (H1N1) 2009 Influenza. Clinical Aspects of Pandemic 2009 Influenza A (H1N1) Virus Infection. *N Engl J Med.* 2010;362:1708-19.
43. Tebruegge M, Pantazidou A, Thorburn K, Riordan A, Round J, De Munter C, et al. Bacterial tracheitis: a multi-centre perspective. *Scand J Infect Dis.* 2009;41:548-57.
44. Rajan S, Emery KC, Sood SK. Bacterial tracheitis. Medscape reference. Drugs, Diseases & Procedures. Available from: http://emedicine.medscape.com/article/961647-overview#a0199. April 2010.
45. Anand D, Kantak AD, McBride JT. Bacterial tracheitis (Pseudomembranous Croup). The Merck Manual for Health Care Professionals. Available at http://www.merckmanuals.com/professional/pediatrics/respiratory_disorders_in_neonates_infants_and_young_children/bacterial_tracheitis.html. March 2009.
46. Pettigrew MM, Gent JF, Pyles RB, Miller AL, Nokso-Koivisto J, Chonmaitree T. Viral-bacterial interactions and risk of acute otitis media complicating upper respiratory tract infection. *J Clin Microbiol.* 2011;49:3750-5.
47. Tomita K, Sano H, Iwanaga T, Ishihara K, Ichinose M, Kawase I, et al. Association between episodes of upper respiratory infection and exacerbations in adult patients with asthma. *J Asthma.* 2012;49:253-9.
48. Braman SS. Postinfectious Cough. ACCP. evidence-based clinical practice guidelines. *Chest.* 2006;129:138S-46S.
49. Schubert CR, Cruickshanks KJ, Wiley TL, Klein R, Klein BE, Tweed TS. Diphtheria and hearing loss. *Public Health Rep.* 2001;116:362-8.

CHAPTER 3

Community Acquired Pneumonia

Adamantia Liapikou, Antoni Torres

ABSTRACT

Community-acquired pneumonia (CAP) remains the leading cause of death from infectious diseases. The use of new molecular techniques holds great promise to increase the etiologic diagnosis and potentially decrease use of inappropriately broad antibiotic therapy. Despite an extensive number of published studies, management controversies remain, which guidelines have addressed, including who to admit to the hospital and intensive care unit, what prognostic scoring systems are best, what diagnostic testing should be done, and which therapies should be used and for how long.

Several prognostic rules have been developed to predict severe CAP (SCAP) and mortality, but extended validation is demanded. A new approach is the evaluation of biomarkers as C-reactive protein, procalcitonin (PCT), and other cytokines on the diagnosis, prognosis, therapy duration and response of CAP with promising results. The challenges to patient management include the emergence of new pathogens as community-acquired methicillin-resistant *Staphylococcus aureus* and the high prevalence of multidrug resistant in CAP, mainly from institutionalizing patients. Interventions for optimizing the management of CAP include shortening antibiotic therapy, early "antibiotic switching" from intravenous to oral and PCT—guided approach. Such interventions have led to reduced antibiotic exposure without evidence of causing patient harm. In hospitalized cases up to 10% of patients do not respond to initial antibiotic therapy. The recent commercialization of the 13-valent conjugate vaccine surely provides important clinical benefits. Its use in the adult population more than 50 years olds with risk factors, already authorized, will assess its impact in the coming years.

INTRODUCTION

Community-acquired pneumonia is an important cause of morbidity and mortality worldwide. CAP accounts for 3–5 cases/1,000 persons/year, particularly in the elderly with a 10-fold increased incidence rate.[1,2] In general, the incidence of pneumonia is age dependent, with the highest incidence at the extremes of age, and it is obvious that mortality rates are mainly driven by age. Studies in elderly patients (usually >65 years of age) reported a mortality of 30%, but may exceed 50% in nursing home residents.[2,3] Up to 75% of patients with CAP are hospitalized and of these, up to 10% require admission to the ICU. The data from the German Community Acquired Pneumonia Competence Network (CAPNETZ) trial showed that the mortality among patients hospitalized with CAP ranged from 5% to 20%, but was up to 50% in patients admitted to the ICU.[2] In addition, influenza and pneumonia together was the seventh cause of death for those aged 1–24 years and for those aged more than 65 years and the most common cause of infection-related mortality.

Community-acquired pneumonia represents an inflammatory condition with not only short term but also significant long-term complications. Evidence suggests that hospitalization for pneumonia is associated with higher long-term mortality than of many other major medical conditions.[4] Aliberti and colleagues,[5] reported an association between a longer duration of reaching clinical stability and an increase of adverse events and deaths after hospital discharge.

The excess mortality observed among CAP patients who survived the initial event could be as high as 50% within 5 years after hospital discharge. The highest impact of CAP on long-term mortality is in the first year after the initial episode of CAP, reaching up to 40%.[6] Yende et al. found that persistent inflammation, defined as increased circulating levels of interleukin (IL)-6 and IL-10 at hospital discharge after CAP were associated with all-cause and cause-specific mortality over 1 year despite the resolution of clinical signs of an acute infection.[7]

CLINICAL PRESENTATION

A patient with CAP usually presents with acute symptoms of lower respiratory tract infection (LRTI), such as fever, productive cough, hemoptysis, malaise, dyspnea, pleuritic chest pain with a consolidation on the chest X-ray.[8] In the elderly, the symptoms present maybe of slower onset, with the major complaint being altered mental status, a failure to thrive, tachypnea, falling and decomposition of a chronic illness.

Historic categorization of CAP as "typical" and "atypical" relying on the causing agents, is now a matter of debate. Atypical pneumonia is caused by atypical pathogens (*Mycoplasma pneumoniae, Legionella pneumophila, Coxiella burnetti,* and *Chlamydia* spp.) and presented with a gradual onset of illness, malaise, low fever, normal white blood cell (WBC) and usually with extra pulmonary manifestations.[9]

Many factors influence the presentation of CAP, apart from the virulence of the microorganism, including age, comorbid conditions and lifestyle habits.[10]

Certain *risk factors* are associated with higher frequency of CAP from specific pathogens, such as chronic obstructive pulmonary disease (COPD), diabetes, excessive consumption of alcohol, smoking, cardiovascular and renal morbidity, malnutrition, institutionalization, and immunocompromising conditions/ medications[11] (Table 1).

The patient history should focus on underlying defects in host defenses and possible exposure to specific pathogens. Patients should be asked about occupation, sexual history and contact with animals including house pets or a recent travel history (within 2 weeks). The history should identify risk factors for drug-resistant *S. pneumoniae* (DRSP) and Gram-negative organisms [Gram-negative enteric bacteria (GNEB)]. The risk factors for infection with DRSP include age less than 2 years or more than 65 years, β-lactam therapy within the previous 3 months, alcoholism, medical comorbidities,

TABLE 1

Risk Factors Related to Specific Pathogens in Community-acquired Pneumonia[3]

Condition	Commonly encountered pathogen(s)
Alcoholism	*Streptococcus pneumoniae*, oral anaerobes, *Klebsiella pneumoniae, Acinetobacter* spp., *Mycobacterium tuberculosis*
COPD and/or smoking	*Haemophilus influenzae, Pseudomonas aeruginosa, Legionella* spp., *S. pneumoniae, Moraxella cararrhalis, Chlamydophila pneumoniae*
Aspiration	Gram-negative enteric pathogens, oral anaerobes
Lung abscess	CA-MRSA, oral anaerobes, endemic fungal pneumonia, *M. tuberculosis*, atypical mycobacteria
Structural lung disease (e.g., bronchiectasis)	*Pseudomonas aeruginosa, Burkholderia cepacia, S. aureus*
Endobronchial obstruction	Anaerobes, *S. pneumoniae, H. influenzae, S. aureus*
Exposure to farm animals or parturient cats	Histoplasma capsulatum
Exposure to birds	*Chlamydophila psittaci* (if poultry: avian influenza)
Hotel or cruise ship stay in previous 2 weeks	*Legionella* spp.
HIV infection (early)	*S. pneumoniae, H. influenzae, M. tuberculosis*
Injection drug use	*S. aureus*, anaerobes, *M. tuberculosis, S. pneumoniae*
Influenza active in community	Influenza, *S. pneumoniae, S. aureus, H. influenzae*

COPD, chronic obstructive pulmonary disease; CA-MRSA, community-acquired methicillin-resistant *Staphylococcus aureus*; HIV, human immunodeficiency virus.

immunosuppressive illness or therapy, and exposure to a child in a daycare center.[8,12]

Gram-negative enteric bacteria pneumonia has been associated with acute clinical symptoms, risk of aspiration, previous hospitalization, recent treatment with antibiotics or corticosteroids, and pulmonary comorbidity.[13]

Radiologic examination: A chest radiograph should be obtained whenever pneumonia is suspected. The extent of radiographic findings may help to identify the severity of illness and assist with initial point-of-care decisions. Some radiographic features as lobar consolidation, cavitation and pleural effusions suggest a bacterial etiology.

MICROBIOLOGICAL ETIOLOGY OF COMMUNITY-ACQUIRED PNEUMONIA

The etiology of CAP can be defined into typical pathogens (*S. pneumoniae, Haemophilus influenzae,* and *Moraxella catarrhalis*), atypical pathogens (*Legionella* spp., *M. pneumoniae, C. pneumoniae,* anaerobics, viruses, and other agents. The likely microbial causes of CAP differ according to the severity of disease at clinical presentation.

Streptococcus pneumoniae continues to be the main cause of CAP regardless of severity.

In mild CAP the most common pathogens are *S. pneumoniae, H. influenzae, M. pneumoniae, C. pneumoniae,* and viruses and in moderate CAP *S. pneumoniae* is the most commonly identified etiologic agent followed by *H. influenzae* and *M. pneumoniae* (Table 2). In a study of Cilloniz et al.[14] from Spain, including 588 outpatients with CAP, the most frequent pathogens isolated were *S. pneumoniae* (n = 66; 35.1%), atypical microbials (n= 63, 33, 5%), *H. influenzae* (n = 9; 4.8%) and respiratory viruses (n = 25; 13.3%). More than one causative agent was found in 17 (9.0%) patients. Gutierrez et al.[15] reported mixed infection in 6% of 493 patients with the most frequent combinations being those of bacteria with an atypical organism (29%) and two bacteria (29%). Additionally, patients with mixed pneumonia are likely to have more comorbidities and a more altered outcome.

The spectrum of causal pathogens in severe pneumonia is broader than that in nonsevere cases. *S. pneumoniae* is still the leading pathogen, followed by *S. aureus, L. pneumophila, Enterobacteriaceae,* especially *Escherichia coli, Klebsiella* spp., and *P. aeruginosa.*[8] CAP caused by GNEB and *P. aeruginosa* has been reported to be associated with excess mortality.[13] Aspiration pneumonia is a common cause of severe CAP and is generally polymicrobial with Gram-positive and Gram-negative anaerobes.

In another study of Torres et al.,[16] including 3,523 patients with CAP, in those admitted in the ICU the most common etiologies were *S. pneumoniae* (42%), mixed etiologies (22%) and atypical pathogens (18%). *S. pneumoniae* had the highest number of deaths, although the relative mortality rates were higher for *S. aureus,* GNEB, *P. aeruginosa,* and mixed etiologies.

TABLE 2

Common Etiologic Agents of Community-acquired Pneumonia

Outpatient	*Streptococcus pneumoniae* *Mycoplasma pneumoniae*
	Haemophilus influenzae *Chlamydophila pneumoniae*
	Respiratory viruses: influenza A and B, adenovirus, RSV, parainfluenza virus
Inpatient (non-ICU)	*Streptococcus pneumoniae*
	Mycoplasma pneumoniae
	Chlamydophila pneumoniae
	Haemophilus influenzae
	Legionella spp.
	Aspiration (anaerobes)
	Respiratory viruses
Inpatient (ICU)	*Streptococcus pneumoniae*
	Staphylococcus aureus
	Legionella spp.
	Enteric Gram-negative bacilli
	Respiratory viruses
	Pseudomonas aeruginosa (relative frequency determined by the presence or absence of specific risk factors)

ICU, intensive care unit; RSV, respiratory syncytial virus.

Although viruses have been identified as an important cause of CAP, only recently, mainly due to the 2009 H1N1 pandemic, there has been a greater interest in the role of these agents. Several recent reports of adult viral pneumonia in which polymerase chain reaction (PCR) was used for diagnosis, viruses accounted for approximately 13.5–30% of the cases of CAP,[17,18] either by themselves or as copathogens with bacteria.[19] Among the main viruses that cause pneumonia in immunocompetent adults are the influenza virus, the respiratory syncytial virus (RSV), the adenovirus, and the human parainfluenza virus (HPIV). A recently described paramyxovirus, human metapneumovirus (hMPV) most commonly cause of CAP of young children and older adults, especially with underlying comorbidities.[20]

Multidrug-resistant organisms (MDROs) that causing pneumonia in the community represent a real and emerging problem, because of the increasing number of residents living in healthcare facilities and the appearance of CA-MRSA. CA-MRSA is characterized by a severe, bilateral, necrotizing pneumonia induced by Panton-Valentine leukocidin and other toxins.[21] In an attempt to evaluate risk factors for acquiring MDR bacteria in CAP, Aliberti et al.[22] found that hospitalization in the preceding 90 days [odds ratio (OR): 4.87, 95% confidence interval (CI): 1.90–12.4); $p < 0.001$] and residency in a nursing home [(OR, 3.55, 95% CI: 1.12–11.24); $p < 0.031$] were independent predictors for an actual infection with a resistant pathogen.

DIAGNOSIS

The causative of the pathogen remains unknown in 30–60% of cases, despite vigorous clinical investigation. Reasons include difficulties in obtaining samples for culture because of the lack of a productive cough and frequent use of antibiotics before diagnosis as well as lack of effective and rapid diagnostic tests.

Routine laboratory testing to establish an etiology in outpatients with CAP is usually unnecessary, because of the good prognosis with the recommended empirical therapy.

Establishing a microbiological diagnosis of hospitalized CAP still relies predominantly on the traditional culture techniques of sputum samples. A valid sputum can be obtained from about 40% of CAP patients. The study of Butler et al. reported that when a purulent sputum was available the Gram stain gave the diagnosis in 80% of patients.[23]

In the study of Anevlavis et al.[24] the sensitivity of sputum Gram stain was 82% for pneumococcal pneumonia, 76% for staphylococcal pneumonia and 79% for *H. influenzae* pneumonia, with specificities ranging from 93% to 96%. Infectious Diseases Society of America/American Thoracic Society (IDSA/ATS) guidelines of 2007 recommend that sputum specimens must be obtained before the initiation of antibiotic therapy in inpatients.[8]

Although the overall yield of blood cultures is probably less than 20% in patients hospitalized for CAP, a positive culture of blood or pleural fluid definitively establishes the etiologic diagnosis of pneumonia. The most common blood isolate in patients with CAP is *S. pneumoniae*. The IDSA/ATS guidelines recommend blood culture testing in hospitalized patients presenting in table 3.

Samples for blood culture should be obtained before antibiotic administration. However, when multiple risk factors for bacteremia are present, as severe CAP, blood culture results after initiation of antibiotic therapy are still positive in up to 15% of cases.[8]

Molecular Testing

Several new molecular diagnostic tests exist today for identification of viruses and some new ones are on the horizon for the diagnosis of bacteria and fungi. These tests

TABLE 3

Clinical Indications for More Extensive Diagnostic Testing[8]

	Blood culture	Sputum culture	Legionella UAT	Pneumococcal UAT	Other
ICU admission	X	X	X	X	X[a]
Failure of outpatient antibiotic therapy		X	X	X	
Cavitary infiltrates	X	X			X[b]
Leucopenia	X			X	
Active alcohol abuse	X	X	X	X	
Chronic severe liver disease	X			X	
COPD		X			
Asplenia	X			X	
Recent travel			X		
Positive Legionella UAT result		X			
Positive Pneumococcal UAT results	x	X			
Pleural effusion	x	x	x	x	

UAT, urinary antigen test; ICU, intensive care unit; COPD, chronic obstructive pulmonary disease.
[a]Endotracheal aspirate if intubated, possibly bronchoscopy or nonbronchoscopic bronchoalveolar lavage.
[b]Fungal and tuberculosis cultures.

are rapid, accurate and can detect multiple pathogens in one assay or a minimum of assays.[25]

Before these, a nonmolecular assay had been developed—the direct fluorescent antibody test (DFA), using monoclonal antibodies for the rapid identification of influenza, with variable sensitivities of (10–70%) and specificities (50–100%).

Nucleic Acid Amplification Tests-Polymerase Chain Reaction

Detection of microbial nucleic acid with nucleic acid amplification tests, such as polymerase chain reaction (PCR) in respiratory samples or blood has improved our diagnostic accuracy in CAP. Real-time PCR is commonly used for certain respiratory viral pathogens (e.g., influenza, RSV, hMPV) and atypical but not yet for bacterial pathogens.[26-28] Reverse transcriptase-PCR (rt-PCR) in respiratory samples or blood combines amplification and detection in one reaction (reducing cross-contamination) allows quantification of the infection load.[29]

As with culture techniques, PCR results cannot distinguish between colonization and infection, although quantification of bacterial deoxyribonucleic acid (DNA) load or relating this to the number of human epithelial cells may help in doing so.[30]

The application of PCR for the detection of *S. pneumoniae*, both in sputum and in blood, may be valuable in CAP patients whom antibiotic therapy has been initiated.[9] Direct testing of blood samples with PCR-based tests for *S. pneumoniae* had reported sensitivities of 50–70% and specificities of 90–100% when compared with blood culture results.

A new molecular technique called multiplex reverse transcriptase-PCR (MRT-PCR) allows for the rapid detection of several respiratory viruses such as *influenza A* and *B*; RSV A and B; HPIV 1, 2, and 3; metapneumovirus; and adenovirus. Its disadvantage is the low sensitivity for H1N1 influenza, described by the method as nontypeable.

As a recent study confirms, the application of PCR-based methods to the conventional microbial techniques improves the yield of etiological agents significantly and indicate that PCR is not only more rapid than conventional methods, but also more sensitive, both in etiological diagnosis of CAP.[17]

Antigen Detection

Antigen determination diagnostics are still largely based on the detection of pneumococcal and *Legionella* antigens in urine, although point-of-care tests have also been established for influenza.[31] For the pneumococcal urinary antigen test, reported specificities and sensitivities ranged from 90% to 100% and from 50% to 80%, respectively, depending on the reference standards that were used. The urinary antigen test may also be applied on pleural fluid with a sensitivity and specificity of almost 100%.[12]

In patients with bacteremia pneumococcal CAP, although, 15–20% had negative urinary antigen tests, which may result from sequestration of antigen-antibody immune complexes with decreased antigen shedding in the urine.[32] The most commonly available *Legionella* urinary antigen assays have a sensitivity of around 80% for serogroup 1 infection [which account for around 85% of infections in the United States (US) and Europe] but do not detect other serotypes.

Serology

Serological assays have several drawbacks—especially sensitivity, specificity, and delays to a detectable serological response—that have generally hampered their utility in direct patient management (as opposed to epidemiological and other studies).

A combination of immunoglobulin M (IgM) antibody detection and PCR may be the most sensitive approach for atypical pathogens, is the suggestion of European Respiratory Society/European Society of Clinical Microbiology and Infectious Diseases (ERS/ESCMID).[12]

Inflammatory Response

Biomarkers CRP and PCT, measured in serum may give an indication for bacterial infection, identifying patients with similar conditions to those with CAP.

The European guidelines suggest that in patients with a suspected pneumonia: a test for serum-level of CRP; a level of more than 100 mg/L makes pneumonia likely.[12]

The value of PCT arises because serum levels are increased in severe bacterial infections, but not in viral illness. Masia et al.[9] found lower PCT and CRP levels in atypicals compared with bacteria, although neither of them was found to predict the etiology. Furthermore, Almirall et al,[33] identified that CRP values are especially high in patients with pneumonias caused by *S. pneumoniae* or *L. pneumophila,* and the level of CRP related to the severity of the disease.

Biomarkers include several proinflammatory cytokines such as placental growth factor, PCT, neopterin, mid-regional proatrial natriuretic peptide (MR-proANP), and hepatocyte growth factor.[34] Endothelin-1 precursor peptides and MR-proANP may have some utility in defining severity, determining prognosis, and assessing initial response to therapy in those with CAP,[35,36] but it is

PCT that is the most researched and validated of these host response assays.

Invasive Diagnostic Techniques

Invasive techniques, specially, bronchoscopy, are suitable for the management of patients with life-threatening CAP in whom diagnostic materials cannot otherwise be obtained rapidly, patients with progressive pneumonia despite seemingly appropriate antimicrobial therapy, immunocompromised patients, especially in the setting of endotracheal intubation.

The diagnostic accuracy is improved by semi-quantitative or quantitative cultures of materials obtained bronchoscopically with a protected brushing specimen (PBS) or through bronchoalveolar lavage (BAL) and by direct lung aspiration.[37] For quantitative cultures of endotracheal aspirate samples, a threshold of more than 10^5 colony-forming units (CFU)/mL is used to distinguish colonization from infection.

SEVERITY ASSESSMENT

An accurate assessment of CAP severity is crucial when making decisions regarding the site of care. The decision of hospital admission depends not only on the severity of pneumonia, the underlying disease, but on social factors and clinical experience of the doctor.

Several prognostics tools have been created to predict prognosis in CAP.

The most widely validated CAP prediction rule is the Pneumonia Severity Index (PSI) developed by Fine et al.[38] in 1997, which was designed to identify CAP patients with a low 30-day mortality risk. It stratifies patients into five risk classes using a scoring system based on a logistic probability model. Its drawback is its complexity and can occasionally underestimate the severity of illness, especially in young patients without comorbid illness because it heavily weighs age and comorbidity.

TABLE 4

Confusion, Urea Nitrogen, Respiratory Rate, Blood Pressure, and Age ≥65 (CURB-65)

Variables:
- Confusion
- Blood urea nitrogen level >20 mg/dL (7.14 mmol/L)
- Respiratory rate ≥30 breaths/minute
- Blood pressure (systolic <90 mmHg or diastolic ≤60 mmHg)
- Age ≥65 years

Score	Inpatient versus outpatient	30-day mortality (%)
0 or 1 point	Treat as outpatient	0.7–2.1
2 points ≥3 points	Treat as inpatient	9.2
>3 points	Treat in intensive care unit	15–40

A more recent alternative model is the CURB-65 (confusion, urea nitrogen, respiratory rate, blood pressure, and age ≥65), derived from the original model of the British Thoracic Society (BTS)[39] (Table 4).

Most recent publications have shown that the CURB-score and its modifications [particularly CRB-65 (confusion, respiratory rate, blood pressure, and age ≥65) score] are comparable to the PSI in terms of prediction of death from pneumonia in both outpatients and inpatients.[12,40] However, both PSI and CURB-65 are poor tools for guidance of decisions about the need for ICU admission.

Severe CAP is best defined as the requirement for ventilator support and/or fluid resuscitation and/or treatment for severe complications. These patients

TABLE 5

Criteria for Intensive Care Unit Admission of American Thoracic Society/Infectious Diseases Society of America[8]

Minor criteria	Major criteria
• Blood urea nitrogen level ≥20 mg/dL (7.14 mmol/L) • Confusion/disorientation • Hypotension requiring aggressive fluid resuscitation • Hypothermia [core temperature < 96.8°F (36°C)] • Leukopenia [WBC <4,000/mm^3 (4.00 × 10^9/L)] • Multilobar infiltrates • PaO_2/FiO_2 ratio ≤250 • Respiratory rate ≥30 breaths/minute • Thrombocytopenia [PLT <100 × 10^3 mm^3 (100 × 10^9/L)]	• Invasive mechanical ventilation • Septic shock with need for vasopressors

WBC, white blood cell; PLT, platelets; PaO_2, partial arterial oxygen pressure; FiO_2, fraction of inspired oxygen.

require intensive care admission for strict monitoring and management. The admission of a patient with CAP to the ICU is a serious and individualized decision, depending on the hospital facilities, ICU availability, disease severity and the patient's medical history.

According to ATS/IDSA rule ICU admission for CAP is warranted for patients who fulfill three minor criteria or one major criterion of those listed in table 5.

This rule has been validated in several studies,[41-44] with widely varied results. In a recent prospective cohort excluding patients with major criteria or therapeutic limitations, ATS-IDSA minor criteria had an area under the curve (AUC) of 0.85 to predict ICU admission.[44] As it stands today, it is possible to predict SCAP with sensitivity of around 70% and specificity of around 80–90% using the ATS rule.

The conceptual problem of the rule is that the major criteria are quite obvious and do not predict for themselves which patients are at risk of respiratory failure (and perhaps the need for mechanical ventilation) and/or shock or worsening comorbidity during development of CAP.

Other prediction scales have been developed, first in Spain, the SCAP with eight variables and will be useful in identifying patients who need more aggressive monitoring and treatment.[45] Validation of this rule on three cohorts totaling 3,402 patients (SCAP, 9%) to predict a composite definition of SCAP (in-hospital death, mechanical ventilation, or shock) result with sensitivity 92% and specificity 64%, showing an AUC of 0.92.

Charles et al. derived SMART-COP (systolic blood pressure, multilobar infiltrates, albumin, respiratory rate, tachycardia, confusion, oxygen and pH) score to predict which patients will require intensive respiratory or vasopressor support (IRVS), with a score more than three identified 92% of patients who needed IRVS. It provided sensitivity of 58–85%, specificity of 46–75%, and AUC of 0.72–0.87 in five independent external validation cohorts.[46]

Renaud et al.[47] in an attempt to identify risk factors for early (<3 days) ICU admission of patients hospitalized with CAP and not requiring immediate ICU admission, created a score [risk of early admission (REA)-ICU index] comprised 11 criteria. The REA-ICU index stratified patients into four risk classes with a risk of ICU admission on days 1–3 ranging from 0.7% to 31%. When this score was validated the AUC was 0.81 on the overall population.

Although the new generation of scores which focuses on the early detection of respiratory and circulatory failure, seems to have enhanced operative characteristics to predict ICU admission but their clinical utility is still being debated. High negative predictive value and low positive predictive value are the most consistent findings among the different studies, suggesting that these scores could be more relevant to exclude the presence of a SCAP than to aid in performing triage in patients for ICU admission.[48]

A list of the new prediction scores for SCAP is presented in table 6.

Several studies concluded that variables as hypoglycemia on admission and thrombocytosis are associated with greater inpatient mortality, unaffected by

TABLE 6

Severe Community-acquired Pneumonia Prediction Scores

Name	Variables/points
1. SMART-COP[46]	Systolic blood pressure <90 mmHg/2
	Multilobar infiltrates/1
	Albumin <2,5 g/dL/1
	RR >25 breaths/minute if <50 years; >30 breaths/minute if >50 years/1
	Heart rate (HR) >125 beats/minute/1
	Confusion/1
	PO_2 <70 mmHg, O_2 saturation <93% or PO_2/FiO_2 <333 if <50 years; PO_2 <60 mmHg, O_2 saturation <90% or PO_2/FiO_2 <250, If >50 years/2
	pH <7,35/2
2. SCAP[45]	pH <7,30/2.38
	Systolic blood pressure < 90 mmHg/2,19
	RR > 30 breaths/minute/1.83
	Altered mental status/0.87
	Blood urea nitrogen > 30 mg/dL/0.92
	PO_2 <540 mmHg or PO_2/FiO_2 <250 mmHg/1.12
	Age >80 years/0.86
	Multilobar infiltrates/0.68
3. REA-ICU[47]	Male/1
	Comorbid condition >1/1
	White blood cell count <3 or ≥20 G/L/1
	HR ≥125 beats/minute/1
	Age <80 years/1
	Multilobar infiltrates or pleural effusion/2
	Oxygen saturation<90% or PaO_2 <60 mmHg/2
	Arterial pH <7.35/2
	Blood urea nitrogen ≥11 mmol/L/2
	Sodium <130 mEq/L/3

PaO_2, partial arterial oxygen pressure; FiO_2, fraction of inspired oxygen; REA-ICU, risk of early admission-intensive care unit.

the presence of diabetes.[49] But in other studies, should be added to thrombocytopenia as a risk for 30-day mortality.[50]

It has also been proposed that biomarkers may either simplify or add greater predictive power to the clinical predictive tools already discussed. Inflammatory markers such as CRP and PCT have been shown to be predictive of short-term (usually 28-day or 30-day) mortality. Huang and colleagues as well as Kruger et al. found, that even in patients identified as high risk using CURB-65 or PSI, a low PCT value predicted a low chance of dying.[51,52] Menendez et al.[53] evaluated the impact of adding biomarkers to prognostic scoring in 453 CAP patients. They found that adding CRP levels to PSI, CURB-65 and CRB-65 scales improves the 30-day mortality prediction. In a study of Ramirez et al.[54] from the same group of investigators, the additive value of PCT was not confirmed. In a study by Bello and collegues.[55] another biomarker, mid-regional pro-adrenomedullin (MR-proADM) levels showed considerable prognostic value with/without clinical severity scores such as PSI and CURB-65 independently of etiology of CAP. The same biomarker (MR-proADM) was identified as the best predictor of long-term mortality in a study of Kruger et al.[56,57]

MANAGEMENT

As shown in a number of studies, the use of guidelines for treating CAP can significantly reduce morbidity and mortality. Guidelines recommend basing initial treatment choices on the severity of disease presentation[8,10,12] resulting in hospital admission.

Because no diagnostic testing can rapidly identify the causal pathogens in a patient with CAP, initial therapy is empiric, based on an epidemiologic assessment of patient risk factors for specific pathogens. However, physicians should consider local microbial resistance patterns and drug safety profiles.

The recommended treatment of ERS/ESCMID and ATS/IDSA guidelines according to the site of care is showed in table 7.

The greatest differences from European guidelines are the recommendation for routine atypical pathogen coverage in North America and a trend to use penicillins and to avoid quinolones in the United Kingdom (UK).[8,12]

- In outpatients, healthy adult patients with no risk factors for DRSP, the treatment includes a macrolide or doxycycline in US but in Europe an amoxicillin or a tetracycline
- In patients with comorbidities or risk factors for penicillin-resistant *Streptococcus pneumoniae* (PRSP), a respiratory fluoroquinolone or a β-lactam antibiotic plus a macrolide or doxycycline is recommended.

In a meta-analysis of Mainon et al, it appears that the outcome of outpatient-treated CAP is generally good regardless of whether or not there is coverage for atypical agents, as long as there is coverage for *Streptococcus pneumonia*.[58] In the face of increasing rates of macrolide-resistant pneumococci, is to no longer recommend macrolides for monotherapy for CAP when effective alternatives are available.[59]

The pharmacokinetically enhanced formulation of amoxicillin/clavulanate (tablets, 2,000/125 mg twice daily) determined a high rate of both bacteriological and clinical efficacy (97.7 and 95.6%, respectively) even in CAP caused by multiple-DRSP.[12]

- For patients admitted to the hospital, but not to the ICU, an IV respiratory fluoroquinolone or a β-lactam plus a macrolide should be used.

For severe cases requiring ICU admission, antimicrobial selection will depend on the presence of risk factors for *P. aeruginosa*. The risk factors for *Pseudomonas pneumonia* include: (1) recent hospitalization, (2) frequent (>4 courses/year) or recent administration of antibiotics (last 3 months), (3) severe disease [forced expiratory volume in 1 second (FEV_1) <30%], and (4) oral steroid use (>10 mg of prednisolone daily in the last 2 weeks).

Combination antimicrobial treatment should be used to treat severe CAP. However, respiratory quinolones may be used as monotherapy in severe pneumonia without septic shock.[60]

- For *Pseudomonas* infection, an antipneumococcal/antipseudomonal β-lactam (piperacillin-tazobactam, cefepime, imipenem, or meropenem) plus either ciprofloxacin or levofloxacin or the above β-lactam plus an aminoglycoside and azithromycin should be used.

In patients with bacteremia (pneumococcal and other), atypical pathogen coverage with a macrolide (monotherapy or combination) improves mortality compared with treatment regimens with a quinolone.[61,62]

Aspiration pneumonia happens in patients with a decrease of consciousness due to neurological diseases, drugs or alcoholism. The recommended therapy is clindamycin or metronidazole plus cefalosporine.[12]

Modification of the initial regimen should be considered once specific pathogens have been identified.

In cases of influenza pneumonia early treatment (within 48 hours of onset of symptoms) with oseltamivir or zanamivir are recommended.[8] Both drugs reduce the duration of symptoms, the risk of hospitalization and lower respiratory tract complications.[63,64] In the cases of viral pneumonia, the superinfections from *S. pneumoniae* and *S. aureus* are frequent and dangerous.

The effort to choose the appropriate antibiotic requires the data of the pharmacokinetic-pharmacodynamic

TABLE 7

Empiric Therapy for Community-acquired Pneumonia According to American Thoracic Society/Infectious Diseases Society of America (ATS/IDSA)[8] and Respiratory Society/European Society of Clinical Microbiology and Infectious Diseases[12]

Patient group	ERS/ESCMID12	ATS/IDSA8
• Previously healthy outpatients; no antibiotic use in past 3 months • Comorbidities*	Amoxicillin or tetracycline	Macrolide† or doxycycline Levofloxacin,§ moxifloxacin or β-lactam + macrolide
Inpatients, non-ICU	Aminopenicillin ± macrolide, (Aminopenicillin/β-lactamase inhibitor Nonantipseudomonal cephalosporin Cefotaxime or ceftriaxone) PLUS macrolide or Levofloxacin,§ moxifloxacin or Penicillin G ± macrolide	Levofloxacin,§ moxifloxacin or β-lactam + macrolide
Inpatients, ICU	Non-antipseudomonal cephalosporin III + macrolide or moxifloxacin or levofloxacin ± non-antipseudomonal cephalosporin III	β-lactam (cefotaxime, ceftriaxone ampicillin-sulbactam) + azithromycin or Levofloxacin,§ moxifloxacin
Special considerations		
Risk factors for Pseudomonas species	Antipseudomonal cephalosporin** or acyl ureidopenicillin/β-lactamase inhibitor or carbapenem (meropenem preferred, up to 6 g possible, 32 in 3-hour infusion) PLUS ciprofloxacin§§ or PLUS macrolide + aminoglycoside (gentamicin, tobramycin or amikacin)	An antipneumococcal, antipseudomonal β-lactam plus either ciprofloxacin or levofloxacin or plus aminoglycoside and azithromycin or plus an aminoglycoside and an antipneumococcal fluoroquinolone
Risk factors for MRSA		Vancomycin or linezolid
Influenza virus		Oseltamivir or zanamivir

ICU, intensive care unit; MRSA, methicillin-resistant *Staphylococcus aureus*.

*Such as chronic heart, lung, liver, or renal disease; diabetes mellitus; alcoholism; malignancies; asplenia; immunosuppressing conditions or use of immunosuppressing drugs; use of antimicrobials within the previous 3 months.

**Ceftazidime has to be combined with penicillin G for coverage of S. pneumoniae.

§Within the fluoroquinolones, moxifloxacin has the highest antipneumococcal activity.

§§Levofloxacin 750 mg/24 hours or 500 mg BID is an alternative and also covers Gram-positive bacteria if treatment is empirical.

(PK/PD) parameters of the drug to ensure bacterial eradication.[65] Based on this, optimizing the dose of ciprofloxacin is 750 mg orally twice daily (instead 500 mg/BID) and levofloxacin to 750 mg/day in 5 days regimen.

The current ATS/IDSA consensus guidelines advise the first antibiotic dose (TFAD) to be administered while the patient is still in the emergency department.

Battleman et al. examined the TFAD in patients hospitalized with pneumonia and concluded that timely antibiotic administration was associated with a shorter length of hospital stay.[66] In contrast, Bordon et al.[67] reported that the TFAD does not associated with mortality or hospital stay but should be considered as a marker of optimal care.

ERS/ESCMID recommends that, only in patients with CAP and septic shock, delay in initiating therapy must not be more than 1 hour after diagnosis.[12] However, the American Medicare has set in 6 hours being the maximum time to administer the first dose of antibiotics in emergency departments.

After the initial clinical improvement, hospitalized patients should be switched from IV to oral antibiotics when they have the ability to tolerate antibiotics by mouth and clinical stability has been achieved (Box 1).

A more recent prospective randomized trial from Spain by Carratala and collegues[68] assessed the safety and effectiveness of employing a three-step critical pathway including early mobilization and use of objective criteria for switching to oral antibiotic therapy in an effort to transition to oral antibiotics earlier in hospitalized adult CAP patients. They managed to reduce the length of stay (LOS) (3, 9 vs. 6 days, $p < 0.001$) and the period of IV antibiotic therapy (2 vs. 4 days, $p < 0.001$) of the three step group.

BOX 1

Criteria for Clinical Stability in Community-acquired Pneumonia[8]

1.	Temperature <37, 8°C
2.	Heart rate <100 beats/minute
3.	Systolic blood pressure >90 mmHg
4.	Respiratory rate <24 breaths/minute
5	SO_2 >90% or PO_2 >60 mmHg

The duration of therapy should be a minimum of 5 days, providing that the patient is afebrile for 48–72 hours, and there is no sign of complication (endocarditis, meningitis) or *Paeruginosa* or *S. aureus* bacteremia.

In a meta-analysis of Dimopoulos et al.,[69] comparing short- (≤7 days) versus long- (≥2 days difference) course therapy for CAP, no difference was found in the effectiveness and safety between the two therapeutic courses.

In CAP patients admitted in the ICU, the right duration is still not known.

Shorter course antibiotic therapy for CAP has been associated with several potential benefits, including increased adherence, reduced adverse events, decreased antimicrobial resistance due to less drug exposure, reduced length of hospital stay, and theoretically overall cost savings.[70-72]

Several studies have investigated the role of serial measurements of PCT in the reduction in antibiotic use of CAP. PCT guidance in CAP antibiotic treatment was first evaluated in a randomized intervention trial consisting of 302 patients with suspected CAP (ProCAP trial).[73] In this study, 151 patients were each randomized to a PCT-guided arm or a control (usual practice) arm. The PCT-guided arm demonstrated a reduction in total antibiotic exposure, as compared with the control arm (15 % vs 1%), as a result of withholding therapy in those with low initial PCT levels.

More recently, Albrich and collegues[74] published a multicenter study, taking place in Switzerland, France and US, including 1,789 patients with LRTI (54% with CAP). They found that antibiotic therapy duration was significantly shorter if the PCT algorithm was followed compared with when it was overruled (5.9 vs 7.4 days; $P < 0.001$).

In the Procalcitonin Guided Antibiotic Therapy and Hospitalisation in Patients with Respiratory Tract Infection (ProHOSP) multicenter study performed on 925 CAP patients, the authors confirmed no side effect on patients and lower antibiotic consumption following the PCT guided pathway.[75] A similar approach has been used in a study of severe CAP patients,[76] leading to reduction of antibiotic duration to 5 days, 5 days comparing to 10 days, 5 days the control group.

ADDITIONAL THERAPIES

Corticoids

Because of the weak evidence of survival benefit of corticosteroids in CAP therapy, their role in pneumonia remains highly controversial.

The best evidence comes from studies showing that corticosteroids reduce mortality in acquired immunodeficiency syndrome (AIDS) patients with *Pneumocystis jirovecii* pneumonia.[77]

Recently published data failed to show any positive impact of steroids on clinical end points in hospitalized patients with mild-to-moderate CAP.[78-80] Prospective, randomized trials referring to corticosteroids in severe CAP are the ones of Confalonieri et al.,[81] Sabry et al.,[82] and Fernandez-Serrano et al.[80] The addition of corticosteroids resulted in improvement in respiratory failure [pressure of arterial oxygen (PO_2)/fractional inspired oxygen concentration (FiO_2) ratio], but not in mortality.

1. Two meta-analysis on this subject,[83,84] confirming the above, suggested that only in severe CAP a prolonged low-dose corticosteroids therapy may result in a beneficial effect on mortality.
2. Low molecular heparin should be given to patients with acute respiratory failure.
3. Several studies indicate that noninvasive ventilation (NIV) may also work in patients with pneumonia, particularly in patients with COPD. NIV has been shown to reduce intubation in patients with acute respiratory distress syndrome (ARDS) in 54% of treated cases.[12]

NONRESPONSE TO TREATMENT

In several multicenter studies, treatment failure ranges between 6% and 24%, and can reach up to 31% in patients with severe CAP.[10,85] There are two patterns of nonresponse to treatment: Progressive pneumonia if clinical deterioration with acute respiratory failure requiring ventilatory support and/or septic shock appears within the first 72 hours of hospital admission; Persistent nonresponding pneumonia is characterized by the absence or delay in achieving clinical stability. The term early failure is similar to progressive pneumonia, but used even before 72 hours of treatment.[86]

It is useful to classify the etiological cause of treatment failure in patients with CAP according to the microbiological approach as infectious (40%) and noninfectious[87] as presented in table 8.

TABLE 8

Causes of Nonresponding Pneumonia

Infectious	Noninfectious
Resistant microorganism	ARDS
Nosocomial superinfection (MRSA, *P. aeruginosa*, *Acinetobacter baumanii*)	Pulmonary embolism Pulmonary hemorrhage Vasculitis (e.g., SLE)
Rare organism (*Mycobacterium tuberculosis*, *Aspergilus fumigatus*, *Nocardia* spp., *Pneumocystis jiroveci*)	Sarcoidosis, BOOP, eosinophilic pneumonia, aspiration pneumonitis
Complications empyema, abscess	Pulmonary edema, renal failure
Metastatic infection (endocarditis, meningitis, arthritis)	Drug induced pneumonitis

ARDS, acute respiratory distress syndrome; MRSA, methicillin-resistant *Staphylococcus aureus*; SLE, systemic lupus erythematosus; BOOP, bronchiolitis obliterans organizing pneumoni.

The most frequent pathogens recognized as causes of treatment failure in CAP are *Streptococcus pneumoniae*, MRSA, *P. aeruginosa*, and Gram-negative enteric bacilli, due to resistance to the administered initial antibiotics.

Other infectious causes of nonresponse to treatment are complications of CAP, such as empyema, endocarditis, arthritis, pericarditis, meningitis, or peritonitis and necrotizing pneumonia. In a study of Menendez et al., found that the incidence of empirical treatment failure was 15% and the independent risk factors associated were multilobar CAP, cavitation on chest radiograph, pleural effusion, liver disease, leucopenia and high PSI.[88]

Noninfectious respiratory diseases have to be considered as an alternative cause of misdiagnosis of CAP. These other diseases may include pulmonary edema, pulmonary hemorrhage, inflammatory diseases, such as bronchiolitis obliterans with organizing pneumonia (BOOP), pulmonary eosinophilia, hypersensitivity pneumonitis, neoplasms and drug induced lung disease.

The measurements of biomarkers (CRP and PCT) may help to predict the patients with nonresponse to treatment.[86,89,90]

In patients with nonresponding or progressive pneumonia, complete re-evaluation of the history, physical examination, and Fuhrer laboratory studies is required. Radiologic evaluation with a pulmonary computed tomography (CT) scans provide a more detailed study of the parenchyma, interstitium, pleura and mediastinum. If simpler procedures do not provide a rapid diagnosis, invasive techniques (i.e., bronchoscopy with BAL) are recommended.

If the patient develops early treatment failure, severe clinical deterioration and/or a worsening of the radiologic infiltrates, broad antibiotic therapy may be administered even before 72 hours. It would be useful to detect microbial resistance to the initially administered antimicrobial treatment. Combinations with three antibiotics may be needed in order to cover MRSA, *P. aeruginosa,* and anaerobes.

PREVENTION

The most important tools in CAPs prevention are the pneumococcal and influenza's vaccines.

Currently, pneumococcal vaccination is available as a 23-valent pneumococcal polysaccharide vaccine (PPSV23) and a 13-valent pneumococcal conjugate vaccine (PCV13) that replaced an earlier PCV7.[91] According to European experts the 23-valent polysaccharide pneumococcal vaccine (PPV23) prevents invasive pneumococcal disease (IPD) in older persons and in other high-risk groups and should be given to all adult persons at risk of pneumococcal disease.[10] Thus, on one hand, antibody levels following vaccination progressively decrease to values prevacunales after a period of 5 and 10 years. Therefore, revaccination is recommended for all persons who are vaccinated before age 65, particularly for those who have a high risk of serious disease, after 5 years. The recommendations for pneumococcal and influenza vaccination are listed in table 9.

Despite its use in many countries worldwide, and its reported 50–80% protection against pneumococcal infection, the efficacy of the PPV23 remains debated.[92] In a study of Huss and collegues concluded that PPV23 only prevented from bacteremic but nonbacteremic pneumococcal pneumonia.[93] A recent double-blind randomized controlled trial among about 1,000 nursing home residents in Japan demonstrated that PPV23 was associated with a reduction of the incidence of all-cause pneumonia by 45% and of pneumococcal pneumonia by 64%.[94] The controversy of the effectiveness of the vaccine persists, especially in the elderly, because the benefit

TABLE 9

Recommendations for Influenza and Pneumococcal Vaccination[12]

Factor	Inactivated influenza vaccine	Pneumococcal polysaccharide vaccine
Route of administration	Intramuscular injection	Intramuscular injection
Risk groups	1. Age >50 years old	1. Age >65 years old
	2. Institutionalization	2. Institutionalization
	3. Chronic cardiac disease	3. Chronic cardiac disease
	4. Chronic pulmonary disease (asthma)	4. Chronic obstructive pulmonary disease
	5. Diabetes mellitus	5. Dementia, seizure disorders
	6. Chronic renal disease	6. Diabetes mellitus
	7. Hemoglobinopathies	7. Chronic renal disease
	8. Women who will be in the second or third trimester of pregnancy during the influenza season	8. Chronic liver disease
		9. Alcoholism
		10. Functional or anatomical asplenia
		11. Chronic cerebrospinal fluid leakage
Revaccination	Annual revaccination	Once after 5 years for (1) adults >65 years old, (2) asplenia, and (3) immunocompromised

of the PPV23 decreases with age. Reports of significant reductions in the incidence of IPD in the elderly after the introduction of large-scale vaccination programs from two European countries support the effectiveness of the vaccine against IPD.[95]

Since the turn of the century, PCV are available, with either seven (serotypes 4, 6B, 9V, 14, 18C, 19F, 23F), 10 (additional serotypes 1, 5, 7F) or 13 (additional serotypes 3, 19A, 6A) polysaccharide capsular antigens conjugated to a protein.

In adults, a single dose of PCV7 yields higher or at least equal immune responses to a single dose of PPV23, both in immune-competent and in immune-compromised adults.[96-98]

Conjugated vaccines have now been implemented in national immunization programs for children across the world, with almost the disappearance of serious disease caused by vaccine strains in children.[99] In the US, the introduction of PCV7 vaccination among children was associated with declines in IPD rates in the elderly, presumably because of vaccine-induced herd immunity.[100]

Up till now, actual efficacy of PCV7 vaccination in adults has only been determined in one study, 496 HIV-infected patients who had recovered from IPD in Blantyre, Malawi.[101] PCV7 shows efficacy of 75% in preventing IPD. The overall value of the vaccine was limited by the finding that 64% of pneumococcal infections were by nonvaccine serotypes.

The study by Smith et al.[102] suggests that PCV13 instead of PPSV23 for routine immunization of adults, favor in the prevention against pneumococcal disease in an economically reasonable fashion.

Since October 2011, PCV13 has been licensed for the prevention of IPD in adults aged more than 50 years in Europe, but in the US only for adults more than 19 years with immunocompromising conditions.[103] Regarding the program of vaccination, Advisory Committee on Immunization Practices (ACIP) recommends that adults aged more than or equal to 19 years with immuno-compromising conditions should receive a dose of PCV13 first, followed by a dose of PPSV23 at least 8 weeks later.[104]

Currently, a large scale clinical trial in 85,000 in individuals aged 65 years and older is underway in the Netherlands to estimate the clinical benefit of PCV13 in preventing pneumococcal pneumonia.[105]

The influenza vaccine is also important for the prevention of CAP. However, its effectiveness is influenced by host factors and how closely the antigens in the vaccine are matched with the circulating influenza strain. It has also been shown to effectively prevent pneumonia, hospitalization, and death in older persons.[106,107] Systematic reviews indicate that vaccination of healthcare personnel against influenza may reduce influenza-like illness and all-cause mortality of elderly people in long-term hospitals, but have not demonstrated an effect on specific outcomes, such as laboratory-proven influenza, pneumonia or deaths from pneumonia.[108]

CONCLUSION

Community-acquired pneumonia remains a significant health problem, despite new antibiotic strategies.

The new techniques for microbiological diagnosis, such as the frequent use of urinary antigen testing for *Legionella* and the rt-PCR may yield a rapid etiologic diagnosis, especially viruses and atypicals or identification of resistance.

The incorporation of the biological markers, PCT and especially CRP, in the PSI and CURB65 prognostic scales and in the modified ATS rule for severe CAP, might improve their mortality prediction value. New scores for prediction of SCAP are needed validation in large cohorts. Our daily clinical approach in patients with CAP has changed in the general approach to base empirical treatment on the severity of disease presentation, and the shorter duration of (IV) antibiotic treatment. Newer dosing regimens are attempting to optimize the PK/PD parameters of agents to ensure successful and more rapid eradication of the bacterial pathogen. The use of corticosteroids in pneumonia remains highly controversial and need further trials.

New preventive recommendation is the approval of the of PCV7 vaccine against *S. pneumoniae,* for patients more than 50 years old with risk factors; its drawbacks are the limited number of serotypes, the much higher cost, and the lack of data on efficacy.

REFERENCES

1. Almirall J, Bolıbar I, Vidal J, et al. Epidemiology of community acquired pneumonia in adults: a population-based study. *Eur Respir J.* 2000;15:757-63.
2. Ewig S, Birkner N, Strauss R, et al. New perspectives on community-acquired pneumonia in 388,406 patients. Results from a nationwide mandatory performance measurement programme in healthcare quality. *Thorax.* 2009;64:1062-9.
3. Zalacain R, Torres A, Celis R, et al. Community-acquired pneumonia in the elderly: Spanish multicentre study. *Eur Respir J.* 2003;21:294-302.
4. Mortensen EM, Kapoor WN, Chang CC, et al. Assessment of mortality after long-term follow-up of patients with community-acquired pneumonia. *Clin Infect Dis.* 2003;37 (12):1617-24.
5. Aliberti S, Peyrani P, Filardo G, et al. Association between time to clinical stability and outcomes after discharge in hospitalized patients with community-acquired pneumonia. *Chest.* 2011;140(2):482-8.
6. Kaplan V, Clermont G, Griffin MF, et al. Pneumonia: still the old man's friend? *Arch Intern Med.* 2003;163:317-23.
7. Yende S, D'Angelo G, Kellum JA, et al. Inflammatory markers at hospital discharge predict subsequent mortality after pneumonia and sepsis. *Am J Respir Crit Care Med.* 2008;177:1242e7.
8. Mandell LA, Wunderink RG, Anzueto A, et al. Infectious Diseases Society of America/American Thoracic Society consensus guidelines on the management of community-acquired pneumonia in adults. *Clin Infect Dis.* 2007; 44(Suppl 2):S27-72.
9. Masiá M, Gutiérrez F, Padilla S, et al. Clinical characterisation of pneumonia caused by atypical pathogens combining classic and novel predictors. *Clin Microbiol Infect.* 2007;13(2):153-61.
10. Torres A, Barberán J, Falguera M, et al. Multidisciplinary guidelines for the management of community-acquired pneumonia. *Med Clin (Barc).* 2013;140(5):223.e1-223.e19.
11. Almirall J, Bolíbar I, Serra-Prat M, et al. Community-Acquired Pneumonia in Catalan Countries (PACAP) Study Group. New evidence of risk factors for community-acquired pneumonia: a population-based study. *Eur Respir J.* 2008;31(6):1274-84.
12. Woodhead M. New guidelines for the management of adult lower respiratory tract infections. *Eur Respir J.* 2011; 38(6):1250-1.
13. Arancibia F, Bauer TT, Ewig S, et al. Community-acquired pneumonia due to gram-negative bacteria and *Pseudomonas aeruginosa*: incidence, risk, and prognosis. *Arch Intern Med.* 2002;162(16):1849-58.
14. Cillóniz C, Ewig S, Polverino E, et al. Community-acquired pneumonia in outpatients: aetiology and outcomes. *Eur Respir J.* 2012;40(4):931-8.
15. Gutierrez F, Masia M, Rodriguez JC, et al. Community-acquired pneumonia of mixed etiology: prevalence, clinical characteristics, and outcome. *Eur J Clin Microbiol Infect Dis.* 2005;24:377-83.
16. Cillóniz C, Ewing S, Polverino E, et al. Microbial aetiology of community-acquired pneumonia and its relation to severity. *Thorax.* 2011;66:340-6.
17. Johansson N, Kalin M, Tiveljung-Lindell A, et al. Etiology of community-acquired pneumonia: increased microbiological yield with new diagnostic methods. *Clin Infect Dis.* 2010;50(2):202-9.
18. Jennings LC, Anderson TP, Beynon KA, et al. Incidence and characteristics of viral community-acquired pneumonia in adults. *Thorax.* 2008;63(1):42-8.
19. Templeton KE, Scheltinga SA, van den Eeden WC, et al. Improved diagnosis of the etiology of community-acquired pneumonia with real-time polymerase chain reaction. *Clin Infect Dis.* 2005;41(3):345-51.
20. Schildgen V, van den Hoogen B, Fouchier R, et al. Human metapneumovirus: lessons learned over the first decade. *Clin Microbiol Rev.* 2011;24(4):734-54.
21. Rubinstein E, Kollef MH, Nathwani D. Pneumonia caused by methicillin-resistant *Staphylococcus aureus. Clin Infect Dis.* 2008;46(Suppl 5):S378-85.
22. Aliberti S, Zanaboni AM, Blasi F. Pneumonia in the community caused by multidrug-resistant organisms: keep working on probabilistic scores. *Clin Infect Dis.* 2012;54(10):1519-20.
23. Butler JC, Bosshardt SC, Phelan M, et al. Classical and latent class analysis evaluation of sputum polymerase chain reaction and urine antigen testing for diagnosis of pneumococcal pneumonia in adults. *J Infect Dis.* 2003;187(9):1416-23.

24. Anevlavis S, Petroglou N, Tzavaras A, et al. A prospective study of the diagnostic utility of sputum Gram stain in pneumonia. *J Infect.* 2009;59:83-9.
25. Gaydos CA. What is the role of newer molecular tests in the management of CAP? *Infect Dis Clin North Am.* 2013;27(1):49-69.
26. Postma DF, van Werkhoven CH, Huijts SM, et al. New trends in the prevention and management of community-acquired pneumonia. *Neth J Med.* 2012;70(8):337-48.
27. Han X, Li S, Lu S, et al. Amplification of 16S rDNA by nested PCR for measurement of *Mycoplasma pneumoniae* DNA over time: clinical application. *J Med Microbiol.* 2011.
28. Lienard J, Croxatto A, Aeby S, et al. Development of a new chlamydial specific real-time PCR and its application to respiratory clinical samples. *J Clin Microbiol.* 2011;49:2637-42.
29. Rello J, Lisboa T, Lujan M, et al. Severity of pneumococcal pneumonia associated with genomic bacterial load. *Chest.* 2009;136:832-40.
30. Hirama T, Yamaguchi T, Miyazawa H, et al. Prediction of the pathogens that are the cause of pneumonia by the battlefield hypothesis. *PLoS One.* 2011;6:e24474.
31. Ginocchio CC, Zhang F, Manji R, et al. Evaluation of multiple test methods for the detection of the novel 2009 influenza A (H1N1) during the New York City outbreak. *J Clin Virol.* 2009;45:191-5.
32. Falguera M, Ruiz-Gonzalez A, Schoenenberger JA, et al. Prospective, randomized study to compare empirical treatment versus targeted treatment on the basis of the urine antigen results in hospitalized patients with community-acquired pneumonia. *Thorax.* 2010;65:101-6.
33. Almirall J, Bolíbar I, Toran P, et al. Contribution of C-reactive protein to the diagnosis and assessment of severity of community-acquired pneumonia. *Chest.* 2004;125(4):1335-42.
34. Higa F, Akamine M, Furugen M, et al. Hepatocyte growth factor levels in Legionella pneumonia: a retrospective study. *BMC Infect Dis.* 2011;11:74.
35. Lacoma A, Rodriguez N, Prat C, et al. Usefulness of consecutive biomarkers measurement in the management of community-acquired pneumonia. *Eur J Clin Microbiol Infect Dis.* 2011.
36. Schuetz P, Christ-Crain M, Zimmerli W, et al. Repeated measurements of endothelin-1 precursor peptides predict the outcome in community acquired pneumonia. *Intensive Care Med.* 2011;37:970-80.
37. Rello J, Bodi M, Mariscal D, et al. Microbiological testing and outcome of patients with severe community-acquired pneumonia. *Chest.* 2003;123:174-80.
38. Fine MJ, Auble TE, Yealy DM, et al. A prediction rule to identify low-risk patients with community-acquired pneumonia. *N Engl J Med.* 1997;336:243-50.
39. Lim WS, van der Eerden MM, Laing R, et al. Defining community acquired pneumonia severity on presentation to hospital: an international derivation and validation study. *Thorax.* 2003;58:377-82.
40. Buising KL, Thursky KA, Black JF, et al. A prospective comparison of severity scores for identifying patients with severe community acquired pneumonia: reconsidering what is meant by severe pneumonia. *Thorax.* 2006;61:419-24.
41. Liapikou A, Ferrer M, Polverino E, et al. Severe community-acquired pneumonia: validation of the Infectious Diseases Society of America/American Thoracic Society guidelines to predict an intensive care unit admission. *Clin Infect Dis.* 2009;48(4):377-85.
42. Brown SM, Jones BE, Jephson AR, et al. Validation of the Infectious Disease Society of America/American Thoracic Society 2007 guidelines for severe community-acquired pneumonia. *Crit Care Med.* 2009;37:3010-6.
43. Phua J, See KC, Chan YH, et al. Validation and clinical implications of implications of the IDSA/ATS minor criteria for severe community-acquired pneumonia. *Thorax.* 2009;64:598-603.
44. Chalmers JD, Taylor JK, Mandal P, et al. Validation of the Infectious Diseases Society of America/American Thoracic Society minor criteria for intensive care unit admission in community-acquired pneumonia patients without major criteria or contraindications to intensive care unit care. *Clin Infect Dis.* 2011;53(6):503-11.
45. España PP, Capelastegui A, Gorordo I, et al. Development and validation of a clinical prediction rule for severe community-acquired pneumonia. *Am J Respir Crit Care Med.* 2006;174:1249-56.
46. Charles PG, Wolfe R, Whitby M, et al. Australian Community-Acquired Pneumonia Study Collaboration, Grayson ML: SMART-COP: a tool for predicting the need for intensive respiratory or vasopressor support in community-acquired pneumonia. *Clin Infect Dis.* 2008; 47(3):375-84.
47. Renaud B, Santin A, Coma E, et al. Association between timing of intensive care unit admission and outcomes for emergency department patients with community-acquired pneumonia. *Crit Care Med.* 2009;37(11):2867-74.
48. Marti C, Garin N, Grosgurin O, et al. Prediction of severe community-acquired pneumonia: a systematic review and meta-analysis. *Crit Care.* 2012;16(4):R141.
49. Gamble JM, Eurich DT, Marrie TJ, et al. Admission hypoglycemia and increased mortality in patients hospitalized with pneumonia. *Am J Med.* 2010;123:556.e11-6.
50. Prina E, Ferrer M, Ranzani OT, et al. Thrombocytosis is a marker of poor outcome in community-acquired pneumonia. *Chest.* 2013;143(3):767-75.
51. Huang DT, Weissfeld LA, Kellum JA, et al. Risk prediction with procalcitonin and clinical rules in community-acquired pneumonia. *Ann Emerg Med.* 2008;52:48-58.
52. Kruger S, Ewig S, Marre R, et al. Procalcitonin predicts patients at low risk of death from community acquired pneumonia across all CRB-65 classes. *Eur Respir J.* 2008; 31:349-55.
53. Menéndez R, Martínez R, Reyes S, et al. Biomarkers improve mortality prediction by prognostic scales in community-acquired pneumonia. *Thorax.* 2009;64(7):587-91.
54. Ramírez P, Ferrer M, Martí V, et al. Inflammatory biomarkers and prediction for intensive care unit admission in severe community-acquired pneumonia. *Crit Care Med.* 2011;39(10):2211-7.
55. Bello S, Lasierra AB, Mincholé E, et al. Prognostic power of proadrenomedullin in community-acquired pneumonia is independent of aetiology. *Eur Respir J.* 2012;39:1144-55.

56. Christ-Crain M, Opal SM. Clinical review: the role of biomarkers in the diagnosis and management of community-acquired pneumonia. *Crit Care.* 2010;14(1): 203.
57. Krüger S, Ewig S, Kunde J, et al. Pro-atrial natriuretic peptide and pro-vasopressin for predicting short-term and long-term survival in community-acquired pneumonia: results from the German Competence Network CAPNETZ. *Thorax.* 2010;65(3):208-14.
58. Maimon N, Nopmaneejumruslers C, Marras TK. Antibacterial class is not obviously important in outpatient pneumonia: a meta-analysis. *Eur Respir J.* 2008;31(5):1068-76.
59. Bébéar C, Pereyre S, Peuchant O. Mycoplasma pneumoniae: susceptibility and resistance to antibiotics. *Future Microbiol.* 2011;6(4):423-31.
60. Leroy O, Saux P, Bédos JP, et al. Comparison of levofloxacin and cefotaxime combined with ofloxacin for ICU patients with community-acquired pneumonia who do not require vasopressors. *Chest.* 2005;128:172-83.
61. Metersky ML, Ma A, Houck PM, et al. Antibiotics for bacteremic pneumonia: improved outcomes with macrolides but not fluoroquinolones. *Chest.* 2007;131:466-73.
62. Baddour LM, Yu VL, Klugman KP, et al. Combination antibiotic therapy lowers mortality among severely ill patients with pneumococcal bacteremia. *Am J Respir Crit Care Med.* 2004;170:440-4.
63. Kaiser L, Wat C, Mills T, et al. Impact of oseltamivir treatment on influenza-related lower respiratory tract complications and hospitalizations. *Arch Intern Med.* 2003;163(14):1667-72.
64. McGeer A, Green KA, Plevneshi A, et al. Toronto Invasive Bacterial Diseases Network. Antiviral therapy and outcomes of influenza requiring hospitalization in Ontario, Canada. *Clin Infect Dis.* 2007;45(12):1568-75.
65. File TM. The science of selecting antimicrobials for community-acquired pneumonia (CAP). *J Manag Care Pharm.* 2009;15(2 Suppl):S5-11.
66. Battleman DS, Callahan M, Thaler HT. Rapid antibiotic delivery and appropriate antibiotic selection reduce length of hospital stay of patients with community-acquired pneumonia: link between quality of care and resource utilization. *Arch Intern Med.* 2002;162:682-8.
67. Bordon J, Aliberti S, Duvvuri P, et al. Early administration of the first antimicrobials should be considered a marker of optimal care of patients with community-acquired pneumonia rather than a predictor of outcomes. *Int J Infect Dis.* 2013;17(5):e293-8.
68. Carratala J, Garcia-Vidal C, Ortega L, et al. Effect of a 3-step critical pathway to reduce duration of intravenous antibiotic therapy and length of stay in community-acquired pneumonia. *Arch Intern Med.* 2012;172(12):922-8.
69. Dimopoulos G, Matthaiou DK, Karageorgopoulos DE, et al. Short- versus long-course antibacterial therapy for community-acquired pneumonia: a meta-analysis. *Drugs.* 2008;68(13):1841-54.
70. Scalera NM, File TM. Determining the duration of therapy for patients with community-acquired pneumonia. *Curr Infect Dis Rep.* 2013;15(2):191-5.
71. el Moussaoui R, de Borgie CA, van den Broek P, et al. Effectiveness of discontinuing antibiotic treatment after three days versus eight days in mild to moderate-severe community acquired pneumonia: randomized, double blind study. *BMJ.* 2006;332(7554):1355.
72. Choudhury G, Mandal P, Singanayagam A, et al. Seven-day antibiotic courses have similar efficacy to prolonged courses in severe community-acquired pneumonia-a propensity-adjusted analysis. *Clin Microbiol Infect.* 2011; 17:1852-8.
73. Christ-Cain M, Stolz D, Bingisser R, et al. Procalcitonin guidance of antibiotic therapy in community-acquired pneumonia: a randomized trial. *Am J Respir Crit Care Med.* 2006;174:84-93.
74. Albrich WC, Dusemund F, Bucher B, et al. Effectiveness and safety of procalcitonin-guided antibiotic therapy in lower respiratory tract infections in "real life": an international, multicenter poststudy survey (ProREAL). *Arch Intern Med.* 2012;172(9):715-22.
75. Schuetz P, Christ-Crain M, Thomann R, et al. Effect of procalcitonin-based guidelines versus standard guidelines on antibiotic use in lower respiratory tract infections: the ProHOSP randomized controlled trial. *JAMA.* 2009; 302(10):1059-66.
76. Bouadma L, Luyt CE, Tubach F, et al. Use of procalcitonin to reduce patients' exposure to antibiotics in intensive care units (PRORATA trial): a multicentre randomized controlled trial. *Lancet.* 2010;375(9713):463-74.
77. Bozzette SA, Sattler FR, Chiu J, et al. A controlled trial of early adjunctive treatment with corticosteroids for pneumocystis carinii pneumonia in the acquired immunodeficiency syndrome. *N Engl J Med.* 1990;323(21):1451-7.
78. Meijvis SC, Hardeman H, Remmelts HH, et al. Dexamethasone and length of hospital stay in patients with community- acquired pneumonia: a randomized, double blind, placebo-controlled trial. *Lancet.* 2011;377:2023-30.
79. Snijders D, Daniels JM, de Graaff CS, et al. Efficacy of corticosteroids in community-acquired pneumonia: a randomized double-blinded clinical trial. *Am J Respir Crit Care Med.* 2010;181:975-82.
80. Fernandez-Serrano S, Dorca J, Garcia-Vidal C, et al. Effect of corticosteroids on the clinical course of community-acquired pneumonia: a randomized controlled trial. *Crit Care.* 2011;15:R96.
81. Confalonieri M, Urbino R, Potena A, et al. Hydrocortisone infusion for severe community-acquired pneumonia: a preliminary randomized study. *Am J Respir Crit Care Med.* 2005;171:242-8.
82. Sabry NA, Omar EE-D. Corticosteroids and ICU course of community acquired pneumonia in Egyptian settings. *Pharmacology & Pharmacy.* 2011;2:73-81.
83. Confalonieri M, Annane D, Antonaglia C, et al. Is prolonged low-dose glucocorticoid treatment beneficial in community-acquired pneumonia? *Curr Infect Dis Rep.* 2013;15(2):158-66.
84. Nie W, Zhang Y, Cheng J, et al. Corticosteroids in the treatment of community-acquired pneumonia in adults: a meta-analysis. *PLoSOne.* 2012;7(10):e47926.
85. Aliberti S, Blasi F. Clinical stability versus clinical failure in patients with community-acquired pneumonia. *Semin Respir Crit Care Med.* 2012;33(3):284-91.

86. Menendez R, Cavalcanti M, Reyes S, et al. Markers of treatment failure in hospitalized community acquired pneumonia. *Thorax.* 2008;63:447-52.
87. Jefferson T, Rivetti D, Rivetti A, et al. Efficacy and effectiveness of influenza vaccines in elderly people: a systematic review. *Lancet.* 2005;366(9492):1165-74.
88. Menéndez R, Torres A, Zalacaín R, et al. Risk factors of treatment failure in community acquired pneumonia: implications for disease outcome. *Thorax.* 2004;59(11): 960-5.
89. Ruiz-Gonzalez A, Falguera M, Porcel JM, et al. C-reactive protein for discriminating treatment failure from slow responding pneumonia. *Eur J Intern Med.* 2010;21(6):548-52.
90. Sialer S, Liapikou A, Torres A. What is the best approach to the nonresponding patient with community-acquired pneumonia? *Infect Dis Clin North Am.* 2013;27(1):189-203.
91. Centers for Disease Control and Prevention (CDC). Use of 13-valent pneunococcal conjugate vaccine and 23-valent pneumococcal polysaccharide vaccine for adults with immunocompromising conditions recommendations of the Advisory Committee on Immunization Practices (ACIP). *MMWR Morb Mortal Wkly Rep.* 2012:61(40):816-9.
92. Fisman DN, Abrutyn E, Spaude KA, et al. Prior pneumococcal vaccination is associated with reduced death, complications and length of stay among hospitalized adults with community-acquired pneumonia. *Clin Infect Dis.* 2006;42:1093-101.
93. Huss A, Scott P, Stuck AE, et al. Efficacy of pneumococcal vaccination in adults: a meta-analysis. *CMAJ.* 2009;180(1): 48-58.
94. Maruyama T, Taguchi O, Niederman MS, et al. Efficacy of 23-valent pneumococcal vaccine in preventing pneumonia and improving survival in nursing home residents: double blind, randomized and placebo controlled trial. *BMJ.* 2010; 340:c1004.
95. Spindler C, Hedlund J, Jasir A, et al. Effects of a large-scale introduction of the pneumococcal polysaccharide vaccine among elderly persons in Stockholm, Sweden. *Vaccine.* 2008;26:5541-6.
96. Goldblatt D, Southern J, Andrews N, et al. The immunogenicity of 7-valent pneumococcal conjugate vaccine versus 23-valent polysaccharide vaccine in adults aged 50–80 years. *Clin Infect Dis.* 2009;49:1318-25.
97. Kapetanovic MC, Roseman C, Jonsson G, et al. Heptavalent pneumococcal conjugate vaccine elicits similar antibody response as standard 23-valent polysaccharide vaccine in adult patients with RA treated with immunomodulating drugs. *Clin Rheumatol.* 2011;30:1555-61.
98. De Roux A, Schmöele-Thoma B, Siber GR, et al. Comparison of pneumococcal conjugate polyssaccharide and free polysaccharide vaccines in elderly adults: conjugate vaccine elicits improved antibacterial immune responses and immunological memory. *Clin Infect Dis.* 2008;46:1015-23.
99. Whitney CG, Pilishvili T, Farley MM, et al. Effectiveness of seven-valent pneumococcal conjugate vaccine against invasive pneumococcal disease: a matched case-control study. *Lancet.* 2006;368(9546):1495-502.
100. Hammitt LL, Bruden DL, Butler JC, et al. Indirect effect of conjugate vaccine on adult carriage of *Streptococcus pneumoniae*: an explanation of trends in invasive pneumococcal disease. *J Infect Dis.* 2006;193(11):1487-94.
101. French N, Gordon SB, Mwalukomo T, et al. A trial of a 7-valent pneumococcal conjugate vaccine in HIV-infected adults. *N Engl J Med.* 2010;362:812-22.
102. Smith KJ, Wateska AR, Nowalk MP, et al. Cost-effectiveness of adult vaccination strategies using pneumococcal conjugate vaccine compared with pneumococcal polysaccharide vaccine. *JAMA.* 2012;307:804-12.
103. US Food and Drug Administration. Approved products: Prevnar 13 [Internet] Silver Spring: US Food and Drug Administration. [online] Available from: www.fda.gov/BiologicsBloodVaccines/Vaccines/ApprovedProducts/ucm201667htm [Accessed February, 2014].
104. Centers for Disease Control and Prevention. Fast Stats. Deaths and mortality. [online] Available from www.cdc.gov/nchs/fastats/pneumonia.htm. [Accessed February, 2014].
105. Food and Drug Administration. FDA expands use of Prevnar 13 vaccine for people ages 50 and older. Silver Spring, MD: US Department of Health and Human Services, Food and Drug Administration; 2011.
106. Ortqvist A, Granath F, Askling J, et al. Influenza vaccination and mortality: prospective cohort study of the elderly in a large geographical area. *Eur Respir J.* 2007;30:414-22.
107. Jefferson T, Rivetti D, Rivetti A, et al. Efficacy and effectiveness of influenza vaccines in elderly people: a systematic review. *Lancet.* 2005;366(9492):1165-74.
108. Thomas RE, Jefferson T, Lasserson TJ. Influenza vaccination for healthcare workers who work with the elderly. *Cochrane Database Syst Rev.* 2010;2:CD005187.

CHAPTER 4

Atypical Pneumonias

Francesco Blasi, Maria Pappalettera, Federico Piffer, Paolo Tarsia

ABSTRACT

The atypical bacteria *Mycoplasma pneumoniae*, *Legionella pneumophila*, and *Chlamydia pneumoniae* are recognized as a common cause of acute respiratory tract infections such as community-acquired pneumonia, being involved in over 20% of cases. Identification of atypical infection has traditionally been largely based on serological methods; however, in recent years, addition of newer diagnostic methods has contributed to a better understanding of the epidemiological role of atypical bacteria. The aim of this review is to discuss relevant aspects of atypical bacterial infections of the respiratory tract.

INTRODUCTION

In its broadest sense, the array of pathogens, which constitute "atypical bacteria" includes both zoonotic and non-zoonotic agents. The former include *Coxiella burnetii* (agent of Q fever), *Francisella tularensis* (involved in tularemia), and *Chlamydia psittaci* (etiologic agent of psittacosis).[1] The present review will, however, focus exclusively on the nonzoonotic atypical bacteria: *Mycoplasma pneumoniae*, *Legionella* spp., and *Chlamydia pneumoniae*. These agents are primarily known as causative agents in community-acquired pneumonia (CAP).

What is currently meant with the terms "typical" and "atypical" in the context of CAP may be confusing and may need some clarification. The traditional clinical notion was that "typical" pathogens present with acute onset of symptoms, high grade fever, high blood leukocyte counts, productive cough, localized rales on auscultation, and infiltrates due to alveolar airspace consolidation on chest X-ray. Conversely, "atypical" pathogens would cause pneumonia, defined clinically as progressive in onset, with moderate general clinical signs, preceded by a sore throat, a paucity of clinical findings, dry non-productive cough, and interstitial involvement on chest X-ray. The above clinical distinction has not stood the test of time and is now considered meaningless, as there is a large degree of overlap between these syndromes.[2,3] The distinction between "typical" and "atypical" pathogens is still retained because the latter are unresponsive to traditional first line β-lactam treatment of CAP cases and require specific antibiotic classes (macrolides, ketolides, tetracyclines, and fluoroquinolones).

CHARACTERISTICS OF ATYPICAL PATHOGENS

Mycoplasma pneumoniae

Mycoplasma pneumoniae is a slowly growing, pleomorphic, non-motile bacteria bound by a single triple-layered membrane that lacks a cell wall and reproduces by binary fission.[4,5] Mycoplasmas represent the smallest self-replicating organisms that are capable of cell-free existence.[6] *M. pneumoniae* cell volume is less than 5% of that of typical bacteria. They have never been found as freely living organisms in nature. They depend on a host cell to supply them with necessary nutrients, particularly sterols that are an essential component of the *Mycoplasma* cell wall providing some structural support to the osmotically fragile *Mycoplasma*.[7] Another structural component of the *M. pneumoniae* cell that is important for extracellular survival is a protein network that provides a cytoskeleton to support the cell membrane.

Legionella pneumophila

Legionella is a small, pleomorphic, Gram-negative bacillus. Water reservoirs are the microorganism's natural habitat in which it may thrive for long time. Man-made niches include air-conditioning systems, thermal habitats, hot water systems, respiratory ventilators, and shower heads of bathroom taps. *Legionella* shows an increased tolerance to common disinfectants, such as chlorine and may thus proliferate in water supply systems.[8,9]

Legionella life cycle consists of two reciprocal phases: replicative and transmissive. Transmissive *L. pneumophila* is engulfed by phagocytic cells within which it establishes vacuoles derived from the endoplasmic reticulum (ER) that provide protection from lysosomal digestion. When conditions are favorable, intracellular bacteria repress transmission traits and activate pathways that promote replication. As conditions deteriorate, the progeny stop dividing and coordinately express traits that promote survival in the environment and transmission to a new phagocytic host.[10]

Legionella pneumophila was first identified following a large outbreak of pneumonia among members of the American Legion in 1976.[11] Since then, at least 16 serogroups of *L. pneumophila* and over 50 additional *Legionella* species have been described. *L. pneumophila* serogroup 1 is the most frequently encountered cause of Legionnaires' disease in most countries. Other *Legionella* species commonly identified include *L. longbeachae, L. bozemanii, L. dumoffii,* and *L. micdadei*.[12,13] *L. longbeachae* is particularly common in Australia and New Zealand.

Chlamydia pneumoniae

Chlamydia is an obligatory intracellular bacteria that present in two developmental forms: infective elementary bodies and reproductive reticulate bodies.[14,15] Elementary bodies are the metabolically-inactive infectious form of the organism. They have a rigid cell wall, allowing survival outside the host cell. After host cell infection, elementary bodies differentiate into reticulate bodies. Reticulate bodies are larger, metabolically active forms of the organism. Inside the host cell, reticulate bodies divide by binary fission, forming a microcolony referred to as a chlamydial inclusion. After a period of growth and division, the reticulate bodies reorganize and condense to form new elementary bodies. Following host cell lysis, the elementary bodies are released to initiate new infectious cycles.[16]

Under suboptimal growth conditions (such as nutrient deficiency, presence of hostile host cytokine profile, or under the influence of antibiotics), completion of the above biphasic cycle is prevented and reticulate bodies do not go on to develop new elementary bodies but transform into aberrant bodies.[15,17] These are non-growing, nonculturable forms, insensitive to antibiotic treatment that are nonetheless vital and may persist for long periods within the infected organism. Persistence in this form allows long-term survival through evasion of the host immunological responses. Aberrant forms also provide a reservoir for new infections, once environmental conditions allow reactivation of normal development to elementary bodies.[14]

In 1999 a new taxonomic classification of *C. pneumoniae* was proposed, renaming the bacterium as *Chlamydophila pneumoniae*.[18] The proposal failed to encounter universal acceptance and both names are currently in use by different authors.

C. pneumoniae infection appears to be uncommon before 5 years of age but is increasingly common thereafter. By 20 years of age, approximately, 50% of persons have detectable levels of antibody to the organism and seroprevalence increases to approximately 75% in the elderly.[19] Reinfection is, therefore, common. Although the exact mode of transmission is not known, spread via droplets has been proposed.

ATYPICAL BACTERIA AS A CAUSE OF COMMUNITY-ACQUIRED PNEUMONIA

The true prevalence of single etiologic agents as a cause of pneumonia is difficult to assess due to variations between epidemiological studies. Studies on the etiology of CAP during the 1990s attributed 20–30% of cases to atypical bacteria both in Europe and the US.[20,21] *C. pneumoniae* and *M. pneumoniae* were reported in just over, or just below, 10% of cases, respectively, and *L. pneumophila* in approximately 5%.[20] Most of these studies were based on the use of serology alone, some of which used a single high IgG antibody titer to establish the diagnosis (a criterion currently considered unsatisfactory). Over the last decade, additional diagnostic tests for atypical bacteria have been made available, such as molecular biology techniques for all 3 pathogens and urinary antigen detection for *L. pneumophila*. More recent reports using more extensive diagnostic testing for atypical bacteria identify *C. pneumoniae* in 0.9–17% of cases, *M. pneumoniae* in 2.1–12.5% of cases, and *Legionella* in 1–5% of patients.[9,35] Similar studies in pediatric populations have identified *C. pneumoniae* in 0–44% of cases and *M. pneumoniae* in 15–40%.[36-47]

There is substantial variation in the rate of identification of these pathogens depending on the site of care. Studies in adult outpatients show high yields of *M. pneumoniae*, whereas studies involving patients with severe CAP who require admission to the intensive care unit almost exclusively identify *Legionella* among atypical bacteria.

Retrospective analysis of a large international CAP database [community-acquired pneumonia organization (CAPO), headed by the University of Louisville, Kentucky] studied 4,337 patients with CAP from 21 countries (Europe, North America, South America, and combined centres in Africa/Asia) to evaluate the distribution of atypical bacteria.[48] A surprisingly similar rate of atypical bacteria retrieval was observed in CAP patients from different regions of the world (Europe 28%, North America 22%, South America 21%, and Asia/Africa 20%). *M. pneumoniae* was identified in 11–15% of cases in the different world regions, *L. pneumophila* in 3–6%, and *C. pneumoniae* in 5–8%. In a different study involving another large computerised database based in Germany [community-acquired pneumonia (CAPNETZ)], *M. pneumoniae* was identified as etiologic agent in 6.8% of 4532 patients with CAP, using serology and polymerase chain reaction (PCR).[49] The true incidence of *M. pneumoniae* may have been underestimated in this paper, as the study design required only one acute serum sample for testing. A similar work by the same network investigating *Legionella* in 2503 patients with pneumonia identified this agent in 3.8% of cases.[50] Children and young adults are the individuals most often involved in *M. pneumoniae* infections, with this agent even ranking above *Streptococcus pneumoniae* as the most common cause of CAP in this age group.[51-53] *M. pneumoniae* infection has, however, also been identified in 11–17% cases of pneumonia in patients of over 40 years of age.[54]

The reported variable incidence of atypical pathogens in different clinical settings is summarised in table 1.

TABLE 1

Range of Incidence of Atypical Pathogens as Causative Agents of Pneumonia in Different Clinical Settings

	M. pneumoniae (%)	*L. pneumophila* (%)	*C. pneumoniae* (%)
Community	1–33	0–13	7–37
Hospital	0–18	1–14	0–18
ICU	0–7	0–30	0–6

ICU, intensive care unit.

CLINICAL CHARACTERISTICS OF ATYPICAL PNEUMONIA INFECTIONS

Mycoplasma pneumoniae

Worldwide, *M. pneumoniae* infections may occur both endemically and epidemically involving persons of all ages. Peaks of incidence of *M. pneumoniae* infection occur every 5–7 years.[55] Long incubation period (up to 3 weeks), relatively low transmission rate, and variable persistence of the microorganism in the respiratory tract of infected subjects may explain prolonged duration of epidemics that may last 6–8 months. Climate, seasonal variations, and geography are not thought to be of major significance. Epidemics have been described in enclosed populations, such as college students, prisoners, military garrisons, religious communities, institutions for the disabled and even hospital workers.[56] Simultaneous involvement of several family members within single household has also been described.

Person-to-person infection transmission is caused by inhalation of droplet nuclei after exposure to an acutely ill actively coughing individual. Following natural human infection, subjects may develop both temporary and prolonged carrier state conditions. *M. pneumoniae* adheres to airway epithelial cells by means of its neuraminic differentiated terminal unit. Attachment induces an interruption of cellular RNA and protein synthesis, resulting in ciliostasis, denudation of cilia, and extensive epithelial cell injury. Inflammatory cell recruitment is also induced.[57] *Mycoplasma* invasion is generally limited to the airways as the organism does not generally penetrate into the lung parenchyma or the bloodstream. Airways inflammation may involve the entire extent of conductive airways, from the trachea and bronchi down to the bronchioles. Histological examination generally reveals acute and chronic bronchiolitis and peribronchiolitis. Mimicry between *M. pneumoniae* and host antigens is felt to mediate immunopathological damage. *M. pneumoniae* infection may be associated with extrapulmonary manifestations, such as hemolytic anemia.

The typical respiratory symptoms include a slowly developing syndrome presenting with pharyngitis, sinus congestion, occasionally otitis media, and eventually, prolonged lower respiratory tract involvement with dry cough and dry rales on chest auscultation.

In a recent CAPNETZ database study[49] on patients with *Mycoplasma* pneumonia, the patients were significantly younger than any other age group of CAP patients (mean age 41 ± 16 years in *Mycoplasma* pneumonia vs. 61 ± 17 years in other CAP patients). The patients also had fewer comorbidities and the severity of their pneumonia was much lower as reflected by low CRB-65 scores and lower inflammatory response. The majority of these patients were treated as outpatients, and those hospitalized had a shorter length of stay compared to CAP caused by other etiologies. The fatality rate was also very low (0.7%) compared to the remaining CAP population (8.7%).

Legionella pneumophila

The traditional view that *L. pneumophila* is considered exclusively as a cause of severe pneumonia cases has been questioned,[50] and the range of clinical severity of legionella pneumonia may vary from mild respiratory disease managed on an outpatient basis to fulminating pneumonia requiring intensive care unit (ICU) treatment. Given its capacity to thrive and proliferate in water supplies, the most likely mode of *L. pneumophila* transmission is direct inhalation from contaminated water systems. Conversely, there is no evidence of person-to-person transmission, and, therefore, patient isolation is not considered mandatory. The reported incubation period varies between 2 and 10 days. Dry cough and fever are the most commonly reported symptoms, with high grade fever (>40°C) being present in about 20% of cases. Similar to *Mycoplasma* infections, *L. pneumophila* may also cause extrapulmonary symptoms, although manifestations are very different in both pathogens. Neurologic complaints, abnormal liver enzymes, diarrhea, hypophosphatemia, hematuria, and hematologic abnormalities are relatively common but nonspecific.[58,59] A distinctive feature of *Legionella* infection is central nervous system involvement, which may be manifested by headache, mental confusion, or lethargy. Fairly dramatic changes in mental status or encephalopathy may be present. Hypophosphatemia is a common finding but may be missed, as it occurs early and generally subsides within 3 days.[60]

In a study specifically evaluating *Legionella* pneumonia in the German CAPNETZ database, it was found to involve elderly men predominantly, with a high incidence of diabetes and heavy smoking as comorbidities.[50] Interestingly, the study found the pathogen in identical frequencies among inpatients and outpatients, challenging the view that *L. pneumophila* is associated with intrinsic pathogenicity and is thus inevitably associated with more severe pneumonia. Conversely, the severity of *Legionella* pneumonia may derive mainly from the interplay of host-pathogen interactions. The study also showed that approximately 10% of infections are caused by species other than *L. pneumophila*. This may have important implications when devising diagnostic strategies for the identification of this pathogen. Considering that non-*L. pneumophila* species are identifiable only by PCR and culture, overreliance on urinary antigen testing may lead to missing out on other *Legionella* species.

Initial radiological involvement is usually unilateral with a frequent rapidly progressive spread to multilobar asymmetrical infiltrates. Pleural effusion is a common finding. Often, control chest X-ray shows worsening pulmonary infiltrates while the patient is receiving seemingly appropriate empirical antimicrobial therapy.

Chlamydia pneumoniae

The incubation period of infection due to *C. pneumoniae* is about 21 days. Upper respiratory signs and symptoms, such as rhinitis, sore throat, or hoarseness may be reported initially.[61] These may then subside over days to weeks, followed by the onset of cough, resulting in a biphasic pattern of illness symptoms.[62] Body temperature seldom increases higher than 38–39°C. In addition to having a gradual onset, symptoms due to *C. pneumoniae* respiratory infections may be of prolonged duration with persistence of cough and malaise for several weeks or months despite appropriate antibiotic therapy.

C. pneumoniae is reported to account for a relatively large number (6–20%) of CAP cases.[63] This agent is part of a coinfection involving other bacterial agents in approximately 30% of adult CAP cases.[64] The clinical course may vary from mild, self-limiting illnesses to severe forms of pneumonia, particularly in elderly patients, and with coexisting cardiopulmonary diseases. Chest X-ray generally reveals small pulmonary infiltrates, sublobar or segmental at presentation. Multiple infiltrates may sometimes be seen and are often bilateral. Extensive lobar involvement is uncommon, whereas pleural effusion may be present in up to 20% of cases.

SEVERITY SCORING SYSTEMS AND BIOMARKERS IN ATYPICAL PNEUMONIA

Distinguishing between atypical and typical CAP based on presenting clinical characteristics is virtually impossible as single clinical, radiological, or laboratory parameters have limited value in predicting the infectious organism.[2,3]

Recently, severity scores, such as the Pneumonia Severity Index (PSI) and Confusion, Urea, Respiratory Rate, Age more than 65 years (CURB-65) and novel biomarkers, such as procalcitonin (PCT), lipopolysaccharide-binding protein (LBP), have been introduced in clinical practice or as research tools. A limited number of studies have addressed the issues whether use of these scores and biomarkers may aid in distinguishing atypical from atypical CAP in presentation. If proved useful, clinicians may acquire a help in deciding whether atypical antibiotic coverage is needed in the single patient or not.

In one of the studies involving 185 CAP patients, Masia et al.[65] found a tendency towards lower PCT and C-reactive protein (CRP) levels in atypical pneumonia compared to typical bacterial CAP, although neither of them reached statistical significance. Differences in PCT levels between typical and atypical etiology, patients were more marked in PSI low class risk subjects (PSI I-II), than among patients with more severe CAP (PSI III-V). Hedlund et al.[66] also reported lower PCT in atypical bacteria. Eight of nine patients with pneumonia caused by atypical agents had PCT levels less than 0.5 µg/L compared with 6/27 patients with pneumonia caused by classic bacterial pathogens, mainly *Streptococcus pneumoniae* ($p = 0.03$). No such correlation between CRP levels and etiology was found.

A more recent and larger study of the German CAPNETZ database investigated 1,337 patients with CAP. Etiological diagnosis was reached in 472 patients (35.3%), with a typical bacterial infection being identified in 185 subjects, and atypical bacterial infection in 190 patients.[67] Patients with typical bacterial pneumonia showed significantly higher levels of PCT, CRP, and white blood cell (WBC) counts compared to patients with atypical etiology. Regarding PCT, using a cutoff level of 0.1 ng/mL showed an odds ratio of 8.3 (95% confidence interval (CI) 4.8–14.5) whereas a cutoff level of 0.25 ng/mL showed an odds ratio (OR) of 3.2 (95% CI 2.1–5.0) in differentiating pneumonia caused by *S. pneumoniae* from CAP due to atypical or viral etiology. However, serum biomarkers were unable to differentiate single etiologic atypical agents, as there were no significant differences in PCT, CRP, and WBC levels between patients with CAP caused by *L. pneumophila, M. pneumoniae,* or *C. pneumoniae*. In this study, CRB-65 scores were unable to differentiate between patients with CAP due to typical pathogens (mean CRB-65 score: 0.98 ± 0.92), and atypical microrganisms (mean: 0.79 ± 0.84). Conversely, in a study on 3,523 patients with CAP that evaluated the distribution of the microbial etiology in relation to severity scores (PSI and CURB-65) the frequency of atypical pathogens was more common in low-risk scores, and atypical frequency decreased with increasing CAP severity scores.[68]

In a Spanish prospective study of 658 subjects, PCT, PCR, and inflammatory cytokines [tumor necrosis factor (TNF)-α, interleukin (IL)-1β, IL-6, IL-8, and IL-10] were measured in all patients admitted with CAP.[69] Different cytokine profiles and biomarkers were found depending on etiology: atypical bacteria (lower PCT and IL-6), viruses (lower PCT and higher IL-10), Enterobacteriaceae (higher IL-8), *S. pneumoniae* (high PCT), and *L. pneumophila* (higher CRP and TNF-α). A cut-off PCT level of less than 0.5 mg/dL was able to predict atypical vs. typical bacteria etiology with 81% sensitivity, 68% specificity, a positive predictive value of 22%, and a negative predictive value of 97%.

LBP has been proposed as a marker for bacterial infection, as high serum concentrations of this protein have been found in sepsis caused by Gram-negative and Gram-positive bacteria.[70] A prospective population-based study investigated CRP and LBP levels in 196 patients with CAP.[71] In this study, the median CRP concentration was significantly higher in patients with pneumonia caused by typical bacteria (26.4 mg/L; range, 3.7–343 mg/L) than in those with atypical pneumonia (3.7 mg/L; range, 3.7–150 mg/L, $p = 0.002$). Serum LBP concentrations were also significantly higher in patients with bacterial pneumonia than in those with pneumonia caused by atypical organisms ($p < 0.001$). A cutoff LBP level of 14 mg/L showed the best discriminatory power in distinguishing atypical from typical pneumonia. Serum LBP concentrations below 14 mg/L and a neutrophil count of less than 8.5×10^{12}/L identified nearly 50% of the patients with pneumonia caused by atypical organisms but was present in only 4% of patients with typical bacterial pneumonia. In patients less than 35 years of age, serum LBP had a sensitivity of 59% and a specificity of 94% for identifying pneumonia caused by atypical organisms, suggesting that the accuracy of LBP was greater in younger subjects.

In a different study based on the CAPNETZ database, IL-6, IL10, and LBP levels were analyzed in 1,000 patients with CAP.[72] Significant differences in the LBP concentrations were found in patients with typical (23.25 µg/mL) and atypical bacterial infections (18.7 µg/mL, $p < 0.012$). However, individual predictions could not be made based on LBP levels. IL-6, and IL-10 levels tended to be greater in typical than atypical pneumonia, although statistical significance was not reached.

The triggering receptor expressed on myeloid cells (TREM)-1 is a cell-surface molecule that has been recently discovered. In the course of infections sustained by bacterial agents, cell surface expression of TREM-1 is upregulated together with the release of a soluble form of this receptor.[73] A recent prospective, noninterventional study of 88 hospitalized CAP patients analyzed soluble TREM-1, PCT, and CRP levels at admission as a tool for differentiating between typical and atypical pneumonia cases.[74] Among patients with CAP caused by typical bacterial pathogens, median plasma soluble TREM-1 levels at admission were 65.2 pg/mL (range, 17.6–138.1 pg/mL), whereas corresponding values in subjects with atypical pneumonia were 25.9 pg/mL (range, 11.5–54.8 pg/mL; $p < 0.001$). Soluble TREM-1 had good discriminative power in differentiating typical from atypical pathogens with an area under the receiver operating characteristic curve of 0.87 (95% CI 0.75–0.98). Using a cutoff level of 44.2 pg/mL as the soluble TREM-1 discriminatory threshold, sensitivity of 81%, a specificity of 79%, a positive likelihood ratio of 3.79, and a negative likelihood ratio of 0.24 were found. No differences were recorded for PCT and CRP levels between patients with typical and atypical pneumonia.

In conclusion, both severity scores and biomarker levels are interesting but as yet unsatisfactory in distinguishing typical from atypical CAP upon presentation, as there is considerable overlap in levels between the two groups. This should lead us to be cautious in order to avoid prescribing insufficient antibiotics based on these parameters. In the future, more effective biomarkers for identifying the etiology of CAP could be derived by unusual intermediate metabolites whose levels are altered by a specific microorganism (as shown for *Pneumocystis*),[75] or a proteomics approach to identify characteristic signature patterns for particular microbial species.

MICROBIOLOGICAL DIAGNOSIS

One of the greatest technical limitations in addressing the role of atypical bacteria in respiratory infections is their lack of growth on common culture media. All 3 organisms are extremely fastidious in growth requirements, and culture is currently clinically available only for *Legionella*, although not in all laboratories. Serological determination of antibody titers to these agents has long been the reference technique. Lately, molecular biology techniques, such as PCR, have been successfully employed in the detection of atypical pathogen DNA within different biological samples (airway secretions, blood, etc.). Urinary *Legionella* antigen detection has now become fairly widespread in clinical use. The clinical relevance of different diagnostic techniques applied in the identification of atypical pathogens is presented in table 2.

Culture

Culture methods for *M. pneumoniae* are relatively insensitive, require specialised media, and are time-consuming, requiring 3-6 weeks for signal detection.[76] This makes it impractical for use in routine patient care. Culture for *L. pneumophila* on respiratory samples is 100% specific and allows for the detection of *Legionella* species other than *L. pneumophila*. It requires selective media, is technically demanding, costly and requires up to 10 days for results (generally 3-7 days).[77] Bronchoscopic samples have a greater diagnostic yield compared with expectorated sputum samples, whereas the diagnostic yield from blood cultures is rather poor.[78]

The procedure for culturing *C. pneumoniae* is slow, time consuming, expensive, and insensitive.[79] So far, successful culture of *C. pneumoniae* has been obtained

TABLE 2

Summary of Clinical Relevance of Diagnostic Techniques for Identification of Atypical Pathogens

Technique	*C. pneumoniae*	*M. pneumoniae*	*L. pneumophila*	Comments
Culture	Sensitivity 50%, Specificity 100%	Sensitivity 50–60%, Specificity 100%	Sensitivity <10–80% Specificity 100%	Useful for *Legionella* species other than *L. pneumophila*
Antigen detection	Sensitivity 20–60%, Specificity 95%	Sensitivity 20–50%, Specificity 60–70%	Sensitivity 33–68% Specificity >95%	Little clinical value except for legionella urinary antigen testing
Serology	Sensitivity 60–80% Specificity 90–100%	Sensitivity 70–90%, Specificity 80–90%	Sensitivity 60–80% Specificity >95%	• MIF is still the gold standard for *C. pneumoniae* and *M. pneumoniae* acute infection diagnosis • Paired serum samples are required
PCR	Sensitivity 85–90%, Specificity 95–100%	Sensitivity 80–90%, Sensitivity 95–100%	Sensitivity 83–100% Specificity 90–100%	• Nested PCR may be prone to contamination • Real-time PCR seems the most promising technique • Multiplex PCR allows testing for multiple pathogens with a single test • May become reference diagnostic test in the near future but is still under evaluation

MIF, microimmunofluroscence; PCR, polymerase chain reaction.

in a limited number of laboratories. Main problems encountered with culture are easy inactivation during transport, collection from anatomical sites devoid of active colonization, and low yield, often requiring repeated blind passages.

Serology

Serology testing is usually not helpful in the initial evaluation of patients with respiratory infections, generally requiring paired determinations (acute phase and convalescent phase specimens) but may provide reliable retrospective diagnosis. Therefore, serology provides useful data primarily for epidemiological surveillance. Serologic evidence of an on-going infection is generally based on a fourfold increase in titer of IgG (or IgG + IgM) antibodies during the evolution of the disease episode based on two serum samples collected with an interval of 7–10 days, and/or the appearance of IgM antibodies during the evolution of the disease at the earliest 8–10 days after the start of the infection.[80] There is a little value in testing single serum samples taken within 7 days of the onset of symptoms, as high titers of IgG and/or IgM above a certain threshold early during the disease are often erroneously interpreted as diagnostic but may indicate a previous infection prior to the present disease. Reinfections do not give rise to increasing IgM titers, particularly in adults.

Serology is currently the mainstay for the diagnosis of *M. pneumoniae* pneumonia. Although serological cold agglutinin testing is reported to be positive in approximately 50–75% of patients with pneumonia due to *M. pneumoniae*, this test is seldom employed in clinical practice.[81] Currently, the most reliable test in identifying acute infection is an enzyme-linked immunosorbent assay (ELISA) that allows both IgG and IgM titration. The test presents 92% sensitivity and 95% specificity on paired samples. Second testing should be performed 6–8 weeks after acute sampling as seroconversion timing may vary between 3 and 8 weeks.[82]

Immunofluorescent antibody (IFA), ELISA, and microagglutination are currently the most reliable serological techniques employed in clinical practice for the diagnosis of legionella infection.[77] IgM titres are an unreliable marker of acute infection because these antibodies may persist for long periods of time. Seroconversion commonly requires 4–8 weeks but may take up to 14 weeks in elderly patients.[83] ELISA is now the most commonly employed antibody detection test. Reported sensitivities range from 41 to 94% with 96% specificity, which however decreases for strains other than serogroup 1.[78]

Serology testing for *C. pneumoniae* currently includes only microimmunofluorescence assay (MIF) and ELISA, given that complement fixation (CF) is not species-specific.[84] Several ELISA kits are commercially available, all giving qualitative but not quantitative information on *C. pneumoniae* antibody levels. Experience with these kits is limited and sensitivity and/or specificity are currently unsatisfactory.[85] The current gold standard for serological diagnosis is MIF testing due to high sensitivity and specificity.[86] Utility of serology for *C. pneumoniae* identification is limited by the high prevalence of antibodies in the general population, particularly in the elderly, and difficulties in reliably distinguishing between acute and chronic infection.

More recently, a rapid and simple immunochromatographic test has been developed that allows the detection of *C. pneumoniae*-specific IgM antibodies. The test requires a drop of blood collected by a finger prick and results may be read in 5–10 minutes. In a study comparing the test and enzyme immunoassay, the reported sensitivity and specificity were 100% and 92.9%, respectively.[87] However, as the immunochromatographic test only detects IgM antibodies, its utility may be limited only to primary infection.

Legionella Urinary Antigen Test

Urinary antigen tests have sensitivities in the range of 70–100% and specificities approaching 100% in detecting *L. pneumophila* serogroup 1.[77] Sensitivities can be increased up to 20% by 25-fold concentration of urine samples before testing.[88] *Legionella* antigenuria can be detected as early as 1 day after onset of symptoms and may persist for days to weeks.

Currently marketed commercial test include the Legionella Urinary Antigen EIA (Binax, Inverness Medical: Scarborough, Maine), which gives results in a couple of hours, and the ICT membrane assay (NOW *Legionella* Urinary Antigen Test: Binax, Inverness Medical: Scarborough, Maine), which needs approximately 20 minutes to operate. One of the main disadvantages of these tests is that they are prevalently (but not exclusively) intended to detect *L. pneumophila* serogroup 1 antigen. Some authors suggest that limiting diagnostic testing to urinary antigen detection alone may result in up to 40% of legionellosis cases being lost.[12] Particularly, it may be less sensitive for nosocomial cases because of the frequent involvement of serogroups other than serogroup 1 in this setting. A recent systematic review analyzed 30 studies on urinary antigen detection.[89] Among the 30 studies analyzed the pooled sensitivity for the test was 0.74 (95% CI 0.68–0.81) and specificity 0.991

(95% CI 0.984–0.997). In essence, this study suggests that the test is better for "ruling in" disease rather than "ruling it out", as 26% of patients with confirmed legionellosis had a negative urinary antigen test result. The sensitivity of the antigen test may also be affected by the course of the infection. In milder cases, the disease may not be sufficiently advanced, such that the amount of antigen in the urine is not detectable.

In addition to urinary antigen test, antigen detection by direct immunofluorescence assay (DFA) stain on respiratory samples has been used with variable sensitivity (18–80%) and good specificity (94%). The technique has the advantage of providing results within 2–4 hours, but is technically demanding. Sensitivity appears to be greater on bronchoalveolar lavage specimens than on sputum samples.[90]

Nucleic Acid Amplification Techniques

In the last decade nucleic acid amplification techniques, mainly PCR, have been developed for the identification of a number of microorganisms. These determinations are potentially very useful as results may be obtained in a matter of hours, technique sensitivity allows the detection of minute amounts of pathogen DNA in specimens, and results are not influenced by previous antibiotic treatment. Initially, the use of PCR techniques involved a number of limitations, including presence of PCR inhibitors leading to false-negative results, contamination leading to false-positive results, equipment expense and personnel training, and lack of standardization. More recently, the development of quantitative real-time PCR has allowed simplification of the process (amplification and detection occur in a single test tube) and involves fluorescent-labeled DNA probes that allow quantification of the number of gene copies. Another advancement has been the development of multiplex PCR systems, in which multiple DNA targets from different microorganisms are assessed in one reaction.

Mycoplasma pneumoniae

DNA and RNA probes have been developed and are commercially available and show high specificity but low sensitivity (22–100%) in pharyngeal specimens.[91-93] Real-time PCR assays have significant advantages over traditional PCR.[94] Use of PCR combined with serology in symptomatic patients may be optimum approach for the diagnosis of *M. pneumoniae* respiratory infections. Benefits of combined testing include providing interpretative guidance in distinguishing colonization from infection.[95]

Legionella pneumophila

PCR-based assays have been repeatedly shown to have sensitivity equal to or greater than culture in identifying *Legionella* in respiratory samples.[96,97] The role of PCR for testing other sample types is less clear. PCR test have the advantage of identifying *Legionella* species other than *L. pneumophila.*[98] The test is rapid, not operator-dependant, being expensive, it has not reached widespread clinical use.

Chlamydia pneumoniae

The development of PCR techniques represents a major step forward in the diagnosis of *C. pneumoniae* infection. It has been successfully employed both on respiratory specimens and blood samples. PCR is currently felt to be a more sensitive and less time consuming technique than culture.[99] Enthusiasm for nested PCR assays has been dampened by the fact that the technique involves a significant risk of contamination. Reliance on this particular assay may be associated with an overestimation of the role of *C. pneumoniae* as a causative agent in pneumonia or other clinical contexts. Real-time assays are currently favored, as they are reported to have distinct advantages over traditional PCR assays.[100,101]

The development of multiple PCR determination techniques has allowed simultaneous testing for *C. pneumoniae, L. pneumophila,* and *M. pneumoniae* on a single respiratory specimen.[102,103] Moreover, multiple PCR determination of all three atypical pathogens in addition to *S. pneumoniae* on a single sample has been proposed.[104] This test alone could potentially identify the agents causing roughly three quarters of pneumonia cases. Should this test receive sufficient clinical validation, they may become an attractive diagnostic opportunity, provided their cost is kept reasonable.

In conclusion, although a number of PCR assays are now available for detection of atypical pathogens in respiratory specimens, few satisfy the optimal criteria for a validated assay. Some are now marketed in Europe, but none has been approved by the US Food and Drug Administration (FDA). Therefore, although PCR techniques may become reference tests in the near future, their current overall diagnostic utility is limited by the lack of standardization of extraction procedures, primer definition, etc.

TREATMENT FOR ATYPICAL BACTERIAL RESPIRATORY INFECTIONS

Compared to traditional bacteria, *Mycoplasma, Legionella,* and *Chlamydia* infections present distinctive pathogenic characteristics, and optimal antimicrobial treatment should combine high levels of drug intrinsic activity with the capability to reach high intracellular concentrations. Table 3 summarizes antibiotic susceptibility of the atypical pathogens.

Specific characteristics of *M. pneumoniae* (such as the absence of a bacterial cell wall) determine the complete inactivity of antibiotics, such as β-lactams, glycopeptides, sulfonamides, and rifampicin. Antibiotic classes that show activity towards *Mycoplasma* include tetracyclines, macrolides, ketolides, lincosamides, streptogramins, chloramphenicol, and fluoroquinolones. Whereas macrolides and tetracyclines are primarily bacteriostatic against *M. pneumoniae,* fluoroquinolones have been shown to possess bactericidal activity.[105,106] Newer fluoroquinolones, such as moxifloxacin, show greater *in vitro* activity compared to older agents, such as ciprofloxacin and ofloxacin.[107]

Newer macrolides are generally preferred over erythromycin due to their greater tolerability; once- or twice-daily dosing requirements, and shorter treatment duration in the case of azithromycin, even though their costs are greater. Erythromycin and tetracyclines are active towards *M. pneumoniae.* Although these agents are effective in abating fever and systemic symptoms associated with *M. pneumoniae* CAP, they do not influence the typical long-lasting, dry, and nonproductive cough that may last for weeks.

Antimicrobial agents that achieve intracellular concentrations higher than the minimal inhibitory concentration (MIC) are more effective than antibiotics with poor intracellular penetration towards *Legionella.*[108] Thus, macrolides, quinolones, tetracyclines, and rifampicin are most likely to be effective. There is debate as to whether rifampin provides additional benefit to patients with *Legionella* infection, and coadministration of this agent is of questionable benefit.[109]

The efficacy of newer and older macrolides has been compared with that of levofloxacin in clinical observational studies of patients with *Legionella* pneumonia.[110-112] Levofloxacin therapy was associated with shorter time to defervescence in two of such studies. Length of hospital stay was significantly shorter for patients treated with levofloxacin in three studies. Although a trend towards lower mortality was observed in levofloxacin-treated patients compared to those receiving a macrolide, it did not reach statistical significance.

A 7–14-day course of therapy is considered sufficient to cure most patients, although clinical judgment is still the best tool to establish the optimal length of treatment. In recent years, mortality for *Legionella* infection has decreased substantially, probably due to increased awareness among physicians, early empirical antimicrobial coverage towards *Legionella,* and the introduction of rapid laboratory tests, such as urinary antigen detection. Specifically, delay in starting appropriate therapy has been associated with increased mortality. Data from a large-scale study observed a decrease in the case-fatality rate for community-acquired *Legionella* pneumonia from 26 to 10% for the period 1980–1998.[113] Similarly, in recent studies of patients who received rapid diagnosis of *Legionella* pneumonia by means of urine antigen testing the reported case-fatality rates varied between 0 and 5.5%.[110,114,115]

TABLE 3

***In vitro* Susceptibility of Atypical Pathogens Towards Commonly Employed Antibiotics**

Drug	*C. pneumoniae*	*M. pneumoniae*	*L. pneumophila*
Tetracycline	0.05–1	0.05–2.0	—
Doxycycline	0.01–0.5	0.06–0.25	0.5–2.0
Minocycline	0.016–0.06	—	0.25–1.0
Erythromycin	0.01–0.5	0.03–0.12	0.06–0.5
Clarithromycin	0.004–0.25	0.004–0.03	0.008–0.03
Azithromycin	0.01–2	0.01–0.02	0.03–0.5
Roxithromycin	0.05–2	0.01–0.02	0.03–0.25
Telithromycin	0.01–2	0.002–0.015	0.015–0.06
Ciprofloxacin	0.25–4	2–4	0.015–0.06
Ofloxacin	0.25–2	0.5–2	0.06–1.0
Levofloxacin	0.125–0.5	0.25–1	0.008–0.03
Moxifloxacin	0.06–0.1	0.06–0.12	0.015–0.06
Gemifloxacin	0.06–0.25	0.05–0.12	0.008–0.03

MIC, minimal inhibitory concentration: ranges of values reported in literature (values are given as range against clinical isolates or against type strains).

Tetracyclines, macrolides, and azalides are active against *C. pneumoniae*. Although older quinolones, such as ofloxacin are not highly active against this agent, the MIC ranges of newer quinolone agents are comparable to macrolide agents.[116,117] Following short or conventional courses of antimicrobials showing activity towards this pathogen, cases of recurrence of symptoms have been described. Persistence of infection following treatment has also been documented by culture. As a consequence, a relatively intensive long-term course of treatment may be advisable.

It is accepted that newer macrolides, such as azithromycin and clarithromycin are at least as effective as doxycycline or erythromycin in the treatment of *C. pneumoniae* respiratory infections.[118] Clarithromycin and azithromycin achieve higher tissue and intracellular concentrations than those found in the bloodstream, have demonstrated *in vitro* efficacy against *C. pneumoniae*, and are better tolerated than erythromycin, with fewer gastrointestinal side effects. These agent may, therefore, be preferable for the treatment of *C. pneumoniae* infections in certain situations.

Atypical bacterial sensitivity to active classes of antibiotics (macrolides, fluoroquinolones, etc.) has traditionally been considered as relatively stable over time, and resistance issues have never posed the threat observed for "typical" pathogens, such as *S. pneumoniae* or *Staphylococcus aureus*. Conversely, in recent years strains of macrolide-resistant *M. pneumoniae* have been identified. The mechanism involved, determines reduced affinity of these agents for ribosomes. In Japan, macrolide-resistant strains have rapidly increased in number over recent years and now may involve 35–40% of *M. pneumoniae* clinical isolates.[121] Resistant strains have also been identified in France,[120] China,[121] and the US.[122] The clinical impact of these finding needs to be closely evaluated in the future, as there are some indications that the presence of resistant strains does associate with treatment failures.

Need for Atypical Coverage in Empirical Treatment of CAP Patients

The precise definition of the true role of atypical bacteria in respiratory infections has been hampered by the difficulties in correctly identifying these agents in the clinical setting. Studies conducted both with traditional techniques (such as serology and culture), and more novel methodologies (such as *Legionella* urinary antigen and molecular biology) are concordant in attributing a remarkable number of acute respiratory tract infections to these pathogens.[123]

It is now well recognized that among CAP patients, distinction of a typical and atypical infection on clinical grounds alone is meaningless, and atypical infections are considered as a group primarily for their lack of clinical response to traditional β-lactam treatment and the need for specific antibiotic classes (macrolides, ketolides, tetracycline, fluoroquinolones, etc.). Given the difficulties in promptly identifying atypical bacteria as the etiologic agents of pneumonia, antibiotic coverage must necessarily be started on empirical grounds alone in most patients. There is considerable variation in current guidelines regarding the indication for atypical antibiotic coverage in patients presenting with CAP. In outpatients, where monotherapy is generally considered sufficient, the North American approach suggests that due to the concomitant presence of atypical pathogens, mostly *M. pneumoniae*, ideal antibiotic treatment in previously healthy patients with no underlying comorbidities, should include a newer macrolide that offers protection both against *S. pneumoniae* and atypical bacteria.[124] Conversely, the European guidelines argue that the true role of atypical pathogens is still debated in patients with mild-to-moderate disease, particularly outside epidemic outbreaks. Given the high levels of macrolide-resistant pneumococci in many countries, the prevailing attitude is that β-lactams, such as penicillin or amoxicillin are still the antibiotics of choice in these patients.[125,126]

At least 3 meta-analyses and 1 Cochrane review of randomized controlled trials comparing monotherapy with atypical coverage (mostly a macrolide or a fluoroquinolone) against monotherapy with no atypical coverage (a β-lactam) in patients with mild-to-moderate CAP have been conducted.[127-130] The fact that these studies found no improvement in clinical outcomes by using antibiotics active against atypical pathogens has been used to demonstrate that β-lactams should remain the antibiotics of choice in non-severe CAP patients.

In hospitalized non-severe CAP patients, the North American guideline suggests that treatment should always include coverage towards atypicals, either with a combination treatment (β-lactam + a macrolide) or monotherapy with a respiratory fluoroquinolone. Conversely, the European guidelines are once again skeptical on the relevance of atypicals in non-severe pneumonia. The evidence that combination treatment or monotherapy with a fluoroquinolone are associated with better outcomes compared to monotherapy with a β-lactam was first suggested by large retrospective and prospective studies,[131-134] totalling over 26,000 patients, one retrospective analysis of prospectively collected data,[135] and 2 prospective trials[136-137] involving just over 3,000 patients. The matter is, however, controversial as other retrospective studies,[138,139] and 2 prospective studies[140,141] provided no evidence of benefits in mortality or length of hospital stay with the addition of atypical coverage to β-lactam monotherapy. In a worldwide study conducted on 4,337 patients with CAP, patients treated with atypical coverage had significantly decreased time to clinical stability, decreased length of stay, decreased total mortality, and decreased CAP-related mortality compared to those with no atypical coverage.[48] It has been suggested that patients that receive combination therapy are probably different *a priori* from those who receive a β-lactam alone, due to physician-related perceptions at the patient bedside. Furthermore, in the above studies, the results (whether positive or negative) were not associated with etiologic demonstration of atypical etiology. It is, therefore, unclear whether potential advantages may be due to coverage towards atypical organisms, or other as yet not fully elucidated effects, such as the immunomodulatory activity of macrolides.[142,143]

European and North American guidelines are concordant regarding the need for combination treatment in patients with severe CAP, with a parenteral cephalosporin plus either a newer macrolide or a respiratory fluoroquinolone as preferred solutions. In this setting, the main concern would be adequate coverage towards *Legionella*, as this agent is among the most common etiologic agents of severe CAP. It is recognized that delay in instituting antibiotic coverage for *Legionella* for more than 24 hours is associated with greater mortality for legionellosis compared to prompt adequate antibiotic treatment.[144]

Decisive information regarding the true need for atypical bacteria coverage in all patients with CAP is needed. This could only be obtained through future trials comparing agents that are active towards atypical agents versus β-lactams in patients with an etiological diagnosis of CAP. The greater availability of diagnostic methods allowing prompt identification of atypical bacteria (such as PCR or urinary antigen test) may render these trials more feasible, although they might be ethically questionable in countries where guidelines suggest routine coverage towards these agents in all patients with CAP (such as the US and Canada). Better standardization of molecular biology techniques and reduced costs may help more diffuse use of PCR both within epidemiological research investigations and "real-life" clinical situations.

CONCLUSION

Atypical bacteria are recognized as an important cause of respiratory tract infections. The primary concern for these agents is their role as a cause of CAP. Both, older studies based mostly on serology, and more recent studies based on newer methodologies, identify these agents cumulatively in over 20% of cases of pneumonia.

Knowledge on the true impact of these bacteria in respiratory tract infections has been hampered by difficulties in their identification through culture and reliance prevalently on serology. Novel microbiological methods now allow prompt identification of these agents although standardization issues regarding molecular biology techniques still need to be addressed.

The need for atypical coverage in the empirical antibiotic treatment of all patients with CAP is still debated. Current major European and North American guidelines diverge substantially on the issue. Among atypical bacteria, *Legionella* infection is certainly associated with greater disease severity and mortality and there is substantial accordance that prompt coverage must be instituted whenever this pathogen is a potential issue.

Antimicrobial resistance within antibiotic classes exerting activity towards atypical bacteria has so far never been a relevant issue. However, recent reports indicate growing numbers of macrolide-resistant *M. pneumoniae* strains. The clinical significance of this phenomenon needs to be further investigated.

Further insights into the genetics determining susceptibility to infection with atypical bacteria, and better knowledge of virulence factors may lead to both novel treatment strategies and vaccine development. Novel virulence factors favoring atypical infection of host cells are being identified. The type III system is a specialized secretion system that translocates bacterial proteins into host cells.[145] Inhibitors of type III secretion proteins are being devised, capable of interfering with intracellular pathogen capacity to thrive within host cells.[146] Should these molecules prove effective, alternative strategies to traditional antibiotic treatment of atypical bacteria may be introduced into clinical practice some day. Alternatively, virulence factor proteins or other immunogenic peptides may be employed as a basis for generating efficient vaccines.[147]

REFERENCES

1. Cunha BA. Atypical pneumonias: current clinical concepts focusing on Legionnaires' disease. *Curr Opin Pulm Med.* 2008;14:183-94.
2. Farr BM, Kaiser DL, Harrison BD, Connolly CK. Prediction of microbial aetiology at admission to hospital for pneumonia from the presenting clinical features. British Thoracic Society Pneumonia Research Subcommittee. *Thorax.* 1989;44:1031-5.
3. Schneeberger PM, Dorigo-Zetsma JW, van der Zee A, van Bon M, van Opstal JL. Diagnosis of atypical pathogens in patients hospitalized with community-acquired respiratory infection. *Scand J Infect Dis.* 2004;36:269-73.

4. Waites KB, Talkington DF. *Mycoplasma pneumoniae* and its role as a human pathogen. *Clin Microbiol Rev.* 2004;17:697-728.
5. Balish, M F, Krause DC. Cytadherence and the cytoskeleton. In: Molecular biology and pathogenicity of mycoplasmas. Razin S, Herrman R, editors. New York, USA: Kluwer Academic/Plenum Publishers; 2002. p. 491-518.
6. Wilson MH, Collier AM. Ultrastructural study of *Mycoplasma pneumoniae* in organ culture. *J Bacteriol.* 1976;125:332-9.
7. Dandekar T, Snel B, Schmidt S, Lathe W, Suyama M, Huynen M, et al. Comparative genome analysis of the mollicutes. In: Molecular biology and pathogenicity of mycoplasmas. Razin S, Herrman R, editors. New York, USA:Kluwer Academic/Plenum Publishers; 2002.p.255-78.
8. Diederen BM. *Legionella* spp. and Legionnaires' disease. *J Infect.* 2008;56:1-12.
9. Stout JE, Yu VL, Yee YC, Vaccarello S, Diven W, Lee TC. *Legionella pneumophila* in residential water supplies: environmental surveillance with clinical assessment for Legionnaires' disease. *Epidemiol Infect.* 1992;109:49-57.
10. Molofsky AB, Swanson MS. Differentiate to thrive: lessons from the *Legionella pneumophila* life cycle. *Mol Microbiol.* 2004;53:29-40.
11. Fraser DW, Tsai TR, Orenstein W, Parkin WE, Beecham HJ, Sharrar RG, et al. Legionnaries' disease: description of an epidemic of pneumonia. *N Engl J Med.* 1977;297:1189-97.
12. Fields BS, Benson RF, Besser RE. *Legionella* and Legionnaires' disease: 25 years of investigation. *Clin Microbiol Rev.* 2002;15:506–26.
13. Stout JE, Yu VL. Legionellosis. *N Engl J Med.* 1997;337:682-7.
14. Hogan RJ, Mathews SA, Mukhopadhyay S, Summersgill JT, Timms P. Chlamydial persistence: beyond the biphasic paradigm. *Infect Immun.* 2004;72:1843-55.
15. Campbell LA, Kuo CC. *Chlamydia pneumoniae* - an infectious risk factor for atherosclerosis? *Nat Rev Microbiol.* 2004;2:23-32.
16. Byrne GI. *Chlamydia* uncloaked. *Proc Natl Acad Sci USA.* 2003;100:8040-2.
17. Belland RJ, Ouellette SP, Gieffers J, Byrne GI. *Chlamydia pneumoniae* and atherosclerosis. *Cell Microbiol.* 2004; 6:117-27.
18. Everett KD, Bush RM, Andersen AA. Emended description of the order Chlamydiales, proposal of Parachlamydiaceae fam. nov. and Simkaniaceae fam. nov., each containing one monotypic genus, revised taxonomy of the family Chlamydiaceae, including a new genus and five new species, and standards for the identification of organisms. *Int J Syst Bacteriol.* 1999;49:415-40.
19. Blasi F, Tarsia P, Aliberti S. *Chlamydophila pneumoniae. Clin Microbiol Infect.* 2009;15:29-35.
20. Woodhead M. Community-acquired pneumonia guidelines – an international comparison: a view from Europe. *Chest.* 1998;113:183S-187S.
21. Niederman MS, Mandell LA, Anzueto A, Bass JB, Broughton WA, Campbell GD, et al; American Thoracic Society.. Guidelines for the management of adults with community-acquired pneumonia. Diagnosis, assessment of severity, antimicrobial therapy, and prevention. *Am J Respir Crit Care Med.* 2001;163:1730-54.
22. Macfarlane J, Holmes W, Gard P, Macfarlane R, Rose D, Weston V, et al. Prospective study of the incidence, aetiology, and outcome of adult lower respiratory tract illness in the community. *Thorax.* 2001;56:109-14.
23. Oosterheert JJ, van Loon AM, Schuurman R, Hoepelman AI, Hak E, Thijsen S, et al. Impact of rapid detection of viral and atypical bacterial pathogens by real-time polymerase chain reaction for patients with lower respiratory tract infection. *Clin Infect Dis.* 2005;41:1438-44.
24. Stralin K, Backman A, Holmberg H, Fredlund H, Olcen P. Design of a multiplex PCR for *Streptococcus pneumoniae, Haemophilus influenzae, Mycoplasma pneumoniae,* and *Chlamydophila pneumoniae* to be used on sputum samples. *APMIS.* 2005;113:99-111.
25. Marrie TJ, Poulin-Costello M, Beecroft MD. Herman-Gnjidic Z. Etiology of community-acquired pneumonia treated in an ambulatory setting. *Resp Med.* 2005;99:60-5.
26. Saito A, Kohno S, Matsushima T, Watanabe A, Oizumi K, Yamaguchi K, et al. Prospective multicenter study of the causative organisms of community acquired pneumonia in adults in Japan. *J Infect Chemother.* 2006;12:63-9.
27. Wellinghausen N, Straube E, Freidank H, Baum HV, Marre R, Essig A. Low prevalence of *Chlamydia pneumoniae* in adults with community-acquired pneumonia. *Int J Med Microbiol.* 2006;296:485-91.
28. Charles PG, Whitby M, Fuller AJ, Stirling R, Wright AA, Korman TM, et al.; Australian CAP Study Collaboration. Australian CAP Study Collaboration. The etiology of community-acquired pneumonia in Australia: why penicillin plus doxycycline or a macrolide is the most appropriate therapy. *Clin Infect Dis.* 2008;46:1513-21.
29. Almirall J, Bolíbar I, Serra-Prat M, Roig J, Hospital I, Carandell E, Agustí M, et al.; Community-Acquired Pneumonia in Catalan Countries (PACAP) Study Group. Community-Acquired Pneumonia in Catalan Countries (PACAP) Study Group. New evidence of risk factors for community-acquired pneumonia: a population-based study. *Eur Respir J.* 2008;31:1274-84.
30. Jennings LC, Anderson TP, Beynon KA, Chua A, Laing RT, Werno AM, et al. Incidence and characteristics of viral community-acquired pneumonia in adults. *Thorax.* 2008;63:658-9.
31. Johnstone J, Majumdar SR, Fox JD, Marrie J. Viral infection in adults hospitalized with community acquired pneumonia: prevalence, pathogens and presentation. *Chest.* 2008;134:1141-8.
32. Song JH, Oh WS, Kang CI, Chung DR, Peck KR, Ko KS, et al; Asian Network for Surveillance of Resistant Pathogens Study Group. Asian Network for Surveillance of Resistant Pathogens Study Group. Epidemiology and clinical outcomes of communityacquired pneumonia in adult patients in Asian countries: a prospective study by the Asian network for surveillance of resistant pathogens. *Int J Antimicrob Agents.* 2008;31:107-14.
33. Lui G, Ip M, Lee N, Rainer TH, Man SY, Cockram CS, et al. Role of 'atypical pathogens' among adult hospitalized patients with community-acquired pneumonia. *Respirology.* 2009;14:1098-105.
34. Johansson N, Kalin M, Tiveljung-Lindell A, Giske CG, Hedlund J. Etiology of community-acquired pneumonia:

increased microbiological yield with new diagnostic methods. *Clin Infect Dis.* 2010;50:202-9 .

35. Roig J, Domingo C, Morera J. Legionnaires' Disease. *Chest.* 1994;105:1817-25.
36. Juvén T, Mertsola J, Waris M, Leinonen M, Meurman O, Roivainen M, et al. Etiology of community-acquired pneumonia in 254 hospitalized children. *Pediatr Infect Dis J.* 2000;19:293-8.
37. Principi N, Esposito S, Blasi F, Allegra L, Mowgli Study Group. Role of *Mycoplasma pneumoniae* and *Chlamydia pneumoniae* in children with community-acquired lower respiratory tract infections. *Clin Infect Dis.* 2001;32:1281-9.
38. Baer G, Engelcke G, Abele-Horn M, Schaad UB, Heininger U. Role of *Chlamydia pneumoniae* and *Mycoplasma pneumoniae* as causative agents of community-acquired pneumonia in hospitalised children and adolescents. *Eur J Clin Microbiol Infect Dis.* 2003;22:742-5.
39. Likitnukul S, Nunthapisud P, Prapphal N. Prevalence of *Chlamydia pneumoniae* infection in Thai children with community-acquired pneumonia. *Pediatr Infect Dis J.* 2003;22:749-50.
40. Korppi M, Heiskanen-Kosma T, Kleemola M. Incidence of community-acquired pneumonia in children caused by *Mycoplasma pneumoniae*: serological results of a prospective, population-based study in primary health care. *Respirology.* 2004;9:109-14.
41. Michelow IC, Olsen K, Lozano J, Rollins NK, Duffy LB, Ziegler T, et al. Epidemiology and clinical characteristics of community-acquired pneumonia in hospitalized children. *Pediatrics.* 2004;113:701-7.
42. Tsolia MN, Psarras S, Bossios A, Audi H, Paldanius M, Gourgiotis D, et al. Etiology of community-acquired pneumonia in hospitalized school-age children: evidence for high prevalence of viral infections. *Clin Infect Dis.* 2004;39:681-6.
43. Liu G, Talkington DF, Fields BS, Levine OS, Yang Y, Tondella ML. *Chlamydia pneumoniae* and *Mycoplasma pneumoniae* in young children from China with community-acquired pneumonia. *Diagn Microbiol Infect Dis.* 2005;52:7-14.
44. Somer A, Salman N, Yalc¸in I, Agacfidan A. Role of *Mycoplasma pneumoniae* and *Chlamydia pneumoniae* in children with community-acquired pneumonia in Istanbul, Turkey. *J Trop Pediatr.* 2006;52:173-8.
45. Kurz H, Göpfrich H, Wabnegger L, Apfalter P. Role of *Chlamydophila pneumoniae* in children hospitalized for community-acquired pneumonia in Vienna, Austria. *Pediatr Pulmonol.* 2009;44:873-6.
46. Carrillo JA, Gutiérrez J, García F, Muñoz A, Villegas E, Rojas J, et al. Clin Development and evaluation of a multiplex test for the detection of atypical bacterial DNA in community-acquired pneumonia during childhood. *Microbiol Infect.* 2009:15:473-80.
47. Hamano-Hasegawa K, Morozumi M, Nakayama E, Chiba N, Murayama SY, Takayanagi R , et al; Acute Respiratory Diseases Study Group. Comprehensive detection of causative pathogens using real-time PCR to diagnose pediatric community-acquired pneumonia. *J Infect Chemother.* 2008;14:424-32.
48. Arnold FW, Summersgill JT, Lajoie AS, Peyrani P, Marrie TJ, Rossi P, et al. A worldwide perspective of atypical pathogens in community-acquired pneumonia. *Am J Respir Crit Care Med.* 2007;175:1086-93.
49. von Baum H, Welte T, Marre R, Suttorp N, Lück C, Ewig S. *Mycoplasma pneumoniae* pneumonia revisited within the German Competence Network for Community-acquired pneumonia (CAPNETZ). *BMC Infect Dis.* 2009;9:62.
50. von Baum H, Ewig S, Marre R, Suttorp N, Gonschior S, Welte T, et al; Competence Network for Community Acquired Pneumonia Study Group. Community-acquired *Legionella* pneumonia: new insights from the German Competence Network for Community Acquired Pneumonia. *Clin Infect Dis.* 2008;46:1356-64.
51. Foy HM, Kenny GE, McMahan R, Mansy AM, Grayston JT. *Mycoplasma pneumoniae* pneumonia in an urban area. *JAMA.* 1970;214:1666-72.
52. Ruiz M, Ewig S, Marcos MA, Martinez JA, Arancibia F, Mensa J, et al. Etiology of community-acquired pneumonia: impact of age, comorbidity, and severity. *Am J Respir Crit Care Med.* 1999;160:397-405.
53. Weigl JA, Puppe W, Meyer CU, Berner R, Forster J, Schmitt HJ, et al. Ten years' experience with year-round active surveillance of up to 19 respiratory pathogens in children. *Eur J Pediatr.* 2007;166:957-66.
54. Murray HW, Masur H, Senterfit LB, Roberts RB. The protean manifestations of *Mycoplasma pneumoniae* infections in adults. *Am J Med.* 1975;58:229-42.
55. Foy HM, Kenny GE, Cooney MK, Allan ID. Long-term epidemiology of infections with *Mycoplasma pneumoniae. J Infect Dis.* 1979;214:1666-72.
56. Levine DP, Lerner AM. The clinical spectrum of *Mycoplasma pneumoniae* infections. *Med Clin North Am.* 1978;62:961-78.
57. Rollins S, Colby T, Clayton F. Open lung biopsy in *Mycoplasma pneumoniae* pneumonia. *Arch Pathol Lab.* 1986;110:34-41.
58. Yu VL, Kroboth FJ, Shonnard J, Brown A, McDearman S, Magnussen M. Legionnaires' disease: new clinical perspectives from a prospective pneumonia study. *Am J Med.* 1982;73:357-61.
59. Masiá M, Gutiérrez F, Padilla S, Soldán B, Mirete C, Shum C, et al. Clinical characterisation of pneumonia caused by atypical pathogens combining classic and novel predictors. *Clin Microbiol Infect.* 2007;13:153-61.
60. Cunha BA. Hypophosphatemia: diagnostic significance in Legionnaires' disease. *Am J Med.* 2006;119:5-6.
61. Grayston JT. *Chlamydia pneumoniae* strain TWAR. *Chest.* 1989;95:664-9.
62. Grayston JT, Campbell LA, Kuo CC, Mordhorst CH, Saikku P, Thom DH, et al. A new respiratory tract pathogen: *Chlamydia pneumoniae* strain TWAR. *J Infect Dis.* 1990; 161:618-25.
63. Hammerschlag MR. *Chlamydia pneumoniae* and the lung. *Eur Respir J.* 2000;16:1001-7.
64. Marrie TJ, Peeling RW, Reid T, De Carolis E; Canadian Community-Acquired Pneumonia Investigators. *Chlamydia* species as a cause of community-acquired pneumonia in Canada. *Eur Respir J.* 2003;21:779-84.
65. Masia M, Gutierrez F, Shum C, Padilla S, Navarro JC, Flores E, et al. Usefulness of procalcitonin levels in community-acquired pneumonia according to the patients outcome

research team pneumonia severity index. *Chest.* 2005;128:2223-9.
66. Hedlund J, Hansson LO. Procalcitonin and C-reactive protein levels in community-acquired pneumonia: correlation with etiology and prognosis. *Infection.* 2000; 28:68-73.
67. Krüger S, Ewig S, Papassotiriou J, Kunde J, Marre R, von Baum H, et al. Inflammatory parameters predict etiologic patterns but do not allow for individual prediction of etiology in patients with CAP - Results from the German competence network CAPNETZ. *Respiratory Research.* 2009;10:65.
68. Cillóniz C, Ewig S, Polverino E, Marcos MA, Esquinas C, Gabarrús A, et al. Microbial aetiology of community-acquired pneumonia and its relation to severity. *Thorax.* 2011;66:340-6.
69. Menendez R, Sahuquillo-Acre JM, Reyes S, Martinez R, Polverino E, Cilloniz C, et al. Cytokine activation patterns and biomarkers are influenced by microrganisms in community-acquired pneumonia. *Chest.* Prepublished online December 2011; DOI 10.1378/chest.11-1446.
70. Blairon L, Wittebole X, Laterre PF. Lipopolysaccharide-binding protein serum levels in patients with severe sepsis due to gram-positive and fungal infections. *J Infect Dis.* 2003;187:287-91.
71. Masia M, Gutierrez F, Llorca B, Navarro JC, Mirete C, Padilla S, et al. Serum concentrations of Lipopolysaccharide-Binding Protein as a biochemical marker to differentiate microbial etiology in patients with community-acquired pneumonia. *Clin Chem.* 2004;50:1661-4.
72. Zobel K, Martus P, Pletz MW, Ewig S, Prediger M, Welte T, et al.; CAPNETZ study group. Interleukin 6, lipopolysaccharide-binding protein and interleukin 10 in the prediction of risk and etiologic patterns in patients with community-acquired pneumonia: results from the German competence network CAPNETZ. *BMC Pulmonary Medicine.* 2012;12:6.
73. Gibot S, Le Renard PE, Bollaert PE, Kolopp-Sarda MN, Béné MC, Faure GC, et al. Surface triggering receptor expressed on myeloid cells 1 expressed patterns in septic shock. *Intensive Care Med.* 2005;31:594-7.
74. How CK, Hou SK, Shih HC, Yen DH, Huang CI, Lee CH, et al. Usefulness of triggering receptor expressed on myeloid cells-1 in differentiating between typical and atypical community-acquired pneumonia. *Am J Emerg Med.* 2011;29:626-31.
75. Skelly M, Hoffman J, Fabbri M, Holzman RS, Clarkson AB Jr, Merali S. S-Adenosylmethionine concentrations in diagnosis of *Pneumocystis carinii* pneumonia. *Lancet.* 2003;361:1267-8.
76. Taylor-Robinson D. Infections due to species of *Mycoplasma* and *Ureaplasma*: an update. *Clin Infect Dis.* 1996;23:671-84.
77. Murdoch DR. Diagnosis of *Legionella* infection. *Clin Infect Dis.* 2003;36:64-9.
78. Den Boer JW, Yzerman EPF. Diagnosis of *Legionella* infection in Legionnaires' disease. *Eur J Clin Microbiol Infect Dis.* 2004;23:871-8.
79. Ramsey KM, deShazo RD. *Chlamydia pneumoniae*: new diagnostic tools for the detection of a common pathogen. *Chest.* 1996;110:593-4.
80. Bartlett JG, Dowell SF, Mandell LA, File Jr TM, Musher DM, Fine MJ. Practice guidelines for the management of community-acquired pneumonia in adults. *Clin Infect Dis.* 2000;31:347-82.
81. Skerrett SJ. Diagnostic testing for community-acquired pneumonia. *Clin Chest Med.* 1999;20:531-48.
82. Smith TF. *Mycoplasma pneumoniae* infection: diagnosis based on immunofluorescence titre of IgG and IgM antibodies. *Mayo Clin Proc.* 1986;61:830-1.
83. Monforte R, Estruch R, Vidal J, Cervera R, Urbano-Marquez A. Delayed seroconversion in Legionnaire's disease. *Lancet.* 1988;2:513.
84. Dowell SF, Peeling RW, Boman J, Carlone GM, Fields BS, Guarner J, et al.; C. pneumoniae Workshop Participants. Standardizing *Chlamydia pneumoniae* assays: recommendations from the Centers for Disease Control and Prevention (USA) and the Laboratory Centre for Disease Control (Canada). *Clin Infect Dis.* 2001;33:492-503.
85. Kutlin A, Tsumura N, Emre U, Roblin PM, Hammerschlag MR. Evaluation of *Chlamydia* immunoglobulin M (IgM), IgG, and IgA rELISAs Medac for diagnosis of *Chlamydia pneumoniae* infection. *Clin Diag Lab Immunol.* 1997;4: 213-6.
86. Tompkins LS, Schachter J, Boman J, Chernesky MA, Dowell S, Gaydos CA, et al. Collaborative multidisciplinary workshop report: detection, culture, serology, and antimicrobial susceptibility testing of *Chlamydia pneumoniae.* *J Infect Dis.* 2000;181: S460-1.
87. Miyashita N, Ouchi K, Kishi F, Tabuchi M, Tsumura N, Bannai H, et al. Rapid and simple diagnosis of *Chlamydophila pneumoniae* pneumonia by an immunochromatographic test for detection of immunoglobulin M antibodies. *Clin Vaccine Immunol.* 2008;15:1128-31.
88. Domínguez JA, Galí N, Pedroso P, Fargas A, Padilla E, Manterola JM, et al. Comparison of the Binax *Legionella* urinary antigen enzyme immunoassay (EIA) with the Biotest *Legionella* urine antigen EIA for detection of *Legionella* antigen in both concentrated and nonconcentrated urine samples. *J Clin Microbiol.* 1998;36:2718-22.
89. Shimada T, Noguchi Y, Jackson JL, Miyashita J, Hayashino Y, Kamiya T, et al. Systematic review and meta-analysis: urinary antigen tests for legionellosis. *Chest.* 2009;136: 1576-85.
90. Kohorst WR, Schonefeld SA, Macklin JE, Whitcombe ME. Rapid diagnosis of Legionnaire's disease by bronchoalveolar lavage. *Chest.* 1983;84:186-90
91. Kleemola M, Jokinen C. Outbreak of *Mycoplasma pneumoniae* infection among hospital personnel studied by a nucleic acid hybridisation test. *J Hosp Infect.* 1992; 21:213-21.
92. Kai M, Kamiya S, Yabe H, Takakura I, Shiozawa K, Ozawa A. Rapid detection of *Mycoplasma pneumoniae* in clinical samples by the polymerase chain reaction. *J Med Microbiol.* 1993;38:166-70.
93. van Kuppeveld FJ, Johansson KE, Galama JM, Kissing J, Bölske G, Hjelm E, et al. 16S rRNA based polymerase chain reaction compared with culture and serological methods for diagnosis of *Mycoplasma pneumoniae* infection. *Eur J Clin Microbiol Infect Dis.* 1994;13:401-5.
94. Saito R, Misawa Y, Moriya K, Koike K, Ubukata K, Okamura N. Development and evaluation of a loop-mediated isothermal amplification assay for rapid

detection of *Mycoplasma pneumoniae. J Med Microbiol.* 2005;54:1037-41.

95. Waites KB, Balish MF, Atkinson TP. New insights into the pathogenesis and detection of *Mycoplasma pneumoniae* infections. *Future Microbiol.* 2008;3:635-48.
96. Ginevra C, Lopez M, Forey F, Reyrolle M, Meugnier H, Vandenesch F, et al. Evaluation of a nested-PCR-derived sequence-based typing method applied directly to respiratory samples for patients with Legionnaires' disease. *J Clin Microbiol.* 2009;47:981-7.
97. Maurin M, Hammer L, Gestin B, Timsit JF, Rogeaux O, Delavena F, et al. Quantitative real-time PCR tests for diagnosis and prognostic purposes in cases of legionellosis. *Clin Microbiol Infect.* 2010;16:379-84.
98. Yang G, Benson R, Pelish T, Brown E, Winchell JM, Fields B. Dual detection of *Legionella pneumophila* and *Legionella* species by real-time PCR targeting the 23S-5S rRNA gene spacer region. *Clin Microbiol Infect.* 2010;16:255-61.
99. Kumar S, Hammerschlag MR. Acute respiratory infection due to *Chlamydia pneumoniae*: current status of diagnostic methods. *Clin Infect Dis.* 2007;44:568-76.
100. Apfalter P, Reischl U, Hammerschlag MR. In-house nucleic acid amplification assays in research: how much quality control is needed before one can rely upon the results? *J Clin Microbiol.* 2005;43:5835-41.
101. Tang YW, Sriram S, Li H, Yao SY, Meng S, Mitchell WM, et al. Qualitative and quantitative detection of *Chlamydophila pneumonia* DNA in cerebrospinal fluid from multiple sclerosis patients and controls. *PloS One.* 2009;4:e5200.
102. Welti M, Jaton K, Altwegg M, Sahli R, Wenger A, Bille J. Development of a multiplex real-time quantitative PCR assay to detect *Chlamydia pneumoniae, Legionella pneumophila* and *Mycoplasma pneumoniae* in respiratory tract secretions. *Diagn Microbiol Infect Dis.* 2003;45:85-95.
103. Loens K, Beck T, Ursi D, Overdijk M, Sillekens P, Goossens H, et al. Development of real-time multiplex nucleic acid sequence-based amplification for detection of *Mycoplasma pneumoniae, Chlamydophila pneumoniae,* and Legionella spp. in respiratory specimens. *J Clin Microbiol.* 2008;46:185-91.
104. Swati Kumar, Lihua Wang, Jiang Fan, Andrea Kraft, Michael E. Bose, Sagarika Tiwari, et al. Detection of 11 common viral and bacterial pathogens causing community-acquired pneumonia or sepsis in asymptomatic patients by using a multiplex reverse transcription-PCR assay with manual (enzyme hybridization) or automated (electronic microarray) detection. *J Clin Microbiol.* 2008;46:3063-72.
105. Bebear CM, Renaudin H, Schaeverbeke T, LeBlanc F, Bebear C. Comparative activities of telithromycin (HMR 3647), levofloxacin and other antimicrobial agents against human mycoplasmas. *Antimicrob Agents Chemother.* 2000;47:1980-2.
106. Waites KB, Crabb DM, Duffy LB. Inhibitory and bactericidal activities of gemifloxacin and other antimicrobials against *Mycoplasma pneumoniae. Int J Antimicrob Agents.* 2003; 21:574-7.
107. Waites KB, Crabb DM, Duffy LB. In vitro activities of ABT-773 and other antimicrobials against human mycoplasmas. *Antimicrob. Agents Chemother.* 2003;47:39-42.
108. Roig J, Rello J. Legionnaires' disease: a rational approach to therapy. *J Antimicrob Chemother.* 2003;51:1119-29.
109. Grau S, Antonio JM, Ribes E, Salvado M, Garces JM, Garau J. Impact of rifampicin addition to clarithromycin in *Legionella pneumophila* pneumonia. *Int. J. Antimicrob. Agents.* 2006;28: 249-52.
110. Mykietiuk A, Carratalà J, Fernández-Sabé N, Dorca J, Verdaguer R, Manresa F, et al. Clinical outcomes for hospitalized patients with Legionella pneumonia in the antigenuria era: the influence of levofloxacin therapy. *Clin Infect Dis.* 2005;40:794-9.
111. Sabrià M, Pedro-Botet ML, Gómez J, Roig J, Vilaseca B, Sopena N, et al.; Legionnaires Disease Therapy Group. LD Therapy Group. Fluoroquinolones vs macrolides in the treatment of Legionnaires' disease. *Chest.* 2005;128:1401-5.
112. Blázquez Garrido RM, Espinosa Parra FJ, Alemany Francés L, Ramos Guevara RM, Sánchez-Nieto JM, Segovia Hernández M, et al. Antimicrobial chemotherapy for legionnaires' disease: levofloxacin versus macrolides. *Clin Infect Dis.* 2005;40:800-6.
113. Benin AL, Benson RF, Besser RE. Trends in Legionnaires' disease, 1980-1998: declining mortality and new patterns of diagnosis. *Clin Infect Dis.* 2002;35:1039-46.
114. Plouffe JF, Breiman RF, Fields BS, Herbert M, Inverso J, Knirsch C, et al. Azithromycin in the treatment of *Legionella* pneumonia requiring hospitalization. *Clin Infect Dis.* 2003;37:1475-80.
115. Yu VL, Greenberg RN, Zadeikis N, Stout JE, Khashab MM, Olson WH, et al. Levofloxacin efficacy in the treatment of community-acquired Legionellosis. *Chest.* 2004;125: 2135-9.
116. Hammerschlag MR. Activity of gemifloxacin and other new quinolones against *Chlamydia pneumoniae*: a review. *J Antimicrobial Chemotherapy.*2000;45:35-9.
117. Roblin PM, Kutlin A, Reznik T, Hammerschlag MR. Activity of grepafloxacin and other fluoroquinolones and new macrolides against recent clinical isolates of *Chlamydia pneumoniae. Int J Antimicrob Agents.* 1999;12;181-4.
118. Kuo CC, Jackson LA, Lee A, Grayston JT. In vitro activities of azithromycin, clarithromycin, and other antibiotics against *Chlamydia pneumoniae. Antimicrob Agents Chemother.* 1996;40:2669-70.
119. Morozumi M, Iwata S, Hasegawa K, Chiba N, Takayanagi R, Matsubara K, et al.; Acute Respiratory Diseases Study Group. Increased macrolide resistance of *Mycoplasma pneumoniae* in pediatric patients with community-acquired pneumonia. *Antimicrob Agents Chemother.* 2008;52:348-50.
120. Pereyre S, Charron A, Renaudin H, Bébéar C, Bébéar CM. First report of macrolide-resistant strains and description of a novel nucleotide sequence variation in the P1 adhesin gene in *Mycoplasma pneumoniae* clinical strains isolated in France over 12 years. *J Clin Microbiol.* 2007;45:3534-9.
121. Xin D, Mi Z, Han X, Qin L, Li J, Wei T, et al. Molecular mechanisms of macrolide resistance in clinical isolates of *Mycoplasma pneumoniae* from China. *Antimicrob. Agents. Chemother.* 2009;53:2158-9.
122. Wolff BJ, Thacker WL, Schwartz SB, Winchell JM. Detection of macrolide resistance in *Mycoplasma pneumoniae* by real-time PCR and high-resolution melt analysis. *Antimicrob Agents Chemother.* 2008;52:3542-9.
123. Blasi F. Atypical pathogens and respiratory tract infections. *Eur Respir J.* 2004;24:171-81.

124. Mandell LA, Wunderink RG, Anzueto A, Bartlett JG, Campbell GD, Dean NC, et al.; Infectious Diseases Society of America; American Thoracic Society. Infectious Diseases Society of America/American Thoracic Society Consensus guidelines on the management of community-acquired pneumonia in adults. *Clin Infect Dis.* 2007;44: S27-S72.
125. Woodhead M, Blasi F, Ewig S, Huchon G, Ieven M, Ortqvist A, et al.; European Respiratory Society; European Society of Clinical Microbiology and Infectious Diseases. Guidelines for the management of adult lower respiratory tract infections. *Eur Respir J.* 2005;26:1138-80.
126. Woodhead M, Blasi F, Ewig S, Garau J, Huchon G, Ieven M, et al.; Joint Taskforce of the European Respiratory Society and European Society for Clinical Microbiology and Infectious Diseases. Guidelines for the management of adult lower respiratory tract infections. *Clin Microbiol Infect.* 2011;17:E1-59.
127. Mills GD, Oehley MR, Arrol B. Effectiveness of β-lactam antibiotics compared with antibiotics active against atypical pathogens in non-severe community acquired pneumonia: meta-analysis. *BMJ.* 2005;doi:10.1136/bmj.38334.591586.82.
128. Shefet D, Robenshtok E, Paul M, Leibovici L. Empirical atypical coverage for inpatients with community-acquired pneumonia. Systematic review of randomized controlled trails. *Arch Intern Med.* 2005;165:1992-2000.
129. Robenshtok E, Shefet D, Gafter-Gvili A, Paul M, Vidal L, Leibovici L. Empiric antibiotic coverage of atypical pathogens for community acquired pneumonia in hospitalized adults. *Cochrane Database Syst Rev.* 2008;(1):CD004418.
130. Maimon N, Nopmaneejumruslers C, Marras TK. Antibacterial class not obviously important in outpatient pneumonia: a meta-analysis. *Eur Respir J.* 2008;31:1068-76.
131. Gleason PP, Meehan TP, Fine JM, Galusha DH, Fine MJ. Associations between initial antimicrobial therapy and medical outcomes for hospitalized elderly patients with pneumonia. *Arch Intern Med.* 1999;159:2562-72.
132. Houck PM, MacLehose RF, Niederman MS, Lowery JK. Empiric antibiotic therapy and mortality among Medicare pneumonia inpatients in 10 western states: 1993, 1995, and 1997. *Chest.* 2001;119:1420-6.
133. Brown RB, Iannini P, Gross P, Kunkel M. Impact of initial antibiotic choice on clinical outcomes in community-acquired pneumonia: analysis of a hospital claims-made database. *Chest.* 2003;123:1503-11.
134. Metersky ML, Ma A, Houck PM, Bratzler DW. Antibiotics for bacteremic pneumonia: improved outcomes with macrolides but not fluoroquinolones. *Chest.* 2007;131: 466-73.
135. García Vázquez E, Mensa J, Martínez JA, Marcos MA, Puig J, Ortega M, et al. Lower mortality among patients with community-acquired pneumonia treated with a macrolide plus a β-lactam agent versus a β-lactam agent alone. *Eur J Clin Microbiol Infect Dis.* 2005;24:190-5.
136. Dudas V, Hoepfl A, Jacobs R, Guglielmo JB. Antimicrobial selection for hospitalized patients with presumed community-acquired pneumonia: a survey of non-teaching US Community Hospitals. *Ann Pharmacother.* 2000;34:446-52.
137. Stahl JE, Barza M, DesJardin J, Martin R, Eckman MH. Effect of macrolides as part of initial empiric therapy on length of stay in patients hospitalized with community-acquired pneumonia. *Arch Intern Med.* 1999;159: 2576-80.
138. Burgess DS, Lewis JS. Effect of macrolides as part of initial empiric therapy on medical outcomes for hospitalized patients with community-acquired pneumonia. *Clin Ther.* 2000;22:872-8.
139. Frei CR, Koeller JM, Burgess DS, Talbert RL, Johnsrud MT. Impact of atypical coverage for patients with community-acquired pneumonia managed on the medical ward: results from the United States Community-Acquired Pneumonia Project. *Pharmacotherapy.* 2003;23:1167-74.
140. Aspa J, Rajas O, Rodriguez de Castro F, Huertas MC, Borderías L, Cabello FJ, et al.; Pneumococcal Pneumonia in Spain Study Group. Impact of initial antibiotic choice on mortality from pneumococcal pneumonia. *Eur Respir J.* 2006;27:1010-9.
141. Loh LC, Quah SY, Khoo SK, Vijayasingham P, Thayaparan T. Addition of macrolide in treating adult hospitalized community-acquired pneumonia. *Respirology.* 2005;10: 371-7.
142. Tamaoki J, The effects of macrolides on inflammatory cells. *Chest.* 2004;125:41S-50S.
143. Rubin B. Immunomodulatory properties of macrolides: overview and historical perspective. *Am J Med.* 2004;117: 2S-4S.
144. Lettinga KD, Verbon A, Weverling GJ, Schellekens JF, Den Boer JW, Yzerman EP, et al. Legionnaires' disease at a Dutch flower show: prognostic factors and impact of therapy. *Emerg Infect Dis.* 2002;8:1448-54.
145. Byrne GI. *Chlamydia trachomatis* strains and virulence: rethinking links to infection prevalence and disease severity. J Infect Dis. 2010;201:126-33.
146. Johnson DL, Stone CB, Bulir DC, Coombes BK, Mahony JB. A novel inhibitor of *Chlamydophila pneumoniae* protein kinase D (PknD) inhibits phosphorylation of CdsD and suppresses bacterial replication. *BMC Microbiol.* 2009;9:218.
147. Heur D, Kneip C, Mäurer AP, Meyer TF. Tackling the intractable - Approaching the genetics of *Chlamydiales*. *Int J Med Microbiol.* 2007;297:569-76.

CHAPTER 5

Healthcare-associated Pneumonia

Muthiah P Muthiah, M Jawad Habib, Ali E Solh

ABSTRACT

Healthcare-associated pneumonia (HCAP) is a relatively new description, occurring in patients who have had recent exposure to the healthcare environment and differs from hospital-acquired pneumonia (HAP), HAP occurs in patients who are currently hospitalized; HCAP is potentially caused by multidrug-resistant pathogens, resulting in increase in length of hospital stay, healthcare cost, as well as loss of lives. These infections are predominantly caused by methicillin-ressitant *Staphylococcus aureus* and *Pseudomonas aeruginosa*, but other organisms can be involved as well. Further research is needed to characterize the distinctions including diagnostic and therapeutic and possible preventive approaches that will improve outcomes. This is especially important, given the rapidly increasing number of people living in nursing homes and other long-term care facilities.

INTRODUCTION

Healthcare-associated pneumonia (HCAP) is a relatively new description, occurring in patients who have had recent exposure to the healthcare environment. HCAP differs from hospital-acquired pneumonia (HAP), in that HAP occurs in patients who are currently hospitalized; HCAP is potentially caused by multidrug-resistant (MDR) pathogens, resulting in increase in length of hospital stay, healthcare cost, as well as loss of lives.

Healthcare-associated pneumonia is a relatively new definition, and there is an insufficient body of literature to suggest evidence-based recommendations, and research in this area is ongoing.

DEFINITION

Healthcare-associated pneumonia refers to pneumonia that develops in patients who have ongoing or prior contact with the healthcare environment. HCAP potentially involves MDR pathogens, inherent to the healthcare environment, resulting in increased morbidity and mortality, as well as a further increase in healthcare expenditure. HCAP includes any patient who was hospitalized in an acute care hospital for 2 or more days within 90 days of the infection; resided in a nursing home or long-term care facility; received recent intravenous antibiotic therapy, chemotherapy, or wound care or attended a hospital or hemodialysis clinic within the past 30 days of the current infection. Box 1 depicts the risk factors MDR pathogens, including risk factors for developing HCAP.[1] There is significant overlap between HCAP, ventilator-associated pneumonia (VAP), and HAP in terms of risk factors, etiologic agents, as well as outcomes.

Figure 1 shows the relationship between community-acquired pneumonia (CAP), HAP, HCAP, and VAP.

The HCAP summit provided further clarity into the definition and laid the ground work for future work to come.[2]

BOX 1

Risk factors for multidrug-resistant pathogens causing healthcare-assiciated pneumonia[1]

- Antimicrobial therapy in preceding 90 days
- Current hospitalization of 5 days or more
- Presence of risk factors for HCAP:
  - Hospitalization for 2 days or more in the preceding 90 days
  - Residence in a nursing home or extended care facility
  - Home infusion therapy (including antibiotics)
  - Chronic dialysis within 30 days
  - Home wound care
  - Family member with multidrug-resistant pathogen
- Immunosuppressive disease and/or therapy

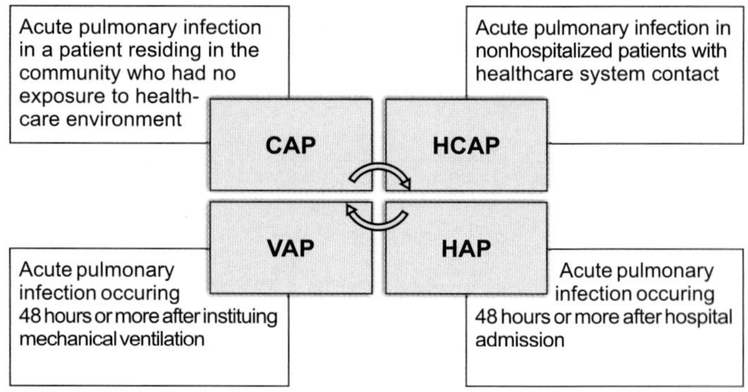

FIGURE 1 Relationship of community-acquired pneumonia, healthcare-assiciated pneumonia, hospital-acquired pneumonia, and ventilator-associated pneumonia.

It is clear, that VAP, HAP, and HCAP occur in similar populations, have higher mortality than CAP, and can be potentially caused by MDR pathogens. VAP obviously happens in intubated patients. It is designated as HAP, when diagnosed 48 hours after hospitalization and is termed HCAP when it occurs in patients with the above risk factors, in those who have had recent contact with the healthcare system, in one of many ways. It is because of their frequent contact with the healthcare environment, these patients become colonized with MDR pathogens. When the circumstances promote multiplication and virulence of organisms, including host immune dysfunction, HCAP occurs.

Excessive antibiotic use may be a major factor contributing to increased frequency of antibiotic-resistant pathogens in the hospital setting. VAP, occurring in the setting of conventional mechanical ventilation with an endotracheal (or tracheostomy) tube interface is described in detail in chapter 16.

EPIDEMIOLOGY

Incidence

Healthcare-associated infections (HAIs) affect an estimated 1.7 million hospitalizations in the United States each year. HCAP is a serious infection that affects approximately 250,000 US hospitalizations each year.[3]

Hospital-acquired pneumonia accounts for up to 25% of all ICU infections and for more than 50% of the antibiotics prescribed. Rates of HAP due to MDR pathogens have increased dramatically in hospitalized patients, especially in intensive care and transplant patients.[4] The actual incidence of HCAP is unknown due to the paucity of data but it is estimated to range between 17.3% and 67.4% depending on the population analyzed and the diagnostic techniques utilized.[5]

A special entity of the HCAP is the population residing in nursing homes. The number of frail older adults living in long-term care (LTC) facilities is expected to rise dramatically over the next 30 years.[6] An estimated 40% of adults will spend some time in an LTC facility before dying. According to several surveys, the estimated incidence of nursing home-acquired pneumonia (NHAP) ranges from 0.3 episodes to 2.5 episodes per 1,000 days of resident care.[7,8] If the incidence of pneumonia in this population remains the same, by the year 2030, there will be an estimated 1.9 million episodes of NHAP annually.

PATHOGENESIS

Pneumonia in general occurs by several mechanisms: inhalation, aspiration of oropharyngeal pathogens, hematogenous seeding of the lungs, as well as by contiguous spread of infection. HCAP arises from aspiration of oropharyngeal secretions that are colonized by pathogenic organisms. Host factors, including mechanical, as well as immune status determine occurrence, or abatement of the pneumonic process. Poor cough reflex will prevent adequate clearance of colonized secretions, resulting in pneumonia; a poor or dysfunctional immune system will fail to clear or contain the aspirated bolus of organisms, leading to an invasive infection of the lower respiratory tract, resulting in pneumonia and sepsis. Pneumonia can also result, when the inoculum size is large, or when the organism is particularly virulent, despite the presence of a robust immune system.

Oropharyngeal Flora in the Hospitalized Patient

The oropharyngeal flora gets replaced by pathogenic Gram-negative bacteria rapidly after being exposed to healthcare environment; this seems to be proportional to severity of illness, and not merely to the exposure to organism.[9] For instance, healthcare workers, who are constantly exposed to these MDR pathogens, may not necessarily be colonized with these organisms, although this needs to be further validated.

Colonization also happens more in the elderly than younger patients. Among the elderly, concomitant respiratory disease and functional limitation are strongly associated with colonization. The prevalence of colonization increases as the level of care increases (6% in healthy elders living in a nursing home versus 40% in acute hospital ward).[10] Following illness or antibiotic therapy, competitive pressures within the oropharynx favor Gram-negative bacterial adherence to epithelial cells, which lead to oropharyngeal colonization.[11] Age-related impairment in mucociliary clearance, thereby decreasing mucus travel velocity may play a role in promoting colonization, as well as the increased susceptibility to pneumonia in the elderly population.[12]

The normal flora serves as a barrier to colonization by pathogenic bacteria. Elimination of this normal flora, for example, due to administration of antibiotics promotes colonization by the pathogenic bacteria.[13]

The presence of several factors such as bed confinement, urinary incontinence, and prior antibiotic usage, has been linked to oropharyngeal colonization by Gram-negative bacteria.[14,15] With increasing severity of illness, changes in epithelial glycoprotein binding characteristics develop along with alterations in the enzymatic content of salivary and tracheal secretions, promoting oropharyngeal colonization.[16]

Sources of Colonization

Colonizing organisms can be derived from endogenous or exogenous sources. Endogenous sources include nasal or sinus carriage, subgingival dental plaque, and the periodontal spaces, oropharynx, gastric, or tracheal colonization, and hematogenous spread. Dental plaque colonization may be a significant risk factor in the development of lower respiratory tract infections. In one study, the amount of dental plaque increased during ICU stay. A positive dental plaque culture during initial hospitalization was significantly associated with subsequent nosocomial infections.[17]

Pathogens are inadvertently transmitted from various sources in the hospital environment. Healthcare providers are the main carriers, who seem to unintentionally carry organisms from different sources, including other patients, healthcare devices, and other fomites, including door knobs, room and hospital surfaces, etc. This nosocomial colonization is most often the result of horizontal cross-transmission from other colonized or infected patients in the ICU and is mediated through contact with the hands of transiently colonized healthcare workers.[18-21] Ambient air and water can also be sources of pathogens.[22]

Continued manipulation of these factors, especially strict hand washing before and after patient contact will go a long way in preventing most of these HAIs, including HCAP.

ETIOLOGY AND RISK FACTORS

Healthcare-associated Pneumonia versus Community-acquired Pneumonia

Healthcare-associated pneumonia is different in various ways compared to CAP. HCAP patients in general are older, have multiple comorbid conditions, have a higher PSI score, and are associated with a higher case fatality rate.[23] Pathogens isolated from patients diagnosed with HCAP are listed in box 2.

There is variation in risk factor definitions between published studies and the ATS-IDSA guidelines. Most of the variations pertain to time interval to hospitalizations, ranging from 30 days, to as long as 360 days.[31] The risk factors are summarized in box 1.

In The United States, the main pathogens associated with HCAP are Pseudomonas and MRSA;[31] however, other pathogens, including MSSA, *S. pneumoniae* and other Gram-negative rods are also significant offenders. *S. pneumoniae* could be isolated from a patient who fits the definition of HCAP, but this is often community acquired, rather than true healthcare associated. The individual factors do not carry equivalent risk; however, some factors may be associated with isolation of MDR pathogens (Box 1). In a study of 190 patients admitted with severe HCAP, Schreiber and colleagues found that immunosuppression, use of prior antibiotics and admission from a LTC facility were associated with MDR pathogens.[25]

BOX 2

Pathogens isolated from patients diagnosed with healthcare-associated pneumonia[24-30]

HCAP Pathogens	
MRSA	*Klebsiella* spp.
MSSA	*Escherichia* spp.
P. aeruginosa	*Acinetobacter* spp.
Haemophilus spp.	*S. pneumoniae*

HCAP, healthcare-associated pneumonia; MRSA, methicillin-resistant *Staphylococcus aureus*; MSSA, methicillin-sensitive *Staphylococcus aureus*.

In a retrospective cohort analysis, Kollef and colleagues characterized culture positive CAP, HCAP, HAP, and VAP. In this cohort study consisting of 4,543 patients, 988 patients fit the definition of HCAP. *S. aureus* (56.8% MRSA) and *Pseudomonas* species were the most predominant organisms, with distribution similar to HAP.[26] This was validated in Schreiber and colleagues cohort, which had *S. aureus* and *P. aeruginosa* as the predominant pathogen isolated in patients with HCAP (33 out of 94 patients grew *S. aureus,* out of which 22 were MRSA); this cohort also showed *E. coli* (12.8%), as well as *K. pneumoniae* (10.6%) among other organisms.[25] Micek and colleagues had similar observations, with MRSA and *Pseudomonas* as the predominant organisms grown in patients with HCAP;[29] however, *S. pneumoniae* was also found to be a common offender in another cohort analysis by the same author.[30] Two studies, however, showed that the definition of HCAP predicted poorly the presence of MDR.[32,25] Indeed, an observational cohort published by Carratala and colleagues from Spain showed *S. pneumoniae* to be the most common pathogen among both CAP and HCAP patients, underlining the variability between different healthcare settings. Of interest, atypical pathogens like *Mycoplasma*, *Chlamydia*, and *Legionella* represented a small fraction of the total pathogens isolated.[23] Among patients admitted from nursing homes, the presence of foreign bodies, chronic wounds, recent hospitalization and dependency on or need for contact care (help with activities of daily living) were found to be risk factors for MDR pathogens.[24,33,34] Box 3 outlines the factors that may indicate a higher likelihood isolating MDR pathogens in HCAP.

BOX 3

Factors that may indicate a higher likelihood of multidrug-resistant pathogens in healthcare-associated pneumonia[1,24,25,33,35-37]

- Elderly age
- Long-term care admission
- Recent hospitalization
- Recent broad spectrum antibiotics
- Immunosuppressive condition
- Functional dependency or need for contact care (lower activities of daily living score)
- Multilobar infiltrates
- Presence of mental status change
- High prevalence of antibiotic resistance in the community
- Admission to the intensive care unit
- Use of acid suppressive medications
- Healthcare worker developing pneumonia

Use of acid suppressive medication in hospitalized patients may increase the risk of developing pneumonia, which is more pronounced in PPI than H2-receptor blockers.[35]

In summary, MRSA, *Pseudomonas aeruginosa,* and pneumococci appear to be predominant organisms causing HCAP; however, local microbial patterns need to be taken into consideration before formulating treatment options at the local level.

Morbidity and Mortality

Healthcare-associated pneumonia mortality evidently will be dictated by comorbid conditions, as well as presence of MDR pathogens. Kollef et al. cohort showed similar mortality in HCAP and HAP (19.8% and 18.8% respectively); this was higher than mortality associated with CAP (10%), and lower than VAP (29.3%).[26] Micek et al. reported a comparable HCAP mortality of 24.6%.[30]

Hsu et al. conducted a retrospective cohort study to evaluate mortality rates and health system costs for patients with CAP or HCAP; among over 50,000 patients admitted to the Veterans affairs (VA) healthcare system, they observed an HCAP hospital mortality of 23.9%, and a 1 year mortality of 54.8% among patients who developed HCAP. These were considerably higher, compared to patients admitted with a diagnosis of CAP (CAP hospital mortality 17.2%, and 1 year mortality 34.6%). A history of aspiration pneumonia was associated with the highest cumulative 1 year mortality of 62.1%. The mortality was also higher in patients with more comorbidities, as measured by the Charlson-Deyo-Quan comorbidity index score.[38]

In summary, comparative (estimated) mortality rates are highest among VAP (>30%), followed by HAP and HCAP (20%), then CAP (10%).

Culture Positive versus Culture Negative Healthcare-Associated Pneumonia

Culture positive HCAP patients may have a higher mortality compared to culture negative patients. In an elegant retrospective cohort analysis, Labelle and colleagues demonstrate higher mortality in HCAP patients who have a pathogen identified by culture; culture positive patients had a 24.6% mortality, compared to 7.4% mortality in culture negative patients. Culture positive patients also had higher severity of illness, longer hospital lengths of stay, were more likely to be treated with an appropriate initial antimicrobial regimen, and were significantly less likely to receive an initial antibiotic regimen directed against

CAP pathogens compared with culture negative patients.[39] Similar observations have been found in other studies as well.[40]

Cost

Healthcare system cost for HCAP is also higher than that of CAP. HCAP length of stays were 1.6 days (23%) longer, with cost $3,640 (31%) more compared to CAP, in the VA cohort evaluated by Hsu et al. Among patients alive at discharge, the estimated cost to VA healthcare in the following year averaged $45,594 for CAP patients and $80,861 for HCAP patients.[38]

DIAGNOSIS

Clinical Presentation

The usual presentation of pneumonia includes fever, chills, cough, etc. Older patients, patients debilitated due to any reason as well as immunocompromised patients may not show the classic signs of infections. Patients who developed NHAP as described by Marrie et al. showed, that compared to patients with CAP, NHAP patients less likely to have a productive cough (61% versus 35%), chills (58% versus 24%), myalgia (33% versus 7%), or arthralgia (10% versus 0%).[41] A retrospective cohort analysis comparing the clinical presentations of NHAP and CAP found similarly that patients with NHAP were more likely to have altered mental status (55.9% versus 11.3%), tachypnea (40.9% versus 22.8%), and hypotension (7.0% versus 1.1%).[42] These atypical findings could be responsible for the delay in diagnosis and treatment, contributing to increased morbidity and mortality in this group of patients.

Diagnostic Testing

There is no gold standard for establishing the diagnosis of HCAP. Some of the recommendations are rather an extrapolation of the data that have emerged over the years with our experience in the treatment of CAP, HAP, and VAP.

Box 4 shows suggestions for evaluation of patients suspected to have HCAP. The diagnosis of HCAP is entertained in a patient who develops a new or progressive lung infiltrate by radiography, and has evidence of infection, such as new onset of fever, leukocytosis, purulent expectoration, tachypnea, declining oxygenation, etc. in the presence of risk factors for HCAP. While at times straightforward diagnosis could be challenging. All patients should have a thorough history and physical examination, which will aid in localization of infection; patients with frank consolidation will have bronchial breath sounds and egophony; however, frank consolidation in HCAP is not commonly seen in our practice. Physical exam in patients with HCAP is more likely to show a febrile, tachypneic patient, who has declining oxygenation status. Crackles may be heard over the involved area of the lung.

A chest radiograph should be obtained, which will help to localize the infiltrate, characterize the severity, as well as show associated complications of HCAP if any, such as pleural effusions.

BOX 4

Evaluation of healthcare-associated pneumonia

- History and physical examination
- CBC with differential
- Chest radiograph
- Blood cultures
- Sputum Gram stain and culture
- BAL or ET aspirate*

CBC, complete blood count; BAL, bronchoalveolar lavage; ET, endotracheal.

*In intubated patients.

Microbiologic Testing

Establishing a microbiologic cause of pneumonia may influence outcome if the information allows change in treatment regimens and could promote antimicrobial de-escalation depending on pathogen and susceptibility patterns.

Sputum and or Lower Respiratory secretion Examination

We favor obtaining lower respiratory secretion examination by way of expectorated sputum for Gram stain and culture, or in intubated patients, bronchoscopic or non-bronchoscopically obtained bronchoalveolar lavage (BAL) examination or at least, an endotracheal aspirate (ETA). Significant colony counts (colony forming units) include, greater than or equal to 10^4 for specimen obtained by BAL, and more than or equal to 10^5 for specimen obtained by ETA. However, the potential value of expectorated sputum Gram stain in nonintubated HCAP patients remains to be determined. The usual limitations of sputum examination include inability to distinguish colonization of the oropharynx from a true representation of a lower respiratory origin of the cultured organism. Moreover, a significant portion of the patients, especially those who are older, having other comorbid conditions such as stroke, other causes of neuromuscular weakness, presence of mental status changes, etc. may not be able to expectorate a good quality sputum. In nonintubated patients, we have advocated obtaining specimen obtained by nasotracheal suctioning in some of our patients with HCAP, who are unable to bring up adequate sputum samples due to various reasons, but this has not been systematically studied. Furthermore, the likelihood of obtaining a positive specimen is reduced further in those who have received prior antibiotics.[43]

Blood Cultures

Blood cultures should be obtained, since a fair portion of patients could be bacteremic as well. In the cohort of patients analyzed by Labelle et al., 30.9% of patients had concomitant bacteremia, with *Escherichia coli* (55.6%), *Streptococcus pneumoniae* (44.4%), *Klebsiella* species (39.3%), *Enterobacteriaceae* (28.2%), and MRSA (25.8%) had the highest rates of bacteremia.[39]

Urinary Antigen Testing and Serology

Urinary antigen testing, as well as serologic testing are of limited value, and generally are of low yield; nevertheless, we continue to advocate urinary antigen testing for patients with HCAP until further recommendations are available.

Diagnostic yield after extensive testing is variable, and obviously not 100%; Labelle and colleagues found a diagnostic yield of about 74%, while Shindo and colleagues observed a diagnostic yield of about 55%.[39,44]

Biomarkers-Procalcitonin

Procalcitonin (PCT) or other biomarkers may help to decrease antibiotic exposure; Biologic markers have been used in an attempt to distinguish between bacterial and nonbacterial causes of pneumonia. PCT is the most promising of all the biomarkers.[45] PCT is a peptide precursor of calcitonin that is released by parenchymal cells in response to bacterial toxins and certain bacterial-specific proinflammatory mediators (i.e., interleukin-1β, tumor necrosis factor-α, and IL-6), leading to elevated serum levels in patients with bacterial infections.[46,47] PCT shows a prompt increase upon initial infection within 6–12 hours and reduces rapidly when the bacterial infection is controlled by the host immune system and antimicrobial therapy. In contrast, PCT is downregulated in patients with viral infections because of the release by cytokines typically associated with viral infections, such as interferon-γ.[45]

Procalcitonin can potentially differentiate between bacterial and nonbacterial infections.[48-50] Several studies, many conducted in Europe seem to indicate that the duration of antibiotics can be reduced without affecting mortality by using the PCT strategy in patients with lower respiratory tract infections.[51] Even though, PCT has not been formally tested specifically in patients with HCAP, future studies need to evaluate PCT toward reducing antibiotic exposure, thereby helping not only better utilize the healthcare resources, but also to decrease antibiotic pressure that creates MDR pathogens.

TREATMENT

Once a diagnosis is strongly suspected, antimicrobial treatment needs to be promptly initiated. Early aggressive, appropriate empiric treatment and de-escalation for HCAP reduces mortality and minimizes resistance.[52]

The provider should be familiar with the patient as well the healthcare environment the patient was/is exposed to, including distribution of MDR pathogens, as well as susceptibility patterns. Antimicrobial therapy applicable to an urban, highly populated busy practice setting may not be applicable to a small community-based hospital.

Observations published by Arancibia et al. and Carratala and colleagues highlight the importance of understanding local or regional variations in pathogen distribution associated with pneumonia. Patients infected with Gram-negative bacilli were more likely to have clinical criteria consistent with HCAP, including probable aspiration, previous hospitalization, previous antimicrobial treatment, and the presence of pulmonary comorbidities.[53,23]

An important distinction of HCAP when compared to CAP is the presence of MDR bacteria, attributed to the risk factors associated with HCAP.[1] Therefore, the initial treatment of HCAP should be similar to that for HAP and VAP.[26] This is especially important in the emergency department, as well as the inpatient and ICU settings, where therapy should be appropriate, meaning the chosen antibiotics should be able to cover all of the likely pathogens. Antibiotics also need to be started promptly, avoiding delays. Several studies have shown increased mortality attributable to delay in appropriate antibiotic therapy. Houck and colleagues, in a Medicare data analysis were able to show a decrease in hospital mortality, 30 day mortality, as well as a decrease in length of stay among patient who received antibiotics within 4 hours of arrival, compared to those who received antibiotics beyond 4 hours of arrival.[54] Iregui and coworkers showed increase in mortality among patients with VAP whose antibiotic administration was delayed, in spite of the fact that the antibiotics were appropriate.[55] A prospective examination of patients admitted to the hospital revealed a much higher mortality of 42% among patients who received inadequate antibiotics, versus 17.7% for patients who received adequate antibiotics. More of the patients who received inadequate antibiotics also required vasopressor, as well as increased duration of mechanical ventilation.[56]

In summary, treatment of HCAP should be early, appropriate, and adequate with prompt de-escalation at the appropriate time, with a good understanding of the local pathogen distribution and susceptibility patterns, in order to achieve the best possible outcome. Multidrug resistant pathogens should be adequately targeted, with attention to pseudomonas and MRSA coverage. Focusing on covering these two common offenders in HCAP will most often, but not always, automatically ensure coverage of the other usual pathogens in majority of the settings. Other troublesome organisms such as ESBL producing enterobacteriacea, or *S. maltophilia* coverage should be considered, depending on the local pathogen and susceptibility patterns.

El Solh and colleagues evaluated factors associated with infections caused by MDR pathogens in patients admitted with NHAP. The factors associated with MDR pathogens include requirement for admission in an ICU, low functional status, and prior exposure to antibiotics for more than 3 days in the preceding 6 months.[36] Altered mental status and multilobar presentation also showed a trend toward a preponderance of MDR pathogens. Interestingly, patients who had cough had less incidence of MDR pathogens in this data set. Therefore, antimicrobial coverage directed against MDR pathogens must be carefully chosen, with consideration given to higher acuity of illness, use of prior antibiotics,

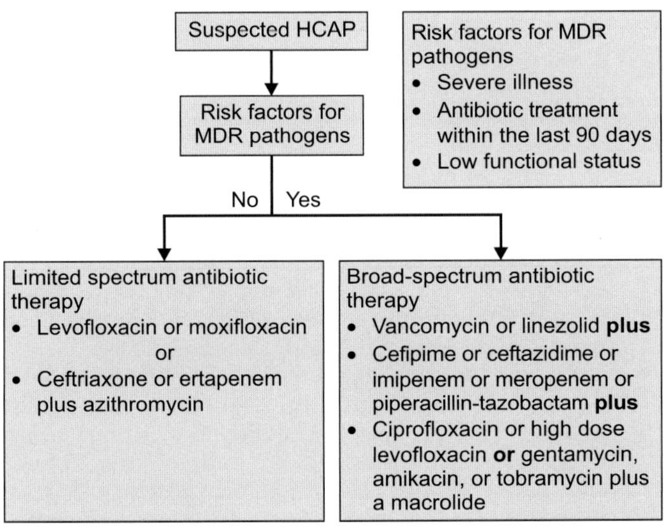

FIGURE 2 Approach to initial empiric antimicrobial therapy of healthcare-associated pneumonia.

presence of altered mental status, poor functional status of patients, presence of wounds, including decubitus ulcers, etc. (Figure 2). Interestingly, two studies have evaluated the impact of guideline concordant therapy on patients' outcomes with HCAP. In a Canadian study comparing the impact of guideline concordant therapy in patients with CAP and HCAP, guideline concordant therapy was associated with lower mortality in CAP but not HCAP.[57] In a comparable study involving more than 150 hospitals in the US Veterans Health Administration including over 15,000 patients, guideline concordant HCAP therapy was an independent predictor of 30-day mortality.[58]

Some of the key practice statements from the HCAP summit include recommendation to have initial empiric therapy that covers MRSA and dual coverage for Gram-negative bacteria in those with risk factors, to ensure coverage for possible MDR pathogens. The summit also recommended against de-escalation when microbiological data are unavailable.[2]

Duration of Antibiotic Treatment in Healthcare-associated Pneumonia

Until about a decade ago, infections such as VAP and HAP were routinely treated with antimicrobials for 2–3 weeks. The current recommendation is to treat patients with HCAP who show a clinical response for 7–8 days except for nonlactose fermenting organisms.[1,2] Most if not all of the evidence for this recommendation comes from patients with VAP.

Consideration for extended therapy may be advocated for patients infected with unique MDR pathogens, especially those who are "slow to respond".

Prevention

Hand hygiene plays an important role in preventing person to person spread of organisms. Hand hygiene should be implemented in every healthcare setting, and this will go a long way in preventing healthcare-associated infections, including HCAP. Plaque reduction, including measures such as maintaining oral hygiene, with modalities as simple as brushing of teeth twice a day, and periodic flossing may dramatically reduce the incidence of HCAP; however, further research is needed to substantiate this.

The eligible population should receive pneumococcal and influenza vaccination at appropriate times and this is also likely to modulate the risk for developing HCAP, by keeping the at risk population away from the healthcare environment.

CONCLUSION AND FUTURE DIRECTIONS

Healthcare-associated pneumonia is a relatively new entity, with the application of this new term to pneumonia occurring outside the hospital in patients who are currently, or recently in contact with the healthcare environment. The pathogenesis of HCAP most commonly involves oropharyngeal colonization followed by aspiration. There is potential for MDR pathogens, predominated by MRSA and *P aeruginosa*, but other organisms can be involved as well. Further research is needed to characterize the distinctions including diagnostic and therapeutic and possible preventive approaches that will improve outcomes. This is especially important, given the rapidly increasing number of people living in nursing homes and other long-term care facilities.

REFERENCES

1. Guidelines for the management of adults with hospital-acquired, ventilator-associated, and healthcare-associated pneumonia. *Am J Respir Crit Care Med.* 2005;171(4):388-416.
2. Kollef MH, Morrow LE, Baughman RP, et al. Health care-associated pneumonia (HCAP): a critical appraisal to improve identification, management, and outcomes-proceedings of the HCAP Summit. *Clin Infect Dis.* 2008;46 Suppl 4:S296-334; quiz 5-8.
3. Klevens RM, Edwards JR, Richards CL, et al. Estimating health care-associated infections and deaths in US hospitals, 2002. *Public Health Rep.* 2007;122(2):160-6.
4. Richards MJ, Edwards JR, Culver DH, et al. Nosocomial infections in medical intensive care units in the United States. National Nosocomial Infections Surveillance System. *Crit Care Med.* 1999;27(5):887-92.
5. Carratala J, Garcia-Vidal C. What is healthcare-associated pneumonia and how is it managed? *Curr Opin Infect Dis.* 2008;21(2):168-73.
6. Richards C. Infections in residents of long-term care facilities: an agenda for research. Report of an expert panel. *J Am Geriatr Soc.* 2002;50(3):570-6.
7. Muder RR. Pneumonia in residents of long-term care facilities: epidemiology, etiology, management, and prevention. *Am J Med.* 1998;105(4):319-30.
8. Loeb M, McGeer A, McArthur M, et al. Risk factors for pneumonia and other lower respiratory tract infections in elderly residents of long-term care facilities. *Arch Intern Med.* 1999;159(17):2058-64.
9. Johanson WG, Pierce AK, Sanford JP. Changing pharyngeal bacterial flora of hospitalized patients. Emergence of gram-negative bacilli. *New Eng J Med.* 1969;281(21):1137-40.
10. Valenti WM, Trudell RG, Bentley DW. Factors predisposing to oropharyngeal colonization with gram-negative bacilli in the aged. *New Eng J Med.* 1978;298(20):1108-11.
11. Estes RJ, Meduri GU. The pathogenesis of ventilator-associated pneumonia: I. Mechanisms of bacterial transcolonization and airway inoculation. *Intens Care Med.* 1995;21(4):365-83.
12. Goodman RM, Yergin BM, Landa JF, et al. Relationship of smoking history and pulmonary function tests to tracheal mucous velocity in nonsmokers, young smokers, ex-smokers, and patients with chronic bronchitis. *Am Rev Respir Dis.* 1978;117(2):205-14.
13. Mackowiak PA. The normal microbial flora. *New Eng J Med.* 1982;307(2):83-93.
14. Cunha BA. Pneumonia in the elderly. *Clin Microbiol Infect.* 2001;7(11):581-8.
15. Quinn MO, Miller VE, Dal Nogare AR. Increased salivary exoglycosidase activity during critical illness. *Am J Respir Critical Care Med.* 1994;150(1):179-83.
16. McDonald DS, Jameson P. Injection pain with propofol. Reduction with aspiration of blood. *Anaesthesia.* 1996;51(9):878-80.
17. Fourrier F, Duvivier B, Boutigny H, et al. Colonization of dental plaque: a source of nosocomial infections in intensive care unit patients. *Critical Care Med.* 1998;26(2):301-8.
18. Lortholary O, Fagon JY, Hoi AB, et al. Nosocomial acquisition of multiresistant Acinetobacter baumannii: risk factors and prognosis. *Clin Infect Dis.* 1995;20(4):790-6.
19. Koeleman JG, Parlevliet GA, Dijkshoorn L, et al. Nosocomial outbreak of multi-resistant Acinetobacter baumannii on a surgical ward: epidemiology and risk factors for acquisition. *J Hosp Infect.* 1997;37(2):113-23.
20. Speijer H, Savelkoul PH, Bonten MJ, et al. Application of different genotyping methods for Pseudomonas aeruginosa in a setting of endemicity in an intensive care unit. *J Clin Microbiol.* 1999;37(11):3654-61.
21. Simor AE, Lee M, Vearncombe M, et al. An outbreak due to multiresistant Acinetobacter baumannii in a burn unit: risk factors for acquisition and management. Infection control and hospital epidemiology: the official journal of the Society of Hospital Epidemiologists of America. 2002;23(5):261-7.
22. Crnich CJ, Safdar N, Maki DG. The role of the intensive care unit environment in the pathogenesis and prevention of ventilator-associated pneumonia. *Respir Care.* 2005;50(6): 813-36; discussion 36-8.
23. Carratala J, Mykietiuk A, Fernandez-Sabe N, et al. Health care-associated pneumonia requiring hospital admission: epidemiology, antibiotic therapy, and clinical outcomes. *Arch Intern Med.* 2007;167(13):1393-9.
24. Drinka PJ, Stemper ME, Gauerke CD, et al. Clustering of multiple endemic strains of methicillin-resistant Staphylococcus aureus in a nursing home: an 8-year study. *Infect Control Hosp Epidemiol.* 2005;26(2):215-8.
25. Schreiber MP, Chan CM, Shorr AF. Resistant pathogens in nonnosocomial pneumonia and respiratory failure: is it time to refine the definition of health-care-associated pneumonia? *Chest.* 2010;137(6):1283-8.
26. Kollef MH, Shorr A, Tabak YP, et al. Epidemiology and outcomes of health-care-associated pneumonia: results from a large US database of culture-positive pneumonia. *Chest.* 2005;128(6):3854-62.
27. O'Donovan CA, Fan-Havard P, Tecson-Tumang FT, et al. Enteric eradication of vancomycin-resistant Enterococcus faecium with oral bacitracin. *Diagn Microbiol Infect Dis.* 1994;18(2):105-9.

28. Tesh VL, O'Brien AD. Adherence and colonization mechanisms of enteropathogenic and enterohemorrhagic Escherichia coli. *Microbial Pathogenesis.* 1992;12(4):245-54.
29. Micek ST, Reichley RM, Kollef MH. Health care-associated pneumonia (HCAP): empiric antibiotics targeting methicillin-resistant Staphylococcus aureus (MRSA) and Pseudomonas aeruginosa predict optimal outcome. *Medicine.* 2011;90(6):390-5.
30. Micek ST, Kollef KE, Reichley RM, et al. Health care-associated pneumonia and community-acquired pneumonia: a single-center experience. *Antimicrobial Agents Chemother.* 2007;51(10):3568-73.
31. Kleemann J, Rincon-Rivera LJ, Takahara H, et al. Sequential delivery of host-induced virulence effectors by appressoria and intracellular hyphae of the phytopathogen colletotrichum higginsianum. *PLoS Pathog.* 2012;8(4): e1002643.
32. Shorr AF, Zilberberg MD, Micek ST, et al. Prediction of infection due to antibiotic-resistant bacteria by select risk factors for health care-associated pneumonia. *Arch Intern Med.* 2008;168(20):2205-10.
33. O'Sullivan NP, Keane CT. Risk factors for colonization with methicillin-resistant Staphylococcus aureus among nursing home residents. *J Hosp Infect.* 2000;45(3):206-10.
34. El-Solh AA, Pietrantoni C, Bhat A, et al. Colonization of dental plaques: a reservoir of respiratory pathogens for hospital-acquired pneumonia in institutionalized elders. *Chest.* 2004;126(5):1575-82.
35. Herzig SJ, Howell MD, Ngo LH, et al. Acid-suppressive medication use and the risk for hospital-acquired pneumonia. *JAMA.* 2009;301(20):2120-8.
36. El Solh AA, Pietrantoni C, Bhat A, et al. Indicators of potentially drug-resistant bacteria in severe nursing home-acquired pneumonia. *Clin Infect Dis.* 2004;39(4):474-80.
37. Scanvic A, Denic L, Gaillon S, et al. Duration of colonization by methicillin-resistant *Staphylococcus aureus* after hospital discharge and risk factors for prolonged carriage. *Clin Infect Dis.* 2001;32(10):1393-8.
38. Hsu JL, Siroka AM, Smith MW, et al. One-year outcomes of community-acquired and healthcare-associated pneumonia in the Veterans Affairs Healthcare System. *Int J Infect Dis.* 2011;15(6):e382-7.
39. Labelle AJ, Arnold H, Reichley RM, et al. A comparison of culture-positive and culture-negative health-care-associated pneumonia. *Chest.* 2010;137(5):1130-7.
40. Venditti M, Falcone M, Corrao S, et al. Outcomes of patients hospitalized with community-acquired, health care-associated, and hospital-acquired pneumonia. *Ann Intern Med.* 2009;150(1):19-26.
41. Marrie TJ, Blanchard W. A comparison of nursing home-acquired pneumonia patients with patients with community-acquired pneumonia and nursing home patients without pneumonia. *J Am Geriatr Soc.* 1997;45(1):50-5.
42. Meehan TP, Chua-Reyes JM, Tate J, et al. Process of care performance, patient characteristics, and outcomes in elderly patients hospitalized with community-acquired or nursing home-acquired pneumonia. *Chest.* 2000;117(5):1378-85.
43. Houck PM, MacLehose RF, Niederman MS, et al. Empiric antibiotic therapy and mortality among medicare pneumonia inpatients in 10 western states: 1993, 1995, and 1997. *Chest.* 2001;119(5):1420-6.
44. Shindo Y, Sato S, Maruyama E, et al. Health-care-associated pneumonia among hospitalized patients in a Japanese community hospital. *Chest.* 2009;135(3):633-40.
45. File TM. New diagnostic tests for pneumonia: what is their role in clinical practice? *Clin Chest Med.* 2011; 32(3):417-30.
46. Niederman MS. Biological markers to determine eligibility in trials for community-acquired pneumonia: a focus on procalcitonin. *Clin. Infect Dis.* 2008;47 Suppl 3:S127-32.
47. Schuetz P, Albrich W, Christ-Crain M, et al. Procalcitonin for guidance of antibiotic therapy. *Exp Rev Anti-infect.* 2010;8(5):575-87.
48. Maisel A, Neath SX, Landsberg J, et al. Use of procalcitonin for the diagnosis of pneumonia in patients presenting with a chief complaint of dyspnoea: results from the BACH (Biomarkers in Acute Heart Failure) trial. *Eur J Heart Fail.* 2012;14(3):278-86.
49. Ahn S, Kim WY, Kim SH, et al. Role of procalcitonin and C-reactive protein in differentiation of mixed bacterial infection from 2009 H1N1 viral pneumonia. *Influenza other Respir viruses.* 2011;5(6):398-403.
50. Cuquemelle E, Soulis F, Villers D, et al. Can procalcitonin help identify associated bacterial infection in patients with severe influenza pneumonia? A multicentre study. *Intensive Care Med.* 2011;37(5):796-800.
51. Bafadhel M, Clark TW, Reid C, et al. Procalcitonin and C-reactive protein in hospitalized adult patients with community-acquired pneumonia or exacerbation of asthma or COPD. *Chest.* 2011;139(6):1410-8.
52. Kollef MH, Napolitano LM, Solomkin JS, et al. Health care-associated infection (HAI): a critical appraisal of the emerging threat-proceedings of the HAI Summit. Clinical infectious diseases : an official publication of the Infectious *Diseases Society of America.* 2008;47 Suppl 2:S55-99; quiz S100-1.
53. Arancibia F, Bauer TT, Ewig S, et al. Community-acquired pneumonia due to gram-negative bacteria and pseudomonas aeruginosa: incidence, risk, and prognosis. *Arch Intern Med.* 2002;162(16):1849-58.
54. Houck PM, Bratzler DW, Nsa W, et al. Timing of antibiotic administration and outcomes for Medicare patients hospitalized with community-acquired pneumonia. *Arch Intern Med.* 2004;164(6):637-44.
55. Iregui M, Ward S, Sherman G, et al. Clinical importance of delays in the initiation of appropriate antibiotic treatment for ventilator-associated pneumonia. *Chest.* 2002;122(1):262-8.
56. Kollef MH, Sherman G, Ward S, et al. Inadequate antimicrobial treatment of infections: a risk factor for hospital mortality among critically ill patients. *Chest.* 1999;115(2):462-74.
57. Grenier C, Pepin J, Nault V, et al. Impact of guideline-consistent therapy on outcome of patients with healthcare-associated and community-acquired pneumonia. J *Antimicrob Chemother.* 2011;66(7):1617-24.
58. Attridge RT, Frei CR, Restrepo MI, et al. Guideline-concordant therapy and outcomes in healthcare-associated pneumonia. *Eur Respir J.* 2011;38(4):878-87.

CHAPTER 6

Community-acquired Methicillin-resistant *Staphylococcus aureus* Pneumonia

Irene D Karampela, Garyphallia Poulakou, Despoina Koulenti, George Dimopoulos

ABSTRACT

Community-acquired methicillin resistant *Staphylococcus aureus* (CA-MRSA) has emerged as a new infectious threat during the last decade, affecting previously healthy individuals. It has been distinguished from the hospital-acquired strains (HA-MRSA) by molecular means, thus providing strong evidence that CA-MRSA strains have not emerged from HA-MRSA strains but rather from the spread of clonally related methicillin-susceptible *S. aureus* strains in the community. It has been established as a cause of severe necrotizing pneumonia, a syndrome of hemoptysis, leukopenia, high fever, and cavitary lung lesions, often requiring mechanical ventilation. Prompt administration of appropriate treatment is of high importance. Although multiple classes of anti-staphylococcal agents retain activity against CA-MRSA strains; linezolid and vancomycin are currently considered as first line treatment. Given its high mortality despite early clinical suspicion, the new anti-MRSA drugs ceftaroline and telavancin, along with possible combinations, have to be urgently evaluated.

INTRODUCTION

Methicillin-resistant *Staphylococcus aureus* (MRSA) has been a major cause of nosocomial infections since the decade of '1960s', and those strains were defined as hospital-acquired MRSA (HA-MRSA).[1] Methicillin resistance results from the acquisition of the staphylococcal cassette chromosome *mec* (SCC*mec*) carrying the *mec*A gene, which mediates resistance to methicillin, penicillins, and other β-lactams. MRSA is the cause of skin and soft tissue infections (SSTIs), sepsis, bacteremia, endovascular infections, endocarditis, pneumonia, septic arthritis, osteomyelitis, and infections of prostheses and implantable devices.[2-4] A changing epidemiology for MRSA infections has been reported over the last 10 years throughout the world with infections affecting children without established risk factors for MRSA acquisition. Numerous other reports of severe infections have also reported the same in otherwise healthy outpatient adults, including sport team members and correctional facility inmates. These strains, in contrast to HA-MRSA, retain susceptibility to various classes of antibiotics except for β-lactams, indicating a different origin. This recent epidemiological trend has been defined as community-acquired MRSA (CA-MRSA).[5,6] Infections by CA-MRSA strains and, particularly, pneumonia have been associated with high mortality rates, often attributed to the production of toxins, such as the Panton-Valentine leukocidin (PVL).[7,8]

EPIDEMIOLOGY

The epidemiology of MRSA changed dramatically since the '1990s' and is characterized by a significant increase in the infection rates in the community. Interestingly, the new MRSA infections affect people lacking the usual risk factors arising from exposure to the health care system. These new MRSA strains responsible for infections in previously healthy individuals have been distinguished from the hospital-acquired strains (HA-MRSA) by molecular means and were named community-acquired (CA-MRSA). Genotypic studies revealed significant differences between community- and hospital-acquired-MRSA strains (genetic lineage, architecture of methicillin-resistance genetic elements, and the presence of PVL) provide strong evidence that CA-MRSA strains have not emerged from HA-MRSA strains but from the spread of clonally related methicillin-susceptible *S. aureus* strains (MSSA) in the community.[9]

On the other hand, CA-MRSA shares common epidemiological features with community-acquired-MSSA, such as racial distribution, age, socioeconomic status, living conditions, site of infection, prior antibiotic use, substance use, and sexual behavior.[10] The primary natural reservoir of *S. aureus* arises from asymptomatic carriage of humans while domestic animals, livestock, and fomites may serve as secondary reservoirs. CA-MRSA is preferentially recovered from the throat, axilla, inguinal area, and perineum whereas the nasal mucosa is the anatomical niche of MSSA and HA-MRSA.[11-13]

Early studies of MRSA colonization in the general US population showed a relatively low prevalence (32.4% for *S. aureus* and 0.8% for MRSA); however, certain medically underserved populations, such as homeless or poor adults had significantly higher asymptomatic MRSA nasal colonization as well as CA-MRSA SSTIs.[14-16] Intravenous drug users had even higher rates of MRSA colonization (6.1%), and most of them were CA-MRSA.[17] Comparison of populations with different socioeconomic status in a US study concluded that CA-MRSA strains were more prevalent in the urban population of lower socioeconomic status.[18] Nonwhite race and people younger than 60 years of age were additional risk factors for CA-MRSA SSTIs.[18]

In a study from Taiwan, 7.8% of healthy children were colonized by MRSA (88% of them being CA-MRSA by molecular typing). Number of children in the family and daycare attendance were independent risk factors for MRSA colonization and CA-MRSA transmission in the community.[19]

Transmission of CA-MRSA was documented in the household setting, among healthcare workers, and after nonoccupational exposure within the community. Transmission is possible by contact with colonized or infected persons or contaminated material (clothing, towels, razors, soaps, bandages, and sports equipment); furthermore, colonization of an individual is a risk factor for infection.[20-23] Sexual activity might represent another way of transmission in the household setting.[24] A history of MRSA infection in any family member poses a risk of transmission to other members of the same family (Table 1).[19,20]

TABLE 1

Risk Groups for CA-MRSA Colonization

- Children <2 years (especially neonates)
- School-aged children
- Military personnel
- Intravenous drug users
- Homosexual males
- Correctional facilities inmates (jails and prisons)
- Residents of skilled nursing facilities
- Shelter residents
- Competitive sports participants (mainly contact sports)
- Veterinarians
- Pig farmers
- Contact with colonized pets
- Family member with history of MRSA infection

CA-MRSA, community-aquired methicillin-resistant *Staphylococcus aureus*.

Transmission from person-to-person through hand carriage had also been shown for HA-MRSA inside the hospital as well as in the household setting.[25-27] The risk of progression to infection was higher for MRSA-colonized individuals, compared to MSSA-colonized counterparts in 2 studies involving soldiers and children, respectively (38% vs. 3% and 31.8% vs. 9.9% risk for an SSTI).[28, 29]

Athletic facilities were demonstrated as a possibly favorable environment for CA-MRSA transmission. Most reports for CA-MRSA SSTIs in the US derive from football teams in high schools and colleges.[30-32] However, several reports were published relating to other athletic activities, such as basketball, wrestling, soccer, and dancing. Modes of transmission among athletes include sharing personal items, such as towels, clothing, and training equipment and close skin contact in certain sports like wrestling.[32] In one report, the implementation of a protocol for improvement of hygiene habits with use of antiseptic soap and disposable towels among other measures showed a drastic decrease of MRSA SSTIs cases in a college football team in the US.[33]

Outbreaks of infections by CA-MRSA have been reported among Alaskan natives, American natives, Pacific islanders, correctional facility inmates, competitive sports participants, homosexual men, military personnel, neonates, and school-aged children.[4] Newborns comprise a well defined high risk population for *S. aureus* infections. Except for MRSA, which can cause hospital outbreaks in neonatal intensive care units (NICUs), there are reports of CA-MRSA infections associated with transmission by colonized or infected visitors or healthcare workers and vertical transmission in the context of peripartum maternal MRSA infections, maternal mastitis, or vaginal colonization. The majority of neonatal infections were SSTIs with rare cases of severe fatal neonatal pneumonia reported in the US.[34]

In a 3-year surveillance study of pediatric otherwise healthy patients with community-onset *S. aureus* infections, the percentage of CA-MRSA increased from 60% in year 2001 to 76.4% in 2004.[35] Community-acquired pneumonia (CAP) ranked second, after osteomyelitis, among invasive CA-MRSA infections in this study, whereas invasive infections represented 4.4% of the infections by *S. aureus* population. In the USA HA-MRSA caused 73% of skin infections in children during a 2-year period (2003–2005) and CA-MRSA ranged from 81 to 85%.[36] Most of the studies indicate that the burden of the CA-MRSA infections affects pediatric and adult populations with SSTIs.[26,37,38]

The epidemiology of CA-MRSA is rapidly evolving. Recently, as a result of the movement of patients between hospitals and the community, the boundaries between hospital- and community-acquired MRSA are becoming blurred.[8,39] An increasing prevalence of CA-MRSA infections has been reported into the healthcare environment suggesting that it might replace the traditional HA-MRSA in the future. Currently, in the US, it is becoming increasingly difficult to distinguish between community- and hospital-acquired MRSA on clinical and epidemiological grounds. This distinction can be made by use of microbiological characteristics or molecular typing.[10] In a study from Brazil, more than 10% of the cases of nosocomial MRSA bacteraemia were caused by CA-MRSA strains in 2003.[40] The investigators reported that age less than 1 year, less frequent use of central venous catheters, no history of surgery, less severe illness, and female sex were identified as risk factors for nosocomial bloodstream infection from CA-MRSA. A similar study from Korea reported that the prevalence of CA-MRSA in hospitals has increased from less than 10% in 2003 to more than 25% in 2007.[41] This increase affected emergency department and general ward patients particularly, while intensive care unit (ICU) patients were affected to a lesser extent. A study from Taiwan reported an incidence rate of 3 per 1,000 patient-days. Prior administration of antipseudomonal penicillins and antifungals and the presence of a nasogastric tube were found to be independent risk factors for acquisition of CA-MRSA during the ICU stay.[42] A recent retrospective study of 16 patients with CA-MRSA pneumonia from Australia has clearly demonstrated a wide distribution of ages along with increased rates of noncavitary infiltrates on the X-ray.[43] Interestingly, evidence of influenza infection was a risk factor encountered in 25% of the cohort patients. Although there was a great fear of increasing prevalence of CA-MRSA infections during the pandemic and post-pandemic H1N1 (2009) influenza A, another recent study from Australia reported very low rates of CA-MRSA infections.[44]

The prevalence of CA-MRSA pneumonia in the community setting was assessed for the first time in a big US population-based study which was published in 2012. During the winter-spring of 2006 and 2007, CA-MRSA was encountered in 2.4% of all adult patients referred to the emergency department of 12 University affiliated hospitals with CAP, whereas it was recovered from 5% of those admitted to the ICU.[45] The recovery of MRSA was associated with more severe presentation: shock, need for vasopressors and/or mechanical ventilation, comatose state, and presence of multiple infiltrates or cavities in the chest X-ray. Mortality was estimated at 14% for the surveyed population with MRSA CAP.[45]

MICROBIOLOGICAL AND MOLECULAR CHARACTERISTICS OF CA-MRSA STRAINS

From the microbiological viewpoint, CA-MRSA strains are typically resistant to β-lactam agents with relatively universal susceptibility to most of the other anti-staphylococcal agents except for clindamycin and erythromycin. For the latter 2 antibiotics, a wide range of susceptibility is reported across the world (Table 2).[46,47]

The molecular markers of CA-MRSA are the SCC*mec* type IV, V, or VII, the *lukF-lukS* genes, and the accessory gene regulator genotype I or III.[48, 49] All of them are responsible for virulence and resistance to antibiotics expressed by the CA-MRSA strains.

The *mec* Gene Complex

Methicillin resistance in *S. aureus* is mediated by the production of a modified low-affinity penicillin-binding protein (PBP) called PBP2a (or PBP2). PBP2a production is encoded by the *mec*A gene and confers resistance to all β-lactam antibiotics. The *mec* gene complex, resides within a mobile genetic island named SCC*mec*. There are at least 8 SCC*mec* types (types I–VII) in *S. aureus*. They contain different genetic elements, which result in variations in susceptibility patterns (i.e., the transposon, Tn554, encodes resistance to macrolides, clindamycin, and streptogramin B, whereas pT181 encodes resistance to tetracyclines).[50] CA-MRSA has almost exclusively been associated with type IV SCC*mec* and rarely, with type V and VII, that do not contain other resistance genes than *mec*A.[51] In contrast, the most commonly encountered SCC*mec* types in HA-MRSA strains are

TABLE 2

Susceptibility Patterns of the Most Prevalent CA-MRSA Strains According to Their Geographic Distribution

Geographic area	Pulsed field type	Susceptibility pattern	Production of PVL toxin	Comments
North America	USA300 (ST8-MRSA-IV)	R: ERY, GATS: TMP-SMX, CLD, TET	+	Predominant
	USA400 (ST1-MRSA-IV)	R: ERY, CLDS: all others	+	Predominant in native Americans
Europe	European ST80-MRSA-IV	R: TETIR or S: FA	+	Prevalent in southern Europe
	USA300 (ST8-MRSA-IV)	as above	+	Present in UK
	Pig-associated ST398-MRSA-IV/V	R: TET, Variable R: ERY, TMP-SMX, AMGS: FQ, FA	–	Prevalent in Netherlands, Denmark, Germany
	ST5-MRSA-I (Geraldine clone)	R:FA, variable R: TOB, ERY S: FQ, CLD, GEN	–	Prevalent in France
Australia	ST1-MRSA-IV (WA-1)	S: ERY, TET, FQ, TMP-SMX,	–	Frequent
	ST93-MRSA-IV (Queensland clone)	S: ERY, TET, FQ, AMG	+	Frequent
	ST30-MRSA-IV (SWP clone)	S: ERY, TET, FQ, FA, AMG	+	Frequent
Asia	ST59-MRSA-V_T/IV	R: ERY, CLDS: TET, FQ, TMP-SMX	+	Frequent

ERY, Erythromycin; GAT, Gatifloxacin; TMP-SMX, trimethoprim-sulphamethoxazole; CLD, clindamycin; TET, tetracycline; FA, Fucidic acid; FQ, fluoroquinolones; AMG, aminoglycosides; GEN, gentamicin; TOB, tobramycin; MRSA, methicillin-resistant *Staphylococcus aureus*; CA-MRSA, community-aquired MRSA; PVL, Panton Valentine leukocidin toxin.

Data from Poulakou G, Souto J, Kmet Lunanek N, Rello J. Pneumonia due to methicilin-resistant *Staphylococcus aureus* (MRSA): A review. *Curr Respir Med Rev.* 2012;8:245-58.

I–III that carry genes mediating resistance to multiple antibiotic classes.[52]

The Accessory Gene Regulator

The accessory gene regulator (agr), also termed agrBCDA, is the *S. aureus* global regulatory system.[53] The expression of its 5 genes mediates a quorum-sensing mechanism and modulate the production of virulence factors. Polymorphism defined as *S. aureus agr* groups I–IV, varies with geographical region and results in variability in biofilm production, expression of virulence factors, and resistance to antibiotics.[54-56] The operon of agr gene has also significant contribution to the resistance to glycopeptides.[57]

Panton-Valentine Leukocidine and the LukS-PV and LukF-PV Genes

PVL is a strong cytolytic factor with high specificity for human polymorhonuclear (PMN) leukocytes, being a principal determinant of the virulence of CA-MRSA. Its ability to lyse leukocytes was first described by Van de Velde in 1894. In 1932 Panton and Valentine first associated the leukotoxin with skin and soft tissue infections.[58] High concentration of PVL causes leukocyte necrosis with the production of inflammatory mediators, whereas lower concentrations induce apoptosis with the release of caspases. The production of PVL is regulated by the lukS-PV and lukF-PV genes. PVL production has been associated with furuncles, ulcers, severe necrotizing skin infections, leukopenia, and hemoptysis. Additionally, in respiratory tract infections, extensive necrosis of respiratory epithelium and necrotizing pneumonia are often attributed to PVL.[7,59] However, only a small percentage of strains causing necrotizing pneumonia contain genes coding for PVL. In such infections, mortality rates are very high.[60] Although the role of PVL has been overemphasized in the past, today we know that it is not the only one nor the most lethal virulence factor of CA-MRSA. Other toxins have been reported with great geographic variation, such as α-hemolysin (αHL) also known as α-toxin, δ-hemolysin, γ-hemolysin, the superantigen enterotoxins B and C, the leukocidin encoded by the lukE–lukD gene, and the recently discovered, α-type phenol-soluble modulin (PSMα) peptides. All of them have been associated with significant virulence.[61-63] Alpha hemolysin binds to susceptible host cells and acts through the formation of heptameric transmembrane pores. Molecular evidence suggests that CA-MRSA strains have evolved as a result of introduction of the SCC*mec* type IV into MSSA strains that had already adapted to the community. Horizontal transfer of several virulence genes has also been demonstrated among different strains.[6,50,63]

MOLECULAR EPIDEMIOLOGY AND EMERGING RESISTANCE

The worldwide spread of CA-MRSA has diverse patterns with a single clone dominating in some countries and multiple clones in other regions. In North America, the dominating community-acquired-MRSA clone is pulsed field type USA300 (ST8-MRSA-IV). USA400 (ST1-MRSA-IV) is the second most prevalent with increasing trends. More rarely, USA1000 (ST59-MRSA-IV) and USA1100 (ST30-MRSA-IV) are reported (Table 1).[64] Although clindamycin resistance rate was reported at 6.5%, resistance to erythromycin can be as high as 92.8%.[65] The Centers for Disease Control and Prevention (CDC) recommends testing for inducible clindamycin resistance (i.e., by the D-test), for all isolates displaying resistance to erythromycin and susceptibility to clindamycin, because there have been reports of clindamycin treatment failures.[66] Typically, USA400 is resistant to erythromycin and clindamycin but susceptible to other agents.[65,67] Multidrug resistant USA300 clones have been recently reported with only cotrimoxazole susceptibility universally preserved. The typical antibiotic profiles of the most prevalent CA-MRSA strains worldwide are shown in table 1.[46]

European community MRSA is very heterogeneous, the predominant clone being the *lukSF-PV*–positive European ST80-MRSA-IV. USA300 (ST8-MRSA-IV) has also been reported throughout the UK and Europe. Four other clones have been reported in northern Europe: the pig-associated ST398-MRSA-IV/V, the Australian WA-1 (ST1-MRSA-IV), the ST5-MRSA-I, and the sporadically *lukSF-PV*–positive ST152-MRSA-V clone.[67] ST80 MRSA-IV has been identified in up to 92% of all CA-MRSA infections and 24% of HA-MRSA infections from Greece.[68,69] Many patients infected with the ST80 clone have epidemiological links to countries south of the Mediterranean (Algeria, Tunisia, Egypt, and Lebanon).[70] ST80 clone is typically resistant to tetracycline and may demonstrate intermediate susceptibility or resistance to fusidic acid (FA).[67,68] Varying patterns of susceptibility are encountered among the other clones. The Geraldine ST5-MRSA-I clone expressing toxic shock syndrome toxin (TSST-1) is now the most prevalent community MRSA clone in France.[67] In Australia and Oceania, more than 100 clones have been reported, the most prevalent of them being *lukSF-PV*-negative.[67] Remote Australian aboriginal communities have very high rates of colonization and infection with MRSA, the clone ST75-MRSA-IV being predominant.

CLINICAL MANIFESTATIONS

The most dreadful manifestation of CA-MRSA infection is necrotizing pneumonia, a syndrome of hemoptysis, leukopenia, high fever, and cavitary lung lesions, often requiring mechanical ventilation (Figure 1).[71] This syndrome has been linked to antecedent respiratory viral infection, particularly influenza. In 2009 during the first 2 waves of the worldwide pandemic of (H1N1) influenza A virus, several published series included cases of MRSA pneumonia complicating influenza in previously healthy people. In a study from Australia, coinfection with CA-MRSA represented 1.2% of admissions with the pandemic flu.[72] Necrotizing pneumonia has a rapidly progressive and fatal course occurring most often in children and young adult patients. CA-MRSA pneumonia has a high mortality rate of 56–63%. Death is independently associated with "airway bleeding", erythroderma (a generalized erythematous exfoliative rash), and leukopenia.[7,73] According to a recent analysis of pooled data of 114 patients (case reports), the most common complication of CA-MRSA pneumonia is shock (56%) followed by multiple organ failure (44%), and acute respiratory distress syndrome (ARDS) (23.5%). Other complications include pneumatoceles, pneumothorax, deep venous thrombosis (DVT), acidosis, digital necrosis, abscesses, Waterhouse-Friderichsen syndrome, secondary hospital infections, cerebral septic emboli, cardiac arrhythmias, and cardiac arrest (Table 3).[74] However, according to a recent population-based study in the US, CA-MRSA accounted for 1.2% of emergency department diagnoses for CAP with a mortality of 14% and a large proportion of cases being treated in the outpatient setting.[45]

DIAGNOSIS

It is well established that CA-MRSA should be suspected when a young, previously healthy, patient is admitted in the emergency or critical care department with community-onset necrotizing pneumonia.[8] Specific features that prompt suspicion of CA-MRSA have been highlighted in the "Guidelines for the management of hospital-acquired pneumonia in the UK. Report of the Working Party on Hospital-acquired Pneumonia of the British Society for Antimicrobial Chemotherapy (BSAC)" as follows:

- Influenza-like prodrome
- Severe respiratory symptoms with a rapidly progressive pneumonia evolving to ARDS
- Fever more than 39°C
- Hemoptysis

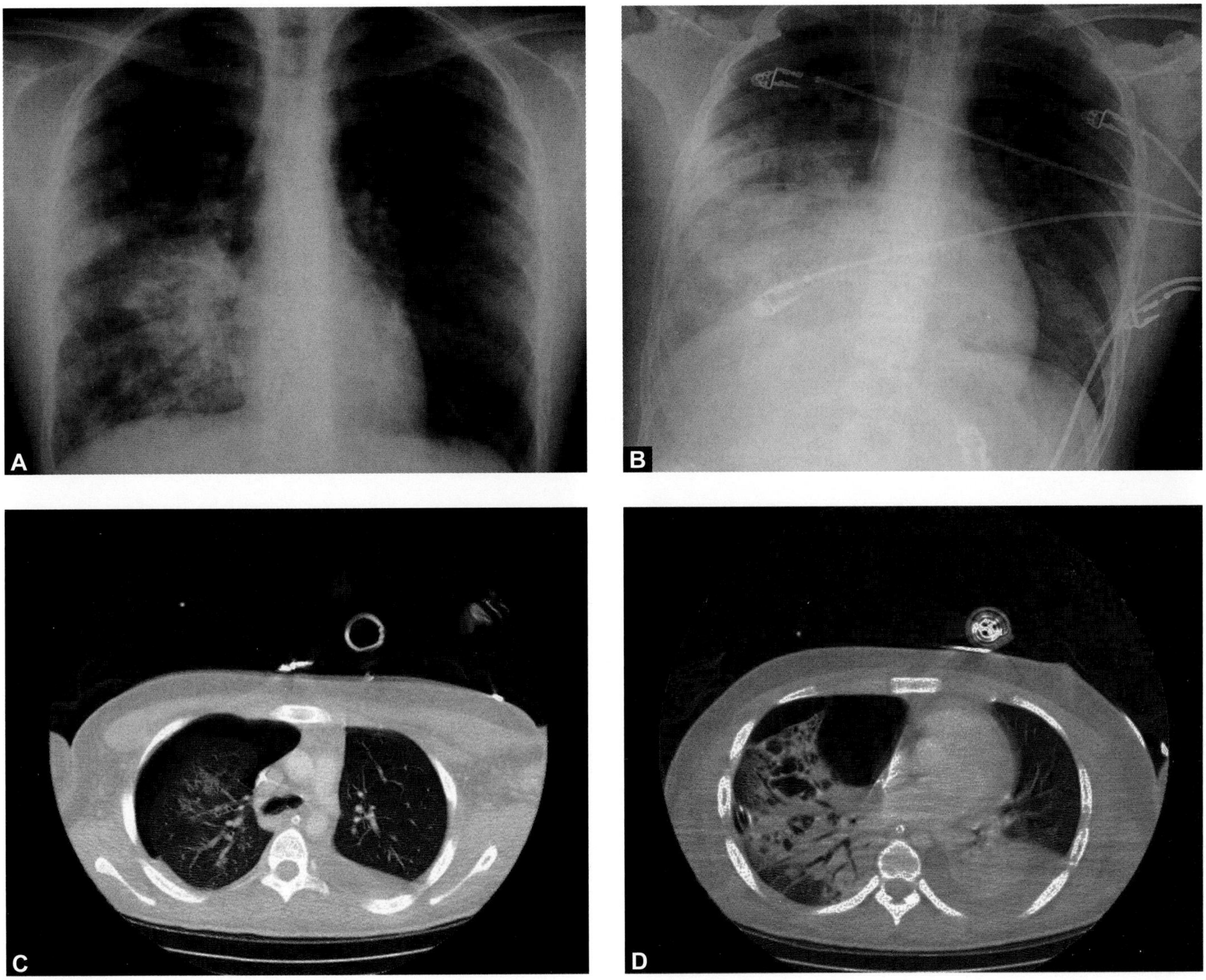

FIGURE 1 Chest X-rays and CT-scan of a 17-year-old male who was admitted to the ICU of 'ATTIKON' hospital immediately after endotracheal intubation. Chest X-rays in the emergency room (ER) show a large lesion of the right lower lobe confirming the diagnosis of community-acquired pneumonia (CAP). Bronchial secretions and bronchoalveolar lavage (BAL) performed at admission in the ICU revealed *Staphylococcus aureus* with a phenotype of CA-MRSA. Molecular study confirmed the isolate as CA-MRSA *meqA* (+), PVL(+). Ten days after ICU admission, chest CT-scan reveals extensive necrotizing lesions and pneumothorax of the right lung.

- Hypotension
- Leukopenia
- Chest radiograph showing multilobar infiltrates, which may have cavitated
- Known to be colonized with CA-MRSA or recent travel to an endemic area, such as North America, and recent contact with CA-MRSA
- Belong to a group associated with increased rates of colonization of CA-MRSA namely, children aged <2 years, athletes (mainly contact sports), injection drug users, homosexual males, military personnel, inmates of correctional facilities, residential homes and shelters, veterinarian surgeons, pig farmers, and contact with colonized pets
- Previous history or family history of recurrent furuncles or skin abscesses (2 or more in past 6 months).[75]

However, a recent retrospective analysis of 16 cases with CA-MRSA pneumonia from Australia has reported a shift towards higher ages and a higher than previously reported rate of noncavitary pulmonary manifestation. This study also stressed the importance of timely-administered appropriate treatment, since none of the reported cases had received anti-MRSA treatment upon admission. Evidently, there is accumulating evidence

TABLE 3

Clinical Features, Laboratory and Radiological Findings of CA-MRSA Pneumonia: Analysis of 114 Case Reports

Clinical features			
Tachypnea	92%	Chest pain	19%
Fever	89%	GI symptoms	18%
Cough	58%	Rash	15%
Shock	56%	Confusion	13%
Hemoptysis	29%		
Laboratory and radiological findings			
Leukopenia	45%	Pleural effusion (including empyema)	34%
Multilobar consolidation or bilateral lung infiltrates (CXR/CT)	75%	Evidence of necrotizing pneumonia in CT and/or lung biopsy	77%

CXR, chest radiograph; CT, computed tomography; GI, gastrointestinal; MRSA, methicillin-resistant *Staphylococcus aureus;* CA-MRSA, community-aquired MRSA.

Data from Vardakas KZ, Matthaiou DK, Falagas ME. Incidence, characteristics, and outcomes of patients with severe community acquired-MRSA pneumonia. *Eur Respir J.* 2009;4:1148-58.

that an expanding range of pulmonary syndromes with various clinical and radiographic pictures, including noncavitary bilateral consolidations could be associated with CA-MRSA infection.[45]

Clinical presentation of MSSA and CA-MRSA pneumonia could be indistinguishable. Specific features indicative of PVL-associated staphylococcal disease include hemoptysis, high respiratory rate, and a low white cell count (leukopenia) in the presence of a high C-reactive protein (CRP) and systemic sepsis in a previously healthy individual.[75] The presence of blood in sputum should alert the clinician to the possibility of PVL production and prompt extended coverage to include *S. aureus*. On the other hand, while *Streptococcus pneumoniae* and *S. pyogenes* will be empirically covered by the same regimen, other possible pathogens, such as *Legionella pneumophila* and viruses, such as influenza should be taken into consideration.

TREATMENT

Given the increasing prevalence of CA-MRSA in some parts of the world, empirical treatment against MRSA should be considered in cases of fulminant CAP according to local epidemiological data.[8] In that context, the most recent Canadian guidelines suggest vancomycin to be considered as empirical therapy for patients with life-threatening pneumonia in communities of high prevalence of CA-MRSA.[76]

Older and more recent reports imply that CA-MRSA pneumonia requires hospitalization and prompt treatment with intravenous antibiotics. Appropriate cultures are essential and should be obtained prior to the initiation of empiric antibiotic therapy. A simple Gram stain of the sputum could prove to be extremely valuable because *S. aureus* has a distinct morphology. Antimicrobial therapy for such severe CA-MRSA infections is generally the same as for invasive HA-MRSA infections (Table 4).[8,77,78] The low prevalence of cases of CA-MRSA pneumonia pose a difficulty for big randomized controlled trials (RCTs); therefore, conclusions have to be drawn from meta-analyses, retrospective analyses of case series, and indirectly, from studies of HA-MRSA pneumonia.

Vancomycin

Vancomycin, the first glycopeptide, is a first line antibiotic for the treatment of MRSA. Within-patient pharmacokinetic variability, narrow therapeutic index, and nephrotoxic potential at high doses mandate therapeutic drug monitoring. Its slow bactericidal activity combined with a slow clinical response and a poor penetration into lung tissue has prompted its role in the treatment of MRSA pneumonia to be questioned.[79,80] Furthermore, there are reports of therapeutic failure of vancomycin in cases of necrotizing pneumonia caused by PVL producing CA-MRSA strains.[79] Recently, there is an evidence of a gradual increase in vancomycin minimum inhibitory concentrations (MICs) in the last few years ("MIC creep"), although within the defined limits of susceptibility. Increases of vancomycin MIC are associated with the phenomenon of heteroresistant vancomycin-intermediate *S. aureus* (hVISA), which is attributed to small subpopulations of cells able to grow at a vancomycin concentration of 4 mg/L, while the MICs of the hVISA isolates remain within the susceptibility range (0.5–1 mg/L). The hVISA phenotype heralds a full-blown VISA; however, full resistance of *S. aureus* to vancomycin remains rare with very few cases reported worldwide.[81] Clinically, MICs more than 1 mg/L are clearly associated with high treatment failure rates and thus high mortality rates when the patients were treated with vancomycin.[82,83] Thus, the "MIC creep" and heteroresistance have triggered a controversy about the optimal MIC breakpoints for vancomycin (currently at ≤2 mg/L). Certainly, there is evidence to support a lower clinical breakpoint, such as 1 mg/L for the E-test. Furthermore, when vancomycin is administered in the treatment of serious MRSA infections it is essential that the MIC of the isolate is reported to the clinician. Recent pharmacokinetic-pharmacodynamic (PK-PD) data call for vancomycin trough serum

TABLE 4

Antibiotics Used for Treatment of Community-acquired MRSA Pneumonia

Antibiotic	Mechanism of action	Dose	Adverse effects	Comments
Vancomycin (glycopeptide)	Slowly bactericidal	15–20 mg/kg every 8–12 hours	"Red man" syndrome, chemical phlebitis, ototoxicity, nephrotoxicity, thrombocytopenia	• First line antibiotic • Usually combined with clindamycin • Therapeutic levels must be monitored
Linezolid (oxazolidinone)	Bacteriostatic	600 mg PO/IV every12 hours	Myelotoxicity, peripheral and optic neuropathy, lactic acidosis, serotonin syndrome	• Reserved for empiric therapy • Preferred over vancomycin when MIC high or renal failure • Resistance rare
Clindamycin (lincozamide)	Bacteriostatic	600 mg PO/IV every 8 hours	Diarrhea up to 20%, pseudomembranous colitis more often	• Excellent tissue penetration • Decreases PVL production • Inducible resistance
Rifampicin (rifamycine)	Bactericidal	600–900 mg IV daily	Nausea,vomiting,diarrhea, hypersensitivity reactions, hepatotoxicity	• Rapid resistance with monotherapy • Usually combined with TMP-SMX. • Drug-drug interactions
Novel glycopeptides				
Telavancine (lipoglycopeptide)	Rapidly bactericidal	10 mg/kg/day IV	Headache, dizziness, nausea, taste disorders, nephrotoxicity	FDA approved for cSSTIs, EMA approved for HAP
Novel cephalosporins				
Ceftaroline	Broad-spectrum bactericidal	600 mg every 12 hours		FDA approved for cSSTIs and CABP

PO, orally; IV, intravenously; MIC, minimal inhibitory concentration; PVL, Panton-Valentine leukocidine; TMP-SMX, trimethoprime-sulfomethoxazole; CPK, creatinophosphokinase; cSSTIs, complicated skin and soft tissue infections; HAP, hospital-acquired pneumonia; FDA, Food and Drug Administration; CABP, community-acquired bacterial pneumonia; MRSA, methicillin-resistant *Staphylococcus aureus.*

concentrations of 15–20 mg/L, when treating MRSA with MIC below 1 mg/L.[79,84-86]

Another issue of controversy related to vancomycin is the type of infusion. Several studies have demonstrated that continuous infusion allows more rapid achievement of therapeutic drug concentrations than intermittent infusion and may optimize its bactericidal activity. Early publications recommended a loading dose of 15 mg/kg of body weight followed by a daily dose of 30 mg/kg.[87] More recent PK studies in critically ill patients suggested that higher loading doses, such as 35 mg/kg and higher than recommended daily doses of vancomycin, depending on creatinine clearance, might be necessary to rapidly achieve therapeutic serum concentrations of 20–25 mg/L.[88,89] A consensus paper by the American Society of Health System Pharmacists (ASHP), the Infectious Diseases Society of America (IDSA), and the Society of Infectious Disease Pharmacists (SDIP), in 2009, recommended a more aggressive vancomycin dosing to achieve the pharmacodynamic index associated with efficacy without, however, any recommendation favoring continuous infusion.[90] Enhancing this aspect, a recent meta-analysis reported that continuous infusion was associated with significantly lower risk of nephrotoxicity; however, no advantages over mortality were demonstrated.[91]

Linezolid

Linezolid is the first oxazolidinone antibiotic. It is bactericidal against streptococci but bacteriostatic against *Staphylococcus* and *Enterococcus* through inhibition of protein synthesis. Linezolid is approved for treatment of SSTIs as well as HA-MRSA pneumonia.[92] It rapidly achieves therapeutic plasma concentrations, has relatively low protein binding, and is well distributed to the tissues, being suitable for invasive MRSA infections. Linezolid is characterized by an excellent penetration into the lung parenchyma, reflecting an appropriate treatment choice especially in cases in which the MIC of vancomycin is high. The main adverse effect of linezolid is myelosuppression (mainly anemia and thrombocytopenia), especially during prolonged administration (more than 2 weeks), but it is reversible after drug discontinuation. Thrombocytopenia rates up to 30% are reported with treatment duration of more than 4 weeks.[84] Optic nerve toxicity and nonreversible peripheral neuropathy have been reported in patients who received linezolid for more than 4 weeks. Finally, linezolid may be toxic when it is coadministered with serotoninergic agents.[92] Linezolid resistance is rare for MRSA, but it has been reported for vancomycin-resistant *Enterococcus* strains after prolonged use.[93,94]

Trimethoprim/Sulfamethoxazole

CA-MRSA strains show high susceptibility rates *in vitro* (95–100%) to trimethoprim/sulfamethoxazole (TMP-SMX), but data regarding its role in CA-MRSA pneumonia are lacking. The efficacy of intravenous TMP-SMX in the treatment of invasive CA-MRSA infections deserves additional evaluation.[95] The effect of bacterial inoculum in severe infections and a theoretic risk of deactivation of TMP-SMX by the thymidine released by MRSA isolates deserve futher investigation.[46]

Clindamycin

Clindamycin is an alternative to vancomycin for the treatment of MRSA pneumonia in children, but there are limited data for its use in adults. It is bacteriostatic and inhibits PVL synthesis. It has excellent tissue penetration, especially in abscesses. Rates of susceptibility to clindamycin are higher among CA-MRSA than HA-MRSA, but there is a great variability worldwide, and European strains are generally less susceptible to clindamycin compared to US circulating clones (Table 1). Diarrhea can occur up to 20%, and *Clostridium difficile* colitis occurs more frequently with clindamycin.[78] Clindamycin is often used in combination to another anti-MRSA agent, because of its potential of inhibiting toxin synthesis. Rifampicin, a potent antistaphylococcal agent with bactericidal activity against intracellular *S. aureus,* may be useful as an adjunctive therapy. When used alone, it easily selects resistant mutants, so it should only be used in combination with a second drug.[78] Finally, fluoroquinolones are not routinely recommended for the treatment of MRSA pneumonia.[77,78]

Newer Agents

The newer available antistaphylococcal agents for parenteral therapy include daptomycin, tigecycline and the 2 newly developed cephalosposrins, ceftaroline and ceftobiprole. Daptomycin is a bactericidal agent, and it is administered once daily to patients with normal renal function. It is effective against SSTIs due to MRSA and in adults with bacteremic infections, but it is not useful for treating pneumonia, because it is inactivated by pulmonary surfactant.[96,97] Tigecycline is a bacteriostatic antimicrobial agent belonging to a new class of antibiotics, the glycylcyclines, which are chemically related to minocycline. It has been approved for use only in patients with intra-abdominal infections and MRSA cSSTIs, indicating a safe and effective profile in hospitalized patients similar to that of vancomycin.[98] Despite being approved in the US for CAP, there are still no convincing data to support its use for the treatment of CA-MRSA pneumonia.[99]

The 2 newly developed cephalosposrins, ceftaroline and ceftobiprole, possess a high affinity for PBP2a correlating well with low minimum inhibitory concentrations for MRSA, a main difference from the other β-lactams. Ceftaroline is a broad-spectrum cephalosporin with bactericidal activity not only against CA-MRSA but also against vancomycin intermediate *S. aureus* (VISA), hVISA, vancomycin-resistant *S. aureus* (VRSA), including daptomycin-resistant strains.[100,101] It is US Food and Drug Administration (FDA) approved for the treatment of cSSTIs (including those caused by MRSA) and CAP.[102] The recommended dose is 600 mg over 1 hour, every 12 hours for 14 days while dosage adjustment is recommended for patients with moderate (creatinine clearance 30–50 mL/min) but not for mild renal impairment.[103]

The novel glycopeptides, dalbavancin, telavancin, and oritavancin act through inhibition of cell wall synthesis like vancomycin, while telavancin also causes depolarization of the bacterial cell membrane enhancing its bactericidal effect.[104-106] The main advantages of dalbavancin and oritavancin over vancomycin are their long half-lives, which allow for infrequent dosing.[107] Telavancin is bactericidal against MRSA and VISA, and it has been shown to be equally effective to vancomycin in the treatment of cSSTIs.[108] The results of the 2 large, double-blinded, randomized ATTAIN (Assesment of Telavancin for Treatment of Hospital Acquired Pneumonia) trials have established telavancin's non-inferiority compared to vancomycin (endpoint of clinical response) in the treatment of hospital-acquired pneumonia due to the Gram-positive bacteria, such as MRSA.[109] In the clinically evaluable population, telavancin achieved cure rates of 82.4% compared to 80.7% of vancomycin. Increases in serum creatinine level were more common in the telavancin group (16% vs. 10%).[109] Telavancin was FDA approved for cSSTIs, whereas for Europe, the European

Medicine Agency (EMA) has recently issued approval only for nosocomial pneumonia.[110] However, the drug's distribution in Europe was halted due to manufacturing and licensure-commercialization issues; therefore, the EMA's Committee for Medicinal Products for Human Use (CHMP) has recommended the suspension of the marketing authorizations until a suitable alternative manufacturing site is approved.[111] Dalbavancin and oritavancin have stepped back from development. Newer antistaphylococcal agents, such as new fluoroquinolones and oxazolidinones are in development for potential use in MRSA infections.[112,113]

APPROACH TO TREATMENT

The classic therapeutic approach for the treatment of CA-MRSA pneumonia is a combination of anti-staphylococcal agents. According to this approach, one of the components, usually clindamycin, should target the inhibition of bacterial protein synthesis in order to eliminate toxin production.[114] This has been tested *in vitro* after exposure of MRSA isolates to sub-inhibitory concentrations of β-lactam antibiotics, where an increased expression of toxin genes, including those for PVL, α-toxin, and TSST-1 has been noted, while the use of clindamycin decreased the production of those toxins.[115,116]

Rifampicin is known to exert bactericidal effect against most Gram-positive organisms, including MRSA.[117] Because of its wide-spectrum antimicrobial activity and its sufficient tissue concentration throughout the body, rifampicin is used to treat patients with inadequate leukocytic bactericidal activity and to eradicate the staphylococcal nasal carrier state. In addition, successful use of rifampicin as an adjunct to vancomycin therapy has been reported in staphylococcal endocarditis, ventriculoperitoneal shunt infections, and bacteremia.[118-120]

The combination of vancomycin (standard dosing 1 g every 12 hours) plus rifampicin has been tested in a RCT of 93 patients with MRSA pneumonia. Although the combination arm performed arithmetically better against all endpoints, clinical cure (63.3% vs. 38.2%), microbiological eradication (69% vs. 63.6%), and 28-day mortality (22% vs. 38.1%) did not differ significantly; however, a marginal statistical difference was in favor of the combination arm on 60-day mortality (26.8% vs. 50%, $p = 0.04$).[121] Probably, larger number of patients and studies with dose optimization of vancomycin would be able to clarify this issue.

A great variability characterizes recommendations coming from different countries. According to the German Sepsis Society (GSS) Recommendations, monotherapy with glycopeptides is not advised for the treatment of pulmonary MRSA infections, based on their limited tissue penetration. In confirmed cases of pulmonary MRSA infections, treatment with linezolid is recommended, as it is superior to vancomycin monotherapy (Recommendation level C).[122] On the other hand, according to the 2008 "Community Acquired MRSA Pneumonia British Society for Antimicrobial Chemotherapy Recommendations" for severe infections with known or suspected CA-MRSA, it is recommended to start treatment in hospital with parenteral vancomycin, teicoplanin, daptomycin (but not for pneumonia), or linezolid, as there is no evidence that one agent is superior to another.[75] Tigecycline may also offer broader polymicrobial coverage, if required. The Guidelines derived from the same UK scientific community for the diagnosis and management of MRSA infections presenting in the community recommend that in case of severe pneumonia, although there is as yet no unequivocal clinical evidence to support the combination of linezolid (intravenous, 600 mg, 12 hourly) plus clindamycin (intravenous, 1.2–1.8 g, 6 hourly). Because of the life-threatening nature of this disease, it is recommended that consideration be given to using this combination for initial therapy. Some experts suggest adding rifampicin 600 mg twice daily, based on synergistic activity and intracellular clearance of staphylococci. Finally, the most recently issued by the IDSA "Guidelines on the treatment of MRSA infections" state that for hospital- or community-acquired MRSA pneumonia, intravenous vancomycin (A-II) or linezolid 600 mg twice daily (A-II) or clindamycin 600 mg thrice daily (B-III) if the strain is susceptible, is recommended for 7–21 days depending on the extent of infection.[78]

It is evident that the ongoing scientific debate has not yet clarified, whether linezolid or vancomycin should be the treatment of choice for MRSA pneumonia and eventually CA-MRSA pneumonia. Linezolid has the ability of suppressing protein synthesis of the bacterial cell and does not require the addition of clindamycin for that purpose.[115] Moreover, the predominant CA-MRSA clones in Europe are clindamycin-resistant.[69] For vancomycin, loading doses in the range of 25–30 mg/kg and therapeutic drug monitoring is required to ensure efficacious concentrations and avoid toxicity in critically ill patients.[88] Even the implementation of strict PK/PD protocols lead to achievement of optimal initial vancomycin exposures, only in 32.3% of patients [area under the curve (AUC)/MIC ratio ≥400] in the first 24 hours of therapy.[123]

The largest RCT comparing linezolid to vancomycin in the treatment of proven HA-MRSA pneumonia (the

ZEPHyR study) showed end of study success rates in 95/165 patients (57.6%) for linezolid and 81/174 patients (46.6%) for vancomycin arm, respectively.[124] Linezolid was non-inferior to vancomycin (95% CI, 0.5–21.6%) and statistically superior (p = 0.042). The same applies for end of treatment clinical outcome and microbiologic outcome at end of treatment and end of study. No significant difference was observed on mortality. In this study, vancomycin use was optimized with therapeutic drug monitoring; however, failures in the arm of vancomycin were not related with the height of trough levels. Although extrapolation of these data cannot be directly done to CA-MRSA pneumonia, linezolid seems to have an advantageous clinical and microbiogical outcome in MRSA pneumonia.

ADJUNCTIVE TREATMENTS AND PREVENTION OF CA-MRSA PNEUMONIA

Treatment with intravenous immunoglobulin has not been evaluated in RCTs. However, based on the recommendation for streptococcal toxic shock, intravenous immunoglobulin has been administered along with antibiotics in several cases of CA-MRSA pneumonia. intravenous immunoglobulin acts through a concentration dependent inhibition of cytopathic effect and pore-formation of PVL *in vitro*.[125] BSAC guidelines suggest a dosage of 2 g/kg as recommended for streptococcal toxic syndrome, repeated at 48 hours if there is still evidence of sepsis or failure to respond.[75] Prevention of CA-MRSA spread within hospitals can be achieved by the implementation of the standard infection control practices and adherence to meticulous hand hygiene and disinfection protocols.[126] Other more specific interventions, such as isolation or cohorting of colonized individuals, active identification of MRSA carriage by surveillance cultures of high-risk populations, decolonization of MRSA carriers, and environmental disinfection have failed to reliably eradicate transmission or spread. There is no evidence for the prophylactic use of any antibiotic against CA-MRSA in the community setting. Mupirocin ointment use to decolonize MRSA carriers has been advocated; however, it fails to produce long-lasting decolonization or reduction of skin infections and is associated with development of resistance.[127,128] In the community, good personal hygiene is essential along with the avoidance of sharing personal items. All infected skin lesions should be covered and special care should be taken to avoid contact with open skin lesions (e.g., during sports, use of pools, or saunas). Although research is focused on the production of an effective anti-staphylococcal vaccine, no product is approaching to the market in the near future.[129] Recently α-hemolysin has acquired increasing interest as a major contributor to the MRSA virulence in lung infections as well as a possible therapeutic target. Recent studies targeting various approaches of α-hemolysin blockade were encouraging in preventing MRSA pneumonia (including CA-MRSA). Those studies certainly indicate a novel promising approach in vaccine strategies to prevent MRSA infections.[130-132]

CONCLUSION

CA-MRSA pneumonia represents a new infectious threat affecting mainly young nonimmunocompromised adults without risk factors. The epidemiology, risk factors, and pathogenesis are unclear and might differ significantly among countries or continents. Although multiple classes of antistaphylococcal agents retain activity against CA-MRSA strains, linezolid, and vancomycin are currently considered as the first line drugs available for the treatment of CA-MRSA pneumonia. The addition of clindamycin to vancomycin is frequently used, aiming to a rapid decrease of PVL production. Given the high mortality of CA-MRSA pneumonia despite early clinical suspicion, the new anti-MRSA drugs ceftaroline and telavancin, along with possible combinations, have to be urgently evaluated.

REFERENCES

1. Brumfitt W, Hamilton-Miller J. Methicillin-resistant *Staphylococcus aureus*. *N Engl J Med* 1989;320:1188-96.
2. Zhang KJ, McClure A, Elsayed S, Louie T, Conly JM. Novel multiplex PCR assay for characterization and concomitant subtyping of staphylococcal cassette chromosome *mec* types I-V in MRSA. *J Clin Microbiol.* 2005;43:5026-33.
3. Oliveira DC, de Lencastre H. Multiplex PCR strategy for rapid identification of structural types and variants of the *mec* element in methicillin-resistant *Staphylococcus aureus*. *Antimicrob Agents Chemother.* 2002;46:2155-61.
4. David MZ, Daum RS. Community-Associated MRSA: Epidemiology and Clinical Consequences of an Emerging Epidemic. *Clin Microb Rev.* 2010;23:616-87.
5. Weber JT. Community-associated MRSA. *Clin Infect Dis.* 2005;41:S269-72.
6. Maltezou HC, Giamarellou H. Community-acquired methicillin-resistant *Staphylococcus aureus* infections. *Int J Antim Agents.* 2006;27:87-96.
7. Gillet Y, Issartel B, Vanhems P, Fournet JC, Lina G, Bes M, et al. Association between *Staphylococcus aureus* strains carrying gene for PVL and highly lethal necrotizing pneumonia in young immunocompetent patients. *Lancet.* 2002;359:753-9.
8. Karampela I, Poulakou G, Dimopoulos G. Community Acquired Methicillin Resistant *Staphylococcus aureus*

pneumonia: an update for the emergency and intensive care physician. *Minerva Anestesiol.* 2012.
9. Boyle-Vavra S, Daum RS. Community-acquired methicillin-resistant *Staphylococcus aureus*: the role of Panton-Valentine leukocidin. *Lab Invest.* 2007;87:3-9.
10. Miller LG, Perdreau-Remington F, Bayer AS, Diep B, Tan N, Bharadwa K, et al. Clinical and epidemiologic characteristics cannot distinguish community associated methicillin-resistant *Staphylococcus aureus* infection from methicillin-susceptible *S. aureus* infection: a prospective investigation. *Clin Infect Dis.* 2007;44:471-82.
11. Bignardi GE, Lowes S. MRSA screening: throat swabs are better than nose swabs. *J Hosp Infect.* 2009;71:373-4.
12. Harbarth S, Schrenzel J, Akakpo C, Renzi G, Ricou B. Is throat screening necessary to detect MRSA colonization upon admission to an intensive care unit? *J Clin Microbiol.* 2007;45:1072-3.
13. Yang ES, Tan J, Eells S, Rieg G, Tagudar G, Miller LG. Body site colonization in patients with community-associated methicillin-resistant *Staphylococcus aureus* and other types of *S. aureus* skin infections. *Clin Microbiol Infect.* 2010;16:425-31.
14. Kluytmans, J, Van Belkum A, Verbrugh H. Nasal carriage of *Staphylococcus aureus*: epidemiology, underlying mechanisms, and associated risks. *Clin Microbiol Rev.* 1997;10:505-20.
15. Kuehnert MJ, Kruszon-Moran D, Hill HA, McQuillan G, McAllister SK, Fosheim G, et al. Prevalence of *Staphylococcus aureus* nasal colonization in the United States. *J Infect Dis.* 2006;193:172-9.
16. Charlebois ED, Bangsberg DR, Moss NJ, Moore MR, Moss AR, Chambers HF, et al. Population-based community prevalence of methicillin-resistant *Staphylococcus aureus* in the urban poor of San Francisco. *Clin Infect Dis.* 2002;34:425-33.
17. Charlebois ED, Perdreau-Remington F, Kreiswirth B, Bangsberg DR, Ciccarone D, Diep BA, et al. Origins of community strains of MRSA. *Clin Infect Dis.* 2004;39:47-54.
18. Bhattacharya D, Carleton H, Tsai CJ, Baron EJ, Perdreau-Remington F. Differences in clinical and molecular characteristics of skin and soft tissue MRSA isolates between two hospitals in northern California. *J Clin Microbiol.* 2007;45:1798-803.
19. Chen CJ, Hsu KH, Lin TY, Hwang KP, Chen PY, Huang YC. Factors associated with nasal colonization of methicillin-resistant *Staphylococcus aureus* among healthy children in Taiwan. *J Clin Microbiol.* 2011;49:131-7.
20. Eveillard M, Martin Y, Hidri N, Boussougant Y, Joly-Guillou M. Carriage of methicillin-resistant *Staphylococcus aureus* among hospital employees: prevalence, duration, and transmission to households. *Infect Control Hosp Epidemiol.* 2004;25:114-20.
21. Crum NF, Lee RU, Thornton MS, Stine OC, Wallace MR, Barrozo C, et al. Fifteen-year study of the changing epidemiology of MRSA. *Am J Med.* 2006;119:943-51.
22. Faden H, Ferguson S. Community-acquired methicillin-resistant *Staphylococcus aureus* and intrafamily spread of pustular disease. *Pediatr Infect Dis J.* 2001;20:554-5.
23. Helgason KO, Jones ME, Edwards G. Panton-Valentine leukocidin positive *Staphylococcus aureus* and foreign travel. *J Clin Microbiol.* 2007;46:832-3.
24. Cook HA, Furuya EY, Larson E, Vasquez G, Lowy FD. Heterosexual transmission of community-associated MRSA. *Clin Infect Dis.* 2007;44:410-3.
25. Tammelin A, Klötz F, Hambræus A, Ståhle E, Ransjö U. Nasal and hand carriage of *Staphylococcus aureus* in staff at a department for thoracic and cardiovascular surgery: endogenous or exogenous source? *Infect Control Hosp Epidemiol.* 2003;24:686-9.
26. Lescure FX, Locher G, Eveillard M, Biendo M, Van Agt S, Le Loup G, et al. Community-acquired infection with healthcare-associated MRSA: the role of nursing care. *Infect Control Hosp Epidemiol.* 2006;27:1213-8.
27. Cookson B, Peters B, Webster M, Phillips I, Rahman M, Noble W. Staff carriage of epidemic MRSA. *J Clin Microbiol.* 1989;27:1471-6.
28. Ellis MW, Hospenthal DR, Dooley DP, Gray PJ, Murray CK. Natural history of CAMRSA colonization and infection in soldiers. *Clin Infect Dis.* 2004;39:971-9.
29. Fritz SA, Epplin EK, Garbutt J, Storch GA. Skin infection in children colonized with community-associated MRSA. *J Infect.* 2009;59:394-401.
30. Centers for Disease Control and Prevention (CDC). MRSA among players on a high school football team—New York City, 2007. *MMWR Morb Mortal Wkly Rep.* 2009;58:52-5.
31. Centers for Disease Control and Prevention. MRSA infections among competitive sports participants—Colorado, Indiana, Pennsylvania, and Los Angeles County, 2000-2003. *MMWR Morb Mortal Wkly Rep.* 2003;52:793-5.
32. Nguyen DM, Mascola L, Bancroft E. Recurring methicillin-resistant *Staphylococcus aureus* infections in a football team. *Emerg Infect Dis.* 2005;11:526-32.
33. Romano R, Lu D, Holtom P. Outbreak of community-acquired MRSA skin infections among a collegiate football team. *J Athl Train.* 2006;41:141-5.
34. Yee-Guardino S, Kumar D, Abughali N, Tuohy M, Hall S, Kumar L. Recognition and treatment of neonatal CAMRSA pneumonia and bacteraemia. *Pediatr Pulm.* 2008;43:203-5.
35. Kaplan SL, Hulten KG, Gonzalez BE, Hammerman WA, Lamberth L, Versalovic J, et al. Three-year surveillance of CAMRSA in children. *Clin Infect Dis.* 2005;40:1785-91.
36. Szczesiul JM, Shermock KM, Murtaza UI, Siberry GK. No decrease in clindamycin susceptibility despite increased use of clindamycin for pediatric community-associated MRSA skin infections. *Pediatr Infect Dis J.* 2007;26:852-4.
37. Moran GJ, Krishnadasan A, Gorwitz RJ, Fosheim GE, McDougal LK, Carey RB, et al.; EMERGEncy ID Net Study Group. Methicillin-resistant *S. aureus* infections among patients in the emergency department. *N Engl J Med.* 2006;355:666-74.
38. Chambers HF. The changing epidemiology of *Staphylococcus aureus*? *Emerg Infect Dis.* 2001;7:178-82.
39. Otter JA, French GL Nosocomial transmission of community-associated methicillin-resistant *Staphylococcus aureus*: an emerging threat. *Lancet Infect Dis.* 2006;6:753-5.
40. Vidal M, Trindade A, Garcia O, Pacheco L, Costa F, Reinert C, et al. Differences between "classical" risk factors for infections caused by MRSA and risk factors for nosocomial bloodstream infections caused by multiple clones of the staphylococcal cassette chromosome mec type IV MRSA strain. *Infect Control Hosp Epidemiol.* 2009;30:139-45.

41. Park SH, Park C, Yoo JH, Choi SM, Choi JH, Shin HH, et al. Emergence of community-associated MRSA strains as a cause of healthcare-associated bloodstream infections in Korea. *Infect Control Hosp Epidemiol.* 2009;30:146-55.
42. Wang JT, Liao CH, Fang CT, Chie WC, Lai MS, Lauderdale T, et al. Incidence of and risk factors for community-associated MRSA acquired infection or colonization in intensive-care-unit patients. *J Clin Microbiol.* 2010;48:4439-44.
43. Thomas R, Ferguson J, Coombs G, Gibson PG. Community-acquired methicillin-resistant *Staphylococcus aureus* pneumonia: a clinical audit. *Respirology.* 2011;16:926-31.
44. Hayashi Y, Vaska VL, Baba H, Nimmo GR, Davis L, Paterson DL. Influenza-associated Bacterial Pathogens in Patients with 2009 Influenza A (H1N1) Infection: Impact of Community-Associated Methicillin Resistant *Staphylococcus aureus* (MRSA) in Queensland, Australia. *Intern Med J.* 2011.
45. Moran G, Krishnadasan A, Gorwitz RJ, Fosheim GE, Albrecht V, Limbaqo B, et al.; EMERGEncy ID NET Study Group. Prevalence of Methicillin-Resistant *Staphylococcus aureus* as an Etiology of Community-Acquired Pneumonia. *Clin Infect Dis.* 2012; 54:1126-33.
46. Poulakou G, Souto J, Kmet Lunanek N, Rello J. Pneumonia due to methicilin-resistant *Staphylococcus aureus* (MRSA): A review. *Curr Respir Med Rev.* 2012;8:245-58.
47. Kowalski TJ, Berbari EF, Osmon DR. Epidemiology, treatment, and prevention of community-acquired MRSA infections. *Mayo Clin Proc.* 2005;80:1201-7.
48. Tristan A, Bes M, Meugnier H, Lina G, Bozdogan B, Courvalin P, et al. Global distribution of Panton–Valentine leukocidin–positive methicillin-resistant *Staphylococcus aureus. Emerg Infect Dis.* 2006;13:594-600.
49. Tenover FC, McDougal LK, Goering VR, Killgore G, Projan SJ, Patel JB, et al. Characterization of a strain of community-associated methicillin-resistant *Staphylococcus aureus* widely disseminated in the United States. *J Clin Microbiol.* 2006;44:108-18.
50. Deresinski S. Methicillin-resistant *Staphylococcus aureus*: an evolutionary, epidemiologic and therapeutic Odyssey. *Clin Infect Dis.* 2005;40:562-73.
51. Baba T, Takeuchi F, Kuroda M, Yuzawa H, Aoki K, Oguchi A, et al. Genome and virulence determinants of high virulence community-acquired MRSA. *Lancet.* 2002;359:1819-27.
52. Eady EA, Cove JH. Staphylococcal resistance revisited: community-acquired methicillin resistant *Staphylococcus aureus*—an emerging problem for the management of skin and soft tissue infections. *Curr Opin Infect Dis.* 2003;16:103-24.
53. Cotter PA, Miller JF. *In vivo* and *ex vivo* regulation of bacterial virulence gene expression. *Curr Opin Microbiol.* 1998;1:17-26.
54. Novick P. Pathogenicity factors and their regulation. In: Fischetti A, Novick P, Ferretti J, Portnoy A, Rood I, editors. Gram-positive pathogens. Washington: ASM; 2000. pp. 392-407.
55. Gomes R, Vinga S, Zavolan M, de Lencastre H. Analysis of the genetic variability of virulence-related loci in epidemic clones of MRSA. *Antim Agents Chem.* 2005;49:366-79.
56. Boles R, Horswill R. *agr*-mediated dispersal of *Staphylococcus aureus* Biofilms. *PLoS Pathog.* 2008;25:4:e1000052.
57. Sakoulas G. The accessory gene regulator (*agr*) in MRSA: role in virulence and reduced susceptibility to glycopeptide antibiotics. *Drug Discov Today.* 2006;3:287-94.
58. Panton PN, Valentine FC. Staphylococcal toxin. *Lancet.* 1932;222:506-8.
59. Gillet Y, Vanhems P, Lina G, Bes M, Vandenesch F, Floret D, et al. Factors predicting mortality in necrotizing community-acquired pneumonia caused by *Staphylococcus aureus* containing Panton-Valentine leukocidin. *Clin Infect Dis.* 2007;45:315-21.
60. Lopez-Aguilar C, Perez-Roth E, Moreno A, Duran MC, Casanova C, Aguirre-Jaime A, et al. Association between the presence of the Panton–Valentine leukocidin-encoding gene and a lower rate of survival among hospitalized pulmonary patients with Staphylococcal disease. *J Clin Microbiol.* 2007;45:274-6.
61. Bubeck Wardenburg J, Bae T, Otto M, DeLeo FR, Schneewind O. Poring over pores: alpha-hemolysin and Panton-Valentine leukocidin in *Staphylococcus aureus* pneumonia. *Nat Med.* 2007;13:1405-6.
62. Vandenesch F, Naimi T, Enright MC, Lina G, Nimmo GR, Heffernan H, et al. Community-acquired methicillin-resistant *Staphylococcus aureus* carrying Panton–Valentine leukocidin genes: worldwide emergence. *Emerg Infect Dis.* 2003;9:978-84.
63. Wielders CL, Vriens MR, Brisse S, de Graaf-Miltenburg LA, Troelstra A, Fleer A, et al. *In vivo* transfer of *mecA* DNA to *Staphylococcus aureus. Lancet.* 2001;357:1674-5.
64. Klevens RM, Morrison MA, Nadle J, et al. Invasive methicillin-resistant *Staphylococcus aureus* infections in the United States. *JAMA.* 2007;298:1763-71.
65. Mendes RE, Sader HS, Deshpande LM, Diep BA, Chambers HF, Jones RN. Characterization of baseline methicillin-resistant *Staphylococcus aureus* isolates recovered from phase IV clinical trial for linezolid. *J Clin Microbiol.* 2010;48:568-74.
66. Gorwitz RJ, Jernigan DB, Powers JH, Jernigan JA and Participants in the CDC- Convened Experts' Meeting on Management of MRSA in the Community. Strategies for clinical management of MRSA in the community: summary of an experts' meeting convened by the CDC and Prevention. 2006. Available from: www.cdc.gov/mrsa/pdf/MRSA-Strategies-ExpMtgSummary-2006.pdf, July 2012.
67. Chua K, Laurent F, Coombs G, Grayson ML, Howden BP. Antimicrobial resistance: Not community-associated methicillin-resistant *Staphylococcus aureus* (CA-MRSA)! A clinician's guide to community MRSA - its evolving antimicrobial resistance and implications for therapy. *Clin Infect Dis.* 2011;52:99-114.
68. Chini V, Petinaki E, Meugnier H, Foka A, Bes M, Etienne J, et al. Emergence of a new clone carrying Panton-Valentine leukocidin genes and staphylococcal cassette chromosome mec type V among MRSA in Greece. *Scand J Infect Dis.* 2008;40:368-72.
69. Chini V, Petinaki E, Foka A, Paratiras S, Dimitracopoulos G, Spiliopoulou I. Spread of *Staphylococcus aureus* clinical isolates carrying Panton-Valentine leukocidin genes

during a 3-year period in Greece. *Clin Microbiol Infect.* 2006;12:29-34.
70. Otter JA, French GL. Molecular epidemiology of community-associated methicillin-resistant *Staphylococcus aureus* in Europe. *Lancet Infect Dis.* 2010;10:227-39.
71. Chi CY, Wong W, Fung P, Yu W, Liu Y. Epidemiology of community-acquired *Staphylococcus aureus* bacteremia. *J Microbiol Immunol Infect.* 2004;37:16-23.
72. Murray RJ, Robinson JQ, White JN, Hughes F, Coombs GW, Pearson JC, et al. Community-acquired pneumonia due to pandemic A(H1N1) 2009 influenza virus and methicillin-resistant *Staphylococcus aureus* co-infection. *PLoS One.* 2010;5:e8705.
73. Vidaur L, Planas K, Sierra R, Dimopoulos G, Ramirez A, Lisboa T, et al. Ventilator-associated pneumonia: impact of organisms on clinical resolution and medical resources utilization. *Chest.* 2008;133:625-32.
74. Vardakas KZ, Matthaiou DK, Falagas ME. Incidence, characteristics and outcomes of patients with severe community acquired-MRSA pneumonia. *Eur Respir J.* 2009;4:1148-58.
75. Nathwani D, Morgan M, Masterton RG, Dryden M, Cookson BD, French G, Lewis D; British Society for Antimicrobial Chemotherapy Working Party on Community-onset MRSA Infections. Guidelines for UK practice for the diagnosis and management of methicillin-resistant *Staphylococcus aureus* (MRSA) infections presenting in the community. *J Antim Chem.* 2008;61:976-94.
76. Barton-Forbes M, Hawkes M, Moore D, Conly J, Nicolle L, Allen U, et al. Guidelines for the prevention and management of community associated methicillin resistant *Staphylococcus aureus* (CA-MRSA): a perspective for Canadian health care practitioners. *Can. J Infect Dis Med Microbiol.* 2006;17:4C-24C.
77. Rubinstein E, Kollef MH, Nathwani D. Pneumonia caused by methicillin-resistant *Staphylococcus aureus. Clin Infect Dis.* 2008;46:S378-85.
78. Liu C, Bayer A, Cosgrove SE, Daum RS, Fridkin SK, Gorwitz RJ, et al. Infectious Diseases Society of America. Clinical Practice Guidelines by the Infectious Diseases Society of America for the Treatment of Methicillin-Resistant *Staphylococcus aureus* Infections in Adults and Children. *Clin Infect Dis.* 2011;52:e18-55.
79. Wargo K, Eliand E.. Appropriate antimicrobial therapy for community-acquired MRSA carrying the PVL genes. *Clin Infect Dis.* 2005;40:1376-8.
80. Steinkraus G, White R, Friedrich L. Vancomycin MIC creep in non-vancomycin-intermediate *Staphylococcus aureus* (VISA), vancomycin-susceptible clinical MRSA blood isolates from 2001-05. *J Antimicrob Chemother.* 2007;60:788-94.
81. Horne KC, Howden BP, Grabsch EA, Graham M, Ward PB, Xie S, et al. Prospective comparison of the clinical impacts of heterogeneous vancomycin-intermediate MRSA and vancomycin-susceptible MRSA. *Antimicr Agents Chem.* 2009;53:3447-52.
82. Bae IG, Federspiel JJ, Miro JM, Woods CW, Park L, Rybak MJ, et al. Heterogeneous vancomycin-intermediate susceptibility phenotype in bloodstream MRSA isolates from an international cohort of patients with infective endocarditis: prevalence, genotype, and clinical significance. *J Infect Dis.* 2009;200:1355-66.
83. Woodford N. Epidemiology of the genetic elements responsible for acquired glycopeptide resistance in enterococci. *Microb Drug Resist.* 2001;7:229-36.
84. Werner G, Coque M, Hammerum M, Hope R, Hryniewicz W, Johnson A, et al. Emergence and spread of vancomycin resistance among enterococci in Europe. *Euro Surveill.* 2008;13:pii: 19046.
85. Hiramatsu K. The emergence of *Staphylococcus aureus* with reduced susceptibility to vancomycin in Japan. *Am J Med.* 1998;104:75-105.
86. Liu C, Chambers H. *Staphylococcus aureus* with heterogeneous resistance to vancomycin: epidemiology, clinical significance, and critical assessment of diagnostic methods. *Antimicrob Agents Chemother.* 2003;47:3040-5.
87. Wysocki M, Delatour F, Faurisson F, Rauss A, Pean Y, Misset B, et al. Continuous versus intermittent infusion of vancomycin in severe Staphylococcal infections: prospective multicenter randomized study. *Antimicrob Agents Chemother.* 2001;45:2460-7.
88. Roberts JA, Taccone FS, Udy AA, Vincent JL, Jacobs F, Lipman J. Vancomycin dosing in critically ill patients: robust methods for improved continuous-infusion regimens. *Antimicrob Agents Chemother.* 2011; 55:2704-9.
89. Jeurissen A, Sluyts I, Rutsaert R. A higher dose of vancomycin in continuous infusion is needed in critically ill patients. *Int J Antimicrob Agents.* 2011;37:75-7.
90. Rybak MJ, Lomaestro BM, Rotschafer JC, Moellering RC, Craig WA, Billeter M et al. Vancomycin therapeutic guidelines: a summary of consensus recommendations from the infectious diseases Society of America, the American Society of Health-System Pharmacists, and the Society of Infectious Diseases Pharmacists. *Clin Infect Dis.* 2009;49:325-7.
91. Cataldo MA, Tacconelli E, Grilli E, Pea F, Petrosillo N. Continuous versus intermittent infusion of vancomycin for the treatment of Gram-positive infections: systematic review and meta-analysis. *J Antimicrob Chemother.* 2012;67:17-24.
92. Paterson DL. Clinical experience with recently approved antibiotics. *Curr Opin Pharmacol.* 2006;6:486-90.
93. Skrupky L, Micek S, Kollef M. Optimizing therapy for MRSA pneumonia. *Semin Respir Crit Care Med.* 2007;28: 615-23.
94. DeGiroami P, Eliopoulos G, Moellering R, Gold H. Linezolid resistance in sequential *Staphylococcus aureus* isolates associated with a T2500A mutation in the 23S rRNA gene and loss of a single copy of rRNA. *J Infect Dis.* 2004;190:311-7.
95. Markowitz N, Quinn L, Saravolatz L. Trimethoprim-sulfamethoxazole vs with vancomycin for the treatment of *Staphylococcus aureus* infection. *Ann Intern Med.* 1992;117:390-8.
96. Carpenter CF, Chambers HF. Daptomycin: another novel agent for treating infections due to drug-resistant Gram-positive pathogens. *Clin Infect Dis.* 2004;38: 994-1000.

97. Arbeit RD, Maki D, Tally FP, Campanaro E, Eisenstein BI and Daptomycin 90-01 and 99-01 Investigators. The safety and efficacy of daptomycin for the treatment of complicated skin and skin-structure infections. *Clin Infect Dis.* 2004;38:1673-81.
98. Stein G, Craig A. Tigecycline: a critical analysis. *Clin Infect Dis.* 2006;43:518-24.
99. Falagas ME, Karageorgopoulos D, Dimopoulos G. Clinical significance of the PK/PD characteristics of tigecycline. *Curr Drugs Metab.* 2009;10:13-21.
100. Zhanel G, Sniezek G, Schweizer F, Zelenitsky S, Lagace-Wiens P, Rubinstein E, et al. Ceftaroline: a novel broad-spectrum cephalosporin with activity against meticillin-resistant *Staphylococcus aureus. Drugs.* 2009;69:809-31.
101. Saravolatz L, Pawlak J, Johnson L. *In vitro* activity of ceftaroline against community-associated methicillin-resistant, vancomycin-intermediate, vancomycin-resistant, and daptomycin-nonsusceptible *Staphylococcus aureus* isolates. *Antimicrob Agents Chemother.* 2010;54:3027-30.
102. U.S. Department of Health & Human Services. FDA Approved Drug Products. Available from: http://www.accessdata.fda.gov/scripts/cder/drugsatfda/index.cfm?fuseaction=Search.DrugDetails. March 2012.
103. Rank DR, Friedland HD, Laudano JB. Integrated safety summary of FOCUS 1 and FOCUS 2 trials: Phase III randomized, double-blind studies evaluating ceftaroline fosamil for the treatment of patients with community-acquired pneumonia. *J Antimicrob Chemother.* 2011; 66:iii53-59.
104. Roecker A, Pope S. Dalbavancin: a lipoglycopeptide antibacterial for Gram-positive infections. *Expert Opin Pharmacother.* 2008;9:1745-54.
105. Charneski L, Patel P, Sym D. Telavancin: a novel lipoglycopeptide antibiotic. *Ann Pharmacother.* 2009;43:928-38.
106. Poulakou, G, Giamarellou H. Oritavancin: a new promising agent in the treatment of infections due to Gram-positive pathogens. *Expert Opin Invest Drugs.* 2008;17:225-43.
107. Van Bambeke F. Glycopeptides and glycodepsipeptides in clinical development: a comparative review of their antibacterial spectrum, pharmacokinetics and clinical efficacy. *Curr Opin Invest Drugs.* 2006;7:740-9.
108. Stryjewski ME, Graham DR, Wilson SE, O'Riordan W, Young D, Lentnek A, et al. Telavancin versus vancomycin for the treatment of complicated skin and skin-structure infections caused by gram-positive organisms. *Clin Infect Dis.* 2008; 46:1683-93.
109. Rubinstein E, Lalani T, Corey GR, Kanafani ZA, Nannini EC, Rocha MG, et al. ATTAIN Study Group. Telavancin versus vancomycin for hospital-acquired pneumonia due to gram-positive pathogens. *Clin Infect Dis.* 2011;52: 31-40.
110. European Medicines Agency. Human Medicines. Vibativ, telavancin. Available at: www.ema.europa.eu/ema/index.jsp?curl=pages/medicines/human/medicines/001240/human_med_001467.jsp&mid=WC0b01ac058001d124&jsenabled=true. March 2012.
111. European Medicines Agency. Press release 22 February 2012. European Medicines Agency gives final recommendations for 12 centrally authorised medicines manufactured at Ben Venue Laboratories. Available at: http://www.ema.europa.eu/docs/en_GB/document_library/Press_release/2012/02/WC500122877.pdf. July 2012.
112. Morrow J, He W, Amsler M, Foleno D, Macielag J, Lynch S, et al. *In vitro* antibacterial activities of JNJ-Q2, a new broad-spectrum fluoroquinolone. *Antimicrob Agents Chemother.* 2010;54:1955-64.
113. Kalia V, Miglani R, Purnapatre KP, Mathur T, Singhal S, Khan S, et al. Mode of action of Ranbezolid against staphylococci and structural modeling studies of its interaction with ribosomes. *Antimicrob Agents Chemother.* 2009;53:1427-33.
114. Micek T, Dunne M, Kollef M. Pleuropulmonary complications of PVL positive community-acquired methicillin-resistant *Staphylococcus aureus*: importance of treatment with antimicrobials inhibiting exotoxin production. *Chest.* 2005;128:2732-8.
115. Stevens L, Ma Y, Salmi D, McIndoo E, Wallace R, Bryant A. Impact of antibiotics on the expression of virulence-associated exotoxin genes in methicillin-sensitive and in methicillin-resistant *Staphylococcus aureus. J Infect Dis.* 2007;195:202-11.
116. Gould FK, Brindle R, Chadwick PR, Fraise AP, Hill S, Nathwani D, et al; MRSA Working Party of the British Society for Antimicrobial Chemotherapy. Guidelines for the prophylaxis and treatment of MRSA infections in the UK. *J Antimicrob Chemother.* 2009;63:849-61.
117. Furesz S: Chemical and biological properties of rifampin. *Antibiot Chemother.* 1970;16:316-51.
118. Wheat LJ, Kohler RB, Luft FC, White A. Long-term studies of the effect of rifampin on nasal carriage of coagulase-positive staphylococci. *Rev Infect Dis.* 1983;5:S459-62.
119. Vichyanond P, Oslan LC. Staphylococcal CNS infections with vancomycin and rifampin. *Arch Neurol.* 1984;41:637-9.
120. Tan TQ, Mason EO Jr, Ou CN, Kaplan SL. Use of intravenous rifampicin in neonates with persistent staphylococcal bacteraemia. *Antimicrob Agents Chemother.* 1993; 37:2401-6.
121. Jung YJ, Koh Y, Hong SB, Chung JW, Ho Choi S, Kim NJ, et al. Effect of vancomycin plus rifampicin in the treatment of nosocomial MRSA pneumonia. *Crit Care Med.* 2010; 38:175-80.
122. Reinhart K, Brunkhorst FM, Bone HG, Bardutzky J, Dempfle CE, Forst H, et al; German Sepsis Society; German Interdisciplinary Association of Intensive Care and Emergency Medicine. Prevention, diagnosis, therapy and follow-up care of sepsis: 1st revision of S-2k guidelines of the German Sepsis Society (Deutsche Sepsis-Gesellschaft e.V. (DSG)) and the German Interdisciplinary Association of Intensive Care and Emergency Medicine (Deutsche Interdisziplinäre Vereinigung für Intensiv- und Notfallmedizin (DIVI) GMS. *Ger Med Sci.* 2010;8:Doc14.
123. Li J, Udy A, Kirkpatrick M, Lipman J, Roberts JA. Improving vancomycin prescription in critical illness through a drug use evaluation process: a weight-based dosing intervention study. *Int J Antimicrob Agents.* 2011.
124. Wunderink RG, Niederman MS, Kollef MH, Shorr AF, Kunkel MJ, Baruch A, et al. Linezolid in methicillin-resistant *Staphylococcus aureus* nosocomial pneumonia:

a randomized, controlled study. *Clin Infect Dis.* 2012;54: 621-9.
125. Gauduchon V, Cozon G, Vandenesch F, Genestier AL, Eyssade N, Peyrol S, et al. Neutralization of *Staphylococcus aureus* Panton-Valentine leukocidin by intravenous immunoglobulin *in vitro*. *J Infect Dis.* 2004;189:346-53.
126. Muto A, Jernigan A, Ostrowsky E, Richet M, Jarvis R, Boyce M, Farr M. SHEA guideline for preventing nosocomial transmission of multidrug-resistant strains of *Staphylococcus aureus* and *Enterococcus*. *Infect Control Hosp Epidemiol.* 2003;24:362-86.
127. Graber J, Schwartz S. Failure of decolonization in patients with infections due to mupirocin-resistant strains of community-associated MRSA *Infect Control Hosp Epidemiol.* 2008;29:284.
128. Upton A, Lang S, Heffernan H. Mupirocin and *Staphylococcus aureus*: a recent paradigm of emerging antibiotic resistance. *J Antimicrob Chemother.* 2003;51:613-7.
129. Robbins B, Schneerson R, Horwith G, Naso R, Fattom A. *Staphylococcus aureus* types 5 and 8 capsular polysaccharide-protein conjugate vaccines. *Am Heart J.* 2004; 147:593-8.
130. Bubeck Wardenburg J, Schneewind O. Vaccine protection against *Staphylococcus aureus* pneumonia. *J Exp Med.* 2008;205:287-94.
131. Karginov VA, Nestorovich EM, Schmidtmann F, Robinson TM, Yohannes A, Fahmi NE, et al. Inhibition of S. aureus alpha-hemolysin and B. anthracis lethal toxin by beta-cyclodextrin derivatives. *Bioorg Med Chem.* 2007;15: 5424-31.
132. Ragle BE, Karginov VA, Bubeck Wardenburg J. Prevention and treatment of *Staphylococcus aureus* pneumonia with a beta-cyclodextrin derivative. *Antimicrob Agents Chemother.* 2010;54:298-304.

CHAPTER 7

Acute Exacerbations of Chronic Bronchitis and Chronic Obstructive Pulmonary Disease

Zinka Matkovic, Marc Miravitlles

ABSTRACT

Acute exacerbations are frequent events in the course of chronic bronchitis and chronic obstructive pulmonary disease (COPD). Individuals with these conditions may suffer a mean of 1–3 episodes/year, some of which lead to hospital admission and may even be a cause of death. The importance of exacerbations of COPD has become increasingly apparent due to the impact of these episodes on the natural history of the disease. It is now known that frequent exacerbations can adversely affect a patient's health-related quality of life and short- and long-term pulmonary function. Costs associated with exacerbations are high, particularly due to relapses and admissions. Advanced age, severe lung function impairment, respiratory insufficiency, and comorbidity are some of the risk factors for frequent exacerbations in COPD.

Bronchial infection is the main cause of exacerbations, but the problem in defining the microbial etiology of a COPD exacerbation is that a great proportion of these patients have bacteria colonizing their lower airways in the stable phase of the disease. However, some studies clearly suggest that the bacterial burden increases during exacerbations, and recent findings indicate that acquisition of new strains of bacteria or antigenic changes in the pre-existing ones are associated with an increased risk of developing an exacerbation. Sputum color has proved to be useful in differentiating infectious from non-infectious exacerbations. Antibiotic treatment of exacerbations must take into account the microorganisms most likely to be the causative agents and their patterns of resistance. Besides antibiotics, systemic corticosteroids and inhaled bronchodilators are mainstay in the treatment of exacerbations.

Optimizing treatment for stable COPD will help to reduce exacerbations. Non-pharmacological interventions such as rehabilitation, self-management plans, and maintaining high levels of physical activity in daily life are useful strategies to prevent exacerbations in patients with COPD.

INTRODUCTION

Chronic lung diseases, particularly chronic bronchitis and chronic obstructive pulmonary disease (COPD), are one of the main causes of morbidity and mortality in developed countries. It is estimated that more than 15 million persons in the US have COPD, and more than 12 million have chronic bronchitis[1] with this numbers having grown over recent decades. The age-adjusted mortality rate from COPD doubled from 1970 to 2002 in the US, whereas rates from stroke and heart disease decreased by 63% and 52%, respectively.[2]

The prevalence of COPD in Spain is 10.2% in adults between 40 and 80 years of age, although only 24% are diagnosed.[3] Regarding chronic bronchitis, an international survey showed that up to 11.8% of subjects aged between 20 and 44 years had chronic bronchitis,[4] which is remarkable considering the young age of the participants. In addition, there has been a change in the characteristics of chronic respiratory patients. Traditionally, chronic bronchitis and COPD were considered diseases of males, but after women started smoking in the 50s and 60s, the prevalence of obstructive lung diseases increased dramatically in women. Nowadays, the mortality due to COPD in women equals that of men in some developed countries.[5]

The chronic and progressive course of COPD is often aggravated by short periods of increasing symptoms, particularly increasing cough, dyspnea, and production of sputum that can become purulent. Exacerbations have demonstrated to accelerate lung function decline and to have a negative impact on the quality of life of patients with COPD.[6-8] Furthermore, acute exacerbations are the most frequent cause of medical visits, hospital admissions, and death among patients with chronic lung disease.[9]

DEFINITION AND FREQUENCY OF EXACERBATIONS

Exacerbations are frequent events in the natural history of patients with chronic bronchitis and COPD. Patients included in clinical trials had a mean of 1–3 exacerbations/year.[10] In an observational study performed in the community, patients had a mean of 2 episodes/year, this number being dependent on the degree of functional impairment at baseline. Patients with forced expiratory volume in 1 second (FEV_1) below 40%, presented 2.3 exacerbations/year and those with FEV_1 above 60% had only 1.6 exacerbations.[11] It is important to underline that many exacerbations remain unreported to the physician (up to two thirds) because they are underestimated by the patient or self-treated at home.[7,12] As a consequence, the frequency of exacerbations depends on the definition used. Studies using diary cards and symptom-based definition provide higher estimates than those following a healthcare use approach and event-based definition of an exacerbation.[13]

Unfortunately, there is no diagnostic test or biological marker that would be self-sufficient to confirm the diagnosis of an exacerbation. In an attempt to select the best biomarker of COPD exacerbation among 36 candidates, Hurst et al.[14] identified C-reactive protein (CRP) as the most selective one, although it was neither sufficiently sensitive nor specific alone, and clinical symptoms provided the best aid in the diagnosis. Serum amyloid A is a possible biomarker of exacerbation identified in recent proteomic studies. It has demonstrated good discrimination between stable and exacerbated states and was significantly better than CRP in determination of exacerbation severity.[15] New, multicenter studies should provide insight into its usefulness in clinical practice.

In an attempt to establish a uniform definition of exacerbation to be used as an outcome measure in clinical trials, the European Respiratory Society (ERS) and the American Thoracic Society (ATS) task force defined exacerbation as an increase in patient's baseline dyspnea, cough, and/or sputum that usually require a change in therapy.[16] It is clear that the increase in respiratory symptoms is a key to identify a COPD exacerbation and no biomarker or physiologic measure can help us yet in the early recognition of its onset. The most important concern in the diagnostic procedure is to exclude alternative diagnosis, since some other cardiopulmonary conditions such as pneumonia and congestive heart failure may provoke an increase in respiratory symptoms in a patient with COPD, which may be easily misdiagnosed as COPD exacerbation.

It is of note that the frequency of exacerbations increases with age and severity of functional impairment.[17-20] Documenting exacerbations through the use of diary cards in a group of 132 patients during almost 3 years, Donaldson et al.[19] have found that patients with severe COPD (FEV_1 <30% predicted) experienced exacerbations more frequently (3.43/year) in comparison to those with moderate disease (FEV_1 >30% and <80% predicted; 2.68/year). Interestingly, the annual exacerbation frequency remained constant throughout the study period, although physiologic and clinical recovery from exacerbations was significantly longer each year.[19] This suggests that the frequent exacerbators have particular characteristics that make them prone to develop recurrent episodes. In a very recent study by Hurst et al.[20] who followed 2,138 COPD patients over 3 years, it was demonstrated again that exacerbations become more frequent when lung function is severely impaired, but frequent exacerbators (patients with ≥2 exacerbations annually) can be found with lower frequency among milder patients as well. There is a group of patients especially susceptible to exacerbations, the so-called frequent exacerbators, in whom main characteristic is the history of previous exacerbations.[20]

OUTCOMES OF EXACERBATIONS AND RISK FACTORS OF ADVERSE OUTCOMES

The most severe exacerbations, those requiring hospital management, have an independent negative impact on patient prognosis and health status.[21] The mortality of patients hospitalized for COPD exacerbation is 2–11%, up to 24% for those admitted to an intensive care unit (ICU), while the mortality in the first year after discharge

TABLE 1

Risk Factors for Frequent COPD Exacerbations, Hospital Admission, Mortality, and Relapse/Readmission[17-37]

Risk factors for frequent COPD exacerbations (>2/year)	Risk factors for hospital admission	Risk factors for mortality during or after hospitalization for COPD exacerbations	Risk factors for relapse/ readmission
• Older age • Lower FEV_1 • Frequent past exacerbation of COPD • Chronic bronchial mucus hypersecretion • Bronchitic symptoms	• Older age • Lower FEV_1 • High admission rate for previous exacerbation of COPD • Comorbidity • Under-prescription of LTOT • Lack or reduction in physical activity	• Older age • Lower FEV_1 • Frequent past exacerbation of COPD/admissions for exacerbation of COPD • Comorbidity • Need for LTOT • Hypoxemia and/or hypercapnia at admission • Cor pulmonale • Hypoalbuminemia • Lower BMI • Increasing dyspnea	• Older age • Lower FEV_1 • Frequent past exacerbations of COPD/ admissions for exacerbation of COPD • Comorbidity, especially cardiopulmonary • Need for LTOT • Hypercapnia • Frequent previous visits to the general practitioner for respiratory problems • Increasing baseline dyspnea • Poor health-related quality of life

COPD, chronic obstructive pulmonary disease; FEV_1, forced expiratory volume in 1 second; LTOT, long-term oxygen therapy; BMI, body mass index.

is as high as 22–43%.[21-33] Some of the most frequently identified predictors of mortality in hospitalized COPD patients are advanced age, lower FEV_1, acute or chronic respiratory failure, comorbidity, cor pulmonale, previous exacerbations and admissions, severity of dyspnea, and lower body mass index (BMI).[21-33] Readmissions after hospitalization for an exacerbation are frequent, ranging from 14 to 16% in the first month after discharge and 25–58% in the first year, with the same predictors as previously mentioned for mortality.[26,27,34-37]

Hospitalizations are crucial events in the course of COPD. In a population-based study, including 20,571 participants with different degree of lung function impairment and 10 years of median follow-up, it has been shown that the risk for COPD-related hospitalizations was the highest in patients with severe and very severe COPD. But at the same time, COPD-related hospitalizations increased the risk of all-cause mortality in all patients irrespective of the severity of the disease.[38]

After the first admission to hospital, the mean survival time has been estimated to be 5.7 years, with COPD together with lung cancer being the main causes of death.[39] Patients with severe disease, with a mean FEV_1 of only 0.8 L, admitted for an exacerbation and hypercapnia, presented a poor prognosis with a mortality of 11% during admission and almost 50% during the first 2 years after hospitalization.[23] Almagro et al.[24] followed a cohort of 135 patients with COPD after being discharged from hospital for an exacerbation and found that 22%, 36%, and 44% died after 1, 2, and 2 and a half years of follow-up, respectively. Besides clinical variables, other newly recognized factors such as quality of life, depressive symptoms, and marital status (living alone) were significantly associated with a reduced survival.[24]

A summary of risk factors for frequent exacerbations, hospital admission, mortality, and relapse/readmission are presented in table 1.

ETIOLOGY OF EXACERBATIONS

Published data suggest that approximately 70% of exacerbations are caused by respiratory infections, including bacteria (40–60%), respiratory viruses (about 30%), and atypical bacteria (5–10%).[40,41] Some investigators have demonstrated polymicrobial etiology in as much as 33% of exacerbations, being particularly important in the most severe cases.[42,43] In patients with a mean age of 70 years admitted to hospital for an exacerbation of COPD, viral, and/or bacterial infection was detected in as high as 78% of cases and more importantly, patients with infective exacerbations had a more severe clinical course demonstrated by a more marked impairment in lung function and longer hospitalization.[42] Despite the importance of infection, other factors may as well provoke the exacerbations.[43] Environmental factors, including low temperature and air pollution (exposure to increased concentrations of black smoke particulate matter, sulphur dioxide, nitrogen dioxide, and ozone) are considered causative for approximately, 10% of exacerbations, depending on season and geographical settings.[44-46] Furthermore, noncompliance with respiratory medication and/or abrupt withdrawal of therapy is responsible for the onset of some exacerbations.[47] Multifactor etiology is not uncommon, e.g., a combination of infective and environmental factors or already mentioned polymicrobial infections.[42,43,49] However, in certain proportion of exacerbations, the etiology remains unknown. A summary of the main causes of exacerbations of COPD, including most important microbial pathogens are presented in table 2.

Concerning bacterial exacerbations, until recently, the accepted gold standard for bacterial etiology of COPD exacerbations has been the isolation of a potentially pathogenic microorganism in sputum during the episode. However, sputum cultures have several limitations. Sputum mostly comes from large airways and is often contaminated by upper airways microbial flora. Additionally, it has been demonstrated that sputum cultures may yield false negative results. In the classic study by Austrian and Gold,[50] *S. pneumoniae* was absent from the sputum in a quarter of the patients with pneumococcal pneumonia whose etiology was unequivocally proven by the presence of bacteremia. Similarly, up to 60% of cases of community-acquired pneumonia (CAP) are classified as caused by an unidentified pathogen even with the aid of invasive diagnostic techniques, such as bronchoscopic protected specimen brush sampling but, no doubt, is raised as to the infectious origin. Furthermore, Murphy et al.[51] observed the presence of bacteria by using polymerase chain reaction (PCR) to detect strain-specific *H. influenzae* DNA in some sputum samples that yielded negative cultures, thus, demonstrating that sputum cultures underestimate the presence of bacteria in sputum in COPD patients. Since bronchoscopic sampling of distal respiratory secretions as well as utilization of nonculture-based techniques, such as PCR in the routine clinical practice is very unpractical and costly, the physicians are facing a lot of difficulties in obtaining a specific microbiologic diagnosis in the respiratory infections in general, thus, making the prescription of antibiotic treatment empirical. Therefore, clinical criteria must be used to aid in the assessment of bacterial etiology of an exacerbation and decision on antibiotic therapy. With the current knowledge, the presence of green or yellow (purulent) sputum as opposed to white (mucoid) is one of the best and easiest methods of predicting a high bacterial load in respiratory tract secretions and the need for antibiotic therapy.[52,53] In a study by Stockley et al.,[52] the presence of green sputum was 94.4% sensitive and 77.0% specific for the yield of a high bacterial load and indicates a clear subset of episodes identified at presentation that is likely to benefit most from antibiotic therapy. In addition, when antibiotic therapy is effective in reducing the bacterial load associated with exacerbation, the color of sputum returns to the baseline, usually white appearance.[54] The production of purulent sputum is a surrogate marker for exaggerated bronchial inflammation associated with the presence of bacterial pathogens in increasing concentrations, both in exacerbated as well as in clinically stable COPD.[55-57] Findings in sputum have been validated using the protected specimen brush (PSB) in a population of exacerbated COPD patients.[58] With good quality sputum samples, the concordance between PSB and sputum cultures was high and self-reporting of sputum purulence was a good predictor of bacterial infection in the distal airways.[58]

TABLE 2

Etiology of COPD Exacerbations[40-49]

Infectious etiology
(accounting for approximately, 70% of all exacerbations)

- Aerobic bacteria (40–60%)
  - Frequently isolated bacteria: *Haemophilus* spp. especially nontypeable *H. influenzae, Streptococcus pneumoniae,* and *Moraxella catarrhalis*
  - Bacteria associated with advanced disease and special risk factors: *Pseudomonas aeruginosa,* members of Enterobacteriaceae family (*Escherichia coli, Proteus mirabilis, Klebsiella pneumoniae, Serratia marcescens, Enterobacter cloacae*), and *Stenotrophomonas maltophilia*
  - Others: *Staphylococcus aureus*
- Viruses (~30%)
  - Frequently detected viruses: picornavirus (especially rhinovirus), influenza, respiratory syncytial virus
  - Infrequently detected viruses: coronavirus, parainfluenza, adenovirus, human metapneumovirus
- Atypical bacteria (5–10%)
  - *Chlamydophila pneumoniae, Mycoplasma pneumoniae, Legionella* spp.
- Polymicrobial infection (20–30%)

Noninfectious etiology
(accounting for 20–40% of all exacerbations)

- Environmental factors (~10%)
  - Cold air
  - Air pollution (black smoke particulate matter, sulfur dioxide, nitrogen dioxide, and ozone)
  - Allergens
- Therapeutical issues
  - Noncompliance with respiratory medication
  - Abrupt withdrawal of respiratory medication

Multifactor etiology

Unknown etiology

The use of biomarkers to differentiate between bacterial and nonbacterial COPD exacerbations and to guide antibiotic therapy has been an area of intense research.[59,60] Since procalcitonin is a relatively specific marker of invasive bacterial infections like pneumonia and sepsis,[61,62] it was expected that it might be useful in discrimination of bacterial exacerbations of COPD as well. Although there is some evidence in favor of procalcitonin,[63] more recent studies give advantage to the CRP as a better biomarker in selection of bacterial exacerbations and patients likely to benefit from antibiotic therapy with consequent reduction in antibiotic overuse.[64] In the study by Daniels et al.[64] in patients with probable bacterial exacerbations, serum levels of procalcitonin were low in the majority (75%) of cases, while CRP was elevated in 83% and higher in the presence of bacteria. The most likely explanation is that in the bacterial exacerbations, mucosal airway infection triggers a local and systemic inflammatory response with subsequent rise in CRP and other acute-phase reactants, but since in most cases there is no invasion of bacteria into the bloodstream, the major stimulus for procalcitonin production is lacking.[64] On the other hand, for identification of viral exacerbations, especially, most frequent human rhinovirus (HRV) associated exacerbations, the most promising biomarker is interferon (IFN)-γ-inducible protein (IP)-10 since its serum concentration rises significantly in HRV-positive exacerbations and correlates with sputum HRV load.[65]

An additional problem in defining the microbial etiology of a COPD exacerbation is that a great proportion of COPD patients have potentially pathogenic microorganisms colonizing their lower airways in the stable phase of the disease. Patients with COPD present significant impairment in lung defence mechanisms, which enables proliferation of potentially pathogenic microorganisms in their bronchial secretions. Different species can be found as colonisers; however, nontypeable *H. influenzae* is the most frequent bacterium found in distal airways of patients with COPD, both in stable periods as well as in exacerbations.[66,67] *H. influenzae* has also been detected intracellularly in bronchial biopsy specimens of patients with COPD, but more frequently during exacerbations than during stable disease.[68] The same pathogen has been detected diffusely in the lung tissue (bronchial and bronchiolar epithelium and submucosa, interstitium, alveolar epithelium, alveoli, and visceral pleura) of patients with end-stage COPD, thus, suggesting a relationship in the pathogenesis of the disease that has yet to be completely understood.[69] The relationship between bronchial colonization and the evolution of COPD has been shown in a study by Wilkinson et al.[70] who observed that patients with higher bronchial bacterial loads and those experiencing changes in colonizing bacterial type over time, presented a faster decline in lung function during a 1-year follow-up.

One of the main mechanisms that explain the onset of an exacerbation is the acquisition of a new strain of bacteria in the lower airways or antigenic changes in the preexisting ones.[71] There is evidence that a change in a strain of most important potentially pathogenic micro-organisms (*H. influenzae, S. pneumoniae, M. catarrhalis, and P. aeruginosa*) leads to the increased bronchial and systemic inflammation and consequently to the development of symptoms of exacerbation.[71-73]

Studies in patients with exacerbations treated in the community[66,74] have shown that around half of these patients have bacteria in their lower airways and that the predominant microorganisms are nontypeable *H. influenzae, S. pneumoniae,* and *M. catarrhalis.* In contrast, studies in patients with the most severe exacerbations requiring mechanical ventilation [mean FEV_1 (% predicted) of 30%][43,75] have shown that the role of these microorganisms is less important and that other bacteria, such as *P. aeruginosa* and enteric Gram-negative bacilli (e.g., *Escherichia coli, Proteus mirabilis, Klebsiella pneumoniae, Serratia marcescens, and Enterobacter cloacae*) may be more frequent. Other observations have shown that the severity of COPD measured by the FEV_1 is an important determinant of the type of microorganism.[76-78] *P.aeruginosa* and enteric Gram-negative bacteria appear more frequently in patients with the most severely impaired lung function (usually FEV_1<35% predicted), with other important risk factors for their isolation being antibiotic therapy within the past three months and the use of systemic corticosteroids.[76-78]

The definition of risk factors for *P. aeruginosa* infection is a potentially important issue because of the difference in the preferred antibiotic treatment and the risk of unfavorable evolution if antipseudomonal antibiotics are not given very early.[43,79] Different studies in the literature[53,76-78,80,81] have identified some of the risk factors associated with *P. aeruginosa* infection (Table 3).

Overall, the percentage of *Pseudomonas* infection is around 10–15% in series of patients with COPD exacerbations with a FEV_1 lower than 50% and requiring hospitalization, and this percentage is increased in patients admitted to ICU needing mechanical ventilation.[43,79] There is certain proportion of COPD patients who develop persistent or chronic bronchial infection with *P. aeruginosa*[73,83] and their isolates have distinct characteristics, similar to those found in patients with cystic fibrosis (CF), e.g., coexistence of isolates with different morphotypes and antibiotic susceptibility, high

TABLE 3

Risk Factors for *Pseudomonas aeruginosa* Infection in COPD

Reference	Risk factors
Allegra et al.[53]	FEV_1 <35%
Eller et al.[76]	FEV_1 <35%
	Pretreatment with antibiotics
Miravitlles et al.[77]	FEV_1 <50%
Lode et al.[78]	FEV_1 <35%
	Use of systemic corticosteroids
	Antibiotics in the previous 3 months
Monsó et al.[80]	Low FEV_1
	Use of oral corticosteroids
	Antibiotics in the previous 3 months
	Protective effect of anti-influenza vaccine
García-Vidal et al.[81]	Use of systemic corticosteroids
	Poor BODE index
	Hospital admissions in the previous year
	Previous isolation of *P. aeruginosa*

COPD, chronic obstructive pulmonary disease; FEV_1, forced expiratory volume in 1 second; BODE,[82] body mass index (B), airflow obstruction (O), severity of dyspnea (D), exacerbation capacity (E).

prevalence of hypermutable strains, increased biofilm production, reduced production of virulence factors, and increased antibiotic resistance rate.[83] The incidence of infections caused by multiresistant *P. aeruginosa* (MDRP) is increasing, especially in critically ill patients. Patients hospitalized for COPD exacerbation who have MDRP isolated from sputum have higher mortality in comparison to patients without isolation of MDRP.[84]

However, the issue of *P. aeruginosa* in COPD exacerbations is far from clear, and no study has investigated whether specific treatment for *P. aeruginosa* on the basis of risk factors (as opposed to isolation of the organism) influences the outcome.

Viruses account for approximately 30% of exacerbations, either alone or as copathogens, with most frequent being picornavirus (especially rhinovirus), influenza virus (prevalence rate depends on vaccination status of population), and respiratory syncytial virus (RSV).[85,86] In a systematic review on prevalence of viral infection in COPD exacerbations,[85] which included 8 studies using PCR and/or reverse transcription PCR for detection of viruses in respiratory secretions (sputum, nasal lavage fluid), weighted mean prevalence of respiratory viral infection was 34%, while in one included study, the prevalence was as high as 56%.[86] In a more recent study, including hospitalized COPD exacerbations, upper respiratory viral infections were detected in 51% of patients, compared with only 11% of them after recovery.[87] The causal relationship between upper respiratory viral infection and COPD exacerbations has been demonstrated by Mallia et al.[88] in a study with experimental rhinovirus infection in COPD patients and healthy subjects. After being infected with rhinovirus, COPD patients developed more severe and prolonged respiratory symptoms, greater lung function impairment, and increased airway inflammation, thus, resembling naturally occurring exacerbations.[88] Considering the clinical presentation, viral exacerbations have been associated with more severe respiratory symptoms, higher rate of additional symptoms (cold, sore throat, increased dyspnea, and fever), slower recovery, and frequent previous exacerbations.[89] Viral infection may facilitate subsequent bacterial infection or increase the number of bacteria already present in the lower airways.[49] Coinfection with viruses and bacteria can be found in 20–30% of hospitalized COPD exacerbations, being particularly important in severe cases.[42,43] Although the viral infection itself may be self-limiting, secondary bacterial infection may prolong the course of an exacerbation.[42,90]

Atypical bacteria (e.g., *Chlamydophila pneumoniae, Mycoplasma pneumonia, Legionella* spp. etc.) are intracellular pathogens that share some characteristics of viruses, but their role in the pathogenesis of COPD exacerbations is less clear. According to published literature, they contribute to the occurrence of 5–10% of exacerbations, either as independent pathogens or more frequently as copathogens.[40,41]

NON-ANTIMICROBIAL TREATMENT OF EXACERBATIONS

Treatment of exacerbations should provide symptomatic relief, prevent transient loss of pulmonary function that may lead to hospitalization and ensure re-evaluation of the disease in a particular patient to determine if the risk of future exacerbations can be reduced. Pharmacological treatment aims at decreasing the work of breathing, reducing airway inflammation, reducing the bacterial burden in the lower airways, and treating any accompanying hypoxemia.[91] An algorithm for ambulatory treatment of exacerbations is shown in figures 1 and 2.

A patient with an exacerbation of COPD must be evaluated for severity to decide if treatment can be ambulatory or hospital assessment is required (Figure 2). Indications for hospital assessment are presented in table 4.

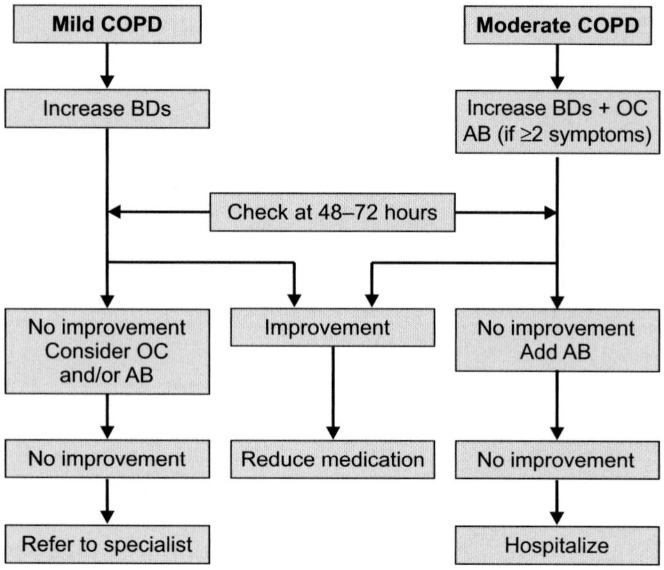

BD, bronchodilator; OC, oral corticosteroid; AB, antibiotic.

FIGURE 1 Algorithm of ambulatory treatment of exacerbations of chronic obstructive pulmonary disease (COPD) in patients with mild or moderate disease.

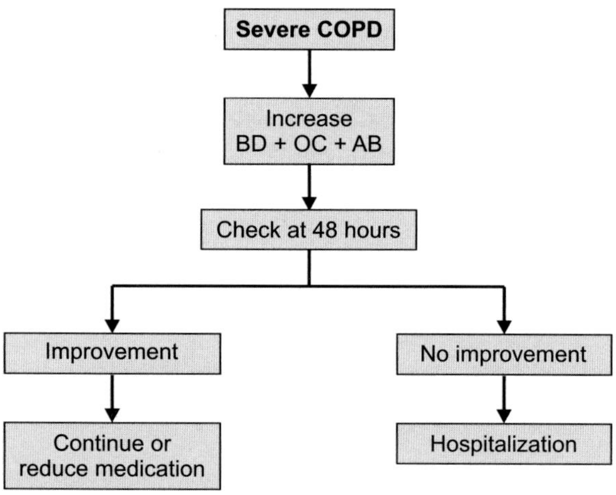

BD, bronchodilator; OC, oral corticosteroid; AB, antibiotic.

FIGURE 2 Algorithm of ambulatory treatment of exacerbations of chronic obstructive pulmonary disease (COPD) in patients with severe COPD.

Short-acting inhaled β2 agonists are usually the preferred bronchodilators for treatment of exacerbations of COPD. If clinical response is insufficient, the addition of a short-acting anticholinergic is recommended. The role of methylxantines in exacerbations is still controversial. The beneficial effect of these drugs in patients admitted for an exacerbation of COPD has not been clearly demonstrated.[93] However, the detrimental effect of withdrawal of methylxantines has been described in patients who were chronically treated with these drugs. Therefore, for patients who are already on an oral methylxantine product, it is reasonable to continue the medication during the exacerbation.[91] It is important to keep the frequent side effects associated with the use of methylxantines in mind as well as the possibility of drug interactions with antibiotics, such as ciprofloxacin and clarithromycin.

TABLE 4

Indications for Hospital Assessment or Admission for Exacerbations of COPD

- Marked increase in intensity of symptoms or change in vital signs
- Severe underlying COPD
- Onset of new physical signs (cyanosis, peripheral edema)
- Failure to respond to initial treatment
- Significant comorbidities (cardiac disease, chronic liver or renal failure)
- Newly occurring arrhythmias
- Diagnostic uncertainty
- Insufficient home support

COPD, chronic obstructive pulmonary disease.

A short course of oral corticosteroids has been demonstrated to accelerate recovery from exacerbation and reduce the rate of relapse in patients with moderate-to-severe COPD.[94-96] Multiple different dose regimens have been proposed and no standard regimen exists. Patients can be treated with 0.5 mg/kg/day of methylprednisolone or equivalent in a single morning dose for 7–14 days. Treatment for more than 14 days has not demonstrated to be of more benefit and increases the likelihood of adverse side effects.[94-96]

Patients with COPD are at risk of developing hypoxemia during an exacerbation. Low-flow oxygen should be administered with the goal of maintaining a partial pressure of oxygen in the arterial blood at or just above 60 mmHg. The use of noninvasive ventilation has been demonstrated to reduce mortality and decrease the need for intubation and mechanical ventilation.[92]

ANTIMICROBIAL TREATMENT OF EXACERBATIONS OF CHRONIC OBSTRUCTIVE PULMONARY DISEASE

Antibiotic treatment is based on 4 premises:

- The probability of a bacterial etiology of the exacerbation, almost always based on the clinical symptoms at presentation
- The severity of the underlying pulmonary disease, which is related to the likelihood of bacterial infection and the presence of more aggressive microorganisms during exacerbations

- The presence of risk factors for treatment failure or relapse that indicate the need for more aggressive therapy
- The patterns of resistance to antibiotics of the micro-organisms involved in the exacerbations.[97]

Placebo-controlled trials involving small numbers of patients have provided conflicting evidence on the efficacy of antibiotics in exacerbations of chronic bronchitis and COPD. However, a meta-analysis of 9 placebo-controlled trials concluded that, overall, there was a small but significant benefit from antibiotic treatment of COPD exacerbations in terms of recovery and change in peak flow.[98] A more recent meta-analysis has demonstrated an improvement in survival in moderate to severe COPD patients treated with antibiotics compared to placebo.[99]

The study by Anthonisen et al.[100] developed a classification system to identify patients more likely to have bacterial exacerbations based on the presentation of clinical symptoms. A type I exacerbation was characterized by the increasing dyspnea, sputum volume and purulence. A type II exacerbation included two of these symptoms, while a type III exacerbation included only one symptom together with at least one additional finding including sore throat or nasal discharge within the past five days, fever, increased wheezing, increased cough, or a 20% increase in respiratory rate or heart rate as compared with baseline. Patients exhibiting type I or II exacerbations obtained significant benefit from antimicrobial therapy, while outcomes in those with a type III exacerbation did not differ from patients receiving placebo.

In another well-designed placebo-controlled trial with a large number of patients with moderate to severe COPD, Allegra et al.[101] demonstrated the clear superiority of amoxicillin/clavulanate to placebo. Superiority in clinical efficacy was demonstrated especially for patients with severe disease, but to a lower extent also for milder disease. There is no doubt as to the importance of the prescription of antibiotics in severe exacerbated COPD patients. A recent placebo-controlled study in mechanically ventilated patients with an exacerbation demonstrated a reduction in mortality with the use of a quinolone compared to placebo.[102] On the other hand, patients with acute bronchitis, i.e., without baseline airflow obstruction, and those without chronic bronchial disease, who present with acute onset of respiratory symptoms such as cough with expectoration, should not receive antibiotics, particularly, if sputum is mucoid.[52,55] Most of these cases of acute bronchitis are of viral etiology, occur in young adults without risk factors, and are self-limiting.[103]

The Canadian guidelines were the first to adapt an approach based on risk factors for poor outcome and the most likely pathogens involved. Their latest edition incorporates the new research on risk factors and etiology of exacerbations and stratifies the patients according to the severity of the baseline pulmonary disease.[91] In their approach, the guidelines do not focus exclusively on patients with COPD, but rather on patients with symptoms of lower, non-pneumonic, respiratory infection. The guidelines cover the entire spectrum, from patients without underlying lung disease to patients with severe COPD and bronchiectasis. According to the Canadian guidelines, the classification system divides patients into 4 groups. Group 0 includes patients without chronic bronchial or pulmonary disease. Group 1 patients have exacerbated chronic bronchitis with worsening cough and increased sputum production that can be purulent but without risk factors of poor outcome. Group 2 includes patients with complicated chronic bronchitis and most patients with COPD belong to this group. Patients tend to be older and have risk factors for treatment failure, such as poor underlying lung function (FEV_1 <50% predicted) (see Table 1). Group 3 patients suffer from chronic bronchial infection with daily production of purulent secretions. They are subject to frequent exacerbations characterized by increased sputum production, sputum purulence, cough, and worsening dyspnea.

As mentioned by the investigators, this stratification scheme had not been prospectively validated, but summarized the best published evidence on the treatment of bronchial infections.[91] It is important to mention that the classification and therapeutic recommendations are based on the prevalence of pathogens and patterns of resistance that apply to Canada. Local patterns of resistance should guide antibiotic therapy in any given territory. As an example, the high degree of penicillin-resistant *S. pneumoniae* in some European countries, such as Spain and France, together with the high prevalence of macrolide-resistant *H. influenzae,* implies that fluoroquinolones or high-dose amoxicillin-clavulanic acid are preferred options instead of cephalosporins or macrolides in these countries. Supporting this approach, a recent meta-analysis indicated that not all antibiotics provide the same clinical outcome. Second-line antibiotics (amoxicillin/clavulanic acid, macrolides, second- or third generation cephalosporins, and quinolones) were more effective compared with first-line agents (amoxicillin, ampicillin, pivampicillin, trimethoprim/sulfamethoxazole, and doxycycline).[104] A recent randomized double-blind clinical trial comparing moxifloxacin with amoxicillin/clavulanate in COPD patients with risk factors of failure demonstrated superiority of moxifloxacin in the subgroup of patients with positive sputum culture at initiation of therapy, with significantly better eradication rates at the end of therapy (66.1% vs. 58.8%; p = 0.026) and higher cure rate at 8 weeks post-therapy (81% vs. 74.6%; p = 0.016).[105] In addition, there was a significant prolongation to the time to the clinical failure or relapse with moxifloxacin compared to amoxicillin-clavulanate (p = 0.015).[105] These results justify the use of moxifloxacin as first-line therapy in patients with bacterial exacerbations of COPD and risk factors for relapse.

Another approach is presented in the current Latin American guidelines, which use FEV_1 impairment as the primary variable to select the choice of antibiotic. Patients with mild COPD are divided into 2 groups according to the presence of risk factors for failure and more active antibiotics are recommended in this group (Table 5).[106]

A similar approach has been adopted by recent joint guidelines among the national medical scientific societies in Spain.[107] The final algorithm of antimicrobial treatment is presented in figure 3.

The European Respiratory Society (ERS) guidelines cover the full spectrum of lower respiratory tract infections. They provide general guidance about the use of antimicrobials in the different patient populations. The recommendations must be adapted to each geographical setting according to resistance patterns of the microorganisms involved.[108]

PREVENTION OF EXACERBATIONS

Repeated exacerbations have an impact on the natural history of the disease. Patients with severe COPD and frequent exacerbations present an excessive decline in lung function over time.[6] Patients are frightened of exacerbations and have important limitations in their daily-life activities because of these episodes.[109,110] The impact of exacerbations on the health status of patients with COPD was first observed by Seemungal et al.[7] in a cohort of patients with severe disease over one year of follow-up. This observation was confirmed in patients with different degrees of severity, both in specialized hospital-based cohorts[8,111] and in milder patients followed in primary care.[112]

Based on this evidence and in the expectations of the patients, for whom the prevention of exacerbations is the first unmet need of treatment of COPD,[109] the prevention of episodes should be one of the main goals of treatment of COPD. In this chapter we refer to those related to the etiology or treatment of exacerbations.

TABLE 5

Risk Classification and Suggested Antimicrobial Therapy

	FEV_1 (% predicted)	More frequent microorganisms	Suggested treatment
Mild-to-moderate COPD without risk factors	>50%	• *H. influenzae* • *M. catarrhalis* • *S. pneumoniae* • *C. pneumoniae* • *M. pneumoniae*	• Amoxicillin-clavulanate • Cefditoren, cefuroxime • In areas of low incidence of resistance: amoxicillin, tetracycline
Mild-to-moderate COPD with risk factors[1]	>50%	• *H. influenzae* • *M. catarrhalis* • PRSP	• Moxifloxacin/levofloxacin • Amoxicillin-clavulanate • Cefditoren, cefuroxime
Severe COPD	30–50%	• *H. influenzae* • *M. catarrhalis* • PRSP • Enteric Gram-negatives	• Moxifloxacin/levofloxacin • Amoxicillin-clavulanate
Very severe COPD	<30%	• *H. influenzae* • PRSP • Enteric Gram-negatives • *P. aeruginosa*	• Moxifloxacin/levofloxacin • Ciprofloxacin if *Pseudomonas* is suspected • Amoxicillin-clavulanate (if allergic to quinolones)[2]

[1]Risk factors are explained in Table 1.

[2]In case of intravenous therapy other antibiotics can be used: piperacillin-tazobactam or imipenem or cefepime.

FEV_1, forced expiratory volume in 1 second; COPD, chronic obstructive pulmonary disease; PRSP, penicillin-resistant *S. pneumoniae*.

Modified from Miravitlles M; Grupo de trabajo de la Asociación Latinoamericana del Tórax (ALAT). Update to the Latin American Thoracic Society (ALAT) recommendations on infectious exacerbations of chronic obstructive pulmonary disease. *Arch Bronconeumol*. 2004;40:315-25.

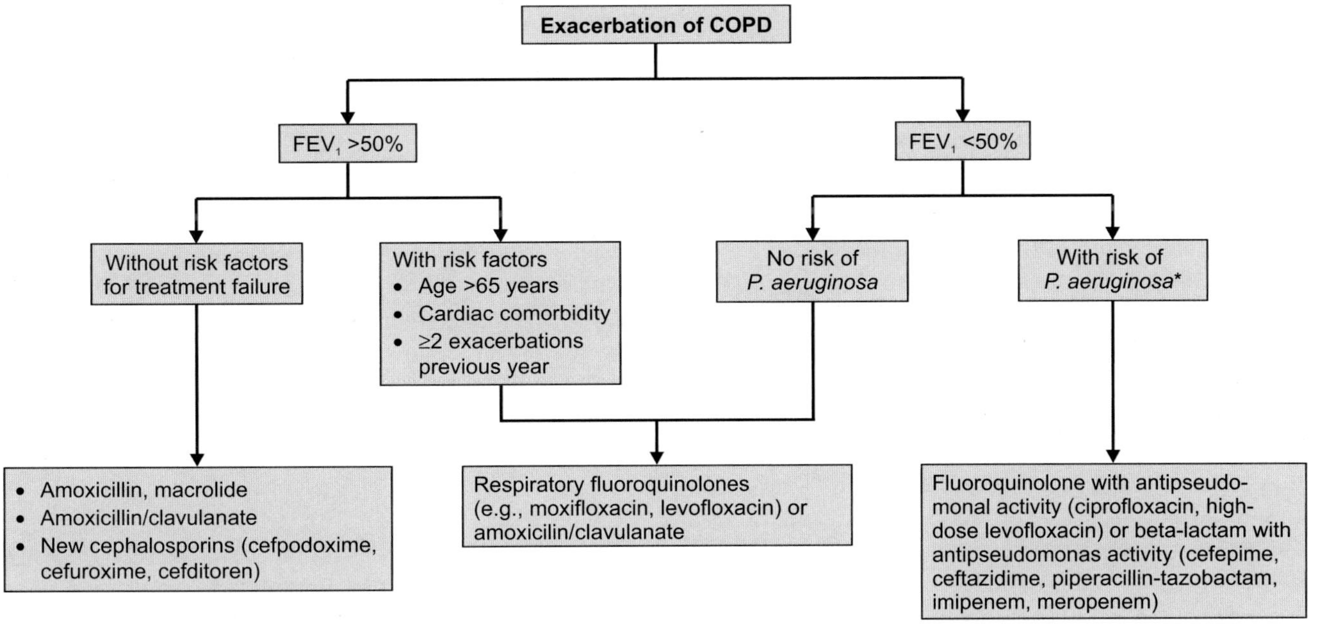

*Antibiotics in the previous 3 months, >4 courses of antibiotics in the previous year, use of systemic corticosteroids, previuos isolation of .

FIGURE 3 Antimicrobial treatment of exacerbations of chronic obstructive pulmonary disease (COPD). The antimicrobial recommendations apply for Spain and countries with similar rates of bacterial resistance to antibiotics, such as France, Italy and others. In countries or areas with lower rates of resistance other antibiotics may be also used as first-line therapy. *Adapted from* Woodhead M, Blasi F, Ewig S, Huchon G, Leven M, Ortqvist A, et al.; European Respiratory Society and European Society of Clinical Microbiology and Infectious Diseases. Guidelines for the management of adult lower respiratory tract infections. *Eur Respir J.* 2005;26:1138-80.

Antimicrobial Treatment of Exacerbations Importance of Eradication

In clinical trials with antibiotics in exacerbations of COPD, a prolonged time to the next exacerbation has been observed in patients who eradicate the bronchial pathogen after an exacerbation.[105,113,114] This suggests that in patients who effectively eradicate bacteria, a longer time is needed to achieve the threshold of bacterial counts required for an exacerbation to occur compared to patients who cure the exacerbation, but in whom bacteria still persist after antibiotic treatment.[115,116] This hypothesis would also explain why patients with acute exacerbations may be clinically cured, even without eradication of the bacterial pathogen.[117] This is not proof that a particular bacterium is not the cause of the exacerbation, it rather demonstrates that the antibiotic only needs to reduce bacterial counts to below the threshold to eliminate symptoms. Nevertheless, if eradication also occurs, the time needed in the future, for a bacterial load to reach above the threshold will be longer.

This quantitative or "fall and rise" hypothesis may explain the mechanism of bacterial exacerbations in patients with chronic bronchial colonization and frequent exacerbations.[116] In this group of patients, the change in a strain of the colonizing bacteria, as demonstrated by Sethi et al.,[71] may act as a trigger that initiates proliferation of microorganisms in some cases. "Fall and rise" may also explain relapses when bacteria have not been eradicated after antibiotic treatment of the exacerbation. In contrast, the change in a strain of the infective bacteria may be crucial in patients who do not suffer frequent exacerbations, i.e., less than 2 in a year. In a recent work, Sethi et al.[118] demonstrated that no increase in bacterial counts was associated with the occurrence of exacerbations. Only *H. influenzae* presented significantly higher concentrations in sputum during exacerbations compared with stable COPD, but the magnitude of the difference was small. These results are against the hypothesis that merely an increase in bacterial counts is enough to initiate an exacerbation. New evidence is required on the complex relationship between microorganisms and the host, particularly considering that important therapeutic implications may derive from these findings. In fact, if the new exacerbation is caused by the regrowth of the same bacteria that remained unkilled, the logical approach to treatment would be to use a different antibiotic and rotation of antibiotics should be recommended to prevent bacteriological failure and the development of resistance. In contrast, if new exacerbations are caused by the acquisition of new strains, the same antibiotic can be used in repeated exacerbations without concern about increased exposure to the same antibiotic.

On the other hand, the restriction in the use of antibiotics for respiratory infections in the community may have serious consequences in elderly patients. A recent survey in the UK using the general practice research database has demonstrated that the risk of pneumonia after chest infection was high, particularly in patients older than 65 years, and was substantially reduced by antibiotic use, with a number needed to treat of 39 in those over the age of 65 years compared with 96–119 in younger age group.[119] Interestingly, only 50% of elderly ambulatory patients with COPD (mean age 75 years) treated by general practitioners in the Netherlands received an antibiotic, and the factors associated with antibiotic prescription were male gender and coexistence of diabetes or heart failure.[120] Considered together, these results suggest that effective and eradicative treatment of bacterial exacerbations may result in what has been called the hypothesis of the "virtuous circle", with reduced bronchial inflammation, prevention of relapse, and preservation of lung function and quality of life (Figure 4).[121]

Antimicrobials in Stable State Treatment of Chronic Bronchial Infection

The use of prophylactic antibiotics in patients with severe COPD to prevent exacerbations was common in the 70s but was not recommended in guidelines due to the controversial efficacy, the risk of side effects, and the potential development of bacterial resistance. New ongoing clinical trials in selected populations of COPD, using the new, more active antibiotics available will provide interesting data about the benefits and risks of this therapeutic strategy.[122,123]

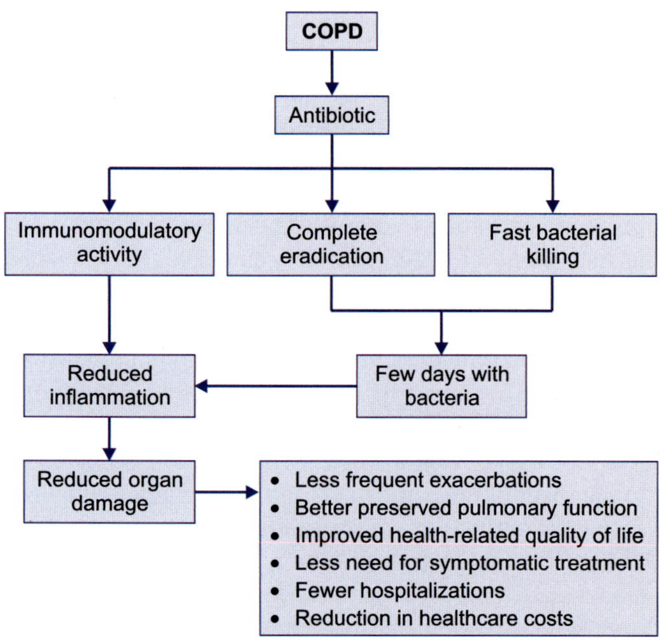

COPD, chronic obstructive pulmonary disease.

FIGURE 4 The "virtuous circle" of antimicrobial treatment of exacerbations of chronic obstructive pulmonary disease.

Other Preventive Treatments

Other treatments may have an effect in reducing exacerbations. The use of anti-influenza[124] and antipneumococcal vaccination[125] are useful in reducing the frequency of lower respiratory tract infections and pneumonia in COPD. In contrast, the use of mucolytics, antioxidants, and immunomodulators is not supported by enough evidence. However, there are studies that suggest an effect in reducing the severity of exacerbations with oral bacterial vaccines[126] or with oral carbocisteine,[127] and a reduction of exacerbations with N-acetyl cysteine in patients not treated with inhaled corticosteroids.[128] These results should be replicated in large trials to evaluate the role of these therapies in patients with COPD and frequent exacerbations.

Other Interventions During Exacerbations

The use of a self-management plan provided by a trained health professional can significantly reduce the utilization of healthcare services and improve health status.[129] The implementation of supported discharge or home hospitalization programs is another strategy to reduce the length of stay and associated complications, as well as the rate of emergency department visits and to improve satisfaction with the treatment.[130-132] These programs must include respiratory nurses that can attend the patients at home and solve their immediate requirements and provide medical education about the disease and its treatment.

There are other strategies aimed at preventing exacerbations which include quitting smoking, optimization of bronchodilator treatment in stable COPD, and rehabilitation, among others. There are excellent recent revisions available about this interesting subject.[133,134] A summary of interventions in presented in table 6.

CONCLUSION

Exacerbations significantly impair both the short- and long-term quality of life of COPD patients, accelerate lung function decline, and produce a reduction in physical activity. Furthermore, the reduction in physical activity is a risk factor for hospitalizations and death in COPD. Older age, impaired lung function, respiratory failure, cor pulmonale, comorbidity, and previous exacerbations are

TABLE 6

Strategies Aimed at Preventing Exacerbations

Proven efficacy	
• Quit smoking	• Antipneumococcal vaccine*
• LABAs: salmeterol, formoterol	• Rehabilitation
• Tiotropium	• Physical exercise
• Combination therapy: LABA/ICS	• Self-management plans
• Anti-influenza vaccine	• LVRS in selected patients
Questionable efficacy	
• Theophyllines	• Mucolytic agents
• Prophylactic antibiotic in selected patients	• Antioxidants
• Immunomodulators	

*Efficacy demonstrated in prevention of pneumonia but not in prevention of exacerbations.

LABA, long-acting β2 agonist; ICS, inhaled corticosteroid; LVRS, lung volume reduction surgery.

the most important risk factors for frequent exacerbations, hospitalizations, prolonged length of hospital stay, and mortality after an exacerbation of COPD.

Treatment of exacerbations consists of adequate ventilatory support and oxygenation when required, bronchodilators, oral corticosteroids, and antibiotics when signs of bacterial infection are present. The use of antibiotics that produce better bacterial eradication may have an effect on reducing the risk of early relapse. Other interventions, such as optimization of treatment for stable COPD, anti-influenza and antipneumococcal vaccination, self-management plans, and rehabilitation programs are effective in reducing the frequency of exacerbations and the impact of these episodes on the natural history of the disease.

REFERENCES

1. Celli BR, MacNee W, ATS/ERS Task Force. Standards for the diagnosis and treatment of patients with COPD: a summary of the American Thoracic Society/European Respiratory Society position paper. *Eur Respir J.* 2004;23:932-46.
2. Jemal A, Ward E, Hao Y, Thun M. Trends in the leading causes of death in the United States, 1970-2002. *JAMA.* 2005;294:1255-9.
3. Miravitlles M, Soriano JB, García-Río F, Muñoz L, Duran-Taulería E, Sánchez G, et al. Prevalence of COPD in Spain: impact of undiagnosed COPD on quality of life and daily life activities. *Thorax.* 2009;64:863-8.
4. De Marco R, Accordini S, Cerveri I, Corsico A, Sunyer J, Neukirch F, et al. An international survey of chronic obstructive pulmonary disease in young adults according to GOLD stages. *Thorax.* 2004;59:120-5.
5. Centers for Disease Control and Prevention. Chronic obstructive pulmonary disease surveillance - United States, 1971-2000. *MMWR.* 2002;51:SS6.
6. Donaldson GC, Seemungal TAR, Bhowmik A, Wedzicha JA. Relationship between exacerbation frequency and lung function decline in chronic obstructive pulmonary disease. *Thorax.* 2002;57:847-52.
7. Seemungal TAR, Donaldson GC, Paul EA, Bestall JC, Jeffries DJ, Wedzicha JA. Effect of exacerbation on quality of life in patients with chronic obstructive pulmonary disease. *Am J Respir Crit Care Med.* 1998;157:1418-22.
8. Miravitlles M, Ferrer M, Pont A, Zalacain R, Alvarez-Sala JL, Masa F, et al, for the IMPAC Study Group. Effect of exacerbations on quality of life in patients with chronic obstructive pulmonary disease: a 2 year follow up study. *Thorax.* 2004;59:387-95.
9. Burrows B, Bloom JW, Traver GA, Cline MG. The course and prognosis of different forms of chronic airways obstruction in a sample from the general population. *N Engl J Med.* 1987; 317:1309-14.
10. Burge PS, Calverley PMA, Jones PW, Spencer S, Anderson JA, Maslen TK. Randomised, double blind, placebo controlled study of fluticasone propionate in patients with moderate to severe chronic obstructive pulmonary disease: the ISOLDE trial. *BMJ.* 2000;320:1297-303.
11. Miravitlles M, Mayordomo C, Artés M, Sánchez-Agudo L, Nicolau F, Segú JL on Behalf of the EOLO Group. Treatment of chronic obstructive pulmonary disease and its exacerbations in general practice. *Respir Med.* 1999;93:173-9.
12. Langsetmo L, Platt RW, Ernst P, Bourbeau J. Underreporting exacerbation of chronic obstructive pulmonary disease in a longitudinal cohort. *Am J Respir Crit Care Med.* 2008;177:396-401.
13. Calverley P, Pauwels Dagger R, Löfdahl CG, Svensson K, Higenbottam T, Carlsson LG, et al. Relationship between respiratory symptoms and medical treatment in exacerbations of COPD. *Eur Respir J.* 2005;26:406-13.
14. Hurst JR, Donaldson GC, Perera WR, Wilkinson TMA, Bilello JA, Hagan GW, et al. Use of plasma biomarkers at exacerbation of chronic obstructive pulmonary disease. *Am J Respir Crit Care Med.* 2006;174:867-74.
15. Bozinovski S, Hutchinson A, Thompson M, MacGregor L, Black J, Giannakis E, et al. Serum amyloid A is a biomarker of acute exacerbations of chronic obstructive pulmonary disease. *Am J Respir Crit Care Med.* 2008;177;269-78.
16. Cazzola M, MacNee W, Martinez FJ, Rabe KF, Franciosi LG, Barnes PJ, et al, on behalf of the American Thoracic Society/European Respiratory Society Task Force on outcomes of COPD. Outcomes for COPD pharmacological trials: from lung function to biomarkers. *Eur Respir J.* 2008;31:416-68.
17. Miravitlles M, Guerrero T, Mayordomo C, Sánchez-Agudo L, Nicolau F, Segú JL on behalf of the EOLO Study Group. Factors associated with increased risk of exacerbation and hospital admission in a cohort of ambulatory COPD patients: a multiple logistic regression analysis. *Respiration.* 2000;67:495-501.
18. Niewoehner DE, Lokhnygina Y, Rice K, Kuschner WG, Sharafkhaneh A, Sarosi GA, et al. Risk indexes for

exacerbations and hospitalizations due to COPD. *Chest.* 2007;131:20-8.
19. Donaldson GC, Seemungal TA, Patel IS, Lloyd-Owen SJ, Wilkinson TM, Wedzicha JA. Longitudinal changes in the nature, severity and frequency of COPD exacerbations. *Eur Respir J.* 2003;22:931-6.
20. Hurst JR, Vestbo J, Anzueto A, Locantore N, Müllerova H, Tal-Singer R, et al. Susceptibility to exacerbation in chronic obstructive pulmonary disease. *N Engl J Med.* 2010;363: 1128-38.
21. Soler-Cataluña JJ, Martinez-García MA, Roman Sánchez P, Salcedo E, Navarro M, Ochando R. Severe acute exacerbations and mortality in patients with chronic obstructive pulmonary disease. *Thorax.* 2005;60:925-31.
22. Seneff MG, Wagner DP, Wagner RP, Zimmerman JE, Knaus WA. Hospital and 1-year survival of patients admitted to intensive care units with acute exacerbation of chronic obstructive pulmonary disease. *JAMA.* 1995;274:1852-7.
23. Connors AF Jr, Dawson NV, Thomas C, Harrell FE Jr, Desbiens N, Fulkerson WJ, et al. Outcomes following acute exacerbation of severe chronic obstructive pulmonary disease. The SUPPORT Investigators. *Am J Respir Crit Care Med.* 1996;154:959-67.
24. Almagro P, Calbo E, Ochoa de Echagüen A, Barreiro B, Quintana S, Heredia JL, et al. Mortality after hospitalization for COPD. *Chest.* 2002;121:1441-8.
25. Patil SP, Krishnan JA, Lechtzin N, Diette GB. In-hospital mortality following acute exacerbations of chronic obstructive pulmonary disease. *Arch Intern Med.* 2003;163: 1180-6.
26. McGhan R, Radcliff T, Fish R, Sutherland ER, Welsh C, Make B. Predictors of rehospitalization and death after a severe exacerbation of COPD. *Chest.* 2007;132:1748-55.
27. Groenewegen KH, Schols AMWJ, Wouters EFM. Mortality and mortality-related factors after hospitalisation for acute exacerbation of COPD. *Chest.* 2003;124:459-67.
28. Roche N, Zureik M, Soussan D, Neukirch F, Perrotin D and the Urgence BPCO (COPD emergency) scientific committee and investigators. Predictors of outcomes in COPD exacerbation cases presenting to the emergency department. *Eur Respir J.* 2008;32:953-61.
29. Antonelli Incalzi R, Fuso L, De Rosa M, Forastiere F, Rapiti E, Nardecchia B, et al. Co-morbidity contributes to predict mortality of patients with chronic obstructive pulmonary disease. *Eur Respir J.* 1997;10:2794-800.
30. Gunen H, Hacievliyagil SS, Kosar F, Mutlu LC, Gulbas G, Pehlivan E, et al. Factors affecting survival of hospitalised patients with COPD. *Eur Respir J.* 2005;26:234-41.
31. Ranieri P, Bianchetti A, Margiotta A, Virgillo A, Clini EM, Trabucchi M. Predictors of 6-month mortality in elderly patients with mild chronic obstructive pulmonary disease discharged from a medical ward after acute nonacidotic exacerbation. *J Am Geriatr Soc.* 2008;56:909-13.
32. Nevins ML, Epstein SK. Predictors of outcome for patients with COPD requiring invasive mechanical ventilation. *Chest.* 2001;119:1840-9.
33. Tsimogianni AM, Papiris SA, Stathopoulos GT, Manali ED, Roussos C, Kotanidou A. Predictors of outcome after exacerbation of chronic obstructive pulmonary disease. *J Gen Intern Med.* 2009;24:1043-8.
34. Almagro P, Barreiro B, Ochoa de Echaguen A, Quintana S, Rodriguez Carballeira M, Heredia JL, et al. Risk factors for hospital readmission in patients with chronic obstructive pulmonary disease. *Respiration.* 2006;73:311-7.
35. Gudmundsson G, Gislason T, Janson C, Lindberg E, Hallin R, Ulrik CS, et al. Risk factors for rehospitalisation in COPD: role of health status, anxiety and depression. *Eur Respir J.* 2005;26:414-9.
36. Vega Reyes JA, Montero Perez-Barquero M, Sanchez Guijo P. Factores pronosticos de reingreso en la enfermedad pulmonar obstructiva cronica. *Med Clin (Barc).* 2004; 122:293-7.
37. Matkovic Z, Huerta A, Soler N, Domingo R, Gabarrús A, Torres A, et al. Predictors of adverse outcome in patients hospitalised for exacerbation of COPD. *Respiration.* 2012.
38. Garcia-Aymerich J, Serra Pons I, Mannino DM, Maas AK, Miller DP, Davis KJ. Lung function impairment, COPD hospitalisations and subsequent mortality. *Thorax.* 2011; 66:585-90.
39. Vilkman S, Keistinen T, Tuuponen T, Kivelä SL. Survival and cause of death among elderly chronic obstructive pulmonary disease patients after first admission to hospital. *Respiration.* 1997;64:281-4.
40. Sethi S. Infectious etiology of acute exacerbations of chronic bronchitis. *Chest.* 2000;117:380S-5S.
41. Sapey E, Stockley RA. COPD exacerbations 2: aetiology. *Thorax.* 2006;61:250-8.
42. Papi A, Bellettato CM, Braccioni F, Romagnoli M, Casolari P, Caramori G, et al. Infections and airway inflammation in chronic obstructive pulmonary disease severe exacerbations. *Am J Respir Crit Care Med.* 2006;173:1114-21.
43. Soler N, Torres A, Ewig S, Gonzalez J, Celis R, El-Ebiary M, et al. Bronchial microbial patterns in severe exacerbations of chronic obstructive pulmonary disease (COPD) requiring mechanical ventilation. *Am J Respir Crit Care Med.* 1998;157:1498-505.
44. Miravitlles M. Epidemiology of chronic obstructive pulmonary disease exacerbations. *Clin Pulm Med.* 2002; 9:191-7.
45. Donaldson GC, Seemungal T, Jeffries DJ, Wedzicha JA. Effect of temperature on lung function and symptoms in chronic obstructive pulmonary disease. *Eur Respir J.* 1999;13:844-9.
46. MacNee W, Donaldson K. Exacerbations of COPD: environmental mechanisms. *Chest.* 2000;117:390S-7S.
47. Anderson HR, Spix C, Medina S, Schouten JP, Castellsague J, Rossi G, et al. Air pollution and daily admissions for chronic obstructive pulmonary disease in 6 European cities: results from the APHEA project. *Eur Respir J.* 1997;10:1064-71.
48. Jarad NA, Wedzicha JA, Burge PS, Calverley PMA, for the ISOLDE study group. An observational study of inhaled corticosteroid withdrawal is stable chronic obstructive pulmonary disease. *Respir Med.* 1999;93:161-6.
49. Wilkinson TMA, Hurst JR, Perera WR, Wilks M, Donaldson GC, Wedzicha JA. Effect of interactions between lower airway bacterial and rhinoviral infection in exacerbations of COPD. *Chest.* 2006;129:317-24.
50. Austrian R, Gold J. Pneumococcal bacteremia with especial reference to bacteremic pneumococcal pneumonia. *Ann Intern Med.* 1964;60:759-76.

51. Murphy TF, Brauer AL, Schiffmacher AT, Sethi S. Persistent colonization by *Haemophilus influenzae* in chronic obstructive pulmonary disease. *Am J Respir Crit Care Med.* 2004;170:266-72.
52. Stockley RA, O'Brien C, Pye A, Hill SL. Relationship of sputum color to nature and outpatient management of acute exacerbations of COPD. *Chest.* 2000;117:1638-45.
53. Allegra L, Blasi F, Diano P, Cosentini R, Tarsia P, Confalonieri M, et al. Sputum color as a marker of acute bacterial exacerbations of chronic obstructive pulmonary disease. *Respir Med.* 2005;99:742-7.
54. White AJ, Gompertz S, Bayley DL, Hill SL, O'Brien C, Unsal I, et al. Resolution of bronchial inflammation is related to bacterial eradication following treatment of exacerbations of chronic bronchitis. *Thorax.* 2003;58:680-5.
55. Gompertz S, O'Brien C, Bayley DL, Hill SL, Stockley RA. Changes in bronchial inflammation during acute exacerbations of chronic bronchitis. *Eur Respir J.* 2001; 17:1112-9.
56. Miravitlles M, Marin A, Monsó E, Vilà S, de la Roza C, Hervás R, et al. Colour of sputum is a marker of bacterial colonization in COPD. *Respir Res.* 2010;11:58.
57. Miravitlles M, Kruesmann F, Haverstock D, Perroncel R, Choudhri SH, Arvis P. Sputum colour and bacteria in chronic bronchitis exacerbations: a pooled analysis. *Eur Respir J.* 2012.
58. Soler N, Agustí C, Angrill J, Puig de la Bellacasa J, Torres A. Bronchoscopic validation of the significance of sputum purulence in severe exacerbations of chronic obstructive pulmonary disease. *Thorax.* 2007;62:29-35.
59. Christ-Crain M, Müller B. Biomarkers in respiratory tract infections: diagnostic guides to antibiotic prescription, prognostic markers and mediators. *Eur Respir J.* 2007; 30:556-73.
60. Bafadhel M, Clark TW, Reid C, Medina MJ, Batham S, Barer MR, et al. Procalcitonin and C-reactive protein in hospitalized adult patients with community-acquired pneumonia or exacerbation of asthma or COPD. *Chest.* 2011;139:1410-8.
61. Niederman MS. Biological markers to determine eligibility in trails for community-acquired pneumonia: a focus on procalcitonin. *Clin Infect Dis.* 2008;47:S127-S132.
62. Becker KL, Snider R, Nylen ES. Procalcitonin assay in systemic inflammation, infection, and sepsis: clinical utility and limitations. *Crit Care Med.* 2008;36:941-52.
63. Stolz D, Christ-Crain M, Bingisser R, Leuppi J, Miedinger D, Muller C, et al. Antibiotic treatment of exacerbations of COPD: a randomized, controlled trial comparing procalcitonin-guidance with standard therapy. *Chest.* 2007;131:9-19.
64. Daniels JMA, Schoorl M, Snijders D, Knol DL, Lutter R, Jansen HM, et al. Procalcitonin vs C-reactive protein as predictive markers of response to antibiotic therapy in acute exacerbations of COPD. *Chest.* 2010;138:1108-15.
65. Quint JK, Donaldson GC, Goldring JJP, Baghai-Ravary R, Hurst JR, Wedzicha JA. Serum IP-10 as a biomarker of human rhinovirus infection at exacerbation of COPD. *Chest.* 2010;137:812-22.
66. Monsó E, Ruiz J, Rosell A, Manterola J, Fiz J, Morera J, et al. Bacterial infection in chronic obstructive pulmonary disease. A study of stable and exacerbated outpatients using the protected specimen brush. *Am J Respir Crit Care Med.* 1995;152:1316-20.
67. Zalacain R, Sobradillo V, Amilibia J, Barrón J, Achótegui V, Pijoan JI, et al. Predisposing factors to bacterial colonization in chronic obstructive pulmonary disease. *Eur Respir J.* 1999;13:343-8.
68. Bandi V, Apicella MA, Mason E, Murphy TF, Siddiqi A, Atmar RL, et al. Nontypeable *Haemophilus influenzae* in the lower respiratory tract of patients with chronic bronchitis. *Am J Respir Crit Care Med.* 2001;164:2114-9.
69. Möller LV, Timens W, van der Bij W, Kooi K, de Wever B, Dankert J, et al. *Haemophilus influenzae* in lung explants of patients with end-stage pulmonary disease. *Am J Respir Crit Care Med.* 1998;157:950-6.
70. Wilkinson TMA, Patel IS, Wilks M, Donaldson GC, Wedzicha JA. Airway bacterial load and FEV_1 decline in patients with chronic obstructive pulmonary disease. *Am J Respir Crit Care Med.* 2003;167:1090-5.
71. Sethi S, Evans N, Grant BJ, Murphy TF. New strains of bacteria and exacerbations of chronic obstructive pulmonary disease. *N Engl J Med.* 2002;347:465-71.
72. Sethi S, Wrona C, Eschberger K, Lobbins P, Cai X, Murphy TF. Inflammatory profile of new bacterial strain exacerbations of chronic obstructive pulmonary disease. *Am J Respir Crit Care Med.* 2008;177:491-7.
73. Murphy TF, Brauer AL, Eschberger K, Lobbins P, Grove L, Cai X, et al. *Pseudomonas aeruginosa* in chronic obstructive pulmonary disease. *Am J Respir Crit Care Med.* 2008;177:853-60.
74. Rosell A, Monso E, Soler N, Torres F, Angrill J, Riise G, et al. Microbiologic determinants of exacerbation in chronic obstructive pulmonary disease. *Arch Intern Med.* 2005;165:891-7.
75. Fagon JY, Chastre J, Trouillet JL, Domart Y, Dombret MC, Bornet M, et al. Characterization of distal bronchial microflora during acute exacerbation of chronic bronchitis. Use of the protected specimen brush technique in 54 mechanically ventilated patients. *Am Rev Respir Dis.* 1990;142:1004-8.
76. Eller J, Ede A, Schaberg T, Niederman MS, Mauch H, Lode H. Infective exacerbations of chronic bronchitis: relation between bacteriologic etiology and lung function. *Chest.* 1998;113:1542-8.
77. Miravitlles M, Espinosa C, Fernández-Laso E, Martos JA, Maldonado JA, Gallego M. Relationship between bacterial flora in sputum and functional impairment in patients with acute exacerbations of COPD. Study Group of Bacterial Infection in COPD. *Chest.* 1999;116:40-6.
78. Lode H, Allewelt M, Balk S, De Roux A, Mauch H, Niederman M, et al. A prediction model for bacterial etiology in acute exacerbations of COPD. *Infection.* 2007; 35:143-9.
79. Ewig S, Soler N, Gonzalez J, Celis R, El-Ebiary M, Torres A. Evaluation of antimicrobial treatment in mechanically ventilated patients with severe chronic obstructive pulmonary disease exacerbations. *Crit Care Med.* 2000; 28:692-7.
80. Monsó E, García-Aymerich J, Soler N, Farrero E, Felez MA, Anto JM, et al; EFRAM Investigators. Bacterial infection in

exacerbated COPD with changes in sputum characteristics. *Epidemiol Infect.* 2003;131:799-804.
81. García-Vidal C, Almagro P, Romaní V, Rodríguez-Carballeira M, Cuchi E, Canales L, et al. *Pseudomonas aeruginosa* in patients hospitalised for COPD exacerbation: a prospective study. *Eur Respir J.* 2009;34:1072-8.
82. Celli BR, Cote CG, Marin JM, Casanova C, Montes de Oca M, Mendez RA, et al. The body-mass index, airflow obstruction, dyspnea, and exercise capacity index in chronic obstructive pulmonary disease. *N Engl J Med.* 2004;350:1005-12.
83. Martínez-Solano L, Macia MD, Fajardo A, Oliver A, Martinez JL. Chronic *Pseudomonas aeruginosa* infection in chronic obstructive pulmonary disease. *Clin Infect Dis.* 2008;47:1526-33.
84. Montero M, Domínguez M, Orozco-Levi M, Salvadó M, Knobel H. Mortality of COPD patients infected with multi-resistant *Pseudomonas aeruginosa*: a case and control study. *Infection.* 2009;37:16-9.
85. Mohan A, Chandra S, Agarwal D, Guleria R, Broor S, Gaur B, et al. Prevalence of viral infection detected by PCR and RT-PCR in patients with acute exacerbation of COPD: A systematic review. *Respirology.* 2010;15:536-42.
86. Rohde G, Wiethege A, Borg I, Kauth M, Bauer TT, Gillissen A, et al. Respiratory viruses in exacerbations of chronic obstructive pulmonary disease requiring hospitalisation: a case-control study. *Thorax.* 2003;58:37-42.
87. Kherad O, Kaiser L, Bridevaux PO, Sarasin F, Thomas Y, Janssens JP, et al. Upper-respiratory viral infection, biomarkers, and COPD exacerbations. *Chest.* 2010; 138:896-904.
88. Mallia P, Message SD, Gielen V, Contoli M, Gray K, Kebadze T, et al. Experimental rhinovirus infection as a human model of chronic obstructive pulmonary disease exacerbation. *Am J Respir Crit Care Med.* 2011;183:734-42.
89. Seemungal T, Harper-Owen R, Bhowmik A, Moric I, Sanderson G, Message S, et al. Respiratory viruses, symptoms, and inflammatory markers in acute exacerbations and stable chronic obstructive pulmonary disease. *Am J Respir Crit Care Med.* 2001;164:1618-23.
90. Mallia P, Johnston SL. How viral infections cause exacerbation of airway diseases. *Chest.* 2006;130:1203-10.
91. Balter MS, La Forge J, Low DE, Mandell L, Grossman RF, and the Chronic Bronchitis Working Group; Canadian Thoracic Society and Canadian Infectious Disease Society. Canadian guidelines for the management of acute exacerbations of chronic bronchitis. *Can Respir J.* 2003; 10:3B-32B.
92. Rabe KF, Hurd S, Anzueto A, Barnes PJ, Buist SA, Calverley P, et al. Global strategy for the diagnosis, management, and prevention of chronic obstructive pulmonary disease: GOLD executive summary. *Am J Respir Crit Care Med.* 2007;176:532-55.
93. Duffy N, Walker P, Diamantea F, Calverley PM, Davies L. Intravenous aminophylline in patients admitted to hospital with non-acidotic exacerbations of chronic obstructive pulmonary disease: a prospective randomised controlled trial. *Thorax.* 2005;60:713-7.
94. Niewoehner DE, Erbland ML, Deupree RH, Collins D, Gross NJ, Light RW, et al. Effect of systemic glucocorticoids on exacerbations of chronic obstructive pulmonary disease. *N Engl J Med.* 1999;340:1941-7.
95. Aaron SD, Vandemheen KL, Hebert P, Dales R, Stiell IG, Ahuja J, et al. Outpatient oral prednisone after emergency treatment of chronic obstructive pulmonary disease. *N Engl J Med.* 2003;348:2618-25.
96. Singh JM, Palda VA, Stanbrook MB, Chapman KR. Corticosteroid therapy for patients with acute exacerbations of chronic obstructive pulmonary disease: a systematic review. *Arch Intern Med.* 2002;162:2527-36.
97. Miravitlles M. Do we need new antibiotics for treating exacerbations of COPD? *Ther Adv Respir Dis.* 2007;1:61-76.
98. Saint S, Bent S, Vittinghoff E, Grady D. Antibiotics in chronic obstructive pulmonary disease exacerbations: a meta-analysis. *JAMA.* 1995;273:957-60.
99. Puhan MA, Vollenweider D, Latshang T, Steurer J, Steurer-Stey C. Exacerbations of chronic obstructive pulmonary disease: When are antibiotics indicated? A systematic review. *Respir Res.* 2007;8:30.
100. Anthonisen NR, Manfreda J, Warren CPW, Hershfield ES, Harding GKM, Nelson NA. Antibiotic therapy in exacerbations of chronic obstructive pulmonary disease. *Ann Intern Med.* 1987;106:196-204.
101. Allegra L, Grassi C, Grossi E, Pozzi E, Blasi F, Frigerio D, et al. Ruolo degli antibiotici nel trattamento delle riacutizzazioni della bronchite cronica: risultati di uno studio italiano multicentrico. *Ital J Chest Dis.* 1991;45:138-148.
102. Nouira S, Marghli S, Belghith M, Besbes L, Elatrous S, Abroug F. Once daily oral ofloxacin in chronic obstructive pulmonary disease exacerbation requiring mechanical ventilation: a randomised placebo-controlled trial. *Lancet.* 2001;358:2020-5.
103. Evans AT, Husain S, Durairaj L, Sadowski LS, Charles-Damte M, Wang Y. Azithromycin for acute bronchitis: a randomised, double-blind, controlled trial. *Lancet.* 2002;359:1648-54.
104. Dimopoulos G, Siempos II, Korbila IP, Manta KG, Falagas ME. Comparison of first-line with second-line antibiotics for acute exacerbations of chronic bronchitis: a metaanalysis of randomized controlled trials. *Chest.* 2007;132:447-55.
105. Wilson R, Anzueto A, Miravitlles M, Arvis P, Alder J, Haverstock D, et al. Moxifloxacin vs amoxicillin/clavulanic acid in outpatient AECOPD: MAESTRAL results. *Eur Respir J.* 2012.
106. Miravitlles M; Grupo de trabajo de la Asociación Latinoamericana del Tórax (ALAT). Update to the Latin American Thoracic Society (ALAT) recommendations on infectious exacerbations of chronic obstructive pulmonary disease. *Arch Bronconeumol.* 2004;40:315-25.
107. Miravitlles M, Monsó E, Mensa J, Aguarón Pérez J, Barberán J, Bárcena Caamaño M, et al. Antimicrobial treatment of exacerbation in chronic obstructive pulmonary disease: 2007 consensus statement. *Arch Bronconeumol.* 2008;44: 100-8.
108. Woodhead M, Blasi F, Ewig S, Huchon G, Leven M, Ortqvist A, et al.; European Respiratory Society and European Society of Clinical Microbiology and Infectious Diseases. Guidelines for the management of adult lower respiratory tract infections. *Eur Respir J.* 2005;26:1138-80.

109. Miravitlles M, Anzueto A, Legnani D, Forstmeier L, Fargel M. Patient's perception of exacerbations of COPD – the PERCEIVE study. *Respir Med.* 2007;101:453-60.
110. Kessler R, Stahl E, Vogelmeier C, Haughney J, Trudeau E, Löfdahl CG, et al. Patient understanding, detection, and experience of COPD exacerbations: an observational, interview-based study. *Chest.* 2006;130:133-42.
111. Miravitlles M, Calle M, Alvarez-Gutierrez F, Gobartt E, López F, Martín A. Exacerbations, hospital admissions and impaired health status in chronic obstructive pulmonary disease. *Qual Life Res.* 2006;15:471-80.
112. Llor C, Molina J, Naberan K, Cots JM, Ros F, Miravitlles M, on behalf of the EVOCA study. Exacerbations worsen the quality of life of chronic obstructive pulmonary disease patients in primary healthcare. *Int J Clin Pract.* 2008;62:585-92.
113. Chodosh S, Schreurs A, Siami G, Barkman HW Jr, Anzueto A, Shan M, et al. Efficacy of oral ciprofloxacin vs. clarithromycin for treatment of acute bacterial exacerbations of chronic bronchitis. *Clin Infect Dis.* 1998; 27:730-8.
114. Wilson R, Allegra L, Huchon G, Izquierdo JL, Jones P, Schaberg T, et al, on behalf of the MOSAIC Study Group. Short-term and long-term outcomes of moxifloxacin compared to standard antibiotic treatment in acute exacerbations of chronic bronchitis. *Chest.* 2004;125: 953-64.
115. Chodosh S. Clinical significance of the infection-free interval in the management of acute bacterial exacerbations of chronic bronchitis. *Chest.* 2005;127:2231-6.
116. Miravitlles M. Exacerbations of chronic obstructive pulmonary disease: when are bacteria important? *Eur Respir J.* 2002;20:9s-19s.
117. Wilson R, Kubin R, Ballin I, Deppermann KM, Bassaris HP, Leophonte P, et al. Five day moxifloxacin therapy compared with 7 day clarithromycin therapy for the treatment of acute exacerbations of chronic bronchitis. *J Antimicrob Chemother.* 1999;44:501-13.
118. Sethi S, Sethi R, Eschberger K, Lobbins P, Cai X, Grant BJB, et al. Airway bacterial concentrations and exacerbations of chronic obstructive pulmonary disease. *Am J Respir Crit Care Med.* 2007;176:356-61.
119. Petersen I, Johnson AM, Islam A, Duckworth G, Livermore DM, Hayward AC. Protective effect of antibiotics against serious complications of common respiratory tract infections: retrospective cohort study with the UK General Practice Research Database. *BMJ.* 2007;335;982-7.
120. Bont J, Hak E, Birkhoff CE, Hoes AW, Verheij TJM. Is co-morbidity taken into account in the antibiotic management of elderly patients with acute bronchitis and COPD exacerbations? *Fam Pract.* 2007;24:317-22.
121. De Benedetto F, Sevieri G. Chronic obstructive pulmonary disease (COPD) exacerbation and inflammation of the respiratory tract: clinical implication, prognostic consequences, and therapeutic strategies. *Multidisciplinary Respiratory Medicine.* 2006;1:36-48.
122. Sethi S, Jones PW, Theron MS, Miravitlles M, Rubinstein E, Wedzicha JA, et al.; PULSE Study group. Pulsed moxifloxacin for the prevention of exacerbations of chronic obstructive pulmonary disease: a randomized controlled trial. *Respir Res.* 2010;11:10.
123. Albert RK, Connett J, Bailey WC, Casaburi R, Cooper JA Jr, Criner GJ, et al; COPD Clinical Research Network. Azithromycin for prevention of exacerbations of COPD. *N Engl J Med.* 2011;365:689-98.
124. Poole PJ, Chacko E, Wood-Baker RW, Cates CJ. Influenza vaccine for patients with chronic obstructive pulmonary disease. *Cochrane Database Syst Rev.* 2006;(1):CD002733.
125. Alfageme I, Vazquez R, Reyes N, Muñoz J, Fernández A, Hernandez M, et al. Clinical efficacy of anti-pneumococcal vaccination in patients with COPD. *Thorax.* 2006;61:189-95.
126. Steurer-Stey C, Bachmann LM, Steurer J, Tramèr MR. Oral purified bacterial extracts in chronic bronchitis and COPD: systematic review. *Chest.* 2004;126:1645-55.
127. Zheng JP, Kang J, Huang SG, Chen P, Yao WZ, Yang L, et al. Effect of carbocisteine on acute exacerbation of chronic obstructive pulmonary disease (PEACE Study): a randomized placebo-controlled study. *Lancet.* 2008; 371:2013-8.
128. Decramer M, Rutten-van Mölken M, Dekhuijzen PN, Troosters T, van Herwaarden C, Pellegrino R, et al. Effects of N-acetylcysteine on outcomes in chronic obstructive pulmonary disease (Bronchitis Randomised on NAC Cost-Utility Study, BRONCUS): a randomised placebo-controlled trial. *Lancet.* 2005;365:1552-60.
129. Bourbeau J, Julien M, Maltais F, Rouleau M, Beaupré A, Bégin R, et al. Reduction of hospital utilization in patients with chronic obstructive pulmonary disease: a disease-specific self-management intervention. *Arch Intern Med.* 2003;163:585-91.
130. Skwarska E, Cohen G, Skwarski KM, Lamb C, Bushell D, Parker S, et al. Randomised controlled trial of supported discharge in patients with exacerbations of chronic obstructive pulmonary disease. *Thorax.* 2000;55:907-12.
131. Sala E, Alegre L, Carrera M, Ibars M, Orriols FJ, Blanco ML, et al. Supported discharge shortens hospital stay in patients hospitalized because of an exacerbation of COPD. *Eur Respir J.* 2001;17:1138-42.
132. Hernandez C, Casas A, Escarrabill J, Alonso J, Puig-Junoy J, Farrero E, et al., on behalf of the CHRONIC project. Home hospitalisation of exacerbated chronic obstructive pulmonary disease patients. *Eur Respir J.* 2003;21:58-67.
133. Scott S, Walker P, Calverley PMA. COPD exacerbations. 4: Prevention. *Thorax.* 2006;61:440-7.
134. Wedzicha JA, Seemungal TAR. COPD exacerbations: defining their cause and prevention. *Lancet.* 2007;370: 786-96.

CHAPTER 8

Viral Respiratory Infections

Ioannis Mastoris, Sotirios Tsiodras

ABSTRACT

Viruses have been increasingly recognized as significant pathogens in both upper and lower respiratory tract infections. In addition they may have a role in the pathogenesis of other diseases like asthma. Herein, we comprehensively describe the epidemiology, pathophysiology, clinical picture, laboratory diagnosis and therapeutic interventions for the most significant respiratory viral pathogens.

INTRODUCTION

The upper respiratory tract in most instances represents the portal of entry of significant bacteria and pathogens including viruses. Traditionally, the infections of respiratory system are classified as either upper or lower respiratory tract infections (LRTIs). Moreover, it is becoming more and more evident that respiratory viruses may have a role in the pathogenesis of other diseases like asthma.[1,2] In this chapter, a comprehensive description of specific respiratory viruses and the associated clinical syndromes has been presented.

RESPIRATORY SYNCYTIAL VIRUS

Basic Knowledge-Epidemiology-Pathophysiology

Respiratory synctical virus (RSV) is a single-stranded, negative sense RNA virus, member of the paramyxoviridae family along with parainfluenza, measles, and mumps. Two subtypes A and B are identified, with the former one producing serious disease.[3-7] Shifting is the mechanism responsible for numerous reinfections.[5,8] Direct contact as well as respiratory droplets are implicated in the transmission.[9] Average time of shedding is 3–8 days but can be extended up to 1 month in infants. Viral dissemination can be facilitated due to viral survival on hands and fomites.[10,11] The virus is inoculated either on nasopharyngeal or ocular mucous membranes. The incubation period ranges 2–8 days (commonly 4–6 days). Subsequent to the initial viral inoculation and the upper respiratory tract infection, the infection can affect the lower respiratory tract. More specifically, the small bronchiolar epithelium is affected, extending then to the type 1 and 2 pneumocytes with clinically obvious disease ensuing 1–3 days after.[12,13] The infection is characterized by an obstructive pattern due to sloughing of the epithelium, occasional proliferation of the residual one, and a monocytic inflammation around the arterioles.[13,14] Neutrophilia is an associated finding in bronchoalveolar lavage (BAL).[15] RSV is typically found in the luminal apical epithelium but occasionally can be recovered from the liver, the cerebrospinal fluid (CSF), the pericardial fluid, or the blood most probably representing inactive genome in immune cells.[16-20] It seems that some cytokines (IL-8, IL-6, TNF-alpha, and IL-1 beta) and chemokines (CCL2, CCL3, CCL5, CCL11) are an integral part in the pathogenicity and severity of disease[21-29] (especially IL-6 and CCL3 levels correlate with the severity[22,30,31]). However, it is not clear whether this is a causative association or whether these represent a higher inflammatory response. Previous RSV infection does not confer immunity even with elevated specific antibody titers, although symptoms in repeated disease tend to be milder.[32,33] Currently no preventive vaccine exists.

The infection follows a seasonal pattern primarily occurring during the winter months.[34,35] The clinical manifestations vary by whether the infection occurs primarily or secondarily, the age group of the patient and his overall medical history.[32,36-42] Typically, it affects children younger than 2 years old with a peak incidence during the period from 2 months to 6 months of age resulting in bronchiolitis or other LRTI.[34,43] Nevertheless, it is increasingly recognized that RSV can also cause severe disease in the elderly and immunocompromised patients accounting for one quarter of deaths attributable to a virus other than influenza during the winter season.[38,44,45] RSV infection can be additionally blamed for recurrent upper respiratory tract infections typically in healthy adults with no other comorbidities.[46] RSV associated disease can also be associated with significant mortality; about 2,700 pediatric and adult deaths can be attributed to RSV pneumonia annually in the USA, according to Centers for Disease Control and Prevention (CDC).[47]

Clinical Picture in Infants and Young Children

Infants and children that are infected with RSV for the first time usually exhibit a LRTI, such as pneumonia (most frequent pneumonia cause in children less than 5 years of age), bronchiolitis, bronchospasm, and acute respiratory failure.[32,48,49] Apnea may be the presenting symptom in up to 20% of infants coming to the hospital suffering from RSV infection.[50-55] Factors that have been identified to contribute to apneic episodes include prematurity (with its own apnea of prematurity) and subsequent severity of hypoxia.[51-54] A loose association with sudden infant death syndrome has been made.[56] However, the underlying mechanisms still remain obscure.[57] LRTI happens more frequently with primary disease although secondary disease may also cause the same symptoms in about half of the affected patients.[32,48]

Bronchiolitis is a well-known cause of illness and hospitalization in infants and young children. It is defined as the first episode of wheezing in a child younger than 1–2 years old with viral infection symptoms and lacking other causes of wheezing.[58] In general, a child less than 2 years old presenting with wheezing and an obstructive pattern due to viral or bacterial infection is thought to suffer from bronchiolitis. Other than RSV, rhinovirus, parainfluenza, human metapneumovirus, influenza, coronavirus, and human bocavirus can cause it and occasionally lab results may show coinfection.[59-67] Normally patients will have prodromal symptoms of nasal congestion and discharge along with mild cough but upon presentation to hospital they will have fever (typically <38.3°C), cough and respiratory distress.[68] Involvement of the sinuses and ear (otitis media), and low levels of fever may be indicative of RSV infection.[69,70] It is necessary to exclude severe disease indicated by symptoms, such as lethargy or restlessness, apneic spells, cyanosis, respiratory distress, and inadequate hydration status.[70] Physical examination may demonstrate tachypnea, intercostal retractions, expiratory wheezing with prolongation of expiratory time. Signs of obstruction, such as hyperresonance to percussion and an increased anteroposterior thoracic diameter, may be evident. Constant pulse oximetry may show mild hypoxemia. Radiologically, sites of patchy atelectasis, peribronchial thickening and hyperinflation are frequent in bronchiolitis.[71-74] Chronic underlying diseases, such as congenital heart disease, pulmonary disease, neurologic conditions, and immunodeficiencies may predispose to severe disease.[75-79] Concomitant bacterial infections are not common although the risk for meningitis and bacteremia is approximately 1–2% and that for urinary tract infections is 1–5%.[80-88] Typically, the disease is self-limited and resolves within 1 month after onset in patients with noncompromising conditions. Complications can occur especially in infants with the aforementioned comorbidities usually resulting in apnea, respiratory failure and secondary bacterial infection.[71,89-93] Long-term prognosis is not well known but there are studies indicating an association between the infection during infancy and bronchospastic disease occurring later in life, though therapy with palivizumab seems to reducc the incidence of reactive airways disease.[94-100] It has also been postulated that there is an increased risk of wheezing until the age of 6 years old, normalizing until 13 years in patients with RSV associated LRTI.[95,101] In this setting, RSV infection can be a predictive factor of asthma development in childhood.[95,96,98,102-105] It remains unclear whether this connection is causative or just predictive.[106] Nonetheless, it seems that children, who develop bronchospastic symptoms or frank asthma, in addition carry a burdened history of maternal atopy and increased immunoglobulin E levels.[100,107-114]

Other Clinical Presentations in Children and Adults

Children and young adults presenting with a constellation of cough, coryza, conjunctivitis along with rhinorrhea and ear involvement may also suffer from RSV infection of the upper respiratory tract.[69] Usually self-limited, these episodes of RSV infection can also result in airway reactivity but with no further pulmonary sequela after 4 months from onset.[115] Data on the effect of an RSV respiratory infection on an asthmatic's or chronic obstructive pulmonary disease (COPD) patients' pulmonary function remains equivocal.[116,117]

The virus can also take the form of a common cold infection but its range may include a viral pneumonia. As much as 5% of common cold cases can be attributed to RSV infection along with parainfluenza virus (PIV).[118,119] RSV associated community acquired pneumonia (CAP) has been recognized in adults.[120] Immunocompromised patients suffering from RSV pneumonia exhibit a very high rate of mortality ranging from 70% to 100% as a result of respiratory failure. The highest risk exists for those patients that have undergone bone marrow transplantation.[121,122] In such populations, RSV may occur as a nosocomial outbreak following nevertheless the seasonal variation in incidence.[39] Radiologic findings include ground glass opacities. Surprisingly these patients do not seem to have any adverse pulmonary outcome after recovery from the initial attack.[123,124]

Diagnosis

Diagnosis of RSV infection is usually made clinically in accordance with and based on the demographic (e.g., age <5 years old), epidemiologic (e.g., winter season, community outbreak), and the clinical (e.g., LRTI or bronchiolitis) evidence with regards to the affected patients. The diagnosis can be supported by additional data provided by radiologic and/or lab studies but these are not routinely performed. There are instances though where etiologic diagnosis is warranted. These include cases where antiviral therapy may be needed (e.g., if an influenza infection is suspected), the need of empirical antibiotic therapy is obvious (according to presenting symptoms and signs), and the prevention of a nosocomial outburst of bronchiolitis is of paramount importance (e.g., in a high-risk unit, such as a BMT ward).[125-130] Under these circumstances, several laboratory evaluations can be helpful. The diagnostic mainstay (screening test) is the rapid antigen test (usually a 30 minute or less procedure) with sensitivity and specificity over 90%, bypassing in this way the more time-consuming viral cultures. Analysis of secretions can yield results with the nasal swab being ideal and pharyngeal/throat ones being adequate for diagnosis.[131] Newer molecular techniques, such as polymerase chain reaction (PCR), can also be used along with the benefit of simultaneously detecting numerous respiratory pathogens responsible for the disease.[132] PCR can be further used as a confirmation to the rapid test, especially in adults where the test has lower sensitivity.[133,134] Serology is not helpful because stable level of antibodies is maintained after subsequent infections in adults, and maternal antibody is present in infants.

Differential Diagnosis

Differential diagnosis is made among the other viral respiratory pathogens including rhinovirus, adenovirus, metapneumovirus, PIV, influenza virus, and bocavirus in infants and children. In the elderly, the RSV associated syndrome must be differentiated from influenza. In immunocompromised patients, PIV remains the main differential. It must be noted that in case of bronchiolitis, coinfections with bacteria should be excluded.[135-137]

Treatment

Treatment is supportive in most cases of disease. Antibiotic therapy may be considered if a comorbid bacterial infection is suspected. Although respiratory synctial virus immune globulin and other monoclonal antibodies do not seem to result in clinical improvement, once the disease is active, they may play a significant role in RSV prevention.[138-141] Palivizumab and motavizumab are new monoclonal antibody agents available for use in RSV prevention with evidence indicating overall reduction in LTRIs and rate of hospitalization.[142-145] These new agents can be particularly advantageous and safe for children with severe underlying diseases, such as congenital heart disease, prematurity, and bronchopulmonary dysplasia.[146-152] Palivizumab has also been shown to decrease recurrent wheezing in children that had already RSV infection.[94,153] Intramuscular home administration of the drug results in higher compliance rates with subsequent reduction of RSV hospitalization and is only indicated for high-risk pediatric patients.[154-156] Some resistant RSV strains to palivizumab have been documented although data is equivocal.[157-159]

PARAINFLUENZA VIRUS
Basic Knowledge-Epidemiology-Pathophysiology

Parainfluenza virus belongs to the paramyxoviridae family, along with mumps, measles, RSV, and human metapneumovirus.[160] It is a single strand negative sense RNA virus, consisting of six viral proteins.[161] The fusion glycoprotein (F) and hemagglutinin-neuraminidase (HN) proteins contribute to the virus' infectivity and are the main site of neutralizing antibody binding.[162-164] Contrary to influenza proteins, the PIV HN protein shows antigenic stability although antigenic drifts have been reported.[165] Transmission of the virus is largely the same as other respiratory viruses with extensive spread being observed within families due to hand-to-hand contact, large droplet inhalation and through fomites.[166] PIV initially attacks the nasal and oropharyngeal epithelium, subsequently spreads downward affecting bronchial and alveolar epithelium (with little direct damaging effect) with the degree of spreading dictating the severity.[167-170] Incubation period ranges from 2 days to 6 days, and detection is possible from day 1 to day 6.[169,171]

Parainfluenza virus infection occurs all year long throughout the world without exhibiting any overall variations. PIV-1 tends to cause outbursts during the autumn of the odd years, PIV-2 peak is during fall annually and PIV-3 does not have a specific pattern; however, it tends to cause spring outbreaks.[172,173] PIV-4 is the least studied due to the associated mild disease.[172] In tropics, no such variation exists.[174] Any of the serotypes can invariably affect children and adults; some clinical syndromes can be attributed to particular serotypes with higher propensity. PIV-3 is the most prevalent in both adults and children leading to pneumonia and bronchiolitis, essentially the same as RSV in young children by the age of 5.[175] PIV-1 and PIV-2 are not that frequent in adults and produce croup or laryngotracheobronchitis in children; PIV-2 infection is typically milder.[176-178] PIV-4 usually produces only mild upper respiratory syndrome (URI) symptoms but serious disease has been reported in patients with burdened medical history, i.e. cardiopulmonary disease and immunosuppression.[179-182] Ethnicity may play a role in the severity of the infection.[170] Breast-fed infants appear to be protected from serious disease.

Clinical Picture

In children, more than half of the PIV infections involve the upper respiratory tract.[183,184] In adults, PIV usually presents with cold symptoms including fever, rhinorrhea, cough, and sore throat.[177] PIV-1 is mainly responsible for croup or laryngotracheobronchitis in children.[178] It is characterized by fever, rhinorrhea, and pharyngitis resulting in barking cough, respiratory distress including stridor, dyspnea, and chest wall retractions with hypoxemia requiring mechanical ventilation. PIV-2 is also implicated in croup with milder course. The most frequent PIV-3 infection is linked with the development of CAP in adults, particularly those who are older, debilitated with cardiac disease compared to those with bacterial pneumonia.[185-187] Children present with bronchiolitis and belong to the same age group of RSV bronchiolitis, i.e., children less than 2 years old and especially in the first 6 months of life. PIV-4 serotype is commonly implicated in mild URI but can cause any type of respiratory disease in patients with chronic underlying conditions.[180,181] Otitis media and sinusitis can be a result of the primary viral infection or secondary bacterial infection.[188] PIV is also blamed for asthma and COPD exacerbations in addition to some extrarespiratory manifestations, such as meningitis, myocarditis, pericarditis, and Guillain-Barré syndrome.[45,189-194]

Outbreaks and sporadic cases of PIV infections have been documented in infants in neonatal ICUs (NICUs).[195-198] PIV-3 is the most common serotype closely mimicking RSV.[196,197,199-202] Symptom severity ranges from mild cough and coryza to severe LTRI with apneic episodes.[196,197,199] Premature babies often present with atypical findings including a sepsis-like syndrome, recurrent apneic episodes and an aggravation of bronchopulmonary dysplasia with escalating oxygen needs.[196,201] Often these infants require mechanical ventilation and prolonged oxygen therapy.[196,199,200,203]

Parainfluenza virus infections are responsible for significant morbidity and mortality in immunocompromised patients.[176] The most severe cases involve hematopoietic cell transplant recipients, leukemic patients and patients with solid organ transplants but milder cases have been reported in HIV and cancer patients.[182,204-210] Available data refer mostly to hospitalized patients presumably overrating the severity.[176] Estimated incidence is 2–7% in hematopoietic cell transplant (HCT) patients and 5% in lung transplant patients.[182,204,205,211,212] Since most PIV infections are community acquired, it is not a surprise that PIV-3 serotype is the most prevalent but outbreaks due to other types have been also reported.[204,213,214] It seems that some immunocompromised patients eventually proceed to LRTI after 3 days of upper respiratory tract infection.[204] Glucocorticoids may exacerbate disease progression in a dose-dependent way;[215] the same is true for neutropenia. APACHE II score more than 15 and other respiratory coinfections.[209] Mortality at 30 days has been estimated to be between 17% and 35%.[209,215] PIV can be asymptomatically shedding among HCT recipients; a fact that can directly contribute to hospital outbreaks.[211] In general, PIV are also associated with pulmonary sequela in both HCT and lung transplant patients. In HCT patients, PIV infection increased 18 times the risk of reduced pulmonary airflow during the first year whereas in lung transplant patients, PIV infections were linked to acute lung rejection or with the development of the bronchiolitis obliterans syndrome.[205,206,216-219]

Diagnosis

Since no pathognomonic findings exist for PIV infections and PIV cocirculates with other respiratory viruses, diagnosis becomes challenging. Viral culture of the nasal washings or swabs or BAL is the gold standard although time consuming. Immunofluorescence of the aforementioned specimens is available for detection of the viral antigen. Its major drawback is limited sensitivity ranging from 70% to 90%. Almost 100% sensitivity is obtained with PCR techniques in addition to the detection opportunity of multiple respiratory viruses.[220,221] A fourfold increase in IgG levels can provide a diagnosis, although serology is not routinely used. Imaging findings include interstitial infiltrates and a ground glass pattern along with peribronchial nodules.[222] However, none of these findings is specific for PIV infection.

Typically infections in immunocompromised patients are managed with glucocorticoid reduction.[176] Case reports and studies have not proven any mortality gain or reduction in viral shedding in patients treated with ribavirin.[204,223-227] Hemagglutinin-neuraminidase inhibitors are available.[228,229] A recombinant sialidase fusion protein, DAS181, has also been proven to inhibit human PIV infection and is available for compassionate use.[230-232] Currently, no preventive vaccine exists but several PIV-1 and PIV-2 candidate vaccines are undergoing trials in children.[233-237]

HUMAN RHINOVIRUS

Basic Knowledge-Epidemiology-Pathophysiology

Rhinovirus, the most common cause of common cold belongs to the *Picornavirus* family; it consists of one RNA strand of the size of a ribosome (pico).[238-240] Other members of the picorna family resulting in respiratory infection are *Enteroviruses* and *Parechovirus*. Currently 99% of human rhinovirus (HRV) genomes have been fully sequenced and potential antiviral drug goals have been identified.[241,242] IgG antibodies bind to the virus surface blunting its capacity to infect the cells and cause clinical disease.[239] HRV as all common cold viruses spreads mainly by direct contact with infectious secretions, subsequently inoculated in the eyes' or the nasal mucosa.[243-245] Their capacity to endure in environmental conditions for a couple of hours, on both hands and fomites, boosts their potential for infection.[245] Porous materials and alcohol disinfectants reduce the rate of transmission.[245-248] Droplet transmission is another possible way but occurs more frequently in influenza and RSV.[118,249] Nasopharyngeal mucosa is the first site of infection that then spreads anteriorly and downward.[239,250] The peak of viral shedding, and thus infectivity, happens on the third day of infection and coincides well with the peak of clinical symptoms.[251-253] HRV can be detected in respiratory secretions up to 7 days after the first insult.[250] Nevertheless, baseline viral replication may continue up to 3 weeks in the nasopharynx until apoptosis of infected cells has occurred.[250,254] Unlike RSV, rhinovirus seems to cause little and limited damage to nasal epithelium.[241,255-261] Kinins, known vasoactive substances, are thought to be responsible for the clinical symptoms of common cold, with their absence coinciding with absence of any symptom confirming this assumption.[256,262,263] HRV genome has been isolated from the bronchial epithelium reinforcing the belief that HRV contributes to asthma exacerbations.[45,264]

Human rhinovirus is characterized by a seasonal pattern of transmission particularly exhibiting a double peak in its outburst periods in autumn and late spring.[118,265] HRV has been identified to cause common cold but has also been documented in LRTIs and asthma exacerbations.[266] It has been found that HRV is responsible for about 50% of the common cold cases with over than 100 serotypes being isolated.[238,262,266,267] Typically adults suffer common cold symptoms about 2–3 times a year while children constituting the main viral pool are affected about 8–12 times a year.[238] It is often implicated in respiratory viral infections in infancy resulting in bronchiolitis and wheezing, but contrary to RSV, its effect (mainly HRV-A, HRV-B, and HRV-C) is more significant in adults and children older than 2 years old.[102,268-273]

Clinical Picture

Rhinovirus is identified as the number one cause globally for the most frequent acute illness in the industrialized world, the common cold.[265] Other viruses causing common cold are coronaviruses, influenza viruses, parainfluenza, and RSV with adenoviruses and *Enteroviruses* being the least prevalent.[118,119] Every age group is affected.[238,274] The severity of symptoms varies among people and age groups and is mainly defined by immune system function rather than virulence of pathogen involved.[119] Except for the age, it is also based on medical history.[119] Nasal stuffiness and secretions are the most common ones. Sore throat initiates the course of the disease but lasts usually only for the first day.[274] Then nasal congestion ensues by day 2 along with sneezing, and cough by day 5 while nasal symptoms wane gradually.[275] Conjunctivitis is an unstable finding. Fever is an unlikely finding in children.

Human rhinovirus has been also found to cause bronchiolitis in infants resulting in the same clinical picture as RSV.[59] The main difference is in seasonal incidence with HRV following its known double-peak pattern (fall and spring).[276] Rhinovirus has been isolated as a potential cause of pneumonia in both children and adults.[120,277,278] However, the great majority of the adults in such reports had a coinfection with another organism pointing to the role of HRV acting as a Trojan horse blunting upper respiratory tract immune defense mechanisms.[279]

In addition to RSV, HRV infection during infancy may be predictive of asthma development without any hard data confirming a causal association.[91,92,94,98-101] Children, who had wheezing during rhinovirus infection, have increased risk for recurrent wheezing and asthma in later years.[268,270] It seems that patients with a history of atopy may exhibit an increased susceptibility in developing asthma.[280-282] Once developed, rhinovirus is identified as the first cause of asthma exacerbation in preschool children (older than 2) and school children-adults accounting for 71% and 60%, respectively, as well as COPD exacerbation in adults.[2,45,107,269,281,283-288] Characteristically, HRV is responsible for the "September asthma epidemic" and the peak in spring hospitalizations due to asthma attacks whereas RSV contributes to the winter peak.[289-292] Other complications include viral sinusitis or acute bacterial sinusitis developing after URI infection.[293] Although acute otitis media is more frequent in children, adults can also be affected after rhinovirus or influenza infection.[294-296]

Diagnosis

Diagnosis of the common cold is predominantly clinical and based on symptoms, season, age, and medical history, but if one needs to isolate the pathogen, antigen tests and PCR-based technologies are available. Common cold has to be differentiated from allergic or seasonal rhinitis, bacterial pharyngitis, sinusitis, influenza, and pertussis. Bronchiolitis and pneumonia are in the differential for LTRI. A recent study using rapid multiviral testing in the emergency room for patients with common cold found that it could result in a reduction of antibiotic prescription in the community after discharge.[297]

Treatment

Provided that common cold is self-limited disease, therapy is largely supportive. Antitussives, expectorants, decongestants, ipratropium, cromolyn sodium, and antihistamines are commonly used. Antibiotics are used in the case of secondary bacterial infections or sinusitis and bronchodilators and steroids in the case of asthma symptoms. Other experimental agents include pleconaril (active against >90% of rhinoviruses serotypes), tremacamra (a recombinant soluble ICAM 1) and 3C protease inhibitors (e.g., nasal spray of ruprintrivir).[298-300]

INFLUENZA VIRUS

Basic Knowledge-Epidemiology-Pathophysiology

Influenza virus belongs to the *Orthomyxoviridae* family, which is divided into three types: influenza A, B, and C. Only influenza A and B are of medical importance. They are spherical enveloped viruses containing eight segments of negative-strand RNA genome. Type A can infect birds, pigs, and humans whereas type B is responsible only for human infections. On their envelope surface, two types of spikes project: one is composed of hemagglutinin (H protein) and the other is neuraminidase (N protein) both of which convey the virus infectivity. Hemagglutinin is involved in fusion and attachment functions and neuraminidase mediates the release of the newly assembled virus from the cell surface by clipping off sialic acid residues. Due to the unique structure the virus has, it possesses some special reassortment mechanisms. Both influenza A and B viruses exhibit antigenic drift.[301-303] This represents slight changes in antigenicity due to mutations in H and/or N proteins. As it is understood this process is responsible for recurrent seasonal influenza infection, epidemics, and outbreaks happening every year.[303,304] Antigenic shift is noticed only in type A influenza virus because it has the ability of infecting cells from multiple species. In this process, two different strains of a segmented RNA virus infect the same cell. When viruses assemble their virion, major new genetic combinations are produced through shuffling, resulting in a stable and dramatic change. The virus generated comes from two different species' viruses and represents an agent to which the population may have no immunity. Influenza shifting is responsible for pandemics with last example being the 2009 pandemic strain of influenza A H1N1 (swine influenza) and the not pandemic strain of the avian influenza A H5N1.[305]

Influenza occurs every year in outbreaks during winter and early spring. Expansion of the infection depends mainly on the susceptibility of the population, the degree of antigenic change, and the herd immunity acquired through vaccination. Transmission of the virus is the same as other respiratory viruses although some minor differences exist. Sneezing and coughing is the principal way of spreading. It seems that large particle droplets are the predominant mechanism through which virus is transmitted.[306,307] Since large droplets cannot stay in the air for long time, close contact between persons is required. Aerosolized small particles are a possible but not well-established way.[308-310] Direct contact with secretions on contaminated objects can transfer the virus but not for long as influenza is an enveloped virus and subsequently sensitive to environmental conditions. Except for the respiratory tree, transocular entry of the virus may happen.[311]

The incubation period is 2 days on average.[312,313] Viral shedding increases 1–2 days before symptoms onset, peaks on day 2 of symptomatic disease and then rapidly declines.[314,315] Most often it is undetected after 6–7 days but in some studies was found to insist until day 10.[314,316-318] It lasts longer in a large number of conditions, such as childhood, senescence, underlying diseases, impaired immunity, glucocorticoid use, lymphopenia and may be lower if antiviral treatment is given.[319-325] In asymptomatic patients, viral load was significantly lower than symptomatic prompting to suggest that asymptomatic individuals do not transmit the flu.[317,318] Despite the systemic symptoms present, it seems that influenza viral replication happens only in the respiratory tract.

Clinical Picture

Following the incubation period, influenza symptoms quickly emerge with sudden onset of fever, headache, myalgia, and malaise being most prevalent.[318,326-328] Non-productive cough, rhinorrhea, and sore throat are usual companions.[329,330] Influenza though has a wide range of clinical expression based on factors of age, previous immunity (vaccination) and impaired immune system. Because of that, symptoms may vary from a benign common cold-like picture to a severe lower respiratory infection, such as pneumonia. However, children may not have these, typical for influenza, symptoms either because of their inability to express symptoms as myalgia and headache, or due to their lack of immunity resulting in high fever, seizures, and gastrointestinal symptoms.[330-333]

Physical findings are commonly few in uncomplicated influenza both in adults and children. In adults, the patient may appear hot and flushed due to fever, and despite sore throat, the nasopharynx may only appear hyperemic. Pulmonary findings are usually absent and lymphadenopathy may be found in young adults. Alterations in gas exchange physiology have been described.[334] In children, fever is a stable finding with cough and rhinitis being relatively stable.[330,335,336] In children older than 13 years, influenza may cause more serious disease with tachypnea, conjunctival erythema, nasal injection, and cervical adenopathy being evident.[330,337]

In healthy individuals, influenza is a self-limited disease. In patients with uncomplicated influenza, symptoms wane over a period of 2–5 days but may not improve until 1 week has passed. Cough may persist after resolution of influenza, and numerous patients may complain of a residual sensation of weakness or easy fatigability, referred as post-influenza asthenia, for up to a month. However, there have been cases where even healthy children develop a fatal disease.[329,338] In high-risk patients, infection may instead results in severe complications and death.[339,340]

Influenza Related Complications

Complications in adults usually involve patients that belong to high-risk groups, but there are numerous cases where no underlying condition was identified.[341] The most common complication is influenza pneumonia or secondary bacterial pneumonia or both. In primary pneumonia, the virus affects directly the lung producing severe symptoms, such as high fever, dyspnea, and cyanosis.[342] It must be suspected when the typical flu symptoms do not abate or worsen. Patients with underlying cardiovascular disease and impaired immunity are in high risk for pneumonia. Imaging typically shows bilateral reticular or reticulonodular opacities.[343] Less commonly focal areas of consolidation may be seen especially in the basal lungs. Ground glass opacities are seen in high-resolution CT.[343] Secondary bacterial infection must be suspected when there is worsening of fever after an initial period of improvement. It is responsible for about a quarter of influenza mortality.[344] These symptoms are of bacterial infection, with productive cough, purulent sputum, and focal radiographic opacities. The most common pathogen is *Streptococcus pneumoniae*, with *S. aureus* following.[345,346] Community-acquired MRSA has been also identified, accounting for high-mortality rates in young previously healthy patients with influenza.[347-349] In addition, influenza virus is implicated in the exacerbation of chronic respiratory diseases, such as COPD and asthma.[45] Central nervous system (CNS) or peripheral nervous system involvement is well documented with encephalitis, transverse myelitis, aseptic meningitis, and Guillain-Barré syndrome reported but without a causal link.[350-356] Transient abnormal ECG findings have been found in previously healthy patients with influenza.[357] Data also indicate an increase in myocardial infarction-linked and ischemic heart disease-linked hospitalization and death during influenza outbreak periods.[358,359] Myocarditis and pericarditis may be included in the cardiac sequela of influenza with increased prevalence in type B fatal cases.[360,361]

In children, the most common complication in up to half of the cases is otitis media starting usually 3 days after influenza symptoms onset.[330,331,362-364] Influenza can cause a wide range of lower respiratory tract disease including pneumonia, laryngotracheitis, bronchitis, and bronchiolitis making the differential diagnosis from RSV and parainfluenza really challenging.[329,365] Tracheitis and tracheobronchitis may be exceptionally severe.[365,366] Asthmatic exacerbations may also occur.[367,368] Influenza pneumonia occurs most commonly in children less than 2 years old, but unlike adults, it has a benign and short course.[329,369,370] Neurologic complications are the same as adults in addition to cerebellar ataxia, encephalopathy, febrile seizures, and acute mental status changes.[371-377] Febrile seizures are the most common.[372] Neurologic complications happen in children aged from 6 months to 4 years and those with neuromuscular disease.[372] Acute myositis and rhabdomyolysis affect children more frequently than adults and happen more commonly with influenza type B.[378,379] Typical symptoms are extreme tenderness, swelling, and heaviness of the calves. CPK is significantly high and renal failure may ensue due to concomitant myoglobinuria.[364,379,380] Other complications include myocarditis, pericarditis, and toxic shock syndrome.[381-387]

Influenza A H1N1—2009 Related Pandemic

In March of 2009, an outbreak of H1N1 influenza virus emerged in Mexico spreading subsequently in many countries.[388] In June of the same year, the World Health Organization raised its pandemic alert at the highest level indicating widespread community transmission on at least two continents. This strain represents a quadruple reassortment of two swine, one human, and one avian strain. Available data show that the pandemic strain carried a higher rate of extrapulmonary complications and/or death than the seasonal strain, although affected patients at the pandemic onset were young and had less comorbidities.[389] Otherwise, and especially later on the course of the pandemic it was recognized that patients suffering from severe influenza disease seemed to be older, obese, have underlying diseases, and have LTRI symptoms upon presentation. In general, symptoms were identical to seasonal strains, although gastrointestinal manifestations were more commonly seen in association with the H1N1 pandemic strain.[390-392]

Diagnosis

Diagnosis of the influenza virus infection is usually clinically made and based on symptoms and signs of the disease. Influenza infection should be suspected in febrile patients with symptoms of common cold presenting in the outpatient office during wintertime. It should also be suspected in patients with chronic underlying disease exacerbation including asthma and COPD.[45] Laboratory diagnosis requires viral identification or viral protein detection or viral genome isolation. Testing should be performed in case of treatment decision, virus-spreading prophylaxis and for differentiation among pathogens.[340] Tests should be performed in the initial 72 hours since symptom onset, based on the fact that viral shedding usually peaks on day 2. Negative tests after day 5 do not exclude influenza infection. Nasopharyngeal specimens along with a throat specimen confer a higher degree of sensitivity and specificity to the procedure.[340,393]

Polymerase chain reaction tests offer the greatest levels of sensitivity and specificity in addition to the ability to distinguish between influenza A and B.[340,364,394,395] Direct and indirect fluorescent tests are also available but are inferior in sensitivity compared to PCR. However, they retain their ability to differentiate between the two types and among respiratory viruses especially in the acute care setting.[340,394,396] Available rapid tests detect virus antigen and neuraminidase.[340] Due to low sensitivity (especially when used out of the influenza season), this test cannot rule out influenza infection.[394,397-399] Rapid tests are recommended for use when influenza activity is high in community.[400,401] However, in the case of negative result during this period, confirmation with culture or PCR is warranted since it frequently represents a false negative result.[340,402] Viral culture is only helpful in confirming results from other tests, but has no role in the acute setting due to the time-consuming procedure.[340] Serology is not used in clinical practice.[340]

Treatment

Treatment consists of two major antiviral drug classes: (i) neuraminidase inhibitors such as oseltamivir, zanamivir and peramivir and (ii) adamantanes, such as amantadine and rimantadine.[403] Treatment with neuraminidase inhibitors has been shown to reduce the duration of disease, to decrease viral shedding and subsequently illness severity and complications rates.[404-411] Data indicate that treatment should be administered promptly within 2 days since symptom onset to result in better outcome.[404,405,412-417] Inhaled zanamivir is contraindicated in patients with underlying respiratory disease.[418,419] Emerging resistant influenza strains to oseltamivir have been reported so that it should be administered with caution.[420-428] An intravenous preparation of zanamivir is under clinical investigation. Adamantanes are not routinely used in clinical practice because of resistance reported.[418] Laminavir and peramivir are only available in Japan.

Prevention

The primary prevention of influenza virus spreading mainly consists of the use of immunization against it programs. Since the virus is characterized by a high frequency of mutations, the human immune system is constantly naïve to new influenza strains.[429] This means that new vaccines have to be produced each year against the most prevalent influenza strains.[430,431] There are two main types of vaccines currently circulating: (i) intramuscular inactivated vaccines and (ii) intranasal live-attenuated vaccines, each type with specific indications and contraindications.[339,432] In general, vaccination should be done every year in autumn, especially in persons who run the risk of severe influenza disease including pregnant women, and immunocompromised hosts and with underlying cardiovascular and respiratory diseases.[339,431] Annual health care worker immunization is of paramount importance.

ADENOVIRUS INFECTIONS

Basic Knowledge-Epidemiology-Pathophysiology

Adenovirus is a double-stranded DNA virus surrounded by a nonenveloped icosahedral virion with fiber-like projections.[433] The majority of adenoviruses, along with coxsackie virus B, bind to the coxsackie-adenovirus receptor through this fiber-like protein.[434] Contrary to that, adenovirus type B fibers bind to CD46, a complement-related protein, initiating in this way the complement cascade (this may be related to the direct cytopathic effect of the virus).[435,436] Many adenoviruses can hemagglutinate rat or rhesus red blood cells, a property that is mainly attributed to the fiber-like protein and helps classify adenoviruses into six subgroups.[437,438] In addition, adenoviruses, besides types 40 and 41, have a direct cytopathic effect on cells usually occurring within 2–7 days, a fact that laboratories use to isolate adenoviruses. Except for infectious capacity, adenoviruses have been intensively studied as a gene vector making it appropriate for gene therapy and immunization against tumors and infections.

Adenoviruses can cause infections worldwide and throughout the year without any seasonal predominance. It is responsible for about 10% of all febrile illnesses in children, who in most instances experience at least one adenoviral infection by the age of ten.[439] Typically, adenoviruses causes disease in places with high rates of contact between people, such as daycare centers, households with young children, military bases and hospitals; they are also responsible for pharyngoconjunctival fever in summer camps (swimming pools), keratoconjunctivitis in hospitals and acute respiratory disease in military recruits.[440-443] Transmission is typical for respiratory viruses occurring via aerosol droplets, contact with contaminated fomites, and the fecal-oral route. There has been data that neonates can acquire the infection via cervical secretions at birth. In addition, transmission has been documented in instances of an infected donor of a kidney or liver transplant.[444-447] It seems that these tissues can foster adenovirus in a latent condition.[447] Viral shedding can last for months in the feces causing persistent infections.[439] More than 50 serotypes of adenovirus have been isolated. These serotypes are further divided in subgroups. Since virus culture in patients with disease is not routinely done, the exact prevalence of adenovirus serotypes is not known. However, one study conducted with specimens from 22 hospitals, showed that serotype 3 was responsible in 35% of the cases, serotype 2 in 24%, and the least prevalent was serotype 1 with 18% of the cases.[448] This distribution, however, does not necessarily represent other groups, such as military recruits or immunocompromised patients.

After discontinuation of the live oral vaccine in military recruits in 1996, infection rates due to adenovirus have increased.[449] Data have shown that in 2004 more than 75% of recruits were susceptible to adenovirus type 4 and type 7. Twenty five percent of them have developed respiratory illness due to adenovirus 4 and almost all were seropositive by the end of the study, indicating that asymptomatic viral pharyngeal shedding can contribute to transmission.[450] Although serotype 4 has been found almost exclusively in recruits until the mid-twenties (1926), subgroup B (types 3, 7, 14, and 21) has become more prevalent since then.[448,450-452] In 2011, a new adenoviral vaccine has become available against serotypes 4 and 7 approved for ages 17 through 50 years.[453] Adenovirus type 14 emerged in the United States in the last decade, often presenting in clusters of severe respiratory disease in numerous States. A report showed that serotype 14 was responsible for 38% of hospitalization and a 5% mortality among those who were infected.[454-456] It seems that previous infection with adenovirus 7 may provide some level of protection against adenovirus 14.[457] Women had higher rates of hospitalization when infected with serotype 14.[458] This serotype has been also identified in other patient groups including health care workers and their homes, in individuals that socialized together in Alaska and health care personnel in military hospitals.[456,459-461]

Clinical Picture

Adenovirus is responsible for a variety of clinical syndromes and manifestations influenced by age group and immune status. Serotypes 5, 7, 14, and 21 are associated with serious disease.[448,454,461-467] As mentioned, they are the most common cause of acute febrile illness in children and infants lasting from 5 days to 7 days, although there are cases that may persist for 2 weeks. Coryza and pharyngitis accompanied by conjunctivitis, laryngitis, tracheitis, and pneumonia are common symptoms. Adenovirus is the most common cause of tonsillitis in young children, and is often accompanied by cervical lymphadenopathy. Otitis media is mostly seen in infants younger than 1 year old.[468,469] One in ten cases of children pneumonia can be attributed to adenoviruses with subgroup B types causing more severe disease.[454,461,470-474] Bronchiectasis can be the outcome of pneumonia in children. In patients with comorbidities in great risk of fatal pneumonia is observed. Infants are at a greater risk than older children for developing other severe symptoms, such as diarrhea and vomiting. Complications may include meningoencephalitis, hepatitis, nephritis, myocarditis, and DIC.[475,476] Fever, headache, malaise, and abdominal pain are frequent during pharyngitis.[477]

Other Adenovirus Related Syndromes

Eyes disease, such as pharyngoconjunctival fever and epidemic keratoconjunctivitis, can result from adenovirus infection. The former is the constellation of follicular conjunctivitis, fever, pharyngitis and adenopathy. It occurs as an outbreak in summer camps and is related to swimming pools.[440] Almost all types can cause it, but subgroup types 3 and 7 are the most prevalent. Epidemic keratoconjunctivitis is a bilateral conjunctivitis accompanied by preauricular adenopathy and corneal opacities. Although self-limited, it can last up to 1 month. Severe pain and blurry vision is the usual presentation. It is caused mainly by subgroup D and transmission occurs through ophthalmologist's hands, contaminated tools, and eye drops.[441,478]

Up to 10% of diarrheal episodes in young children can be attributed to adenoviruses types 40 and 41 of subgroup F and rarely type 31 subgroup A.[479] However, in immunocompromised patients, a wide range of serotypes can be found, and are frequently complicated with hepatitis.[480] Episodes can last up to 12 days, or the infection may have an asymptomatic course despite the detection of antigen in stool.[481,482] Stool antigen may also persist for months making it a useless tool in identifying the etiology of the diarrhea. Diarrhea can be accompanied by mesenteric adenopathy mimicking appendicitis and complicated by intussusception.[483]

Adenoviruses subgroup D types 19 and 37 have been linked to hemorrhagic cystitis in children without any further sequela, but must be differentiated from other kidney diseases that cause hematuria.[484] Urethritis has been associated with infection due to subgroup B types 19 and 37.[485,486] The nervous system can be also affected by adenoviruses with meningitis and encephalitis being reported.[487] These can be a primary target of the virus or can occur secondarily.[475] Interestingly, adenovirus is more prevalent than coxsackie B in provoking myocarditis in children.[488,489] Myositis followed by rhabdomyolysis and arthritis has also been reported.[490-493]

Adenovirus and Immunocompromised Subjects

Adenovirus infections may cause severe disease in immunocompromised patients; this represents either a reactivation of a latent infection or prolonged harboring possibly inside immune system cells, such as lymphocytes, or a primary infection of the patient.[447,494] Transplant patients exhibit a wide range of clinical symptoms and disease, severity.[495,496] In hematopoietic transplant patients syndromes may include pneumonia, colitis, hepatitis, hemorrhagic cystitis, tubulo-intestitial nephritis, encephalitis, and disseminated disease.[495,497-500] Except for the usual serotypes, subgroup B types 11, 34, and 35 have been implicated.[497,498] One study showed that infection occurred about 1.6 months post transplantation (consistent with the reactivation theory) and that overall mortality affected exclusively the HCT patients compared to solid organ transplant patients.[501] Data from another study showed a higher incidence of adenoviral infection and disease in HCT patients who received T-cell depleted bone marrow and intensive immunosuppressive therapy[497,498] strengthening the observation that severe disease is associated with severe immune dysfunction. In addition to that, children in pediatric HCT units acquired adenoviral infection more frequently than adults.[499,502] Contrary to HCT patients, adenoviral infections involve only the donor organ in transplant patients. This is seen in kidney transplantation resulting in acute hemorrhagic cystitis, sometimes progressing to interstitial nephritis (in general with benign course although exceptions are observed[503,504]). Cases in lung transplantation with, usually, benign course have been recorded.[505] Hepatitis is the most common finding in patients with invasive adenoviral disease, who have undergone liver transplantation.[506] Outcomes are not favorable with 43% mortality and 28.5% requiring retransplantation.[506] Adenovirus infection has been also implicated in graft loss and coronary vasculopathy in cardiac transplant patients when found in cardiac biopsies with PCR.[507] In patients with acquired immunodeficiency as in

HIV cases, uncommon serotypes have been collected from stool or urine including subgroup B types 11, 34, and 35 in urine and subgroup D in stools.[508,509] Although recovered from specimens, they rarely cause significant disease with some fatal cases been reported due to hepatitis, pneumonia, encephalitis, and tubulo-intestitial nephritis.[510-512]

Diagnosis

Adenovirus infection can cause a variety of clinical syndromes thus diagnosis based only on manifestations can be arduous. It is crucial to identify the virus in outbreaks and in groups running the risk of serious or fatal disease, such as children and immunocompromised patients. Diagnosis will lead to better treatment and preventive measures to inhibit further spread of the infection. Because adenovirus lacks envelope, it is relatively stable and an assortment of specimens can be used; nasopharyngeal aspirates or swabs, throat swabs, sputum, tracheal aspirates, BAL fluid, conjunctival swabs, stool specimen, urine, CSF, and tissue samples can all be sent for viral culture. The virus can be found in stool specimens or the urine of immunocompromised individuals for months representing asymptomatic shedding of the virus.

Direct detection of viral antigen can be used for types 40 and 41 in stool specimens in cases of infant diarrhea.[513] These rapid assays lack sensitivity and are not used in immunocompromised patients.[514,515] They can be also used in epidemic keratoconjunctivitis, with the limitation of having to use them early in course to achieve maximum sensitivity.[516] Polymerase chain reaction can also be used and is predominantly helpful in normally sterile tissues, such as blood, CSF, and tissues. Its results must be interpreted with caution and in the context of clinical symptoms as it may otherwise represent asymptomatic shedding.[517,518] Quantitative PCR is helpful in immunocompromised patients in predicting disseminated disease and mortality as well as monitoring response to treatment.[517,519-525] Together with sequencing, it helps by genotyping the specific adenovirus.[448] In order to make an ultimate diagnosis, tissue biopsy may be necessary. Both pathology and culture/PCR may be needed on the tissue specimen. Adenovirus infection is characterized by intranuclear basophilic inclusions, making cells seem like "smudge cells" and eosinophilic inclusions in postinfectious stages.[526,527] If findings are equivocal, culture/PCR are warranted. A fourfold increase in antibody titers confirms the diagnosis of active infection. Identification of hemagglutination inhibition or inhibition antibodies is more sensitive and helpful in serotype isolation. Restriction endonuclease analysis helps to identify whether clinical isolates of the same serotype have a common source.[528]

Differential Diagnosis

Due to the wide variety of clinical symptoms that adenoviruses can cause, differential diagnosis is equally large and challenging. When upper respiratory system is involved, then adenovirus must be differentiated from rhinovirus, influenza, RSV, and parainfluenza. It usually causes acute febrile illness in children and is identified as a common cause of exudative tonsillitis. Outbreaks in swimming pools and summer camps also involve adenoviruses. When epidemic keratoconjunctivitis is suspected, bacterial conjunctivitis, *Enterovirus,* and HSV must be excluded. Pneumonia associated morbidity is well documented among children, military recruits, and adults in chronic care facilities. Differential diagnosis in this case includes RSV, influenza, parainfluenza, and *Human metapneumovirus*. Although rotavirus is the leading cause of diarrhea in infants, adenovirus infection has been found to cause a prolonged diarrheal syndrome. Taking into consideration the fact that adenovirus infection frequently causes disease in immunocompromised patients, PCR is warranted for immediate diagnosis in these individuals.

Treatment

Antiviral therapy for adenovirus is currently approved for severe cases and immunocompromised patients. Cidofovir is preferred from ganciclovir for the treatment of adenovirus.[522,523,529] Despite being scarce, data from case reports and nonrandomized studies are encouraging showing better outcomes and increased survival in HCT and immunocompromised patients.[498,499,522,523,530-536] Nephrotoxicity is a major drawback and may require dose modification.[532] IVIG may be used as an adjunct in adenovirus disease. It contains high levels of pooled neutralizing antibodies against common adenoviral serotypes.[537-539]

Prevention

In 2011, a new live oral adenoviral vaccine against serotypes 4 and 7 was approved for military personnel aged 17–50 years in the United States.[453] Since adenovirus is stable in environmental conditions and resistant to alcohol and ether, decontamination is arduous and special agents are required, such as chlorine, formaldehyde, and heat.[540] Fastidious water chlorination in swimming pools can prevent outbreaks in summer camps.[541]

CORONAVIRUS

Basic Knowledge-Epidemiology-Pathophysiology

Coronaviruses are enveloped positive sense single-stranded RNA viruses with the largest RNA genome ever found. Their name, deriving from the Latin word *corona* which means crown, is suggestive of their look under electronic microscopy.[542] The S protein found on the surface of the virus is responsible for this effect as well as the host tropism since it is heavily glycosylated and resides on the membrane that the virus took from the previously infected host cell.[543] Two genera infecting human beings have been identified; namely, alphacoronaviruses and betacoronaviruses.[542] These genera contain four non-SARS and one *SARS* viruses.[542] Coronavirus is also a member of the *Nidovirales* order,[544] i.e., viruses with RNA genome that is structurally close to the eukaryotic mRNA so that they can use the host replicating mechanisms in order to produce new virions. As an example, the coronavirus genome does not code for a polymerase, rather it codes for some proteins regulating viral replication and some structural proteins (S, M, HE, and E).[544] The hemagglutinin-esterase protein in concordance to influenza and parainfluenza HN helps in absorption and release of the virus to and from the host cell.[545]

Coronavirus infections are universal; although infections may have winter predominance as influenza does, illness can occur round the year.[546-548] Since testing for corona infections still remains unreliable, it is difficult to identify the prevalence and frequency of each strain. Direct contact with contaminated surfaces and aerosol droplets is implicated in viral transmission. Some antigenic variation may result in reinfection with the virus.[549]

Clinical Picture

Coronavirus infections result in most instances in common cold symptoms, such as nasal congestion, rhinorrhea, sore throat, sneezing, cough, and watery eyes.[118,119,550,551] Other respiratory viruses, such as rhinovirus, coxsackie virus, and RSV can cause the same symptoms.[118,119] Asymptomatic shedding of the virus occurs and is probably responsible for reported transmission in hospitalized pediatric patients.[552] The percentage of people with common cold hosting the virus may range from 1% to 35%.[553] In children, coronavirus infection can be complicated by serous otitis media and the virus can be easily detected in the ear fluid, although there is data that the infection may run an asymptomatic course in children.[554,555] Other than common cold, coronavirus can be responsible for significant cases of LTRI infections, such as community-acquired pneumonia in adults and bronchiolitis and croup in children.[556-564] In addition to primary disease, as already described, it can also cause exacerbation of underlying pulmonary diseases including asthma and COPD in the elderly.[1,565]

Novel Coronaviruses

In November 2002, in China, a new member of the *betacoronavirus* genus emerged.[566,567] Termed as severe acute respiratory syndrome coronavirus (SARS CoV) due to the disease associated with it, it is thought to use palm civets, an animal resembling to cat, as an intermediate link before infection is passed to humans.[568,569] Contrary to non-SARS coronavirus, SARS CoV presents with an initial period of flu-like symptoms and fever in almost all cases.[570] After 5–7 days, a nonproductive cough starts along with dyspnea that may proceed to respiratory failure requiring mechanical ventilation.[567,571-576] Frequent laboratory findings included lymphopenia, an increased LDH and an elevated SGPT.[567,577] The virus transmission was halted at a global level through intense infection control measures; however, not before resulting in a near pandemic with 8,273 cases and 775 deaths worldwide (9.6% fatality rate) according to the World Health Organization.

More recently a novel coronavirus was first identified in September 2012 in a patient who died from a severe respiratory infection in June 2012. The virus has so far (March 27th 2014) been identified in 206 cases resulting in 86 deaths. Thus far, the affected countries in the Middle East include Jordan, Kuwait, Oman, Qatar, Saudi Arabia and the United Arab Emirates (UAE), all of which appear to have had primary transmission events from non-human sources. Other affected countries include France, Germany, Italy, and the United Kingdom, in Europe; and Tunisia, in North Africa. In these countries, cases have been imported from the Middle East with some secondary transmission (dataavailable at http://www.who.int/csr/disease/coronavirus_infections/MERS_CoV_Update_27_March_2014.pdf?ua=1). Patients exhibit an acute, serious respiratory illness with fever, cough, shortness of breath, and breathing difficulties. Dromedary camels maybe the host for the virus in the natural environment in the Arabian peninsula.

Coronaviruses and Other Clinical Associations

There has been some loose association between coronavirus infection and gastrointestinal (GI) tract pathology including gastroenteritis and necrotizing hemorrhagic enterocolitis in newborns, as it was suggested by the detection of coronavirus-like particles in stool.[578-581] However, these findings occurred with concomitant detection of other diarrhea causing pathogens, such as rotavirus or norovirus.[582] Coronavirus has been identified as a potential cause of multiple sclerosis based on data indicating the presence of cross-reactive T-cells for myelin as well as for the virus itself during persistent virus infection of oligodendroglia and neuroglia.[583-585]

Diagnosis

Diagnosis can be based on clinical suspicion when common cold symptoms ensue, but for definite virus diagnosis, PCR techniques are warranted as they carry higher levels of sensitivity-specificity than other rapid techniques.[586-588]

Treatment

Treatment, as in most cases of respiratory viruses, is largely supportive, while in SARS several experimental protocols were tried including interferon plus corticosteroids, protease inhibitors, intravenous immunoglobulin, and convalescent plasma.[589-591] The development of specific monoclonal antibodies may hold promise for the future.[592]

HUMAN METAPNEUMOVIRUS

Basic Knowledge-Epidemiology-Pathophysiology

Human metapneumovirus (HMPV) is an enveloped, nonsegmented negative-sense RNA virus. It belongs to the *Paramyxoviridae* family along with other viruses including RSV and parainfluenza. Virus analysis has identified two types, HMPV A and B, circulating concurrently in the community, although some type predominance may be observed each year.[593,594] HMPV is phylogenetically close to the avian metapneumovirus but a direct link has not been established.[595-598] In experiments conducted in species other than humans, HMPV is linked to upper respiratory tract insult with prolonged airway inflammation.[599] It seems that the inflammation results in airway epithelium hyperresponsiveness and an obstructive respiratory pattern due to epithelium hyperplasia and mucus overproduction.[600,601] Transmission occurs through direct contact with contaminated surfaces, droplets, and large particle aerosols.[602-604]

Human metapneumovirus has been causing respiratory infections universally for more than 60 years, although infections up till the discovery of the virus where attributed to other known respiratory viruses with higher prevalence.[595-598,605-607] It can affect all ages resulting in asymptomatic or mild upper or lower respiratory infection. Symptomatic disease usually affects the extremes of age, i.e., young children and the elderly.[608,609] It exhibits a seasonal variation, identical to that of RSV, causing disease during winter and early spring.[595,602,608,610] Nevertheless, summer outbreaks have been also reported.[611] HMPV, infection is responsible for about 8–25% of URI, 12% of LTRI and 6% of respiratory infections requiring hospitalization in children.[608,609,612-615] Almost all children have at least one episode of infection by the age of 5 years old.[595] In adults, the infection prevalence seems to be lower accounting for 4.5% of both URI and LTRI and 11% in patients requiring admission.[616]

Clinical Picture

Incubation period ranges from 3–5 days. Viral peak shedding is thought to occur two days after incubation but symptoms reach their height two days later. In children, URI symptoms are relatively unstable with cough and fever being more common followed by rhinitis and wheezing.[608-610] Rhinopharyngitis and laryngitis can also occur.[608-610] LRTI manifestations include bronchiolitis, croup, and pneumonia.[608] HMPV is also implicated in wheezing as well as in asthma exacerbation.[606,609,610,617] Coinfection with RSV increases significantly the severity of bronchiolitis, and pneumonia requiring hospitalization, and mechanical ventilation.[135,618,619] There have been rare reports of severe/fatal encephalitis in children, but causal relationship remains equivocal.[620,621] Adult patients present with symptoms resembling the common cold infection, that is with cough, nasal congestion and rhinorrhea in addition to dyspnea, hoarseness and wheezing.[616] HMPV infection can cause asthma exacerbation, but an association with COPD exacerbations remains unclear.[622-625] Immunocompromised individuals are more prone to severe complicated infections.[626-630]

Diagnosis

Diagnosis of HMPV virus on clinical grounds is extremely difficult and HMPV frequency may be underestimated provided that symptomatology is essentially the same as with other, more common viruses. Viral cultures are difficult to be processed, as virus isolation requires inoculation onto special cell lines available only in research laboratories.[608] Since all individuals are infected until the age of 5, serologic diagnosis requires recent seroconversion, i.e., a fourfold increase in antibody titers.[595,616,631] Immunofluorescence testing has not yet been widely used in the clinical setting. PCR techniques remain the most reliable means of virus isolation of metapneumovirus and other respiratory viral pathogens. Diagnostic testing to exclude invasive bacterial disease is necessary.

Treatment

Therapy is exclusively supportive and based upon clinical manifestations. Ribavirin has shown activity against pneumovirus but is not used due to the toxicity it causes.[600,632] Specific monoclonal antibodies have been developed but have not been tested in clinical trials yet. Antibiotic treatment can be used in cases of bacterial superinfection.

ENTEROVIRUS INFECTION

Basic Knowledge-Epidemiology-Pathophysiology

Although *Enterovirus* does not belong to the respiratory viruses, a brief description is provided in this section since it might be associated with respiratory symptoms. *Enterovirus* genus belongs to the picornavirus family along with rhinovirus and hepatitis A virus and consists of poliovirus, coxsackie A and B viruses, and echovirus.[633] Collectively, they are called *Enteroviruses*.

Enteroviruses are small, nonenveloped, icosahedral viruses that contain a single-stranded, nonsegmented RNA genome.[633] Individuals are infected by ingestion of contaminated food or water.[633] Due to the lack of an envelope, *Enteroviruses* are stable in stomach pH, replicate in GI tract, and can be detected in stool. As a result, they exhibit a fecal-oral pattern of transmission.[634] The GI system function as an entry portal and then viruses are spread in multiple organs via the bloodstream. The vast majority of *Enteroviruses* (>90%) run an asymptomatic course of disease.[635] However, when symptomatic, they cause significant and severe disease varying according to age, gender, and immune status of the host.[636-642]

Clinical Picture

Enteroviruses may cause an undifferentiated febrile illness or illness with symptoms identical to common cold. Usually this illness is self-limited and does not cause any complications. It is vital to be able to differentiate them from other respiratory viruses, since they can have increased morbidity and mortality.

Enterovirus infections are associated with some characteristic symptoms that can assist in this differential diagnosis. Maculopapular eruptions are common with *Enteroviruses*[643-645] and usually appear 24–36 hours after fever onset; as the temperature declines simultaneously, a discrete, non-pruritic, salmon-pink rash in the face and upper chest appears.[646,647] Hand-foot-mouth (HFM) syndrome is an acute illness characterized by fever, oral vesicles on the buccal mucosa and tongue, accompanied by tender cutaneous lesions of the hands, feet, buttocks, and rarely genitalia.[648] When caused by *Enterovirus 71*, it can result in CNS disease, pulmonary edema, and hemorrhage and heart failure.[649-653] Coxsackie A, except from HFM syndrome, can also cause a vesicular enanthem of the tonsils and soft palate in young children resulting in sore throat and odynophagia, known as herpangina.[654] Summer outbreaks are typical for the disease.[654]

Manifestations from the CNS include mostly aseptic meningitis and less commonly encephalitis. Viral meningitis affects infants more frequently than adults.[655,656] Coxsackie B and echovirus are involved in the majority of cases.[657] Fever and irritability are usually the symptoms. Complete recovery occurs in almost all cases in 3–7 days. Encephalitis can also occur but cases caused by *Enteroviruses* are usually milder than arboviruses and HSV.[658] Poliomyelitis is an acute febrile disease along with aseptic meningitis resulting in weakness and paralysis of one or more extremities. Brainstem encephalitis and pulmonary edema caused by *Enterovirus 71* can rapidly lead to death.[659-661]

Pleurodynia is another acute illness caused by coxsackie B virus that is characterized by fever and muscle spasms of the chest and abdomen.[662-664] It takes the form of outbreaks during summer in adults and adolescents. Pain caused by pleurodynia can mimic pneumonia, myocardial infarction, acute abdomen, pulmonary embolism, and herpes zoster infection. Myopericarditis can also be a manifestation of *Enterovirus* infection with various degrees of either pericardial or myocardial inflammation, and symptoms ranging from mild disease to acute heart failure.[665-667] Acute hemorrhagic conjunctivitis is an ocular infection presenting with pain, lid edema, and subconjunctival hemorrhage.[668] It is commonly self-limited and must be differentiated from adenovirus caused disease, such as pharyngoconjunctival fever and epidemic keratoconjunctivitis.

Neonates are particularly susceptible to severe infection by *Enterovirus*.[669] The virus can be acquired either in the NICU or directly from the mother.[670-675] Initial symptoms are vague and mild, such as anorexia and minimal respiratory distress.[670,676] More serious disease can ensue with myocarditis, encephalitis, and fulminant hepatitis being common.[677-683]

Diagnosis

Enteroviruses can be responsible for severe morbidity and mortality in the community. Thus it is critical to include them in our differential diagnosis in the early stages of an apparent respiratory infection. The diagnosis is obtained either by serology (for diagnosis fourfold increase in antibodies to *Enteroviruses* between the acute and convalescent phases of illness) needs to be demonstrated or by culture (characteristic cytopathic in samples from CSF, blood, or feces) or by newer molecular techniques such as PCR.

Treatment

Management is largely supportive. Symptomatic treatment is necessary and IV immune globulin and pleconaril have been used in small case series.[684,685]

HUMAN BOCAVIRUS

Basic Knowledge-Epidemiology-Pathophysiology

Human bocavirus (HBoV) is a viral pathogen belonging to the *Parvoviridae* family that was first identified in Sweden in 2005 from respiratory tract samples.[66] It shares many similarities to parvovirus B19 and exhibits a direct pathogenic effect on bronchial cells.[686-688] HBoV is a small, nonenveloped, negative-sense or positive-sense, single stranded DNA virus.[689] Since its identification, four bocavirus types have been documented.[690]

Bocavirus is ubiquitous.[691,692] It seems that it has no specific seasonal variation with slight winter predominance and causes about 5–10% of respiratory infections during this season with newer data suggesting an even higher incidence.[693-699] All of the children become exposed to the virus until 6 years of age indicating that it may run an asymptomatic course when in low viral load.[700-703] The virus causes upper or LRTIs (when in high viral loads) in pediatric patients, with children less than 2 years old running the greatest risk.[694,704-707] High rates of coinfection with other viruses have been documented including RSV, rhinovirus, and adenovirus making pathogenicity difficult to define.[708-712] It seems though that this happens due to HBoV persistence in the respiratory tract.[713,714] Spread of the virus is thought to occur in the classic ways of transmission, but there is some data suggesting that river and sewage contaminated water may play an additional role.[715,716]

Clinical Picture

Manifestations from the upper respiratory tract include cough, fever, rhinorrhea, sore throat, persistent otitis media, and a pertussis like syndrome due to paroxysmal cough.[693,717-719] LTRI in young children may be present as bronchitis, bronchiolitis, and pneumonia.[720-726] Petechial rash, hypoxia, and neutrophilia are associated findings.[727,728] Life-threatening disease with severe respiratory disease necessitating the use of extracorporeal membrane oxygenation (ECMO) has been documented.[729,730] It has been also associated with wheezing with possible asthma sequela and asthmatic exacerbation.[708,709,731-733] Except for community CAP, bocavirus may be responsible for hospital-acquired pneumonia in children.[734] There is evidence that HBoV can additionally cause gastroenteritis presenting as diarrhea and abdominal pain with subsequent isolation of the virus in stool, but causal relation remains to be proven.[735-740] A loose association with Kawasaki disease and encephalitis may exist.[741-745]

Immunocompromised children experience the same symptoms as normal ones, but viral reactivation and prolonged shedding might occur producing persistent symptoms.[746,747] Incidence seems to be the same as in immunocompetent children.[748] However, in rare cases disseminated disease may ensue along with hepatitis and severe diarrhea.[749-751]

Diagnosis

Classic and real-time quantative PCR techniques using nasopharyngeal aspirates and swabs are available for HBoV detection.[689,752-754] Serologic testing from nasopharyngeal specimen is also helpful.[755-757]

Treatment

Management of bocavirus infections is largely supportive as there is no known effective antiviral against this virus.

REFERENCES

1. Nicholson KG, Kent J, Ireland DC. Respiratory viruses and exacerbations of asthma in adults. *BMJ.* 1993;307(6910):982-6.
2. Johnston SL, Pattemore PK, Sanderson G, et al. Community study of role of viral infections in exacerbations of asthma in 9-11 year old children. *BMJ.* 1995;310(6989):1225-9.
3. Gilca R, De Serres G, Tremblay M, et al. Distribution and clinical impact of human respiratory syncytial virus genotypes in hospitalized children over 2 winter seasons. *J Infect Dis.* 2006;193(1):54-8.
4. Papadopoulos NG, Gourgiotis D, Javadyan A, et al. Does respiratory syncytial virus subtype influences the severity of acute bronchiolitis in hospitalized infants? *Respir Med.* 2004;98(9):879-82.
5. Hall CB, Walsh EE, Schnabel KC, et al. Occurrence of groups A and B of respiratory syncytial virus over 15 years:

associated epidemiologic and clinical characteristics in hospitalized and ambulatory children. *J Infect Dis.* 1990; 162(6):1283-90.
6. McConnochie KM, Hall CB, Walsh EE, et al. Variation in severity of respiratory syncytial virus infections with subtype. *J Pediatr.* 1990;117(1 Pt 1):52-62.
7. Walsh EE, McConnochie KM, Long CE, et al. Severity of respiratory syncytial virus infection is related to virus strain. *J Infect Dis.* 1997;175(4):814-20.
8. Peret TC, Hall CB, Schnabel KC, et al. Circulation patterns of genetically distinct group A and B strains of human respiratory syncytial virus in a community. *J Gen Virol.* 1998;79(Pt 9):2221-9.
9. Hall CB, Douglas RG, Geiman JM. Quantitative shedding patterns of respiratory syncytial virus in infants. *J Infect Dis.* 1975;132(2):151-6.
10. Hall CB, Douglas RG. Modes of transmission of respiratory syncytial virus. *J Pediatr.* 1981;99(1):100-3.
11. Hall CB, Douglas RG, Schnabel KC, et al. Infectivity of respiratory syncytial virus by various routes of inoculation. *Infect Immun.* 1981;33(3):779-83.
12. Hoffman SJ, Laham FR, Polack FP. Mechanisms of illness during respiratory syncytial virus infection: the lungs, the virus and the immune response. *Microbes Infect.* 2004;6(8):767-72.
13. Johnson JE, Gonzales RA, Olson SJ, et al. The histopathology of fatal untreated human respiratory syncytial virus infection. *Mod Pathol.* 2007;20(1):108-19.
14. Aherne W, Bird T, Court SD, et al. Pathological changes in virus infections of the lower respiratory tract in children. *J Clin Pathol.* 1970;23(1):7-18.
15. Everard ML, Swarbrick A, Wrightham M, et al. Analysis of cells obtained by bronchial lavage of infants with respiratory syncytial virus infection. *Arch Dis Child.* 1994;71(5):428-32.
16. Nadal D, Wunderli W, Meurmann O, et al. Isolation of respiratory syncytial virus from liver tissue and extrahepatic biliary atresia material. *Scand J Infect Dis.* 1990;22(1):91-3.
17. Zlateva KT, Van Ranst M. Detection of subgroup B respiratory syncytial virus in the cerebrospinal fluid of a patient with respiratory syncytial virus pneumonia. *Pediatr Infect Dis J.* 2004;23(11):1065-6.
18. Fishaut M, Tubergen D, McIntosh K. Cellular response to respiratory viruses with particular reference to children with disorders of cell-mediated immunity. *J Pediatr.* 1980; 96(2):179-86.
19. Rohwedder A, Keminer O, Forster J, et al. Detection of respiratory syncytial virus RNA in blood of neonates by polymerase chain reaction. *J Med Virol.* 1998;54(4):320-7.
20. O'Donnell DR, McGarvey MJ, Tully JM, et al. Respiratory syncytial virus RNA in cells from the peripheral blood during acute infection. *J Pediatr.* 1998;133(2):272-4.
21. Legg JP, Hussain IR, Warner JA, et al. Type 1 and type 2 cytokine imbalance in acute respiratory syncytial virus bronchiolitis. *Am J Respir Crit Care Med.* 2003;168(6):633-9.
22. Garofalo RP, Patti J, Hintz KA, et al. Macrophage inflammatory protein-1alpha (not T helper type 2 cytokines) is associated with severe forms of respiratory syncytial virus bronchiolitis. *J Infect Dis.* 2001;184(4):393-9.
23. Tripp RA, Moore D, Barskey A, et al. Peripheral blood mononuclear cells from infants hospitalized because of respiratory syncytial virus infection express T helper-1 and T helper-2 cytokines and CC chemokine messenger RNA. *J Infect Dis.* 2002;185(10):1388-94.
24. Van Benten IJ, van Drunen CM, Koopman LP, et al. RSV-induced bronchiolitis but not upper respiratory tract infection is accompanied by an increased nasal IL-18 response. *J Med Virol.* 2003;71(2):290-7.
25. Einarsson O, Geba GP, Zhu Z, et al. Interleukin-11: stimulation in vivo and in vitro by respiratory viruses and induction of airways hyperresponsiveness. *J Clin Invest.* 1996;97(4):915-24.
26. Puthothu B, Krueger M, Forster J, et al. Interleukin (IL)-18 polymorphism 133C/G is associated with severe respiratory syncytial virus infection. *Pediatr Infect Dis J.* 2007;26(12):1094-8.
27. Noah TL, Henderson FW, Wortman IA, et al. Nasal cytokine production in viral acute upper respiratory infection of childhood. *J Infect Dis.* 1995;171(3):584-92.
28. Matsuda K, Tsutsumi H, Okamoto Y, et al. Development of interleukin 6 and tumor necrosis factor alpha activity in nasopharyngeal secretions of infants and children during infection with respiratory syncytial virus. *Clin Diagn Lab Immunol.* 1995;2(3):322-4.
29. Smyth RL, Fletcher JN, Thomas HM, et al. Immunological responses to respiratory syncytial virus infection in infancy. *Arch Dis Child.* 1997;76(3):210-4.
30. Welliver RC, Garofalo RP, Ogra PL. Beta-chemokines, but neither T helper type 1 nor T helper type 2 cytokines, correlate with severity of illness during respiratory syncytial virus infection. *Pediatr Infect Dis J.* 2002;21(5):457-61.
31. Garofalo RP, Hintz KH, Hill V, et al. A comparison of epidemiologic and immunologic features of bronchiolitis caused by influenza virus and respiratory syncytial virus. *J Med Virol.* 2005;75(2):282-9.
32. Henderson FW, Collier AM, Clyde WA, et al. Respiratory-syncytial-virus-infections, reinfections and immunity. A prospective, longitudinal study in young children. *N Engl J Med.* 1979;300(10):530-4.
33. Hall CB, Walsh EE, Long CE, et al. Immunity to and frequency of reinfection with respiratory syncytial virus. *J Infect Dis.* 1991;163(4):693-8.
34. Hall CB, Weinberg GA, Iwane MK, et al. The burden of respiratory syncytial virus infection in young children. *N Engl J Med.* 2009;360(6):588-98.
35. Agoti CN, Mbisa JL, Bett A, et al. Intrapatient variation of the respiratory syncytial virus attachment protein gene. *J Virol.* 2010;84(19):10425-8.
36. Boyce TG, Mellen BG, Mitchel EF, et al. Rates of hospitalization for respiratory syncytial virus infection among children in medicaid. *J Pediatr.* 2000;137(6):865-70.
37. Falsey AR, Walsh EE. Respiratory syncytial virus infection in adults. *Clin Microbiol Rev.* 2000;13(3):371-84.
38. Englund JA, Sullivan CJ, Jordan MC, et al. Respiratory syncytial virus infection in immunocompromised adults. *Ann Inter Med.* 1988;109(3):203-8.
39. Harrington RD, Hooton TM, Hackman RC, et al. An outbreak of respiratory syncytial virus in a bone marrow transplant center. *J Infect Dis.* 1992;165(6):987-93.

40. Glezen WP, Paredes A, Allison JE, et al. Risk of respiratory syncytial virus infection for infants from low-income families in relationship to age, sex, ethnic group, and maternal antibody level. *J Pediatr.* 1981;98(5):708-15.
41. Walsh EE, Falsey AR. Age related differences in humoral immune response to respiratory syncytial virus infection in adults. *J Med Virol.* 2004;73(2):295-9.
42. Stensballe LG, Ravn H, Kristensen K, et al. Seasonal variation of maternally derived respiratory syncytial virus antibodies and association with infant hospitalizations for respiratory syncytial virus. *J Pediatr.* 2009;154(2):296-8.
43. Shay DK, Holman RC, Newman RD, et al. Bronchiolitis-associated hospitalizations among US children, 1980-1996. *JAMA.* 1999;282(15):1440-6.
44. Zacharoula Oikonomopoulou M, Petros Karakitsos, Archontis Zampogiannis, et al. Changes in the clinical & molecular epidemiology of respiratory viruses in a tertiary care center during the 2009-2012 consecutive winter seasons. ID Week 2012. San Diego, CA; 2012.
45. Dimopoulos G, Lerikou M, Tsiodras S, et al. Viral epidemiology of acute exacerbations of chronic obstructive pulmonary disease. *Pulm Pharmacol Ther.* 2012;25(1):12-8.
46. O'Shea MK, Ryan MA, Hawksworth AW, et al. Symptomatic respiratory syncytial virus infection in previously healthy young adults living in a crowded military environment. *Clin Infect Dis.* 2005;41(3):311-7.
47. Thompson WW, Shay DK, Weintraub E, et al. Mortality associated with influenza and respiratory syncytial virus in the United States. *JAMA.* 2003;289(2):179-86.
48. Glezen WP, Taber LH, Frank AL, et al. Risk of primary infection and reinfection with respiratory syncytial virus. *Am J Dis Child.* 1986;140(6):543-6.
49. Heiskanen-Kosma T, Korppi M, Jokinen C, et al. Etiology of childhood pneumonia: serologic results of a prospective, population-based study. *Pediatr Infect Dis J.* 1998;17(11):986-91.
50. Anas N, Boettrich C, Hall CB, et al. The association of apnea and respiratory syncytial virus infection in infants. *J Pediatr.* 1982;101(1):65-8.
51. Bruhn FW, Mokrohisky ST, McIntosh K. Apnea associated with respiratory syncytial virus infection in young infants. *J Pediatr.* 1977;90(3):382-6.
52. Church NR, Anas NG, Hall CB, et al. Respiratory syncytial virus-related apnea in infants. Demographics and outcome. *Am J Dis Child.* 1984;138(3):247-50.
53. Hall CB, Hall WJ, Speers DM. Clinical and physiological manifestations of bronchiolitis and pneumonia. Outcome of respiratory syncytial virus. *Am J Dis Child.* 1979; 133(8):798-802.
54. Arms JL, Ortega H, Reid S. Chronological and clinical characteristics of apnea associated with respiratory syncytial virus infection: a retrospective case series. *Clin Pediatr.* 2008;47(9):953-8.
55. Ralston S, Hill V. Incidence of apnea in infants hospitalized with respiratory syncytial virus bronchiolitis: a systematic review. *J Pediatr.* 2009;155(5):728-33.
56. Uren EC, Williams AL, Jack I, et al. Association of respiratory virus infections with sudden infant death syndrome. *Med J Aust.* 1980;1(9):417-9.
57. Rayyan M, Naulaers G, Daniels H, et al. Characteristics of respiratory syncytial virus-related apnoea in three infants. *Acta Paediatr.* 2004;93(6):847-9.
58. McConnochie KM, Roghmann KJ. Predicting clinically significant lower respiratory tract illness in childhood following mild bronchiolitis. *Am J Dis Child.* 1985;139(6): 625-31.
59. Mansbach JM, Piedra PA, Teach SJ, et al. Prospective multicenter study of viral etiology and hospital length of stay in children with severe bronchiolitis. *Arch Pediatr Adolesc Med.* 2012;166(8):700-6.
60. Richard N, Komurian-Pradel F, Javouhey E, et al. The impact of dual viral infection in infants admitted to a pediatric intensive care unit associated with severe bronchiolitis. *Pediatr Infect Dis J.* 2008;27(3):213-7.
61. Stempel HE, Martin ET, Kuypers J, et al. Multiple viral respiratory pathogens in children with bronchiolitis. *Acta Paediatr.* 2009;98(1):123-6.
62. Miron D, Srugo I, Kra-Oz Z, et al. Sole pathogen in acute bronchiolitis: is there a role for other organisms apart from respiratory syncytial virus? *Pediatr Infect Dis J.* 2010;29(1):e7-10.
63. Midulla F, Scagnolari C, Bonci E, et al. Respiratory syncytial virus, human bocavirus and rhinovirus bronchiolitis in infants. *Arch Dis Child.* 2010;95(1):35-41.
64. Calvo C, Garcia-Garcia ML, Blanco C, et al. Multiple simultaneous viral infections in infants with acute respiratory tract infections in Spain. *J Clin Virol.* 2008;42(3): 268-72.
65. Calvo C, Garcia-Garcia ML, Pozo F, et al. Clinical characteristics of human bocavirus infections compared with other respiratory viruses in Spanish children. *Pediatr Infect Dis J.* 2008;27(8):677-80.
66. Allander T, Tammi MT, Eriksson M, et al. Cloning of a human parvovirus by molecular screening of respiratory tract samples. *Proc Natl Acad Sci USA.* 2005;102(36):12891-6.
67. Mansbach JM, McAdam AJ, Clark S, et al. Prospective multicenter study of the viral etiology of bronchiolitis in the emergency department. *Acad Emerg Med.* 2008;15(2):111-8.
68. Lina B, Valette M, Foray S, et al. Surveillance of community-acquired viral infections due to respiratory viruses in Rhone-Alpes (France) during winter 1994 to 1995. *J Clin Microbiol.* 1996;34(12):3007-11.
69. Hall CB, Long CE, Schnabel KC. Respiratory syncytial virus infections in previously healthy working adults. *Clin Infect Dis.* 2001;33(6):792-6.
70. American Academy of Pediatrics Subcommittee on Diagnosis and Management of Bronchiolitis. Diagnosis and management of bronchiolitis. *Pediatrics.* 2006; 118(4): 1774-93.
71. Hall CB, Powell KR, Schnabel KC, et al. Risk of secondary bacterial infection in infants hospitalized with respiratory syncytial viral infection. *J Pediatr.* 1988;113(2):266-71.
72. Swingler GH, Hussey GD, Zwarenstein M. Randomised controlled trial of clinical outcome after chest radiograph in ambulatory acute lower-respiratory infection in children. *Lancet.* 1998;351(9100):404-8.
73. Dawson KP, Long A, Kennedy J, et al. The chest radiograph in acute bronchiolitis. *J Paediatr Child Health.* 1990; 26(4):209-11.
74. Wang EE, Law BJ, Stephens D. Pediatric Investigators Collaborative Network on Infections in Canada (PICNIC) prospective study of risk factors and outcomes in patients hospitalized with respiratory syncytial viral lower respiratory tract infection. *J Pediatr.* 1995;126(2):212-9.

75. Shaw KN, Bell LM, Sherman NH. Outpatient assessment of infants with bronchiolitis. *Am J Dis Child.* 1991;145(2):151-5.
76. Wang EE, Law BJ, Boucher FD, et al. Pediatric Investigators Collaborative Network on Infections in Canada (PICNIC) study of admission and management variation in patients hospitalized with respiratory syncytial viral lower respiratory tract infection. *J Pediatr.* 1996;129(3):390-5.
77. MacDonald NE, Hall CB, Suffin SC, et al. Respiratory syncytial viral infection in infants with congenital heart disease. *N Engl J Med.* 1982;307(7):397-400.
78. Hall CB, Powell KR, MacDonald NE, et al. Respiratory syncytial viral infection in children with compromised immune function. *N Engl J Med.* 1986;315(2):77-81.
79. Meissner HC. Selected populations at increased risk from respiratory syncytial virus infection. *Pediatr Infect Dis J.* 2003;22(2 Suppl):S40-4.
80. Levine DA, Platt SL, Dayan PS, et al. Risk of serious bacterial infection in young febrile infants with respiratory syncytial virus infections. *Pediatrics.* 2004;113(6):1728-34.
81. Bilavsky E, Shouval DS, Yarden-Bilavsky H, et al. A prospective study of the risk for serious bacterial infections in hospitalized febrile infants with or without bronchiolitis. *Pediatr Infect Dis J.* 2008;27(3):269-70.
82. Kuppermann N, Bank DE, Walton EA, et al. Risks for bacteremia and urinary tract infections in young febrile children with bronchiolitis. *Arch Pediatr & Adolesc Med.* 1997;151(12):1207-14.
83. Melendez E, Harper MB. Utility of sepsis evaluation in infants 90 days of age or younger with fever and clinical bronchiolitis. *Pediatr Infect Dis J.* 2003;22(12):1053-6.
84. Purcell K, Fergie J. Concurrent serious bacterial infections in 2396 infants and children hospitalized with respiratory syncytial virus lower respiratory tract infections. *Arch Pediatr Adolesc Med.* 2002;156(4):322-4.
85. Bloomfield P, Dalton D, Karleka A, et al. Bacteraemia and antibiotic use in respiratory syncytial virus infections. *Arch Dis Child.* 2004;89(4):363-7.
86. Titus MO, Wright SW. Prevalence of serious bacterial infections in febrile infants with respiratory syncytial virus infection. *Pediatrics.* 2003;112(2):282-4.
87. Purcell K, Fergie J. Lack of usefulness of an abnormal white blood cell count for predicting a concurrent serious bacterial infection in infants and young children hospitalized with respiratory syncytial virus lower respiratory tract infection. *Pediatr Infect Dis J.* 2007; 26(4):311-5.
88. Ralston S, Hill V, Waters A. Occult serious bacterial infection in infants younger than 60 to 90 days with bronchiolitis: a systematic review. *Arch Pediatr Adolesc Med.* 2011;165(10):951-6.
89. Willson DF, Landrigan CP, Horn SD, et al. Complications in infants hospitalized for bronchiolitis or respiratory syncytial virus pneumonia. *J Pediatr.* 2003;143(5 Suppl): S142-9.
90. Kneyber MC, Brandenburg AH, de Groot R, et al. Risk factors for respiratory syncytial virus associated apnoea. *Eur J Pediatr.* 1998;157(4):331-5.
91. Thorburn K, Harigopal S, Reddy V, et al. High incidence of pulmonary bacterial co-infection in children with severe respiratory syncytial virus (RSV) bronchiolitis. *Thorax.* 2006;61(7):611-5.
92. Duttweiler L, Nadal D, Frey B. Pulmonary and systemic bacterial co-infections in severe RSV bronchiolitis. *Arch Dis Child.* 2004;89(12):1155-7.
93. Willwerth BM, Harper MB, Greenes DS. Identifying hospitalized infants who have bronchiolitis and are at high risk for apnea. *Ann Emerg Med.* 2006;48(4):441-7.
94. Simoes EA, Groothuis JR, Carbonell-Estrany X, et al. Palivizumab prophylaxis, respiratory syncytial virus, and subsequent recurrent wheezing. *J Pediatr.* 2007;151(1):34-42.
95. Stein RT, Sherrill D, Morgan WJ, et al. Respiratory syncytial virus in early life and risk of wheeze and allergy by age 13 years. *Lancet.* 1999;354(9178):541-5.
96. Sigurs N, Bjarnason R, Sigurbergsson F, et al. Respiratory syncytial virus bronchiolitis in infancy is an important risk factor for asthma and allergy at age 7. *Am J Respir Crit Care Med.* 2000;161(5):1501-7.
97. Hall CB, Hall WJ, Gala CL, et al. Long-term prospective study in children after respiratory syncytial virus infection. *J Pediatr.* 1984;105(3):358-64.
98. Sigurs N, Gustafsson PM, Bjarnason R, et al. Severe respiratory syncytial virus bronchiolitis in infancy and asthma and allergy at age 13. *AmJ Respir Crit Care Med.* 2005;171(2):137-41.
99. Henderson J, Hilliard TN, Sherriff A, et al. Hospitalization for RSV bronchiolitis before 12 months of age and subsequent asthma, atopy and wheeze: a longitudinal birth cohort study. *Pediatric Allergy Immunol.* 2005;16(5):386-92.
100. Sigurs N, Bjarnason R, Sigurbergsson F, et al. Asthma and immunoglobulin E antibodies after respiratory syncytial virus bronchiolitis: a prospective cohort study with matched controls. *Pediatrics.* 1995;95(4):500-5.
101. Martinez FD. Respiratory syncytial virus bronchiolitis and the pathogenesis of childhood asthma. *Pediatr Infect Dis J.* 2003;22(2 Suppl):S76-82.
102. Jackson DJ, Gangnon RE, Evans MD, et al. Wheezing rhinovirus illnesses in early life predict asthma development in high-risk children. *Am J Respir Crit Care Med.* 2008;178(7):667-72.
103. Gern JE. Viral respiratory infection and the link to asthma. *Pediatr Infect Dis J.* 2008;27(10 Suppl):S97-103.
104. Kotaniemi-Syrjanen A, Vainionpaa R, Reijonen TM, et al. Rhinovirus-induced wheezing in infancy—the first sign of childhood asthma? *J Allergy Clin Immunol.* 2003;111(1):66-71.
105. Carroll KN, Wu P, Gebretsadik T, et al. Season of infant bronchiolitis and estimates of subsequent risk and burden of early childhood asthma. *J Allergy Clin Immunol.* 2009; 123(4):964-6.
106. Bartlett NW, McLean GR, Chang YS, et al. Genetics and epidemiology: asthma and infection. *Curr Opin Allergy Clin Immunol.* 2009;9(5):395-400.
107. Pattemore PK, Johnston SL, Bardin PG. Viruses as precipitants of asthma symptoms. I. Epidemiology. *Clin Exp Allergy.* 1992;22(3):325-36.
108. Martinez FD, Morgan WJ, Wright AL, et al. Diminished lung function as a predisposing factor for wheezing respiratory illness in infants. *N Engl J Med.* 1988;319(17):1112-7.
109. Martinez FD, Wright AL, Taussig LM, et al. Asthma and wheezing in the first six years of life. The Group Health Medical Associates. *N Engl J Med.* 1995;332(3):133-8.

110. Shaheen SO. Changing patterns of childhood infection and the rise in allergic disease. *Clin Exp Allergy.* 1995;25(11): 1034-7.
111. Busse WW. Role and contribution of viral respiratory infections to asthma. *Allergy.* 1993;48(17 Suppl):57-61.
112. Cogswell JJ, Halliday DF, Alexander JR. Respiratory infections in the first year of life in children at risk of developing atopy. *Br Med J.* 1982;284(6321):1011-3.
113. Welliver RC. RSV and chronic asthma. *Lancet.* 1995; 346(8978):789-90.
114. Bacharier LB, Cohen R, Schweiger T, et al. Determinants of asthma after severe respiratory syncytial virus bronchiolitis. *J Allergy Clin Immunol.* 2012;130(1):91-100.
115. Hall WJ, Hall CB, Speers DM. Respiratory syncytial virus infection in adults: clinical, virologic, and serial pulmonary function studies. *Ann Intern Med.* 1978;88(2):203-5.
116. Wilkinson TM, Donaldson GC, Johnston SL, et al. Respiratory syncytial virus, airway inflammation, and FEV1 decline in patients with chronic obstructive pulmonary disease. *Am J Respir Crit Care Med.* 2006; 173(8):871-6.
117. Falsey AR, Formica MA, Hennessey PA, et al. Detection of respiratory syncytial virus in adults with chronic obstructive pulmonary disease. *Am J Respir Crit Care Med.* 2006;173(6):639-43.
118. Heikkinen T, Jarvinen A. The common cold. *Lancet.* 2003;361(9351):51-9.
119. Eccles R. Understanding the symptoms of the common cold and influenza. *Lancet Infect Dis.* 2005;5(11):718-25.
120. Ruuskanen O, Lahti E, Jennings LC, et al. Viral pneumonia. *Lancet.* 2011;377(9773):1264-75.
121. Hertz MI, Englund JA, Snover D, et al. Respiratory syncytial virus-induced acute lung injury in adult patients with bone marrow transplants: a clinical approach and review of the literature. *Medicine.* 1989;68(5):269-81.
122. Whimbey E, Champlin RE, Englund JA, et al. Combination therapy with aerosolized ribavirin and intravenous immunoglobulin for respiratory syncytial virus disease in adult bone marrow transplant recipients. *Bone Marrow Transplant.* 1995;16(3):393-9.
123. Wendt CH, Fox JM, Hertz MI. Paramyxovirus infection in lung transplant recipients. *J Heart Lung Transplant.* 1995; 14(3):479-85.
124. Miller RB, Chavers BM. Respiratory syncytial virus infections in pediatric renal transplant recipients. *Pediatr Nephrol.* 1996; 10(2):213-5.
125. Bordley WC, Viswanathan M, King VJ, et al. Diagnosis and testing in bronchiolitis: a systematic review. *Arch Pediatr Adolesc Med.* 2004;158(2):119-26.
126. Harris JA, Huskins WC, Langley JM. Health care epidemiology perspective on the October 2006 recommendations of the Subcommittee on Diagnosis and Management of Bronchiolitis. *Pediatrics.* 2007;120(4):890-2.
127. Smyth RL, Openshaw PJ. Bronchiolitis. *Lancet.* 2006; 368(9532):312-22.
128. Vogel AM, Lennon DR, Harding JE, et al. Variations in bronchiolitis management between five New Zealand hospitals: can we do better? *J Pediatr Child Health.* 2003; 39(1):40-5.
129. Adcock PM, Stout GG, Hauck MA, et al. Effect of rapid viral diagnosis on the management of children hospitalized with lower respiratory tract infection. *Pediatr Infect Dis J.* 1997;16(9):842-6.
130. Doan QH, Kissoon N, Dobson S, et al. A randomized, controlled trial of the impact of early and rapid diagnosis of viral infections in children brought to an emergency department with febrile respiratory tract illnesses. *J Pediatr.* 2009;154(1):91-5.
131. Ahluwalia G, Embree J, McNicol P, et al. Comparison of nasopharyngeal aspirate and nasopharyngeal swab specimens for respiratory syncytial virus diagnosis by cell culture, indirect immunofluorescence assay, and enzyme-linked immunosorbent assay. *J Clin Microbiol.* 1987;25(5):763-7.
132. Puppe W, Weigl JA, Aron G, et al. Evaluation of a multiplex reverse transcriptase PCR ELISA for the detection of nine respiratory tract pathogens. *J Clin Virol.* 2004;30(2):165-74.
133. Casiano-Colon AE, Hulbert BB, Mayer TK, et al. Lack of sensitivity of rapid antigen tests for the diagnosis of respiratory syncytial virus infection in adults. *J Clin Virol.* 2003;28(2):169-74.
134. Moore C, Valappil M, Corden S, et al. Enhanced clinical utility of the NucliSens EasyQ RSV A+B Assay for rapid detection of respiratory syncytial virus in clinical samples. *Eur J Clin Microbiol Infect Dis.* 2006;25(3):167-74.
135. Greensill J, McNamara PS, Dove W, et al. Human metapneumovirus in severe respiratory syncytial virus bronchiolitis. *Emerg Infect Dis.* 2003;9(3):372-5.
136. Crowcroft NS, Booy R, Harrison T, et al. Severe and unrecognised: pertussis in UK infants. *Arch Dis Child.* 2003;88(9):802-6.
137. Nuolivirta K, Koponen P, He Q, et al. Bordetella pertussis infection is common in nonvaccinated infants admitted for bronchiolitis. *Pediatr Infect Dis J.* 2010;29(11):1013-5.
138. Fuller H, Del Mar C. Immunoglobulin treatment for respiratory syncytial virus infection. *Cochrane Database Syst Rev.* 2006;(4):CD004883.
139. Hemming VG, Rodriguez W, Kim HW, et al. Intravenous immunoglobulin treatment of respiratory syncytial virus infections in infants and young children. *Antimicrob Agents and Chemother.* 1987;31(12):1882-6.
140. Rodriguez WJ, Gruber WC, Groothuis JR, et al. Respiratory syncytial virus immune globulin treatment of RSV lower respiratory tract infection in previously healthy children. *Pediatrics.* 1997;100(6):937-42.
141. Saez-Llorens X, Moreno MT, Ramilo O, et al. Safety and pharmacokinetics of palivizumab therapy in children hospitalized with respiratory syncytial virus infection. *Pediatr Infect Dis J.* 2004;23(8):707-12.
142. Carbonell-Estrany X, Simoes EA, Dagan R, et al. Motavizumab for prophylaxis of respiratory syncytial virus in high-risk children: a noninferiority trial. *Pediatrics.* 2010;125(1):e35-51.
143. Venkatesh MP, Weisman LE. Prevention and treatment of respiratory syncytial virus infection in infants: an update. *Expert Rev Vaccines.* 2006;5(2):261-8.
144. Frogel M, Nerwen C, Cohen A, et al. Prevention of hospitalization due to respiratory syncytial virus: results

from the Palivizumab Outcomes Registry. *J Perinatol.* 2008;28(7):511-7.
145. Palivizumab, a humanized respiratory syncytial virus monoclonal antibody, reduces hospitalization from respiratory syncytial virus infection in high-risk infants. The IMpact-RSV Study Group. *Pediatrics.* 1998;102(3 Pt 1): 531-7.
146. Null D, Pollara B, Dennehy PH, et al. Safety and immunogenicity of palivizumab (Synagis) administered for two seasons. *Pediatr Infect Dis J.* 2005;24(11):1021-3.
147. Oh PI, Lanctjt KL, Yoon A, et al. Palivizumab prophylaxis for respiratory syncytial virus in Canada: utilization and outcomes. *Pediatr Infect Dis J.* 2002;21(6):512-8.
148. Sorrentino M, Powers T. Effectiveness of palivizumab: evaluation of outcomes from the 1998 to 1999 respiratory syncytial virus season. The Palivizumab Outcomes Study Group. *Pediatr Infect Dis J.* 2000;19(11):1068-71.
149. Feltes TF, Sondheimer HM, Tulloh RM, et al. A randomized controlled trial of motavizumab versus palivizumab for the prophylaxis of serious respiratory syncytial virus disease in children with hemodynamically significant congenital heart disease. *Pediatr Res.* 2011;70(2):186-91.
150. Reduction of respiratory syncytial virus hospitalization among premature infants and infants with bronchopulmonary dysplasia using respiratory syncytial virus immune globulin prophylaxis. The PREVENT Study Group. *Pediatrics.* 1997;99(1):93-9.
151. Harkensee C, Brodlie M, Embleton ND, et al. Passive immunisation of preterm infants with palivizumab against RSV infection. *J Infect.* 2006;52(1):2-8.
152. Tulloh R, Marsh M, Blackburn M, et al. Recommendations for the use of palivizumab as prophylaxis against respiratory syncytial virus in infants with congenital cardiac disease. *Cardiol Young.* 2003;13(5):420-3.
153. Simoes EA, Carbonell-Estrany X, Rieger CH, et al. The effect of respiratory syncytial virus on subsequent recurrent wheezing in atopic and nonatopic children. *J Allergy Clin Immunol.* 2010;126(2):256-62.
154. Golombek SG, Berning F, Lagamma EF. Compliance with prophylaxis for respiratory syncytial virus infection in a home setting. *Pediatr Infect Dis J.* 2004;23(4):318-22.
155. Frogel M, Nerwen C, Boron M, et al. Improved outcomes with home-based administration of palivizumab: results from the 2000-2004 Palivizumab Outcomes Registry. *Pediatr Infect Dis J.* 2008;27(10):870-3.
156. American Academy of Pediatrics Committee on Infectious Diseases, Committee on Fetus and Newborn. Revised indications for the use of palivizumab and respiratory syncytial virus immune globulin intravenous for the prevention of respiratory syncytial virus infections. *Pediatrics.* 2003;112(6 Pt 1):1442-6.
157. DeVincenzo JP, Hall CB, Kimberlin DW, et al. Surveillance of clinical isolates of respiratory syncytial virus for palivizumab (Synagis)-resistant mutants. *J Infect Dis.* 2004; 190(5):975-8.
158. Adams O, Bonzel L, Kovacevic A, et al. Palivizumab-resistant human respiratory syncytial virus infection in infancy. *Clin Infect Dis.* 2010;51(2):185-8.
159. Zhao X, Sullender WM. In vivo selection of respiratory syncytial viruses resistant to palivizumab. *J Virol.* 2005; 79(7):3962-8.
160. Lambert DM, Barney S, Lambert AL, et al. Peptides from conserved regions of paramyxovirus fusion (F) proteins are potent inhibitors of viral fusion. *Proc Natl Acad Sci U S A.* 1996;93(5):2186-91.
161. Murphy BR, Hall SL, Kulkarni AB, et al. An update on approaches to the development of respiratory syncytial virus (RSV) and parainfluenza virus type 3 (PIV3) vaccines. *Virus Res.* 1994;32(1):13-36.
162. Tao T, Durbin AP, Whitehead SS, et al. Recovery of a fully viable chimeric human parainfluenza virus (PIV) type 3 in which the hemagglutinin-neuraminidase and fusion glycoproteins have been replaced by those of PIV type 1. *J Virol.* 1998;72(4):2955-61.
163. Moscona A. Interaction of human parainfluenza virus type 3 with the host cell surface. *Pediatr Infect Dis J.* 1997;16(10): 917-24.
164. Huberman K, Peluso RW, Moscona A. Hemagglutinin-neuraminidase of human parainfluenza 3: role of the neuraminidase in the viral life cycle. *Virology.* 1995;214(1): 294-300.
165. Henrickson KJ, Savatski LL. Genetic variation and evolution of human parainfluenza virus type 1 hemagglutinin neuraminidase: analysis of 12 clinical isolates. *J Infect Dis.* 1992;166(5):995-1005.
166. Ansari SA, Springthorpe VS, Sattar SA, et al. Potential role of hands in the spread of respiratory viral infections: studies with human parainfluenza virus 3 and rhinovirus 14. *J Clinical Microbiol.* 1991;29(10):2115-9.
167. Castleman WL, Brundage-Anguish LJ, Kreitzer L, et al. Pathogenesis of bronchiolitis and pneumonia induced in neonatal and weanling rats by parainfluenza (Sendai) virus. *Am J Pathol.* 1987;129(2):277-86.
168. Zhang L, Bukreyev A, Thompson CI, et al. Infection of ciliated cells by human parainfluenza virus type 3 in an in vitro model of human airway epithelium. *J Virol.* 2005;79(2):1113-24.
169. Porter DD, Prince GA, Hemming VG, etal. Pathogenesis of human parainfluenza virus 3 infection in two species of cotton rats: Sigmodon hispidus develops bronchiolitis, while Sigmodon fulviventer develops interstitial pneumonia. *J Virol.* 1991;65(1):103-11.
170. Welliver RC, Wong DT, Sun M, et al. Parainfluenza virus bronchiolitis. Epidemiology and pathogenesis. *Am J Dis Child.* 1986;140(1):34-40.
171. Prince GA, Porter DD. Treatment of parainfluenza virus type 3 bronchiolitis and pneumonia in a cotton rat model using topical antibody and glucocorticosteroid. *J Infect Dis.* 1996;173(3):598-608.
172. Fry AM, Curns AT, Harbour K, et al. Seasonal trends of human parainfluenza viral infections: United States, 1990-2004. *Clin Infect Dis.* 2006;43(8):1016-22.
173. Marx A, Torok TJ, Holman RC, et al. Pediatric hospitalizations for croup (laryngotracheobronchitis): biennial increases associated with human parainfluenza virus 1 epidemics. *J Infect Dis.* 1997;176(6):1423-7.
174. Chew FT, Doraisingham S, Ling AE, et al. Seasonal trends of viral respiratory tract infections in the tropics. *Epidemiol Infect.* 1998;121(1):121-8.
175. Walker TA, Khurana S, Tilden SJ. Viral respiratory infections. *Pediatr Clin North Am.* 1994;41(6):1365-81.

176. Ison MG. Respiratory viral infections in transplant recipients. *Antivir Ther.* 2007;12(4 Pt B):627-38.
177. Falsey AR, Walsh EE. Viral pneumonia in older adults. *Clin Infect Dis.* 2006;42(4):518-24.
178. Denny FW. The clinical impact of human respiratory virus infections. *Am J Respir Crit Care Med.* 1995;152(4 Pt 2):S4-12.
179. Rubin EE, Quennec P, McDonald JC. Infections due to parainfluenza virus type 4 in children. *Clin Infect Dis.* 1993; 17(6):998-1002.
180. Slavin KA, Passaro DJ, Hacker JK, et al. Parainfluenza virus type 4: case report and review of the literature. *Pediatr Infect Dis J.* 2000;19(9):893-6.
181. Lau SK, To WK, Tse PW, et al. Human parainfluenza virus 4 outbreak and the role of diagnostic tests. *J Clin Microbiol.* 2005;43(9):4515-21.
182. Kim YJ, Boeckh M, Englund JA. Community respiratory virus infections in immunocompromised patients: hematopoietic stem cell and solid organ transplant recipients, and individuals with human immunodeficiency virus infection. *Semin Respir Crit Care Med.* 2007;28(2):222-42.
183. Reed G, Jewett PH, Thompson J, et al. Epidemiology and clinical impact of parainfluenza virus infections in otherwise healthy infants and young children < 5 years old. *J Infect Dis.* 1997;175(4):807-13.
184. Vesa S, Kleemola M, Blomqvist S, et al. Epidemiology of documented viral respiratory infections and acute otitis media in a cohort of children followed from two to twenty-four months of age. *Pediatr Infect Dis J.* 2001;20(6):574-81.
185. Johnstone J, Majumdar SR, Fox JD, et al. Viral infection in adults hospitalized with community-acquired pneumonia: prevalence, pathogens, and presentation. *Chest.* 2008; 134(6):1141-8.
186. Angeles Marcos M, Camps M, Pumarola T, et al. The role of viruses in the aetiology of community-acquired pneumonia in adults. *Antivir Ther.* 2006;11(3):351-9.
187. Diederen BM, Van Der Eerden MM, Vlaspolder F, et al. Detection of respiratory viruses and *Legionella* spp. by real-time polymerase chain reaction in patients with community acquired pneumonia. *Scand J Infect Dis.* 2009; 41(1):45-50.
188. Gwaltney JM, Scheld WM, Sande MA, et al. The microbial etiology and antimicrobial therapy of adults with acute community-acquired sinusitis: a fifteen-year experience at the University of Virginia and review of other selected studies. *J Allergy Clin Immunol.* 1992;90(3 Pt 2):457-61.
189. Matsuse H, Kondo Y, Saeki S, et al. Naturally occurring parainfluenza virus 3 infection in adults induces mild exacerbation of asthma associated with increased sputum concentrations of cysteinyl leukotrienes. *Int Archiv Allergy Immunol.* 2005;138(3):267-72.
190. Johnston NW. The similarities and differences of epidemic cycles of chronic obstructive pulmonary disease and asthma exacerbations. *Proc Am Thorac Soc.* 2007;4(8):591-6.
191. Hansbro NG, Horvat JC, Wark PA, et al. Understanding the mechanisms of viral induced asthma: new therapeutic directions. *Pharmacol Ther.* 2008;117(3):313-53.
192. Arisoy ES, Demmler GJ, Thakar S, et al. Meningitis due to parainfluenza virus type 3: report of two cases and review. *Clin Infect Dis.* 1993;17(6):995-7.
193. Wilks D, Burns SM. Myopericarditis associated with parainfluenza virus type 3 infection. *Eur J Clin Microbiol Infect Dis.* 1998;17(5):363-5.
194. Roman G, Phillips CA, Poser CM. Parainfluenza virus type 3: isolation from CSF of a patient with Guillain-Barré syndrome. *JAMA.* 1978;240(15):1613-5.
195. Verboon-Maciolek MA, Krediet TG, Gerards LJ, et al. Clinical and epidemiologic characteristics of viral infections in a neonatal intensive care unit during a 12-year period. *Pediatr Infect Dis J.* 2005;24(10):901-4.
196. Ng W, Rajadurai VS, Pradeepkumar VK, et al. Parainfluenza type 3 viral outbreak in a neonatal nursery. *Ann Acad Med Singapore.* 1999;28(4):471-5.
197. Moisiuk SE, Robson D, Klass L, et al. Outbreak of parainfluenza virus type 3 in an intermediate care neonatal nursery. *Pediatr Infect Dis J.* 1998;17(1):49-53.
198. Simmonds A, Munoz J, Montecalvo M, et al. Outbreak of parainfluenza virus type 3 in a neonatal intensive care unit. *Am J Perinatol.* 2009;26(5):361-4.
199. Meissner HC, Murray SA, Kiernan MA, et al. A simultaneous outbreak of respiratory syncytial virus and parainfluenza virus type 3 in a newborn nursery. *J Pediatr.* 1984;104(5):680-4.
200. McCarthy VP, Carlile JR, Reichelderfer PS, et al. Parainfluenza type 3 in newborns. *Pediatr Infect Dis J.* 1987;6(2): 217-8.
201. Singh-Naz N, Willy M, Riggs N. Outbreak of parainfluenza virus type 3 in a neonatal nursery. *Pediatr Infect Dis J.* 1990;9(1):31-3.
202. Abzug MJ, Beam AC, Gyorkos EA, et al. Viral pneumonia in the first month of life. *Pediatr Infect Dis J.* 1990;9(12):881-5.
203. Heidemann SM. Clinical characteristics of parainfluenza virus infection in hospitalized children. *Pediatr Pulmonol.* 1992;13(2):86-9.
204. Nichols WG, Corey L, Gooley T, et al. Parainfluenza virus infections after hematopoietic stem cell transplantation: risk factors, response to antiviral therapy, and effect on transplant outcome. *Blood.* 2001;98(3):573-8.
205. Vilchez RA, Dauber J, McCurry K, et al. Parainfluenza virus infection in adult lung transplant recipients: an emergent clinical syndrome with implications on allograft function. *Am J Transplant.* 2003;3(2):116-20.
206. Kumar D, Husain S, Chen MH, et al. A prospective molecular surveillance study evaluating the clinical impact of community-acquired respiratory viruses in lung transplant recipients. *Transplantation.* 2010;89(8):1028-33.
207. Campbell AP, Chien JW, Kuypers J, et al. Respiratory virus pneumonia after hematopoietic cell transplantation (HCT): associations between viral load in bronchoalveolar lavage samples, viral RNA detection in serum samples, and clinical outcomes of HCT. *J Infect Dis.* 2010;201(9):1404-13.
208. Weinberg A, Lyu DM, Li S, et al. Incidence and morbidity of human metapneumovirus and other community-acquired respiratory viruses in lung transplant recipients. *Transpl Infect Dis.* 2010;12(4):330-5.
209. Chemaly RF, Hanmod SS, Rathod DB, et al. The characteristics and outcomes of parainfluenza virus infections in 200 patients with leukemia or recipients of

hematopoietic stem cell transplantation. *Blood.* 2012; 119(12):2738-45.
210. Whimbey E, Bodey GP. Viral pneumonia in the immunocompromised adult with neoplastic disease: the role of common community respiratory viruses. *Semin Respir Infect.* 1992;7(2):122-31.
211. Peck AJ, Englund JA, Kuypers J, et al. Respiratory virus infection among hematopoietic cell transplant recipients: evidence for asymptomatic parainfluenza virus infection. *Blood.* 2007;110(5):1681-8.
212. Nichols WG, Gooley T, Boeckh M. Community-acquired respiratory syncytial virus and parainfluenza virus infections after hematopoietic stem cell transplantation: the Fred Hutchinson Cancer Research Center experience. *Biol Blood Marrow Transplant.* 2001;7(Suppl):11S-5S.
213. Nichols WG, Erdman DD, Han A, et al. Prolonged outbreak of human parainfluenza virus 3 infection in a stem cell transplant outpatient department: insights from molecular epidemiologic analysis. *Biol Blood Marrow Transplant.* 2004;10(1):58-64.
214. Zambon M, Bull T, Sadler CJ, et al. Molecular epidemiology of two consecutive outbreaks of parainfluenza 3 in a bone marrow transplant unit. *J Clin Microbiol.* 1998;36(8):2289-93.
215. Frampton MW, Boscia J, Roberts NJ, et al. Nitrogen dioxide exposure: effects on airway and blood cells. *Am J Physiol Lung Cell Mol Physiol.* 2002;282(1):L155-65.
216. Vilchez R, McCurry K, Dauber J, et al. Influenza and parainfluenza respiratory viral infection requiring admission in adult lung transplant recipients. *Transplantation.* 2002;73(7):1075-8.
217. Billings JL, Hertz MI, Savik K, et al. Respiratory viruses and chronic rejection in lung transplant recipients. *J Heart Lung Transplant.* 2002;21(5):559-66.
218. Garbino J, Gerbase MW, Wunderli W, et al. Respiratory viruses and severe lower respiratory tract complications in hospitalized patients. *Chest.* 2004;125(3):1033-9.
219. Erard V, Chien JW, Kim HW, et al. Airflow decline after myeloablative allogeneic hematopoietic cell transplantation: the role of community respiratory viruses. *J Infect Dis.* 2006;193(12):1619-25.
220. Fan J, Henrickson KJ. Rapid diagnosis of human parainfluenza virus type 1 infection by quantitative reverse transcription-PCR-enzyme hybridization assay. *J Clinl Microbiol.* 1996;34(8):1914-7.
221. Fan J, Henrickson KJ, Savatski LL. Rapid simultaneous diagnosis of infections with respiratory syncytial viruses A and B, influenza viruses A and B, and human parainfluenza virus types 1, 2, and 3 by multiplex quantitative reverse transcription-polymerase chain reaction-enzyme hybridization assay (Hexaplex). *Clin Infect Dis.* 1998;26(6): 1397-402.
222. Ferguson PE, Sorrell TC, Bradstock KF, et al. Parainfluenza virus type 3 pneumonia in bone marrow transplant recipients: multiple small nodules in high-resolution lung computed tomography scans provide a radiological clue to diagnosis. *Clin Infect Dis.* 2009.
223. Wendt CH, Weisdorf DJ, Jordan MC, et al. Parainfluenza virus respiratory infection after bone marrow transplantation. *New Engl J Med.* 1992;326(14):921-6.
224. Elizaga J, Olavarria E, Apperley J, et al. Parainfluenza virus 3 infection after stem cell transplant: relevance to outcome of rapid diagnosis and ribavirin treatment. *Clin Infect Dis.* 2001;32(3):413-8.
225. Chakrabarti S, Collingham KE, Holder K, et al. Parainfluenza virus type 3 infections in hematopoetic stem cell transplant recipients: response to ribavirin therapy. *Clin Infect Dis.* 2000;31(6):1516-8.
226. Cobian L, Houston S, Greene J, et al. Parainfluenza virus respiratory infection after heart transplantation: successful treatment with ribavirin. *Clin Infect Dis.* 1995;21(4):1040-1.
227. Wright JJ, O'driscoll G. Treatment of parainfluenza virus 3 pneumonia in a cardiac transplant recipient with intravenous ribavirin and methylprednisolone. *J Heart Lung Transplant.* 2005;24(3):343-6.
228. Alymova IV, Portner A, Takimoto T, et al. The novel parainfluenza virus hemagglutinin-neuraminidase inhibitor BCX 2798 prevents lethal synergism between a paramyxovirus and Streptococcus pneumoniae. *Antimicrob Agents Chemother.* 2005;49(1):398-405.
229. Alymova IV, Taylor G, Takimoto T, et al. Efficacy of novel hemagglutinin-neuraminidase inhibitors BCX 2798 and BCX 2855 against human parainfluenza viruses in vitro and in vivo. *Antimicrob Agents Chemother.* 2004;48(5):1495-502.
230. Moscona A, Porotto M, Palmer S, et al. A recombinant sialidase fusion protein effectively inhibits human parainfluenza viral infection in vitro and in vivo. *J Infect Dis.* 2010;202(2):234-41.
231. Chen YB, Driscoll JP, McAfee SL, et al. Treatment of parainfluenza 3 infection with DAS181 in a patient after allogeneic stem cell transplantation. *Clin Infect Dis.* 2011; 53(7):e77-80.
232. Guzman-Suarez BB, Buckley MW, Gilmore ET, et al. Clinical potential of DAS181 for treatment of parainfluenza-3 infections in transplant recipients. *Transplant Infect Dis.* 2012;14(4):427-33.
233. Bartlett EJ, Cruz AM, Boonyaratanakornkit J, et al. A novel human parainfluenza virus type 1 (HPIV1) with separated P and C genes is useful for generating C gene mutants for evaluation as live-attenuated virus vaccine candidates. *Vaccine.* 2010;28(3):767-79.
234. Schmidt AC. Progress in respiratory virus vaccine development. *Semin Respir Crit Care Med.* 2007;28(2):243-52.
235. Bartlett EJ, Amaro-Carambot E, Surman SR, et al. Human parainfluenza virus type I (HPIV1) vaccine candidates designed by reverse genetics are attenuated and efficacious in African green monkeys. *Vaccine.* 2005;23(38):4631-46.
236. Nolan SM, Surman SR, Amaro-Carambot E, et al. Live-attenuated intranasal parainfluenza virus type 2 vaccine candidates developed by reverse genetics containing L polymerase protein mutations imported from heterologous paramyxoviruses. *Vaccine.* 2005;23(39):4765-74.
237. Bartlett EJ, Castano A, Surman SR, et al. Attenuation and efficacy of human parainfluenza virus type 1 (HPIV1) vaccine candidates containing stabilized mutations in the P/C and L genes. *Virol J.* 2007;4:67.
238. Winther B, Gwaltney JM, Mygind N, et al. Viral-induced rhinitis. *Am J Rhinol.* 1998;12(1):17-20.
239. Hendley JO. Clin virol rhinoviruses. *Adv Virus Res.* 1999;54: 453-66.

240. Hendley JO. Rhinovirus colds: immunology and pathogenesis. *Eur J Respir Dis Suppl.* 1983;128(Pt 1):340-4.
241. Palmenberg AC, Spiro D, Kuzmickas R, et al. Sequencing and analyses of all known human rhinovirus genomes reveal structure and evolution. *Science.* 2009;324(5923):55-9.
242. Poland GA, Barry MA. Common cold, uncommon variation. *New Engl J Med.* 2009;360(21):2245-6.
243. Sung RY, Murray HG, Chan RC, et al. Seasonal patterns of respiratory syncytial virus infection in Hong Kong: a preliminary report. *J Infect Dis.* 1987;156(3):527-8.
244. Hendley JO, Gwaltney JM. Mechanisms of transmission of rhinovirus infections. *Epidemiol Rev.* 1988;10:243-58.
245. Gwaltney JM, Hendley JO. Transmission of experimental rhinovirus infection by contaminated surfaces. *Am J Epidemiol.* 1982;116(5):828-33.
246. Dick EC, Hossain SU, Mink KA, et al. Interruption of transmission of rhinovirus colds among human volunteers using virucidal paper handkerchiefs. *J Infect Dis.* 1986;153(2):352-6.
247. Hendley JO, Wenzel RP, Gwaltney JM. Transmission of rhinovirus colds by self-inoculation. *New Engl J Med.* 1973; 288(26):1361-4.
248. Lee GM, Salomon JA, Friedman JF, et al. Illness transmission in the home: a possible role for alcohol-based hand gels. *Pediatrics.* 2005;115(4):852-60.
249. Wendt CH, Hertz MI. Respiratory syncytial virus and parainfluenza virus infections in the immunocompromised host. *Semin Respir Infect.* 1995;10(4):224-31.
250. Winther B, Gwaltney JM, Mygind N, et al. Sites of rhinovirus recovery after point inoculation of the upper airway. *JAMA.* 1986;256(13):1763-7.
251. Hendley JO, Gwaltney JM. Viral titers in nasal lining fluid compared to viral titers in nasal washes during experimental rhinovirus infection. *J Clin Virol.* 2004;30(4): 326-8.
252. Douglas RG, Cate TR, Gerone PJ, et al. Quantitative rhinovirus shedding patterns in volunteers. *Am Rev Respir Dis.* 1966;94(2):159-67.
253. D'Alessio DJ, Peterson JA, Dick CR, et al. Transmission of experimental rhinovirus colds in volunteer married couples. *J Infect Dis.* 1976;133(1):28-36.
254. Wark PA, Johnston SL, Bucchieri F, et al. Asthmatic bronchial epithelial cells have a deficient innate immune response to infection with rhinovirus. *J Exp Med.* 2005; 201(6):937-47.
255. Winther B, Brofeldt S, Christensen B, et al. Light and scanning electron microscopy of nasal biopsy material from patients with naturally acquired common colds. *Acta Otolaryngol.* 1984;97(3-4):309-18.
256. Naclerio RM, Proud D, Lichtenstein LM, et al. Kinins are generated during experimental rhinovirus colds. *J Infect Dis.* 1988;157(1):133-42.
257. Arruda E, Boyle TR, Winther B, et al. Localization of human rhinovirus replication in the upper respiratory tract by in situ hybridization. *J Infect Dis.* 1995;171(5):1329-33.
258. Bardin PG, Johnston SL, Sanderson G, et al. Detection of rhinovirus infection of the nasal mucosa by oligonucleotide in situ hybridization. *Am J Respir Cell Mol Biol.* 1994; 10(2):207-13.
259. Turner RB, Hendley JO, Gwaltney JM. Shedding of infected ciliated epithelial cells in rhinovirus colds. *J Infect Dis.* 1982; 145(6):849-53.
260. Douglass JA, Dhami D, Gurr CE, et al. Influence of interleukin-8 challenge in the nasal mucosa in atopic and nonatopic subjects. *Am J Respir Crit Care Med.* 1994; 150(4):1108-13.
261. Zhu Z, Tang W, Gwaltney JM, et al. Rhinovirus stimulation of interleukin-8 in vivo and in vitro: role of NF-kappa B. *Am J Physiol.* 1997;273(4 Pt 1):L814-24.
262. Proud D, Naclerio RM, Gwaltney JM, et al. Kinins are generated in nasal secretions during natural rhinovirus colds. *J Infect Dis.* 1990;161(1):120-3.
263. Proud D, Reynolds CJ, Lacapra S, et al. Nasal provocation with bradykinin induces symptoms of rhinitis and a sore throat. *Am Rev Respir Dis.* 1988;137(3):613-6.
264. Papadopoulos NG, Bates PJ, Bardin PG, et al. Rhinoviruses infect the lower airways. *J Infect Dis.* 2000;181(6):1875-84.
265. Kirkpatrick GL. The common cold. *Prim Care.* 1996;23(4): 657-75.
266. Heymann PW, Platts-Mills TA, Johnston SL. Role of viral infections, atopy and antiviral immunity in the etiology of wheezing exacerbations among children and young adults. *Pediatr Infect Dis J.* 2005;24(11 Suppl):S217-22.
267. Hendley JO. The host response, not the virus, causes the symptoms of the common cold. *Clin Infect Dis.* 1998;26(4): 847-8.
268. Kusel MM, de Klerk NH, Kebadze T, et al. Early-life respiratory viral infections, atopic sensitization, and risk of subsequent development of persistent asthma. *J Allergy Clin Immunol.* 2007;119(5):1105-10.
269. Jackson DJ. The role of rhinovirus infections in the development of early childhood asthma. *Curr Opin Allergy Clin Immunol.* 2010;10(2):133-8.
270. Lemanske RF, Jackson DJ, Gangnon RE, et al. Rhinovirus illnesses during infancy predict subsequent childhood wheezing. *J Allergy Clin Immunol.* 2005;116(3):571-7.
271. Rosenthal LA, Avila PC, Heymann PW, et al. Viral respiratory tract infections and asthma: the course ahead. *J Allergy lin Immunol.* 2010;125(6):1212-7.
272. Miller EK, Khuri-Bulos N, Williams JV, et al. Human rhinovirus C associated with wheezing in hospitalised children in the Middle East. *J Clin Virol.* 2009;46(1):85-9.
273. Lee WM, Kiesner C, Pappas T, et al. A diverse group of previously unrecognized human rhinoviruses are common causes of respiratory illnesses in infants. *PLoS One.* 2007;2(10):e966.
274. Turner RB. Epidemiology, pathogenesis, and treatment of the common cold. *Ann Allergy, Asthma & Immunol.* 1997; 78(6):531-9.
275. Tyrrell DA, Cohen S, Schlarb JE. Signs and symptoms in common colds. *Epidemiol Infect.* 1993;111(1):143-56.
276. Jacques J, Bouscambert-Duchamp M, Moret H, et al. Association of respiratory picornaviruses with acute bronchiolitis in French infants. *Clin Virol.* 2006;35(4): 463-6.
277. Juven T, Mertsola J, Waris M, et al. Etiology of community-acquired pneumonia in 254 hospitalized children. *Pediatr Infect Dis J.* 2000;19(4):293-8.

278. McIntosh K. Community-acquired pneumonia in children. *N Engl J Med.* 2002;346(6):429-37.
279. Templeton KE, Scheltinga SA, van den Eeden WC, et al. Improved diagnosis of the etiology of community-acquired pneumonia with real-time polymerase chain reaction. *Clin Infect Dis.* 2005;41(3):345-51.
280. Calhoun WJ, Dick EC, Schwartz LB, et al. A common cold virus, rhinovirus 16, potentiates airway inflammation after segmental antigen bronchoprovocation in allergic subjects. *J Clin Invest.* 1994;94(6):2200-8.
281. Rakes GP, Arruda E, Ingram JM, et al. Rhinovirus and respiratory syncytial virus in wheezing children requiring emergency care. IgE and eosinophil analyses. *Am J Respir Crit Care Med.* 1999;159(3):785-90.
282. Jartti T, Kuusipalo H, Vuorinen T, et al. Allergic sensitization is associated with rhinovirus-, but not other virus-, induced wheezing in children. *Pediatr Allergy Immunol.* 2010;21(7):1008-14.
283. Bizzintino J, Lee WM, Laing IA, et al. Association between human rhinovirus C and severity of acute asthma in children. *Eur Respir J.* 2011;37(5):1037-42.
284. Mak RK, Tse LY, Lam WY, et al. Clinical spectrum of human rhinovirus infections in hospitalized Hong Kong children. *Pediatr Infect Dis J.* 2011;30(9):749-53.
285. Iwane MK, Prill MM, Lu X, et al. Human rhinovirus species associated with hospitalizations for acute respiratory illness in young US children. *J Infect Dis.* 2011;204(11):1702-10.
286. Sterk PJ. Virus-induced airway hyperresponsiveness in man. *Eur Respir J.* 1993;6(6):894-902.
287. Duff AL, Pomeranz ES, Gelber LE, et al. Risk factors for acute wheezing in infants and children: viruses, passive smoke, and IgE antibodies to inhalant allergens. *Pediatrics.* 1993;92(4):535-40.
288. Johnston SL, Bardin PG, Pattemore PK. Viruses as precipitants of asthma symptoms. III. Rhinoviruses: molecular biology and prospects for future intervention. *Clin Exp Allergy.* 1993;23(4):237-46.
289. Bates DV, Baker-Anderson M, Sizto R. Asthma attack periodicity: a study of hospital emergency visits in Vancouver. *Environ Res.* 1990;51(1):51-70.
290. Weiss KB. Seasonal trends in US asthma hospitalizations and mortality. *JAMA.* 1990;263(17):2323-8.
291. Kimes D, Levine E, Timmins S, et al. Temporal dynamics of emergency department and hospital admissions of pediatric asthmatics. *Environ Res.* 2004;94(1):7-17.
292. Johnston NW, Johnston SL, Norman GR, et al. The September epidemic of asthma hospitalization: school children as disease vectors. *J Allergy Clin Immunol.* 2006; 117(3):557-62.
293. Puhakka T, Makela MJ, Alanen A, et al. Sinusitis in the common cold. *J Allergy Clin Immunol.* 1998;102(3):403-8.
294. Rovers MM, Schilder AG, Zielhuis GA, et al. Otitis media. *Lancet.* 2004;363(9407):465-73.
295. McBride TP, Doyle WJ, Hayden FG, et al. Alterations of the eustachian tube, middle ear, and nose in rhinovirus infection. *Arch Otolaryngol Head Neck Surg.* 1989;115(9):1054-9.
296. Heikkinen T, Thint M, Chonmaitree T. Prevalence of various respiratory viruses in the middle ear during acute otitis media. *N Engl J Med.* 1999;340(4):260-4.
297. Gambarino S, Costa C, Elia M, et al. Development of a RT real-time PCR for the detection and quantification of human rhinoviruses. *Mol Biotechnol.* 2009;42(3):350-7.
298. Hayden FG, Herrington DT, Coats TL, et al. Efficacy and safety of oral pleconaril for treatment of colds due to picornaviruses in adults: results of 2 double-blind, randomized, placebo-controlled trials. *Clin Infect Dis.* 2003; 36(12):1523-32.
299. Turner RB, Wecker MT, Pohl G, et al. Efficacy of tremacamra, a soluble intercellular adhesion molecule 1, for experimental rhinovirus infection: a randomized clinical trial. *JAMA.* 1999;281(19):1797-804.
300. Hayden FG, Turner RB, Gwaltney JM, et al. Phase II, randomized, double-blind, placebo-controlled studies of ruprintrivir nasal spray 2-percent suspension for prevention and treatment of experimentally induced rhinovirus colds in healthy volunteers. *Antimicrob Agents Chemother.* 2003;47(12):3907-16.
301. de Jong JC, van Nieuwstadt AP, Kimman TG, et al. Antigenic drift in swine influenza H3 haemagglutinins with implications for vaccination policy. *Vaccine.* 1999;17(11-12):1321-8.
302. Antigenic shift and drift. *Nature.* 1980;283(5747):524-5.
303. Boni MF. Vaccination and antigenic drift in influenza. *Vaccine.* 2008;26(Suppl 3):C8-14.
304. Boni MF, Gog JR, Andreasen V, et al. Influenza drift and epidemic size: the race between generating and escaping immunity. *Theor Popul Biol.* 2004;65(2):179-91.
305. Capua I, Alexander DJ. Avian influenza and human health. *Acta Trop.* 2002;83(1):1-6.
306. Mubareka S, Lowen AC, Steel J, et al. Transmission of influenza virus via aerosols and fomites in the guinea pig model. *J Infect Dis.* 2009;199(6):858-65.
307. Brankston G, Gitterman L, Hirji Z, et al. Transmission of influenza A in human beings. *Lancet Infect Dis.* 2007;7(4): 257-65.
308. Blachere FM, Lindsley WG, Pearce TA, et al. Measurement of airborne influenza virus in a hospital emergency department. *Clin Infect Dis.* 2009;48(4):438-40.
309. Wong BC, Lee N, Li Y, et al. Possible role of aerosol transmission in a hospital outbreak of influenza. *Clinical Infect Dis.* 2010;51(10):1176-83.
310. Noti JD, Lindsley WG, Blachere FM, et al. Detection of infectious influenza virus in cough aerosols generated in a simulated patient examination room. *Clin Infect Dis.* 2012;54(11):1569-77.
311. Bischoff WE, Reid T, Russell GB, et al. Transocular entry of seasonal influenza-attenuated virus aerosols and the efficacy of n95 respirators, surgical masks, and eye protection in humans. *J Infect Dis.* 2011;204(2):193-9.
312. Cox NJ, Subbarao K. Influenza. *Lancet.* 1999;354(9186): 1277-82.
313. Cowling BJ, Chan KH, Fang VJ, et al. Comparative epidemiology of pandemic and seasonal influenza A in households. *N Engl J Med.* 2010;362(23):2175-84.
314. Bell DM, World Health Organization Writing G. Nonpharmaceutical interventions for pandemic influenza, international measures. *Emerg Infect Dis.* 2006;12(1): 81-7.

315. Carrat F, Vergu E, Ferguson NM, et al. Time lines of infection and disease in human influenza: a review of volunteer challenge studies. *Am J Epidemiol.* 2008;167(7):775-85.
316. Aoki FY, Boivin G. Influenza virus shedding: excretion patterns and effects of antiviral treatment. *J Clin Virol.* 2009;44(4):255-61.
317. Lau LL, Cowling BJ, Fang VJ, et al. Viral shedding and clinical illness in naturally acquired influenza virus infections. *J Infect Dis.* 2010;201(10):1509-16.
318. Loeb M, Singh PK, Fox J, et al. Longitudinal study of influenza molecular viral shedding in Hutterite communities. *J Infect Dis.* 2012;206(7):1078-84.
319. Leekha S, Zitterkopf NL, Espy MJ, et al. Duration of influenza A virus shedding in hospitalized patients and implications for infection control. *Infect Control Hospit Epidemiol.* 2007;28(9):1071-6.
320. Lee N, Chan PK, Hui DS, et al. Viral loads and duration of viral shedding in adult patients hospitalized with influenza. *J Infect Dis.* 2009;200(4):492-500.
321. Klimov AI, Rocha E, Hayden FG, et al. Prolonged shedding of amantadine-resistant influenzae A viruses by immunodeficient patients: detection by polymerase chain reaction-restriction analysis. *J Infect Dis.* 1995;172(5):1352-5.
322. Englund JA, Champlin RE, Wyde PR, et al. Common emergence of amantadine- and rimantadine-resistant influenza A viruses in symptomatic immunocompromised adults. *Clin Infect Dis.* 1998;26(6): 1418-24.
323. Boivin G, Goyette N, Bernatchez H. Prolonged excretion of amantadine-resistant influenza a virus quasi species after cessation of antiviral therapy in an immunocompromised patient. *Clin Infect Dis.* 2002;34(5):E23-5.
324. Nichols WG, Guthrie KA, Corey L, et al. Influenza infections after hematopoietic stem cell transplantation: risk factors, mortality, and the effect of antiviral therapy. *Clin Infect Dis.* 2004;39(9):1300-6.
325. Gooskens J, Jonges M, Claas EC, et al. Prolonged influenza virus infection during lymphocytopenia and frequent detection of drug-resistant viruses. *J Infect Dis.* 2009;199(10):1435-41.
326. Nicholson KG. Clinical features of influenza. *Semin Respir-Infect.* 1992;7(1):26-37.
327. Dolin R. Influenza: current concepts. *Am Fam Physician.* 1976;14(3):72-7.
328. Kilbourne ED, Loge JP. Influenza A prime: a clinical study of an epidemic caused by a new strain of virus. *Ann Intern Med.* 1950;33(2):371-9.
329. Poehling KA, Edwards KM, Weinberg GA, et al. The underrecognized burden of influenza in young children. *N Engl J Med.* 2006;355(1):31-40.
330. Silvennoinen H, Peltola V, Lehtinen P, et al. Clinical presentation of influenza in unselected children treated as outpatients. *Pediatr Infect Dis J.* 2009;28(5):372-5.
331. Neuzil KM, Zhu Y, Griffin MR, et al. Burden of inter-pandemic influenza in children younger than 5 years: a 25-year prospective study. *J Infect Dis.* 2002;185(2):147-52.
332. Peltola V, Ziegler T, Ruuskanen O. Influenza A and B virus infections in children. *Clin Infect Dis.* 2003;36(3):299-305.
333. Chiu SS, Tse CY, Lau YL, et al. Influenza A infection is an important cause of febrile seizures. *Pediatrics.* 2001; 108(4):E63.
334. Hall WJ, Douglas RG, Hyde RW, et al. Pulmonary mechanics after uncomplicated influenza A infection. *Am Rev Respir Dis.* 1976;113(2):141-8.
335. Hall CB, Douglas RG. Nosocomial influenza infection as a cause of intercurrent fevers in infants. *Pediatrics.* 1975;55(5):673-7.
336. Dagan R, Hall CB. Influenza A virus infection imitating bacterial sepsis in early infancy. *Pediatr Infect Dis.* 1984; 3(3):218-21.
337. Monto AS. Epidemiology of influenza. *Vaccine.* 2008; 26(Suppl 4):D45-8.
338. Kumar S, Havens PL, Chusid MJ, et al. Clinical and epidemiologic characteristics of children hospitalized with 2009 pandemic H1N1 influenza A infection. *Pediatr Infect Dis J.* 2010;29(7):591-4.
339. Fiore AE, Uyeki TM, Broder K, et al. Prevention and control of influenza with vaccines: recommendations of the Advisory Committee on Immunization Practices (ACIP), 2010. *MMWR Recomm Rep.* 2010;59(RR-8):1-62.
340. Harper SA, Bradley JS, Englund JA, et al. Seasonal influenza in adults and children—diagnosis, treatment, chemoprophylaxis, and institutional outbreak management: clinical practice guidelines of the Infectious Diseases Society of America. *Clin Infect Dis.* 2009;48(8):1003-32.
341. Lyytikäinen O, Hoffmann E, Timm H, et al. Influenza A outbreak among adolescents in a ski hostel. *Eur J Clin Microbiol Infect Dis.* 1998;17(2):128-30.
342. Martin CM, Kunin CM, Gottlieb LS, et al. Asian influenza A in Boston, 1957-1958. I. Observations in thirty-two influenza-associated fatal cases. *AMA Arch Intern Med.* 1959;103(4):515-31.
343. Kim EA, Lee KS, Primack SL, et al. Viral pneumonias in adults: radiologic and pathologic findings. *Radiographics.* 2002;22(Spec No):S137-49.
344. Simonsen L. The global impact of influenza on morbidity and mortality. *Vaccine.* 1999;17(Suppl 1):S3-10.
345. Schwarzmann SW, Adler JL, Sullivan RJ, et al. Bacterial pneumonia during the Hong Kong influenza epidemic of 1968-1969. *Arch Intern Med.* 1971;127(6):1037-41.
346. Bisno AL, Griffin JP, Van Epps KA, et al. Pneumonia and Hong Kong influenza: a prospective study of the 1968-1969 epidemic. *Am J Med Sci.* 1971;261(5):251-63.
347. Kallen AJ, Brunkard J, Moore Z, et al. *Staphylococcus aureus* community-acquired pneumonia during the 2006 to 2007 influenza season. *Ann Emerg Med.* 2009;53(3):358-65.
348. Hageman JC, Uyeki TM, Francis JS, et al. Severe community-acquired pneumonia due to *Staphylococcus aureus*, 2003-04 influenza season. *Emerg Infect Dis.* 2006;12(6):894-9.
349. Centers for Disease Control and Prevention (CDC). Severe methicillin-resistant Staphylococcus aureus community-acquired pneumonia associated with influenza—Louisiana and Georgia, December 2006-January 2007. *MMWR Morb Mortal Wkly Rep.* 2007;56(14):325-9.
350. Bayer WH. Influenza B encephalitis. *West J Med.* 1987; 147(4):466.
351. Fujimoto S, Kobayashi M, Uemura O, et al. PCR on cerebrospinal fluid to show influenza-associated acute encephalopathy or encephalitis. *Lancet.* 1998; 352(9131): 873-5.

352. Steininger C, Popow-Kraupp T, Laferl H, et al. Acute encephalopathy associated with influenza A virus infection. *Clin Infect Dis.* 2003;36(5):567-74.
353. Hjalmarsson A, Blomqvist P, Brytting M, et al. Encephalitis after influenza in Sweden 1987-1998: a rare complication of a common infection. *Eur Neurol.* 2009;61(5):289-94.
354. Salonen O, Koshkiniemi M, Saari A, et al. Myelitis associated with influenza A virus infection. *J Neurovirol.* 1997;3(1):83-5.
355. Rotbart HA. Viral meningitis. Semin *Neurol.* 2000;20(3): 277-92.
356. Sivadon-Tardy V, Orlikowski D, Porcher R, et al. Guillain-Barré syndrome and influenza virus infection. *Clin Infect Dis.* 2009;48(1):48-56.
357. Ison MG, Campbell V, Rembold C, et al. Cardiac findings during uncomplicated acute influenza in ambulatory adults. *Clin Infect Dis.* 2005;40(3):415-22.
358. Warren-Gash C, Bhaskaran K, Hayward A, et al. Circulating influenza virus, climatic factors, and acute myocardial infarction: a time series study in England and Wales and Hong Kong. *J Infect Dis.* 2011;203(12):1710-8.
359. Lichenstein R, Magder LS, King RE, et al. The relationship between influenza outbreaks and acute ischemic heart disease in Maryland residents over a 7-year period. *J Infect Dis.* 2012;206(6):821-7.
360. Mamas MA, Fraser D, Neyses L. Cardiovascular manifestations associated with influenza virus infection. *Int J Cardiol.* 2008;130(3):304-9.
361. Paddock CD, Liu L, Denison AM, et al. Myocardial injury and bacterial pneumonia contribute to the pathogenesis of fatal influenza B virus infection. *J Infect Dis.* 2012;205(6): 895-905.
362. Heikkinen T, Silvennoinen H, Peltola V, et al. Burden of influenza in children in the community. *J Infect Dis.* 2004;190(8):1369-73.
363. Henderson FW, Collier AM, Sanyal MA, et al. A longitudinal study of respiratory viruses and bacteria in the etiology of acute otitis media with effusion. *N Engl J Med.* 1982;306(23):1377-83.
364. Rennels MB, Meissner HC, Committee on Infectious D. Technical report: reduction of the influenza burden in children. *Pediatrics.* 2002;110(6):e80.
365. Rihkanen H, Ronkko E, Nieminen T, et al. Respiratory viruses in laryngeal croup of young children. *J Pediatr.* 2008;152(5):661-5.
366. Peltola V, Heikkinen T, Ruuskanen O. Clinical courses of croup caused by influenza and parainfluenza viruses. *Pediatr Infect Dis J.* 2002;21(1):76-8.
367. Neuzil KM, Wright PF, Mitchel EF, et al. The burden of influenza illness in children with asthma and other chronic medical conditions. *J Pediatr.* 2000;137(6):856-64.
368. Miller EK, Griffin MR, Edwards KM, et al. Influenza burden for children with asthma. *Pediatrics.* 2008;121(1):1-8.
369. Lahti E, Peltola V, Virkki R, et al. Influenza pneumonia. *Pediatr Infect Dis J.* 2006;25(2):160-4.
370. Dawood FS, Fiore A, Kamimoto L, et al. Influenza-associated pneumonia in children hospitalized with laboratory-confirmed influenza, 2003-2008. *Pediatr Infect Dis J.* 2010;29(7):585-90.
371. Ekstrand JJ, Herbener A, Rawlings J, et al. Heightened neurologic complications in children with pandemic H1N1 influenza. *Ann Neurol.* 2010;68(5):762-6.
372. Newland JG, Laurich VM, Rosenquist AW, et al. Neurologic complications in children hospitalized with influenza: characteristics, incidence, and risk factors. *J Pediatr.* 2007; 150(3):306-10.
373. Maricich SM, Neul JL, Lotze TE, et al. Neurologic complications associated with influenza A in children during the 2003-2004 influenza season in Houston, Texas. *Pediatrics.* 2004;114(5):e626-33.
374. Lin CH, Huang YC, Chiu CH, et al. Neurologic manifestations in children with influenza B virus infection. *Pediatr Infect Dis J.* 2006;25(11):1081-3.
375. Amin R, Ford-Jones E, Richardson SE, et al. Acute childhood encephalitis and encephalopathy associated with influenza: a prospective 11-year review. *Pediatr Infect Dis J.* 2008;27(5):390-5.
376. Haber P, DeStefano F, Angulo FJ, et al. Guillain-Barré syndrome following influenza vaccination. *JAMA.* 2004; 292(20):2478-81.
377. Huang YC, Li WC, Tsao KC, et al. Influenza-associated central nervous system dysfunction in Taiwanese children: clinical characteristics and outcomes with and without administration of oseltamivir. *Pediatr Infect Dis J.* 2009;28(7):647-8.
378. Hu JJ, Kao CL, Lee PI, et al. Clinical features of influenza A and B in children and association with myositis. *J Microbiol Immunol Infect.* 2004;37(2):95-8.
379. Agyeman P, Duppenthaler A, Heininger U, et al. Influenza-associated myositis in children. *Infection.* 2004;32(4):199-203.
380. Hall CB, Douglas RG, Geiman JM, et al. Viral shedding patterns of children with influenza B infection. *J Infect Dis.* 1979;140(4):610-3.
381. Tolan RW. Toxic shock syndrome complicating influenza A in a child: case report and review. *Clin Infect Dis.* 1993;17(1):43-5.
382. Rothberg MB, Haessler SD. Complications of seasonal and pandemic influenza. *Crit Care Med.* 2010;38(4 Suppl):e91-7.
383. Kumar K, Guirgis M, Zieroth S, et al. Influenza myocarditis and myositis: case presentation and review of the literature. *Can J Cardiol.* 2011;27(4):514-22.
384. Sion ML, Hatzitolios AI, Toulis EN, et al. Toxic shock syndrome complicating influenza A infection: a two-case report with one case of bacteremia and endocarditis. *Intensive Care Med.* 2001;27(2):443.
385. Sharkey R, Mulloy E, O'Neill G, et al. Toxic shock syndrome following influenza A infection. *Intensive Care Med.* 1999; 25(3):335-6.
386. Conway EE, Haber RS, Gumprecht J, et al. Toxic shock syndrome following influenza A in a child. *Crit Care Med.* 1991;19(1):123-5.
387. Prechter GC, Gerhard AK. Postinfluenza toxic shock syndrome. *Chest.* 1989;95(5):1153-4.
388. Centers for Disease Control and Prevention(CDC). Outbreak of swine-origin influenza A (H1N1) virus infection—Mexico, March-April 2009. *MMWR Morb Mortal Wkly Rep.* 2009;58(17):467-70.
389. Lee N, Chan PK, Lui GC, et al. Complications and outcomes of pandemic 2009 Influenza A (H1N1) virus infection in hospitalized adults: how do they differ from those in seasonal influenza? *J Infect Dis.* 2011;203(12):1739-47.

390. Novel Swine-Origin Influenza AVIT, Dawood FS, Jain S, et al. Emergence of a novel swine-origin influenza A (H1N1) virus in humans. *N Engl J Med.* 2009;360(25):2605-15.
391. Writing Committee of the WHOCoCAoPI, Bautista E, Chotpitayasunondh T, et al. Clinical aspects of pandemic 2009 influenza A (H1N1) virus infection. *New Engl J Med.* 2010;362(18):1708-19.
392. Belongia EA, Irving SA, Waring SC, et al. Clinical characteristics and 30-day outcomes for influenza A 2009 (H1N1), 2008-2009 (H1N1), and 2007-2008 (H3N2) infections. *JAMA.* 2010;304(10):1091-8.
393. Robinson JL, Lee BE, Kothapalli S, et al. Use of throat swab or saliva specimens for detection of respiratory viruses in children. *Clin Infect Dis.* 2008;46(7):e61-4.
394. Ginocchio CC, Zhang F, Manji R, et al. Evaluation of multiple test methods for the detection of the novel 2009 influenza A (H1N1) during the New York City outbreak. *J Clin Virol.* 2009;45(3):191-5.
395. Daum LT, Canas LC, Schadler CA, et al. A rapid, single-step multiplex reverse transcription-PCR assay for the detection of human H1N1, H3N2, and B influenza viruses. *J Clin Virol.* 2002;25(3):345-50.
396. Uyeki TM. Influenza diagnosis and treatment in children: a review of studies on clinically useful tests and antiviral treatment for influenza. *Pediatr Infect Dis J.* 2003;22(2):164-77.
397. Chartrand C, Leeflang MM, Minion J, et al. Accuracy of rapid influenza diagnostic tests: a meta-analysis. *Ann Intern Med.* 2012;156(7):500-11.
398. Centers for Disease Control and Prevention (CDC). Performance of rapid influenza diagnostic tests during two school outbreaks of 2009 pandemic influenza A (H1N1) virus infection—Connecticut, 2009. *MMWR Morb Mortal Wkly Rep.* 2009;58(37):1029-32.
399. Cruz AT, Cazacu AC, Greer JM, et al. Rapid assays for the diagnosis of influenza A and B viruses in patients evaluated at a large tertiary care children's hospital during two consecutive winter seasons. *J Clin Virol.* 2008;41(2):143-7.
400. Glezen WP. Modifying clinical practices to manage influenza in children effectively. *Pediatr Infect Dis J.* 2008; 27(8):738-43.
401. Grijalva CG, Poehling KA, Edwards KM, et al. Accuracy and interpretation of rapid influenza tests in children. *Pediatrics.* 2007;119(1):e6-11.
402. Chan KH, Lam SY, Puthavathana P, et al. Comparative analytical sensitivities of six rapid influenza A antigen detection test kits for detection of influenza A subtypes H1N1, H3N2 and H5N1. *J Clin Virol.* 2007;38(2):169-71.
403. Tsiodras S, Nikolopoulos G, Bonovas S. Antivirals used for influenza chemoprophylaxis. *Curr Med Chem.* 2012;19(35): 5947-56.
404. Jefferson T, Demicheli V, Rivetti D, et al. Antivirals for influenza in healthy adults: systematic review. *Lancet.* 2006;367(9507):303-13.
405. Randomised trial of efficacy and safety of inhaled zanamivir in treatment of influenza A and B virus infections. The MIST (Management of Influenza in the Southern Hemisphere Trialists) Study Group. *Lancet.* 1998;352(9144):1877-81.
406. Treanor JJ, Hayden FG, Vrooman PS, et al. Efficacy and safety of the oral neuraminidase inhibitor oseltamivir in treating acute influenza: a randomized controlled trial. US Oral Neuraminidase Study Group. *JAMA.* 2000;283(8):1016-24.
407. Kaiser L, Wat C, Mills T, et al. Impact of oseltamivir treatment on influenza-related lower respiratory tract complications and hospitalizations. *Arch Intern Med.* 2003; 163(14):1667-72.
408. Hernan MA, Lipsitch M. Oseltamivir and risk of lower respiratory tract complications in patients with flu symptoms: a meta-analysis of eleven randomized clinical trials. *Clin Infect Dis.* 2011;53(3):277-9.
409. Lee N, Chan PK, Choi KW, et al. Factors associated with early hospital discharge of adult influenza patients. *Antivir Ther.* 2007;12(4):501-8.
410. McGeer A, Green KA, Plevneshi A, et al. Antiviral therapy and outcomes of influenza requiring hospitalization in Ontario, Canada. *Clin Infect Dis.* 2007;45(12):1568-75.
411. Bowles SK, Lee W, Simor AE, et al. Use of oseltamivir during influenza outbreaks in Ontario nursing homes, 1999-2000. *J Am Geriatrics Soc.* 2002;50(4):608-16.
412. Fiore AE, Shay DK, Broder K, et al. Prevention and control of influenza: recommendations of the Advisory Committee on Immunization Practices (ACIP), 2008. *MMWR Recomm Rep.* 2008;57(RR-7):1-60.
413. Cooper NJ, Sutton AJ, Abrams KR, et al. Effectiveness of neuraminidase inhibitors in treatment and prevention of influenza A and B: systematic review and meta-analyses of randomised controlled trials. *BMJ.* 2003;326(7401):1235.
414. Nicholson KG, Aoki FY, Osterhaus AD, et al. Efficacy and safety of oseltamivir in treatment of acute influenza: a randomised controlled trial. Neuraminidase Inhibitor Flu Treatment Investigator Group. *Lancet.* 2000;355(9218): 1845-50.
415. Hayden FG, Osterhaus AD, Treanor JJ, et al. Efficacy and safety of the neuraminidase inhibitor zanamivir in the treatment of influenzavirus infections. GG167 Influenza Study Group. *N Engl J Med.* 1997;337(13):874-80.
416. Jefferson T, Jones M, Doshi P, et al. Neuraminidase inhibitors for preventing and treating influenza in healthy adults: systematic review and meta-analysis. *BMJ.* 2009;339:b5106.
417. Gaglia MA, Cook RL, Kraemer KL, et al. Patient knowledge and attitudes about antiviral medication and vaccination for influenza in an internal medicine clinic. *Clin Infect Dis.* 2007;45(9):1182-8.
418. Fiore AE, Fry A, Shay D, et al. Antiviral agents for the treatment and chemoprophylaxis of influenza—recommendations of the Advisory Committee on Immunization Practices (ACIP). *MMWR Recomm Rep.* 2011;60(1):1-24.
419. Kiatboonsri S, Kiatboonsri C, Theerawit P. Fatal respiratory events caused by zanamivir nebulization. *Clin Infect Dis.* 2010;50(4):620.
420. Lee VJ, Yap J, Cook AR, et al. Oseltamivir ring prophylaxis for containment of 2009 H1N1 influenza outbreaks. *N Engl J Med.* 2010;362(23):2166-74.
421. Iuliano AD, Reed C, Guh A, et al. Notes from the field: outbreak of 2009 pandemic influenza A (H1N1) virus at a large public university in Delaware, April-May 2009. *Clin Infect Dis.* 2009;49(12):1811-20.

422. Centers for Disease Control and Prevention (CDC). Update: influenza activity—United States, August 30-October 31, 2009. *MMWR Morb Mortal Wkly Rep.* 2009;58(44): 1236-41.
423. Centers for Disease Control and Prevention. Oseltamivir-resistant novel influenza A (H1N1) virus infection in two immunosuppressed patients—Seattle, Washington, 2009. *MMWR Morb Mortal Wkly Rep.* 2009;58(32):893-6.
424. Centers for Disease Control and Prevention. Oseltamivir-resistant 2009 pandemic influenza A (H1N1) virus infection in two summer campers receiving prophylaxis—North Carolina, 2009. *MMWR Morb Mortal Wkly Rep.* 2009; 58(35):969-72.
425. Baz M, Abed Y, Papenburg J, et al. Emergence of oseltamivir-resistant pandemic H1N1 virus during prophylaxis. *N Engl J Med.* 2009;361(23):2296-7.
426. Le QM, Wertheim HF, Tran ND, et al. A community cluster of oseltamivir-resistant cases of 2009 H1N1 influenza. *N Engl J Med.* 2010;362(1):86-7.
427. Memoli MJ, Hrabal RJ, Hassantoufighi A, et al. Rapid selection of oseltamivir- and peramivir-resistant pandemic H1N1 virus during therapy in 2 immunocompromised hosts. *Clin Infect Dis.* 2010;50(9):1252-5.
428. Inoue M, Barkham T, Leo YS, et al. Emergence of oseltamivir-resistant pandemic (H1N1) 2009 virus within 48 hours. *Emerg Infect Dis.* 2010;16(10):1633-6.
429. Kilbourne ED. Influenza immunity: new insights from old studies. *J Infect Dis.* 2006;193(1):7-8.
430. Glezen WP. Clinical practice. Prevention and treatment of seasonal influenza. *N Engl J Med.* 2008;359(24):2579-85.
431. Centers for Disease Control and Prevention. Prevention and control of influenza with vaccines: recommendations of the Advisory Committee on Immunization Practices (ACIP)—United States, 2012-13 influenza season. *MMWR Morb Mortal Wkly Rep.* 2012;61(32):613-8.
432. Influenza vaccine 2007-2008. *Med Lett Drugs Ther.* 2007; 49(1271):81-3.
433. Wadell G, Norrby E. Immunological and other biological characteristics of pentons of human adenoviruses. *J Virol.* 1969;4(5):671-80.
434. Roelvink PW, Lizonova A, Lee JG, et al. The coxsackievirus-adenovirus receptor protein can function as a cellular attachment protein for adenovirus serotypes from subgroups A, C, D, E, and F. *J Virol.* 1998;72(10):7909-15.
435. Segerman A, Atkinson JP, Marttila M, et al. Adenovirus type 11 uses CD46 as a cellular receptor. *J Virol.* 2003; 77(17):9183-91.
436. Gaggar A, Shayakhmetov DM, Lieber A. CD46 is a cellular receptor for group B adenoviruses. *Nat Med.* 2003; 9(11):1408-12.
437. Madisch I, Harste G, Pommer H, et al. Phylogenetic analysis of the main neutralization and hemagglutination determinants of all human adenovirus prototypes as a basis for molecular classification and taxonomy. *J Virol.* 2005;79(24):15265-76.
438. Dre⊠zin RS, Zolotarskaia EE. Division of adenoviruses into subgroups according to their hemagglutinating activity and properties of the hemagglutinins. *Vopr Virusol.* 1967;12(5):577-81.
439. Fox JP, Hall CE, Cooney MK. The Seattle Virus Watch. VII. Observations of adenovirus infections. *Am J Epidemiol.* 1977;105(4):362-86.
440. Foy HM, Cooney MK, Hatlen JB. Adenovirus type 3 epidemic associated with intermittent chlorination of a swimming pool. *Arch Environ Health.* 1968;17(5): 795-802.
441. Birenbaum E, Linder N, Varsano N, et al. Adenovirus type 8 conjunctivitis outbreak in a neonatal intensive care unit. *Arch of Dis Child.* 1993;68(5 Spec No):610-1.
442. Dingle JH, Langmuir AD. Epidemiology of acute, respiratory disease in military recruits. *Am Rev Respir Dis.* 1968;97(6):Suppl:1-65.
443. Kolavic-Gray SA, Binn LN, Sanchez JL, et al. Large epidemic of adenovirus type 4 infection among military trainees: epidemiological, clinical, and laboratory studies. *Clin Infect Dis.* 2002;35(7):808-18.
444. Montone KT, Furth EE, Pietra GG, et al. Neonatal adenovirus infection: a case report with in situ hybridization confirmation of ascending intrauterine infection. *Diagnostic Cytopathology.* 1995;12(4):341-4.
445. Pinto A, Beck R, Jadavji T. Fatal neonatal pneumonia caused by adenovirus type 35. Report of one case and review of the literature. *Arch Pathol Lab Med.* 1992;116(1):95-9.
446. Osamura T, Mizuta R, Yoshioka H, et al. Isolation of adenovirus type 11 from the brain of a neonate with pneumonia and encephalitis. *Eur J Pediatr.* 1993; 152(6): 496-9.
447. Koneru B, Atchison R, Jaffe R, et al. Serological studies of adenoviral hepatitis following pediatric liver transplantation. *Transplantat Proc.* 1990;22(4):1547-8.
448. Gray GC, McCarthy T, Lebeck MG, et al. Genotype prevalence and risk factors for severe clinical adenovirus infection, United States 2004-2006. *Clin Infect Dis.* 2007; 45(9):1120-31.
449. Centers for Disease Control and Prevention. Two fatal cases of adenovirus-related illness in previously healthy young adults—Illinois, 2000. *MMWR Morb Mortal Wkly Rep.* 2001;50(26):553-5.
450. Russell KL, Broderick MP, Franklin SE, et al. Transmission dynamics and prospective environmental sampling of adenovirus in a military recruit setting. *J Infect Dis.* 2006;194(7):877-85.
451. Metzgar D, Osuna M, Kajon AE, et al. Abrupt emergence of diverse species B adenoviruses at US military recruit training centers. *J Infect Dis.* 2007;196(10):1465-73.
452. Binn LN, Sanchez JL, Gaydos JC. Emergence of adenovirus type 14 in US military recruits—a new challenge. *J Infect Dis.* 2007;196(10):1436-7.
453. Lyons A, Longfield J, Kuschner R, et al. A double-blind, placebo-controlled study of the safety and immunogenicity of live, oral type 4 and type 7 adenovirus vaccines in adults. *Vaccine.* 2008;26(23):2890-8.
454. Centers for Disease Control and Prevention. Acute respiratory disease associated with adenovirus serotype 14—four states, 2006-2007. *MMWR Morb Mortal Wkly Rep.* 2007;56(45):1181-4.
455. Centers for Disease Control and Prevention. Outbreak of adenovirus 14 respiratory illness—Prince of Wales Island, Alaska, 2008. *MMWR Morb Mortal Weekly Rep.* 2010; 59(1):6-10.
456. Esposito DH, Gardner TJ, Schneider E, et al. Outbreak of pneumonia associated with emergent human adenovirus serotype 14—Southeast Alaska, 2008. *J Infect Dis.* 2010; 202(2):214-22.

457. Tate JE, Bunning ML, Lott L, et al. Outbreak of severe respiratory disease associated with emergent human adenovirus serotype 14 at a US air force training facility in 2007. *J Infect Dis.* 2009;199(10):1419-26.
458. Vento TJ, Prakash V, Murray CK, et al. Pneumonia in military trainees: a comparison study based on adenovirus serotype 14 infection. *J Infect Dis.* 2011;203(10):1388-95.
459. Yun HC, Prakash V. Transmission of adenovirus serotype 14 in the health care setting. *Clin Infect Dis.* 2008;46(12):1935-6.
460. Lessa FC, Gould PL, Pascoe N, et al. Health care transmission of a newly emergent adenovirus serotype in health care personnel at a military hospital in Texas, 2007. *J Infect Dis.* 2009;200(11):1759-65.
461. Louie JK, Kajon AE, Holodniy M, et al. Severe pneumonia due to adenovirus serotype 14: a new respiratory threat? *Clin Infect Dis.* 2008;46(3):421-5.
462. Centers for Disease Control. Adenovirus type 7 outbreak in a pediatric chronic-care facility—Pennsylvania, 1982. *MMWR Morb Mortal Wkly Rep.* 1983;32(19):258-60.
463. Straube RC, Thompson MA, Van Dyke RB, et al. Adenovirus type 7b in a children's hospital. *J Infect Dis.* 1983;147(5):814-9.
464. de Silva LM, Colditz P, Wadell G. Adenovirus type 7 infections in children in New South Wales, Australia. *J Med Virol.* 1989;29(1):28-32.
465. Porter JD, Teter M, Traister V, et al. Outbreak of adenoviral infections in a long-term pediatric facility, New Jersey, 1986/87. *J Hosp Infect.* 1991;18(3):201-10.
466. Mitchell LS, Taylor B, Reimels W, et al. Adenovirus 7a: a community-acquired outbreak in a children's hospital. *Pediatr Infect Dis J.* 2000;19(10):996-1000.
467. Becroft DM. Bronchiolitis obliterans, bronchiectasis, and other sequelae of adenovirus type 21 infection in young children. *J Clin Pathol.* 1971;24(1):72-82.
468. Edwards KM, Thompson J, Paolini J, et al. Adenovirus infections in young children. *Pediatrics.* 1985;76(3):420-4.
469. Pacini DL, Collier AM, Henderson FW. Adenovirus infections and respiratory illnesses in children in group day care. *J Infect Dis.* 1987;156(6):920-7.
470. Tabain I, Ljubin-Sternak S, Cepin-Bogovi⊠ J, et al. Adenovirus respiratory infections in hospitalized children: clinical findings in relation to species and serotypes. *Pediatr Infect Dis J.* 2012;31(7):680-4.
471. Chuang Yu, Chiu CH, Wong KS, et al. Severe adenovirus infection in children. *J Microbiol, Immunol Infect.* 2003; 36(1):37-40.
472. Carballal G, Videla C, Misirlian A, et al. Adenovirus type 7 associated with severe and fatal acute lower respiratory infections in Argentine children. *BMC Pediatr.* 2002;2:6.
473. Lang WR, Howden CW, Laws J, et al. Bronchopneumonia with serious sequelae in children with evidence of adenovirus type 21 infection. *Br Med J.* 1969;1(5636):73-9.
474. Levy Y, Nitzan M, Beharab A, et al. Adenovirus type 3 infection with systemic manifestation in apparently normal children. *Isr J Med Sci.* 1986;22(11):774-8.
475. Simila S, Jouppila R, Salmi A, et al. Encephaloningitis in children associated with an adenovirus type 7 epidemic. *Acta Pediatr Scand.* 1970;59(3):310-6.
476. Wadell G, Varsányi TM, Lord A, et al. Epidemic outbreaks of adenovirus 7 with special reference to the pathogenicity of adenovirus genome type 7b. *Am J Epidemiol.* 1980; 112(5):619-28.
477. Dominguez O, Rojo P, de Las Heras S, et al. Clinical presentation and characteristics of pharyngeal adenovirus infections. *Pediatr Infect Dis J.* 2005;24(8):733-4.
478. Azar MJ, Dhaliwal DK, Bower KS, et al. Possible consequences of shaking hands with your patients with epidemic keratoconjunctivitis. *Am J Ophthalmol.* 1996; 121(6):711-2.
479. Krajden M, Brown M, Petrasek A, et al. Clinical features of adenovirus enteritis: a review of 127 cases. *Pediatr Infect Dis J.* 1990;9(9):636-41.
480. South MA, Dolen J, Beach DK, et al. Fatal adenovirus hepatic necrosis in severe combined immune deficiency. *Pediatr Infect Dis.* 1982;1(6):416-9.
481. Uhnoo I, Wadell G, Svensson L, et al. Importance of enteric adenoviruses 40 and 41 in acute gastroenteritis in infants and young children. *J Clin Microbiol.* 1984;20(3):365-72.
482. Van R, Wun CC, O'Ryan ML, et al. Outbreaks of human enteric adenovirus types 40 and 41 in Houston day care centers. *J Pediatr.* 1992;120(4 Pt 1):516-21.
483. Bines JE, Liem NT, Justice FA, et al. Risk factors for intussusception in infants in Vietnam and Australia: adenovirus implicated, but not rotavirus. *J Pediatr.* 2006; 149(4):452-60.
484. Mufson MA, Belshe RB. A review of adenoviruses in the etiology of acute hemorrhagic cystitis. *J Urol.* 1976; 115(2):191-4.
485. Harnett GB, Phillips PA, Gollow MM. Association of genital adenovirus infection with urethritis in men. *Med J Aust.* 1984;141(6):337-8.
486. Swenson PD, Lowens MS, Celum CL, et al. Adenovirus types 2, 8, and 37 associated with genital infections in patients attending a sexually transmitted disease clinic. *J Clin Microbiol.* 1995;33(10):2728-31.
487. Frange P, Peffault de Latour R, Arnaud C, et al. Adenoviral infection presenting as an isolated central nervous system disease without detectable viremia in two children after stem cell transplantation. *J Clin Microbiol.* 2011;49(6):2361-4.
488. Martin AB, Webber S, Fricker FJ, et al. Acute myocarditis. Rapid diagnosis by PCR in children. *Circulation.* 1994; 90(1):330-9.
489. Bowles NE, Ni J, Kearney DL, et al. Detection of viruses in myocardial tissues by polymerase chain reaction. Evidence of adenovirus as a common cause of myocarditis in children and adults. *J Am Coll Cardiol.* 2003;42(3):466-72.
490. Wright J, Couchonnal G, Hodges GR. Adenovirus type 21 infection. Occurrence with pneumonia, rhabdomyolysis, and myoglobinuria in an adult. *JAMA.* 1979;241(22):2420-1.
491. Meshkinpour H, Vaziri ND. Association of myoglobinuria with adenovirus infection. *West J Med.* 1982;137(2):130-2.
492. Rahal JJ, Millian SJ, Noriega ER. Coxsackievirus and adenovirus infection. Association with acute febrile and juvenile rheumatoid arthritis. *JAMA.* 1976;235(23):2496-501.
493. Fraser KJ, Clarris BJ, Muirden KD, et al. A persistent adenovirus type 1 infection in synovial tissue from an immunodeficient patient with chronic, rheumatoid-like polyarthritis. *Arthritis Rheum.* 1985;28(4):455-8.
494. Garnett CT, Erdman D, Xu W, et al. Prevalence and quantitation of species C adenovirus DNA in human mucosal lymphocytes. *J Virol.* 2002;76(21):10608-16.

495. Ison MG. Adenovirus infections in transplant recipients. *Clin Infect Dis.* 2006;43(3):331-9.
496. Kojaoghlanian T, Flomenberg P, Horwitz MS. The impact of adenovirus infection on the immunocompromised host. *Rev Med Virol.* 2003;13(3):155-71.
497. Shields AF, Hackman RC, Fife KH, et al. Adenovirus infections in patients undergoing bone-marrow transplantation. *N Engl J Med.* 1985;312(9):529-33.
498. Flomenberg P, Babbitt J, Drobyski WR, et al. Increasing incidence of adenovirus disease in bone marrow transplant recipients. *J Infect Dis.* 1994;169(4):775-81.
499. Baldwin A, Kingman H, Darville M, et al. Outcome and clinical course of 100 patients with adenovirus infection following bone marrow transplantation. *Bone Marrow Transplant.* 2000;26(12):1333-8.
500. Vyas JM, Marasco WA. Fatal fulminant hepatic failure from adenovirus in allogeneic bone marrow transplant patients. *Case Rep Infect Dis.* 2012;2012:463569.
501. de Mezerville MH, Tellier R, Richardson S, et al. Adenoviral infections in pediatric transplant recipients: a hospital-based study. *Pediatr Infect Dis J.* 2006;25(9):815-8.
502. Müller WJ, Levin MJ, Shin YK, et al. Clinical and in vitro evaluation of cidofovir for treatment of adenovirus infection in pediatric hematopoietic stem cell transplant recipients. *Clin Infect Dis.* 2005;41(12):1812-6.
503. Ito M, Hirabayashi N, Uno Y, et al. Necrotizing tubulo-interstitial nephritis associated with adenovirus infection. *Hum Pathol.* 1991;22(12):1225-31.
504. Myerowitz RL, Stalder H, Oxman MN, et al. Fatal disseminated adenovirus infection in a renal transplant recipient. *Am J Med.* 1975;59(4):591-8.
505. Ohori NP, Michaels MG, Jaffe R, et al. Adenovirus pneumonia in lung transplant recipients. *Hum Pathol.* 1995;26(10):1073-9.
506. Michaels MG, Green M, Wald ER, et al. Adenovirus infection in pediatric liver transplant recipients. *J Infect Dis.* 1992;165(1):170-4.
507. Shirali GS, Ni J, Chinnock RE, et al. Association of viral genome with graft loss in children after cardiac transplantation. *N Engl JMed.* 2001;344(20):1498-503.
508. Hierholzer JC, Wigand R, Anderson LJ, et al. Adenoviruses from patients with AIDS: a plethora of serotypes and a description of five new serotypes of subgenus D (types 43-47). *J Infect Dis.* 1988;158(4):804-13.
509. De Jong JC, Wermenbol AG, Verweij-Uijterwaal MW, et al. Adenoviruses from human immunodeficiency virus-infected individuals, including two strains that represent new candidate serotypes Ad50 and Ad51 of species B1 and D, respectively. *J Clin Microbiol.* 1999; 37(12):3940-5.
510. Krilov LR, Rubin LG, Frogel M, et al. Disseminated adenovirus infection with hepatic necrosis in patients with human immunodeficiency virus infection and other immunodeficiency states. *Rev Infect Dis.* 1990;12(2):303-7.
511. Anders KH, Park CS, Cornford ME, et al. Adenovirus encephalitis and widespread ependymitis in a child with AIDS. *Pediatr Neurosurg.* 1990-1991;16(6):316-20.
512. Shintaku M, Nasu K, Ito M. Necrotizing tubulo-interstitial nephritis induced by adenovirus in an AIDS patient. *Histopathology.* 1993;23(6):588-90.
513. Herrmann JE, Perron-Henry DM, Blacklow NR. Antigen detection with monoclonal antibodies for the diagnosis of adenovirus gastroenteritis. *J Infect Dis.* 1987;155(6):1167-71.
514. Levent F, Greer JM, Snider M, et al. Performance of a new immunochromatographic assay for detection of adenoviruses in children. *J Clin Virol.* 2009;44(2):173-5.
515. Raboni SM, Nogueira MB, Tsuchiya LR, et al. Respiratory tract viral infections in bone marrow transplant patients. *Transplant.* 2003;76(1):142-6.
516. Wiley LA, Roba LA, Kowalski RP, et al. A 5-year evaluation of the adenoclone test for the rapid diagnosis of adenovirus from conjunctival swabs. *Cornea.* 1996;15(4):363-7.
517. Claas EC, Schilham MW, de Brouwer CS, et al. Internally controlled real-time PCR monitoring of adenovirus DNA load in serum or plasma of transplant recipients. *J Clin Microbiol.* 2005;43(4):1738-44.
518. Damen M, Minnaar R, Glasius P, et al. Real-time PCR with an internal control for detection of all known human adenovirus serotypes. *J Clin Microbiol.* 2008;46(12):3997-4003.
519. Heim A, Ebnet C, Harste G, et al. Rapid and quantitative detection of human adenovirus DNA by real-time PCR. *J Med Virol.* 2003;70(2):228-39.
520. Echavarria M, Forman M, van Tol MJ, et al. Prediction of severe disseminated adenovirus infection by serum PCR. *Lancet.* 2001;358(9279):384-5.
521. Lion T, Baumgartinger R, Watzinger F, et al. Molecular monitoring of adenovirus in peripheral blood after allogeneic bone marrow transplantation permits early diagnosis of disseminated disease. *Blood.* 2003; 102(3):1114-20.
522. Leruez-Ville M, Minard V, Lacaille F, et al. Real-time blood plasma polymerase chain reaction for management of disseminated adenovirus infection. *Clin Infect Dis.* 2004; 38(1):45-52.
523. Neofytos D, Ojha A, Mookerjee B, et al. Treatment of adenovirus disease in stem cell transplant recipients with cidofovir. *Biol Blood Marrow Transplant.* 2007;13(1):74-81.
524. Lankester AC, Heemskerk B, Claas EC, et al. Effect of ribavirin on the plasma viral DNA load in patients with disseminating adenovirus infection. *Clin Infect Dis.* 2004; 38(11):1521-5.
525. Lankester AC, van Tol MJ, Claas EC, et al. Quantification of adenovirus DNA in plasma for management of infection in stem cell graft recipients. *Clin Infect Dis.* 2002;34(6):864-7.
526. Becroft DM. Histopathology of fatal adenovirus infection of the respiratory tract in young children. *J Clin Pathol.* 1967;20(4):561-9.
527. Landry ML, Fong CK, Neddermann K, et al. Disseminated adenovirus infection in an immunocompromised host. Pitfalls in diagnosis. *Am J Med.* 1987;83(3):555-9.
528. McMinn PC, Stewart J, Burrell CJ. A community outbreak of epidemic keratoconjunctivitis in central Australia due to adenovirus type 8. *J Infect Dis.* 1991;164(6):1113-8.
529. Kodama E, Shigeta S, Suzuki T, et al. Application of a gastric cancer cell line (MKN-28) for anti-adenovirus screening using the MTT method. *Antiviral Res.* 1996;31(3):159-64.
530. Legrand F, Berrebi D, Houhou N, et al. Early diagnosis of adenovirus infection and treatment with cidofovir after bone marrow transplantation in children. *Bone Marrow Transplant.* 2001;27(6):621-6.

531. Ljungman P, Ribaud P, Eyrich M, et al. Cidofovir for adenovirus infections after allogeneic hematopoietic stem cell transplantation: a survey by the Infectious Diseases Working Party of the European Group for Blood and Marrow Transplantation. *Bone Marrow Transplant.* 2003;31(6):481-6.
532. Doan ML, Mallory GB, Kaplan SL, et al. Treatment of adenovirus pneumonia with cidofovir in pediatric lung transplant recipients. *J Heart Lung Transplant.* 2007; 26(9):883-9.
533. Hoffman JA, Shah AJ, Ross LA, et al. Adenoviral infections and a prospective trial of cidofovir in pediatric hematopoietic stem cell transplantation. *Biol Blood Marrow Transplant.* 2001;7(7):388-94.
534. La Rosa AM, Champlin RE, Mirza N, et al. Adenovirus infections in adult recipients of blood and marrow transplants. *Clin Infect Dis.* 2001;32(6):871-6.
535. Symeonidis N, Jakubowski A, Pierre-Louis S, et al. Invasive adenoviral infections in T-cell-depleted allogeneic hematopoietic stem cell transplantation: high mortality in the era of cidofovir. *Transpl Infect Dis.* 2007;9(2):108-13.
536. Heemskerk B, Lankester AC, van Vreeswijk T, et al. Immune reconstitution and clearance of human adenovirus viremia in pediatric stem-cell recipients. *J Infect Dis.* 2005;191(4):520-30.
537. Flomenberg PR, Chen M, Munk G, et al. Molecular epidemiology of adenovirus type 35 infections in immunocompromised hosts. *J Infect Dis.* 1987;155(6):1127-34.
538. Dagan R, Schwartz RH, Insel RA, et al. Severe diffuse adenovirus 7a pneumonia in a child with combined immunodeficiency: possible therapeutic effect of human immune serum globulin containing specific neutralizing antibody. *Pediatr Infect Dis.* 1984;3(3):246-51.
539. Lenaerts L, Kelchtermans H, Geboes L, et al. Recovery of humoral immunity is critical for successful antiviral therapy in disseminated mouse adenovirus type 1 infection. *Antimicrob Agents Chemother.* 2008;52(4):1462-71.
540. Buehler JW, Finton RJ, Goodman RA, et al. Epidemic keratoconjunctivitis: report of an outbreak in an ophthalmology practice and recommendations for prevention. *Infect Control.* 1984;5(8):390-4.
541. D'Angelo LJ, Hierholzer JC, Keenlyside RA, et al. Pharyngoconjunctival fever caused by adenovirus type 4: report of a swimming pool-related outbreak with recovery of virus from pool water. *J Infect Dis.* 1979;140(1):42-7.
542. Carstens EB. Ratification vote on taxonomic proposals to the International Committee on Taxonomy of Viruses (2009). *Arch Virol.* 2010;155(1):133-46.
543. McIntosh KPJ. Coronaviruses. In: Richman D, Whitley RJ, Hayden FG, editors. Clinical Virology 3rd ed. Washington, DC: ASM Press; 2009.
544. Nidovirales. 09/27/2012 2012 (accessed 02/13/2013).
545. Luytjes W, Bredenbeek PJ, Noten AF, et al. Sequence of mouse hepatitis virus A59 mRNA 2: indications for RNA recombination between coronaviruses and influenza C virus. *Virology.* 1988;166(2):415-22.
546. McIntosh K, Kapikian AZ, Turner HC, et al. Seroepidemiologic studies of coronavirus infection in adults and children. *Am J Epidemiol.* 1970;91(6):585-92.
547. Vabret A, Dina J, Gouarin S, et al. Human (non-severe acute respiratory syndrome) coronavirus infections in hospitalised children in France. *J Paediatr Child Health.* 2008;44(4):176-81.
548. Gaunt ER, Hardie A, Claas EC, et al. Epidemiology and clinical presentations of the four human coronaviruses 229E, HKU1, NL63, and OC43 detected over 3 years using a novel multiplex real-time PCR method. *J Clin Microbiol.* 2010;48(8):2940-7.
549. Reed SE. The behaviour of recent isolates of human respiratory coronavirus in vitro and in volunteers: evidence of heterogeneity among 229E-related strains. *J Med Virol.* 1984;13(2):179-92.
550. Bradburne AF, Bynoe ML, Tyrrell DA. Effects of a "new" human respiratory virus in volunteers. *Br Med J.* 1967;3(5568):767-9.
551. Bradburne AF, Somerset BA. Coronative antibody tires in sera of healthy adults and experimentally infected volunteers. *J Hyg (Lond).* 1972;70(2):235-44.
552. Gagneur A, Vallet S, Talbot PJ, et al. Outbreaks of human coronavirus in a pediatric and neonatal intensive care unit. *Eur J Pediatr.* 2008;167(12):1427-34.
553. Monto AS. Medical reviews. Coronaviruses. *Yale J Biol Med.* 1974;47(4):234-51.
554. Prill MM, Iwane MK, Edwards KM, et al. Human coronavirus in young children hospitalized for acute respiratory illness and asymptomatic controls. *Pediatr Infect Dis J.* 2012;31(3):235-40.
555. Chonmaitree T, Revai K, Grady JJ, et al. Viral upper respiratory tract infection and otitis media complication in young children. *Clin Infect Dis.* 2008;46(6):815-23.
556. Bastien N, Anderson K, Hart L, et al. Human coronavirus NL63 infection in Canada. *J Infect Dis.* 2005;191(4):503-6.
557. Woo PC, Lau SK, Tsoi HW, et al. Clinical and molecular epidemiological features of coronavirus HKU1-associated community-acquired pneumonia. *J Infect Dis.* 2005;192(11):1898-907.
558. McIntosh K, Chao RK, Krause HE, et al. Coronavirus infection in acute lower respiratory tract disease of infants. *J Infect Dis.* 1974;130(5):502-7.
559. Kuypers J, Martin ET, Heugel J, et al. Clinical disease in children associated with newly described coronavirus subtypes. *Pediatrics.* 2007;119(1):e70-6.
560. Talbot HK, Shepherd BE, Crowe JE, et al. The pediatric burden of human coronaviruses evaluated for twenty years. *Pediatr Infect Dis J.* 2009;28(8):682-7.
561. Talbot HK, Crowe JE, Edwards KM, et al. Coronavirus infection and hospitalizations for acute respiratory illness in young children. *J Med Virol.* 2009;81(5):853-6.
562. Kristoffersen AW, Nordbø SA, Rognlien AG, et al. Coronavirus causes lower respiratory tract infections less frequently than RSV in hospitalized Norwegian children. *Pediatr Infect Dis J.* 2011;30(4):279-83.
563. Van der Hoek L, Sure K, Ihorst G, et al. Croup is associated with the novel coronavirus NL63. *PLoS Med.* 2005;2(8): e240.
564. Sung JY, Lee HJ, Eun BW, et al. Role of human coronavirus NL63 in hospitalized children with croup. *Pediatr Infect Dis J.* 2010;29(9):822-6.

565. McIntosh K, Ellis EF, Hoffman LS, et al. The association of viral and bacterial respiratory infections with exacerbations of wheezing in young asthmatic children. *J Pediatr.* 1973;82(4):578-90.
566. Christian MD, Poutanen SM, Loutfy MR, et al. Severe acute respiratory syndrome. *Clin Infect Dis.* 2004;38(10):1420-7.
567. Peiris JS, Yuen KY, Osterhaus AD, et al. The severe acute respiratory syndrome. *N Engl J Med.* 2003;349(25):2431-41.
568. He Y, Li J, Li W, et al. Cross-neutralization of human and palm civet severe acute respiratory syndrome coronaviruses by antibodies targeting the receptor-binding domain of spike protein. *J Immunol.* 2006;176(10):6085-92.
569. Tu C, Crameri G, Kong X, et al. Antibodies to SARS coronavirus in civets. *Emerg Infect Dis.* 2004;10(12):2244-8.
570. Koley TK. Severe acute respiratory syndrome: a preliminary review. *J Indian Med Assoc.* 2003;101(5):308-10.
571. Hsueh PR, Yang PC. Severe acute respiratory syndrome epidemic in Taiwan, 2003. *J Microbiol Immunol Infect.* 2005;38(2):82-8.
572. Tsang KW, Mok TY, Wong PC, et al. Severe acute respiratory syndrome (SARS) in Hong Kong. *Respirology.* 2003;8(3):259-65.
573. Peiris JS, Chu CM, Cheng VC, et al. Clinical progression and viral load in a community outbreak of coronavirus-associated SARS pneumonia: a prospective study. *Lancet.* 2003;361(9371):1767-72.
574. Booth CM, Matukas LM, Tomlinson GA, et al. Clinical features and short-term outcomes of 144 patients with SARS in the greater Toronto area. *JAMA.* 2003;289(21):2801-9.
575. Chan JW, Ng CK, Chan YH, et al. Short term outcome and risk factors for adverse clinical outcomes in adults with severe acute respiratory syndrome (SARS). *Thorax.* 2003;58(8):686-9.
576. Hsu LY, Lee CC, Green JA, et al. Severe acute respiratory syndrome (SARS) in Singapore: clinical features of index patient and initial contacts. *Emerg Infect Dis.* 2003;9(6):713-7.
577. Choi KW, Chau TN, Tsang O, et al. Outcomes and prognostic factors in 267 patients with severe acute respiratory syndrome in Hong Kong. *Ann Intern Med.* 2003;139(9):715-23.
578. Gerna G, Passarani N, Battaglia M, et al. Human enteric coronaviruses: antigenic relatedness to human coronavirus OC43 and possible etiologic role in viral gastroenteritis. *J Infect Dis.* 1985;151(5):796-803.
579. Chany C, Moscovici O, Lebon P, et al. Association of coronavirus infection with neonatal necrotizing enterocolitis. *Pediatrics.* 1982;69(2):209-14.
580. Rousset S, Moscovici O, Lebon P, et al. Intestinal lesions containing coronavirus-like particles in neonatal necrotizing enterocolitis: an ultrastructural analysis. *Pediatrics.* 1984;73(2):218-24.
581. Moscovici O, Chany C, Lebon P, et al. Association of coronavirus infection with hemorrhagic entercolitis in newborn infants. *C R Seances Acad Sci D.* 1980;290(13):869-72.
582. Risku M, Lappalainen S, Räsänen S, et al. Detection of human coronaviruses in children with acute gastroenteritis. *J Clin Virol.* 2010;48(1):27-30.
583. Boucher A, Desforges M, Duquette P, et al. Long-term human coronavirus-myelin cross-reactive T-cell clones derived from multiple sclerosis patients. *Clin Immunol.* 2007;123(3):258-67.
584. Arbour N, Ekandé S, Côté G, et al. Persistent infection of human oligodendrocytic and neuroglial cell lines by human coronavirus 229E. *J Virol.* 1999;73(4):3326-37.
585. Arbour N, Day R, Newcombe J, et al. Neuroinvasion by human respiratory coronaviruses. *J Virol.* 2000;74(19):8913-21.
586. Gerna G, Campanini G, Rovida F, et al. Genetic variability of human coronavirus OC43-, 229E-, and NL63-like strains and their association with lower respiratory tract infections of hospitalized infants and immunocompromised patients. *J Med Virol.* 2006;78(7):938-49.
587. Gerna G, Percivalle E, Sarasini A, et al. Human respiratory coronavirus HKU1 versus other coronavirus infections in Italian hospitalised patients. *J Clin Virol.* 2007;38(3):244-50.
588. Sizun J, Arbour N, Talbot PJ. Comparison of immunofluorescence with monoclonal antibodies and RT-PCR for the detection of human coronaviruses 229E and OC43 in cell culture. *J Virol Methods.* 1998;72(2):145-52.
589. Loutfy MR, Blatt LM, Siminovitch KA, et al. Interferon alfacon-1 plus corticosteroids in severe acute respiratory syndrome: a preliminary study. *JAMA.* 2003;290(24):3222-8.
590. Chan KS, Lai ST, Chu CM, et al. Treatment of severe acute respiratory syndrome with lopinavir/ritonavir: a multicentre retrospective matched cohort study. *Hong Kong Med J.* 2003;9(6):399-406.
591. Cheng Y, Wong R, Soo YO, et al. Use of convalescent plasma therapy in SARS patients in Hong Kong. *Eur J Clin Microbiol Infect Dis.* 2005;24(1):44-6.
592. Ter Meulen J, Bakker AB, van den Brink EN, et al. Human monoclonal antibody as prophylaxis for SARS coronavirus infection in ferrets. *Lancet.* 2004;363(9427):2139-41.
593. Boivin G, Mackay I, Sloots TP, et al. Global genetic diversity of human metapneumovirus fusion gene. *Emerg Infect Dis.* 2004;10(6):1154-7.
594. Mackay IM, Bialasiewicz S, Jacob KC, et al. Genetic diversity of human metapneumovirus over 4 consecutive years in Australia. *J Infect Dis.* 2006;193(12):1630-3.
595. Van den Hoogen BG, de Jong JC, Groen J, et al. A newly discovered human pneumovirus isolated from young children with respiratory tract disease. *Nature Med.* 2001; 7(6):719-24.
596. Boivin G, Abed Y, Pelletier G, et al. Virological features and clinical manifestations associated with human metapneumovirus: a new paramyxovirus responsible for acute respiratory-tract infections in all age groups. *J Infect Dis.* 2002;186(9):1330-4.
597. Nissen MD, Siebert DJ, Mackay IM, et al. Evidence of human metapneumovirus in Australian children. *Med J Aust.* 2002;176(4):188.
598. Peret TC, Boivin G, Li Y, et al. Characterization of human metapneumoviruses isolated from patients in North America. *J Infect Dis.* 2002;185(11):1660-3.
599. Kuiken T, van den Hoogen BG, van Riel DA, et al. Experimental human metapneumovirus infection of cynomolgus macaques (Macaca fascicularis) results in virus replication in ciliated epithelial cells and pneumocytes with associated lesions throughout the respiratory tract. *Am J Pathol.* 2004;164(6):1893-900.

600. Hamelin ME, Prince GA, Gomez AM, et al. Human metapneumovirus infection induces long-term pulmonary inflammation associated with airway obstruction and hyperresponsiveness in mice. *J Infect Dis.* 2006;193(12):1634-42.
601. Openshaw PJ, Dean GS, Culley FJ. Links between respiratory syncytial virus bronchiolitis and childhood asthma: clinical and research approaches. *Pediatr Infect Dis J.* 2003;22(2 Suppl):S58-64.
602. Peiris JS, Tang WH, Chan KH, et al. Children with respiratory disease associated with metapneumovirus in Hong Kong. *Emerg Infect Dis.* 2003;9(6):628-33.
603. Kim S, Sung H, Im HJ, et al. Molecular epidemiological investigation of a nosocomial outbreak of human metapneumovirus infection in a pediatric hemato-oncology patient population. *J Clin Microbiol.* 2009;47(4):1221-4.
604. Tu CC, Chen LK, Lee YS, et al. An outbreak of human metapneumovirus infection in hospitalized psychiatric adult patients in Taiwan. *Scand J Infect Dis.* 2009;41(5):363-7.
605. Stockton J, Stephenson I, Fleming D, et al. Human metapneumovirus as a cause of community-acquired respiratory illness. *Emerg Infect Dis.* 2002;8(9):897-901.
606. Jartti T, van den Hoogen B, Garofalo RP, et al. Metapneumovirus and acute wheezing in children. *Lancet.* 2002;360(9343):1393-4.
607. Osterhaus A, Fouchier R. Human metapneumovirus in the community. *Lancet.* 2003;361(9361):890-1.
608. Williams JV, Harris PA, Tollefson SJ, et al. Human metapneumovirus and lower respiratory tract disease in otherwise healthy infants and children. *N Engl J Med.* 2004;350(5):443-50.
609. Esper F, Martinello RA, Boucher D, et al. A 1-year experience with human metapneumovirus in children aged <5 years. *J Infect Dis.* 2004;189(8):1388-96.
610. Døllner H, Risnes K, Radtke A, et al. Outbreak of human metapneumovirus infection in norwegian children. *Pediatr Infect Dis J.* 2004;23(5):436-40.
611. Louie JK, Schnurr DP, Pan CY, et al. A summer outbreak of human metapneumovirus infection in a long-term-care facility. *J Infect Dis.* 2007;196(5):705-8.
612. Williams JV, Edwards KM, Weinberg GA, et al. Population-based incidence of human metapneumovirus infection among hospitalized children. *J Infect Dis.* 2010;201(12):1890-8.
613. Williams JV, Wang CK, Yang CF, et al. The role of human metapneumovirus in upper respiratory tract infections in children: a 20-year experience. *J Infect Dis.* 2006;193(3):387-95.
614. Boivin G, De Serres G, Côté S, et al. Human metapneumovirus infections in hospitalized children. *Emerg Infect Dis.* 2003;9(6):634-40.
615. Mullins JA, Erdman DD, Weinberg GA, et al. Human metapneumovirus infection among children hospitalized with acute respiratory illness. *Emerg Infect Dis.* 2004;10(4):700-5.
616. Falsey AR, Erdman D, Anderson LJ, et al. Human metapneumovirus infections in young and elderly adults. *J Infect Dis.* 2003;187(5):785-90.
617. Wolf DG, Greenberg D, Shemer-Avni Y, et al. Association of human metapneumovirus with radiologically diagnosed community-acquired alveolar pneumonia in young children. *J Pediatr.* 2010;156(1):115-20.
618. Semple MG, Cowell A, Dove W, et al. Dual infection of infants by human metapneumovirus and human respiratory syncytial virus is strongly associated with severe bronchiolitis. *J Infect Dis.* 2005;191(3):382-6.
619. König B, König W, Arnold R, et al. Prospective study of human metapneumovirus infection in children less than 3 years of age. *J Clin Microbiol.* 2004;42(10):4632-5.
620. Schildgen O, Glatzel T, Geikowski T, et al. Human metapneumovirus RNA in encephalitis patient. *Emerg Infect Dis.* 2005;11(3):467-70.
621. Sánchez Fernández I, Rebollo Polo M, Muñoz-Almagro C, et al. Human metapneumovirus in the cerebrospinal fluid of a patient with acute encephalitis. *Archiv Neurol.* 2012;69(5):649-52.
622. Williams JV, Crowe JE, Enriquez R, et al. Human metapneumovirus infection plays an etiologic role in acute asthma exacerbations requiring hospitalization in adults. *J Infect Dis.* 2005;192(7):1149-53.
623. Boivin G, De Serres G, Hamelin ME, et al. An outbreak of severe respiratory tract infection due to human metapneumovirus in a long-term care facility. *Clin Infect Dis.* 2007;44(9):1152-8.
624. Vicente D, Montes M, Cilla G, et al. Human metapneumovirus and chronic obstructive pulmonary disease. *Emerg Infect Dis.* 2004;10(7):1338-9.
625. Beckham JD, Cadena A, Lin J, et al. Respiratory viral infections in patients with chronic, obstructive pulmonary disease. *J Infect.* 2005;50(4):322-30.
626. Sumino KC, Agapov E, Pierce RA, et al. Detection of severe human metapneumovirus infection by real-time polymerase chain reaction and histopathological assessment. *J Infect Dis.* 2005;192(6):1052-60.
627. Williams JV, Martino R, Rabella N, et al. A prospective study comparing human metapneumovirus with other respiratory viruses in adults with hematologic malignancies and respiratory tract infections. *J Infect Dis.* 2005;192(6):1061-5.
628. Englund JA, Boeckh M, Kuypers J, et al. Brief communication: fatal human metapneumovirus infection in stem-cell transplant recipients. *Ann Intern Med.* 2006;144(5):344-9.
629. Debiaggi M, Canducci F, Sampaolo M, et al. Persistent symptomless human metapneumovirus infection in hematopoietic stem cell transplant recipients. *J Infect Dis.* 2006;194(4):474-8.
630. Larcher C, Geltner C, Fischer H, et al. Human metapneumovirus infection in lung transplant recipients: clinical presentation and epidemiology. *J Heart Lung Transplant.* 2005;24(11):1891-901.
631. Hamelin ME, Boivin G. Development and validation of an enzyme-linked immunosorbent assay for human metapneumovirus serology based on a recombinant viral protein. *Clin Diagn Lab Immunol.* 2005;12(2):249-53.
632. Wyde PR, Chetty SN, Jewell AM, et al. Comparison of the inhibition of human metapneumovirus and respiratory syncytial virus by ribavirin and immune serum globulin in vitro. *Antiviral Res.* 2003;60(1):51-9.

633. Harvey R, Champe P, Fisher B. Positive-strand RNA viruses. Microbiology, 2nd edition. Baltimore: Lippincott Williams & Wilkins; 2007.
634. Ooi MH, Wong SC, Lewthwaite P, et al. Clinical features, diagnosis, and management of enterovirus 71. *Lancet Neurol.* 2010;9(11):1097-105.
635. Kogon A, Spigland I, Frothingham TE, et al. The virus watch program: a continuing surveillance of viral infections in metropolitan New York families. VII. Observations on viral excretion, seroimmunity, intrafamilial spread and illness association in coxsackie and echovirus infections. *Am J Epidemiol.* 1969;89(1):51-61.
636. Joki-Korpela P, Hyypiä T. Parechoviruses, a novel group of human picornaviruses. *Ann Med.* 2001;33(7):466-71.
637. Harvala H, McLeish N, Kondracka J, et al. Comparison of human parechovirus and enterovirus detection frequencies in cerebrospinal fluid samples collected over a 5-year period in edinburgh: HPeV type 3 identified as the most common picornavirus type. *J Med Virol.* 2011; 83(5):889-96.
638. Verboon-Maciolek MA, Krediet TG, Gerards LJ, et al. Severe neonatal parechovirus infection and similarity with enterovirus infection. *Pediatr Infect Dis J.* 2008;27(3):241-5.
639. Wolthers KC, Benschop KS, Schinkel J, et al. Human parechoviruses as an important viral cause of sepsislike illness and meningitis in young children. *Clin Infect Dis.* 2008;47(3):358-63.
640. Abed Y, Boivin G. Human parechovirus types 1, 2 and 3 infections in Canada. *Emerg Infect Dis.* 2006;12(6):969-75.
641. Harvala H, Wolthers KC, Simmonds P. Parechoviruses in children: understanding a new infection. *Curr Opin Infect Dis.* 2010;23(3):224-30.
642. Levorson RE, Jantausch BA. Human parechoviruses. *Pediatr Infect Dis J.* 2009;28(9):831-2.
643. Bell EJ, Ross CA, Grist NR. ECHO 9 infection in pregnant women with suspected rubella. *J Clinl Pathol.* 1975;28(4):267-9.
644. Lerner AM, Klein JO, Levin HS, et al. Infections due to Coxsackie virus group A, type 9, in Boston, 1959, with special reference to exanthems and pneumonia. *N Engl J Med.* 1960;263:1265-72.
645. Sabin AB, Krumbiegel ER, Wigand R. ECHO type 9 virus disease. *AMA J Dis Child.* 1958;96(2):197-219.
646. Neva FA, Feemster RF, Gorbach IJ. Clinical and epidemiological features of an usual epidemic exanthem. *J Am Med Assoc.* 1954;155(6):544-8.
647. Neva FA. A second outbreak of Boston exanthem disease in Pittsburgh during 1954. *N Engl J Med.* 1956;254(18):838-43.
648. Adler JL, Mostow SR, Mellin H, et al. Epidemiologic investigation of hand, foot, and mouth disease. Infection caused by coxsackievirus A 16 in Baltimore, June through September 1968. *Am J Dis Child.* 1970;120(4):309-14.
649. Alexander JP, Baden L, Pallansch MA, et al. Enterovirus 71 infections and neurologic disease—United States, 1977-1991. *J Infect Dis.* 1994;169(4):905-8.
650. Lum LC, Wong KT, Lam SK, et al. Fatal enterovirus 71 encephalomyelitis. *J Pediatr.* 1998;133(6):795-8.
651. Huang CC, Liu CC, Chang YC, et al. Neurologic complications in children with enterovirus 71 infection. *N Engl J Med.* 1999;341(13):936-42.
652. Chan KP, Goh KT, Chong CY, et al. Epidemic hand, foot and mouth disease caused by human enterovirus 71, Singapore. *Emerg Infect Dis.* 2003;9(1):78-85.
653. Jiang M, Wei D, Ou WL, et al. Autopsy findings in children with hand, foot, and mouth disease. *New Engl J Med.* 2012;367(1):91-2.
654. Cherry JD, Jahn CL. Herpangina: the etiologic spectrum. *Pediatrics.* 1965;36(4):632-4.
655. Marier R, Rodriguez W, Chloupek RJ, et al. Coxsackievirus B5 infection and aseptic meningitis in neonates and children. *Am J Dis Child.* 1975;129(3):321-5.
656. Wilfert CM, Lauer BA, Cohen M, et al. An epidemic of echovirus 18 meningitis. *J Infect Dis.* 1975;131(1):75-8.
657. Berlin LE, Rorabaugh ML, Heldrich F, et al. Aseptic meningitis in infants < 2 years of age: diagnosis and etiology. *J Infect Dis.* 1993;168(4):888-92.
658. Fowlkes AL, Honarmand S, Glaser C, et al. Enterovirus-associated encephalitis in the California encephalitis project, 1998-2005. *J Infect Dis.* 2008;198(11):1685-91.
659. McMinn P, Stratov I, Nagarajan L, et al. Neurological manifestations of enterovirus 71 infection in children during an outbreak of hand, foot, and mouth disease in Western Australia. *Clin Infect Dis.* 2001;32(2):236-42.
660. Chang LY, Tsao KC, Hsia SH, et al. Transmission and clinical features of enterovirus 71 infections in household contacts in Taiwan. *JAMA.* 2004;291(2):222-7.
661. Chang LY, Huang LM, Gau SS, et al. Neurodevelopment and cognition in children after enterovirus 71 infection. *N Engl J Med.* 2007;356(12):1226-34.
662. Warin JF, Davies JB, Sanders FK, et al. Oxford epidemic of Bornholm disease, 1951. *Br Med J.* 1953;1(4824):1345-51.
663. Curnen EC, Shaw EW, Melnick JL. Disease resembling non-paralytic poliomyelitis associated with a virus pathogenic for infant mice. *J Am Med Assoc.* 1949;141(13):894-901.
664. Weller TH, Enders JF, Buckingham M, et al. The etiology of epidemic pleurodynia: a study of two viruses isolated from a typical outbreak. *J Immunol.* 1950;65(3):337-46.
665. Smith WG. Adult heart disease due to the Coxsackie virus group B. *Br Heart J.* 1966;28(2):204-20.
666. Verma NA, Zheng XT, Harris MU, et al. Outbreak of life-threatening coxsackievirus B1 myocarditis in neonates. *Clin Infect Dis.* 2009;49(5):759-63.
667. Freund MW, Kleinveld G, Krediet TG, et al. Prognosis for neonates with enterovirus myocarditis. *Archiv Dis Child Fetal Neonatal Ed.* 2010;95(3):F206-12.
668. Sklar VE, Patriarca PA, Onorato IM, et al. Clinical findings and results of treatment in an outbreak of acute hemorrhagic conjunctivitis in southern Florida. *Am J Ophthalmol.* 1983;95(1):45-54.
669. Kinney JS, McCray E, Kaplan JE, et al. Risk factors associated with echovirus 11′ infection in a hospital nursery. *Pediatri Infect Dis.* 1986;5(2):192-7.
670. Modlin JF. Perinatal echovirus infection: insights from a literature review of 61 cases of serious infection and 16 outbreaks in nurseries. *Rev Infect Dis.* 1986;8(6):918-26.
671. Lake AM, Lauer BA, Clark JC, et al. Enterovirus infections in neonates. *J Pediatr.* 1976;89(5):787-91.
672. Cherry JD, Soriano F, Jahn CL. Search for perinatal viral infection. A prospective, clinical, virologic, and serologic study. *Am J Dis Child.* 1968;116(3):245-50.

673. Modlin JF, Polk BF, Horton P, et al. Perinatal echovirus infection: risk of transmission during a community outbreak. *N Engl J Med.* 1981;305(7):368-71.

674. Jones MJ, Kolb M, Votava HJ, et al. Case reports. Intrauterine echovirus type II infection. Mayo Clin Proc. 1980;55(8):509-12.

675. Reyes MP, Ostrea EM, Roskamp J, et al. Disseminated neonatal echovirus 11 disease following antenatal maternal infection with a virus-positive cervix and virus-negative gastrointestinal tract. *J Med Virol.* 1983;12(2):155-9.

676. Kaplan MH, Klein SW, McPhee J, et al. Group B coxsackievirus infections in infants younger than three months of age: a serious childhood illness. *Rev Infect Dis.* 1983;5(6):1019-32.

677. Kibrick S. Current status of coxsackie and echo viruses in human disease. *Prog Med Virol.* 1964;6:27-70.

678. Gear JH, Measroch V. Coxsackievirus infections of the newborn. *Prog Med Virol.* 1973;15:42-62.

679. Chambon M, Delage C, Bailly JL, et al. Fatal hepatic necrosis in a neonate with echovirus 20 infection: use of the polymerase chain reaction to detect enterovirus in liver tissue. *Clin Infect Dis.* 1997;24(3):523-4.

680. Georgieff MK, Johnson DE, Thompson TR, et al. Fulminant hepatic necrosis in an infant with perinatally acquired echovirus 21 infection. *Pediatr Infect Dis J.* 1987;6(1):71-3.

681. Spector SA, Straube RC. Protean manifestations of perinatal enterovirus infections. *West J Med.* 1983;138(6):847-51.

682. Speer ME, Yawn DH. Fatal hepatoadrenal necrosis in the neonate associated with echovirus types 11 and 12 presenting as a surgical emergency. *J Pediatr Surg.* 1984; 19(5):591-3.

683. Wreghitt TG, Gandy GM, King A, et al. Fatal neonatal echo 7 virus infection. *Lancet.* 1984;2(8400):465.

684. Rotbart HA, Webster AD, Pleconaril Treatment Registry Group. Treatment of potentially life-threatening enterovirus infections with pleconaril. *Clin Infect Dis.* 2001;32(2): 228-35.

685. Goland S, Czer LS, Siegel RJ, et al. Intravenous immunoglobulin treatment for acute fulminant inflammatory cardiomyopathy: series of six patients and review of literature. *Can J Cardiol.* 2008;24(7):571-4.

686. Qi ZY, Qu XW, Liu WP, et al. Genome cloning and phylogenetic analysis of human bocavirus capsid gene. *Bing Du Xue Bao.* 2007;23(6):447-53.

687. Lin F, Hou JY, Zheng MQ, et al. Characterization of the cytopathic effect in human bronchial epithelial cell after Human Bocavirus Infection (HBoV). *Zhonghua Shi Yan He Lin Chuang Bing Du Xue Za Zhi.* 2008;22(2):107-9.

688. Deng X, Yan Z, Luo Y, et al. In vitro modeling of human bocavirus 1 infection of polarized primary human airway epithelia. *J Virol.* 2013.

689. Lüsebrink J, Wittleben F, Schildgen V, et al. Human bocavirus—insights into a newly identified respiratory virus. *Viruses.* 2009;1(1):3-12.

690. Wang Y, Gonzalez R, Zhou H, et al. Detection of human bocavirus 3 in China. *Eur J Clin Microbiol Infect Dis.* 2011;30(6):799-805.

691. Naghipour M, Cuevas LE, Bakhshinejad T, et al. Human bocavirus in Iranian children with acute respiratory infections. *J Med Virol.* 2007;79(5):539-43.

692. Völz S, Schildgen O, Müller A, et al. The human bocavirus: pathogen in airway infections? *Dtsch Med Wochenschr.* 2007;132(28-29):1529-33.

693. Arnold JC, Singh KK, Spector SA, et al. Human bocavirus: prevalence and clinical spectrum at a children's hospital. *Clin Infect Dis.* 2006;43(3):283-8.

694. Sloots TP, McErlean P, Speicher DJ, et al. Evidence of human coronavirus HKU1 and human bocavirus in Australian children. *J Clin Virol.* 2006;35(1):99-102.

695. Kesebir D, Vazquez M, Weibel C, et al. Human bocavirus infection in young children in the United States: molecular epidemiological profile and clinical characteristics of a newly emerging respiratory virus. *J Infect Dis.* 2006; 194(9):1276-82.

696. Pozo F, García-García ML, Calvo C, et al. High incidence of human bocavirus infection in children in Spain. *J Clin Virol.* 2007;40(3):224-8.

697. Bharaj P, Sullender WM, Kabra SK, et al. Human bocavirus infection in children with acute respiratory tract infection in India. *J Med Virol.* 2010;82(5):812-6.

698. Ghietto LM, Cámara A, Cámara J, et al. High frequency of human bocavirus 1 DNA in infants and adults with lower acute respiratory infection. *J Med Microbiol.* 2012;61(Pt 4): 548-51.

699. Garcia-Garcia ML, Calvo C, Pozo F, et al. Spectrum of respiratory viruses in children with community-acquired pneumonia. *Pediatr Infect Dis J.* 2012; 31(8):808-13.

700. García-García ML, Calvo C, Pozo F, et al. Human bocavirus detection in nasopharyngeal aspirates of children without clinical symptoms of respiratory infection. *Pediatr Infect Dis J.* 2008; 27(4):358-60.

701. Endo R, Ishiguro N, Kikuta H, et al. Seroepidemiology of human bocavirus in Hokkaido prefecture, Japan. *J Clin Microbiol.* 2007;45(10):3218-23.

702. Von Linstow ML, Høgh M, Høgh B. Clinical and epidemiologic characteristics of human bocavirus in Danish infants: results from a prospective birth cohort study. *Pediatr Infect Dis J.* 2008;27(10):897-902.

703. Martin ET, Taylor J, Kuypers J, et al. Detection of bocavirus in saliva of children with and without respiratory illness. *J Clin Microbiol.* 2009;47(12):4131-2.

704. Ma X, Endo R, Ishiguro N, et al. Detection of human bocavirus in Japanese children with lower respiratory tract infections. *J Clin Microbiol.* 2006;44(3):1132-4.

705. Arden KE, McErlean P, Nissen MD, et al. Frequent detection of human rhinoviruses, paramyxoviruses, coronaviruses, and bocavirus during acute respiratory tract infections. *J Med Virol.* 2006;78(9):1232-40.

706. Foulongne V, Olejnik Y, Perez V, et al. Human bocavirus in French children. *Emerg Infect Dis.* 2006;12(8):1251-3.

707. Kim JS, Lim CS, Kim YK, et al. Human bocavirus in patients with respiratory tract infection. *Korean J Lab Med.* 2011;31(3):179-84.

708. Allander T, Jartti T, Gupta S, et al. Human bocavirus and acute wheezing in children. *Clin Infect Dis.* 2007; 44(7):904-10.

709. Chung JY, Han TH, Kim SW, et al. Detection of viruses identified recently in children with acute wheezing. *J Med Virol.* 2007;79(8):1238-43.

710. Christensen A, Nordbø SA, Krokstad S, et al. Human bocavirus commonly involved in multiple viral airway infections. *J Clin Virol.* 2008;41(1):34-7.
711. Gerna G, Piralla A, Campanini G, et al. The human bocavirus role in acute respiratory tract infections of pediatric patients as defined by viral load quantification. *New Microbiol.* 2007;30(4):383-92.
712. Esposito S, Bosis S, Niesters HG, et al. Impact of human bocavirus on children and their families. *J Clin Microbiol.* 2008;46(4):1337-42.
713. Brieu N, Guyon G, Rodière M, et al. Human bocavirus infection in children with respiratory tract disease. *Pediatr Infect Dis J.* 2008;27(11):969-73.
714. Blessing K, Neske F, Herre U, et al. Prolonged detection of human bocavirus DNA in nasopharyngeal aspirates of children with respiratory tract disease. *Pediatr Infect Dis J.* 2009;28(11):1018-9.
715. Hamza IA, Jurzik L, Wilhelm M, et al. Detection and quantification of human bocavirus in river water. *J Gen Virol.* 2009;90(Pt 11):2634-7.
716. Räsänen S, Lappalainen S, Kaikkonen S, et al. Mixed viral infections causing acute gastroenteritis in children in a waterborne outbreak. *Epidemiol Infect.* 2010;138(9):1227-34.
717. Arnold JC, Singh KK, Spector SA, et al. Undiagnosed respiratory viruses in children. *Pediatrics.* 2008;121(3): e631-7.
718. Beder LB, Hotomi M, Ogami M, et al. Clinical and microbiological impact of human bocavirus on children with acute otitis media. *Eur J Pediatr.* 2009;168(11):1365-72.
719. Pettigrew MM, Gent JF, Pyles RB, et al. Viral-bacterial interactions and risk of acute otitis media complicating upper respiratory tract infection. *J Clin Microbiol.* 2011; 49(11):3750-5.
720. Simon A, Groneck P, Kupfer B, et al. Detection of bocavirus DNA in nasopharyngeal aspirates of a child with bronchiolitis. *J Infect.* 2007;54(3):e125-7.
721. Maggi F, Andreoli E, Pifferi M, et al. Human bocavirus in Italian patients with respiratory diseases. *J Clin Virol.* 2007;38(4):321-5.
722. Bastien N, Chui N, Robinson JL, et al. Detection of human bocavirus in Canadian children in a 1-year study. *J Clin Microbiol.* 2007;45(2):610-3.
723. Fry AM, Lu X, Chittaganpitch M, et al. Human bocavirus: a novel parvovirus epidemiologically associated with pneumonia requiring hospitalization in Thailand. *J Infect Dis.* 2007;195(7):1038-45.
724. García-García ML, Calvo Rey C, Pozo Sánchez F, et al. Human bocavirus infections in Spanish 0-14 year-old: clinical and epidemiological characteristics of an emerging respiratory virus. *An Pediatr (Barc).* 2007;67(3):212-9.
725. Hengst M, Häusler M, Honnef D, et al. Human Bocavirus-infection (HBoV): an important cause of severe viral obstructive bronchitis in children. *Klin Padiatr.* 2008; 220(5):296-301.
726. Don M, Söderlund-Venermo M, Valent F, et al. Serologically verified human bocavirus pneumonia in children. *Pediatr Pulmonol.* 2010;45(2):120-6.
727. Moriyama Y, Hamada H, Okada M, et al. Distinctive clinical features of human bocavirus in children younger than 2 years. *Eur J Pediatr.* 2010;169(9):1087-92.
728. Schneider H, Adams O, Weiss C, et al. Clinical characteristics of children with viral single- and co-infections and a petechial rash. *Pediatr Infect Dis J.* 2013;32(5): e186-91.
729. Edner N, Castillo-Rodas P, Falk L, et al. Life-threatening respiratory tract disease with human bocavirus-1 infection in a 4-year-old child. *J Clin Microbiol.* 2012;50(2):531-2.
730. Korner RW, Söderlund-Venermo M, Van Koningsbruggen-Rietschel S, et al. Severe human bocavirus infection, Germany. *Emerg Infect Dis.* 2011;17(12):2303-5.
731. Terrosi C, Fabbiani M, Cellesi C, et al. Human bocavirus detection in an atopic child affected by pneumonia associated with wheezing. *J Clin Virol.* 2007;40(1):43-5.
732. Deng Y, Liu EM, Zhao XD, et al. Clinical characteristics of 12 persistently wheezing children with human bocavirus infection. *Zhonghua Er Ke Za Zhi.* 2007;45(10):732-5.
733. Vallet C, Pons-Catalano C, Mandelcwajg A, et al. Human bocavirus: a cause of severe asthma exacerbation in children. *J Pediatr.* 2009;155(2):286-8.
734. Durigon GS, Oliveira DB, Vollet SB, et al. Hospital-acquired human bocavirus in infants. *J Hosp Infect.* 2010;76(2): 171-3.
735. Cheng WX, Jin Y, Duan ZJ, et al. Human bocavirus in children hospitalized for acute gastroenteritis: a case-control study. *Clin Infect Dis.* 2008;47(2):161-7.
736. Vicente D, Cilla G, Montes M, et al. Human bocavirus, a respiratory and enteric virus. *Emerg Infect Dis.* 2007;13(4): 636-7.
737. Lau SK, Yip CC, Que TL, et al. Clinical and molecular epidemiology of human bocavirus in respiratory and fecal samples from children in Hong Kong. *J Infect Dis.* 2007;196(7):986-93.
738. Lee JI, Chung JY, Han TH, et al. Detection of human bocavirus in children hospitalized because of acute gastroenteritis. *J Infect Dis.* 2007;196(7):994-7.
739. Huang Y, Mao P, Wang H. Detection of, and frequent co-infection with, human bocavirus in faecal specimens from children in Wuhan, China. *Clin Microbiol Infect.* 2010;16(5):490-2.
740. Zeng M, Wang XH, Yu H, et al. Clinical relevance of human bocavirus with acute respiratory tract infection and diarrhea in children: a prospective case-control study. *Zhonghua Er Ke Za Zhi.* 2010;48(8):580-4.
741. Catalano-Pons C, Giraud C, Rozenberg F, et al. Detection of human bocavirus in children with Kawasaki disease. *Clin Microbiol Infect.* 2007;13(12):1220-2.
742. Bowles NE, Hirono K, Yu X, et al. Absence of parvoviral genomes in endothelial cells of Kawasaki disease patients with coronary artery lesions. *Pediatr Infect Dis J.* 2009; 28(4):345.
743. Lehmann C, Klar R, Lindner J, et al. Kawasaki disease lacks association with human coronavirus NL63 and human bocavirus. *Pediatr Infect Dis J.* 2009;28(6):553-4.
744. Santos RA, Nogueira CS, Granja S, et al. Kawasaki disease and human bocavirus—potential association? *J Microbiol Immunol Infect.* 2011;44(3):235-7.
745. Mitui MT, Tabib SM, Matsumoto T, et al. Detection of human bocavirus in the cerebrospinal fluid of children with encephalitis. *Clin Infect Dis.* 2012;54(7):964-7.
746. Koskenvuo M, Möttönen M, Waris M, et al. Human bocavirus in children with acute lymphoblastic leukemia. *Eur J Pediatr.* 2008;167(9):1011-5.

747. Schenk T, Maier B, Hufnagel M, et al. Persistence of human bocavirus DNA in immunocompromised children. *Pediatr Infect Dis J.* 2011;30(1):82-4.
748. Koskenvuo M, Möttönen M, Rahiala J, et al. Respiratory viral infections in children with leukemia. *Pediatr Infect Dis J.* 2008;27(11):974-80.
749. Schenk T, Strahm B, Kontny U, et al. Disseminated bocavirus infection after stem cell transplant. *Emerg Infect Dis.* 2007;13(9):1425-7.
750. Kainulainen L, Waris M, Söderlund-Venermo M, et al. Hepatitis and human bocavirus primary infection in a child with T-cell deficiency. *J Clin Microbiol.* 2008;46(12): 4104-5.
751. De Vries JJ, Bredius RG, Van Rheenen PF, et al. Human bocavirus in an immunocompromised child presenting with severe diarrhea. *J Clin Microbiol.* 2009;47(4):1241-3.
752. Choi JH, Chung YS, Kim KS, et al. Development of real-time PCR assays for detection and quantification of human bocavirus. *J Clin Virol.* 2008;42(3):249-53.
753. Schenk T, Huck B, Forster J, et al. Human bocavirus DNA detected by quantitative real-time PCR in two children hospitalized for lower respiratory tract infection. *Eur J Clin Microbiol Infect Dis.* 2007;26(2):147-9.
754. Lin F, Zeng A, Yang N, et al. Quantification of human bocavirus in lower respiratory tract infections in China. *Infect Agent Cancer.* 2007;2:3.
755. Kantola K, Hedman L, Allander T, et al. Serodiagnosis of human bocavirus infection. *Clin Infect Dis.* 2008;46(4):540-6.
756. Don M, Söderlund-Venermo M, Hedman K, et al. Don't forget serum in the diagnosis of human bocavirus infection. *J Infect Dis.* 2011;203(7):1031-2.
757. Nascimento-Carvalho CM, Cardoso MR, Meriluoto M, et al. Human bocavirus infection diagnosed serologically among children admitted to hospital with community-acquired pneumonia in a tropical region. *J Med Virol.* 2012;84(2):253-8.

CHAPTER 9

Respiratory Infections in Specific Populations: HIV Patients

Charles Feldman, Ronald Anderson

ABSTRACT

Respiratory diseases constitute a major source of morbidity and mortality in HIV-infected persons and of these, the opportunistic infections play a major role. These infections include the entire spectrum of respiratory pathogens, including bacteria, mycobacteria, viruses, fungi, and parasites/protozoa. The use of prophylaxis (e.g., cotrimoxazole prophylaxis) and the introduction of highly active antiretroviral therapy (HAART) have been associated with changes in the epidemiology of these infections; however, foremost among them are those of bacterial, mycobacterial, and fungal origin. The introduction of HAART has itself been associated with unusual manifestations of these opportunistic infections with the development of the immune reconstitution inflammatory syndrome (IRIS), which is associated with the worsening of existing (paradoxical) or unmasking of latent opportunistic infections. This chapter highlights the occurrence of respiratory infections in the population of HIV-infected persons.

INTRODUCTION

The lungs are the principal site of human immunodeficiency virus (HIV)-associated complications in patients who are HIV-infected, and foremost amongst these complications are the opportunistic pneumonias, which encompass the complete spectrum of bacterial, mycobacterial, fungal, viral, and parasitic/protozoal infections.[1-4] These infections, associated with considerable morbidity and mortality in HIV-infected persons, may be the primary complication heralding the presence of underlying HIV disease and are also the most common reasons for referral of such patients for respiratory and/or infectious disease specialist consultation.[2] In the early years of the HIV epidemic, *Pneumocystis jirovecii* infection was the most common opportunistic respiratory infection. It has declined in prevalence as a consequence of the use of cotrimoxazole prophylaxis, as well as the roll-out of highly active antiretroviral therapy (HAART). Thus community-acquired bacterial pneumonia is the most common opportunistic respiratory infection, followed by *P. jirovecii*, and then tuberculosis in developed countries, such as those in North America and Western Europe.[4,5] However, in the developing world and, especially in countries in sub-Saharan Africa, tuberculosis is the predominant infection, followed by bacterial pneumonia, and *P. jirovecii* infection.[2,4,6] Fungal pneumonias occur particularly in endemic regions, unless the infection is due to reactivation of latent disease; a myriad of parasitic diseases may also cause chest infections.[2] Combined infections, often including tuberculosis, may also occur.[6] The mechanisms of susceptibility to these lung diseases and an approach to the overall evaluation of an HIV-infected patient presenting with a chest disease, particularly due to infection, have been described in the literature.[2,4,7-9] This chapter will review the more common respiratory infections in HIV-infected patients (Table 1), occurring either as a new opportunistic infection or in the setting of the immune reconstitution inflammatory syndrome.

TABLE 1
Common Opportunistic Pneumonias in HIV-infected Patients

Bacterial infections	
• *Streptococcus pneumoniae*	• *Pseudomonas aeruginosa*
• *Haemophilus influenzae*	• *Rhodococcus equi*
• *Staphylococcus aureus*	• *Moraxella catarrhalis*
• *Klebsiella pneumoniae*	• Nocardiosis
• Atypical pathogens	
Mycobacterial infections	
• *Mycobacterium tuberculosis*	• Nontuberculous mycobacteria
Viral infections	
• Varicella-zoster virus	• Cytomegalovirus
• Influenza virus	
Fungal infections	
• *Pneumocystis jirovecii*	• Histoplasmosis
• Cryptococcosis	• Zygomycosis
• Coccidioidomycosis	• Aspergillosis
Parasitic infections	

BACTERIAL INFECTIONS

Bacterial pneumonia is a common opportunistic disease in patients with HIV infection, and its occurrence in a young patient without any apparent additional risk factors should alert the clinician to the possibility of HIV positivity.[2] In HIV-infected persons, bacterial pneumonia is more common than in uninfected persons, and while it may occur at all levels of the CD4 cell count, there is an inverse relationship between the CD4 cell count and the occurence of bacterial pneumonia, which occurs most commonly, once the CD4 cell count falls below 200 cells/μL.[1,2,8,10] Risk factors for community-acquired pneumonia (CAP) in HIV-infected individuals include general risk factors, which are also applicable to HIV-uninfected patients, including low socioeconomic status, cigarette smoking, alcohol abuse, injection drug use, other comorbidities, and malnutrition.[8] An etiological diagnosis is obtained in some 35% (range, 21–55%) of HIV-infected patients with CAP.[8]

The spectrum of bacterial pathogens causing CAP in HIV-infected patients is very similar to that in HIV-uninfected persons and foremost among these are *Streptococcus pneumoniae, pneumococcus,* and *Haemophilus influenzae.*[1,2,8,10] Pneumococcal infections are described in more detail below. Microorganisms, such as *Staphylococcus aureus, Klebsiella pneumoniae,* and the so-called "atypical pathogens" are encountered less frequently and rather more unusually, community-acquired infections with *Pseudomonas aeruginosa* and occassionally, *Rhodococcus equi* are encountered.[1] Pseudomonal infections, including CAP as well as infections in other sites, occur more commonly in HIV-infected patients, particularly in those with advanced disease (e.g., prior acquired immunodeficiency syndrome (AIDS) diagnosis, low CD4 cell count, and neutropenia).[11,12] The microorganisms tend to have a more favorable spectrum of antimicrobial susceptibility than the nosocomial infection counterparts,[11] and the infection has a reasonably favorable outcome and low mortality, if treated "appropriately".[11] Empiric treatment recommendations for suspected pseudomonal infections include the use, of 2 or more antimicrobial agents, at least initially, such as an antipneumococcal, antipseudomonal β-lactam, and a fluoroquinolone that covers Gram-negative pathogens (ciprofloxacin/levofloxacin), or the same type of β-lactam agent plus an aminoglycoside together with either a macrolide or an antipneumococcal fluoroquinolone.[10] *Rhodococcus equi* is a Gram-positive coryneform bacterium that causes zoonotic infections (horses, foals), but sometimes infects humans, particularly in the presence of immunocompromised state, such as HIV infection.[13] It classically presents as a cavitatory pneumonia, although other systemic manifestations have been described. Prompt diagnosis with early institution of combined antimicrobial therapy and antiretroviral treatment may be effective in eradicating the infection.[13] The correct antibiotic treatment of this conditions is uncertain, although it has been suggested that combined antibiotic treatment, including a drug with intracellular activity, for at least 2 months, should be instituted. Surgery is sometimes required. Some studies have indicated that the prevalence of "atypical" infections in HIV-infected persons is very low, possibly even negligible, although others have indicated that infections with *Mycoplasma pneumoniae* may be higher than in HIV-negative patients.[14] With regard to *Legionella* spp. infections, some investigators have indicated that while such infections are not that common, they are more severe in HIV-infected patients with an associated higher mortality, which is greater than that of pneumococcal infections.[15,16] There are also few reported cases of *Moraxella catarrhalis* infection, but when these occur, they may be associated with a significant morbidity in patients with advanced HIV infection, occurring as they do in association with a low CD4 cell count and, particularly in the presence of coexisting lung disease.[17]

Nocardiosis is a relatively uncommon pulmonary infection that infects both immunosuppressed and immunocompetent individuals, although some 60% of infections are associated with underlying immunocompromised states, including HIV infection.[18] *Nocardia asteroides* is commonly considered the predominant pathogen, although other species have been documented to be the cause of either colonization or active infection. Although the organism acts like a fungus, it is truly a bacterium.[18] Most HIV-infected patients with *Nocardia* infection have advanced immunosuppression.[18] Much of the literature regarding this pathogen consists of relatively small cases series.[18] *Nocardia* infections may involve different organ systems, including the lungs, the skin, and the central nervous system; disseminated infections also occur, which are associated with a significant mortality.[18,19] Pulmonary infection is difficult to diagnose, is often delayed, and clinicians should maintain a high index of suspicion for such infections.[19] Antimicrobial therapy needs to be instituted with agents to which the microorganism remains susceptible, which may include the carbapenems, linezolid, amikacin, and cotrimoxazole. Although some recommend combination therapy with agents that have proven synergy against this microorganism, not all support this approach.[18,19]

In general terms, the clinical features of CAP in HIV-infected persons are similar to those occurring in HIV-uninfected persons, and usually the classical signs and symptoms are found.[1,2,6,10] However, it is not always clinically apparent what the likely microbial cause of CAP infection is, and dual infections and even infections with multiple pathogens occur. For example, concomitant infection with both *S. pneumoniae* and *Mycobacterium tuberculosis* has been documented in HIV-infected patients making clinical diagnosis difficult,[20] and to this end, studies have investigated the potential role of procalcitonin (PCT) to differentiate bacterial (pneumococcal) infection from infection with *M. tuberculosis* and also *Pneumocystis* infection.[21,22]

Similarly, the chest radiographic features are also similar when comparing HIV-infected and -uninfected persons, although in *Haemophilus influenzae* infections, a diffuse bilateral interstitial pattern, similar to that of *Pneumocystis* pneumonia, may occur. In infections with *P. aeruginosa* and *S. aureus,* lung cavitation may occur, while infections with both *S. pneumoniae* and *S. aureus* are more commonly associated with complicated parapneumonic infections.[2] Standard diagnostic procedures are recommended in most guidelines for the management of CAP in HIV-infected persons and because of the greater spectrum of possible bacterial causes, and the inclusion of more unusual pathogens, sputum Gram's stain, special staining (e.g., for *Pneumocystis* pneumonia and tuberculosis) and culture, in addition to blood cultures, are considered to be important, particularly in hospitalized cases.[2,23,24] Induced sputum has been found in a number of studies to be helpful in the evaluation of a likely microbial cause of infection.[25] For many years, it has been suggested that routine fiberoptic bronchoscopy contributed little to the overall treatment and final outcome of these infections and, therefore, is limited in use, for specific indications.[26]

No specific guidelines for the management of CAP in HIV-infected patients have been developed.[8] However, in general terms, the management and antibiotic treatment recommendations for CAP in HIV-infected persons are identical to those in uninfected persons.[10] In some CAP guidelines and, particularly, to cover for the potentially broader spectrum of bacterial pathogens more commonly found in HIV-infected persons, the recommendations for antibiotic treatment would be similar to those used for the elderly and/or those with comorbid illness, because of the somewhat broader spectrum of likely pathogens.[27] Clearly, for pathogens, such as *S. aureus* and *P. aeruginosa* more specific therapy needs to be instituted.[10]

Studies have suggested that the time to clinical stability, length of hospital stay, and mortality of all-cause CAP are similar to HIV-infected and -uninfected persons, indicating that clinical outcomes may not be influenced by HIV infection.[28,29] However, in HIV-infected women, the high rates of bacterial pneumonia have persisted in the HAART era, and although there is a decreased risk with the use of HAART and cotrimoxazole prophylaxis, bacterial pneumonia is associated with an accelerated decline in progression to death.[30] Prevention of CAP in HIV-infected persons is, therefore, very important, and this may be acomplished by multiple strategies, many of which are routinely recommended in various countries such as the US.[2,31,32] These may include increasing HAART utilization and smoking cessation strategies.[30] With regard to vaccination, yearly influenza vaccination and also, vaccination with the pneumococcal 23-valent polysaccharide vaccination (PPV), approximately every 5 years in patients with a CD4 cell count above 200 cells/μL and especially, once they are on HAART, are recommended to prevent these infections. However, vaccine strategies are still controversial.[8]

Cotrimoxazole prophylaxis against *Pneumocystis* pneumonia also prevents some bacterial infections. The prevalence of cigarette smoking is high among HIV-infected persons with many smoking more than 1 pack per day, and cigarette smoking attenuates the immunological and virological response to HAART.[3] Very importantly, since it is well recognized that cigarette smoking is a major risk factor not only for bacterial CAP, and in particular, for pneumococcal infections and *Pneumocystis* pneumonia, but also tuberculosis and other infections, smoking cessation strategies should be encouraged in HIV-infected persons who continue to smoke.[33] The introduction of HAART has been associated with a decrease in the incidence of CAP,[8] and absence of HAART use has been found among other factors to increase the risk of bacteremia, which is associated with a poor outcome in HIV-infected patients with CAP.[34]

Streptococcus pneumoniae

The burden of pneumococcal disease, especially CAP, and also meningitis and bacteremia, in HIV-infected persons is considerable in both the developed and developing worlds, and although it decreases after the introduction of HAART, it still remains higher than in age-matched uninfected persons.[35-37] Pneumococcal infections are among the most common infections in HIV-infected persons.[36] The *pneumococcus* is also by far the most common cause of CAP, accounting for some 70% of cases.[8,38] Risk factors for bacteremia in the HAART era are similar to those reported in HIV-noninfected persons and include underlying comorbid illnesses, alcoholism, prior hospitalization, and current smoking, in addition to a low CD4 cell count in the HIV-infected cases.[38,39] Similarly with pneumonia, older age and smoking are considerable risk factors.[37] A number of studies have addressed the pathogenesis of pneumococcal infections.[35-37,40]

While the clinical presentation of pneumococcal pneumonia in HIV-infected persons was initially said to be similar to that in HIV-uninfected persons; more recently, some differences have been noted including a higher frequency of respiratory symptoms and unusual presentations.[35,36,38,41] The radiological pattern is often similar, when comparing HIV-infected and -uninfected cases, demonstrating the typical lobar pattern of consolidation, but sometimes, bilateral infiltrates occur.[38]

In general, the recommended diagnostic approach is no different when comparing HIV-infected and -uninfected cases, nor is the treatment.[36,38] However, there is an increase in the likelihood of antimicrobial resistance among the pneumococcal isolates causing infection in HIV-infected persons, at least partly, due to an increase in infections with so-called childhood serotypes.[37] Furthermore, bacteremia appears to be more common in HIV-infected compared to HIV-uninfected cases.[35,42]

It remains very important to try and prevent CAP occurring in HIV-infected persons, of which *pneumococcus* is the most common cause, and this may encompass a number of stategies, including lifestyle modifications with cessation of smoking, alcohol abuse, and intravenous drug use, as well as pneumococcal vaccination.[38] The conjugate pneumococcal vaccine has been shown to be efficacious in HIV-infected children in preventing not only vaccine serotype-related invasive disease but also the burden of clinical pneumonia and may secondarily benefit adults indirectly through herd immunity in communities where children have been vaccinated.[37,43] However, a randomized controlled study of the PPV in adults in sub-Saharan Africa with HIV infection and a low CD4 cell count showed an increase in pneumonia among the vaccinees initially, while on a 6-year follow-up, there was no further increase in pneumonia, but paradoxically, a decrease in mortality in the vaccinated group. Subsequent studies in HIV-infected persons on HAART showed moderate-to-good efficacy of the PPV in HIV-infected adults, although further investigation of the potential value of the pneumococcal conjugate vaccines in HIV-infected adults is still recommended.[37,38,44] In the sub-Saharan African study, which showed a higher rate of invasive pneumococcal disease in the vaccinated group, the patients were not on HAART; however, the use of HAART and PPV has been shown to be associated with a decreased risk of pneumococcal infections even in a patient with a CD4 count below 200 cells/μL.[5,39] In some studies, while prior vaccination with the PPV failed to prevent invasive pneumococcal disease, it did have beneficial effects on the clinical outcome by decreasing both illness severity and mortality.[45] Further investigation of the potential value of the pneumococcal conjugate vaccines in HIV-infected adults, as recommended in the literature previously, is currently beginning to show good promise.[37,38,44]

The outcome of pneumococcal pneumonia in HIV-infected persons was initially considered to be similar to that of HIV-uninfected persons, although recurrent infections were recognized to occur either from relapse or reinfection.[35,36] Similarly, in the HAART era, the prognosis of pneumococal bacteremia has been said to be more similar to that in HIV-uninfected persons.[39] However, more recently, in a study of 768 cases of bacteremic pneumococcal pneumonia, when the cases were stratified according to age and severity of illness, HIV-infected patients were found to have a significantly higher 14-day mortality with a trend for increasing mortality as the CD4 cell count decreased.[41] One South African study on HIV-infected patients with pneumococcal CAP who were not on HAART indicated that there was a significant depression of the the CD4 cell count during the acute phase of the infection with a subsequent increase in 90% of the patients on resolution of the infection.[46] The investigators urged caution in the use of the CD4 cell counts during the acute infection as an indicator of stage of HIV disease or to prognosticate on the course of the HIV infection.

VIRAL INFECTIONS

Viral infections are a major cause of opportunistic infections in HIV-infected adults and are a cause of considerable morbidity and mortality. Such infections include cytomegalovirus (CMV), John Cunningham virus, varicella-zoster virus, herpes-simplex virus, and human papillomavirus (HPV). The varicella zoster virus produces 2 clinically distinct diseases, namely chickenpox and shingles.[47,48] In adults, complications of chickenpox include varicella pneumonia, which may be very severe and also has a high mortality rate.[49] Furthermore, HIV infection increases the risk of varicella-zoster virus reactivation 7-fold, which may be complicated by disseminated disease, including pneumonia, particularly in immunocompromised patients.[48] Zoster is not considered to be an AIDS-defining illness and may occur at both low and higher CD4 cell counts. While earlier studies suggested that patients with varicella-zoster virus infection may be more likely to progress to AIDS, other investigators indicated that when controlling the CD4 cell counts, there was no indication that varicella-zoster virus was an independent cofactor for HIV progression, although episodes of varicella-zoster virus infection with fever may predict more rapid progression to AIDS.[48] Increasing incidences of HIV infection continue to make safe and effective treatments for immunocompromised patients with chickenpox and shingles infections necessary, particularly with the rise of acyclovir-resistant varicella-zoster virus strains and increasing the use of Oka vaccine may decrease the incidence of the virus.[47]

The influenza virus is one of the most common human respiratory viruses, and there is good evidence that immunosuppressed patients, such as those with HIV infection, are at increased risk of influenza and influenza-related complications, such that yearly vaccination is recommended for these cases even though the efficacy of the vaccine may be compromised.[50] It appears that institution of HAART may be associated with a reduction in the need for hospitalization as a consequence of influenza infection in HIV-infected persons, but clearly, further research is required to fully understand the interaction of influenza virus and HIV infection.[50] One recent systematic review of the epidemiology of seasonal influenza in sub-Saharan Africa indicated the presence of significant gaps in the understanding of this infection and its interaction with HIV.[51] Interestingly, one recent study also indicated that HIV infection did not increase the severity of H1N1 infection, which itself did not have a major effect on HIV infection.[52]

While CMV infection is a major cause of morbidity and mortality in patients with other forms of immunocompromise, its exact role as a cause of lung disease in HIV-infected patients is uncertain, and most HIV-infected adults have latent infection in the lungs and other organs.[53,54] Extrapulmonary infections, such as eye infections are, however, well characterized. When pneumonia occurs, it is believed to be reactivation of the virus in very immunocompromised individuals and to have a similar presentation to that of *Pneumocystis* pneumonia with fever, cough, hypoxemia, and a diffuse pulmonary infiltration.[1,2,54] The chest radiograph in CMV pneumonia varies and may show reticular or ground-glass opacities, alveolar infiltrates, nodules, nodular opacities, and, sometimes, pleural effusion.[2] Several studies indicate that the occurrence of CMV in HIV-infected patients is most commonly in association with other infections rather than as the sole infecting agent, although such cases have, infrequently, been described.[53,55] It is said that when pulmonary infections occur, they frequently respond initially to anti-CMV therapy, although disease progression and high early mortality occur.[54] Ganciclovir and foscarnet have been used to treat CMV pneumonia.[2]

FUNGAL INFECTIONS

It is clearly being recognized that fungal infections are increasing in prevalence worldwide, primarily due to the increased number of susceptible patient groups, which include both critically ill patients as well as those that are immunocompromised, such as by way of HIV/AIDS.[56-58] *Pneumocystis* pneumonia remains the most common opportunistic fungal infection in HIV-infected persons, while cryptococcal meningitis, with or without pneumonia and severe cases of the various endemic mycoses, such as coccidioidomycosis and histoplasmosis are always significant threats. However, while *Aspergillus* pneumonia sometimes occurs in cases with very advanced immunosuppression, it is currently said to be an uncommon complication of HIV infection. It is no longer considered to be an AIDS-defining illness, and when it occurs, additional risk factors are often present.[58] The profound effects of HIV infection on various aspects of the immune system are recognized to be associated with the increased risk of fungal infections, which are fortunately reversed by the use of HAART such that many of these infections are currently decreasing.[58] The epidemiology, clinical features, diagnostic approach, and therapy of the various fungal infections have been described in the literature.[56-62] Different fungi respond to different antifungal treatments and treatment regimens, and there is emerging data for the use of combination therapy in some circumstances.[57,62] Occasionally, surgery is required, for example, for solitary lung lesions or chest wall invasion. New drugs and immunotherapy and vaccines hold hope for the future.[61,62]

Pneumocystis jirovecii

Pneumocystis pneumonia is a common opportunistic pneumonia, now considered to be of fungal origin, occurring especially among severely immunocompromised patients.[63] While in the earlier years, it was the most common opportunistic respiratory infection in HIV-infected persons, as a consequence of cotrimoxazole prophylaxis, and subsequently, by the introduction of HAART, it has become less common, being second only to CAP in the developed world and third after *M. tuberculosis* and CAP in sub-Saharan Africa.[64] It occurs, especially in HIV-infected patients at a low CD4 cell count, and therefore, prophylaxis is recommended in an HIV-infected person at a CD4 count below 200 cells/μL, at which level the risk is significant.[63]

While the organism is widespread across the world, it has not been possible to clearly identify an environmental niche for the pathogen, and there are no data supporting either an environmental or human reservoir for this pathogen.[65,66] However, there is considerable support for the co-called colonization hypothesis in that polymerase chain reaction (PCR) studies of nasopharyngeal specimens, even in nonimmunocompromised individuals, have shown these specimens to harbour Pneumocystis DNA, suggesting that even immunocompromised individuals may act as a transient, or even sustained, reservoir for the organisms, with similar conclusions in various other studies.[65-67] One study, which was an autopsy study of HIV-infected persons dying from causes other than *Pneumocystis* pneumonia, demonstrated a high rate of *Pneumocystis* colonization based on PCR of extracted lung tissue, with only cigarette smoking and city of residence being independent risk factors for such colonization.[68] However, the mode of acquisition of this microorganism is still uncertain and furthermore, there is also uncertainty of the likely consequences of such colonization.[67] While there is a possibility that reactivation of latent infection and/or colonization is causing active infection, there is also increasing evidence for airborne transmission with cases of transmission from infected persons causing colonization of immunocompromised individuals being suggested.[65-67] It has also been suggested that *Pneumocystis* colonization may stimulate pulmonary inflammation and lead to lung damage, which may, at least partly, explain the association between HIV infection and diseases, such as sudden infant death syndrome (SIDS), chronic obstructive pulmonary disease (COPD), and lung cancer. Colonization may also act as a copromoter for the progression of certain lung diseases.[67]

The classical presentation of *Pneumocystis* pneumonia is with fever, nonproductive cough, and progressive dyspnea, while physical examination is nonspecific.[66,69-71] Less commonly, chest pain, productive cough, and occasionally hemoptysis and bronchospasm may occur.[69] Rarely, patients may be asymptomatic.[71] There is said to be a difference in *Pneumocystis* pneumonia presentation in AIDS patients compared with those in whom the immunocompromise is due to another cause. In such cases, the AIDS patients are said to present less acutely.[69] While chest auscultation may be normal, it frequently detects diffuse discrete crackles.[66,70] Tachycardia, tachypnea, and cyanosis can occur in advanced cases. Extrapulmonary pneumocystosis is rare but has been reported.

The chest radiograph has been said to be the cornerstone of diagnostic evaluation, and while it sometimes may be normal, it classically demonstrates bilateral, symmetrical, reticular (interstitial), or granular (ground-glass) opacities especially in the perihilar and lower zones and, sometimes, a complicating pneumothorax.[69,70] Thin-walled cysts can be seen in 10–20% of cases.[65] Atypical presentations (unilateral diseases, nodules, and pleural effusion) occasionally occur. High-resolution computed tomography (CT) scanning of the chest may add to the diagnosis in cases with unhelpful findings on a chest radiograph.[69]

An important diagnostic tool for *Pneumocystis* pneumonia is a high clinical suspicion.[71] The definitive diagnosis of *Pneumocystis* pneumonia requires the detection of the pathogen in respiratory secretions by one or other available staining techniques, or by newer molecular techniques, involving DNA amplification by PCR.[65,70] While bronchoscopy and bronchoalveolar lavage (BAL) for obtaining specimens of respiratory tract secretions yield the greatest sensitivity for isolation and may be considered the gold standard, induced sputum yields reasonable sensitivies of between 74 and 83% and is safer with lesser risks.[65,70] An investigation of cost-effective diagnostic options in *Pneumocystis* pneumonia advocated the use of PCR technologies combined with less invasive techniques, such as expectorated or induced sputum. This was more cost-effective than diagnostic procedures, such as BAL or chest radiographs alone.[72] Other laboratory investigations include blood-gas analysis, serum lactate dehydrogenase (LDH) levels, plasma S-adenosylmethionine (SAM or AdoMET) levels. More recently, serum (1-3)-β-D-glucan and serum KL-6 antigen have been studied and these are either too non-specific or need more evaluation and further validation prior to routine use.[70] It is also important to remember that concomitant infections with *Pneumocystis* and other pathogens, including *M. tuberculosis*, have been documented, not infrequently.[73]

The treatment of choice for *Pneumocystis* pneumonia remains trimethoprim-sulfamethoxazole (TMP-SMX).[65,66,70,71] Choice of first- and second-line agents has been described in the literature.[63,65,66,71,74] Intravenous pentamidine is a second-line agent for patients with severe disease or those who fail primary therapy with TMP-SMX, and other second line regimens tested include dapsone-TMP (inconvenient dosing), primaquine and clindamycin combination (no intravenous form of primaquine), atovaquone (less effective than TMP-SMX but less side effects), trimetrexate (less effective intravenous alternative agent), and inhaled pentamidine (less effective than intravenous pentamidine).[65] There has been considerable debate as to whether *Pneumocystis* pneumonia responds to echinocandins, such as caspofungin, and no recommendations are possible with regard to its use.[71] Adjunctive corticosteroids should be used in severe *Pneumocystis* pneumonia, and should be initiated within 24–72 hours of anti-*Pneumocystis* therapy.[65] While the number of studies investigating adjunctive corticosteroids in patients with *Pneumocystis* pneumonia is small, evidence clearly suggests benefit in patients with substantial hypoxemia.[75] A common dosing regimen recommended is prednisone 40 mg twice daily for 5 days, followed by 40 mg daily for 5 days and then, 20 mg daily, for 11 days.[65] Meta-analyses have confirmed the benefit of corticosteroids. An additional consideration in HIV-infected patients with *Pneumocystis* pneumonia is the timing of initiation of HAART.[65]

TMP-SMX is also considered the treatment of choice for *Pneumocystis* pneumonia prophylaxis, because of superiority above other regimens tested, which is commonly recommended to be initiated in HIV-infected persons when the CD4 cell count falls below 200 cells/μL and/or in the presence of oral thrush.[65] Prophylaxis can be discontinued in cases after initiation of HAART, once there is a sustained increase in CD4 cell count above 200 cells/μL for at least 3 months.[65] Other prophylactic regimens have been described in the literature.[63,65,66,71] A considerable body of literature has been published, detailing the presence of genetic mutations within the dihydrofolate reductase (DHFR) and dihydropteroate reductase (DHPS) genes, which are the enzymatic targets of TMP-SMX and dapsone, as well as, the possible associations between such mutations and clinical outcomes.[70] Such genetic mutations have been shown to cause resistance among other pathogens, such as *Plasmodium falciparum*. Interestingly, a number of studies have suggested that most patients with *Pneumocystis* pneumonia and DHPS mutations respond well to treatment with TMP-SMX, while patients with DHPS mutations alone, similarly treated, tend to have a worse outcome than those treated with a nonsulfa-containing regimen.[70] Thus, while the explanation for these findings is unclear and no studies have examined all the postulated factors at the same time in patients with *Pneumocystis* pneumonia, the recommended first line treatment still remains TMP-SMX.[70]

Cryptococcal Lung Disease

Cryptococcosis is an important opportunistic infection in HIV-infected persons, and although meningitis is the most common manifestation, lung infections do occur and are considerably underdiagnosed.[76,77] That cryptococcal pneumonia occurs quite commonly, is not surprising, given that the portal of entry of this fungus into the body is through inhalation of the encapsulated yeast.[78] Furthermore, while treatment of cryptococcal meningitis has been extensively studied, much less well studied has been the antifungal management of cryptococcal pneumonia. Pulmonary involvement in patients with cryptococcal meningitis may occur in more than 50% of patients with advanced HIV infection and CD4 cell count below 100 cells/μL and despite antifungal therapy, the mortality remains between 10 and 25% in AIDS patients.[77,78] Fortunately, with HAART, there has been a dramatic decline in the prevalence of the infection.[77]

Most infections are due to *Cryptococcus neoformans*, although *C. gattii* accounts for some cases, particularly among those that are immunocompromised.[76] Depending on the site of the infection and the degree of immunosuppression, the manifestations of the infection vary from asymptomatic to life-threatening disease.[78] The lung manifestations are often those of nonspecific respiratory symptoms, although severe respiratory failure has been documented in both immunocompromised and immunocompetent patients.[76] Radiological manifestations are nonspecific and do vary, especially in relation to the degree of immunosuppression.[76] Cryptococcal pneumonia commonly presents with diffuse bilateral interstitial infiltrates and may mimic *Pneumocystis* pneumonia, although unilateral interstitial infiltrates, focal consolidation, nodules, nodular opacities, cavitation, pleural effusion, and hilar adenopathy have all been reported.[2] The clinical manifestations, pathogenesis, diagnosis, and therapy of cryptococcal infections have been described in the literature.[76-79] Amphotericin B and fluconazole, with or without flucytosine, remain the mainstays of therapy for these infections, and the final choice depends on what is available in that region.[61,79] Mortality attributable to cryptococcal infections remains high and various independent risk factors have been identified for mortality within 30 days of diagnosis, two of them being pneumonia and respiratory failure.[80]

Coccidioidomycosis

Coccidioides is one of the recognized opportunistic pathogens in patients with HIV infection and has been described in the literature.[81] It is apparent that there is a dearth of studies regarding this infection. It occurs particularly with more advanced HIV infection and especially once the CD4 count decreases below 250 cells/μL. While some of the cases occurring in the early parts of the HIV epidemic were out of the endemic regions and, therefore, probably represented reactivation of previous infection, most subsequent infections occurred in coccidioidal endemic areas. The infection may manifest in a number of ways, including focal primary pneumonia in those with higher peripheral CD4 cell counts, diffuse reticulonodular pneumonia in those with more advanced immunosuppression, as well as disseminated disease beyond the chest. Liver disease, extrathoracic lymphadenopathy, and meningitis may be found, but bone and/or joint involvement are uncommon. Chest radiograph most commonly demonstrates a diffuse reticulonodular infiltrate in cases with pneumonia, although other findings are also described.[2] Diagnosis may be made on the basis of serology, culture, and histopathological confirmation. Therapy may be undertaken with amphotericin B or the triazole antifungals, such as fluconazole and itraconazole. Some drug interactions may occur between azole antifungal and antiretroviral agents. The duration of therapy is uncertain, and it needs to be prolonged or even life-long. HAART adherence is essential to prevent recurrence.

Histoplasmosis

HIV-infected patients in endemic areas are at an increased risk of histoplasmosis, which is said to be the most common endemic mycosis in immunocompromised patients, probably because it is the most common endemic mycosis worldwide.[82] While it commonly occurs due to direct exposure to the organism, it can also occur as a consequence of reactivation of a latent, prior focus of infection. Initial infection is pulmonary, but widespread asymptomatic infection with hematogenous dissemination is common, which may lead to progressive life-threatening infection. Lung presentation is commonly that of an acute CAP, particularly in those with lesser degrees of immunosuppression, while extensive pneumonia with severe hypoxemia and acute respiratory distress syndrome (ARDS) may occur in those with more advanced immunosuppression.[82] Once disseminated infection occurs, systemic symptoms, septic shock, multiorgan failure, and ARDS commonly ensue. Adrenal insufficiency can occur as a consequence of direct adrenal involvement. Skin lesions of various types may occur, as may mucous membrane lesions, hepatosplenomegaly, and bone marrow involvement, while gastrointestinal and central nervous system involvement occurs in more advanced immunosuppression. Diagnosis is increasingly being made by *Histoplasma* antigen detection, while detection of the yeast phase of *Histoplasma capsulatum* in tissue biopsy specimens or, uncommonly, in circulating blood phagocytes, is helpful in rapid diagnosis.[82] PCR techniques have yet to prove useful and serology is often negative in immunocompromised cases. Culture of the organism remains the definitive diagnostic technique, and while it is always recommended that cultures should be done, treatment initiation, particularly in immunocompromised cases, cannot await confirmation of the culture results.[82] When the diagnosis is made early and therapy is instituted appropriately, the prognosis, even in immunosuppressed patients is good, but often the diagnosis is delayed, and therefore, the infection may be associated with high mortality.

Guidelines for the management of patients with histoplasmosis were updated by the Infectious Diseases Society of America (IDSA) in 2007.[83] Treatment is often undertaken with amphotericin B, although itraconazole may also be used and has been shown to be more effective than ketoconazole.[83] There is no evidence recommending the use of echinocandins.[83] The newer azoles, including posaconazole and voriconazole, have *in vitro* activity against *H. capsulatum.*[83]

Zygomycosis

Zygomycosis (formerly called mucormycosis) is an infection caused by fungi of the order *Mucorales* including *Mucor*, *Rhizopus*, or other species of fungi that share a specific common morphology.[84,85] Morphology allows a specific diagnosis on frozen section or smear prior to growth and identification that would allow specific treatment to be initiated early.[85] The most common form of presentation is with rhinocerebral disease, with or without pulmonary involvement, and pulmonary infection is more common in cases with profound and prolonged neutropenia, presenting as segmental or lobar infiltrates, isolated nodules, cavitary lesions, hemorrhage, or infarction.[84] Zygomycosis is a rare opportunistic infection in patients whose only risk factor is HIV infection.[85] Clinical and radiological features may be similar to those of *Aspergillus* infection. The infection has been described in the literature.[84] Amphotericin B is commonly used for the treatment of zygomycosis, while polyenes, and posaconazole have also been shown to have good activity against these organisms.[61,62] Combination therapy is not recommended.

Aspergillosis

Aspergillosis is an uncommon infection among HIV-infected persons, with invasive pulmonary aspergillosis occurring mostly in patients with a CD4 cell count below 50 cells/μL; however, when it does occur, it is very frequently fatal.[86-88] This infection is no longer considered to be an AIDS-defining illness. The incidence is relatively low and appears to differ in different parts of the world, with neutropenia and corticosteroid use appearing to be major additional predisposing factors.[87,88] The lung has been found to be the most common site of infection in some studies, but central nervous system involvement and disseminated disease may also occur.[89] It appears that previous opportunistic infections involving the lungs, such as *Pneumocystis* pneumonia and CMV infections, may predispose to the development of pulmonary aspergillosis. Common manifestations of pulmonary disease are fever, cough, and dyspnea. However, since pulmonary disease has variable clinical manifestations, which together with nonspecific symptoms make diagnosis difficult, an aggressive diagnostic approach is commonly needed.[87]

While cultures of lower respiratory tract specimens may yield *Aspergillus*, the organism identified in this way may simply be a colonizer. Although the diagnosis cannot be based on culture alone, the presence of positive cultures in the setting of HIV infection with a radiograph showing a new cavity or an infiltrate in a previously normal lung and particularly in the presence of neutropenia and/or low CD4 cell count should not be dismissed, but it warrants institution of antifungal therapy, while awaiting further evaluation.[87] Bronchoscopic transbronchial biopsy assists in diagnosis.[89] Serological testing needs further evaluation, while magnetic resonance imaging (MRI) scanning is a promising diagnostic technique. Treatments that may be used for this infection include amphotericin B, voriconazole, and echinocandins.[62] Voriconazole is currently considered the treatment of choice, but alternative choices are given, and there are insufficient data to recommend combination therapy for primary or salvage therapy.[61] The prognosis is generally poor.[88,89]

PARASITIC INFECTIONS

Protozoal and helminthic lung infections are prevalent throughout the world, although more common in tropical regions, and their prevalence has increased as a consequence of immunosuppression, including that due to HIV infections/AIDS, as a consequence of either de novo infection from the environment or recrudescence from dormant infections.[90] A number of important pathogens may cause pulmonary disease and these have been described in the literature,[90] and a full description of all of these is clearly beyond the capacity of this section. Toxoplasmosis is an infection caused by *Toxoplasma gondii*, which is an obligate intracellular protozoan. It is the most common parasitic pneumonia in HIV-infected persons.[2] Pulmonary toxoplasmosis may occur on its own or in association with central nervous system and/or disseminated disease and when it occurs, it usually presents with nonproductive cough, dyspnea, and fever, with a chest radiograph demonstrating bilateral infiltrates of either a fine reticular or coarse nodular type. Patients almost invariably have a positive IgG antibody, without which the diagnosis is unlikely, but the diagnosis should be confirmed by bronchoscopy with BAL. Treatment with sulfadiazine plus pyrimethamine is recommended as first-line therapy, with clindamycin plus pyrimethamine and TMP-SMX as the main alternatives.

Pulmonary amebiasis is an emerging, parasitic disorder in patients with HIV infection and in homosexual males. Leishmaniasis and HIV infection exist in a deadly synergy and leishmaniasis accelerates the onset of AIDS in patients with HIV infection. Malaria is a common and serious infection and a similar interaction between the malarial parasite and HIV infection can be seen.

Pulmonary babesiosis may also occur in HIV-infected cases and there are various other protozoal organisms that may also represent true emerging pulmonary infestations in HIV-infected persons. Furthermore, a myriad of pulmonary helminthic infections may occur, both established and emerging as a consequence of various factors, including HIV infection, and these have been described in the literature.[90]

MYCOBACTERIAL INFECTIONS

These infections include both *M. tuberculosis* and non-tuberculous mycobacteria (NTM).

Mycobacterium tuberculosis

In sub-Saharan Africa, tuberculosis is by far, the most common and the most serious opportunistic pneumonia occurring in HIV-infected persons.[6]

Frequency of Tuberculosis and Its Clinical Presentation in HIV-endemic Settings

In 2010, the World Health Organization (WHO) reported that one-third of the world's population was currently infected with *M. tuberculosis* of which 5–10% would become ill or infectious at some time during their life, with those coinfected with HIV and *M. tuberculosis* being much more likely to develop tuberculosis.[91] In 2008, the estimated tuberculosis incidence rate in sub-Saharan Africa was over 350 cases per 100 000 population, almost double that of South-east Asia, while an estimated 1.7 million people died from tuberculosis in 2009.[91] Not unexpectedly, the highest number of deaths occurred in sub-Saharan Africa.[91] The estimated worldwide prevalence of tuberculosis in 2009 was a total of 14 million cases with 3.9 and 4.9 million cases occurring in sub-Saharan Africa and South-east Asia, respectively.[91]

While "traditional" tuberculosis is well controlled in industrialized countries with low HIV-infection rates with easily accessible and sophisticated healthcare services, this disease, as mentioned above, has become rampant in developing countries with a high burden of HIV infection, particularly in many countries in sub-Saharan Africa.[91,92] In this geographical region, tuberculosis is frequently the first AIDS-defining opportunistic infection, becoming evident when the circulating CD4+ T-cell count drops to around 350/μL blood.[93,94] As HIV-related immunosuppression progresses, not only does the incidence of tuberculosis coinfection increase but the disease also becomes more difficult to diagnose due to altered clinical, immunological, and microbiological presentation.

Diagnosis of Tuberculosis in HIV-infected Individuals

In HIV-infected patients with circulating CD4+ T-cell counts of 300/μL blood or higher, the clinical presentation may not differ substantially from that of individuals without immunodeficiency. In this setting, there is a history of chronicity of symptoms, such as cough, hemoptysis, dyspnea, chest pain, fever, malaise, apical pulmonary involvement on radiological investigation, and presence of acid-fast bacilli in sputum, which can be detected by microbiological and molecular (PCR) procedures. These are associated with skin-test reactivity to tuberculin and the presence of *M. tuberculosis* -specific circulating CD4+ T-cells, which can be detected using interferon (IFN)-γ release procedures.

On the other hand, when the circulating CD4+ T-cell count declines to less than 200/μL blood, the clinical, radiological, microbiological, and immunological features of the disease may become atypical.[95-97] For example, acid-fast bacilli sputum positivity, as well as cavitation and upper lobe infiltrates on chest X-ray are less frequently encountered in HIV-positive individuals, while changes, such as pleural effusion, mediastinal lymphadenopathy, lobar and miliary disease, or even a normal chest X-ray are evident.[95-98] Recently, Chamie et al. reported on the variation in presentation of pulmonary tuberculosis across a spectrum of circulating CD4+ T-cell counts in HIV-infected African patients (n = 873), all of whom were culture confirmed cases.[98] They observed that 21% of patients with CD4+ T-cell counts of less than 50 cells/μL had normal chest X-rays in comparison with 2% of patients with counts of more than 500/μL with a clear continuum across the spectrum of CD4+ T-cell counts.[98] The corresponding findings for acid-fast bacilli sputum negativity were 23% and 1%, respectively.[98]

Clearly, more sensitive diagnostic procedures are required for the rapid detection of *M. tuberculosis* in smear-negative sputum or other samples from HIV-infected patients with advanced immunosuppression. The most promising of these is the automated molecular diagnostic procedure known as GeneXpert *M. tuberculosis*/resistance to rifampicin (RIF),[99] and possibly, detection of mycolic acids by monoclonal antibody capture methods.[100]

Tuberculosis Presenting as Community-acquired Pneumonia

CAP generally presents with an acute onset of symptoms, while, tuberculosis, as mentioned above, is most frequently characterized by an insidious, smoldering onset. Nonetheless, in regions with a high burden of tuberculosis, especially in association with a high incidence of HIV infection, tuberculosis, usually primary or reactivation disease, may present as an acute pneumonia with respiratory failure and radiographic features, which are compatible with a diagnosis of CAP.[101,102] As recently stated by Schlossberg "tuberculosis can present as an acute process and should be included in the differential diagnosis of CAP....... it may mimic classical bacterial pneumonia or masquerade as atypical pneumonia with non-productive cough and systemic symptomatology."[101] In areas where tuberculosis is relatively uncommon, it may go undetected as a cause of CAP, largely due to its acute clinical presentation.[101] Accordingly, in countries, such as Canada, Malaysia, US, and UK, heightened awareness of the possibility of tuberculosis as a differential diagnosis in patients presenting with CAP has been strongly advocated.[103-106] Warning signs include being alert to patients who:

- Are immigrants from countries with a high tuberculosis prevalence
- Have a history of intravenous drug abuse
- Are HIV-seropositive irrespective of circulating CD4+ T-cell count
- Have a known history of a positive tuberculin skin-test, or previous or recent exposure to tuberculosis
- Have an upper lobe infiltrate, cavitation or miliary pattern on chest X-ray
- A low white blood cell count or lymphopenia
- Have the symptoms of tuberculosis mentioned above in the preceding 4 week period prior to presentation.

In sub-Saharan Africa, which has the highest prevalence of HIV/AIDS, associated with an extremely high incidence of tuberculosis as mentioned above, tuberculosis presenting as CAP is much more common. This is underscored by the study of Nyamande et al. who investigated the etiology of CAP, as well as the associated mortality in HIV-infected and -noninfected adults admitted to a teaching hospital in the KwaZulu-Natal Province of South Africa over a period of 17 months.[102] They reported that out of 430 patients admitted with CAP, 81.4% (n = 311) were infected with HIV. Causative pathogens were identified in 52% of patients (n = 222), the most frequent being *M. tuberculosis* (39.6%) and *S. pneumoniae* (34.5%) with the former being the most common infective agent in both HIV-infected and -noninfected patients (40% and 35%, respectively). The overall in-hospital mortality was 17%, with mortality rates of 15.9% and 25% in the HIV-infected and -non-infected patients respectively, and 38% in patients with polymicrobial infections.[107] The investigators concluded that *M. tuberculosis* is the leading cause of CAP in this region, clearly reflecting the magnitude of the tuberculosis epidemic in sub-Saharan Africa.[102]

If not detected at an early stage, which is most likely to happen in regions with a low tuberculosis prevalence, patients with tuberculosis masquerading as CAP will, in all probability, receive traditional therapy for CAP. Most frequently, this is a β-lactam antibiotic without or with a macrolide, or alternatively, monotherapy with a respiratory fluoroquinolone. Warning signs of misdiagnosis include persistence of symptoms for 2–3 weeks after initiation of antimicrobial therapy, failure to respond, or an initial favorable response followed by relapse, usually in the case of a respiratory fluoroquinolone, all of which are suggestive of tuberculosis.[101,105,107,108] Delayed suspicion and diagnosis of CAP have recently been highlighted in the overview of acute tuberculosis by Schlossberg[101] in which he refers to "one review of unsuspected tuberculosis in a community hospital (in the US), which established that 60% of cases of tuberculosis as a cause of CAP were reported after the patient's death; 92% of the patients were elderly."[109]

The use of respiratory fluoroquinolone monotherapy in the management of tuberculosis misdiagnosed as CAP, as mentioned above, is of particular concern. This is because of the fact that the inappropriate use of this class of antimicrobial agent in this setting may favor the development of fluoroquinolone resistance and emergence of multidrug-resistant strains of *M. tuberculosis*, underscoring the importance of avoidance of these agents as first-line therapy in patients with CAP in whom there is a high index of suspicion of tuberculosis.[105]

If they are available, laboratory tests, which may assist in the early identification of tuberculosis presenting as CAP include rapid molecular diagnostic procedures such as the GeneXpert *M. tuberculosis*/RIF mentioned above, or multiplex molecular procedures, which use multiple primers to detect the nucleic acid of a range of microbial pathogens in a single assay.[99,110] Measurement of PCT may also facilitate the distinction between CAP due to *M. tuberculosis* or other pathogens,[21,22] while measurement of soluble triggering receptor expressed on myeloid cells-1 (TREM-1) or C-reactive protein (CRP) have no discriminatory value.[111,112]

Nontuberculous Mycobacteria

These are nontransmissible, environmental, uncommon, and opportunistic mycobacterial pathogens, which are distinct from *M. tuberculosis* and *M. leprae*. They include, amongst others, *M. avium* complex (MAC), *M. kansasii, M. xenopi, M. malmoense,* and *M. abscessus*, with MAC being the most common cause of both NTM lung disease and disseminated disease.[113] Although NTM disease is of increasing significance in developed countries, such as the US[113,114] and France[115] coincident with the decline in the prevalence of tuberculosis, there is a relative paucity of data on the frequency of NTM lung infections in high HIV-tuberculosis coendemic regions, where the etiologic role of these uncommon pathogens may have been underestimated.[116] There are several reasons for this. Firstly, and most importantly, there appears to be a perception in these regions that disseminated NTM disease in HIV-infected individuals typically occurs when the circulating CD4+ T-cell count falls below 50/μL.[116] Accordingly, in HIV-tuberculosis coendemic regions, it is often reasoned that AIDS patients will succumb to tuberculosis or other HIV-associated infections or malignancies before the circulating CD4+ T-cell count is low enough to result in NTM disease. Other reasons mentioned by Gopinath et al.[116] which may account for underestimating the frequency of NTM disease in tuberculosis-endemic regions include lack of:

- Awareness amongst clinicians and microbiologists
- Standardized criteria for the definition of NTM lung disease
- Expertise and laboratory facilities for the detection and characterization of NTM.[116]

Documented NTM pathogens in HIV-infected persons include MAC, *M. xenopi*, and *M. kansasii.* The two former pathogens frequently cause disseminated disease, while patients coinfected with HIV and *M. kansasii* are more likely to have lung disease without dissemination.[113] As stated by Field et al., "*M. kansasii* is more common in patients with HIV infection than in the non-HIV population, and an isolate from a respiratory specimen is more likely to represent infection and should be treated."[113,117] Interestingly, in HIV-infected South African gold miners presenting with pulmonary disease associated with *M. kansasii* infection, the median circulating CD4+ T-cell count was 381/μL,[118-120] underscoring the possibility that NTM may be underestimated as the causative pathogens in lung disease in tuberculosis-endemic regions.

NTM lung disease may, however, be extremely difficult to distinguish from tuberculosis. According to Field et al. in their 2006 review on the topic,[113] NTM should be considered in patients with:

- Bronchiectasis, especially in the setting of involvement of the right middle lobe and lingula
- Those who, even when receiving therapy, remain symptomatic in association with radiographic deterioration.[113]

The current diagnostic criteria for confirmation of NTM lung disease are those recommended by the American Thoracic Society (ATS) in 2007.[121] They are based primarily on microbiological, radiographic, and histological criteria, which may be complemented by recent innovations in molecular diagnostic procedures.[116] These criteria are applicable to "symptomatic patients with pulmonary symptoms, nodular or cavitary opacities, or a high resolution CT scan that shows multifocal bronchiectasis with multiple small nodules."[121]

Because of the very poor prognosis of NTM infections, early diagnosis is critical.

IMMUNE RECONSTITUTION INFLAMMATORY SYNDROME

This is a generic term encompassing harmful, tissue-damaging inflammatory responses activated by alloantigens, autoantigens, or microbial and viral antigens which occur on restoration of cell-mediated immunity following removal of either primary or acquired (iatrogenic or due to chronic infection) immunosuppression. In the case of immune dysfunction associated with chronic infection, the underlying immunosuppression may be generalized as in HIV/AIDS, or pathogen-specific as in lepromatous leprosy, advanced tuberculosis, or other chronic infections.

Initiation of HAART in patients with HIV/AIDS is the most common cause of IRIS and has been the subject of several recent reviews.[122-124] Two types of IRIS exist in this setting; unmasking IRIS is a reaction to a covert infection, while paradoxical IRIS refers to the deterioration of a recognized infection in the face of appropriate therapy.[122-124] The reported incidence of IRIS in the setting of HIV infection is largely based on retrospective studies and varies from 8 to 43%,[125,126] while in a recent prospective study conducted in South Africa, Murdoch et al. reported an incidence of 10.4% and a median time to onset of 48 days following initiation of HAART.[123] However, as recently stated by Tappuni, due to the lack of widely-recognized diagnostic criteria together with regional differences in incidence, treatment strategies, and endemic infections, the true global incidence of IRIS is difficult to estimate.[124]

Fortunately, mortality is low, although hospitalization may be necessary in some cases (4.5% and 27.3%, respectively, as reported by Murdoch et al.[127]), while discontinuation of therapy is rarely necessary.[122-127] Important exceptions include neurologic tuberculosis-IRIS cases and severe cryptococcal IRIS-related meningitis.[122,126]

Immune Mechanisms in the Pathogenesis of Immune Reconstitution Inflammatory Syndrome

The risk for development of IRIS is known to be closely related to the circulating CD4+ T-cell count at the start of HAART, with highest risk associated with counts of less than 50/μL. Presumably, patients who fall into this category have very poorly controlled opportunistic infections with markedly attenuated inflammatory responses. They are, therefore, likely to be asymptomatic and to present with covert or subdued disease with a high antigen load. Moreover, they are likely to experience the most significant relative increments in circulating CD4+ T-cell counts following initiation of HAART, favoring the development of unmasking or paradoxical IRIS. Recovery of cell-mediated immunity is associated with a resultant inflammatory response at the site of the covert or documented infection, causing bystander, inflammation-mediated tissue damage, which may be severe and which underpins the symptoms of IRIS.[122,124]

The immunopathogenesis of IRIS following initiation of HAART, therefore, results from the therapy-related increase in both the numbers and functions of CD4+ T-cells, with the initial rapid recovery in cell-mediated immunity resulting from the increase in circulating memory CD4+ T-cells recruited from the gut and secondary lymphoid organs.[124,128] These cells can migrate out of the circulation to sites of infection. This is followed by a recovery in the numbers of naïve CD4+ T-cells. The Th1 and Th17 T-cell subsets are likely to contribute most significantly to IRIS, promoting macrophage and monocyte/macrophage/neutrophil recruitment and activation respectively, while innate immune mechanisms involving natural killer (NK) cells have also been implicated.[129] Other mechanisms, which may contribute to the immunopathogenesis of IRIS include sustained high levels of the T-cell growth factor, interleukin (IL)-7, in the setting of abnormal function of circulating, anti-inflammatory regulatory T-cells following initiation of HAART.[130]

Immune activation in HAART-treated AIDS patients may be exacerbated by the concomitant administration of antimicrobial chemotherapy, resulting in the release of proinflammatory cell wall and cytoplasmic components and toxins from disintegrating microorganisms. Nonetheless, this does not justify withholding either type of therapy.[131]

Immune Reconstitution Inflammatory Syndrome and Pulmonary Disease

Pulmonary manifestations of IRIS have recently been reviewed by Calligaro et al., specifically IRIS associated with the more common opportunistic infections caused by *M. tuberculosis*, *P. jirovecii*, and *C. neoformans*, as well as those caused by NTM.[131] Other causes of pulmonary IRIS include Kaposi's sarcoma caused by human herpesvirus-8 (HHV-8) and sarcoidosis.[122,131,132]

Tuberculosis Immune Reconstitution Inflammatory Syndrome

Because HIV-tuberculosis coinfection is overwhelming in regions with the highest prevalence of HIV infection, it is hardly surprising that tuberculosis-IRIS of both the paradoxical and unmasking types is the most common cause of IRIS.[122,131,132] This situation is compounded by both the high rate of pre-HAART undiagnosed tuberculosis in these regions, as well as the often late presentation of HIV-tuberculosis coinfected patients who require prompt administration of dual HIV/tuberculosis therapy.[131]

TABLE 2

Clinical and Radiographic Features of Patients Presenting with Paradoxical Tuberculosis—Immune Reconstitution Inflammatory Syndrome

- High fever
- Recurrence of tuberculosis symptoms
- Lymph node enlargement
- New lymphadenopathy
- New pulmonary infiltrates
- Consolidation, cavitation, miliary infiltrate
- Increasing pleural effusions
- Respiratory failure (uncommon)

The clinical and radiographic features of patients presenting with paradoxical tuberculosis-IRIS are shown in table 2. As mentioned above, central nervous system involvement is the most serious complication, being associated with higher mortality, sometimes necessitating discontinuation of HAART.[122,126,131]

As defined by the International Network for the Study of HIV-Associated IRIS (INSHI), unmasking of tuberculosis-IRIS occurs in a subgroup of patients within the first 3 months of initiation of HAART and results from restoration of *M. tuberculosis*-specific immune responses. The consequence is an over-exuberant inflammatory response and a resultant "flare" in clinical disease. As stated by Calligaro et al., the pulmonary complications are less well characterized than those of paradoxical tuberculosis-IRIS, but may present as rapid-onset pulmonary tuberculosis, ARDS, or bronchiolitis obliterans organizing pneumonia.[131] This condition should be treated using conventional tuberculosis antimicrobial agents, while the potential role of adjunctive anti-inflammatory therapy is mentioned below.

Nontuberculous Mycobacteria Immune Reconstitution Inflammatory Syndrome

Pulmonary IRIS due to NTM occurs much less frequently than tuberculosis-IRIS, possibly for the reasons mentioned above. Nonetheless isolated cases have been described involving pathogens such as *M. kansasii, M. xenopi,* and *M. parascrofulaceum* (recently reviewed by Calligaro et al.[131]). These NTM-IRIS cases may be of the unmasking or paradoxical types and as mentioned above, are associated with endobronchial inflammation.

Cryptococcus neoformans Immune Reconstitution Inflammatory Syndrome

Cryptococcus neoformans like *M. tuberculosis*, is a significant cause of morbidity and mortality in HIV patients with advanced immunosuppression.[122,131] Although it may be localized to the central nervous system, multiorgan disease exists, affecting the central nervous system, lungs, skin, and lymph nodes. The estimated frequencies of paradoxical and unmasking cryptococcal-IRIS are 30% and 1%, respectively.[133] Unlike IRIS due to M. tuberculosis, NTM and *P. jirovecii*, the onset of cryptococcal-IRIS following initiation of HAART is slower, with median time to onset usually ranging from 1 to 10 months, although on rare occasions it may occur within several days of commencement of HAART.[133] The major pulmonary manifestations, recently reviewed by Calligaro et al., are nodular or cavitating lesions with or without mediastinal lymphadenopathy.[131] As mentioned by Haddow et al. in their recent review, cryptococcal-IRIS, which primarily affects the central nervous system, carries a high mortality, especially in Africa, where mortality rates vary from 0 to 83%.[133] Calligaro and colleagues emphasize the urgency of early detection of HAART-associated cryptococcal disease to enable prompt initiation of anti-fungal therapy.[131] They also emphasize the importance of biopsy, histology, and culture in patient management as pulmonary cryptococcal-IRIS may be difficult to distinguish from other types of IRIS in HIV-infected patients.[131]

Pneumocystis jirovecii Immune Reconstitution Inflammatory Syndrome

Pneumocystis pneumonia-IRIS occurring within weeks following initiation of HAART in HIV-infected patients with advanced immunosuppression is well-recognized, but is rarely life-threatening and may be of either the paradoxical or unmasking types. The pulmonary manifestations of *Pneumocystis* pneumonia-IRIS include dry cough, dyspnea, hypoxia, and acute respiratory failure, as well as organizing pneumonia in some cases.[131]

Kaposi's Sarcoma Immune Reconstitution Inflammatory Syndrome

Although the incidence of Kaposi's sarcoma has decreased since the introduction of HAART, some patients experience emergence or relapse of Kaposi's sarcoma after initiation of HAART with a reported frequency of IRIS-related Kaposi's sarcoma of 7% in 1 study, occurring at a median of 3 months.[134] Although clinical presentation is usually limited to skin and mucosal manifestations, pulmonary involvement may occur and is a potentially serious, sometimes fatal, complication requiring chemotherapy and/or radiotherapy in approximately 50% of patients.[131] According to Calligaro et al., radiographic findings associated with pulmonary involvement in Kaposi's sarcoma-IRIS include "worsening or recurrent reticular and reticulonodular opacities, consolidation, ground-glass opacities, lymphadenopathy, and new or enlarging pleural effusion."[131,135] The major risk factors for development of Kaposi's sarcoma-IRIS in HIV-infected African patients are documented Kaposi's sarcoma prior to initiation of HAART, detectable HHV-8 nucleic acid, a high HIV-1 RNA viral load, and a hematocrit of less than 30%.[136]

Sarcoidosis Immune Reconstitution Inflammatory Syndrome

Sarcoidosis is very uncommon in HIV-infected patients with advanced immunosuppression presumably, because there are too few CD4+ T-cells to initiate granuloma formation. Nonetheless, development of sarcoidosis, usually at around 12 months, has been reported, albeit infrequently, following administration of HAART to HIV-infected patients, usually when the circulating CD4+ T-cell count exceeds 200/μL.[131] Whether this represents true IRIS or reactivation of quiescent disease remains to be established.

Clinical and Laboratory Predictors of Future Development of Immune Reconstitution Inflammatory Syndrome

Clinical warning signs of possible development of IRIS have been covered in several recent articles and reviews[122,123,131,132,137] and are shown in table 3. In the absence of IRIS-specific biomarkers, circulating inflammatory biomarkers which may be predictive of predisposition for development of IRIS following initiation of HAART include C-reactive protein (CRP), IL-6, D-dimers, IFN-γ, and IFN-γ inducible protein (IP)-10.[137-141]

Diagnosis and Treatment of Immune Reconstitution Inflammatory Syndrome

Pre-HAART clinical evaluation and post-HAART monitoring of patients according to the clinical and laboratory criteria mentioned in the preceding section, together with prior counseling of patients, are useful strategies to facilitate early detection and control of IRIS. However, the definitive diagnosis of IRIS can only be made when factors such as noncompliance, drug toxicity

TABLE 3
Predictors of Future Development of IRIS

- Male gender
- Younger age
- Low BMI (<18.5)
- Shorter interval between initiation of therapy for opportunistic infections and HAART
- ART naïve at the time of diagnosis of opportunistic infections
- Subclinical infection at the time of initiation of HAART
- genetic factors
- Lower circulating CD4+ T-cell count (<50 μL) at time of initiation of HAART
- Lower CD4+ T-cell percentage and CD4+: CD8+ T-cell ratio at the time of initiation of HAART
- Higher HIV RNA viral load at time of initiation of HAART
- More rapid initial decrease in viral load on initiation of HAART

IRIS, immune reconstitution inflammatory syndrome; ART, antiretroviral therapy; HIV, human immunodeficiency virus; BMI, body mass index; HAART, highly active antiretroviral therapy.

and HIV drug resistance have been excluded.[124] On reaching the diagnosis of IRIS, several approaches can be considered, including temporary withdrawal of HAART. However, as mentioned above, with the exception of severe cases such as tuberculosis-IRIS with central nervous system involvement and IRIS associated with cryptococcal meningitis, this should be avoided as the benefits of continuation of HAART clearly outweigh the risks.[122-131]

Paradoxical IRIS usually resolves spontaneously without the requirement for adjunctive therapy, while in the case of unmasking IRIS, the causative pathogen should be identified and the condition treated.[122,124] Nonsteroidal anti-inflammatory drugs (NSAIDs) may provide symptomatic relief.[122,124,125,131,142] These agents should, however, be used discerningly in the treatment of IRIS, as they may, somewhat counterintuitively, exacerbate inflammatory responses. This is because NSAIDs potentiate both innate and adaptive immune mechanisms.[143,144] This results from interference with the production of the immunosuppressive prostaglandins (PGs)—PGE_2, and PGD_2, which, via their interactions with EP_2/EP_4 and DP_2 receptors on immune and inflammatory cells, activate the synthesis of the broad-spectrum, biological anti-inflammatory cyclic nucleotide, 3'-5'-cyclic adenosine monophosphate (cAMP).[145,146]

Corticosteroids appear to have a niche role in the treatment of mild-to-moderate paradoxical tuberculosis-IRIS.[131] This contention is based on the results of a recently reported randomized clinical trial (RCT) in which administration of prednisone (1.5 mg/kg/day for 2 weeks, followed by 0.75 mg/kg/day for 2 weeks) to patients with tuberculosis-IRIS was found to significantly reduce morbidity according to reductions in duration of hospitalization and frequency of outpatient procedures (aspiration of lymph nodes, cold abscesses, or serous effusions).[147] The investigators however emphasized, that corticosteroid therapy must be used discerningly in the setting of tuberculosis-IRIS to avoid exacerbating other underlying opportunistic infections, drug-resistant tuberculosis, or Kaposi's sarcoma.[131,147] The efficacy of corticosteroid therapy in other types of IRIS remains to be established and similar concerns exist, although Calligaro et al. suggest that there may be a role for these agents in unmasking tuberculosis-IRIS complicated by respiratory failure.[131]

Marais et al. have reported that several other agents, such as hydroxychloroquine, montelukast, pentoxyfylline, and thalidomide are of potential benefit in the therapy of IRIS, but the evidence is limited and largely anecdotal.[142] Other types of anti-inflammatory agents of potential benefit, but for which no supporting evidence currently exists, include macrolides,[40] clofazimine,[148] and ibudilast.[149] The latter, like montelukast, is an agent with a combination of anti-inflammatory activities, these being antagonism of cysteinyl leukotriene receptors on immune and inflammatory cells, as well as nonspecific cyclic nucleotide phosphodiesterase activity.[149]

CONCLUSION

The data clearly indicate that opportunistic respiratory infections remain extremely common and important causes of morbidity and mortality among HIV-infected persons, including those that have been initiated on HAART. One remaining consideration is the timing of initiation of antiviral therapy during the course of an HIV-associated opportunistic infection in patients who have not previously been initiated on such treatment.[150] The literature has recently been reviewed with regard to this decision, and the conclusion reached by the authors based on the currently available evidence was that initiation of HAART should take place during the first 2 weeks of a serious opportunistic infection, and that this appeared to be associated with improved patient survival, except in patients with tuberculous meningitis and cryptococcal meningitis.[150] The collective findings in the literature were that in patients with a CD4 count less than 200 cells/μL, initiation of antiretroviral therapy (ART) within 2 weeks of treatment for *P. jirovecii*, a serious bacterial infection, or pulmonary tuberculosis, there was a lower mortality than in patients initiated at a later time point. However, immediate initiation of HAART had no survival benefit in patients with tubercular meningitis and was associated with a significantly higher mortality in patients with cryptococcal meningitis.[150] Additional studies are ongoing at the current time.

REFERENCES

1. Rosen MJ. Pulmonary complications of HIV infection. *Respirology.* 2008;13:181-90.
2. Huang L, Crothers K. HIV-associated opportunistic pneumonias. *Respirology.* 2009;14:474-85.
3. Morris A, Crothers K, Beck JM, Huang L; American Thoracic Society Committee on HIV Pulmonary Disease. An official ATS workshop report: emerging issues and current controversies in HIV–associated pulmonary diseases. *Proc Am Thorac Soc.* 2011;8:17-26.
4. Benito N, Moreno A, Miro JM, Torres A. Pulmonary infections in HIV-infected patients: an update in the 21st century. *Eur Respir J.* 2011.
5. Davis JL, Fei M, Huang L. Respiratory infection complicating HIV infection. *Curr Opin Infect Dis.* 2008;21:184-90.
6. Murray JF. Pulmonary complications of HIV-1 among adults living in sub-Saharan Africa. *Int J Tuberc Lung Dis.* 2005;9:826-35.
7. Huang L. Pulmonary manifestations of HIV. *HIV InSite.* 2009;1-12.
8. Madeddu G, Fiori ML, Mura MS. Bacterial community-acquired pneumonia in HIV-infected patients. *Curr Opin Pulm Med.* 2010;16:201-7.
9. Segal LN, Methe BA, Nolan A, Hoshino Y, Rom WN, Dawson R, et al. HIV-1 and bacterial pneumonia in the era of antiretroviral therapy. *Proc Am Thorac Soc.* 2011;8:282-7.
10. Bacterial respiratory disease. Guidelines for Prevention and Treatment of Opportunistic Infections in HIV-Infected Adults and Adolescents. National Institutes of Health, the Centers for Disease Control and Prevention, and the HIV Medicine Association of the Infectious Diseases Society of America. *MMWR.* 2009;58.
11. Manfredi R, Nanetti A, Ferri M, Chiodo F. *Pseudomonas* spp. complications in patients with HIV disease: An eight-year clinical and microbiological survey. *Eur J Epidemiol.* 2000;16:111-8.
12. Afessa B, Green B. Bacterial pneumonia in hospitalized patients with HIV infection: The Pulmonary Complications, ICU Support, and Prognostic Factors of Hospitalized Patients with HIV (PIP) Study. *Chest.* 2000;117:1017-22.
13. Topino S, Galati V, Grilli E, Petrosillo N. *Rhodococcus equi* infection in HIV- infected individuals: case reports and review of the literature. *AIDS Patient Care STDS.* 2010;24: 211-22.
14. Shankar EM, Kumarasamy N, Vignesh R, Balakrishnan P, Solomon SS, Murugavel KG, et al. Epidemiological studies on pulmonary pathogens in HIV-positive and –negative subjects with or without community-acquired pneumonia with special emphasis on *Mycoplasma pneumoniae. Jpn J Infect Dis.* 2007;60:337-41.
15. Pedro-Botet ML, Sabrià M, Sopena N, Garcia-Nunez M, Dominquez MJ, Reynaga E, et al. Legionnaires disease and HIV infection. *Chest.* 2003;124:543-7.
16. Pedro-Botet ML, Sopena N, Garcia-Cruz A, Mateu L, Garcia-Nunez M, Rey-Joly C, et al. *Streptococcus pneumoniae* and *Legionella pneumophila* pneumonia in HIV–infected patients. *Scand J Infect Dis.* 2007;39:122-8.
17. Manfredi R, Naneti A, Valentini R, Chiodo F. *Moraxella catarrhalis* pneumonia during HIV disease. *J Chemother.* 2000;12:406-11.
18. Minero MV, Marin M, Cercenado E, Rabadan PM, Bouza E, Munoz P. Nocardiosis at the turn of the century. *Medicine.* 2009; 88:250-61.
19. Menéndez R, Cordero PJ, Santos M, Gobernado M, Marco V. Pulmonary infection with *Nocardia* species: a report of 10 cases and review. *Eur Respir J.* 1997;10:1542-6.
20. Schleicher GK, Feldman C. Dual infection with *Streptococcus pneumoniae* and *Mycobacterium tuberculosis* in HIV-seropositive patients with community-acquired pneumonia. *Int J Tuberc Lung Dis.* 2003;7:1207-8.
21. Nyamande K, Lalloo UG. Serum procalcitonin distinguishes CAP due to bacteria, *Mycobacterium tuberculosis* and PJP. *Int J Tuberc Lung Dis.* 2006;10:510-5.
22. Schleicher GK, Herbert V, Brink A, Martin S, Maraj R, Galpin JS, et al. Procalcitonin and C-reactive protein levels in HIV-positive subjects with tuberculosis and pneumonia. *Eur Respir J.* 2005;25:688-92.
23. Cordero E, Pachón J, Rivero A, Giron-Gonzalez JA, Gomez-Mateos J, Merino MD, et al. Usefulness of sputum culture for diagnosis of bacterial pneumonia in HIV-infected patients. *Eur J Clin Microbiol Infect Dis.* 2002; 21:362-7.
24. De Oliveira GM, Cordeiro AM, Marsico GA, Renteria JM, Guimaraes CA. Induced sputum in HIV-infected patients: diagnosis of acute pulmonary diseases. *Rev Assoc Med Bras.* 2009;55:617-20.
25. Da Silva RM, Teixeira PJ, Moreira Jda S. The clinical utility of induced sputum for the diagnosis of bacterial community-acquired pneumonia in HIV-infected patients: a prospective cross-sectional study. *Braz J Infect Dis.* 2006;10:89-93.
26. Gardner TD, Youle M, Hanson PJV, Griffiths PD, Collins JV, Gazzard BG. Diagnosis, treatment and outcome of pneumonia in the acquired immune deficiency syndrome. *J Infect.* 1989;18:111-7.
27. Feldman C, Brink AJ, Richards GA, Maartens G, Bateman ED. Management of community-acquired pneumonia in adults. Working Group of the South African Thoracic Society. *S Afr Med J.* 2007;97:1295-306.
28. Christensen D, Feldman C, Rossi P, Marrie T, Blasi F, Luna C, et al. HIV infection does not influence clinical outcomes in hospitalized patients with bacterial community-acquired pneumonia: results from the CAPO International Cohort Study. *Clin Infect Dis.* 2005;41:554-6.
29. Malinis M, Myers J, Bordon J, Peyrani P, Kapoor R, Nakamatzu R, et al. Clinical outcomes of HIV-infected patients hospitalized with bacterial community-acquired pneumonia. *Int J Infect Dis.* 2010;14: e22-e27.
30. Kohli R, Lo Y, Homel P, Flanigan TP, Gardner LI, Howard AA, et al. Bacterial pneumonia, HIV therapy, and disease progression among HIV-infected women in the HIV Epidemiologic Research (HER) Study. *Clin Infect Dis.* 2006;43:90-8.

31. Feikin DR, Feldman C, Schuchat A, Janoff EN. Global strategies to prevent bacterial pneumonia in adults with HIV disease. *Lancet Infect Dis.* 2004;4:445-55.
32. Cohen AL, Harrison LH, Farley MM, Reingold AL, Hadler J, Schaffner W, et al. Prevention of invasive pneumococcal disease among HIV-infected adults in the era of childhood pneumococcal immunization. *AIDS.* 2010;24:2253-62.
33. Miguez-Burbano MJ, Ashkin D, Rodriguez A, Duncan R, Pitchenik A, Quintero N, et al. Increased risk of *Pneumocystis carinii* and community-acquired pneumonia with tobacco use in HIV disease. *Int J Infect Dis.* 2005;9:208-7.
34. Perelló R, Miró O, Marcos MA, Almela M, Bragulat E, Sánchez M, et al. Predicting bacteremic pneumonia in HIV-1-infected patients consulting the ED. *Am J Emerg Med.* 2010;28:454-9.
35. Janoff EN, Breiman RF, Daley CL, Hopewell P. Pneumococcal disease during HIV infection. Epidemiologic, clinical, and immunologic perspectives. *Ann Intern Med.* 1992;117:314-24.
36. Daley CL. Pneumococcal infection and HIV. *HIV InSite.* 1998;1-8.
37. Klugman KP, Madhi SA, Feldman C. HIV and pneumococcal disease. *Curr Opin Infect Dis.* 2007;20:11-5.
38. Madeddu G, Fois AG, Pirina P, Mura MS. Pneumococcal pneumonia: clinical features, diagnosis and management in HIV-infected and HIV non-infected patients. *Curr Opin Pulm Med.* 2009;15:236-42.
39. Grau I, Pallares R, Tubau F, Schulze MH, Llopis F, Podzamkzer D, et al. Epidemiologic changes in bacteremic pneumococcal disease in patients with human immunodeficiency virus in the era of highly active antiretroviral therapy. *Arch Intern Med.* 2005;165:1533-40.
40. Feldman C, Anderson R. Bacteraemic pneumococcal pneumonia. Current therapeutic options. *Drugs.* 2011;71:131-53.
41. Feldman C, Klugman KP, Yu VL, Ortqvist A, Choiu CCC, Chedid MBF, et al. Bacteraemic pneumococcal pneumonia: impact of HIV on clinical presentation and outcome. *J Infect.* 2007;55:125-35.
42. Jover F, Cuadrado J-M, Andreu L, Martinez S, Canizares R, Ortiz de la Tabla V, et al. A comparative study of bacteremic and non-bacteremic pneumococcal pneumonia. *Eur J Intern Med.* 2008;19:15-21.
43. Bliss SJ, O'Brien KL, Janoff EN, Cotton MF, Musoke P, Coovadia H, et al. The evidence for using conjugate vaccines to protect HIV-infected children against pneumococcal disease. *Lancet Infect Dis.* 2007;8:67-80.
44. Pedersen RH, Lohse N, Ostergaard L, Sogaard OS. The effectiveness of pneumococcal polysaccharide vaccination in HIV-infected adults: a systematic review. *HIV Medicine.* 2011;12:323-33.
45. Imaz A, Falcó V, Peñaranda M, Jordano Q, Martinez X, Nadal C, *et al.* Impact of prior pneumococcal vaccination on clinical outcomes in HIV-infected adult patients hospitalized with invasive pneumococcal disease. *HIV Medicine.* 2009;10:356-63.
46. Schleicher GK, Hopley MJ, Feldman C. CD4 T-lymphocyte subset counts in HIV-seropositive patients during the course of community-acquired pneumonia caused by *Streptococcus pneumoniae. CMI.* 2004;10:574-92.
47. McCrary ML, Severson J, Tyring SK. Varicella zoster virus. *J Am Acad Dermatol.* 1999;41:1-14.
48. Vafai A, Berger M. Zoster in patients infected with HIV: A review. *Am J Med Sci.* 2001;321:372-80.
49. Popara M, Pendle S, Sacks L, Smego RA, Jr., Mer M. Varicella pneumonia in patients with HIV/AIDS. *Int J Infect Dis.* 2002;6:6-8.
50. Kunisaki KM, Janoff EN. Influenza in immunosuppressed populations: a review of infection frequency, morbidity, mortality, and vaccine responses. *Lancet Infect Dis.* 2009; 9:493-504.
51. Gessner BD, Shindo N, Briand S. Seasonal influenza epidemiology in sub-saharan Africa: a systematic review. *Lancet Infect Dis.* 2011;11:223-35.
52. Martinez E, Marcos MA, Hoyo-Ulloa I, Anton A, Sanchez M, Vilella A, et al. Influenza A H1N1 in HIV-infected adults. *HIV Medicine.* 2011;12:236-45.
53. Millar AB, Patou G, Miller RF, Grundy JE, Katz DR, Weller IV, et al. Cytomegalovirus in the lungs of patients with AIDS. Respiratory pathogen or passenger? *Am Rev Respir Dis.* 1990;141:1474-7.
54. Salomon N, Perlman DC. Cytomegalovirus pneumonia. *Semin Respir Infect.* 1999;14:353-8.
55. Barry SM, Johnson MA, Janossy G. Cytopathology or immunopathology? The puzzle of cytomegalovirus pneumonitis revisited. *Bone Marrow Transplantion.* 2000; 26;591-7.
56. Enoch DA, Ludlam HA, Brown NM. Invasive fungal infections: a review of epidemiology and management options. *J Med Microbiol.* 2006;55:809-18.
57. Lai CC, Tan CK, Huang YT, Shao PL, Hsueh PR. Current challenges in the management of invasive fungal infections. *J Infect Chemother.* 2008;14:77-85.
58. Limper AH. The changing spectrum of fungal infections in pulmonary and critical care practice. *Proc Am Thorac Soc.* 2010;7:163-8.
59. Shao PL, Huang LM, Hsueh PR. Recent advances and challenges in the treatment of invasive fungal infections. *Int J Antimicrob Agents.* 2007;30:487-95.
60. Hsu LY, Ng ES, Koh LP. Common and emerging fungal pulmonary infections. *Infect Dis Clin N Am.* 2010;24:557-77.
61. Chen SC-A, Playford EG, Sorrell TC. Antifungal therapy in invasive fungal infections. *Curr Opin Pharmacol.* 2010; 10:522-30.
62. Kriengkauykiat J, Ito JI, Dadwal SS. Epidemiology and treatment approaches in management of invasive fungal infections. *Clin Epidemiol.* 2011;3:175-91.
63. Leoung GS. Pneumocystosis and HIV. *HIV InSite.* 2006;1-32.
64. Huang L, Morris A, Limper AH, Beck JM; ATS Pneumocystis Workshop Participants. An official ATS workshop summary: Recent advances and future directions in *Pneumocystis* pneumonia (PCP). *Proc Am Thorac Soc.* 2006;3:655-64.
65. D'Avignon LC, Schofield CM, Hospenthal DR. *Pneumocystis* pneumonia. *Semin Respir Crit Care Med.* 2008;29:132-40.
66. Catherinot E, Lanternier F, Bougnoux ME, Lecuit M, Couderc LJ, Lortholary O. *Pneumocystis jirovecii* pneumonia. *Infect Dis Clin N Am.* 2010;24:107-38.
67. Morris A, Wei K, Afshar K, Huang L. Epidemiology and clinical significance of *Pneumocystis* colonization. *J Infect Dis.* 2008;197:10-7.

68. Morris A, Kingsley LA, Groner G, Lebedeva IP, Beard CB, Norris KA. Prevalence and clinical predictors of *Pneumocystis* colonization among HIV-infected men. *AIDS.* 2004;18:793-8.
69. Fujii T, Nakamura T, Iwamoto A. *Pneumocystis* pneumonia in patients with HIV infection: clinical manifestations, laboratory findings, and radiological features. *J Infect Chemother.* 2007;13:1-7.
70. Huang L, Cattamanchi A, Davis JL, den Boon S, Kovacs J, Meshnick S, et al.; International HIV-associated Opportunistic Pneumonias (IHOP) Study and the Lung HIV Study. HIV-associated *Pneumocystis* pneumonia. *Proc Am Thorac Soc.* 2011;8:294-300.
71. Carmona EM, Limper AH. Update on the diagnosis and treatment of *Pneumocystis* pneumonia. *Ther Adv Respir Dis.* 2011;5:41-59.
72. Harris JR, Marston BJ, Sangrujee N, DuPlessis D, Park B. Cost-effectiveness analysis of diagnostic options for *Pneumocystis* pneumonia (PCP). *PLoS One.* 2011;6:e23158.
73. Castro JG, Manzi G, Espinoza L, Campos M, Boulanger C. Concurrent PCP and TB pneumonia in HIV infected patients. *Scand J Infect Dis.* 2007;39:1054-8.
74. Helweg-Larsen J, Benfield T, Atzori C, Miller RF. Clinical efficacy of first- and second-line treatment for HIV-associated *Pneumocystis jirovecii* pneumonia: a tri-centre cohort study. *J Antimicrob Chemother.* 2009;64:1282-90.
75. Briel M, Bucher BM, Boscacci R, Furrer H. Adjunctive corticosteroids for *Pneumocystis jirovecii* pneumonia in patients with HIV-infection (Review). *Cochrane Database Syst Rev.* 2006:(3):CD006150.
76. Jarvis JN, Harrison TS. Pulmonary cryptococcosis. *Semin Respir Crit Care Med.* 2008;29:141-50.
77. Shirley RM, Baddley JW. Cryptococcal lung disease. *Curr Opin Pulmon Med.* 2009;15:254-60.
78. Li SS, Mody CH. *Cryptococcus. Proc Am Thorac Soc.* 2010; 7:186-96.
79. Warkentien T, Crum-Cianflone NF. An update on *Cryptococcus* among HIV-infected patients. *Int J STD AIDS.* 2010;21:679-84.
80. Sajadi MM, Roddy KM, Chan-Tack KM, Forrest GN. Risk factors for mortality from primary cryptococcosis in patients with HIV. *Postgrad Med.* 2009;121:107-13.
81. Ampel NM. Coccidioidomycosis in persons infected with HIV-1. *Ann N Y Acad Sci.* 2007;1111:336-42.
82. Kauffman CA. Diagnosis of histoplasmosis in immuno-suppressed patients. *Curr Opin Infect Dis.* 2008;21:421-5.
83. Wheat LJ, Freifeld AG, Kleiman MB, Baddley JW, McKinsey DS, Loyd JE, et al. Clinical Practice Guidelines for the Management of Patients with Histoplasmosis: 2007 Update by the Infectious Diseases Society of America. *Clin Infect Dis.* 2007;45:807-25.
84. Severo CB, Guazelli LS, Severo LC. Zygomycosis. *J Bras Pneumol.* 2010;36:134-41.
85. Nichols L, Ocque RZ, Daly I. Zygomycosis associated with HIV infection and liver transplantation. *Patholog Res Int.* 2011;545981.
86. Keating JJ, Rogers T, Petrou M, Cartledge JD, Woodrow D, Nelson M, et al. Management of pulmonary aspergillosis in AIDS: an emerging clinical problem. *J Clin Pathol.* 1994;47: 805-9.
87. Mylonakis E, Flanigan T, Rich JD, Barlam TF. Pulmonary aspergillosis and invasive disease in AIDS: Review of 342 cases. *Chest.* 1998;114:251-62.
88. Holding KJ, Dworkin MS, Wan P-C J, Hanson DL, Klevens RM, Jones JL, et al. Aspergillosis among people infected with human immunodeficiency virus: incidence and survival. *Clin Infect Dis.* 2000;31:1253-7.
89. Singh N, Yu VL, Rihs JD. Invasive aspergillosis in AIDS. *South Med J.* 1991;84:822-7.
90. Vijayan VK, Kilani T. Emerging and established parasitic lung infestations. *Infect Dis Clin N Am.* 2010;24:579-602.
91. World Health Organization. Tuberculosis. Fact sheet No 104. Available from: http://www.who.int/mediacentre/factsheets/fs104/en/. March 2012.
92. Corbett EL, Marston B, Churchyard GJ, De Cock KM. Tuberculosis in sub-Saharan Africa: opportunities, challenges, and change in the era of antiretroviral treatment. *Lancet.* 2006;367:926-37.
93. Holmes CB, Wood R, Badri M, Zilber S, Wang B, Maartens G, et al. CD4 decline and incidence of opportunistic infections in Cape Town, South Africa: implications for prophylaxis and treatment. *J Aquir Immune Defic Syndr.* 2006;42;464-9.
94. World Health Organization. Global tuberculosis control-surveillance, planning, financing. WHO Report 2005. WHO/HTM/TB/2005. 349. Geneva: World Health Organization, 2005. Available from: http://library.cphs.chula.ac.th/Ebooks/Annual%20Report/WHO%20Report/WHO%20REPORT%202005.pdf
95. Lawson L, Yassin MA, Thacher TD, Olatunji OO, Lawson JO, Akingbogun TI, et al. Clinical presentation of adults with pulmonary tuberculosis with and without HIV infection in Nigeria. *Scand J Infect Dis.* 2008;40:30-5.
96. Kassu A, Mengistu G, Ayele B, Diro E, Mekonnen F, Ketema D, et al. Coinfection and clinical manifestations of tuberculosis in human immunodeficiency virus-infected and -uninfected adults at a teaching hospital, northwest Ethiopia. *J Microbiol Immunol Infect.* 2007;40:116-22.
97. Pepper T, Joseph P, Mwenya C, McKee GS, Haushalter A, Carter A, et al. Normal chest radiography in pulmonary tuberculosis: implications for obtaining respiratory specimen cultures. *Int J Tuberc Lung Dis.* 2008;12:397-403.
98. Chamie G, Luetkemeyer A, Walusimbi-Nanteza M, Okwera A, Whalen CC, Mugerwa RD, et al. Significant variation in presentation of pulmonary tuberculosis across a high resolution of CD4 strata. *Int J Tuberc Lung Dis.* 2010;14:1295-302.
99. Theron G, Peter J, van Zyl-Smit R, Mishra H, Streicher E, Murray S, et al. Evaluation of the Xpert M. TUBERCULOSIS/RIF assay for the diagnosis of pulmonary tuberculosis in a high HIV prevalence setting. *Am J Respir Crit Care Med.* 2011;184:132-40.
100. Beukes M, Lemmer Y, Deysel M, Al Dulayymi JR, Baird MS, Koza G, et al. Structure-function relationships of the antigenicity of mycolic acids in tuberculosis patients. *Chem Phys Lipids.* 2010;163:800-8.
101. Schlossberg D. Acute tuberculosis. *Infect Dis Clin North Am.* 2010;24:139-46.
102. Nyamande K, Lalloo UG, John M. TB presenting as community-acquired pneumonia in a setting of high TB

incidence and high HIV prevalence. *Int J Tuberc Lung Dis.* 2007;11:1308-13.
103. Kunimoto D, Long R. Tuberculosis: still overlooked as a cause of community-acquired pneumonia - how not to miss it. *Respir Care Clin N Am.* 2005;11:25-34.
104. Liam CK, Pang YK, Poosparajah S. Pulmonary tuberculosis presenting as community-acquired pneumonia. *Respirology.* 2006;11:786-92.
105. Asnis DS, Cherian S, Sun T, Shrestha S, Santucci T Jr. Pulmonary tuberculosis presenting as community-acquired pneumonia. *Clin Infect Dis.* 2002;35:1574-5.
106. Wootton D. Review diagnosis, aetiology, and severity in adult community-acquired pneumonia. Africa Journal of Respiratory Medicine. Available from: http://www.africanjournalofrespiratorymedicine.com/articles/march_2010/AJRM%20MARCH%20pp%205-7.pdf. March 2010.
107. Pinto LM, Shah AC, Shah KD, Udwadia F. Pulmonary tuberculosis masquerading as community acquired pneumonia. *Resp Med CME.* 2010, doi:10.1016/j.rmedc.2010.11.004.
108. Dooley KE, Golub J, Goes FS, Merz WG, Sterling TR. Empiric treatment of community-acquired pneumonia with fluoroquinolones, and delays in the treatment of tuberculosis. *Clin Infect Dis.* 2002;34:1607-12.
109. Counsell SR, Tan JS, Dittus RS. Unsuspected pulmonary tuberculosis in a community teaching hospital. *Arch Intern Med.* 1989;149:1274-8.
110. Bezerra PG, Britto MC, Correia JB, Duarte Mdo C, Fonceca AM, Rose K, et al. Viral and atypical bacterial detection in acute respiratory infection in children under five years. *PLoS One.* 2011;6:e18928.
111. Plit ML, Theron AJ, Fickl H, van Rensburg CE, Pendel S, Anderson R. Influence of antimicrobial chemotherapy and smoking status on the plasma concentrations of vitamin C, vitamin E, beta-carotene, acute phase reactants, iron and lipid peroxides in patients with pulmonary tuberculosis. *Int J Tuberc Lung Dis.* 1998;2:590-6.
112. Tintinger GR, van der Merwe JJ, Fickl H, Rheeder P, Feldman C, Anderson R. Soluble triggering receptor expressed on myeloid cells in sputum of patients with community-acquired pneumonia or pulmonary tuberculosis: a pilot study. *Eur J Clin Microbiol Infect Dis.* 2012;31:73-6
113. Field SK, Cowie RL. Lung disease due to the more common nontuberculous mycobacteria. *Chest.* 2006;129:1653-72.
114. Billinger ME, Olivier KN, Viboud C, de Oca RM, Stiner C, Holland SM, et al. Nontuberculous mycobacteria-associated lung disease in hospitalized persons, United States, 1998-2005. *Emerg Infect Dis.* 2009;15:1562-9.
115. Andréjak C, Lescure FX, Douadi Y, Laurans G, Smail A, Duhaut P, et al. Non-tuberculous mycobacteria pulmonary infection: management and follow-up of 31 infected patients. *J Infect.* 2007;55:34-40.
116. Gopinath K, Singh S. Non-tuberculous mycobacteria in TB-endemic countries: are we neglecting the danger? *PLoS Negl Trop Dis.* 2010:4:e615.
117. Bloch KC, Zwerling L, Pletcher MJ, Hahn JA, Gerberding JL, Ostroff SM, et al. Incidence and clinical implications of isolation of Mycobacterium kansasii: results of a 5-year, population-based study. *Ann Intern Med.* 1998; 129:698-704.
118. Corbett EL, Blumberg L, Churchyard GJ, Moloi N, Mallory K, Clayton T, et al. Nontuberculous mycobacteria: defining disease in a prospective cohort of South African Miners. *Am J Respir Crit Care Med.* 1999;160:15-21.
119. Corbett EL, Churchyard GJ, Clayton T, Herselman P, Williams B, Hayes R, et al. Risk factors for pulmonary mycobacterial disease in South African gold miners. A case-control study. *Am J Respir Crit Care Med.* 1999;159:94-9.
120. Corbett EL, Churchyard GJ, Hay M, Herselman P, Clayton T, Williams B, et al. The impact of HIV infection on Mycobacterium kansasii disease in South African gold miners. *Am J Respir Crit Care Med.* 1999;160:10-4.
121. Griffith DE, Aksamit T, Brown-Elliott BA, Cantanzaro A, Daley C, Gordin F, et al. An official ATS/IDSA statement: diagnosis, treatment, and prevention of nontuberculous mycobacterial diseases. *Am J Respir Crit Care Med.* 2007; 175:367-416.
122. Murdoch DM, Venter WD, Van Rie A, Feldman C. Immune reconstitution inflammatory syndrome (IRIS): review of common infectious manifestations and treatment options. *AIDS Res Ther.* 2007;4:9.
123. Müller M, Wandel S, Colebunders R, Attia S, Furrer H, Egger M, et al. Immune reconstitution inflammatory syndrome in patients starting antiretroviral therapy for HIV infection: a systematic review and meta-analysis. *Lancet Infect Dis.* 2010;10:251-61.
124. Tappuni AR. Immune reconstitution inflammatory syndrome. *Adv Dent Res.* 2011;23:90-6.
125. Beishuizen SJ, Geerlings SE. Immune reconstitution inflammatory syndrome: immunopathogenesis, risk factors, diagnosis, treatment and prevention. *Neth J Med.* 2009;67:327-31.
126. Cohen K, Meintjes G. Management of individuals requiring antiretroviral and TB treatment. *Curr Opin HIV AIDS.* 2010;5:61-9.
127. Murdoch DM, Venter WD, Feldman C, Van Rie A. Incidence and risk factors for the immune reconstitution inflammatory syndrome in HIV patients in South Africa: a prospective study. *AIDS.* 2008;22:601-10.
128. Autran B, Carcelain G, Li TS, Blanc C, Mathez D, Tubiana R, et al. Positive effects of combined antiretroviral therapy on CD4+ T cell homeostasis and function in advanced HIV disease. *Science.* 1997;277:112-6.
129. Conradie F, Foulkes AS, Ive P, Yin X, Roussos K, Glencross DK, et al. Natural killer cell activation distinguishes M. tuberculosis-mediated Immune reconstitution syndrome (IRIS) from chronic HIV and HIV-MTB co-infection. *J Acquir Immune Defic Syndr.* 2011;58:309-18.
130. Seddiki N, Sasson SC, Santner-Nanan B, Munier M, van Bockel D, Ip S, et al. Proliferation of weakly suppressive regulatory CD4+ T cells is associated with over-active CD4+ T-cell responses in HIV-positive patients with mycobacterial immune restoration disease. *Eur J Immunol.* 2009;39:391-403.
131. Calligaro G, Meintjes G, Mendelson M. Pulmonary manifestations of the immune reconstitution inflammatory syndrome. *Curr Opin Pulm Med.* 2011;17:180-8.
132. Grant PM, Komarow L, Andersen J, Sereti I, Pahwa S, Lederman MM, et al. Risk factor analyses for immune reconstitution inflammatory syndrome in a randomized

study of early vs. deferred ART during an opportunistic infection. *PLoS ONE*. 2010;5: e11416.

133. Haddow LJ, Colebunders R, Meintjes G, Lawn SD, Elliott JH, Manabe YC, et al. Cryptococcal immune reconstitution inflammatory syndrome in HIV-1-infected individuals: proposed clinical case definitions. *Lancet Infect Dis*. 2010; 10:791-802.
134. Bower M, Nelson M, Young AM, Thirlwell C, Newsom-Davis T, Mandalia S, et al. Immune reconstitution inflammatory syndrome associated with Kaposi's sarcoma. *J Clin Oncol*. 2005;23:5224-8.
135. Godoy MC, Rouse H, Brown JA, Phillips P, Forrest DM, Müller NL. Imaging features of pulmonary Kaposi sarcoma-associated immune reconstitution syndrome. *AJR Am J Roentgenol*. 2007;189:956-65.
136. Letang E, Almeida JM, Miró JM, Ayala E, White IE, Carrilho C, et al. Predictors of immune reconstitution inflammatory syndrome associated with Kaposi's sarcoma in Mozambique: a prospective study. *J Acquir Immune Defic Syndr*. 2010;53:589-97.
137. Letang E, Miró JM, Nhampossa T, Ayala E, Gascon J, Menéndez C, et al. Incidence and predictors of immune reconstitution inflammatory syndrome in a rural area of Mozambique. *PLoS ONE*. 2011;6:e16946.
138. Sereti I, Rodger AJ, French MA. Biomarkers in immune reconstitution inflammatory syndrome: signals from pathogenesis. *Curr Opin HIV AIDS*. 2010;5:504-10.
139. Boulware DR, Hullsiek KH, Puronen CE, Rupert A, Baker JV, French MA, et al. Higher levels of CRP, D-dimer, IL-6, and hyaluronic acid before initiation of antiretroviral therapy (ART) are associated with increased risk of AIDS or death. *J Infect Dis*. 2011;203:1637-46.
140. Haddow LJ, Dibben O, Moosa MY, Borrow P, Easterbrook PJ. Circulating inflammatory biomarkers can predict and characterize tuberculosis-associated immune reconstitution inflammatory syndrome. *AIDS*. 2011;25:1163-74.
141. French MA, Oliver BG, Elliott JH, Price P. Plasma biomarkers in the prediction and diagnosis of tuberculosis-associated immune reconstitution inflammatory syndrome. *AIDS*. 2011;25:1676-7.
142. Marais S, Wilkinson RJ, Pepper DJ, Meintjes G. Management of patients with the immune reconstitution inflammatory syndrome. *Curr HIV/AIDS Rep*. 2009;6:162-71.
143. Spinas GA, Bloesch D, Keller U, Zimmerli W, Cammisuli S. Pretreatment with ibuprofen augments circulating tumor necrosis factor-alpha, interleukin-6, and elastase during acute endotoxinemia. *J Infect Dis*. 1991;163: 89-95.
144. Stables MJ, Newson J, Ayoub SS, Brown J, Hyams CJ, Gilroy DW. Priming innate immune responses to infection by cyclooxygenase inhibition kills antibiotic-susceptible and -resistant bacteria. *Blood*. 2010;116:2950-9.
145. Moore AR, Willoughby DA. The role of cAMP regulation in controlling inflammation. *Clin Exp Immunol*. 1995; 101:387-9.
146. Serezani CH, Ballinger MN, Aronoff DM, Peters-Golden M. Cyclic AMP: master regulator of innate immune cell function. *Am J Respir Cell Mol Biol*. 2008;39:127-32.
147. Meintjes G, Wilkinson RJ, Morroni C, Pepper DJ, Rebe K, Rangaka MX, et al. Randomized placebo-controlled trial of prednisone for paradoxical tuberculosis-associated immune reconstitution inflammatory syndrome. *AIDS*. 2010;24:2381-90.
148. Cholo MC, Steel HC, Fourie PB, Germishuizen WA, Anderson R. Clofazimine: Current status and future prospects. J Antimicrob Chemother. 2012;67:290-8.
149. Tintinger GR, Feldman C, Theron AJ, Anderson R. Montelukast: more than a cysteinyl leukotriene receptor antagonist? *ScientificWorldJournal*. 2010;10:2403-13.
150. Lawn SD, Török ME, Wood R. Optimum time to start antiretroviral therapy during HIV-associated opportunistic infections. *Curr Opin Infect Dis*. 2011;24:34-42.

CHAPTER 10

Respiratory Infections in Specific Populations: Transplant Patients

Robert P Baughman, Lisa A Haglund, Gautham Mogilishetty

ABSTRACT

Lower respiratory tract infections are one of the most common infectious complications of a patient undergoing either hematopoietic stem cell transplantation or solid organ transplant. In a patient with presumed pneumonia, several respiratory samples can be obtained to help direct therapy. However, empiric therapy is usually initiated while awaiting results of testing. Epidemiologic studies have helped identify which infections are likely to be encountered in the transplant patient. These epidemiologic studies also help to determine which prophylactic regimens should be used and for how long an individual transplant should receive them.

INTRODUCTION

Lower respiratory tract infections (LRTIs) are one of the most common infectious complications of a patient undergoing either hematopoietic stem cell transplantation (HSCT) or solid organ transplant (SOT). While prophylactic regimens have reduced the rate and mortality from such infections, there still remain a major complication. In this chapter, we will review the diagnosis and treatment of LRTI in transplant. We will also summarize some of the prophylaxis regimens, which have proved useful in preventing specific infections.

EPIDEMIOLOGY OF LOWER RESPIRATORY TRACT INFECTIONS IN TRANSPLANT PATIENTS

In evaluating a transplant patient with a potential LRTI, one has to determine the type of transplant, time from transplant, and any prior LRTI immediately before and after transplantation. This information will provide a useful guide into the potential organism the patient may have acquired. It will also assist in determining which diagnostic tests may be most useful.

Figure 1 summarizes the relationship, the time of transplant, and types of organisms noted to cause infection in HSCT.[1] Most patients undergoing HSCT have an underlying hematologic malignancy and as a result of their disease or prior treatment are neutropenic. The patient undergoing transplant is already ill from their under lying illness. This can lead to colonization with resistant bacteria. In a patient who has had prolonged hospitalization prior to transplant, nosocomial infections with multidrug-resistant bacteria can be a major problem. As the patient starts to recover from the transplant, and engraftment leads to resolution of neutropenia, then risk for bacterial infection falls. In some cases, T-cell defects may occur, making the patient susceptible to T-cell mediated infections, such as cytomegalovirus (CMV) and pneumocystis.[2] However, the risk of these types of infections in HSCT is much less than in SOT.

For the SOT, the most common cause of LRTI in a transplant patient is bacterial. This is especially true in the first few weeks after the transplant.[3] This is not only due to the overall condition of the patient prior to the transplant,[4] but also because of the various immunosuppressants begun immediately after transplant. However, a

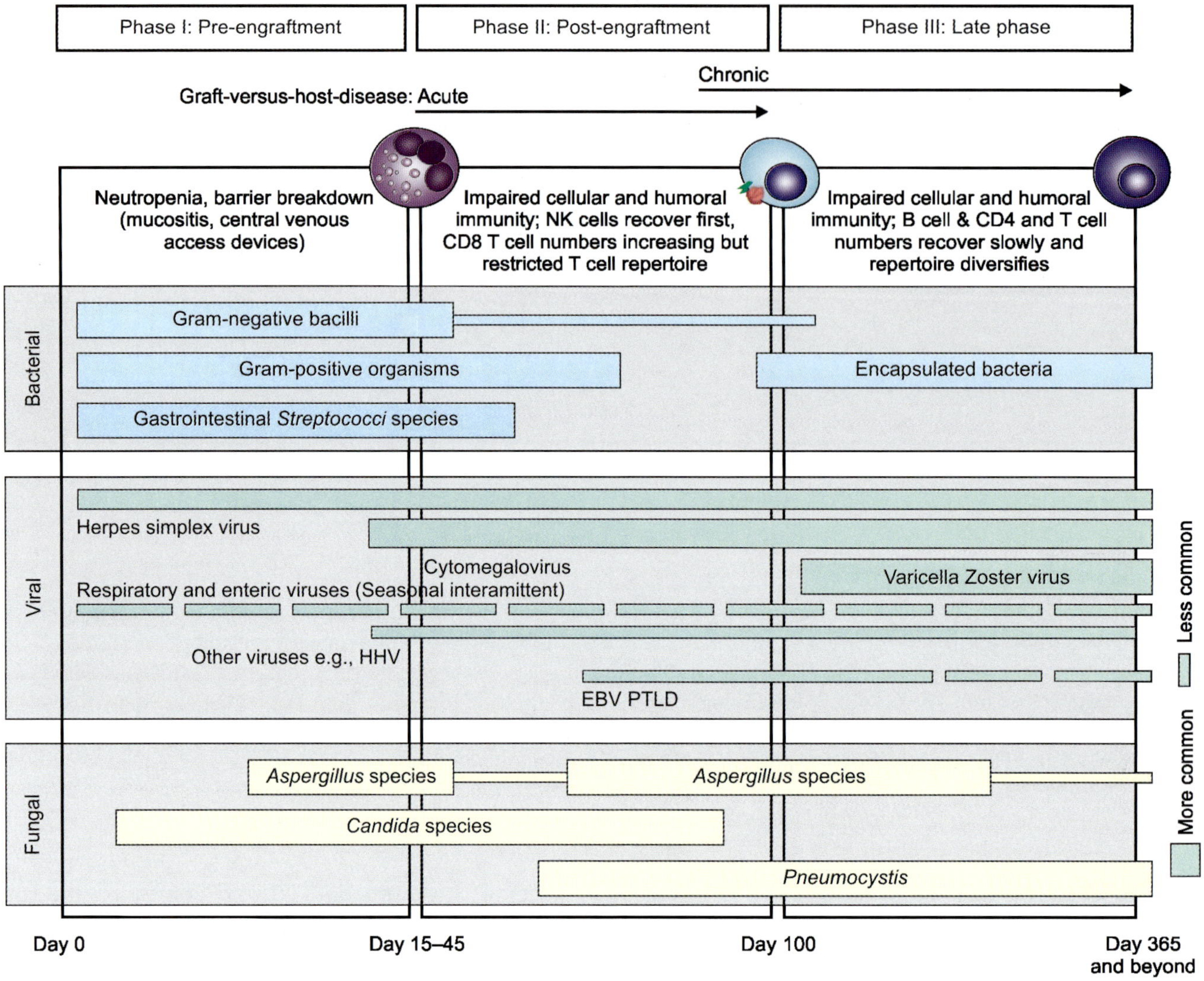

NK, natural killer; CD8, cluster of differentiation 8; HHV, human herpes virus; EBV; Epstein-Barr virus; PTLD, post-transplant lymphoproliferative disorder.

FIGURE 1 Types of organisms causing infection hematopoietic cell transplants in relation to time of transplant. *Source:* Center for International Blood and Marrow Transplant Research (CIBMTR), National Marrow Donor Program (NMDP), European Blood and Marrow Transplant Group (EBMT), et al. Guidelines for preventing infectious complications among hematopoietic cell transplant recipients: a global perspective. *Bone Marrow Transplant.* 2009;44:453-558. .

SOT may also be immunocompromised prior to the transplant. This is especially true for lung transplant, where patients may have recurrent pneumonia and have been on corticosteroids. In addition, conditions such as cystic fibrosis patient are often colonized with *Pseudomonas* and other multidrug-resistant bacteria, including *Burkholderia cepacia* and methicillin-resistant *S. aureus* (MRSA).[5-7] About 5% of cystic fibrosis patients have nontuberculous mycobacteria, such as *M. avium.*[8] Aspergillus infections can occur in cystic fibrosis patients, but also commonly colonizes patients with long-standing bronchiectasis.[9] A double lung transplant may remove the major foci of infection in these patients. However, multi-resistant organisms may still reside in the upper airway. For the cystic fibrosis patient, sinus infection with resistant Gram-negative and fungal organisms is common.

The types of bacteria encountered in first few months following either a SCT or SOT are those organisms that have colonized the upper respiratory tract. Therefore pneumonia in these patients should be considered a healthcare-associated pneumonia (HCAP). Appropriate empiric antibiotics should be adjusted for local epidemiology and include both Gram-positive and Gram-negative organisms.[10]

For SOT, the goal of immunosuppressive therapy is to block cell-mediated immunity. This is usually done using one or more agent that blocks T helper cell function and cause the depletion of CD4 positive lymphocytes.

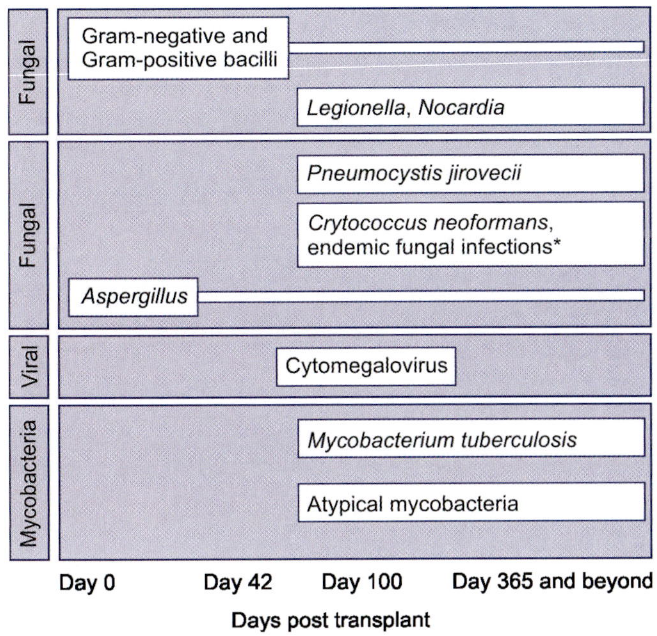

*Endemic fungal infections include *Histoplasmosis capsulatum*, *Blastomyces dermatitidis*, and *Coccidioides immitis*.

FIGURE 2 Types of organisms causing pneumonia in solid organ transplant in relation to time from transplant. The risk for *Aspergillus* infection is related to level of neutropenia. Gram- negative and positive *bacilli* risk depends on neutropenia and prior antibiotic exposure.

One can measure the CD4 count in the same way one measures CD4 count in HIV-infected patients. The lower the CD4 count the more likely one is to encounter unusual opportunistic infections. Figure 2 shows the timing and type of opportunistic infections encountered in SOT. The peak effect of CD4 depletion is usually 6 weeks after beginning immunosuppressive therapy. At this point, one may encounter infections from organisms that have colonized the patient, such as CMV and *Pneumocystis jiroveci* pneumonia (PcP). Usually by 6 months, the level of immunosuppression can be reduced and the patient is no longer at risk for these types of infection.[11] The risk for CMV and PcP rises for those patients treated for rejection.[12,13] These are useful guidelines not only for making empiric choices regarding empiric therapy for initial treatment of pneumonia, but also in deciding when and what prophylaxis agents to be used.

There are some organisms which are an increased risk for the patient for the lifetime of the transplant of the patient. For a SOT, reduced cell-mediated immunity means the patient will have limited ability to control *M. tuberculosis*. In a patient with latent tuberculosis, reactivation of the *M. tuberculosis* may occur as little as 2 weeks after transplant. However, reinfection or reactivation can occur anytime in the life of the patient. In treating renal transplant patient in China, where tuberculosis is endemic, active tuberculosis was encountered in 1.4% of patients. The median was 32 months, but infection was diagnosed anywhere between 2 weeks to 10 years.[14] Other infections that are T-cell mediated and occur more frequently in transplant patients are *Legionella*,[15] *Nocardia*,[16,17] and *Cryptococcus*.[18]

Figures 3 and 4 summarize the pathogens recovered by bronchoscopy from patients undergoing either solid organ or bone marrow/stem cell transplant. There are several trends that are apparent from viewing the results over time. The percentage of patients with bacteria as the cause of pneumonia has risen over time. This may be related to bronchoscopy earlier in the course of the pneumonia, which is associated with a higher yield for the procedure.[19] For those patients undergoing earlier bronchoscopy, one would anticipate less antibiotic use and, therefore, a higher yield of bronchoalveolar lavage (BAL).[20,21] PcP was less commonly diagnosed in the

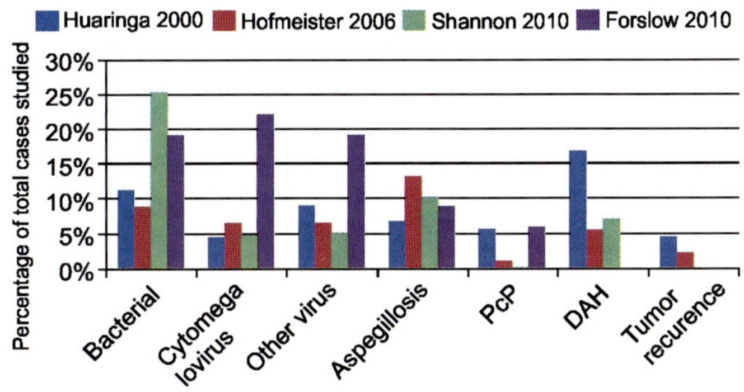

PcP, *Pneumocystis carinii* pneumonia; DAH, diffuse alveolar hemorrhage; BAL, bronchoalnestar lavage.

FIGURE 3 Etiology of acute pulmonary infiltrates as determined by bronchoscopy and BAL, from bone marrow and stem cell transplant patients from various series over a 10 year period of reporting.[19,22,27,28] The yield of bronchoscopy and BAL averaged more than 50% in these studies.

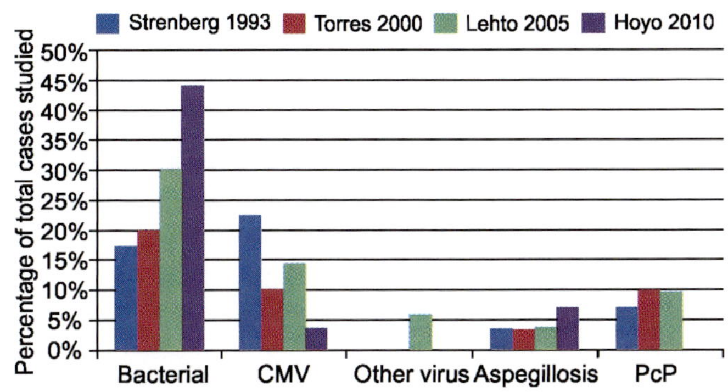

CMV, cytomegalovirus; PcP, *Pneumocystis carinii* pneumonia; BAL, bronchoalnestar lavage.

FIGURE 4 Etiology of acute pulmonary infiltrates as determined by bronchoscopy and BAL, from solid organ transplant patients from various series over a 17-year-period of reporting.[3,23,68,128] The yield of bronchoscopy and BAL was more than 50% in these studies.

past few years, with no cases diagnosed from the three series reported in 2010.[19,22,23] This may be a reflection of more widespread use of pneumocystis prophylaxis. However, this may also reflect the relatively low rate of PcP now encountered in post-transplant patients.[24] However, given the high mortality of PcP, prophylaxis against pneumocystis infection still seems reasonable. This is especially true for patients at increased risk, such as older patients, those with CMV pneumonia, or those having received increased immunosuppression either initially or after episodes of rejection.[11,25] The rate of viral pneumonia other than CMV has risen in the past 10 years. This may be a reflection of increased infections, but also could be because of more routine techniques to detect viruses other than CMV in BAL and other samples.[26] For stem cell transplant patients, diffuse alveolar hemorrhage (DAH) and recurrence of tumor can be diagnosis made by bronchoscopy.[19,27,28] These are not likely to be encountered in SOTs.

DIAGNOSIS OF PNEUMONIA IN TRANSPLANT PATIENT

The diagnosis of pneumonia is usually based on the clinical features, presence of infiltrate on chest X-ray, and identification of an appropriate organism. However, the majority of transplant patients lack one or more of these criteria.

The classic clinical findings of pneumonia include fever, dyspnea, cough, and purulent sputum. For the immunosuppressed patients, these features may be blunted or totally absent.[29] While the presence of fever is a useful clinical clue separating bronchitis from pneumonia, transplant patients with pneumonia may have no fever. An increased respiratory rate may be a good indicator of respiratory distress. It has also proved a more reliable indicator of morbidity and mortality for pneumonia.[30] However, the transplant may have tachypnea for many reasons.

Radiology can be a useful indication of not only the presence of pneumonia, but may also help indicate the causative organism. Table 1 shows several different radiologic patterns seen on chest X-ray and CT scan and the common organisms often associated with these patterns.[31] However, abnormalities on chest X-ray may be due to other causes and the chest X-ray may be normal in patients with lower respiratory infection.[29,32] The CT scan may identify infiltrates not appreciated on plain chest roentgenogram.[31,33]

Examination of respiratory secretions can be performed using a variety of techniques. One can identify by direct examination or culture a variety of potential pathogens in a patient with a potential LRTI. The presence of a particular organism does not guarantee that it is the cause of the LRTI. Figure 5 summarizes the type of organisms and the chances that it represents a pathogen in both the normal host as well as the transplant patient. For example, the identification of *M. tuberculosis* is felt to almost always be a pathogen requiring specific therapy. Aspergillus can colonize the lower respiratory tract of a normal host and not require therapy. However, its presence in the transplant patient usually either implies infection

TABLE 1

Radiographic findings in transplant pneumonia patients

- Lobar infiltrates
  - *S. pneumonia*
- Diffuse multi lobar infiltrates
  - *M. pneumonia*
  - *Chlamydia*
  - *Cytomegalovirus*
  - *Pneumocystis*
- Upper lobe predominant infiltrates
  - *M. tuberculosis*
  - Pneumocystis carinii gneumonia
- Lower lobe predominant infiltrates
  - Aspiration
- Cavitary lesions
  - *Aspergillosis**
  - *S. aureus*
  - Tuberculosis
  - *Pseudomonas*

*Halo sign

	Bacteria		
S. Pneumonia *P. Aureginosa*	*S. aureus* Anaerobes	*E. coli*	Diptheroids
	Fungal		
Cryptococcus *Histoplasmosis* *Coccidiomycosis* *Pneumocystis*	*Aspergillus*		*Candida*
	Mycobacteria		
M. tuberculosis		*M. avium* complex	*M. gordonae*
	Normal Host		
Definite	Possible	Unlikely	Not likely
	Transplant		
Definite	Definite	Usualy	Possible

FIGURE 5 Relationship between organism and possible cause of pneumonia depends on both the virulence of the organism and the underlying immunosuppression of the host. Examples of the interaction are shown for bacterial, fungal, mycobacterial, and viral infections.

TABLE 2

Respiratory samples

Type of sample	Direct examination: common studies	Direct examination: possible further studies	Culture common studies	Culture: possible further studies	PCR
Sputum	Gram stain, AFB smear	Papanicolaou stain, modified silver stain	Bacterial, AFB, fungal	Viral	AFB
Bronchial wash	Gram stain, AFB smear, Papanicolaou stain, modified silver stain		Bacterial, AFB, fungal	Viral	AFB, viral
Bronchoalveolar lavage	Gram stain, AFB smear, Papanicolaou stain, modified silver stain		Bacterial*, AFB, fungal	Viral	AFB, viral
Bronchial brush	Gram stain, Papanicolaou stain, modified silver stain	AFB smear	Bacterial*		
Trans bronchial biopsy	Hematoxylin and eosin stain, Gram stain, AFB smear, modified silver stain	Papanicolaou stain	Bacterial, AFB, fungal		
Trans bronchial needle aspirate	Gram stain, AFB smear, Papanicolaou stain, Modified silver stain			Bacterial, AFB, fungal	
Trans cutaneous needle aspirate	Gram stain, AFB smear, Papanicolaou stain, modified silver stain			Bacterial, AFB, fungal	
Open lung biopsy	Hematoxylin eosin stain, Gram stain, AFB smear, modified silver stain	Papanicolaou stain	AFB, fungal	Bacterial, viral	

PCR, polymerase chain reaction; AFB, acid fast bacilli.

*Semiquantitative culture.

or there is enough risk for future infection, that treatment is indicated.[34] The more intense the immunosuppression, the more likely *Aspergillus* is likely to be invasive.[35] The diagnosis of cryptococcal pneumonia in a normal host is associated with a low rate of dissemination. However, cryptococcal pneumonia in an immunocompromised host may lead to dissemination.[36,37]

Several types of respiratory samples may be obtained and are summarized in table 2. Sputum is the easiest and most commonly acquired respiratory sample. A good sputum sample may prove useful for directing initial therapy.[38] However, there are several well-known limitations of sputum sampling.[20,39] These include mixing of mouth and throat secretions with the lower respiratory sample. The amount of contamination of the lower respiratory secretion varies, with the production of more sputum leading to a better sampling. Also, the ability to expectorate the sputum is key, with some patients unable to provide a good lower respiratory sample. Frustration about obtaining a good respiratory sample can be summarized by the maxim offered by some patients that "nice women don't spit." Also, the patient who has a limited amount of lower respiratory secretions (nonproductive cough) can lead to inadequate sample. In this case, hypertonic saline may enhance the amount of lower respiratory secretions. Any expectorated sputum sample should be evaluated for adequacy. The presence of moderate number of squamous cells implies upper airway contamination. The presence of more than 25 neutrophils per low power field is consistent with purulent sputum. Figure 6 summarizes a prospective study of 533 patients with potential community-acquired pneumonia; only 40% had adequate sputum using Gram-stain criteria.[40]

Organism	% total
GPDC	48.8%
GNCB	16.9%
GPCC	6.1%
GNDC	4.2%
GNR	7.5%
No organism	4.2%
Mixed flora	12.2%

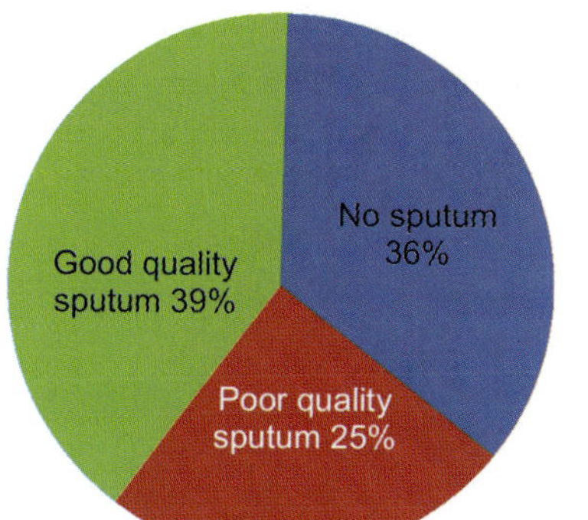

GPDCs, Gram-positive diplococci; GNCBs, Gram-negative coccobacilli; GPCCs, Gram-positive cocci in chains; GNDCs, Gram-negative diplococci; GNRs, Gram-negative rods.

FIGURE 6 The results of Gram stain analysis of sputum in 533 patients with suspected community-acquired pneumonia. The pie diagram demonstrates the overall results. The table gives the proportion of organisms seen in the Gram stain:

Source: Roson B, Carratala J, Verdaguer R, et al. Prospective study of the usefulness of sputum Gram stain in the initial approach to community-acquired pneumonia requiring hospitalization. *Clin Infect Dis.* 2000;31:869-74.

Of these in whom a pathogen was identified by Gram stain, subsequent cultures confirmed the presence of a pathogen in 71% of cases. Therefore, the overall value of Gram stain was 28%. Sputum analysis was most useful for patients with *S. pneumonia* and there was a significantly lower yield if the patient had been on prior antibiotic.

Sputum can also be examined for the presence of acid fast bacilli (AFB). A sample with an AFB positive organism has to be considered as positive, regardless of how inadequate the sample. However, confirmation of the type of organism which is AFB positive is key. There is a range of mycobacterium which can be found in the respiratory secretions, including *M. tuberculosis, M. kansasii,* as well as *M. avium* complex and other atypical mycobacteria. Also, several other microorganisms can be AFB positive, including nocardia and actinomycosis. Cultures and sometime polymerase chain reaction (PCR) can be useful in resolving this situation.[41]

One particular example of sputum examination is PcP. To date, pneumocystis cannot be cultured, so the presence of pneumocystis by smear can only be confirmed by immunohistochemistry or PCR.[42,43] In HIV-infected patients who have not received anti-PcP prophylaxis, the burden of pneumocystis can be quite high. In that situation, sputum examination has a high yield for positive samples. The yield can be enhanced by using immunofluorescent staining.[44] For the non-HIV patient, the pneumocystis burden is not nearly as high and sputum analysis is a much lower yield.[45] In that situation, false positive interpretation may also occur.

Bronchoscopy provides a range of samples from the lower respiratory tract. It has become the standard way to assess an immunocompromised patient with possible pneumonia.[46] There are a range of samples, as indicated in table 2. During any bronchoscopy, one collects bronchial secretions (bronchial washings) and these can be sent for routine bacterial, AFB, and fungal cultures. The bronchial wash sample is similar to sputum examination, since there can be upper airway contamination. Also, bronchial colonization may be present, with organisms in the airway which are not the cause of pneumonia. In most COPD patients not on antibiotics, the lower respiratory tract is not sterile and, therefore, a range of bacteria can be cultured, including normal pharyngeal flora.[47] The presence of these bacteria in the airway does not mean that these organisms are a cause of the pneumonia. However, the presence of bacteria in the airway is more likely to be the cause of pneumonia.

Using a protected specimen brush (PSB), one can obtain a relatively clean sample of the lower respiratory tract.[48] Using a semiquantitative culture, there is usually a 100-fold or greater concentration of bacteria in the lung sample versus the bronchial sample in patients with pneumonia.[49] The PSB provides a good sample for bacterial cultures and is more specific but less sensitive than the bronchoalveolar lavage sample.[50,51] Gram staining of the sample can also identify potential pathogens. The presence of intracellular organisms is a reliable indicator of infection.[50] Unfortunately, the volume of the PSB is limited and, therefore, AFB and fungal cultures as well as cytologic evaluation are not usually performed.

Examination of BAL fluid for infection was introduced in 1980s.[52] At the time, it was most commonly employed to diagnose pneumonia in HIV-infected patients.[53,54] However, it was also found to be useful in diagnosing infection in transplant patients.[3] Cytologic evaluation of the BAL specimen with Papanicolaou and silver staining can identify a variety of microorganisms including pneumocystis, fungal organisms, and viral changes.[55] The Gram stain can be used to identify bacteria. AFB can also be identified by appropriate staining. Most laboratories will use these stains routinely to evaluate the BAL sample. Additional stains are available for identification of pathogens. For patients with possible PcP, fluorescent antibody kits are available.[43,44] One can also use PCR to detect PcP, but this technique is usually applied when there is a low pneumocystis burden, such as in oral washings.[56] Bacteria can easily be cultured from fresh BAL samples. Several studies have demonstrated that the use of semiquantitative bacterial culture techniques can detect pneumonia, even in patients with airway colonization, such as occuring during mechanical ventilation.[20,50,57] The use of the semiquantitative culture allows one to determine the probability of a recovered pathogen being the cause of pneumonia. For example, *S. pneumonia* recovered at 10–100,000 colony forming units cfu/mL of BAL fluid has a 50-50 chance of being just colonization, while if it is recovered at more than 100,000 cfu/mL it has a more than 95% chance of being the cause of pneumonia. Likewise, if recovered at less than 1,000 cfu/mL BAL fluid, it is unlikely to be the cause of pneumonia.[20] There are some modifications of this interpretation. The recovery of diphtheroids, even at high concentrations, may only represent airway contamination.[57] Also, the presence of intracellular organisms on Gram stain of the BAL sample further enhances the specificity of the diagnosis of pneumonia.[50] In ventilator-associated pneumonia, it was found that failure to treat bacteria recovered at more than 10,000 cfu/mL BAL fluid was associated with an increased mortality.[58,59] Viral cultures can also be done of the BAL sample, but semiquantitative cultures have not been routinely applied. The most common viruses identified are CMV, other herpes viruses, adeno virus, and influenza.[60]

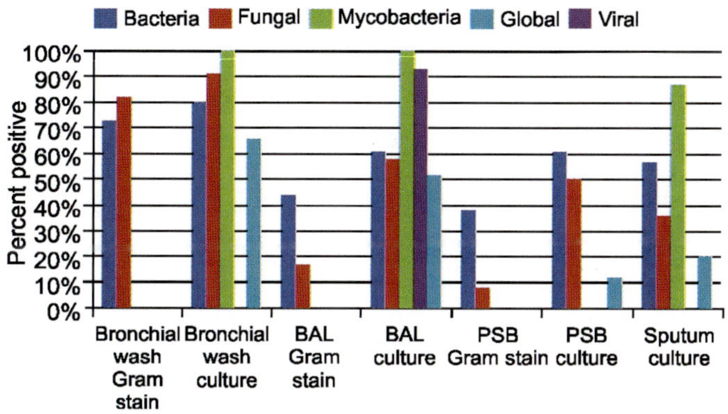

FIGURE 7 The comparative yield of bronchial wash, bronchoalveolar lavage (BAL), protected specimen brush (PSB), and sputum for various types of pathogens in immunosuppressed patients undergoing evaluation at one institution.[46]

Bronchial washings provide a sample that is a mixture of secretions from the airways and lower lung. As such, it can be contaminated by upper respiratory flora. Therefore, bacteria which could be colonizing the upper respiratory tract are easily recovered from bronchial washings. Since the amount of upper airway contamination varies, the use of semiquantitative cultures is not a useful way to correct for this contamination. On the other hand, the broad sampling of bronchial washings versus the targeted sampling of BAL makes the recovery of tuberculosis higher for bronchial washing than BAL.[61]

Figure 7 compares the relative yield of the various bronchoscopic procedures for a group of immunosuppressed patients evaluated at one institution.[46] The overall yield for BAL and bronchial wash was higher than 50%, while it was significantly lower for sputum and PSB. In this study, bronchial washes were routine cultured for bacteria and no semiquantitation was performed. Therefore the sensitivity for bronchial wash was high, but the specificity was low. The authors did not report on PcP. It has been shown that BAL has a higher yield for PcP than bronchial wash.[43]

Needle aspirate provides a small sample, usually for cytology. The use of endobronchial ultrasound has allowed for directed sampling of lymph nodes. While this technique is not usually used in evaluating possible pneumonia in the transplant patient, it may prove useful if new adenopathy is part of the pattern seen on chest imaging. The technique can be useful to detect tuberculosis, fungal infection, and malignancy.[62] The technique can also be used to sample non-lymph node thoracic lesions.[63]

Bronchial and transbronchial biopsy are also useful in identifying pathologic changes. For the most part, cultures are not done of the biopsy samples because of contamination of the sample as it is withdrawn through the channel of the bronchoscope. However, cultures for tuberculosis and fungus may still be of value. The tissue can also be studied with PCR for specific organisms.

Larger samples of lung tissue can be obtained surgically by either open lung biopsy or video-assisted thoracoscopy. While the samples are less likely to be contaminated by routine bacteria than biopsy samples obtained via bronchoscopy, there is still some contamination. These large sample biopsies provide more definitive diagnosis of pneumonia.[64] However, the histologic examination may still fail to recover a specific pathogen. In most cases, this may be because of preceding and ongoing antibiotic therapy. The surgical biopsy may lead to more directed therapy in a significant proportion of patients.[65,66] For many patients, the recovery of a pathogen in the open lung sample does not change the clinical outcome of the patient.[67] This is in part because the most important factor in treating pneumonia is the shortest duration of time onset of pneumonia to appropriate therapy. In cases in whom adequate treatment is delayed by more than 2 days, the mortality is higher.[58,59]

Common Pathogens

Bacteria: The most common identified cause of pneumonia remains bacterial infection. Almost all pneumonias in transplant patients represent a HCAP.[10] This is because of the underlying immunosuppression, repeat hospitalizations prior to pneumonia, and the routine use of prophylactic antibiotics, which selects for resistant bacteria. The most common bacteria reported are MRSA and Gram-negative bacteria.[19,22,23,68] This is in part because invasive testing, such as bronchoscopy, is usually reserved until after initial empiric therapy has been given. The patient with routine bacterial pneumonia tends to have localized rather than diffuse infiltrates. Since many of the other pathogens tend to cause diffuse infiltrates, the patient who presents with a localized infiltrate can be assumed to have a bacterial infection until proven otherwise. In HCAP, the use of aggressive empiric therapy may reduce morbidity and mortality. The recommendations are, therefore, to begin empiric broad spectrum therapy and to deescalate once a pathogen has been identified (if possible).[69] For the transplant patients there are specific pathogens that need to be considered.

Legionella pneumophila is much more common in SOT patients than the general population.[15] The timing of *Legionella* is usually late summer, but outbreaks can occur at other times. The diagnosis can be made with PCR and fluorescent antibody.[70,71] In addition, *Legionella* can be grown from BAL specimens, but that will take several days.[72] Nocardia is similarly more common in SOTs.[16,17] It can be identified by AFB smear, but often is not confirmed until cultures are available.

Virus: The most important post-transplant viral infection is CMV.[22,73,74] In addition, CMV load appears to correlate with long-term outcome.[75] In lung transplantation, CMV infection is related to development of bronchiolitis obliterans.[76] Most middle age adults have been infected with CMV. Therefore, transplant patients can acquire CMV infection either by reactivation of latent virus in the host or new infection from the CMV from the graft into the CMV-naïve host.[77] The mode of infection leads a different prognosis, since reactivation of CMV has a much better prognosis than new infection. For many transplant candidates, prior CMV infection has occurred at the time of evaluation. One of the major methods for transmission of CMV is through blood products. In a transplant candidate who is CMV negative, one can use CMV negative blood products and, therefore, avoid altogether the risk of CMV infection.[78]

Cytomegalovirus recovered from the lung is associated with a range of manifestations, from no symptoms to respiratory failure and death.[79] In HIV-infected patients, recovery is associated with level of immunosuppression, with CMV more likely present in the more immunosuppressed patient. In studies trying to evaluate the impact of CMV infection in HIV patients with possible pneumonia, it appears that CMV does not change the natural course of the HIV condition.[80,81] However, CMV is a marker for increased short-term mortality,[82,83] especially those with PcP.[83] The recovery of CMV from a transplant is associated with morbidity and increased mortality.[18,84] Early treatment with antiviral therapy is associated with improved survival.[85,86] Appropriate use of prophylactic antiviral therapy also reduces the risk of developing respiratory symptoms.[86]

Because of the importance of CMV, several methods have been employed to detect CMV in bronchoscopy samples. These include using PCR, immune fluorescent, and rapid shell viral cultures.[70,87] These techniques are quite sensitive to the presence of CMV. As noted above, the presence of CMV does not always mean CMV-associated disease. Cytopathic changes can be seen with CMV and are diagnostic of disease ("owl's eye").[88] These can be seen in examination of BAL samples or in biopsy samples. While more specific, they are not as sensitive.

The use of BAL and nasal washings has been useful in detecting known pathogens, such as influenza and RSV.[89] In evaluating SCT, it has become clear that viruses other than CMV and influenza may cause pneumonia (Figure 2).[26,68] Detection of viral infection can be enhanced by using PCR, and viral loads can be determined.[26]

Fungal infections: Aspergillus remains an important fungal infection encountered in both SCT and SOTs.[70,74] The fungus is commonly encountered in the real world, so infection and colonization often occurs. Outbreaks of *Aspergillus* have been documented to occur within medical centers when construction is occurring.[90,91] These outbreaks can have major impact on transplant centers. Use of prophylactic amphotericin[90] or azoles[92] as well as high-efficiency particulate absorption filters[90,91] have been shown to reduce the rate of infection. Detection of *Aspergillus* can be made with routine cytology as well as PCR.[34,93] Detection of galactomannan in BAL has been reported as superior to PCR in detecting *Aspergillus*.[94] Subsequent studies have demonstrated that measurement of galactomannan in BAL is useful in detection of invasive *Aspergillus*.[95,96] Antigen detection has also proved useful in detecting other fungal such as *Histoplasma capsulatum* and *Cryptococcus neofromans*.[37,97,98]

Pneumocystis jirovecii is a fungal infection which has been associated with significant morbidity and mortality in transplant patients.[11] In the 1980s, there was a marked increase in the number of cases of PcP diagnosed in many transplant centers. A major cause appeared to be the high number of cases of PcP being diagnosed in AIDS patients.[53,54] Epidemiologic studies supported the transmission of *P. jirovecii* from HIV-infected patients to SOT patients.[99] Also clusters of PcP were observed in transplant units.[100] Genetic analysis of PcP cases identified that patients could have relapse of disease or reinfection with a new strain of *P. jirovecci*.[101] In one report of a cluster of 27 cases PcP in a transplant center, molecular analysis found that all cases were due to the same strain of *P. jiroveci* and human to human contact were documented in 22 cases.[102]

Prophylaxis

A major impact on the rate of pneumonia in transplant patients has been the use of prophylaxis regimens to prevent infection. Table 3 summarizes the approach to prophylaxis for the major infections encountered after transplant.[1,103] Prophylaxis regimens have been made for HSCT and SOT, but are also used for other transplants, including stem cell ocular transplants.[104] The prophylaxis recommendations are based on the effectiveness of these treatment schedules in treating and preventing infection. Most of these recommendations are based on experiences in transplant populations, but in some cases are based on experiences in other at risk groups, such as HIV infected or chemotherapy-induced neutropenic patients.

As noted above, PcP had been a major cause of morbidity and mortality in transplant patients in the past.

TABLE 3
Prophylaxis to prevent pneumonia in transplant patients

Organism	Usual prophylaxis	Alternative prophylaxis	Solid organ	Stem cell
Pneumocystis jiroveci	Trim sulfa	• Inhaled pentamidine (monthly) • Dapsone • Atovaquone	First 6–12 months	6 months after HCT Continue prophylaxis beyond 6 months for the duration of immune suppression
Cytomegalovirus	Ganciclovir	Valganciclovir*	First 6–12 months	From engraftment until at least 100 days
Herpes virus	• Acyclovir • Valacyclovir		Prior infection	Prior infection
Aspergillus spp.	• Inhaled nebulized amphotericin B • Imidazoles (itraconazole, voriconazole)	Caspofungin	During hospitalization	From the start of conditioning/transplant until engraftment (i.e., approximately 30 days after HCT) or until 7 days after the absolute neutrophil count >1,000 cells/mm^3
Candida spp.	• Clotrimazole (topical, troches) Ketoconazole (oral, IV)†	Other imidazole	During hospitalization	During prolonged neutropenia

HCT, hematopoietic cell transplantation; IV, intravenous.
*Use only for ganciclovir resistant cytomegalovirus.
†Not needed if other imidazoles active against Aspergillus are being given.
Source Baughman RP, Meyer KC, Nathanson I, et al. Monitoring of nonsteroidal immunosuppressive drugs in patients with lung disease and lung transplant recipients: american college of chest physicians evidence-based clinical practice guidelines. *Chest.* 2012;142:e1S-e111S.
Center for International Blood and Marrow Transplant Research (CIBMTR), National Marrow Donor Program (NMDP), European Blood and Marrow Transplant Group (EBMT), et al. Guidelines for preventing infectious complications among hematopoietic cell transplant recipients: a global perspective. *Bone Marrow Transplant.* 2009;44:453-558.

However, the reported rate has dropped considerably, although outbreaks of PcP still do occur.[102] For example, one center found the rate of PcP fell from 33% of cases of pneumonia in their transplant patients during the years of 1992–1996 to 8% for the years 1997–2003.[79] The drop in rate of PcP has been attributed to the use of prophylaxis regimens, usually with trimethoprim/sulfamethoxazole (trim/sulfa). Therefore, use of PcP prophylaxis is recommended after SOT. However, not all centers now use PcP prophylaxis.[24] This is because the information regarding effectiveness of PcP prophylaxis is not as robust in the transplant population as it is in the AIDS population. In AIDS patients, trim/sulfa prophylaxis is clearly effective in those with CD4 count of less than 200 cells/mm^3.[105] While trim/sulfa may lead to renal dysfunction and neutropenia, it is not clear how frequently this is encountered with prophylaxis doses.[106] Alternatives, such as atovaquone and aerosolized pentamidine have been used as prophylaxis agents.[107-109] While these agents may have some benefit, trim/sulfa appears to be the most effective.[110,111] In one renal transplant center, analysis of prior cases of PcP led to a proposed targeted approach of prophylaxis to limit prophylaxis only for the first 6 months post-transplant and for a year in those more than 55 years age.[25] The risk of PcP increases the more intense the immunosuppression and with the use of corticosteroids.[112]

The uses of acyclovir, ganciclovir, and valacyclovir have all been shown to reduce the rate of symptomatic CMV pneumonitis in HSCT.[86,113,114] The recommended duration of prophylaxis varies depending on the type of HSCT.[1] In SOT, CMV prophylaxis is commonly used but the duration ranges from 3 months to indefinite.[115] There has been concern about toxicity from the medications and development resistance. In a prospective study of oral valganciclovir treatment as CMV prophylaxis in lung transplant patients, there was a significant reduction in the rate of CMV pneumonia associated with 12 months versus 3 months of therapy without any increased resistance or medication toxicity.[116]

Noninfectious Causes of Pulmonary Disease

Patients may develop respiratory symptoms and infiltrates for noninfectious reasons. In HSCT, this may be the result of DAH.[117] This condition was considered the cause of respiratory event in 5–18% of patients in various series.[19,27,28] DAH can be diagnosed by BAL, with the presence of blood in the latter portion of the BAL process a visual clue of DAH.[118] The diagnosis can be confirmed by identifying a high proportion of hemosiderin laden macrophages in the BAL sample.[119] In SOT, DAH may be seen as a result of toxicity from drugs, such as sirolimus and everolimus.[120,121]

In HSCT, noninfectious lung injury can lead to an idiopathic pneumonia syndrome (IPS).[122] This syndrome has a specific definition (Table 4).[122,123] The diagnosis relies heavily on ruling out other causes, especially infection. While initial encounter in 3–15% of HSCT, the rate of IPS is not nearly as high when nonmyeloablative conditioning is used.[124] However, the condition is still associated with significant mortality.[122,124] Even with recovery, the patient may have severe persistent fibrosis and bronchiolitis.[125]

TABLE 4

Definition of idiopathic pneumonia syndrome

I: Evidence of widespread alveolar injury:

- Multilobar infiltrates on routine chest radiographs or computed tomography
- Symptoms and signs of pneumonia (cough, dyspnea, tachypnea, and rales)
- Evidence of abnormal pulmonary physiology
  - Increased alveolar to arterial oxygen difference
  - New or increased restrictive pulmonary function test abnormality

II: Absence of active lower respiratory tract infection based upon:

- Bronchoalveolar lavage negative for significant bacterial pathogens including acid-fast bacilli, *Nocardia*, and *Legionella* species
- Bronchoalveolar lavage negative for pathogenic nonbacterial microorganisms:
  - Routine culture for viruses and fungi
  - Shell vial culture for CMV and respiratory RSV
  - Cytology for CMV inclusions, fungi, and *Pneumocystis jirovecii* (carinii)
  - Direct fluorescence staining with antibodies against CMV, RSV, HSV,VZV, influenza virus, parainfluenza virus, adenovirus, and other organisms
- Other organisms/tests to also consider:
  - Polymerase chain reaction for human metapneumovirus, rhinovirus, coronavirus, and HHV6
  - Polymerase chain reaction for *Chlamydia*, *Mycoplasma*, and *Aspergillus* species
  - Serum galactomannan ELISA for *Aspergillus* species
  - Transbronchial biopsy if condition of the patient permits

III: Absence of cardiac dysfunction, acute renal failure, or iatrogenic fluid overload as etiology for pulmonary dysfunction

CMV, cytomegalovirus; HSV, herpes simplex virus; RSV, respiratory syncytial virus; CMV, cytomegalovirus; RSV, respiratory syncytial virus; HSV, herpes simplex virus; VZV, varicella–zoster virus; HHV6, human herpesvirus 6; ELISA, enzyme-linked immunosorbent assay.

Source: Panoskaltsis-Mortari A, Griese M, Madtes DK, et al. An official American Thoracic Society research statement: noninfectious lung injury after hematopoietic stem cell transplantation: idiopathic pneumonia syndrome. *Am J Respir Crit Care Med.* 2011;183:1262-79.
Clark JG, Hansen JA, Hertz MI, et al. NHLBI workshop summary. Idiopathic pneumonia syndrome after bone marrow transplantation. *Am Rev Respir Dis.* 1993;147:1601-6.

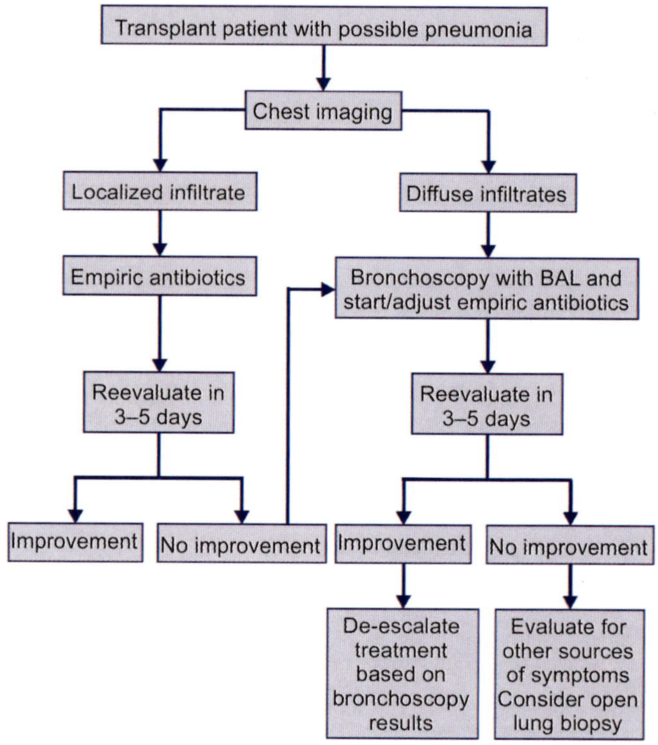

FIGURE 8 Approach to transplant patient with possible pneumonia. Initial evaluation includes chest imaging. If a patient has localized infiltrate, initial therapy with empiric antibiotics based on patient's risk for bacterial infections is appropriate. For the patient with diffuse infiltrate or with localized infiltrate who fails to improve within 3–5 days, bronchoscopy with bronchoalveolar lavage should be considered. After 3–5 days, patient should be evaluated for response to treatment as well as for consideration of de-escalating empiric therapy based on bronchoscopy and other tests.

Approach to Diagnosis and Therapy

An overall approach to diagnosis of treatment of possible pneumonia in transplant patients is shown in figure 8. This figure provides a general approach and should be modified based on patient's individual risk factors. Initial evaluation should include chest imaging. This will determine whether pneumonia is localized or diffuse.[126] For those with localized infiltrate, an empiric antibiotic approach may be an appropriate first step.[10] However, in a patient with diffuse infiltrate, bronchoscopy with BAL should be considered. While this will provide a good sample, the results will not be available for 48–72 hours. Empiric therapy of potential pathogens should be initiated, since delay of appropriate therapy for pneumonia has been associated with increased mortality.[58,59,127] Also, early bronchoscopy is associated with a higher yield of pathogens.[19]

REFERENCES

1. Center for International Blood and Marrow Transplant Research (CIBMTR), National Marrow Donor Program (NMDP), European Blood and Marrow Transplant Group (EBMT), et al. Guidelines for preventing infectious complications among hematopoietic cell transplant recipients: a global perspective. *Bone Marrow Transplant.* 2009;44:453-558.
2. Larsson K, Lonnqvist B, Ringden O, et al. CMV retinitis after allogeneic bone marrow transplantation: a report of five cases. *Transpl Infect Dis.* 2002;4:75-9.
3. Sternberg RI, Baughman RP, Dohn MN, et al. Utility of bronchoalveolar lavage in assessing pneumonia in immunosuppressed renal transplant recipients. *Am J Med.* 1993;95:358-64.
4. Fernandez-Ruiz M, Lopez-Medrano F, Romo EM, et al. Pretransplant lymphocyte count predicts the incidence of infection during the first two years after liver transplantation. *Liver Transpl.* 2009;15:1209-16.
5. De SA, Meachery G, Hester KL, et al. Lung transplantation for patients with cystic fibrosis and Burkholderia cepacia complex infection: a single-center experience. *J Heart Lung Transplant.* 2009;29:1395-404.
6. Samano MN, Pego-Fernandes PM, Fonseca Ribeiro AK, et al. Lung transplantation in patients with cystic fibrosis. Transplant Proc. 2013;45:1137-41.
7. Baughman RP, Keeton DA, Perez C, et al. Use of bronchoalveolar lavage semiquantitative cultures in cystic fibrosis. *Am J Respir Crit Care Med.* 1997;156:286-91.
8. Seddon PK, Fidler S, Raman H, et al. Prevalence of nontuberculous mycobacteria in cystic fibrosis clinics, United kingdom, 2009. *Emerg Infect Dis.* 2013;19:1128-30.
9. Middleton PG, Chen SC, Meyer W. Fungal infections and treatment in cystic fibrosis. *Curr Opin Pulm Med.* 2013;19:670-5.
10. Kollef MH, Morrow LE, Baughman RP, et al. Health care-associated pneumonia (HCAP): a critical appraisal to improve identification, management, and outcomes--proceedings of the HCAP Summit. *Clin Infect Dis.* 2008;46 Suppl 4:S296-334; quiz 335-8.:S296-S334.
11. Goto N, Oka S. Pneumocystis jirovecii pneumonia in kidney transplantation. *Transpl Infect Dis.* 2011;13:551-8.
12. Radisic MR, Lattes JF, Chapman RM, et al. Risk factors for Pneumocystis carinii pneumonia in kidney transplant recipients: a case-control study. *Transpl Infect Dis.* 2003;5:84-93.
13. Arend SM, Westendorp RG, Kroon FP, et al. Rejection treatment and cytomegalovirus infection as risk factors for Pneumocystis carinii pneumonia in renal transplant recipients. *Clin Infect Dis.* 1996;22:920-5.
14. Zhang XF, Lv Y, Xue WJ, et al. Mycobacterium tuberculosis infection in solid organ transplant recipients: experience from a single center in China. *Transplant Proc.* 2008;40:1382-5.
15. Mazieri NA, de Godoy CV, Alves SF, et al. Legionnaires' disease in the renal transplant unit of "Hospital das Clinicas, FMUSP". During a five year period (1988-1993). 1994. *Rev Inst Med Trop Sao Paulo.* 1994;36:231-6.
16. Wilson JP, Turner HR, Kirchner KA, et al. Nocardial infections in renal transplant recipients. *Medicine (Baltimore).* 1989;68:38-57.
17. Khan BA, Duncan M, Reynolds J, et al. Nocardia infection in lung transplant recipients. *Clin Transplant.* 2008;22:562-6.
18. Reis MA, Costa RS, Ferraz AS. Causes of death in renal transplant recipients: a study of 102 autopsies from 1968 to 1991. *J R Soc Med.* 1995;88:24-7.
19. Shannon VR, Andersson BS, Lei X, et al. Utility of early versus late fiberoptic bronchoscopy in the evaluation of new pulmonary infiltrates following hematopoietic stem cell transplantation. *Bone Marrow Transplant.* 2010;45:647-55.
20. Thorpe JE, Baughman RP, Frame PT, et al. Bronchoalveolar lavage for diagnosing acute bacterial pneumonia. *J Infect Dis.* 1987;155:855-61.
21. Torres A, El-Ebiary M. Bronchoscopic BAL in the diagnosis of ventilator-associated pneumonia. *Chest.* 2000;117:198S-202S.
22. Forslow U, Remberger M, Nordlander A, et al. The clinical importance of bronchoalveolar lavage in allogeneic SCT patients with pneumonia. *Bone Marrow Transplant.* 2010;45:945-50.
23. Hoyo I, Linares L, Cervera C, et al. Epidemiology of pneumonia in kidney transplantation. *Transplant Proc.* 2010;42:2938-40.
24. Sarwar S, Carey B, Hegarty JE, et al. Low incidence of Pneumocystis jirovecii pneumonia in an unprophylaxed liver transplant cohort. *Transpl Infect Dis.* 2013;15(5):510-5.
25. de Boer MG, Kroon FP, le CS, et al. Risk factors for Pneumocystis jirovecii pneumonia in kidney transplant recipients and appraisal of strategies for selective use of chemoprophylaxis. *Transpl Infect Dis.* 2011;13:559-69.
26. Campbell AP, Chien JW, Kuypers J, et al. Respiratory virus pneumonia after hematopoietic cell transplantation (HCT): associations between viral load in bronchoalveolar lavage samples, viral RNA detection in serum samples, and clinical outcomes of HCT. *J Infect Dis.* 2010;201: 1404-13.
27. Huaringa AJ, Leyva FJ, Signes-Costa J, Morice RC, et al. Bronchoalveolar lavage in the diagnosis of pulmonary complications of bone marrow transplant patients. *Bone Marrow Transplant.* 2000;25:975-9.
28. Hofmeister C, Czerlanis CC, Forsythe S, et al. Retrospective utility of bronchoscopy after hematopoietic stem cell transplant. *Bone Marrow Transplant.* 2006;38:693-98.
29. Mabie M, Wunderink RG. Use and limitations of clinical and radiologic diagnosis of pneumonia. *Semin Respir Infect.* 2003;18:72-9.
30. Fine MJ, Smith MA, Carson CA, et al. Prognosis and outcomes of patients with community-acquired pneumonia. A meta-analysis. *JAMA.* 1996;275:134-41.
31. Qin J, Xu J, Dong Y, . High-resolution CT findings of pulmonary infections after orthotopic liver transplantation in 453 patients. *Br J Radiol.* 2012;85:e959-e965.

32. Cox J, DeMasi AJ, McCollom S, et al. The diagnostic utility of routine chest radiography in the evaluation of the initial fever in patients undergoing hematopoietic stem cell. *Pediatr Blood Cancer.* 2011;57:666-8.
33. Gulati MR, Kaur V, Jha N, et al. High-resolution CT in renal transplant patients with suspected pulmonary infections. *Acta Radiol.* 2000;41:37-241.
34. Sherif R, Segal BH. Pulmonary aspergillosis: clinical presentation, diagnostic tests, management and complications. *Curr Opin Pulm Med.* 2010;16:242-50.
35. Morgan JK, Wannemuehler A, Marr KA, et al. Incidence of invasive aspergillosis following hematopoietic stem cell and solid organ transplantation: interim results of a prospective multicenter surveillance program. *Med Mycol.* 2005;43 Suppl 1:S49-58.:S49-S58.
36. Kerkering TM, Duma RJ, Shadomy S. The evolution of pulmonary cryptococcosis: clinical implications from a study of 41 patients with and without compromising host factors. *Ann Intern Med.* 1981;94:611-6.
37. Baughman RP, Rhodes JC, Dohn MN, et al. Detection of cryptococcal antigen in bronchoalveolar lavage fluid: a prospective study of diagnostic utility. *Am Rev Respir Dis.* 1992;145:1226-9.
38. Anevlavis S, Petroglou N, Tzavaras A, et al. A prospective study of the diagnostic utility of sputum Gram stain in pneumonia. *J Infect.* 2009;59:83-9.
39. Skerrett SJ. Diagnostic testing to establish a microbial cause is helpful in the management of community-acquired pneumonia. *Semin Respir Infect.* 1997;12:308-21.
40. Roson B, Carratala J, Verdaguer R, et al. Prospective study of the usefulness of sputum Gram stain in the initial approach to community-acquired pneumonia requiring hospitalization. *Clin Infect Dis.* 2000;31:869-74.
41. Chia JH, Wu TH, Su LH, et al. Direct identification of mycobacteria from smear-positive sputum samples using an improved multiplex polymerase chain reaction assay. *Diagn Microbiol Infect Dis.* 2012;72:340-9.
42. Huang SN, Fischer SH, 'Shaughnessy EO, et al. Development of a PCR assay for diagnosis of Pneumocystis carinii pneumonia based on amplification of the multicopy major surface glycoprotein gene family. *Diagn Microbiol Infect Dis.* 1999;35:27-32.
43. Baughman RP, Strohofer SS, Clinton BA, et al. The use of an indirect fluorescent antibody test for detecting Pneumocystis carinii. *Arch Pathol Lab Med.* 1989;113:1062-5.
44. Levine SJ, Kennedy D, Shelhamer JH, , et al. Diagnosis of Pneumocystis carinii pneumonia by multiple lobe, site-directed bronchoalveolar lavage with immunofluorescent monoclonal antibody staining in human immuno-deficiency virus-infected patients receiving aerosolized pentamidine chemoprophylaxis. *Am Rev Respir Dis.* 1992;146:838-43.
45. Limper AH, Offord KP, Smith TF, et al. Pneumocystis carinii pneumonia. Differences in lung parasite number and inflammation in patients with and without AIDS. *Am Rev Respir Dis.* 1989;140:1204-9.
46. Danes C, Gonzalez-Martin J, Pumarola T, et al. Pulmonary infiltrates in immunosuppressed patients: analysis of a diagnostic protocol. *J Clin Microbiol.* 2002;40:2134-40.
47. Soler N, Torres A, Ewig S, et al. Bronchial microbial patterns in severe exacerbations of chronic obstructive pulmonary disease (COPD) requiring mechanical ventilation. *Am J Respir Crit Care Med.* 1998;157:1498-505.
48. Wimberley N, Faling LJ, Bartlett JG. A fiberoptic bronchoscopy technique to obtain uncontaminated lower airway secretions for bacterial culture. *Am Rev Respir Dis.* 1979;119:337-43.
49. Baughman RP, Thorpe JE, Staneck J, et al. Use of the protected specimen brush in patients with endotracheal or tracheostomy tubes. *Chest.* 1987;91:233-6.
50. Chastre J, Fagon JY, Soler P, et al. Diagnosis of nosocomial bacterial pneumonia in intubated patients undergoing ventilation: comparison of the usefulness of bronchoalveolar lavage and the protected specimen brush. *Am J Med.* 1988;85:499-506.
51. Baughman RP. Ventilator-associated pneumonia: use of protected brush technique. *Chest.* 2000;117:203S-6S.
52. Stover DE, Zaman MB, Hajdu SI, et al. Bronchoalveolar lavage in the diagnosis of diffuse pulmonary infiltrates in the immunosuppressed host. *Ann Intern Med.* 1984;101:1-7.
53. Baughman RP, Dohn MN, Frame PT. The continuing utility of bronchoalveolar lavage to diagnose opportunistic infection in AIDS patients. *Am J Med.* 1994;97:515-22.
54. Ognibene FP, Shelhamer J, Gill V, et al. The diagnosis of Pneumocystis carinii pneumonia in patients with the acquired immunodeficiency syndrome using subsegmental bronchoalveolar lavage. *Am Rev Respir Dis.* 1984; 129:929-32.
55. Armbruster C, Pokieser L, Hassl A. Diagnosis of Pneumocystis carinii pneumonia by bronchoalveolar lavage in AIDS patients. Comparison of Diff-Quik, fungifluor stain, direct immunofluorescence test and polymerase chain reaction. *Acta Cytol.* 1995;39:1089-93.
56. Fischer S, Gill VJ, Kovacs J, et al. The use of oral washes to diagnose Pneumocystis carinii pneumonia: a blinded prospective study using a polymerase chain reaction-based detection system. *J Infect Dis.* 2001;184:1485-8.
57. Cantral DE, Tape TG, Reed EC, et al. Quantitative culture of bronchoalveolar lavage fluid for the diagnosis of bacterial pneumonia. *Am J Med.* 1993;95:601-7.
58. Kollef MH, Bock KR, Richards RD, et al. The safety and diagnostic accuracy of minibronchoalveolar lavage in patients with suspected ventilator-associated pneumonia. *Ann Intern Med 1995. 1996;*122:743-8.
59. Luna CM, Vujacich P, Niederman MS, et al. Impact of BAL data on the therapy and outcome of ventilator-associated pneumonia. *Chest.* 1997;111:676-85.
60. Connolly MG, Baughman P, Dohn MN, et al. Recovery of viruses other than cytomegalovirus from bronchoalveolar lavage fluid [see comments]. *Chest.* 1994;105:1775-81.
61. Baughman RP, Dohn MN, Loudon RG, et al. Bronchoscopy with bronchoalveolar lavage in tuberculosis and fungal infections. *Chest.* 1991;99:92-7.
62. Navani N, Molyneaux PL, Breen RA, et al. Utility of endobronchial ultrasound-guided transbronchial needle aspiration in patients with tuberculous intrathoracic lymphadenopathy: a multicentre study. *Thorax.* 2011;66: 889-93.
63. Yang H, Zhao H, Garfield DH, et al. Endobronchial ultrasound-guided transbronchial needle aspiration in the

diagnosis of non-lymph node thoracic lesions. *Ann Thorac Med.* 2013;8:14-21.

64. Chastre J, Fagon JY, Bornet-Lecso M, et al. Evaluation of bronchoscopic techniques for the diagnosis of nosocomial pneumonia. *Am J Respir Crit Care Med.* 1995;152:231-40.
65. Weill D, McGiffin DC, Zorn GL, et al. The utility of open lung biopsy following lung transplantation. *J Heart Lung Transplant.* 2000;19:852-7.
66. Wang JY, Chang YL, Lee LN, et al. Diffuse pulmonary infiltrates after bone marrow transplantation: the role of open lung biopsy. *Ann Thorac Surg.* 2004;78:267-72.
67. Hayes-Jordan A, Benaim E, Richardson S, et alet al. Open lung biopsy in pediatric bone marrow transplant patients. *J Pediatr Surg.* 2002;37:446-52.
68. Lehto JT, Koskinen PK, Anttila VJ, et al. Bronchoscopy in the diagnosis and surveillance of respiratory infections in lung and heart-lung transplant recipients. *Transpl Int.* 2005;18:562-71.
69. American Thoracic Society; Infectious Diseases Society of America. Guidelines for the management of adults with hospital-acquired, ventilator-associated, and healthcare-associated pneumonia. *Am J Respir Crit Care Med.* 2005;171:388-416.
70. Hohenthal U, Itala M, Salonen J, et al. Bronchoalveolar lavage in immunocompromised patients with haematological malignancy--value of new microbiological methods. *Eur J Haematol.* 2005;74:203-11.
71. Sethi S, Gore MT, Sethi KK. Increased sensitivity of a direct fluorescent antibody test for Legionella pneumophila in bronchoalveolar lavage samples by immunomagnetic separation based on BioMags. *J Microbiol Methods.* 2007; 70:328-35.
72. Hayden RT, Uhl JR, Qian X, et al. Direct detection of Legionella species from bronchoalveolar lavage and open lung biopsy specimens: comparison of LightCycler PCR, in situ hybridization, direct fluorescence antigen detection, and culture. *J Clin Microbiol.* 2001;39:2618-26.
73. Schlischewsky E, Fuehner T, Warnecke G, et al. Clinical significance of quantitative cytomegalovirus detection in bronchoalveolar lavage fluid in lung transplant recipients. *Transpl Infect Dis.* 2013;15:60-9.
74. Lease ED, Zaas DW. Update on infectious complications following lung transplantation. *Curr Opin Pulm Med.* 2001;17:206-9.
75. Chemaly RF, Yen-Lieberman B, Chapman J, et al. Clinical utility of cytomegalovirus viral load in bronchoalveolar lavage in lung transplant recipients. *Am J Transplant.* 2005;5:544-8.
76. Snyder LD, Finlen-Copeland CA, Turbyfill WJ, et al. Cytomegalovirus pneumonitis is a risk for bronchiolitis obliterans syndrome in lung transplantation. *Am J Respir Crit Care Med.* 2010;181:1391-6.
77. Atabani SF, Smith C, Atkinson C, et al. Cytomegalovirus replication kinetics in solid organ transplant recipients managed by preemptive therapy. *Am J Transplant.* 2012;12:2457-64.
78. Nichols WG, Price TH, Gooley T, et al. Transfusion-transmitted cytomegalovirus infection after receipt of leukoreduced blood products. *Blood.* 2003;101:4195-200.
79. Joos L, Chhajed PN, Wallner J, et al. Pulmonary infections diagnosed by BAL: a 12-year experience in 1066 immunocompromised patients. *Respir Med.* 2007;101:93-7.
80. Miles PR, Baughman RP, Linnemann CC. Cytomegalovirus in the bronchoalveolar lavage fluid of patients with AIDS. *Chest.* 1990;97:1072-6.
81. Mann M, Shelhamer JH, Masur H, et al. Lack of clinical utility of bronchoalveolar lavage cultures for cytomegalovirus in HIV infection. *Am J Respir Crit Care Med.* 1997;155:1723-8.
82. Hayner CE, Baughman RP, Linnemann CC, et al. The relationship between cytomegalovirus retrieved by bronchoalveolar lavage and mortality in patients with HIV. *Chest.* 1995;107:735-40.
83. Benfield TL, Helweg-Larsen J, Bang D, et al. Prognostic markers of short-term mortality in AIDS-associated Pneumocystis carinii pneumonia. *Chest.* 2001;119:844-51.
84. Kerschner H, Jaksch P, Karigl G, et al. Cytomegalovirus DNA load patterns developing after lung transplantation are significantly correlated with long-term patient survival. *Transplantation.* 2009;87:1720-6.
85. Goodrich JM, Mori M, Gleaves CA, et al. Early treatment with ganciclovir to prevent cytomegalovirus disease after allogeneic bone marrow transplantation. *N Engl J Med.* 1991;325:1601-7.
86. Winston DJ, Ho WG, Bartoni K, et al. Ganciclovir prophylaxis of cytomegalovirus infection and disease in allogeneic bone marrow transplant recipients. Results of a placebo-controlled, double-blind trial. *Ann Intern Med.* 1993;118:179-84.
87. Costa C, Libertucci D, Solidoro P, et al. Rapid shell vial culture for the detection of respiratory viruses from bronchoalveolar lavage in immunocompromised patients. *Panminerva Med.* 2007;49:1-6.
88. Lemert CM, Baughman RP, Hayner CE, et al. Relationship between cytomegalovirus cells and survival in acquired immunodeficiency syndrome patients. *Acta Cytol.* 1996;40:205-10.
89. Connolly MG, Baughman RP, Dohn MN, et al. Recovery of viruses other than cytomegalovirus from bronchoalveolar lavage fluid. *Chest.* 1994;105:1775-81.
90. Oren I, Haddad N, Finkelstein R, et al. Invasive pulmonary aspergillosis in neutropenic patients during hospital construction: before and after chemoprophylaxis and institution of HEPA filters. *Am J Hematol.* 2001;66:257-62.
91. Loo VG, Bertrand C, Dixon C, et al. Control of construction-associated nosocomial aspergillosis in an antiquated hematology unit. *Infect Control Hosp Epidemiol.* 1996;17:360-4.
92. Pechlivanoglou P, Le HH, Daenen S, et al. Mixed treatment comparison of prophylaxis against invasive fungal infections in neutropenic patients receiving therapy for haematological malignancies: a systematic review. *J Antimicrob Chemother.* 2014;69(1):1.
93. Raad I, Hanna H, Huaringa A, et al. Diagnosis of invasive pulmonary aspergillosis using polymerase chain reaction-based detection of aspergillus in BAL. *Chest.* 2002;121:1171-6.
94. Becker MJ, de MS, Willemse D, et al. Quantitative galactomannan detection is superior to PCR in diagnosing

and monitoring invasive pulmonary aspergillosis in an experimental rat model. *J Clin Microbiol.* 2000;38:1434-8.
95. D'Haese J, Theunissen K, Vermeulen E, et al. Detection of galactomannan in bronchoalveolar lavage fluid samples of patients at risk for invasive pulmonary aspergillosis: analytical and clinical validity. *J Clin Microbiol.* 2012;50:1258-63.
96. Hsu LY, Ding Y, Phua J, et al. Galactomannan testing of bronchoalveolar lavage fluid is useful for diagnosis of invasive pulmonary aspergillosis in hematology patients. *BMC Infect Dis.* 2010;10:44.
97. Hage CA, Davis TE, Fuller D, et al. Diagnosis of histoplasmosis by antigen detection in BAL fluid. *Chest.* 2010;137:623-8.
98. Hage CA, Knox KS, Davis TE, et al. Antigen detection in bronchoalveolar lavage fluid for diagnosis of fungal pneumonia. *Curr Opin Pulm Med.* 2011;17:167-71.
99. Chave JP, David S, Wauters JP, et al. Transmission of Pneumocystis carinii from AIDS patients to other immunosuppressed patients: a cluster of Pneumocystis carinii pneumonia in renal transplant recipients. *AIDS.* 1991;5:927-32.
100. Hennequin C, Page B, Roux P, et al. Outbreak of Pneumocystis carinii pneumonia in a renal transplant unit. *Eur J Clin Microbiol Infect Dis.* 1995;14:122-6.
101. Baughman RP, Keely SP, Dohn MN, et al. The use of genetic markers to characterize transmission of Pneumocystis carinii. *AIDS Patient Care STDS.* 1997;11:131-8.
102. Yazaki H, Goto N, Uchida K, et al. Outbreak of Pneumocystis jiroveci pneumonia in renal transplant recipients: P. jiroveci is contagious to the susceptible host. *Transplantation.* 2009;88:380-5.
103. Baughman RP, Meyer KC, Nathanson I, , et al. Monitoring of nonsteroidal immunosuppressive drugs in patients with lung disease and lung transplant recipients: american college of chest physicians evidence-based clinical practice guidelines. *Chest.* 2012;142:e1S-e111S.
104. Holland EJ, Mogilishetty G, Skeens HM et al. Systemic immunosuppression in ocular surface stem cell transplantation: results of a 10-year experience. *Cornea.* 2012;31:655-61.
105. Lopez Bernaldo de Quiros JC, Miro JM, Pena JM, et al. A randomized trial of the discontinuation of primary and secondary prophylaxis against *Pneumocystis carinii* pneumonia after highly active antiretroviral therapy in patients with HIV infection. Grupo de Estudio del SIDA 04/98. *N Engl J Med.* 2001;344:159-67.
106. Maki DG, Fox BC, Kuntz J, et al. A prospective, randomized, double-blind study of trimethoprim-sulfamethoxazole for prophylaxis of infection in renal transplantation. Side effects of trimethoprim-sulfamethoxazole, interaction with cyclosporine. *J Lab Clin Med.* 1992;119:11-24.
107. Gabardi S, Millen P, Hurwitz S, et al. Atovaquone versus trimethoprim-sulfamethoxazole as Pneumocystis jirovecii pneumonia prophylaxis following renal transplantation. *Clin Transplant.* 2012;26:E184-90.
108. Chan C, Montaner J, Lefebvre EA, et al. Atovaquone suspension compared with aerosolized pentamidine for prevention of Pneumocystis carinii pneumonia in human immunodeficiency virus-infected subjects intolerant of trimethoprim or sulfonamides. *J Infect Dis.* 1999;180:369-76.
109. Leoung GS, Feigal DW, Montgomery AB, et al. Aerosolized pentamidine for prophylaxis against Pneumocystis carinii pneumonia. The San Francisco community prophylaxis trial. *N Engl J Med.* 1990;323:769-75.
110. Kimura M, Tanaka S, Ishikawa A, et al. Comparison of trimethoprim-sulfamethoxazole and aerosolized pentamidine for primary prophylaxis of *Pneumocystis jiroveci* pneumonia in immunocompromised patients with connective tissue disease. *Rheumatol Int.* 2008;28:673-6.
111. Vasconcelles MJ, Bernardo MV, King C, et al. Aerosolized pentamidine as pneumocystis prophylaxis after bone marrow transplantation is inferior to other regimens and is associated with decreased survival and an increased risk of other infections. *Biol Blood Marrow Transplant.* 2000;6:35-43.
112. Lufft V, Kliem V, Behrend M, et al. Incidence of *Pneumocystis carinii* pneumonia after renal transplantation. Impact of immunosuppression. *Transplantation.* 1996;62:421-3.
113. Ljungman P, de La CR, Milpied N, et al. Randomized study of valacyclovir as prophylaxis against cytomegalovirus reactivation in recipients of allogeneic bone marrow transplants. *Blood.* 2002;99:3050-6.
114. Prentice HG, Gluckman E, Powles RL, et al. Impact of long-term acyclovir on cytomegalovirus infection and survival after allogeneic bone marrow transplantation. European Acyclovir for CMV Prophylaxis Study Group. *Lancet.* 1994;343:749-53.
115. Zuk DM, Humar A, Weinkauf JG, et al. An international survey of cytomegalovirus management practices in lung transplantation. *Transplantation.* 2010;90:672-6.
116. Palmer SM, Limaye AP, Banks M, et al. Extended valganciclovir prophylaxis to prevent cytomegalovirus after lung transplantation: a randomized, controlled trial. *Ann Intern Med.* 2010;152:761-9.
117. Majhail NS, Parks K, Defor TE, et al. Diffuse alveolar hemorrhage and infection-associated alveolar hemorrhage following hematopoietic stem cell transplantation: related and high-risk clinical syndromes. *Biol Blood Marrow Transplant.* 2006;12:1038-46.
118. Baughman RP, Drent M. Role of bronchoalveolar lavage in interstitial lung disease. *Clin Chest Med.* 2001;22:331-41.
119. Perez-Arellano JL, Losa Garcia JE, Garcia Macias MC, et al. Hemosiderin-laden macrophages in bronchoalveolar lavage fluid. *Acta Cytol.* 1992;36:26-30.
120. Vlahakis NE, Rickman OB, Morgenthaler T. Sirolimus-associated diffuse alveolar hemorrhage. *Mayo Clin Proc.* 2004;79:541-5.
121. Vandewiele B, Vandecasteele SJ, Vanwalleghem L, et al. Diffuse alveolar hemorrhage induced by everolimus. *Chest.* 2010;137:456-9.
122. Panoskaltsis-Mortari A, Griese M, Madtes DK, et al. An official American Thoracic Society research statement: noninfectious lung injury after hematopoietic stem cell transplantation: idiopathic pneumonia syndrome. *Am J Respir Crit Care Med.* 2011;183:1262-79.

123. Clark JG, Hansen JA, Hertz MI, et al. NHLBI workshop summary. Idiopathic pneumonia syndrome after bone marrow transplantation. *Am Rev Respir Dis.* 1993;147:1601-6.
124. Fukuda T, Hackman RC, Guthrie KA, et al. Risks and outcomes of idiopathic pneumonia syndrome after nonmyeloablative and conventional conditioning regimens for allogeneic hematopoietic stem cell transplantation. *Blood.* 2003;102:2777-85.
125. Song I, Yi CA, Han J, et al. CT findings of late-onset noninfectious pulmonary complications in patients with pathologically proven graft-versus-host disease after allogeneic stem cell transplant. *AJR Am J Roentgenol.* 2012;199:581-7.
126. Walsh FW, Rolfe MW, Rumbak MJ. The initial pulmonary evaluation of the immunocompromised patient. *Chest Surg Clin N Am.* 1999;9:19-38.
127. Iregui M, Ward S, Sherman G, et al. Clinical importance of delays in the initiation of appropriate antibiotic treatment for ventilator-associated pneumonia. *Chest.* 2002;122:262-8.
128. Torres A, Ewig S, Insausti J, et al. Etiology and microbial patterns of pulmonary infiltrates in patients with orthotopic liver transplantation. *Chest.* 2000;117:494-502.

CHAPTER 11

Respiratory Infections in Specific Populations: Lung Cancer Patients

Eleftherios Zervas, Athanasios Thomopoulos, Angelos Pefanis, Theoplasti Grigoratou, Ilias Athanasiadis, Mina Gaga

ABSTRACT

Lung cancer patients are particularly prone to infections, which can be life-threatening, particularly when chemotherapy-induced neutropenia is present. Although the most common site of infection for patients with lung cancer is the lung, patients with febrile neutropenia should be thoroughly assessed for other common sites of infection. Infections have been documented in up to 84% of lung cancer patients and are the cause of death in up to 50% of cancer patients. Most infections are caused by bacteriae (especially Gram-negative bacteriae), but viruses are being increasingly identified. The diagnostic evaluation should focus on determining the potential sites and causative organisms of infection. All neutropenic patients should be treated empirically with broad-spectrum antibiotics at the first sign of infection, according to clinical practice guidelines. Prophylactic administration of granulocyte colony stimulating factor (G-CSF) and antibiotics has been shown to reduce the mortality associated with infections and also, to prevent the reduction in chemotherapy doses, which is linked to poorer long-term outcomes. However, due to the high cost of G-CSF treatment, prophylactic use is warranted in patients at high-risk of febrile neutropenia and patients who have experienced neutropenia after a previous dose of chemotherapy.

INTRODUCTION

During the course of their disease, patients with cancer frequently present with an infection and, moreover, this is the cause of death in up to 50% of cases. Infection, therefore, is a very important event in cancer patients and leads to death much more frequently than organ failure or carcinomatosis, which lead to death in 25% and 10% of cases, respectively.[1] In patients with lung cancer, infections of the tracheobronchial tree and the lungs have been documented in up to 84% of cases.[2,3] Lung cancer patients are particularly prone to infections, because they are more often than not smokers and have a number of comorbidities, such as chronic obstructive pulmonary disease (COPD), diabetes, and ischemic heart disease. Tumors that grow rapidly may become necrotic, thus, forming a nidus for infection. Moreover, lung cancer often causes obstruction of the bronchi, leading to accumulation of secretions and pulmonary infection. Patients with advanced malignancy are also commonly malnourished, which further increases the risk of infection. But the most important risk factor for infection in cancer patients is chemotherapy, which dramatically reduces the immune responses and often leads to neutropenia. The National Comprehensive Cancer Network (NCCN) guidelines[4] define *neutropenia* as either an absolute neutrophil count (ANC) less than 500/μL, or an ANC less than 1000/μL, and a predicted decline to 500/μL or less over the next 46 hours. The longer the duration of neutropenia, the higher the risk of infection. A major concern is that signs and symptoms of infection are often blunted or even absent in the absence of neutrophils, but fever remains an early, although nonspecific sign. Fever is defined as a single temperature

38.3°C or more, or 38°C or more over 1 hour in the absence of an obvious cause. Febrile neutropenia constitutes a frequently fatal risk to the patient. Approximately half of the patients with neutropenia who become febrile have an established or occult infection.[5] Patients who develop infections should be treated promptly, and therefore, empirically at first, although every effort should be made to establish a specific diagnosis of the pathogen or pathogens. Moreover, patients at high risk of infection and febrile neutropenia should be treated prophylactically. This chapter will deal with epidemiological data regarding the prevalence of infection in lung cancer patients and the pathogens usually associated with it, preventive measures, such as the prophylactic use of antibiotics and granulocyte colony stimulating factor (G-CSF) to prevent neutropenia and infection in high-risk patients, and with the management of infection.

EPIDEMIOLOGY

Prevalence

In a prospective study conducted in Belgium between January 1997 and February 2001 by Berghmans et al.,[6] 275 of 442 patients with lung cancer (62.2%) acquired 435 episodes of fever and/or microbiologically or otherwise documented infection. 79% of patients had a nonsmall cell lung carcinoma (NSCLC), while 18% patients had small cell lung carcinoma (SCLC) and only 8 patients (roughly, 2%) had other types of thoracic tumors. The following comorbidities and/or potentially predisposing conditions were found at the diagnosis of the infectious episode: 102 patients had COPD, 100 were receiving corticosteroid therapy, 76 had neutropenia; 69, 21, 53 patients had a peripheral, central, totally implantable venous catheter, respectively and 27 had a bladder catheter. In 204 infectious episodes (47% of the total episodes), chemotherapy had been administered in the 15 days preceding the episode. Bacteremia was associated with neutropenia [odd's ratio (OR), 3.24; $p = 0.0001$) and catheter use (OR, 4.84; $p = 0.001$), and urinary infections were associated with the presence of a bladder catheter (OR, 3.99; $p = 0.0001$).

In another retrospective study, multivariate analysis in a large sample of patients (n = 58,053) from the Medicare database (1994–2005)[7] showed that factors associated with febrile neutropenia in older people with lung, breast, prostate, and colorectal cancer included advanced stage at diagnosis, number of associated comorbid conditions, receipt of myelosuppressive chemotherapy, and receipt of chemotherapy within 1 month of diagnosis.

In an older study published in 1990, Perlin et al. examined respiratory infections in patients with lung cancer and reported that the median survival of the patients who developed an infection, was 4.2 months.[8] This was significantly shorter than that of the patients who did not develop an infection and had a median survival of 12.9 months ($p < 0.05$). When stage III patients were analyzed separately, patients with an infection lived a median of 5.8 months and patients without one, lived a median of 13.4 months ($p < 0.05$). This study indicated that pulmonary infections frequently occur in patients with lung cancer and suggested that they may adversely affect survival. In a more recent study, Lyman et al.[9] reported that the adjusted risk of mortality in patients who experienced febrile neutropenia was at least 15% higher than in comparably matched patients without febrile neutropenia, supporting the idea that chemotherapy-induced neutropenia and accompanying infection are clinical important events.

PATHOGENS

In the study conducted by Berghmans et al.,[6] microbiologically documented infections accounted for 70% of the 435 infectious episodes. There were 37 documented polymicrobial infections, including 32 infections with 2 pathogens, 3 infections with 3 pathogens, and 2 infections with 4 pathogens. The most frequent pathogens were Gram-negative bacteria (n = 201, 64%) followed by Gram-positive bacteria (n = 78, 25%), and fungi (n = 25; 8%). When only pathogens documented in blood cultures were considered, Gram-positive bacteria were most frequently observed.

In patients with COPD, the most frequently documented pathogens were *Haemophilus influenzae* (n = 29), *Streptococcus pneumoniae* (n = 12), *Staphylococcus aureus* (n = 12), *Moraxella catarrhalis* (n = 11), *Escherichia coli* (n = 9), and *Pseudomonas aeruginosa* (n = 9). The distribution of microorganisms differed if the infection was acquired in the hospital and there was more *S. pneumoniae* (15 of 21 patients) isolated from patients at home or during the first 48 hours after hospital admission and more *S. aureus* (16 of 27 patients), *Enterobacter* species (10 of 13 patients), and *Proteus* species (8 of 10 patients) when the hospital stay was more than 48 hours.[6]

A review published in the Lancet in 2008[10] reported that in lung cancer patients, most infections are caused by bacteria (especially Gram-negative), but viruses are being increasingly identified. Etiological causes of bacterial infection included most commonly *P. aeruginosa*, *Stenotrophomonas maltophilia*, and *Nocardia* species, of viral infections, respiratory syncytial virus (RSV), parainfluenza virus, influenza virus A and B, and cytomegalovirus (CMV), while fungal infections are often caused by *Aspergillus* species, *Fusarium* species, *Mucorales* species, and *Pneumocystis jirovecii.*

In lung cancer patients the majority of clinically documented infections are due to respiratory germs. In a retrospective study by Lanoix et al.,[11] which was conducted between January 2000 and July 2006 and included 87 lung cancer patients, hospitalized due to febrile neutropenia, the isolates detected predominantly by blood culture were mainly, urinary and digestive tract bacteria (46%). This suggests that respiratory pathogens rarely cause bacteremia. 59% of the identified pathogens were Gram-negative bacteria and most of them were enterobacteriaceae (especially, *E. coli* n = 11 out of 16). Most of the Gram-positive bacteria were *Staphylococcus* species (above all *S. aureus,* n = 6 out of 9). Of the isolated bacteria, 14.6% were multidrug-resistant (i.e., resistant to 2 or more antibiotic families, including β-lactams).

PREVENTION

Infections and, more importantly, febrile neutropenia as a major dose-limiting toxicity of systemic chemotherapy, are both associated with delays in treatment, increased hospitalization rate, higher costs,[12,13] and mortality, ranging from 4 to 21%.[9,13,14]

Hand hygiene is the most effective means of preventing transmission of infection in the hospital, but, also at home. Plants and dried or fresh flowers should not be allowed in the rooms of neutropenic patients. Healthcare workers should be encouraged to report their illnesses or exposures to infections. Standard barrier precautions should be followed for all patients and infection-specific isolation should be used for patients with certain signs or symptoms.

Prophylactic administration of a G-CSF and antibiotics has been shown to reduce the mortality associated with infections and the reductions in chemotherapy doses, which have been linked to poorer long-term outcomes.

Granulocyte Colony-stimulating Factors

Prophylactic administration of G-CSF has been shown to reduce the rates of febrile neutropenia, infection-related mortality, frequency of hospitalization, and frequency of infections,[15-18] although no influence on overall survival has been observed. Given the significant costs associated with G-CSF administration, it is neither practical nor clinically appropriate to administer this agent to all patients receiving chemotherapy. The American Society of Clinical Oncology (ASCO) guidelines recommend G-CSF prophylaxis when the risk of febrile neutropenia is approximately 20% or higher.[19] These guidelines recommend that primary prophylaxis should be considered in patients at increased risk due to advanced age (>65 years), medical history, disease characteristics, and myelotoxicity of the chemotherapy regimen. Other factors associated with increased risk of febrile neutropenia include poor performance status, preexisting neutropenia, extensive prior chemotherapy, irradiation to a significant amount of bone marrow, a history of recurrent febrile neutropenia, and comorbid conditions.

Similarly, in 2006, the European Guidelines Working Party by the European Organisation for Research and Treatment of Cancer (EORTC) published guidelines for the use of G-CSF in adult cancer patients at risk of chemotherapy-induced febrile neutropenia. These guidelines have been updated in 2010[20] and the current guidelines recommend that patient-related adverse risk factors, such as elderly age (≥65 years) and neutrophil count be taken into account in the overall assessment of febrile neutropenia risk before administering each cycle of chemotherapy. It is important that after a previous episode of febrile neutropenia, patients receive prophylactic administration of G-CSF in subsequent cycles. Prophylactic G-CSF continues to be recommended in patients receiving a chemotherapy regimen with high risk of febrile neutropenia (>20%) (Table 1).[21-90] When using a chemotherapy regimen associated with febrile neutropenia in 10–20% of patients, particular attention should be given to patient-related risk factors that may increase the overall risk of febrile neutropenia. In situations where dose-dense or dose-intense chemotherapy strategies have survival benefits, prophylactic G-CSF support is recommended. Filgrastim, lenograstim, and pegfilgrastim, and also filgrastim biosimilars are approved in Europe and may be used when indicated.[91] Table 1 summarizes literature reported risk of grades 3 and 4 neutropenia and of febrile neutropenia related to the most commonly used chemotherapy agents and combination regimens in lung cancer treatment.[21-90]

The use of these agents, however, is associated with a significant increase in cost.[92] A cost effectiveness study was performed in the Netherlands and was published in 2006. For the first cycle, the mean incremental costs of adding G-CSF amounted to €681 (95% confidence interval (CI) €36–1,397)/patient. For the entire treatment period, the mean incremental costs amounted to €5,123/patient; (95% CI €3,908–6,337). This substantial increase in cost was observed despite a significant reduction in the incidence of febrile neutropenia and related savings in medical care utilization.

TABLE 1

Literature-reported Risk of Grade 3/4 Neutropenia and Febrile Neutropenia Related to the Most Commonly Used Chemotherapy Agents and Combination Regimen for Lung Cancer Treatment (Alphabetic Order)

Therapeutic regimen	Neutropenia grade 3/4	Febrile neutropenia
Platinum-based regimen		
Carboplatin plus paclitaxel plus bevacizumab[21-23]	25–27%	5–5.6%
Carboplatin plus pemetrexed plus bevacizumab[24]	4%	0%
Cisplatin plus gemcitabine plus bevacizumab[25]	40%	2%
Carboplatin-based doublets		
Carboplatin plus docetaxel[26-28]	14–74%	5–26%
Carboplatin plus etoposide[29-31]	47–69%	17–20%
Carboplatin plus gemcitabine[32-35]	30–51%	2.8–9%
Carboplatin plus paclitaxel[21,32,36-39]	11.9–54%	0,4–6%
Carboplatin plus pemetrexed[30,40-42]	11–25.6%	0–3%
Carboplatin plus vinorelbine[43-46]	45–68%	0–7.1%
Cisplatin-based doublets		
Cisplatin plus docetaxel[26,47-49]	56.6–74,8%	4.2–11%
Cisplatin plus etoposide[30,37,50-52]	47–85%	4.5–10.4%
Cisplatin plus gemcitabine[25,38,53-56]	26.7–51%	1–4%
Cisplatin plus paclitaxel[39,56-58]	14.6–51%	1,3–8.6%
Cisplatin plus pemetrexed[41,55]	15–15.8%	1.3–2.5%
Cisplatin plus vinorelbine[38,48,59,60]	37–83.3%	3–22.4%
Non-platinum based doublets		
Docetaxel plus gemcitabine[59-62]	16–52.3%	3.9–8.4%
Paclitaxel plus gemcitabine[56,63,64]	13–30.4	1.9–3%
Monotherapy		
Docetaxel[65-69]	43–82.9%	3–12.7%
Gemcitabine[70-72]	6–16.9%	0%
Pemetrexed[73-77]	4–7%	1–2%
Topotecan[65,78-81]	50–87%	2–6.6%
Tyrosine kinase inhibitors (TKIs): erlotinib/gefitinib[82-86]	0–5%	0%
Vinorelbine i.v[64,69,87]	31–69.3%	1–11%
Vinorelbine oral[88-90]	0.2–6%	0%

Antibiotics

According to the Infectious Diseases Society of America (IDSA) guidelines, antibiotic prophylaxis should be considered for high-risk patients with expected durations of profound neutropenia (ANC <100 cells/mm^3) for more than 7 days.[93] A systematic review and meta-analysis of randomized controlled trials (RCTs) including patients with cancer of any type demonstrated that death from all causes was reduced by 34% in neutropenic patients who received any antibiotic prophylaxis and by 40% in patients who received quinolones for prophylaxis.[94] However, most patients receiving chemotherapy for lung cancer have neutropenia lasting less than 7 days.

A recent review of the studies on prophylactic antibiotic treatment[95] showed that fluoroquinolones or cotrimoxazole were the antibiotics most frequently used and that lung cancer patients who received prophylactic antibiotics, exhibited significantly fewer episodes of febrile neutropenia, fewer, documented infections, as well as shorter duration of related hospitalizations.

The IDSA guidelines[93] recommend antibiotic prophylaxis with a fluoroquinolone, and state that both levofloxacin and ciprofloxacin have been evaluated comprehensively and that these antibiotics are considered to be roughly equivalent. However, levofloxacin is preferred in situations with increased risk for oral mucositis-related invasive viridans streptococcal infection. Of note, clinicians should give due consideration to the prevalence of fluoroquinolone resistance in *E. coli*. Fluoroquinolone prophylaxis is unlikely to be effective when the level of resistance within *E. coli* isolated from patients at an institution approaches 20%.

According to the IDSA[93] as well as the NCCN guidelines,[4] antibiotic prophylaxis is not recommended for low-risk patients with neutropenia lasting less than 7 days (a category that includes most patients with solid tumors, such as the lung cancer patients).

Vaccination

Yearly influenza vaccination with inactivated vaccine is recommended for all patients being treated for cancer. Serologic responses may be best between chemotherapy cycles (>7 days after the last treatment) or more than 2 weeks before chemotherapy starts. Vaccination against *S. pneumoniae* is also recommended in cancer patients.

DIAGNOSTIC EVALUATION

The diagnostic evaluation should focus on determining the potential sites and causative organisms of infection. The first step should be a site-specific history and physical examination. The most common site of infection for patients with lung cancer is the lung, but patients with febrile neutropenia should be also thoroughly assessed for other common sites of infection (such as the alimentary tract, groin, skin, sinuses, ears, perivagina, perirectum, and intravascular access device sites). Laboratory tests should include a complete blood cell (CBC) count with differential leukocyte count and platelet count, measurement of serum levels of creatinine and blood urea nitrogen, and measurement of electrolytes, hepatic transaminase enzymes, and total bilirubin. A chest radiograph is indicated for patients with respiratory signs or symptoms; however, radiographic findings may be absent in neutropenic patients with pulmonary infection.[96] At least 2 sets of blood cultures are recommended, with a set collected simultaneously from each lumen of an existing central venous catheter, if present and from a peripheral vein site. Two blood culture sets from separate venipuncture should be sent if no central catheter is present. Culture specimens from other sites of suspected infection should be obtained as clinically indicated.

In patients with symptoms of respiratory viral infection, viral cultures and rapid viral antigen testing of the nasopharyngeal secretions can be useful during outbreaks.

TREATMENT

The important points regarding treatment of infection and febrile neutropenia in cancer patients is that treatment should be started promptly, and that the severity of the infection and the patient's general health status, immune status, and comorbidities should be evaluated thoroughly. All neutropenic patients should be treated empirically with broad-spectrum antibiotics at the first sign of infection (i.e., fever).

As part of the initial evaluation, patients with neutropenia may be divided into either a high- or low-risk group, using criteria from validated clinical prediction rules. This assessment is important for 2 reasons: it helps the clinician predict the probability that a neutropenic patient will experience serious complications during a febrile episode, and it may determine whether the patient may safely receive treatment as an outpatient or not. A widely used and validated prediction rule is the Multinational Association for Supportive Care in Cancer (MASCC) risk index (Table 2). According to MASCC, a score of more than 21 identifies low-risk patients with a positive predictive value of 91%, specificity of 68%, and

TABLE 2

MASCC Risk Index for Febrile Neutropenia[97]

Characteristics	Points attributed
Burden of illness: no or mild symptoms	5
No hypotension	5
No chronic obstructive pulmonary disease	4
Solid tumor or no previous fungal infection	4
No dehydration	3
Burden of illness: moderate symptoms	3
Outpatient status	3
Age <60 years	2

- Points attributed to the variable "burden of illness" are not cumulative. Therefore, the maximum theoretical score is 26.
- Score >21 identifies low-risk patients with a positive predictive value of 91%, specificity of 68%, and sensitivity of 71%.

MASCC, Multinational Association for Supportive Care in Cancer.

sensitivity of 71%.[97] A disadvantage of MASCC prediction rule is that it does not consider the duration of neutropenia to be a deciding factor that influences the clinical course during the febrile episode.

According to clinical practice guidelines for the use of antimicrobial agents in neutropenic patients with cancer (2010 update by the IDSA),[93] low-risk patients should receive initial oral or intravenous (IV) empirical antibiotic doses in a clinic or hospital setting, and then, they may be transitioned to outpatient oral or IV treatment [outpatient parenteral antibiotic therapy, (OPAT)]. Ciprofloxacin in combination with amoxicillin-clavulanate is recommended for oral empirical treatment. Levofloxacin or ciprofloxacin monotherapy or ciprofloxacin and clindamycin, are less well-studied but are commonly used. It is important to remember that patients receiving fluoroquinolone prophylaxis should not receive empirical therapy with a fluoroquinolone. For low risk patients with solid tumor, the median time to defervescence occurs at a median of 2 days.

High-risk patients require hospitalization for IV empirical antibiotic therapy. Monotherapy with an anti-pseudomonal β-lactam, such as cefepime, a carbapenem (meropenem or imipenem), or piperacillin/tazobactam is recommended. Aminoglycosides, fluoroquinolones, and/or vancomycin may be added to the initial regimen for the management of complications (e.g., hypotension and pneumonia) or if antimicrobial resistance is suspected or proven. Vancomycin or other antimicrobials active against aerobic Gram-positive cocci are not recommended as a standard part of the initial antibiotic regimen for fever and neutropenia.

Modifications to initial empirical therapy may be considered for patients at risk of infection with antibiotic-resistant microorganisms, such as methicillin-resistant *S. aureus* (MRSA), vancomycin-resistant enterococci (VRE), extended-spectrum β-lactamase (ESBL)-producing Gram-negative bacteria, and microorganisms producing carbapenemases, including *Klebsiella pneumoniae* carbapenemases (KPCs).

Risk factors for infection with antibiotic-resistant microorganisms are previous infection or colonization with them and treatment in a hospital with high rates of endemicity. Early addition of vancomycin or daptomycin for MRSA and of linezolid or daptomycin for VRE should be considered. For ESBLs, early use of a carbapenem and for KPCs, early use of colistin or tigecycline, should be considered.

Most penicillin-allergic patients tolerate cephalosporins except those with a history of an immediate-type hypersensitivity reaction who should be treated with a regimen that avoids β-lactams or carbapenems, such as ciprofloxacin and clindamycin or aztreonam and vancomycin.

Unexplained persistent fever in an otherwise stable patient rarely requires an empirical change of the initial antibiotic regimen. If an anti-Gram-positive regimen was started initially, it may be stopped after 2 days if there is no evidence for a Gram-positive infection and the patient remains stable. Empirical addition of vancomycin in the case of persistent or recrudescent fever and neutropenia is not recommended. The same is true for the addition of an aminoglycoside to the treatment regimen, unless this is dictated by clinical or microbiologic data.

Patients who remain hemodynamically unstable after the initial doses of a standard regimen for neutropenic fever should be treated with a broader regimen, active against multiresistant Gram-negative, Gram-positive and anerobic bacteria and/or fungi.

Pneumonia in neutropenic patients should be treated as a healthcare-acquired infection with combinations of a β-lactam or carbapenem plus an aminoglycoside or antipseudomonal fluoroquinolone. In severe cases of pneumonia, associated with hypoxia or extensive infiltrates, or if MRSA infection is suspected, the addition of vancomycin or linezolid to the treatment regimen is recommended. When possible, pneumonia should be evaluated with more invasive procedures, such as bronchoscopy with bronchoalveolar lavage (BAL) and biopsy sampling.

An intravenous-to-oral switch in antibiotic regimen may be considered, if patients are clinically stable and gastrointestinal absorption is adequate. Treatment with broad-spectrum antibiotics must be continued until the patient has been afebrile for at least 2 days and the neutrophil count is more than 500 cells/mm^3, with a consistent, increasing trend. The duration of therapy depends also on the particular organism and site. If an appropriate treatment course has been completed and all signs and symptoms of infection have resolved, patients who remain neutropenic may resume oral fluoroquinolone prophylaxis until marrow recovery. For all *S. aureus* bloodstream infections, a transesophageal echocardiogram is recommended to determine the absence or presence of heart valve vegetations and, thus, to help define the duration of therapy.[98]

Empirical antifungal therapy and investigation for invasive fungal infections should be considered for patients with persistent or recurrent fever after 4–7 days of antibiotics and no identified source of fever, or whenever the overall duration of neutropenia is expected to be more than 7 days. Antifungal agents may be withheld, if the patient remains febrile after 4–7 days of broad-spectrum antibiotics but is clinically stable, has no clinical or chest and computed tomography (CT) signs of fungal infection, has negative serological tests for invasive fungal infection, and has no recovery of fungi from any body site. Patients already receiving antifungal prophylaxis should be switched to a different class of IV antifungal. On the contrary, antifungal therapy should be instituted, if the patient is clinically unstable, has clinical or radiological (chest X-ray and CT) signs of fungal infection, has positive fungal serologic assay results, and fungi (such as *Candida* or *Aspergillus* species) are isolated from any body site. In low-risk patients, routine use of empirical antifungal therapy is not recommended, as the risk of invasive fungal infection is low.

Antiviral treatment for herpes simplex virus or varicella-zoster virus infection is only indicated, if there is clinical or laboratory evidence of active viral disease. For patients with upper respiratory symptoms, chest radiography and testing for influenza, parainfluenza, adenovirus, RSV, and human metapneumovirus are indicated. In the setting of an influenza exposure or outbreak, neutropenic patients presenting with influenza-like illness should receive treatment empirically with neuraminidase inhibitors.

CONCLUSION

Infections are common in lung cancer patients and constitute a significant morbidity and mortality risk. Chemotherapy remains the most important risk factor for febrile neutropenia and infection, but other factors, such as older age and the presence of comorbidities further increase the risk. Infections should be recognized and treated promptly while high-risk patients should be treated prophylactically according to the guidelines.

REFERENCES

1. Inagaki J, Rodriguez V, Bodey GP. Proceedings: Causes of death in cancer patients. *Cancer.* 1974;33:568-73.
2. Brambilla C, Romand P, Vanderkerckhove C, Moro D. Respiratory infection and bronchial cancer. *Rev Mal Respir.* 1992;9:R49-52.
3. Klastersky J. The infectious complications of bronchial cancer. *Rev Mal Respir.* 1998;15:451-9.
4. NCCN Clinical Practice Guidelines in Oncology. Prevention and Treatment of Cancer-Related Infections. Version 2.2011. Available from: http://www.medicine.wisc.edu/~williams/infections.pdf. 2011.
5. Hughes WT, Armstrong D, Bodey GP, Bow EJ, Brown AE, Calandra T, et al. 2002 guidelines for the use of antimicrobial agents in neutropenic patients with cancer. *Clin Infect Dis.* 2002;34:730-51.
6. Berghmans T, Sculier JP, Klastersky J. A prospective study of infections in lung cancer patients admitted to the hospital. *Chest.* 2003;124:114-20.
7. Hosmer W, Malin J, Wong M. Development and validation of a prediction model for the risk of developing febrile neutropenia in the first cycle of chemotherapy among elderly patients with breast, lung, colorectal, and prostate cancer. *Support Care Cancer.* 2011;19:333-41.
8. Perlin E, Bang KM, Shah A, Hursey PD, Whittingham WL, Hashmi K, et al. The impact of pulmonary infections on the survival of lung cancer patients. *Cancer.* 1990;66:593-6.
9. Lyman GH, Michels SL, Reynolds MW, Barron R, Tomic KS, Yu J. Risk of mortality in patients with cancer who experience febrile neutropenia. *Cancer.* 2010;116:5555-63.
10. Vento S, Cainelli F, Temesgen Z. Lung infections after cancer chemotherapy. *Lancet Oncol.* 2008;9:982-92.
11. Lanoix JP, Pluquet E, Lescure FX, Bentayeb H, Lecuyer E, Boutemy M, et al. Bacterial infection profiles in lung cancer patients with febrile neutropenia. *BMC Infect Dis.* 2011;11:183.
12. Hardy D, Cormier JN, Xing Y, Liu CC, Xia R, Du XL. Chemotherapy-associated toxicity in a large cohort of elderly patients with non-small cell lung cancer. *J Thorac Oncol.* 2010;5:90-8.
13. Kuderer NM, Dale DC, Crawford J, Cosler LE, Lyman GH. Mortality, morbidity, and cost associated with febrile neutropenia in adult cancer patients. *Cancer.* 2006;106:2258-66.
14. Talcott JA, Siegel RD, Finberg R, Goldman L. Risk assessment in cancer patients with fever and neutropenia: a prospective, two-center validation of a prediction rule. *J Clin Oncol.* 1992;10:316-22.
15. Kuderer NM, Dale DC, Crawford J, Lyman GH. Impact of primary prophylaxis with granulocyte colony-stimulating factor on febrile neutropenia and mortality in adult cancer patients receiving chemotherapy: a systematic review. *J Clin Oncol.* 2007;25:3158-67.
16. Timmer-Bonte JN, de Boo TM, Smit HJ, Biesma B, Wilschut FA, Cheragwandi SA, et al. Prevention of chemotherapy-induced febrile neutropenia by prophylactic antibiotics plus or minus granulocyte colony-stimulating factor in small-cell lung cancer: a Dutch Randomized Phase III Study. *J Clin Oncol.* 2005;23:7974-84.
17. Vogel CL, Wojtukiewicz MZ, Carroll RR, Tjulandin SA, Barajas-Figueroa LJ, Wiens BL, et al. First and subsequent cycle use of pegfilgrastim prevents febrile neutropenia in patients with breast cancer: a multicenter, double-blind, placebo-controlled phase III study. *J Clin Oncol.* 2005;23:1178-84.
18. Crawford J, Ozer H, Stoller R, Johnson D, Lyman G, Tabbara I, et al. Reduction by granulocyte colony-stimulating factor of fever and neutropenia induced by chemotherapy in patients with small-cell lung cancer. *N Engl J Med.* 1991;325:164-70.
19. Smith TJ, Khatcheressian J, Lyman GH, Ozer H, Armitage JO, Balducci L, et al. 2006 update of recommendations for the use of white blood cell growth factors: an evidence-based clinical practice guideline. *J Clin Oncol.* 2006;24:3187-205.
20. Aapro MS, Bohlius J, Cameron DA, Dal Lago L, Donnelly JP, Kearney N, et al.; European Organisation for Research and Treatment of Cancer.. 2010 update of EORTC guidelines for the use of granulocyte-colony stimulating

factor to reduce the incidence of chemotherapy-induced febrile neutropenia in adult patients with lymphoproliferative disorders and solid tumours. *Eur J Cancer.* 2011;47:8-32.

21. Sandler A, Gray R, Perry MC, Brahmer J, Schiller JH, Dowlati A, et al. Paclitaxel-carboplatin alone or with bevacizumab for non-small-cell lung cancer. *N Engl J Med.* 2006;355:2542-50.
22. Brahmer JR, Dahlberg SE, Gray RJ, Schiller JH, Perry MC, Sandler A, et al. Sex differences in outcome with bevacizumab therapy: analysis of patients with advanced-stage non-small cell lung cancer treated with or without bevacizumab in combination with paclitaxel and carboplatin in the Eastern Cooperative Oncology Group Trial 4599. *J Thorac Oncol.* 2011;6:103-8.
23. Johnson DH, Fehrenbacher L, Novotny WF, Herbst RS, Nemunaitis JJ, Jablons DM, et al. Randomized phase II trial comparing bevacizumab plus carboplatin and paclitaxel with carboplatin and paclitaxel alone in previously untreated locally advanced or metastatic non-small-cell lung cancer. *J Clin Oncol.* 2004;22:2184-91.
24. Patel JD, Hensing TA, Rademaker A, Hart EM, Blum MG, Milton DT, et al. Phase II study of pemetrexed and carboplatin plus bevacizumab with maintenance pemetrexed and bevacizumab as first-line therapy for nonsquamous non-small-cell lung cancer. *J Clin Oncol.* 2009;27:3284-9.
25. Reck M, von Pawel J, Zatloukal P, Ramlau R, Gorbounova V, Hirsh V, et al. Phase III trial of cisplatin plus gemcitabine with either placebo or bevacizumab as first-line therapy for nonsquamous non-small-cell lung cancer: AVAil. *J Clin Oncol.* 2009;27:1227-34.
26. Fossella F, Pereira JR, von Pawel J, Pluzanska A, Gorbounova V, Kaukel E, et al. Randomized, multinational, phase III study of docetaxel plus platinum combinations versus vinorelbine plus cisplatin for advanced non-small-cell lung cancer: the TAX 326 study group. *J Clin Oncol.* 2003;21:3016-24.
27. Giannakakis T, Ziras N, Kakolyris S, Mavroudis D, Androulakis N, Agelaki S, et al. Docetaxel in combination with carboplatin for the treatment of advanced non-small cell lung carcinoma: a multicentre phase I study. *Eur J Cancer.* 2000;36:742-7.
28. Millward MJ, Boyer MJ, Lehnert M, Clarke S, Rischin D, Goh BC, et al. Docetaxel and carboplatin is an active regimen in advanced non-small-cell lung cancer: a phase II study in Caucasian and Asian patients. *Ann Oncol.* 2003;14:449-54.
29. Heigener DF, Manegold C, Jager E, Saal JG, Zuna I, Gatzemeier U. Multicenter randomized open-label phase III study comparing efficacy, safety, and tolerability of conventional carboplatin plus etoposide versus dose-intensified carboplatin plus etoposide plus lenograstim in small-cell lung cancer in "extensive disease" stage. *Am J Clin Oncol.* 2009;32:61-4.
30. Socinski MA, Smit EF, Lorigan P, Konduri K, Reck M, Szczesna A, et al. Phase III study of pemetrexed plus carboplatin compared with etoposide plus carboplatin in chemotherapy-naive patients with extensive-stage small-cell lung cancer. *J Clin Oncol.* 2009;27:4787-92.
31. Schmittel A, Fischer von Weikersthal L, Sebastian M, Martus P, Schulze K, Hortig P, et al. A randomized phase II trial of irinotecan plus carboplatin versus etoposide plus carboplatin treatment in patients with extended disease small-cell lung cancer. *Ann Oncol.* 2006;17:663-7.
32. Treat JA, Gonin R, Socinski MA, Edelman MJ, Catalano RB, Marinucci DM, et al.; Alpha Oncology Research Network. A randomized, phase III multicenter trial of gemcitabine in combination with carboplatin or paclitaxel versus paclitaxel plus carboplatin in patients with advanced or metastatic non-small-cell lung cancer. *Ann Oncol.* 2010; 21:540-7.
33. Grønberg BH, Bremnes RM, Fløtten O, Amundsen T, Brunsvig PF, Hjelde HH, et al. Phase III study by the Norwegian lung cancer study group: pemetrexed plus carboplatin compared with gemcitabine plus carboplatin as first-line chemotherapy in advanced non-small-cell lung cancer. *J Clin Oncol.* 2009;27:3217-24.
34. Kosmidis PA, Kalofonos HP, Christodoulou C, Syrigos K, Makatsoris T, Skarlos D, et al. Paclitaxel and gemcitabine versus carboplatin and gemcitabine in patients with advanced non-small-cell lung cancer. A phase III study of the Hellenic Cooperative Oncology Group. *Ann Oncol.* 2008;19:115-22.
35. Rudd RM, Gower NH, Spiro SG, Eisen TG, Harper PG, Littler JA, et al. Gemcitabine plus carboplatin versus mitomycin, ifosfamide, and cisplatin in patients with stage IIIB or IV non-small-cell lung cancer: a phase III randomized study of the London Lung Cancer Group. *J Clin Oncol.* 2005;23:142-53.
36. Scagliotti G, Novello S, von Pawel J, Reck M, Pereira JR, Thomas M, et al. Phase III study of carboplatin and paclitaxel alone or with sorafenib in advanced non-small-cell lung cancer. *J Clin Oncol.* 2010;28:1835-42.
37. Belani CP, Lee JS, Socinski MA, Robert F, Waterhouse D, Rowland K, et al. Randomized phase III trial comparing cisplatin-etoposide to carboplatin-paclitaxel in advanced or metastatic non-small cell lung cancer. *Ann Oncol.* 2005;16:1069-75.
38. Scagliotti GV, De Marinis F, Rinaldi M, Crinò L, Gridelli C, Ricci S, et al.; Italian Lung Cancer Project. Phase III randomized trial comparing three platinum-based doublets in advanced non-small-cell lung cancer. *J Clin Oncol.* 2002;20:4285-91.
39. Rosell R, Gatzemeier U, Betticher DC, Keppler U, Macha HN, Pirker R, et al. Phase III randomised trial comparing paclitaxel/carboplatin with paclitaxel/cisplatin in patients with advanced non-small-cell lung cancer: a cooperative multinational trial. *Ann Oncol.* 2002;13:1539-49.
40. Zinner RG, Fossella FV, Gladish GW, Glisson BS, Blumenschein GR Jr, Papadimitrakopoulou VA, et al. Phase II study of pemetrexed in combination with carboplatin in the first-line treatment of advanced nonsmall cell lung cancer. *Cancer.* 2005;104:2449-56.
41. Socinski MA, Weissman C, Hart LL, Beck JT, Choksi JK, Hanson JP, et al. Randomized phase II trial of pemetrexed combined with either cisplatin or carboplatin in untreated extensive-stage small-cell lung cancer. *J Clin Oncol.* 2006; 24:4840-7.

42. Scagliotti GV, Kortsik C, Dark GG, Price A, Manegold C, Rosell R, et al. Pemetrexed combined with oxaliplatin or carboplatin as first-line treatment in advanced non-small cell lung cancer: a multicenter, randomized, phase II trial. *Clin Cancer Res.* 2005;11:690-6.
43. Reck M, Macha HN, Del Barco S, Cornes P, Vaissière N, Morand M, et al. Phase II study of oral vinorelbine in combination with carboplatin followed by consolidation therapy with oral vinorelbine as single-agent in unresectable localized or metastatic non-small cell lung carcinoma. *Lung Cancer.* 2009;64:319-25.
44. Helbekkmo N, Sundstrøm SH, Aasebø U, Brunsvig PF, von Plessen C, Hjelde HH, et al.; Norwegian Lung Cancer Study Group. Vinorelbine/carboplatin vs gemcitabine/carboplatin in advanced NSCLC shows similar efficacy, but different impact of toxicity. *Br J Cancer.* 2007;97:283-9.
45. O'Brien ME, Szczesna A, Karnicka H, Zatloukal P, Eisen T, Hartmann W, et al. Vinorelbine alternating oral and intravenous plus carboplatin in advanced non-small-cell lung cancer: results of a multicentre phase II study. *Ann Oncol.* 2004;15:921-7.
46. Cremonesi M, Mandala M, Cazzaniga M, Rezzani C, Gambera M, Barni S. Vinorelbine and carboplatin in inoperable non-small cell lung cancer: a monoinstitutional phase II study. *Oncology.* 2003;64:97-101.
47. Schiller JH, Harrington D, Belani CP, Langer C, Sandler A, Krook J, et al.; Eastern Cooperative Oncology Group. Comparison of four chemotherapy regimens for advanced non-small-cell lung cancer. *N Engl J Med.* 2002;346:92-8.
48. Tan EH, Rolski J, Grodzki T, Schneider CP, Gatzemeier U, Zatloukal P, et al. Global Lung Oncology Branch trial 3 (GLOB3): final results of a randomised multinational phase III study alternating oral and i.v. vinorelbine plus cisplatin versus docetaxel plus cisplatin as first-line treatment of advanced non-small-cell lung cancer. *Ann Oncol.* 2009;20:1249-56.
49. Kubota K, Watanabe K, Kunitoh H, Noda K, Ichinose Y, Katakami N, et al.; Japanese Taxotere Lung Cancer Study Group. Phase III randomized trial of docetaxel plus cisplatin versus vindesine plus cisplatin in patients with stage IV non-small-cell lung cancer: the Japanese Taxotere Lung Cancer Study Group. *J Clin Oncol.* 2004;22: 254-61.
50. Zatloukal P, Cardenal F, Szczesna A, Gorbunova V, Moiseyenko V, Zhang X, et al. A multicenter international randomized phase III study comparing cisplatin in combination with irinotecan or etoposide in previously untreated small-cell lung cancer patients with extensive disease. *Ann Oncol.* 2010;21:1810-6.
51. Lara PN Jr, Natale R, Crowley J, Lenz HJ, Redman MW, Carleton JE, et al. Phase III trial of irinotecan/cisplatin compared with etoposide/cisplatin in extensive-stage small-cell lung cancer: clinical and pharmacogenomic results from SWOG S0124. *J Clin Oncol.* 2009;27:2530-5.
52. Hanna N, Bunn PA Jr, Langer C, Einhorn L, Guthrie T Jr, Beck T, et al. Randomized phase III trial comparing irinotecan/cisplatin with etoposide/cisplatin in patients with previously untreated extensive-stage disease small-cell lung cancer. *J Clin Oncol.* 2006;24:2038-43.
53. Ohe Y, Ohashi Y, Kubota K, Tamura T, Nakagawa K, Negoro S, et al. Randomized phase III study of cisplatin plus irinotecan versus carboplatin plus paclitaxel, cisplatin plus gemcitabine, and cisplatin plus vinorelbine for advanced non-small-cell lung cancer: Four-Arm Cooperative Study in Japan. *Ann Oncol.* 2007;18:317-23.
54. Paz-Ares L, Douillard JY, Koralewski P, Manegold C, Smit EF, Reyes JM, et al. Phase III study of gemcitabine and cisplatin with or without aprinocarsen, a protein kinase C-alpha antisense oligonucleotide, in patients with advanced-stage non-small-cell lung cancer. *J Clin Oncol.* 2006;24:1428-34.
55. Scagliotti GV, Parikh P, von Pawel J, Biesma B, Vansteenkiste J, Manegold C, et al. Phase III study comparing cisplatin plus gemcitabine with cisplatin plus pemetrexed in chemotherapy-naive patients with advanced-stage non-small-cell lung cancer. *J Clin Oncol.* 2008;26:3543-51.
56. Smit EF, van Meerbeeck JP, Lianes P, Debruyne C, Legrand C, Schramel F, et al.; European Organization for Research and Treatment of Cancer Lung Cancer Group. Three-arm randomized study of two cisplatin-based regimens and paclitaxel plus gemcitabine in advanced non-small-cell lung cancer: a phase III trial of the European Organization for Research and Treatment of Cancer Lung Cancer Group—EORTC 08975. *J Clin Oncol.* 2003;21:3909-17.
57. Arrieta O, González-De la Rosa CH, Aréchaga-Ocampo E, Villanueva-Rodríguez G, Cerón-Lizárraga TL, Martínez-Barrera L, et al. Randomized phase II trial of All-trans-retinoic acid with chemotherapy based on paclitaxel and cisplatin as first-line treatment in patients with advanced non-small-cell lung cancer. *J Clin Oncol.* 2010;28:3463-71.
58. Stathopoulos GP, Antoniou D, Dimitroulis J, Michalopoulou P, Bastas A, Marosis K, et al. Liposomal cisplatin combined with paclitaxel versus cisplatin and paclitaxel in non-small-cell lung cancer: a randomized phase III multicenter trial. *Ann Oncol.* 2010;21:2227-32.
59. Georgoulias V, Ardavanis A, Tsiafaki X, Agelidou A, Mixalopoulou P, Anagnostopoulou O, et al. Vinorelbine plus cisplatin versus docetaxel plus gemcitabine in advanced non-small-cell lung cancer: a phase III randomized trial. *J Clin Oncol.* 2005;23:2937-45.
60. Pujol JL, Breton JL, Gervais R, Rebattu P, Depierre A, Morère JF, et al. Gemcitabine-docetaxel versus cisplatin-vinorelbine in advanced or metastatic non-small-cell lung cancer: a phase III study addressing the case for cisplatin. *Ann Oncol.* 2005;16:602-10.
61. Boukovinas I, Souglakos J, Hatzidaki D, Kakolyris S, Ziras N, Vamvakas L, et al. Docetaxel plus gemcitabine as front-line chemotherapy in elderly patients with lung adenocarcinomas: a multicenter phase II study. *Lung Cancer.* 2009;63:77-82.
62. Casal J, Amenedo M, Mel JR, Antón LM, Rodríguez-López R, López-López R, et al. Gemcitabine plus docetaxel as first-line chemotherapy in patients with advanced non-small cell lung cancer: a lung cancer Galician group phase II study. *Cancer Chemother Pharmacol.* 2007;60:725-32.
63. Comella P, Filippelli G, De Cataldis G, Massidda B, Frasci G, Maiorino L, et al.; Southern Italy Cooperative

Oncology Group.. Efficacy of the combination of cisplatin with either gemcitabine and vinorelbine or gemcitabine and paclitaxel in the treatment of locally advanced or metastatic non-small-cell lung cancer: a phase III randomised trial of the Southern Italy Cooperative Oncology Group (SICOG 0101). *Ann Oncol.* 2007;18: 324-30.

64. Kosmidis P, Mylonakis N, Nicolaides C, Kalophonos C, Samantas E, Boukovinas J, et al. Paclitaxel plus carboplatin versus gemcitabine plus paclitaxel in advanced non-small-cell lung cancer: a phase III randomized trial. *J Clin Oncol.* 2002;20:3578-85.
65. Ramlau R, Gervais R, Krzakowski M, von Pawel J, Kaukel E, Abratt RP, et al. Phase III study comparing oral topotecan to intravenous docetaxel in patients with pretreated advanced non-small-cell lung cancer. *J Clin Oncol.* 2006; 24:2800-7.
66. Kudoh S, Takeda K, Nakagawa K, Takada M, Katakami N, Matsui K, et al. Phase III study of docetaxel compared with vinorelbine in elderly patients with advanced non-small-cell lung cancer: results of the West Japan Thoracic Oncology Group Trial (WJTOG 9904). *J Clin Oncol.* 2006; 24:3657-63.
67. Pectasides D, Pectasides M, Farmakis D, Kostopoulou V, Nikolaou M, Gaglia A, et al. Comparison of docetaxel and docetaxel-irinotecan combination as second-line chemotherapy in advanced non-small-cell lung cancer: a randomized phase II trial. *Ann Oncol.* 2005;16:294-9.
68. Quoix E, Lebeau B, Depierre A, Ducolone A, Moro-Sibilot D, Milleron B, et al. Randomised, multicentre phase II study assessing two doses of docetaxel (75 or 100 mg/m^2) as second-line monotherapy for non-small-cell lung cancer. *Ann Oncol.* 2004;15:38-44.
69. Fossella FV, DeVore R, Kerr RN, Crawford J, Natale RR, Dunphy F, et al. Randomized phase III trial of docetaxel versus vinorelbine or ifosfamide in patients with advanced non-small-cell lung cancer previously treated with platinum-containing chemotherapy regimens. The TAX 320 Non-Small Cell Lung Cancer Study Group. *J Clin Oncol.* 2000;18:2354-62.
70. Sederholm C, Hillerdal G, Lamberg K, Kölbeck K, Dufmats M, Westberg R, et al. Phase III trial of gemcitabine plus carboplatin versus single-agent gemcitabine in the treatment of locally advanced or metastatic non-small-cell lung cancer: the Swedish Lung Cancer Study Group. *J Clin Oncol.* 2005;23:8380-8.
71. Vansteenkiste JF, Vandebroek JE, Nackaerts KL, Weynants P, Valcke YJ, Verresen DA, et al.; Leuven Lung Cancer Group. Clinical-benefit response in advanced non-small-cell lung cancer: A multicentre prospective randomised phase III study of single agent gemcitabine versus cisplatin-vindesine. *Ann Oncol.* 2001;12:1221-30.
72. Manegold C, Bergman B, Chemaissani A, Dornoff W, Drings P, Kellokumpu-Lehtinen P, et al. Single-agent gemcitabine versus cisplatin-etoposide: early results of a randomised phase II study in locally advanced or metastatic non-small-cell lung cancer. *Ann Oncol.* 1997;8:525-9.
73. Paz-Ares L, de Marinis F, Dediu M, Thomas M, Pujol JL, Bidoli P, et al. Maintenance therapy with pemetrexed plus best supportive care versus placebo plus best supportive care after induction therapy with pemetrexed plus cisplatin for advanced non-squamous non-small-cell lung cancer (PARAMOUNT): a double-blind, phase 3, randomised controlled trial. *Lancet Oncol.* 2012;13:247-55.
74. Smit EF, Burgers SA, Biesma B, Smit HJ, Eppinga P, Dingemans AM, et al. Randomized phase II and pharmacogenetic study of pemetrexed compared with pemetrexed plus carboplatin in pretreated patients with advanced non-small-cell lung cancer. *J Clin Oncol.* 2009;27:2038-45.
75. Cullen MH, Zatloukal P, Sörenson S, Novello S, Fischer JR, Joy AA, et al. A randomized phase III trial comparing standard and high-dose pemetrexed as second-line treatment in patients with locally advanced or metastatic non-small-cell lung cancer. *Ann Oncol.* 2008;19:939-45.
76. Bearz A, Garassino I, Cavina R, Favaretto A, Boccalon M, Talamini R, et al. Pemetrexed single agent in previously treated non-small cell lung cancer: a multi-institutional observational study. *Lung Cancer.* 2008;60:240-5.
77. Hanna N, Shepherd FA, Fossella FV, Pereira JR, De Marinis F, von Pawel J, et al. Randomized phase III trial of pemetrexed versus docetaxel in patients with non-small-cell lung cancer previously treated with chemotherapy. *J Clin Oncol.* 2004;22:1589-97.
78. Jotte R, Conkling P, Reynolds C, Galsky MD, Klein L, Fitzgibbons JF, et al. Randomized phase II trial of single-agent amrubicin or topotecan as second-line treatment in patients with small-cell lung cancer sensitive to first-line platinum-based chemotherapy. *J Clin Oncol.* 2011; 29:287-93.
79. Inoue A, Sugawara S, Yamazaki K, Maemondo M, Suzuki T, Gomi K, et al. Randomized phase II trial comparing amrubicin with topotecan in patients with previously treated small-cell lung cancer: North Japan Lung Cancer Study Group Trial 0402. *J Clin Oncol.* 2008;26:5401-06.
80. Eckardt JR, von Pawel J, Pujol JL, Papai Z, Quoix E, Ardizzoni A, et al. Phase III study of oral compared with intravenous topotecan as second-line therapy in small-cell lung cancer. *J Clin Oncol.* 2007;25:2086-92.
81. O'Brien MF, Ciuleanu TE, Tsekov H, Shparyk Y, Cuceviá B, Juhasz G, et al. Phase III trial comparing supportive care alone with supportive care with oral topotecan in patients with relapsed small-cell lung cancer. *J Clin Oncol.* 2006;24:5441-7.
82. Rosell R, Carcereny E, Gervais R, Vergnenegre A, Massuti B, Felip E, et al.; Spanish Lung Cancer Group in collaboration with Groupe Français de Pneumo-Cancérologie and Associazione Italiana Oncologia Toracica. Erlotinib versus standard chemotherapy as first-line treatment for European patients with advanced EGFR mutation-positive non-small-cell lung cancer (EURTAC): a multicentre, open-label, randomised phase 3 trial. *Lancet Oncol.* 2012;13:239-46.
83. Ciuleanu T, Stelmakh L, Cicenas S, Miliauskas S, Grigorescu AC, Hillenbach C, et al. Efficacy and safety of erlotinib versus chemotherapy in second-line treatment of patients with advanced, non-small-cell lung cancer with poor prognosis (TITAN): a randomised multicentre, open-label, phase 3 study. *Lancet Oncol.* 2012;13:300-8.

84. Reck M, van Zandwijk N, Gridelli C, Baliko Z, Rischin D, Allan S, et al. Erlotinib in advanced non-small cell lung cancer: efficacy and safety findings of the global phase IV Tarceva Lung Cancer Survival Treatment study. *J Thorac Oncol.* 2010;5:1616-22.
85. Maemondo M, Inoue A, Kobayashi K, Sugawara S, Oizumi S, Isobe H, et al.; North-East Japan Study Group. Gefitinib or chemotherapy for non-small-cell lung cancer with mutated EGFR. *N Engl J Med.* 2010;362:2380-8.
86. Kong MF, Nayyar V, Jogia R, Berrington R, Jackson S. A swollen knee: and the father of hysteria. *Lancet.* 2008; 372:1854.
87. Douillard JY, Gervais R, Dabouis G, Le Groumellec A, D'Arlhac M, Spaeth D, et al. Sequential two-line strategy for stage IV non-small-cell lung cancer: docetaxel-cisplatin versus vinorelbine-cisplatin followed by cross-over to single-agent docetaxel or vinorelbine at progression: final results of a randomised phase II study. *Ann Oncol.* 2005;16:81-9.
88. Kosmidis PA, Syrigos K, Kalofonos HP, Dimopoulos MA, Skarlos D, Pavlidis N, et al. Vinorelbine versus paclitaxel for patients with advanced non-small cell lung cancer (NSCLC) and a performance status of 2. *Anticancer Res.* 2012;32:175-81.
89. Camerini A, Valsuani C, Mazzoni F, Siclari O, Puccetti C, Donati S, et al. Phase II trial of single-agent oral vinorelbine in elderly (> or =70 years) patients with advanced non-small-cell lung cancer and poor performance status. *Ann Oncol.* 2010;21:1290-5.
90. Rossi D, Catalano V, Alessandroni P, Fedeli A, Fedeli SL, Giordani P, et al. A phase II study of single-agent oral vinorelbine in patients with pretreated advanced non-small-cell lung cancer. *Clin Lung Cancer.* 2007;8:382-5.
91. Cooper KL, Madan J, Whyte S, Stevenson MD, Akehurst RL. Granulocyte colony-stimulating factors for febrile neutropenia prophylaxis following chemotherapy: systematic review and meta-analysis. *BMC Cancer.* 2011;11:404.
92. Timmer-Bonte JN, Adang EM, Smit HJ, Biesma B, Wilschut FA, Bootsma GP, et al. Cost-effectiveness of adding granulocyte colony-stimulating factor to primary prophylaxis with antibiotics in small-cell lung cancer. *J Clin Oncol.* 2006;24:2991-7.
93. Freifeld AG, Bow EJ, Sepkowitz KA, Boeckh MJ, Ito JI, Mullen CA, et al. Clinical practice guideline for the use of antimicrobial agents in neutropenic patients with cancer: 2010 Update by the Infectious Diseases Society of America. *Clin Infect Dis.* 2011;52:427-31.
94. Gafter-Gvili A, Fraser A, Paul M, Leibovici L. Meta-analysis: antibiotic prophylaxis reduces mortality in neutropenic patients. *Ann Intern Med.* 2005;142:979-95.
95. Kouranos V, Dimopoulos G, Vassias A, Syrigos KN. Chemotherapy-induced neutropenia in lung cancer patients: the role of antibiotic prophylaxis. *Cancer Lett.* 2011;313:9-14.
96. Donowitz GR, Harman C, Pope T, Stewart FM. The role of the chest roentgenogram in febrile neutropenic patients. *Arch Intern Med.* 1991;151:701-4.
97. Klastersky J, Paesmans M, Rubenstein EB, Boyer M, Elting L, Feld R, et al. The Multinational Association for Supportive Care in Cancer risk index: A multinational scoring system for identifying low-risk febrile neutropenic cancer patients. *J Clin Oncol.* 2000;18:3038-51.
98. Mermel LA, Allon M, Bouza E, Craven DE, Flynn P, O'Grady NP, et al. Clinical practice guidelines for the diagnosis and management of intravascular catheter-related infection: 2009 Update by the Infectious Diseases Society of America. *Clin Infect Dis.* 2009;49:1-45.

CHAPTER 12

Respiratory Infections In Specific Populations: Drug Users

Georgios Kouliatsis, Vasileios Papaioannou, Ioannis Pneumatikos

ABSTRACT

Illicit drug use is a worldwide public health problem with high prevalence rate. Drug users often suffer from poor hygiene, malnutrition, or acquired immunodeficiency syndrome while most illicit drugs have direct immunosuppressive and/or immunomodulating properties. Thus, drug abuse increases risk for viral, bacterial, and fungal infections. Community-acquired pneumonia, aspiration pneumonia, necrotic pneumonia due to septic pulmonary emboli, and pulmonary tuberculosis are the most common respiratory infections in this group of patients. The physician in-charge faces a lot of challenges regarding diagnostic and therapeutic alternatives since differential diagnosis includes many different scenarios. Moreover, these patients often present late in the course of illness, commonly fail to comply with treatment, and frequently suffer from complications, relapses, and serious comorbidities.

INTRODUCTION

Illicit drug use is a worldwide health problem. Cannabis, amphetamine-type stimulants, opioids (including opium, heroin, and prescription opioids), and cocaine are the most widely used drugs and dominate the global illicit drug market. Other synthetic drugs, such as lysergic acid diethylamide, phencyclidine, and ketamine are still consumed but their use is limited to a relative small percentage of drug users at the present time. For the purposes of this chapter, we shall consider drug users as people who consume one of the above substances.

According to statistical data provided by the United Nations Office on Drugs and Crime (UNODC) 2011 World Drug Report, it is estimated that in 2009 3.3–6.1% of the population aged between 15 years and 64 years used illicit substances at least once in the previous year.[1] This corresponds to an approximate number of 272 million illicit drug users, half of which are believed to be current drug users. Problem drug users are loosely defined as those who regularly use illicit substances and can be considered dependent on them, as long as those who inject drugs and are estimated to be between 15 million and 39 million. While the total number of drug users and problem drug users shows an increase, the prevalence rates seem to remain stable since the late 90's.

In terms of specific drug prevalence, cannabis is by far the most widely used illicit drug. Cannabis is estimated to be consumed by approximately 125–203 million people. This corresponds to an annual prevalence rate of 2.8–4.5%. In terms of worldwide prevalence, cannabis is followed by amphetamine-type stimulants, opioids, and cocaine. It should be noted that prescription opioid analgesic abuse is the fastest growing form of drug abuse in the United States.

According to UNODC 2011 World Drug Report for Europe, the best estimates suggest that there are between 25,000 and 27,000 drug-related deaths annually, with a rate between 46 deaths and 48 deaths per 1 million people aged 15–64. There are estimates that these numbers could be twice as high. North America seems to experience a large proportion of drug-related deaths and the highest drug-related mortality rate (148 deaths per million population aged 15-64). For the United States, the numbers are even higher as they are estimated up to 182 deaths per 1 million inhabitants aged 15–64. Opioids, mainly heroin, are ranked as the main cause of death in Europe and they are followed by cocaine, at much lower rates. In United States, a significant proportion of drug-related mortality is attributed to prescription opioids. The overdose syndrome-related mortality is a worldwide problem, although actual prevalence does not lack geographical variations.

The possession and trading of most commonly used substances is still a criminal offence in most countries of the world. As a result, only a small proportion of illicit drug users stay in contact with healthcare providing services or other government agencies and, therefore, the numbers reported above can only provide an uncertain estimation of the problem, which is reflected in the wide range of the estimated prevalence rates. In addition, lack of information regarding use of illicit drugs in populous countries, such as China, India, and most African countries generate uncertainty regarding the estimation of the global number of users.

DRUG USE AND INFECTIONS: GENERAL CONCEPTS

Infections are among the most serious complications of drug abuse.[2-4] Illicit drug use is a well-established risk factor for transmission of human immunodeficiency virus (HIV), sexually transmitted diseases, and viral hepatitis.[1] In addition to these infections, drug users risk acquiring a variety of bacterial infections. The most common bacterial infections in drug users include skin and soft tissue infections, such as abscesses and cellulitis, musculoskeletal infections, e.g., septic arthritis and osteomyelitis, tetanus, endovascular infections, such as bloodstream infection, infective endocarditis, septic thrombophlebitis, mycotic aneurysms and, last but not least, respiratory tract infections, which will be discussed in this chapter.[4] The nature of these bacterial infections depends highly on the drug and its interaction with the drug user, the method of administration, social, and hygiene factors.

The drug user's own commensal flora, such as *Staphylococcus* spp. and *Streptococcus* spp. are responsible for the majority of bacterial infections but other organisms such as Gram-negative bacteria contaminating the drugs, drug adulterants, or paraphernalia seem to play an important role as well. *Staphylococcus aureus* and *Streptococcus* species have been identified as major responsible pathogens and have been shown to colonize the skin and nose of drug users. *Staphylococcus aureus* colonization is a well-known risk factor for infection.[5]

Skin damage due to intravenous injection and nasal epithelium damage due to drug inhalation are thought to be two of the most important pathogenetic mechanisms. Insufficient skin and hand cleaning prior to injection,[6] injection at heavily colonized sites, such as the femoral vein,[7] and different drug administration practices and techniques that lack any sense of hygiene rules are also responsible for bacterial infection. Among others, drug users are known to crush capsules or tablets in their mouth while preparing for intravenous injection, blow out needle clots, lick needles to facilitate injection, and share needles for intravenous injections with other drug users. Shared needles and other drug paraphernalia are often rinsed with saliva, running water, or even toilet water.[7,8]

Black tar heroin has been associated with clostridium infections as it is contaminated with spores when mixed with adulterants or diluted with other substances, such as dextrose or dyed paper. Clostridium spores are known to survive from boiling so the typical heating of heroin before injection does not offer any protection against clostridium infection. Additionally, local soft tissue ischemia from repeated injections provide an appropriate environment for infections from anaerobic pathogens, such as clostridium.[9] Other types of drug preparations have been associated with specific infectious complications, such as the outbreak of infective endocarditis caused by *Pseudomonas aeruginosa* associated with the intravenous combination of pentazocine and tripelennamine.[10]

Malnutrition

Apart from the role of hygiene, living conditions, and tissue trauma, there are several other factors that predispose drug users to infections. Malnutrition has a high prevalence among drug users. Malnutrition seems to be multifactorial. Social and economic issues, the drug of choice, and the level of addiction seem to play an important role in the development of malnutrition.[11] Injecting drug users usually have a low body mass index (BMI) and they are often fed a protein-depletion diet. Drug users usually present with kwashiorkor due to severe protein depletion and less frequently with mixed marasmus and kwashiorkor. Illicit drug users should be screened for malnutrition. The Malnutrition Universal Screening Tool is sufficient for use in the community,[12] while Nutritional Risk Screening (NRS-2002) is more suitable for hospitalized individuals.[13]

Malnutrition is an undisputed risk factor of immune suppression and although it has not been extensively studied as an independent risk factor for infection in the population of illicit drug users, its high prevalence allows us to safely assume that it has an important role in the impairment of host responses and the exacerbation of the risk of infection.[14-22] Malnutrition is associated with a spectrum of immune defects including cutaneous anergy, decreased T cell mitogen responses, and decreased phagocytic cell function. Additional abnormalities include the decline of the number of circulating T cells, impaired specific antibody responses in spite of normal or increased levels of serum immunoglobulin, sparse lymphoid follicles and a relative depletion of cells in primary and secondary lymphoid organs.[14-22] Malnutrition predisposes to a greater incidence of infection and increased morbidity and mortality due to infection. It is estimated that malnutrition leads to 10- and 30-fold increased mortality from pneumonia and gastroenteritis, respectively.[23]

Human Immunodeficiency Virus Infection

Human immunodeficiency virus infection is a common coexisting medical condition among drug users. According to UNODC 2011 World Drug Report, the global average prevalence of HIV among injecting drug users is estimated at 17.9%, or equivalently, 2.8 million people who inject drugs are living with HIV.[1] High level of HIV infections are, in general, found among marginalized populations of drug users as well as among those in prison settings. There seem to be large geographical variations in the prevalence of HIV among injecting drug users. Latin America, East Europe, and East and South-East Asia account for 73% of the global number of injecting drug users living with HIV. The prevalence of HIV among injecting drug users is extremely high in certain countries, such as Estonia (72%), Argentina (50%), and Brazil (48%).[1] HIV infection is responsible for acquired immunodeficiency syndrome (AIDS). AIDS is characterized by a reduction in CD4 cell count that progressively causes profound immunosuppression, thus leaving the patient vulnerable to opportunistic infections. Opportunistic pulmonary infections can be caused by bacteria (*Streptococcus pneumoniae, Haemophilus Influenzae, Staphylococcus aureus, Pseudomonas aeruginosa, Nocardia asteroides,* and *Rochalimaea henselae*), fungi (*Pneumocystis jirovecii, Candida albicans, Aspergillus* spp., *Histoplasma capsulatum, Cryptococcus neoformans,* and *Penicillium marneffei*), parasites (*Toxoplasma gondii, Microsporidium, Leishmania, Cryptosporidium,* and *Strongyloides stercoralis*), viruses (cytomegalovirus, hepatitis B virus, hepatitis C virus and others) and mycobacteria (*Mycobacterium tuberculosis, Mycobacterium avium-intracellulare,* and *Mycobacterium kansasii*). HIV-infected drug users carry an increased risk of death from bacterial infection when compared to the general HIV positive population.[24-27] The detailed discussion of HIV-related opportunistic infections is beyond the scope of this chapter. It is worth noting, however, that, given the high prevalence rates, testing for HIV infection is considered mandatory at least for all injecting drug users that seek medical help for any health problem, and especially when they present with recurrent infections.

Immunomodulation

There is a relationship between addictive drugs of abuse and increased susceptibility to infections. Cannabis, opiates, amphetamine-type stimulants, and cocaine have all been shown to cause immunomodulation with a great variety of pathophysiologic pathways.[28]

More than 60 different cannabinoids have already been identified to be contained in the smoke of burning cannabis. Δ-9-tetrahydrocannabinol (Δ-9-THC) is considered to be the major compound and produces most of the characteristic pharmacological effects of smoked cannabis. Numerous studies during the last decades have shown that cannabinoid components have significant immunomodulatory effects.[28-36] Cannabinoids seem to have an effect on the normal function of T and B lymphocytes, natural killer (NK) cells, and macrophages in both *in vivo* and *in vitro* experimental models. Although the mechanisms for this effect seem to be multifactorial, they mostly include cannabinoid receptors (CBRs). There are two major CBRs, CB1, and CB2. CB1 receptor is expressed mainly in the central nervous system and is responsible for the neurologic and euphoric effects of cannabis. CB2 receptor is expressed mainly in the periphery and especially in the immune cells.[37,38] Binding of both CBRs and especially CB2 receptors seems to cause decreased host resistance to bacterial and viral infections. A number of studies have shown that cannabinoids increase susceptibility to intracellular bacteria, such as *Listeria* spp., *Legionella* spp., and even *Treponema pallidum* as well as to the herpes simplex virus. Some data also indicate that cannabinoids are responsible for increased susceptibility to opportunistic microbial infections in HIV patients.[33,36,39-44] It seems that one of the mechanisms responsible for the increased susceptibility to *Legionella* spp. and other intracellular bacteria is inhibition of Th1 cell development and involves both CB1 and CB2 receptors.[45]

Opiates and opioids are now recognized to enhance susceptibility to various infectious agents as well.[46] Opiate users are known to suffer more frequently from pneumonia caused by *Staphylococcus* spp., *Streptococcus* spp. *and* Haemophilus spp. and other more or less common pathogens, such as *Mycobacterium Tuberculosis* and atypical mycobacteria.[29,47] Intravenous drug abuse is a known risk factor for HIV infection and immunomodulation seems to be a reason in addition to contaminated shared needles.[48,49] Phagocytosis, NK cells activity, immune cytotoxicity, chemotaxis, and chemokine production has been shown to be decreased in opiate users. The mechanisms are again multifactorial. Multiple opiate receptors have been recognized and extensively studied. Mu (M), kappa (κ), and gamma (γ) subtypes seem to be the most important ones. Opiate receptors are expressed, among others, by central nervous system and immune cells. Opiates directly bind to these receptors, causing a cascade of effects associated with immunomodulation.[50-53] Again, a shift of Th cells from Th1 toward Th2 differentiation seems to play a central role, similarly to the effects cannabinoids have on immune response.[53,54] Apart from these direct effects, opiates cause immunomodulation indirectly through interaction with the central nervous system. Opiates increase the production of corticotropin-releasing hormone and adrenocorticotropic hormone, thus causing an increase in serum levels of glucocorticoid and corticosterone.[55] Glucocorticoids have well-documented immunoregulatory and actually immunosuppressive effects.

Cocaine-induced immunomodulation seems to be related to receptors in the periphery as well as the central nervous system. Cocaine has been found to decrease lymphocyte proliferation, cytokine production, NK activity, antibody activity and various aspects of both humoral and cellular immunity. The mechanisms of cocaine-induced immunosuppression have been studied mainly *in vitro* lymphoid cells cultures as long as rodent models.[56-65]

Amphetamine-type stimulants effect on immune response has also been investigated. Mice experiments with amphetamine showed a dose-related suppression of the NK cells activity, a reduction in thymus and spleen cellularity and in peripheral T lymphocyte population.[66,67] Treatment with amphetamine has been shown to change hypothalamo-pituitary-adrenal axis responsiveness to stress in experimental models and decrease lung and blood leukocytes cellularity via corticosterone effects.[68]

Cigarette smoking is common in illicit drug users. Nicotine is an agonist for nicotinic acetylene receptors which are found on central nervous system cells as well as other cells in the periphery, including immune cells. Nicotine and cigarette smoke have marked effects on the immune system. Nicotine has been shown to induce glucocorticoid release, decrease the production of cytokines and cause depressed alveolar macrophage function after infection. Nicotine seems to affect lymphocyte proliferation, inhibit antibody formation, and induce T cell anergy.[69-72] Nicotine may have a clinically important effect on the cholinergic anti-inflammatory pathway which signals through the efferent vagus nerve.[73] This pathway is mediated by nicotinic acetylcholine receptors on macrophages and the spleen and is a part of the so-called vagal immune reflex.[74] More studies are warranted regarding the exact mechanisms involved in nicotine-induced immunomodulation.

Alcohol abuse is also common among illicit drug users. Alcohol abusers are known to experience a variety of health problems, including decreased liver function and increased rates of infectious diseases.[75-77] Ethanol, unlike other previously mentioned addictive drugs, does not appear to bind to a specific receptor. Alcohol has been shown to decrease NK activity, antibody formulation, T-cell proliferation, and production of cytokines, such as TNF-α secreted by macrophages.[78-81]

DRUG USE-ASSOCIATED RESPIRATORY INFECTIONS

Aspiration Pneumonia

Illicit drug use and especially intravenous drug abuse is an independent risk factor for aspiration pneumonia and is mainly attributed to neurologic impairment. Most intravenous opioids users will experience drug overdose, aspiration and coma at least once. This complication is among the most common ones in intravenous drug users and kills an estimated 1% of intravenous drug addicts each year, thus accounting for a significant part of intravenous drug abuse-related mortality.[82,83] The usual cause of overdose syndrome is unawareness of the necessary dose that produces the desired effect, also referred to as "fix". Overdose could lead to acute respiratory distress syndrome (ARDS) or impairment of respiratory pump function due to central nervous system depression and subsequent hypercapnic (type II) respiratory failure. Aspiration of gastric content due to neurological impairment is a fearful complication of overdose. Ischemic or hemorrhagic stroke or even drug-induced seizures (e.g., abuse of cocaine) could also be responsible for aspiration.

Aspiration of significant volumes of gastric content will initially cause a chemical pneumonitis attributed to the usually acidic gastric content. This chemical pneumonitis is characterized by hypoxemic respiratory failure, radiographic parenchymal infiltrates, diffuse crackles, fever, purulent secretions, commonly atelectasis and leukocytosis. Aspiration could lead to ARDS or be complicated by bacterial infection. The responsible pathogens encountered usually include anaerobic bacteria, such as *Streptococci* spp. and *Fusobacterium* spp. and Gram-negative enteric bacilli. Dental and periodontal disease is frequent in drug users and could be the source of these pathogens.[84]

Differential diagnoses between aspiration pneumonitis and bacterial aspiration-associated pneumonia could be difficult. The decision when to begin antibiotic treatment is, therefore, based on mainly clinical suspicion. Aspiration pneumonia tends to have a relatively insidious course when compared to community-acquired pneumonia. As a result, the patient may have a parapneumonic effusion, empyema, necrotizing pneumonia, or lung abscesses at the time of the first clinical examination (Figure 1).[84-89]

Community-acquired Pneumonia

Both HIV negative and HIV positive illicit drug users are at high risk of community-acquired pneumonia and aspiration pneumonia. It has been estimated that intravenous drug users have a tenfold increased risk for community-acquired pneumonia.[90] In one case series, pneumonia accounted for 38% of hospital admissions of intravenous drug users with fever. The range and frequency of the responsible pathogens in HIV negative

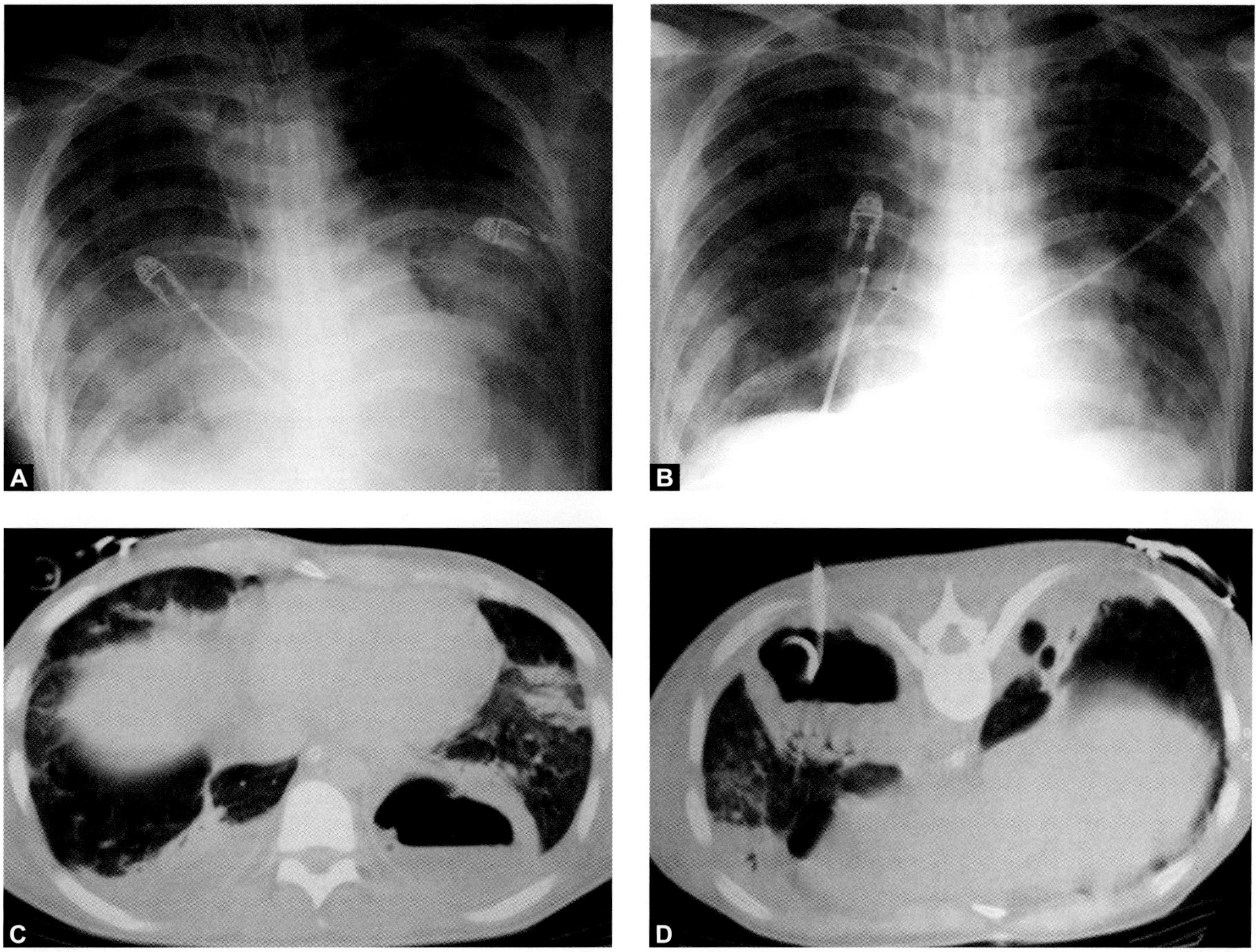

FIGURE 1 Lung abscess in a 23-year-old intravenous drug user. The patient was admitted in intensive care unit (ICU) with fever, severe hypoxemia and altered mental status. He was treated with intravenous clindamycin and ceftriaxone but his condition deteriorated. **A,** The chest X-ray on day 3 showed bilateral pulmonary infiltrates; Ceftriaxone-resistant *Klebsiella pneumoniae* was isolated from bronchial aspirations, so imipenem and amikacin were added to the antibiotic regimen. **B,** The patient remained septic for the next 6 days in spite of the minor improvement in the chest radiograph; **C** and **D,** The chest CT showed a left lower lobe lung abscess which was drained with a chest tube. The patient's condition was significantly improved and he left ICU after 18 days of treatment.

drug users and HIV positive drug users without AIDS are similar to those found in community-acquired pneumonia in the general population, with the exception of *Staphylococcus aureus*.[91] Staphylococcus aureus has been shown to colonize the nose of inhalation drug users. This colonization increases the risk of pneumonia caused by *Staphylococcus aureus*.[5] A 7-year study of hospitalized drug abusers in Switzerland by Scheidegger et al. has recorded *Streptococcus pneumoniae, Haemophilus influenzae, Staphylococcus aureus,* and *Klebsiella pneumonia* as the most common pathogens that cause community-acquired pneumonia leading to hospital admission.[2] A large prospective study of community-acquired pneumonia in institutionalized former drug users by Boschini et al. showed that *Streptococcus pneumoniae, Chlamydia pneumoniae*, and *Haemophilus influenzae* were the most commonly isolated responsible pathogens, followed by *Moraxella catarrhalis, Coxiella burnetii,* and *Pseudomonas aeruginosa* at much lower rates.[92] Intravenous drug users can present with both typical and atypical clinical and radiographic presentation of pneumonia although the typical presentation with fever, chills, productive cough with purulent sputum, inspiratory crackles, leukocytosis, and radiographic consolidation is the most common in patients without AIDS. Intravenous cefuroxime, ampicillin-sulbactam, and fluoroquinolones are commonly used in the setting of community-acquired pneumonia in illicit drug users without AIDS, although serious consideration of *Staphylococcus* should prompt the use of oxacillin or even vancomycin or linezolid. Local antibiotic data regarding methicillin-resistant *Staphylococcus aureus* (MRSA) and Gram-negative bacteria should always be taken under consideration prior to the selection of empiric antibiotic treatment.[93-95] The Pneumonia Severity Index clinical prediction rule could be used for the decision of hospitalization.[96] However, injecting drug users often show poor adherence to therapy and this should be considered before the decision for outpatient treatment. Acute respiratory failure, lung abscess, empyema, severe sepsis, and septic shock may complicate bacterial pneumonia in drug users with comorbidities, such as HIV infection, severe malnutrition, and poor hygiene or, due to late seeking of medical consult and significantly raised morbidity and mortality rates (Fig. 1).

Septic Pulmonary Emboli

Hematogenous spread septic pulmonary infracts in intravenous drug users are the result of recurrent emboli of infected material. The source could be directly from the injection site, tricuspid endocarditis, or both. The responsible pathogens are most commonly *Staphylococcus* spp., with *Staphylococcus aureus* accounting for more than 80% of the septic pulmonary emboli case. MRSA is an already emerged problem among intravenous drug users. Other *Staphylococcus* species, Gram-negative bacteria and, rarely, *Candida* species account for the rest of the cases.

Patients present with symptoms of recurrent pulmonary emboli, such as chest pain, dyspnea, hemoptysis, and high fever and often acute respiratory failure. Common clinical findings characterizing tricuspid endocarditis (e.g., murmurs) may be absent as tricuspid murmurs are often absent. Blood cultures are often positive and usually confirm *Staphylococcus septicemia*. The chest radiograph will show diffuse infiltrates and sometimes peripheral nodules, mediastinal lymphadenopathy, cavities, and pleural infusion. The infection may be complicated by lung abscess, empyema, and pneumothorax with or without bronchopleural fistula and may lead to ARDS.[97-108]

Tricuspid endocarditis is suggested by the sequential appearance of radiographically evident lesions in diverse lung sections and the absence of deep venous thrombosis. Tricuspid endocarditis can be confirmed with transesophageal echocardiography. The diagnosis is important as tricuspid endocarditis requires a conventional 4–6 weeks intravenous antibiotic treatment and carries a significant mortality rate of up to 16%. Drug users quite often refuse to compile with the extended period of intravenous treatment as it requires hospitalization and, therefore, difficult or impossible access to the drug of abuse. Such patients could be treated with a combination of oral antibiotics provided the pathogen is not resistant to the agents prescribed. Dworkin et al. conducted a study in 1989 of per os treatment of right-sided *Staphylococcus aureus* endocarditis in intravenous drug abusers with ciprofloxacin and rifampicin for 4 weeks and showed that it was equally effective to conventional intravenous antibiotic treatment.[109] Nowadays with the increasing rate of MRSA colonization among drug users,[4] such a therapeutic option obviously requires microbiologic evidence of sensitivity to the agents of choice before it is considered as an alternative.[4,97,98,104,108,110-113]

Fungal Pneumonia

There are many cases of pulmonary candidiasis that have been reported among mainly intravenous drug users and these are not confined to patients with AIDS. It seems that the infection is the result of contamination of the lemon used to acidify the injected solution by *Candida albicans*. The clinical symptoms of pneumonia may appear several days after the last injection. The presentation can mimic classic bacterial lobar pneumonia or present as part of systemic candidiasis, thus including ocular infection, endocarditis, arthritis, hepatitis, as long as several other sites of infection. ARDS is a possible complication. Other fungi, such as *Aspergillus* have been also found to contaminate "street" drugs, such as heroin and could potentially cause infection as well.[114-118]

Pulmonary Tuberculosis

Tuberculosis (TB) is more common in intravenous drug users than in the general population.[119] Illicit drug use has a central role in the epidemiology of tuberculosis in both developed and developing countries.[120-122] A number of studies has been conducted in an effort to estimate latent and active tuberculosis infection rates among drug users. Latent TB infection (LTBI) is reported at rates ranging from 10% to 59% of illicit drug users.[119] A longer duration of drug use and an older age have been recognized as independent risk factors for LTBI.[123,124] A study of 11,000 intravenous drug users in the US-border Mexican city of Tijuana, which is a region of TB endemicity, found a prevalence of 67% LTBI.[125] A prospective study was performed from 1986 to 1996 as part of an ongoing cohort study of HIV infection in Amsterdam drug users and showed that 24 persons out of 872 participants developed culture confirmed tuberculosis during the total follow-up period. HIV infection and age above 33 years increased the risk for tuberculosis substantially with a relative risk of 12.9 and 6.8, respectively. The incidence of culture confirmed tuberculosis in HIV negative drug users was still six times higher than in the overall Amsterdam population.[126]

Multiple drug-resistant tuberculosis and extensive drug-resistant tuberculosis (XDR-TB) is nowadays a worldwide problem, although there are still great geographical variations. The World Health Organization issues tactical world reports regarding surveillance of M/XDR-TB.[127] The prevalence of M/XDR-TB among illicit drug users is increasing. Prior exposure to anti-TB drugs, incomplete therapy for LTBI and TB infection and high transmission rates due to lifestyle issues, immunosuppression, and poor medical care are considered to be the most important causes for the increasing M/XDR-TB rates among drug users.[127,128]

Human immunodeficiency virus-induced immunosuppression is the most important reason for the high TB prevalence among intravenous drug users.[129] In recognition of the extension of the problem the World Health Organization, the Joint United Nations Programme on HIV/AIDS, and the UNODC have issued "Policy guidelines for collaborative TB and HIV services for injecting and other drug users" in 2008.[130] Apart from the high prevalence of HIV infection among these patients, high TB prevalence is owned to risk factors discussed above and is associated to lifestyle issues, close contact, malnutrition, depressed immunity, and alcoholism. The high prevalence of LTBI contributes to increased rates of transmission. Cluster analysis of DNA samples during TB outbreaks shows the presence of identical DNA patterns, which is evidence of recent transmission.[131]

Both prevention and treatment of TB in drug users are problematic. Intravenous drug users tend to seek medical attention late in the course of disease. They also seem to have difficulty attending medical re-evaluation and adhering to treatment for LTBI or TB infection. Opiates may depress symptoms of infection, such as cough and this could be another reason for the delay of seeking medical care. Social factors, such as fear of withdrawal symptoms if hospitalized, lack of health insurance, fear of being stigmatized, or having law problems raise even more barriers to proper medical care.[132-135]

Tuberculin skin testing (TST) is the most common test for LTBI. TST is considered positive if the induration is greater than 10 mm in intravenous drug users and 5 mm in HIV-positive individuals. TST has several limitations including the booster phenomenon, potential cross-reactivity with bacilli Calmette-Guérin-vaccination, and anergic response in immunocompromised individuals, such as HIV-positive patients. Regarding intravenous drug users, perhaps the most problematic feature of TST is the requirement for a return visit as many drug users fail to return for the evaluation of the test.[136] IFN-release assays (IGRAs) present a relatively recent development in the diagnosis of LTBI and are free of most TST limitations. IGRAs present insensitivity to bacilli Calmette-Guérin vaccination, lack of requirement of a return visit and there is no need for boosting. The Centers for Disease Control and Prevention has recommended the use of an IGRA for all circumstances in which TST is currently used.[137] However, the diagnostic value of IGRAs in immunocompromised individuals remains unproven.

A detailed discussion regarding the treatment of LTBI and TB infection is beyond the scope of this chapter. However, TB and LTBI treatment in the population of drug users present with some challenges. First of all, it is important for the responsible health service to seek methods for improving TB treatment adherence and completion of therapy among drug users. Individuals actively abusing drugs or alcohol may have impaired cognition and distorted priorities and often face severe financial and social problems. Directly observed treatment (DOT), especially when combined with methadone or monetary incentives seems to achieve adherence and is still cost effective. Regimens may also be modified so that medication is given only 2–3 times per week, thus improving adherence and decreasing the cost of DOT. It should be noted, however, that the once-weekly continuation phase regimen of isoniazid and rifapentine is only indicated in HIV-negative patients who have negative sputum smears at the time of completion of 2 months of therapy and do not have cavitation on initial radiograph.[138]

Conventional TB treatment with isoniazid, rifampin, and pyrazinamide can be hepatotoxic. This could be problematic for the population of drug users because they have a high prevalence of chronic viral hepatitis and alcohol abuse.[1] Studies have established the safety of anti-TB drugs among patients with viral hepatitis who undergo treatment for LTBI and TB disease, regarding the potential risk for drug-induced hepatitis.[139,140] Alcohol consumption, on the other hand, has been consistently recognized as an independent risk factor for drug-induced hepatitis in patients receiving anti-TB treatment.[141] Alcohol consumption and, even more, alcohol abuse is considered as a vital issue that needs to be urgently addressed when receiving anti-TB treatment.

Another issue regarding anti-TB treatment in drug users concerns individuals under therapy with methadone. Rifampin induces hepatic microsomal enzymes that increase clearance and reduce the half-life of barbiturates and methadone.[142] Therefore, patients receiving methadone could need a dose increase in order to deal with withdrawal symptoms. Rifabutin is an alternative agent that seems to lack this side-effect, although patients still refer some withdrawal symptoms.[143,144]

DIFFERENTIAL DIAGNOSIS

The attending physician who is called to treat an illicit drug user that presents with dyspnea, hypoxemic respiratory failure, and an abnormal chest radiograph should bear in mind that illicit drug use is associated with a variety of diseases and syndromes apart from infections that involve lung pathology and usually present with this clinical scenario. Differential diagnosis could be challenging. Both inhaled and intravenously delivered drugs, including opiates, cocaine, and crack, may cause acute lung injury and ARDS. ARDS is sometimes difficult and even impossible to differentiate from bilateral, diffuse pneumonia. Bronchial aspirates cultures, quantitative cultures of protective pulmonary specimens, and bronchoalveolar lavage cultures are neither sensitive nor specific enough to help with the differential diagnoses;[145,146] and the clinician feels often obliged to treat with antibiotics. Cocaine smoking may cause pulmonary hemorrhage[147] and so does crack abuse. Illicit drugs with sympathomimetic properties, such as cocaine, may cause cardiogenic pulmonary edema with high pulmonary artery wedge pressure by inducing myocardial ischemia, arrhythmias, or severe peripheral vasoconstriction with left ventricular failure.[148]Pulmonary vascular granulomatosis is currently a rare lung disease that could be encountered when treating injecting drug users. Some drug users inject aqueous suspensions of medications intended for oral use. The insoluble particles (usually fillers and binders used for the formulation of the tablet) enter the circulation and embolize in the pulmonary arteries, causing the formation of foreign body granulomas. Talc (magnesium trisilicate) is the most commonly associated particle. Cotton, starch, mercury, and even pieces of needles have been reported as embolized material as well. Pulmonary vascular talk granulomatosis is typically a subacute or chronic disease and often remains undiagnosed for a long time until the patient develops symptoms severe enough to seek medical attention. The patient typically complains for progressively deteriorating breathlessness, slightly productive cough, less commonly for wheezing shortly after the injection and, rarely, for symptoms consistent with pulmonary embolism.[149,150] The chest radiograph may show diffuse reticular-nodular infiltrates usually more prominent in the lung base but may also be normal. There is no specific treatment although some cases in the past have shown some responsiveness to prednisolone. The severity of the disease mainly depends on the total amount of talk injected throughout the years of drug injection. Pulmonary hypertension and death from *cor pulmonale* is a frequent sequel of the disease.[151]

A FINAL WORD

There are some key points in the treatment of illicit drug users with respiratory infections:

- Always test for HIV infection
- Always test for HBV and HCV infection
- Always test for LTBI. Know that your patient will probably not come back for TST evaluation
- Always assess the patient's nutritional status
- Illicit drug abuse is not that uncommon among young patients with infections of the lower respiratory tract
- An illicit drug user will probably strongly deny any illicit drug use if he is interviewed by a government employee, including doctors or nurses
- An illicit drug user might not show adherence to therapy and might not follow doctor's instructions. The physician should bear that in mind before deciding outpatient treatment or asking an illicit drug user to return for re-evaluation

- Intravenous drug users are strongly addicted. They will probably try to find a way to gain access to the drug of abuse even when hospitalized
- Drug detoxification and enrollment in a drug rehabilitation program is probably the patient's best chance to obtain an acceptable level of health-related quality of life. However, acute illness may not provide the proper timeframe for such a discussion. Do not hesitate to ask for psychiatric consultation
- Drug addiction is a complex issue. A multidisciplinary approach is often warranted. Refer the patient to a designated health or social service or, preferably, ask them to come and talk to your patient.

REFERENCES

1. United Nations Office on Drugs and Crime. (2011). World Drug Report. [online]. Available from: www.unodc.org/documents/data-and-analysis/WDR2011/World_Drug_Report_2011_ebook.pdf [Accessed February 2013].
2. Scheidegger C, Zimmerli W. Infectious complications in drug addicts: seven-year review of 269 hospitalized narcotics abusers in Switzerland. *Rev Infect Dis.* 1989;11(3):486-93.
3. Palepu A, Tyndall MW, Leon H, et al. Hospital utilization and costs in a cohort of injection drug users. *CMAJ.* 2001;165(4):415-20.
4. Gordon RJ, Lowy FD. Bacterial infections in drug users. *N Engl J Med.* 2005;353(18):1945-54.
5. Kluytmans J, van Belkum A, Verbrugh H. Nasal carriage of *Staphylococcus aureus:* epidemiology, underlying mechanisms, and associated risks. *Clin Microbiol Rev.* 1997;10(3):505-20.
6. Vlahov D, Sullivan M, Astemborski J, et al. Bacterial infections and skin cleaning prior to injection among intravenous drug users. *Public Health Rep.* 1992;107(5):595-8.
7. Binswanger IA, Kral AH, Bluthenthal RN, et al. High prevalence of abscesses and cellulitis among community-recruited injection drug users in San Francisco. *Clin Infect Dis.* 2000;30(3):579-81.
8. Stein MD. Medical complications of intravenous drug use. *J Gen Intern Med.* 1990;5(3):249-57.
9. Passaro DJ, Werner SB, McGee J, et al. Wound botulism associated with black tar heroin among injecting drug users. *JAMA.* 1998;279(11):859-63.
10. Shekar R, Rice TW, Zierdt CH, et al. Outbreak of endocarditis caused by Pseudomonas aeruginosa serotype O11 among pentazocine and tripelennamine abusers in Chicago. *J Infect Dis.* 1985;151(2):203-8.
11. Nazrul Islam SK, Jahangir Hossain K, Ahmed A, et al. Nutritional status of drug addicts undergoing detoxification: prevalence of malnutrition and influence of illicit drugs and lifestyle. *Br J Nutr.* 2002;88(5):507-13.
12. Karsegard VL, Ferlay O, Maisonneuve N, et al. Simplified malnutrition screening tool: Malnutrition Universal Screening Tool (MUST). *Rev Med Suisse Romande.* 2004;124(10):601-5.
13. Kondrup J, Rasmussen HH, Hamberg O, et al. Nutritional risk screening (NRS 2002): a new method based on an analysis of controlled clinical trials. *Clin Nutr.* 2003;22(3):321-36.
14. Bentdal OH, Froland SS, Djoseland O. Alterations in serum cortisol, CD4+ CD8+ lymphocyte sub-population ration and T cell mediated suppression of immune responses in the malnutrition of anorexia nervosa. *Clin Nutr.* 1991;10(3):167-72.
15. Hudgens J, Langkamp-Henken B, Stechmiller JK, et al. Immune function is impaired with a mini nutritional assessment score indicative of malnutrition in nursing home elders with pressure ulcers. *JPEN J Parenter Enteral Nutr.* 2004;28(6):416-22.
16. Marcos A. Eating disorders: a situation of malnutrition with peculiar changes in the immune system. *Eur J Clin Nutr.* 2000;54 Suppl 1:S61-4.
17. Lesourd BM, Mazari L. Immune responses during recovery from protein-energy malnutrition. *Clin Nutr.* 1997;16 Suppl 1:37-46.
18. Shetty PS, James WP, Ferro-Luzzi A. Malnutrition and the immune response. 1. Malnutrition in the community: recent concepts. *Trans R Soc Trop Med Hyg.* 1994;88(6):612-4.
19. Grimble RF. Malnutrition and the immune response. 2. Impact of nutrients on cytokine biology in infection. *Trans R Soc Trop Med Hyg.* 1994;88(6):615-9.
20. Nimmanwudipong T, Cheadle WG, Appel SH, et al. Effect of protein malnutrition and immunomodulation on immune cell populations. *J Surg Res.* 1992;52(3):233-8.
21. Koster F, Gaffar A, Jackson TM. Recovery of cellular immune competence during treatment of protein-calorie malnutrition. *Am J Clin Nutr.* 1981;34(5):887-91.
22. Walker WA. Cellular and immune changes in the gastrointestinal tract in malnutrition. *Curr Concepts Nutr.* 1980;9:197-218.
23. Santos J. Nutrition, infection, and immunocompetence. *Infect Dis Clin North Am.* 1994;8(1):243-67.
24. Stoneburner RL, Des Jarlais DC, Benezra D, et al. A larger spectrum of severe HIV-1--related disease in intravenous drug users in New York City. *Science.* 1988;242(4880):916-9.
25. O'Connor PG, Selwyn PA, Schottenfeld RS. Medical care for injection-drug users with human immunodeficiency virus infection. *N Engl J Med.* 1994;331(7):450-9.
26. Alcabes P, Friedland G. Injection drug use and human immunodeficiency virus infection. *Clin Infect Dis.* 1995;20(6):1467-79.
27. Benson CA, Kaplan JE, Masur H, et al. Treating opportunistic infections among HIV-infected adults and adolescents: recommendations from CDC, the National Institutes of Health, and the HIV Medicine Association/Infectious Diseases Society of America. *MMWR Recomm Rep.* 2004;53(RR-15):1-112.
28. Friedman H, Pross S, Klein TW. Addictive drugs and their relationship with infectious diseases. *FEMS Immunol Med Microbiol.* 2006;47(3):330-42.
29. Friedman H, Newton C, Klein TW. Microbial infections, immunomodulation, and drugs of abuse. *Clin Microbiol Rev.* 2003;16(2):209-19.
30. Baczynsky WO, Zimmerman AM. Effects of delta 9-tetrahydrocannabinol, cannabinol and cannabidiol on

the immune system in mice. I. In vivo investigation of the primary and secondary immune response. *Pharmacology.* 1983;26(1):1-11.
31. Klein TW, Newton CA, Widen R, et al. The effect of delta-9-tetrahydrocannabinol and 11-hydroxy-delta-9-tetrahydrocannabinol on T-lymphocyte and B-lymphocyte mitogen responses. *J Immunopharmacol.* 1985;7(4):451-66.
32. Klein TW, Newton C, Friedman H. Inhibition of natural killer cell function by marijuana components. *J Toxicol Environ Health.* 1987;20(4):321-32.
33. Djeu JY, Wang M, Friedman H. Adverse effect of delta 9-tetrahydrocannabinol on human neutrophil function. *Adv Exp Med Biol.* 1991;288:57-62.
34. Kaminski NE, Koh WS, Yang KH, Lee M, Kessler FK. Suppression of the humoral immune response by cannabinoids is partially mediated through inhibition of adenylate cyclase by a pertussis toxin-sensitive G-protein coupled mechanism. *Biochem Pharmacol.* 1994;48(10):1899-908.
35. Kawakami Y, Klein TW, Newton C, et al. Suppression by cannabinoids of a cloned cell line with natural killer cell activity. *Proc Soc Exp Biol Med.* 1988;187(3):355-9.
36. Friedman H. AIDS, drugs of abuse and the neuroimmune axis: introduction and perspectives. *Adv Exp Med Biol.* 1996;402:1-3.
37. Munro S, Thomas KL, Abu-Shaar M. Molecular characterization of a peripheral receptor for cannabinoids. *Nature.* 1993;365(6441):61-5.
38. Matsuda LA, Lolait SJ, Brownstein MJ, et al. Structure of a cannabinoid receptor and functional expression of the cloned cDNA. *Nature.* 1990;346(6284):561-4.
39. Klein TW, Newton C, Widen R, et al. Delta 9-tetrahydrocannabinol injection induces cytokine-mediated mortality of mice infected with Legionella pneumophila. *J Pharmacol Exp Ther.* 1993;267(2):635-40.
40. Specter S, Lancz G, Westrich G, et al. Delta-9-tetrahydrocannabinol augments murine retroviral induced immunosuppression and infection. *Int J Immunopharmacol.* 1991;13(4):411-7.
41. Morahan PS, Klykken PC, Smith SH, et al. Effects of cannabinoids on host resistance to Listeria monocytogenes and herpes simplex virus. *Infect Immun.* 1979;23(3):670-4.
42. Cabral GA, McNerney PJ, Mishkin EM. Delta-9-tetrahydrocannabinol enhances release of herpes simplex virus type 2. *J Gen Virol.* 1986;67 (Pt 9):2017-22.
43. Paradise LJ, Friedman H. Syphilis and drugs of abuse. *Adv Exp Med Biol.* 1993;335:81-7.
44. Friedman H. Drugs of abuse as possible co-factors in AIDS progression: summary of panel discussion. *Adv Exp Med Biol.* 1996;402:225-8.
45. Newton CA, Klein TW, Friedman H. Secondary immunity to Legionella pneumophila and Th1 activity are suppressed by delta-9-tetrahydrocannabinol injection. *Infect Immun.* 1994;62(9):4015-20.
46. Risdahl JM, Khanna KV, Peterson PK, et al. Opiates and infection. *J Neuroimmunol.* 1998;83(1-2):4-18.
47. Almirall J, Bolibar I, Balanzo X, et al. Risk factors for community-acquired pneumonia in adults: a population-based case-control study. *Eur Respir J.* 1999;13(2):349-55.
48. Battjes RJ, Leukefeld CG, Pickens RW, et al. The acquired immunodeficiency syndrome and intravenous drug abuse. *Bull Narc.* 1988;40(1):21-34.
49. Donahoe RM, Falek A. Neuroimmunomodulation by opiates and other drugs of abuse: relationship to HIV infection and AIDS. *Adv Biochem Psychopharmacol.* 1988;44:145-58.
50. Roy S, Barke RA, Loh HH. MU-opioid receptor-knockout mice: role of mu-opioid receptor in morphine mediated immune functions. *Brain Res Mol Brain Res.* 1998;61 (1-2):190-4.
51. Bryant HU, Roudebush RE. Suppressive effects of morphine pellet implants on in vivo parameters of immune function. *J Pharmacol Exp Ther.* 1990;255(2):410-4.
52. Adler MW, Geller EB, Rogers TJ, et al. Opioids, receptors, and immunity. *Adv Exp Med Biol.* 1993;335:13-20.
53. Roy S, Wang J, Charboneau R, et al. Morphine induces CD4+ T cell IL-4 expression through an adenylyl cyclase mechanism independent of the protein kinase A pathway. *J Immunol.* 2005;175(10):6361-7.
54. Roy S, Balasubramanian S, Sumandeep S, et al. Morphine directs T cells toward T(H2) differentiation. *Surgery.* 2001; 130(2):304-9.
55. Allolio B, Schulte HM, Deuss U, et al. Effect of oral morphine and naloxone on pituitary-adrenal response in man induced by human corticotropin-releasing hormone. *Acta Endocrinol (Copenh).* 1987;114(4):509-14.
56. Rofael HZ, Turkall RM, Abdel-Rahman MS. Immunomodulation by cocaine and ketamine in postnatal rats. *Toxicology.* 2003;188(1):101-14.
57. Watson RR. LP-BM5, a murine model of acquired immunodeficiency syndrome: role of cocaine, morphine, alcohol and carotenoids in nutritional immunomodulation. *J Nutr.* 1992;122(3 Suppl):744-8.
58. Watzl B, Watson RR. Immunomodulation by cocaine--a neuroendocrine mediated response. *Life Sci.* 1990;46(19): 1319-29.
59. Ruiz P, Berho M, Steele BW, et al. Peripheral human T lymphocyte maintenance of immune functional capacity and phenotypic characteristics following in vivo cocaine exposure. *Clin Immunol Immunopathol.* 1998;88(3):271-6.
60. Pellegrino T, Bayer BM. *In vivo* effects of cocaine on immune cell function. *J Neuroimmunol.* 1998;83(1-2):139-47.
61. Baldwin GC, Roth MD, Tashkin DP. Acute and chronic effects of cocaine on the immune system and the possible link to AIDS. *J Neuroimmunol.* 1998;83:(1-2):133-8.
62. Xu W, Bai F, Tummalapalli CM, et al. The interactive effects of cocaine/gender on immune function in mice. An observation of in vivo acute cocaine exposure. *Int J Immunopharmacol.* 1997;19(6):333-40.
63. Di Francesco P, Marini S, Pica F, et al. *In vivo* cocaine administration influences lymphokine production and humoral immune response. *Immunol Res.* 1992;11(1):74-9.
64. Donahoe RM, Falek A, Madden JJ, et al. Effects of cocaine and other drugs of abuse on immune function. *Adv Exp Med Biol.* 1991;288:143-50.
65. Di Francesco P, Pica F, Croce C, et al. Effect of acute or daily cocaine administration on cellular immune response and virus infection in mice. *Nat Immun Cell Growth Regul.* 1990;9(6):397-405.

66. Nunez-Iglesias MJ, Castro-Bolano C, Losada C, et al. Effects of amphetamine on cell mediated immune response in mice. *Life Sci.* 1996;58(2):PL 29-33.
67. Freire-Garabal M, Balboa JL, Nunez MJ, et al. Effects of amphetamine on T-cell immune response in mice. *Life Sci.* 1991;49(16):PL107-12.
68. Ligeiro-Oliveira AP, Fialho de Araujo AM, Lazzarini R, et al. Effects of amphetamine on immune-mediated lung inflammatory response in rats. *Neuroimmunomodulation.* 2004;11(3):181-90.
69. Sopori ML, Kozak W, Savage SM, et al. Nicotine-induced modulation of T Cell function. Implications for inflammation and infection. *Adv Exp Med Biol.* 1998;437:279-89.
70. Sopori ML, Kozak W, Savage SM, et al. Effect of nicotine on the immune system: possible regulation of immune responses by central and peripheral mechanisms. *Psychoneuroendocrinology.* 1998;23(2):189-204.
71. Sopori ML, Kozak W. Immunomodulatory effects of cigarette smoke. *J Neuroimmunol.* 1998;83(1-2):148-56.
72. Hallquist N, Hakki A, Wecker L, et al. Differential effects of nicotine and aging on splenocyte proliferation and the production of Th1- versus Th2-type cytokines. *Proc Soc Exp Biol Med.* 2000;224(3):141-6.
73. Matthay MA, Ware LB. Can nicotine treat sepsis? *Nat Med.* 2004;10(11):1161-2.
74. Tracey KJ. Reflex control of immunity. *Nat Rev Immunol.* 2009;9(6):418-28.
75. Cook RL, Pollock NK, Rao AK, et al. Increased prevalence of herpes simplex virus type 2 among adolescent women with alcohol use disorders. *J Adolesc Health.* 2002;30(3):169-74.
76. Adams HG, Jordan C. Infections in the alcoholic. *Med Clin North Am.* 1984;68(1):179-200.
77. Bermudez LE, Young LS. Ethanol augments intracellular survival of *Mycobacterium avium* complex and impairs macrophage responses to cytokines. *J Infect Dis.* 1991; 163(6):1286-92.
78. Sibley DA, Osna N, Kusynski C, et al. Alcohol consumption is associated with alterations in macrophage responses to interferon-gamma and infection by Salmonella typhimurium. *FEMS Immunol Med Microbiol.* 2001;32(1): 73-83.
79. Bermudez LE, Wu M, Martinelli J, et al. Ethanol affects release of TNF and GM-CSF and membrane expression of TNF receptors by human macrophages. *Lymphokine Cytokine Res.* 1991;10(5):413-9.
80. Nelson S, Kolls JK. Alcohol, host defence and society. *Nat Rev Immunol.* 2002;2(3):205-9.
81. Stoltz DA, Nelson S, Kolls JK, et al. *In vitro* ethanol suppresses alveolar macrophage TNF-alpha during simian immunodeficiency virus infection. *Am J Respir Crit Care Med.* 2000;161(1):135-40.
82. Cherubin CE. The medical sequelae of narcotic addiction. *Ann Intern Med.* 1967;67(1):23-33.
83. Glassroth J, Adams GD, Schnoll S. The impact of substance abuse on the respiratory system. *Chest.* 1987;91(4):596-602.
84. Musola L, Beltrame M, Baldin C, et al. [Clinical case study of the dental and periodontal lesions in heroin addicts]. *Minerva Stomatol.* 1986;35(3):131-5.
85. Johnson JL, Hirsch CS. Aspiration pneumonia. Recognizing and managing a potentially growing disorder. *Postgrad Med.* 2003;113(3):99-102, 5-6, 11-2.
86. Mendelson CL. The aspiration of stomach contents into the lungs during obstetric anesthesia. *Am J Obstet Gynecol.* 1946;52:191-205.
87. Blanksma CJ, Brand HS. [Effects of cocaine use on oral health and implications for dental treatment]. *Ned Tijdschr Tandheelkd.* 2004;111(12):486-9.
88. Marik PE. Aspiration syndromes: aspiration pneumonia and pneumonitis. *Hosp Pract (Minneap).* 2010;38(1):35-42.
89. Marik PE. Pulmonary aspiration syndromes. *Curr Opin Pulm Med.* 2011;17(3):148-54.
90. Hind CR. Pulmonary complications of intravenous drug misuse. 2. Infective and HIV related complications. *Thorax.* 1990;45(12):957-61.
91. Woodhead MA, Macfarlane JT, McCracken JS, et al. Prospective study of the aetiology and outcome of pneumonia in the community. *Lancet.* 1987;1(8534):671-4.
92. Boschini A, Smacchia C, Di Fine M, et al. Community-acquired pneumonia in a cohort of former injection drug users with and without human immunodeficiency virus infection: incidence, etiologies, and clinical aspects. *Clin Infect Dis.* 1996;23(1):107-13.
93. File TM. Community-acquired pneumonia. *Lancet.* 2003; 362(9400):1991-2001.
94. Mandell LA, Wunderink RG, Anzueto A, et al. Infectious Diseases Society of America/American Thoracic Society consensus guidelines on the management of community-acquired pneumonia in adults. *Clin Infect Dis.* 2007;44 Suppl 2:S27-72.
95. Arancibia F, Bauer TT, Ewig S, et al. Community-acquired pneumonia due to gram-negative bacteria and pseudomonas aeruginosa: incidence, risk, and prognosis. *Arch Intern Med.* 2002;162(16):1849-58.
96. Fine MJ, Auble TE, Yealy DM, et al. A prediction rule to identify low-risk patients with community-acquired pneumonia. *N Engl J Med.* 1997;336(4):243-50.
97. Tsai HC, Chao PJ, Sy CL, et al. Community-associated methicillin-resistant Staphylococcus aureus infective endocarditis with Panton-Valentine leukocidin gene in an injection drug user with HIV infection. *Intern Med.* 2008;47(16):1485-9.
98. Chambers HF, Korzeniowski OM, Sande MA. Staphylococcus aureus endocarditis: clinical manifestations in addicts and nonaddicts. *Medicine (Baltimore).* 1983; 62(3):170-7.
99. Alafify AA, Al-Khuwaitir TS, Wani BA, et al. *Staphylococcus aureus* endocarditis complicated by bilateral pneumothorax. *Saudi Med J.* 2006;27(5):707-10.
100. Fleisch F, Oechslin EC, Gujer AR, et al. Transregional spread of a single clone of methicillin-resistant *Staphylococcus aureus* between groups of drug users in Switzerland. *Infection.* 2005;33(4):273-7.
101. Gonzalez C, Rubio M, Romero-Vivas J, et al. *Staphylococcus aureus* bacteremic pneumonia: differences between community and nosocomial acquisition. *Int J Infect Dis.* 2003; 7(2):102-8.
102. Gosbell IB. Epidemiology, clinical features and management of infections due to community methicillin-resistant *Staphylococcus aureus* (cMRSA). *Intern Med J.* 2005;35 Suppl 2:S120-35.

103. Johnston BL. Methicillin-resistant *Staphylococcus aureus* as a cause of community-acquired pneumonia--a critical review. *Semin Respir Infect.* 1994;9(3):199-206.
104. Lodise TP, McKinnon PS, Levine DP, et al. Impact of empirical-therapy selection on outcomes of intravenous drug users with infective endocarditis caused by methicillin-susceptible *Staphylococcus aureus. Antimicrob Agents Chemother.* 2007;51(10):3731-3.
105. Mofredj A, Guerin JM, Leibinger F, et al. Primary sternal osteomyelitis and septicaemia due to *Staphylococcus aureus. Scand J Infect Dis.* 1999;31(1):98-100.
106. Rubio M, Romero J, Corral O, et al. [Bacteremia by *Staphylococcus aureus:* analysis of 311 episodes]. *Enferm Infecc Microbiol Clin.* 1999;17(2):56-64.
107. Sanchez-Porto A, Casanova-Roman M, Casas-Ciria J, et al. In vitro activity of daptomycin and comparator agents against *Staphylococcus aureus* isolates from intravenous drug users with right endocarditis. *Infez Med.* 2010;18(2):108-12.
108. Small PM, Chambers HF. Vancomycin for *Staphylococcus aureus* endocarditis in intravenous drug users. *Antimicrob Agents Chemother.* 1990;34(6):1227-31.
109. Dworkin RJ, Lee BL, Sande MA, et al. Treatment of right-sided *Staphylococcus aureus* endocarditis in intravenous drug users with ciprofloxacin and rifampicin. *Lancet.* 1989;2(8671):1071-3.
110. Bassetti S, Battegay M. *Staphylococcus aureus* infections in injection drug users: risk factors and prevention strategies. *Infection.* 2004;32(3):163-9.
111. Lagier JC, Letranchant L, Selton-Suty C, et al. [Staphylococcus aureus bacteremia and endocarditis]. *Ann Cardiol Angeiol (Paris).* 2008;57(2):71-7.
112. Ribera E, Gomez-Jimenez J, Cortes E, et al. Effectiveness of cloxacillin with and without gentamicin in short-term therapy for right-sided Staphylococcus aureus endocarditis. A randomized, controlled trial. *Ann Intern Med.* 1996;125(12):969-74.
113. Ruotsalainen E, Sammalkorpi K, Laine J, et al. Clinical manifestations and outcome in Staphylococcus aureus endocarditis among injection drug users and nonaddicts: a prospective study of 74 patients. *BMC Infect Dis.* 2006;6:137.
114. Carretero Hernandez G, Cardenes Santana MA, et al. [Disseminated candidiasis in intravenous drug addicts (brown heroin)]. *Rev Clin Esp.* 1992;190(3):159-60.
115. Collignon PJ, Sorrell T. Disseminated candidiasis in drug abusers. *Arch Intern Med.* 1987;147(2):195.
116. Collignon PJ, Sorrell T. Candidiasis in heroin abusers. *J Infect Dis.* 1987;155(3):595.
117. Newton-John HF, Wise K, Looke DF. Role of the lemon in disseminated candidiasis of heroin abusers. *Med J Aust.* 1984;140(13):780-1.
118. Mellinger M, De Beauchamp O, Gallien C, et al. Epidemiological and clinical approach to the study of candidiasis caused by Candida albicans in heroin addicts in the Paris region: analysis of 35 observations. *Bull Narc.* 1982;34(3-4):61-81.
119. Deiss RG, Rodwell TC, Garfein RS. Tuberculosis and illicit drug use: review and update. *Clin Infect Dis.* 2009;48(1):72-82.
120. de Vries G, van Hest RA. From contact investigation to tuberculosis screening of drug addicts and homeless persons in Rotterdam. *Eur J Public Health.* 2006;16(2):133-6.
121. Story A, Murad S, Roberts W, et al. Tuberculosis in London: the importance of homelessness, problem drug use and prison. *Thorax.* 2007;62(8):667-71.
122. Rhodes T, Ball A, Stimson GV, et al. HIV infection associated with drug injecting in the newly independent states, eastern Europe: the social and economic context of epidemics. *Addiction.* 1999;94(9):1323-36.
123. Salomon N, Perlman DC, Friedmann P, et al. Prevalence and risk factors for positive tuberculin skin tests among active drug users at a syringe exchange program. *Int J Tuberc Lung Dis.* 2000;4(1):47-54.
124. Durante AJ, Selwyn PA, O'Connor PG. Risk factors for and knowledge of Mycobacterium tuberculosis infection among drug users in substance abuse treatment. *Addiction.* 1998;93(9):1393-401.
125. Garfein RS, Lozada R, Liu L, et al. High prevalence of latent tuberculosis infection among injection drug users in Tijuana, Mexico. *Int J Tuberc Lung Dis.* 2009;13(5):626-32.
126. Keizer ST, Langendam MM, van Deutekom H, et al. How does tuberculosis relate to HIV positive and HIV negative drug users? *J Epidemiol Community Health.* 2000;54(1):64-8.
127. Multidrug and extensively drug-resistant TB (M/XDR-TB). (2010). Global report on surveillance and respond. [online]. World Health Organization; 2010. Available from: www.whqlibdoc.who.int/publications/2010/9789241599191_eng.pdf.[Accessed Febraury 2014].
128. Prasad R. Multidrug and extensively drug-resistant TB (M/XDR-TB): problems and solutions. *Indian J Tuberc.* 2010;57(4):180-91.
129. Selwyn PA, Hartel D, Lewis VA, et al. A prospective study of the risk of tuberculosis among intravenous drug users with human immunodeficiency virus infection. *N Engl J Med.* 1989;320(9):545-50.
130. World Health Organization, United Nations Programme on HIV/AIDS, and United Nations Office of Drugs and Crime. Policy guidelines for collaborative TB and HIV services for injecting and other drug users—an integrated approach. Geneva. 2008. [online] Available from: http://whqlibdoc.who.int/publications/2008/9789241596930_eng.pdf [Accessed February 2013].
131. Alland D, Kalkut GE, Moss AR, et al. Transmission of tuberculosis in New York City. An analysis by DNA fingerprinting and conventional epidemiologic methods. *N Engl J Med.* 1994;330(24):1710-6.
132. Brassard P, Bruneau J, Schwartzman K, et al. Yield of tuberculin screening among injection drug users. *Int J Tuberc Lung Dis.* 2004;8(8):988-93.
133. Golub JE, Bur S, Cronin WA, et al. Delayed tuberculosis diagnosis and tuberculosis transmission. *Int J Tuberc Lung Dis.* 2006;10(1):24-30.
134. Morice AH, Menon MS, Mulrennan SA, Everett CF, Wright C, Jackson J, et al. Opiate therapy in chronic cough. *Am J Respir Crit Care Med.* 2007;175(4):312-5.
135. Edlin BR, Kresina TF, Raymond DB, Carden MR, Gourevitch MN, Rich JD, et al. Overcoming barriers to prevention, care, and treatment of hepatitis C in illicit drug users. *Clin Infect Dis.* 2005;40 Suppl 5:S276-85.
136. Malotte CK, Rhodes F, Mais KE. Tuberculosis screening and compliance with return for skin test reading among active drug users. *Am J Public Health.* 1998;88(5):792-6.

137. Mazurek GH, Jereb J, Lobue P, et al. Guidelines for using the QuantiFERON-TB Gold test for detecting Mycobacterium tuberculosis infection, United States. *MMWR Recomm Rep.* 2005;54(RR-15):49-55.
138. Blumberg HM, Burman WJ, Chaisson RE, et al. American Thoracic Society/Centers for Disease Control and Prevention/Infectious Diseases Society of America: treatment of tuberculosis. *Am J Respir Crit Care Med.* 2003;167(4):603-62.
139. Ungo JR, Jones D, Ashkin D, et al. Antituberculosis drug-induced hepatotoxicity. The role of hepatitis C virus and the human immunodeficiency virus. *Am J Respir Crit Care Med.* 1998;157(6 Pt 1):1871-6.
140. Fernandez-Villar A, Sopena B, Vazquez R, et al. Isoniazid hepatotoxicity among drug users: the role of hepatitis C. *Clin Infect Dis.* 2003;36:293-8.
141. Sadaphal P, Astemborski J, Graham NM, et al. Isoniazid preventive therapy, hepatitis C virus infection, and hepatotoxicity among injection drug users infected with Mycobacterium tuberculosis. *Clin Infect Dis.* 2001; 33(10):1687-91.
142. Kreek MJ, Garfield JW, Gutjahr CL, et al. Rifampin-induced methadone withdrawal. *N Engl J Med.* 1976; 294(20):1104-6.
143. Blaschke TF, Skinner MH. The clinical pharmacokinetics of rifabutin. *Clin Infect Dis.* 1996;22 Suppl 1:S15-21.
144. Brown LS, Sawyer RC, Li R, et al. Lack of a pharmacologic interaction between rifabutin and methadone in HIV-infected former injecting drug users. *Drug Alcohol Depend.* 1996;43(1-2):71-7.
145. McCarroll KA, Roszler MH. Lung disorders due to drug abuse. *J Thorac Imaging.* 1991;6(1):30-5.
146. Craven DE, Hudcova J, Lei Y. Diagnosis of ventilator-associated respiratory infections (VARI): microbiologic clues for tracheobronchitis (VAT) and pneumonia (VAP). *Clin Chest Med.* 2011;32(3):547-57.
147. Murray RJ, Albin RJ, Mergner W, et al. Diffuse alveolar hemorrhage temporally related to cocaine smoking. *Chest.* 1988;93(2):427-9.
148. Cregler LL, Mark H. Cardiovascular dangers of cocaine abuse. *Am J Cardiol.* 1986;57(13):1185-6.
149. Genereux GP, Emson HE. Talc granulomatosis and angiothrombotic pulmonary hypertension in drug addicts. *J Can Assoc Radiol.* 1974;25(2):87-93.
150. Hopkins GB, Taylor DG. Pulmonary talc granulomatosis. A complication of drug abuse. *Am Rev Respir Dis.* 1970; 101(1):101-4.
151. Hind CR. Pulmonary complications of intravenous drug misuse. 1. Epidemiology and non-infective complications. *Thorax.* 1990;45(11):891-8.

CHAPTER 13

Tuberculosis

Giovanni Sotgiu, Giovanni B Migliori

ABSTRACT

Tuberculosis is an airborne bacterial disease caused by *Mycobacterium tuberculosis*. Several clinical outcomes can follow the biological interaction between mycobacteria and the host—latent tuberculosis infection, pulmonary and/or extra-pulmonary disease, and death. The probability of the last two conditions is relatively low, particularly if the estimates of disease and death are compared with the estimated pool of individuals with latent tuberculosis infection. The global incidence was estimated to be 128/100,000 inhabitants, with a higher proportion of cases in Asia and Africa. More than 10% of the total cases are HIV-positive. In the recent years, it has been described that the spread of new forms of tuberculosis are resistant to the most potent drugs [multidrug-resistant-tuberculosis and extensively drug-resistant-tuberculosis]. The target of the elimination seems difficult to be met in the following years and new multi-disciplinary efforts are required to improve the epidemiological scenario in developed and developing countries.

INTRODUCTION

Tuberculosis is an ancient disease caused by a bacterial infection. *Mycobacterium tuberculosis* is the responsible infectious agent, which originated approximately 400 centuries ago in the African continent.[1] Every human organ can be infected by it; however, in the majority of cases, the respiratory system is the most affected target of the mycobacterial infectious process.

Tuberculosis, causing more than one million deaths annually, represents as one of the main public health concerns along with human immunodeficiency virus (HIV)/acquired immunodeficiency syndrome (AIDS) and malaria worldwide.[2]

ETIOLOGY

Mycobacterium tuberculosis is the most frequently detected bacterial species in humans affected by tuberculosis. It belongs to the *M. tuberculosis* complex, which includes *M. africanum, M. bovis, M. canetti, M. caprae, M. microti,* and *M. pinnipedii.*[3] Although there is an elevated genetic similarity, the host variability can be relevant.

M. tuberculosis is usually 2–4 μm long and 0.2–5 μm wide; it is aerobic, non-motile, and does not form spores.[4]

The constitution of the envelope of *M. tuberculosis* is characteristic if compared to that of other Gram-positive and -negative bacteria. Several biochemical compounds can be found in the envelope, including glycolipids, long-chain fatty acids, proteins (for instance, catalase-peroxidase and superoxide dismutase, useful for survival during infection), and peptidoglycan.[5,6]

Two structures constitute the envelope: the cell wall and the capsule-like outermost structure.[7,8] The latter is characterised by non-covalently bound lipids and proteins linked to the mycolyl-arabinogalactan-peptidoglycan of the cell wall. Furthermore, a high density of carbohydrates on the surface can be detected, functional to interact with host cell receptors (for instance, toll-like receptors (TLRs), intercellular adhesion molecule-3, macrophage mannose receptor) and to help mycobacteria to fight the environmental stress.[7,8] In particular, it is worthwhile to mention the role of mannose-capped lipoarabinomannan, lipomannan, arabinomannan, mannan, mannoglycoproteins, and phosphatidyl-myo-inositol mannosides in the mycobacterial physiology, whose location is quantitatively variable.[7]

Numerous lipids embedding the envelope (e.g., phthiocerol dimycocerosate) are relevant virulence factors.[9,10] Their contribution to the dry weight of the mycobacterium is consistent, being approximately, 40%. On the other side, the sulpholipids seems to play a role in the growth pathways.[9]

Glycolipids containing mycolic acid, a high weight fatty acid, can interfere with the immune system of the host and can confer resistance to anti-tuberculosis drugs owing to their hydrophobic content.[9]

The genome is characterised by 4.4×10^6 bp, with almost 4,000 genes.[6]

Numerous genes (more than 200) are involved in the codification of enzymes included in the metabolism of the fatty acids, particularly in the β-oxidation process. This feature can explain the relevant mycobacterial ability to survive in the host, that is using lipids as the main energetic source.

Another important aspect of *M. tuberculosis* genome is the relative weight of genes encoding the proline-glutamic acid and the proline-proline-glutamic acid families of acidic, glycine-rich proteins (4%): they are 172 genes (104 and 68 genes of the proline-glutamic acid and the proline-proline-glutamic acid family, respectively).[6] The activity of their products is not well known, even if several experimental models proved their virulence and their role in the antigenic changeability during the infection in host tissues.

Its duplication time is about one day (i.e., 18–24 hours), slower than other Gram-positive and -negative bacteria, probably due to the complexity of its structure and metabolism.[5]

PATHOGENESIS

Tuberculosis does not represent the more frequent outcome following the interaction between the human host and the *M. tuberculosis* strains. Environmental, mycobacterial, and host variables can play major/minor roles in the transition from a healthy condition to one or more of the subsequent conditions: latent tuberculosis infection, pulmonary and/or extra-pulmonary disease, and death. An additive and/or synergistic effect between the above-mentioned factors can increase or decrease the probability of the transition from one status to another.[4,11,12]

Tuberculosis is mainly an airborne disease; mycobacteria are transmitted from contagious to susceptible individuals by inhalation of droplet nuclei, which are aerosolized particles produced when an infectious human being coughs, sings, sneezes, or talks. Other routes of transmission have been described but their impact on the incidence of tuberculosis are negligible; they include foodborne transmission (through the ingestion of unpasteurized milk, contaminated by *M. bovis* and collected from cow with tuberculous mastitis), sexual transmission, and direct transmission (mucous or cutaneous unintentional inoculation of mycobacteria in laboratory workers and pathologists).[4,11]

Usually, a prolonged and/or recurrent exposure, like a close contact with a pulmonary source (i.e., a patient with a pulmonary disease who transmits mycobacteria in the environment) is crucial to significantly increase the probability of infection; staying in a small environment with an inadequate ventilation can further augment that risk.[4,11]

The number of prevalent contagious individuals in a specific geographical area, related to the number of incident tuberculosis cases and on the duration of their infectiousness, represents one of the main variables contributing to the probability of exposure.[11] It is relevant to highlight that the duration of infectiousness is significantly influenced by the ability of the local health system to early diagnose and cure a tuberculosis patient.[11,12] Following the bacteriological identification of the responsible mycobacterial strains and their phenotypic characterization in terms of sensitivity to anti-tuberculosis drugs, a tailored therapy based on a combination of antibiotics should be immediately administered.[13] Non-adherence to a correct medical prescription, following the long duration of anti-tuberculosis treatment and/or its adverse effects, or inadequate dosages, incorrect drug combinations, and treatment durations can reduce the probability of treatment success and then, can favor the persistence of contagiousness. Early diagnosis and treatment can significantly reduce the incidence of infected subjects, who can subsequently develop tuberculosis disease; typically 1 out of 2 (~40%) of the close contacts of a highly contagious patient is infected at the time of the case detection.[11,14,15] Patients adequately treated are not infectious after 2–3 weeks; nevertheless, not all patients are similarly contagious, considering a correlation between the number of mycobacteria in an mL of sputum and the efficiency of transmission. At least 5,000 mycobacteria in 1 mL of sputum should be present in a sputum sample to obtain a positive smear microbiological examination. Sputum smear positive patients are significantly more contagious than those who are sputum smear negative and culture positive. Furthermore, the latter are not greatly more infectious than tuberculosis patients who have a negative smear and culture examination.[11,12]

Moreover, the human density (urban vs. rural areas, household crowding) and the climatic conditions (cold vs. warm geographical areas) can affect the quality and the quantity of human relationships and consequently, the probability of close contacts. Social variables related to the age (elderly patients are more frequently diagnosed in high income countries vs. young adults in low income countries), gender, and customs can modify the risk of interaction with a contagious patient.[11]

Following the exposure to a contagious patient, the size of the droplet nuclei containing mycobacterial strains represents a relevant pathogenetic feature influencing the risk of infection: it should range between 1 and 5 μm to be inhaled in the respiratory airways and retained in the pulmonary alveoli; a droplet nucleus sized above 5 μm can be entrapped by the nasal vibrissae and by the mucociliary system, whereas if the diameter is less than 1 μm it can reach the alveoli but is not retained. Physical factors like humidity and temperature, can modify the size of the particles, as well as the ventilation can decrease its density and the probability of exposure with susceptible individuals.[4,11] In particular, natural, mixed-mode, or mechanical ventilation can be important in a household or nosocomial setting to reduce the chance of being infected. Natural ventilation may be enhanced by increasing the size of windows and positioning them on opposite walls but can be hindered by outdoor cold conditions and low air quality (i.e., pollution).[11,16] Fans can improve the airflow direction from a contagious case to an air exhaust area when natural ventilation is not satisfactory. The World Health Organization (WHO) recommends more than 11 air changes/hour for an isolation room of 24 m^3.

This environmental intervention should be supported by preventive measures like education on cough etiquette and respiratory hygiene and personal protective equipment; in particular, high-efficiency particulate air-filter respirators have to be worn in critical situations. They should be able to filter out droplet nuclei whose size range from 1 to 5 μm, that is meeting or exceeding the N95 standards set by the US Centers for Disease Control and Prevention (CDC)/National Institute for Occupational Safety and Health (NIOSH) or the Conformité Européenne (CE) certified free flight phase 2 (FFP2) standards. They should be worn by susceptible individuals (healthcare workers or visitors in a nosocomial setting), while surgical masks should be worn by patients. Health education on the importance of respirators in communities at risk should be carried out in order to avoid stigma; in addition, continuous training of healthcare providers on the correct use (fit testing) and indications of respirators should be organized.[16]

If droplet nuclei can bypass the upper airways and lodge in the alveoli spaces, alveolar macrophages engulf *M. tuberculosis* strains and start a chronic inflammatory process. It includes the enrolment of other mononuclear and non-mononuclear cells, following the release of pro-inflammatory cytokines like interleukin (IL)-12, IL-1β, and tumor necrosis factor (TNF) by infected macrophages.[4,5,17] Interactions between mycobacterial antigens and host cells involve several molecules like TLRs, nucleotide-binding oligomerization domain (NOD)-like receptors and C-type lectins;[3] in the majority of cases, *M. tuberculosis*-host cell receptor contact starts an intracellular signaling cascade oriented to trigger inflammatory events.

Dendritic cells transfer to pulmonary lymph nodes, where mycobacterial antigens are presented to naïve T and B lymphocytes, which are primed and migrate to the original infectious focus in the lung parenchyma. This early inflammatory response, characterized by the pulmonary recruitment of neutrophils, macrophages, dendritic cells, and lymphocytes lasts 12–30 days and culminates in the development of caseous granuloma, acknowledged as the histological feature of the mycobacterial infection and so labeled owing to the gross cheese-like look of its centre.[1,3,10,17-20] Different macrophage phenotypes form the granuloma: they can have anti-mycobacterial activity, can secrete pro- and anti-inflammatory cytokines as well as proteins useful to rebuild the damaged tissues. Only those macrophages activated by T-helper (Th) 1 lymphocytes with IL-12 and TNF (classically activated macrophages) can kill mycobacteria and can recruit T lymphocytes, whereas those macrophages responding to Th2 lymphocyte signals, like IL-4 and -10, decrease the intensity of the inflammation process (alternatively activated macrophages).[5,17] The prevalence of macrophages infected by mycobacteria (i.e., not growing in the extracellular environment) is indirectly linked to their ability of containing *M. tuberculosis* replication.

The granuloma sized between 1 mm and 2 cm cannot eliminate the mycobacterial strains but contain their replication. Some physical and chemical environmental characteristics of the granuloma (i.e., low pH, hypoxia, increased concentration of carbon monoxide, and nitric oxide) favor the induction of *M. tuberculosis* dormancy genes; in case of immunodepression, the transcriptional activity of those genes is inhibited and the mycobacterial replication rate augments, with subsequent shift from latent tuberculosis infection to tuberculosis disease.[5,17]

On the other hand, a crucial role in the pathogenesis of the mycobacterial infection is played by T lymphocytes [particularly, cytotoxic T cells, Th1, and Th17 cells, and T-regulatory (Treg) cells].[10,20]

CD4+ T lymphocytes produce mainly Th1 cytokines (interferon (IFN)-γ, IL-2, and TNF) and coordinate the acquired immune response, principally enhancing cytotoxic CD8+ T lymphocyte function with IL-15. Furthermore, they decrease the intracellular growth of mycobacterial strains through IFN-γ or nitric oxide-dependent mechanisms. Their qualitative and quantitative impairment can increase the probability of transition from latent tuberculosis infection to tuberculosis disease.

Treg cells seem to play a relevant role in the latent tuberculosis infection and in the shift from latent tuberculosis infection to tuberculosis disease.

The activity of humoral immunity is nopt well known. Several studies denied their importance but recently, the role of B-cell mediated responses has been pointed out in several critical steps of the inflammatory process: modulation of susceptibility, recruitment of neutrophils, activation of macrophages, and of T cells and secretion of cytokines.[10,17,18,21]

EPIDEMIOLOGY

The WHO annually evaluates the impact of tuberculosis in developing and developed countries worldwide.[2] Epidemiological indicators are commonly used to compare the temporal and spatial trends of the disease as well as to analyze the efficacy of the adopted public health interventions; in particular, 3 indicators are regularly estimated: annual incidence of the disease (i.e., number of new tuberculosis cases/100,000 population), annual prevalence of the disease (i.e., number of tuberculosis cases/100,000 population), and annual mortality among tuberculosis cases (i.e., number of deaths/100,000 population).

The number of new tuberculosis cases estimated in 2010 globally, was 8.8 million (range: 8.5–9.2 million), equivalent to 128 patients/100,000 population. The proportional spatial distribution of the incident cases was unequal, with Asia and Africa characterized by the higher estimates (59% and 26%, respectively).

The most affected countries were India (range: 2.0–2.5 million), China (range: 900,000–1.2 million), South-Africa (range: 400,000–590,000), Indonesia (range: 370,000–540,000), and Pakistan (range: 330,000–480,000).

An estimated 1.1 million (range: 1.0–1.2 million)/8.8 million (12–14%) incident cases were HIV-positive, mainly living in the WHO African Region, where 82% of the tuberculosis/HIV co-infected patients has been diagnosed.

Annual tuberculosis incidence rate is decreasing worldwide, with different regional declining rates (from <1% to 3.7% in the eastern Mediterranean region and region of the Americas, respectively). Among 22 countries with a relevant burden of disease, only 10 (45.5%) showed a positive decreasing incidence trend in 2010.

The estimated incidence of women affected by tuberculosis is 3.2 million (range: 3–3.5 million); however, the confidence on estimates related to children and women should be significantly improved, particularly, in developing countries.

The global prevalence of tuberculosis was 12 million (range: 11–14 million) in 2010, equivalent to 178 tuberculosis patients/100,000 population. Prevalence started to decline in 1990 worldwide, with a faster declining rate after 1997. The majority of the WHO regions have halved or almost halved their prevalence since 1990; nevertheless, the African Region is considerably far from this target.

Mortality rate was 20/100,000 population in 2010, equivalent to 1.4 million deaths (range: 1.2–1.5 million); it was 15/100,000 population in the HIV-negative patients (equivalent to 1.1 million deaths; range: 900,000–1.2 million); 350,000 patients who died in 2010 were tuberculosis/HIV co-infected (range: 320,000–390,000).

Mortality estimates significantly decreased since 1990 (by more than one third). It is expected that the goal of reducing the mortality by 50% in 2015, compared with the estimates computed in 1990, will be met.

The spatial declining trend of the mortality indicator is similar in all WHO regions but in African region, which is far from the scheduled target of 2015. This situation is comparable to that described for the tuberculosis prevalence: the HIV/AIDS epidemic, not adequately managed by the National Health Systems, is supposed to play a relevant role in this epidemiological context.

In the last decade, the WHO has strictly monitored another relevant epidemiological issue: the global spread of multidrug-resistant (MDR) tuberculosis.[22-30] It is a disease caused by *M. tuberculosis* strains resistant to at least isoniazid and rifampicin—2 of the most effective anti-tuberculosis drugs. A more severe form of MDR-tuberculosis was described in 2006 and was defined extensively drug-resistant (XDR) tuberculosis. It is the MDR-tuberculosis due to strains resistant to any fluoroquinolone and to at least one injectable second-line drug (amikacin, capreomycin, and kanamycin).

Several epidemiological and demographic, clinical factors can favor the emergence and the spread of MDR/XDR-tuberculosis, which can be defined as a man-made product: non- or poor implementation of national public health strategies (for instance, inadequate or lacking clinical and public health guidelines, poor training of the healthcare workers, and poor political commitment), inadequate supply of drugs, administration or poor quality of anti-tuberculosis drugs, inadequate drug intake by the patient due to several reasons (for instance, stigma, adverse events, poor adherence, psychiatric comorbidities, and poor economic support), and poor preventive measures (for instance, inadequate infection control interventions in hospital settings).[31-36]

Cure rates in MDR-tuberculosis are significantly lower if compared with those of tuberculosis caused by drug-susceptible strains (40–80% vs. >90%). Furthermore, they are worse in XDR-tuberculosis compared with MDR-tuberculosis.[22,37-40]

The prevalent cases of MDR-tuberculosis estimated in 2010 were 650,000, whereas the incident cases were 290,000 (range: 210,000–380,000).[2] Twenty-seven countries were defined "high MDR-tuberculosis burden countries" by the WHO, almost half belonging to the former Soviet Union. Belarus and Moldova recorded the highest prevalence among new and previously treated patients (26% and 65%, respectively).

The estimates on MDR-tuberculosis are not representative of the true figures in some countries, particularly those located in the African Region. The drug susceptibility testing is carried out only in less than 2% and 6% among new and previously treated tuberculosis patients worldwide, respectively. Additionally, treatment accounting drug susceptibility testing results was performed in 16% of the 290,000 incident MDR-tuberculosis patients in 2010.

CLINICAL FEATURES

Tuberculosis disease development is favored by a qualitative and/or quantitative impairment of the immune system.[4,11,12,17] It can follow the status "infection" and its probability of occurrence varies, being highest in the first 1–2 years after the mycobacterial entry (5%) and lower as time passes by (lifetime risk: 5–10%).[4,11,12]

The cumulative risk of developing tuberculosis is directly correlated with the age of the primary infection: it is highest in younger subjects (35–50% in children who are in close contact of a contagious patient).[11,12]

Several medical conditions are acknowledged as relevant risk factors for tuberculosis development. One of the most significant factor, from a clinical and public health perspective, is the HIV/AIDS. HIV impairs the innate and the adaptive immune responses, particularly decreasing the CD4+ cells, which play a crucial role in the response to mycobacteria.[4,11,12,41-43] The estimated annual risk of tuberculosis is 5–15% in tuberculosis/HIV co-infected when *M. tuberculosis* infection precedes HIV infection; it could be significantly higher if the mycobacterial infection develops in a severely immunocompromised patients.

Prospective studies showed that HIV-positive patients have a statistically significant highest relative risk (RR) of developing tuberculosis if compared with HIV-negative patients; nevertheless, quantitative differences were demonstrated on the basis of the impact of HIV epidemic in the population. The estimated RR is 36.7 in low HIV/AIDS prevalence areas, 26.7 in areas with concentrated epidemics, and 20.6 in areas with a generalized epidemic.[4,11,12,41-44]

Diabetes mellitus, one of the most frequent chronic diseases worldwide, can affect native and acquired immunity, particularly decreasing the chemotaxis, the oxidative killing ability of neutrophils, and the production of IFN-γ and IL-12.[45-47] The global prevalence of diabetes in people aged 20–79 years was 6.4% in 2010, equivalent to 285 million individuals; it is expected to rise to 7.7% in 2030 (equivalent to 439 million patients), particularly in low-income than in high-income countries (69% vs. 20%, respectively).[48]

The risk of developing tuberculosis in diabetic patients is 2–9 times lower than HIV/AIDS, but the global prevalence of diabetes is significantly higher. The probability of tuberculosis in diabetic patients is 1.5–8 higher than in healthy people.[43,45,47,49-53]

Chronic renal failure and the hemodialytic therapy increase the probability of tuberculosis if compared with the risk of tuberculosis among the healthy subjects (6.9–52.5 times higher than the baseline risk) owing to immunodepression (i.e., declined production of IFN-γ and IL-12), malnutrition (decreased vitamin D intake), and hyperparathyroidism.[11,54,55]

Exposure to crystalline silica dust, associated to a reduced function of macrophages, favors the probability of developing tuberculosis; in particular, silicosis increases the probability of pulmonary and extra-pulmonary tuberculosis of 2.8–39 and 3.7 times, respectively.[4,11,43,56-58] It has been shown that the risk of disease is significantly increased in HIV-positive patients. Several occupational activities are associated to a different likelihood; in particular, drilling seems one of the most hazardous activities.[11,56-58]

Less scientific evidence for tuberculosis risk has been obtained for other chronic conditions like neoplasias (for instance, lymphoma, lung, head/neck cancers), gastrectomy, and jejunoileal by-pass.[11,43]

Exposure to toxic substances or drugs can modify the baseline risk of developing tuberculosis after mycobacterial infection. Anti-TNF-α therapies with monoclonal antibodies (adalimumab, certolizumab pegol, golimumab, and infliximab), prescribed for chronic diseases like rheumatoid arthritis, psoriasis, ankylosing spondylitis, and inflammatory bowel disease rise the probability of tuberculosis from 1.6 to 25.1 times and a preventive chemotherapy is usually prescribed before treating patients with those immunosuppressive drugs.[59,60]

Tobacco smoking is proved to have a role in the susceptibility to latent tuberculosis infection and tuberculosis, damaging the mucociliary system, alveolar macrophages, and CD4+ lymphocytes. The risk of disease is increased from 2.3 to 2.7 times and is directly associated to the daily number of smoked cigarettes. However, it is complicated to separate the effect of smoking from that of other confounding socio-economic factors (for instance, alcohol consumption, intra-venous drug abuse etc.).[4,11,43,61,62]

In the majority of cases, patients develop a pulmonary form; only in a few cases, particularly in those severely immunocompromised (for instance, AIDS patients with less than 100 CD4+ cell counts/μL), an extra-pulmonary tuberculosis may occur, with or without pulmonary involvement.[4]

From a clinical perspective, it can be identified a primary tuberculosis, following the entry of the mycobacteria in the lower respiratory airways and a post-primary tuberculosis, following a latent tuberculosis infection.

Generally, primary tuberculosis occurs without clinical signs and symptoms in adults whereas several age-related clinical syndromes can be described in the pediatric population. In children aged less than 4 years, a regional lymphadenitis may be the cause of cough due to the mechanical compression of main or lobar bronchi; occasionally, a lymphohematogenous spread can cause a systemic disease (the so called miliary tuberculosis from its pathological lesions similar to millet seeds) or a meningoencephalitis.[4,63,64]

Post-primary tuberculosis is characterized by systemic symptoms like low-grade fever, anorexia or inappetence followed by weight loss, asthenia, and night sweats. A persistent mucopurulent cough, lasting more than 21 days, may represent a typical clinical feature. Chest pain can be the consequence of a pleuritic process with or without pleural effusion. Hemoptysis is an infrequent and late clinical sign of progressive illness, following the damage of a pulmonary artery by a tuberculosis cavity (Rasmussen's aneurysm). Physical examination does not reveal specific findings and is frequently negative; only in a few patients, rales, dullness, and signs of consolidation can be detected.[4,65]

Extra-pulmonary tuberculosis, which accounts for 15–20% of all tuberculosis cases in HIV-negative population, is classified in 3 groups on the basis of the pathogenesis: mucosal forms (dissemination of infectious secretions in the gastrointestinal or respiratory tracts), lymphohematogenous forms, and contiguous forms to a primary focus. The most frequently detected conditions are: miliary tuberculosis, tuberculous meningitis, tuberculous pleurisy, skeletal tuberculosis, genitourinary tuberculosis, and tuberculous lymphadenitis.[4,66]

Military tuberculosis could be classified in acute, chronic (or cryptic), and non-reactive. Acute (or usual) miliary tuberculosis is more prevalent in older individuals with co-morbidities or young patients with severe immunodepression and is characterized by non-specific, systemic symptoms like fever, anorexia, weakness, and weight loss. Chronic miliary tuberculosis is diagnosed in elderly patients and is habitually asymptomatic (postmortem examination often allows to diagnose it). Patients with non-reactive miliary tuberculosis show a severe sepsis with splenomegaly and scattered necrotic tissues.[4,67,68]

Meningitis is usually the consequence of the rupture of a subependymal tubercle into the subarachnoid space. The more frequently detected clinical signs and symptoms are: headache, fever, meningismus, vomiting, confusion, and sometimes, focal neurological signs.[4,68-71]

Tuberculous pleurisy typically occurs in several forms of tuberculosis and is characterised by high-grade fever, chest pain, and cough .[4,72,73]

Skeletal tuberculosis is in more than 30% of the skeletal cases located in the spine (tuberculous spondylitis or Pott's disease). The inflammation process involves more vertebral bodies and intervertebral discs. It is often asymptomatic in the early stages and then, patients complain of back pain or stiffness. It occurs in the elderly and in young individuals in high- and low-income countries, respectively.[4,74,75]

Genitourinary tuberculosis usually starts from the kidney and then, can involve testicles, endometrium, or ovaries.[4,68,76]

Tuberculous lymphadenitis (scrofula) frequently involves cervical lymph nodes and is clinically characterized by a red and painless mass. It is multilateral in HIV-positive patients and associated with systemic symptoms. Lymphadenitis can involve even mediastinal or mesenteric lymph nodes.[4,77]

DIAGNOSIS

Pulmonary tuberculosis disease should be suspected in individuals with a persistent, chronic cough, which lasts for more than 14–21 days.[33,78,79] At least 2 sputum specimens should be submitted for a microscopic examination in a quality-assured laboratory; at least 1 sample should be obtained in early morning.[4,33,78,79] The first specimen is positive in 85.8% of the sputum smear positive individuals; the average incremental yield of the second specimen is 11.1%.[14,78,79] Mycobacteria are defined as acid-fast bacilli because of the characteristic reaction of their membrane to the Ziehl-Neelsen staining. The smear is covered with carbol-fuchsin, then heated, rinsed, and decolorized with acid-alcohol and counterstained with methylene blue. More than 5,000–10,000/mL bacilli should be located in the sample in order to obtain a positive result. In the last decades, several laboratories have used a fluorochrome stain with auramine-rhodamine. It was recently proved that fluorescence microscopy has a 10% higher sensitivity than conventional microscopy, whose sensitivity is 50–60% when compared with culture. A 10–20% higher sensitivity was shown after centrifugation and/or sedimentation, although specificity is comparable to conventional light microscopy both for the fluorescence microscopy and after treatment of the sample (i.e., centrifugation and/or sedimentation).[78,79]

Samples can be evaluated directly or after sedimentation by centrifugation.[4] Instead of sputum, gastric aspiration material can be collected for children who are unable to expectorate.[4,33,63,78,79]

Samples are then cultured in solid and/or liquid media; they should be initially liquefied or decontaminated using N-acetyl-L-cysteine in 1% sodium hydroxide solution. After centrifugation, the sediment is inoculated onto solid culture agar-based (for instance, Middlebrook 7H11) or egg-based (for instance, Lowenstein-Jensen) media in 5–10% carbon dioxide. Another option is represented by a liquid culture system (BACTEC) that detects mycobacterial growth through the identification of carbon dioxide from radioactive palmitic acid. Its sensitivity is higher than the sensitivity of the solid media and identifies mycobacteria rapidly (in <3 weeks). Another liquid system, mycobacteria growth indicator tube (MGIT), detects mycobacteria using a fluorescence technique, reducing disadvantages related to the handling of radioactive compounds.[33,78,79]

On the basis of the microscopic positivity, tuberculosis patients are classified as sputum smear-positive or -negative.[78,79] In those who are sputum smear-negative (for instance, some HIV-positives), it is required that a culture as well as chest radiography should be done and a complete course of a broad-spectrum antibiotic should be started in order to falsify the hypothesis of tuberculosis.

M. tuberculosis can be discriminated from other mycobacteria because it reduces nitrates, produces niacin, as well as heat-sensitive catalase in small quantities, but does not produce any pigments. Drug sensitivity testing is performed on both solid and liquid media to evaluate the resistance to first- and second-line drugs helpful to tailor anti-tuberculosis treatment.

More rapid, molecular diagnostic methods were recently introduced [nucleic acid amplification techniques (NAAT)] and can identify even a few mycobacteria in the collected sample.[4] Nevertheless, they cannot replace conventional bacteriological diagnosis because of the lower diagnostic accuracy. The sensitivity is highly variable (lowest in sputum smear-negatives and in extra-pulmonary cases) and the negative predictive value is low.[78,79] In the last few years, the WHO endorsed a new molecular technique [Xpert mycobacterium tubrculosis (Mtb)/resistance to rifampicin(RIF)] for the rapid diagnosis of rifampicin resistance, surrogate marker of MDR-tuberculosis.[80,81]

In case of suspected extra-pulmonary tuberculosis, biological samples of the infected organ should be collected for microscopy, culture, and histopathology.[78,79]

Chest radiography has a good sensitivity but a low specificity to diagnose tuberculosis. There is the risk of over-detection and missed diagnosis using this technique only.[78,79] It can be helpful because it increases the pre-diagnosis sensitivity, specific patterns being suggestive of tuberculosis (for instance, patchy or nodular infiltrates associated to cavitary lesions located in the upper lobes). However, small cavities can be better described by computed tomography (CT) or magnetic resonance imaging (MRI).[4]

Although a microbiological diagnosis of tuberculosis disease is feasible, it is not possible to diagnose latent tuberculosis infection directly. Almost a century ago, tuberculin skin test (TST) was introduced to evaluate the adaptive immunological response to mycobacterial antigens, injecting intradermally in the volar part of the forearm an extract of a boiled culture of *M. tuberculosis* (the so called Mantoux test). In 1934, a protein precipitate [purified protein derivative (PPD)] of that extract was prepared; 7 years later, the standardization of a lot of PPD (PPD-S) was carried out. A 5-tuberculin unit dose of PPD is equivalent to 0.0001 mg of standardized PPD in 0.1 mL solution.[4]

Although indirectly, this technique has been considered as the gold standard for the diagnosis of latent tuberculosis infection. However, several technical issues can reduce the sensitivity and specificity of the test. False negative results may be obtained in case of a deeper injection, interpretation of the test after 48–72 hours, tuberculosis disease (in more than 20% of the patients), HIV/AIDS, viral infections, and corticosteroids exposure. False positive results can be detected after mycobacterial sensitization than *M. tuberculosis* or after vaccination with *M. bovis* Bacillus Calmette-Guerin (BCG).[4,82]

A new diagnostic tool for the *ex vivo* diagnosis of latent tuberculosis infection was marketed a few years ago. It was based on the detection of adaptive immunity (production of IFN-γ by primed lymphocytes) against specific *M. tuberculosis* antigens – 6KDa early secreted antigenic target (ESAT-6), culture filtrate protein 10 (CFP-10), and TB7.7. This reaction allows discriminating individuals immunized with BCG or exposed to environmental mycobacteria and those with latent tuberculosis infection.[83,84]

Two commercial versions are available: QuantiFERONTB Gold In Tube (QFTIT; Cellestis Ltd., Chadstone, Australia) and TSPOT.TB (Oxford Immunotec, Abingdon, UK), an enzyme-linked immunosorbent assay (ELISA) and an enzyme-linked immunosorbent spot (ELISPOT) method, respectively.[85,86]

Unfortunately, they do not discriminate between latent tuberculosis infection and tuberculosis disease using lymphocytes collected from the peripheral blood.

The negative predictive value for progression from latent tuberculosis infection to tuberculosis disease is 97.8–99.8% within 2 years.[83,84]

On the contrary, the sensitivity and the specificity for the diagnosis of tuberculosis disease are almost 80% and 59–79% analyzing blood samples, respectively. Their diagnostic performance for the detection of tuberculosis patients seem to improve when extra-sanguinous fluids are analyzed.[87-89]

TREATMENT

Treatment of tuberculosis disease has a relevant importance from a clinical and public health point of view. It eliminates mycobacteria, avoiding clinical progression and contagiousness, and then, infection of the close contacts.

Different mechanisms of action for the currently available anti-tuberculosis drugs are recognized.[90]

Killing of growing mycobacteria (isoniazid, rifampicin, and streptomycin), killing of semi-dormant mycobacteria (rifampicin and pyrazinamide), prevention of emergence of drug-resistant strains (isoniazid, rifampicin, streptomycin, ethambutol, pyrazinamide, thiacetazone, and para-aminosalicylic acid) (Table 1).

At least 2 drugs should be administered in order to avoid treatment failure and relapse.

Anti-tuberculosis treatment is characterized by an intensive and a continuation phase; the former is aimed at killing rapidly growing and semi-dormant bacteria and the latter is aimed at killing the residual mycobacteria. The number of prescribed drugs should be directly correlated to the presumed bacillary burden; from 3 to 5 in the intensive phase whereas a lower number in the continuation phase. In the intensive phase, at least 2 drugs should be bactericidal (for instance, isoniazid and streptomycin or isoniazid and rifampicin); the

TABLE 1
Anti-tuberculosis Drugs, Dosages, and Adverse Events

Anti-tuberculosis drugs	Recommended daily dosage	Frequent adverse events
Isoniazid	5 mg/kg OD	• CNS toxicity • Elevation of liver enzymes • Gastrointestinal intolerance • Hepatitis • Peripheral neuropathy
Rifampicin	10 mg/kg OD	• Discoloration of body fluids • Elevation of liver enzymes • Fever • Gastrointestinal intolerance • Hepatitis • Hypersensitivity • Thrombocytopenia

Continued

Table 1 *continued*

Anti-tuberculosis drugs	Recommended daily dosage	Frequent adverse events
Ethambutol	15–25 mg/kg OD	Optic neuritis
Pyrazinamide	30 mg/kg OD	• Arthralgia • Gastrointestinal intolerance • Hepatitis • Hyperuricemia
Streptomycin Amikacin Capreomycin Kanamycin	0.75–1 g OD	• Allergy • Auditory and vestibular nerve damage • Nausea • Neuromuscular blockade • Renal failure • Skin rash
Ofloxacin Levofloxacin	750 (800)–1000 mg OD	• CNS toxicity • GI intolerance • Hypersensitivity
Moxifloxacin	400 mg OD	• Dizziness • Elevation of liver enzymes • Gastrointestinal intolerance • Hallucinations • Headache • QT prolongation
Ethionamide Protionamide	500 mg for BW <50 kg OD 750 mg for BW >50 kg OD 1,000 mg for BW >70 kg OD	• CNS toxicity • Gastrointestinal intolerance • Hepatitis
Cycloserine	500 mg for BW <50 kg OD 750 mg for BW >50 kg OD 1,000 mg for BW >70 kg OD	• CNS toxicity • Dizziness • Psychosis
Terizidone	600 mg for BW <70 kg OD 900 mg for BW >70 kg OD	• CNS toxicity • Dizziness • Psychosis
Para-aminosalicylic acid	8 g for BW <70 kg OD 8–12 g for BW >70 kg OD	• Gastrointestinal intolerance • Hypersensitivity
Thiacetazone	150 mg OD	• Gastrointestinal intolerance • Hepatitis • Hypersensitivity • Vertigo
Linezolid	600 mg OD	• Anaemia • Neuropathy • Thrombocytopenia
Clofazimine	100–300 mg OD	• Discoloration of the skin • Gastrointestinal intolerance • Ichthyosis
Amoxicillin-clavulanic	875/125 mg BID or 500/250 mg TID	• Gastrointestinal intolerance • Rash
Clarithromycin	500 mg BID	Gastrointestinal intolerance

OD, once a day; BID, twice a day; TID, thrice a day; BW, body weight; CNS, central nervous system.

combination with pyrazinamide reduces the length of treatment to 6 months. Ethambutol is combined when the probability of resistance to one drug is elevated or when the mycobacterial load is elevated.

For new tuberculosis patients the duration of therapy is 6 months, combining isoniazid, rifampicin, ethambutol, and pyrazinamide for 2 months, followed by isoniazid and rifampicin for 4 months.[91-95]

Fixed-dose combinations are strongly suggested because they improve the patient's adherence, reduce the pill burden, and prescription errors.[91]

Treatment duration in HIV-infected patients is equal to that described for the HIV-negatives.[91]

It is recommended to start anti-tuberculosis treatment before anti-retroviral therapy. There is no clear evidence on the timing of the anti-retroviral therapy; a clear advantage of an early administration of anti-retroviral drugs is the reduction of mortality, particularly high in the first 2 months. On the opposite side, the disadvantages are represented by the pharmacological interactions (particularly, with the protease inhibitors and the non-nucleoside reverse transcriptase inhibitors), the higher risk of adverse events and of immune reconstitution inflammatory syndrome (IRIS), and the pill burden.[96-98] However, the anti-retroviral therapy has to be administered as soon as possible, irrespective of the CD4 cell counts.

Previously-treated patients (i.e., individuals treated for more than 1 month with anti-tuberculosis drugs) should submit a specimen for the drug sensitivity testing, who are being at higher risk of infection with drug-resistant mycobacterial strains; a standard regimen can be recommended before obtaining the drug sensitivity testing results (for instance, 2 HRZES/1 HRZE/5 HRE).[91]

Second-line drugs should be prescribed in case of MDR-tuberculosis, although they are more expensive, more toxic, and less efficacious, with the consequence of increasing the probability of non-adherence. Drug combinations should contain more than 3 second-line drugs, with an injectable administered for 8 months. Treatment duration should be of at least 20 months.[24,99] Strict supervision by skilled healthcare workers should be performed in order to monitor patient's adherence and the potential occurrence of adverse events. Recently, community surveillance activities have been successfully implemented in low-income countries.[100]

Surgery has been performed for the treatment of tuberculosis, particularly in the past; in the last decade, the evidence of poor efficacy of drug combination regimens against some MDR/XDR-tuberculosis forms raised the attention on surgical interventions. Findings related to high success rates and tolerable morbidity suggested their role as adjunctive therapy, even if the quality of the studies is poor, particularly for selection bias due to the exclusion of individuals with severe tuberculosis.[101]

Tuberculosis cases have to be treated to avoid further transmission and new infections, but unfortunately, WHO estimates that almost one third of the global population is infected and new cases of tuberculosis will continuously to emerge from this group.[2,102]

There is a scientific consensus on the individuals who have to be screened to ascertain a mycobacterial infection. They are children and adults having close contact with a contagious tuberculosis patient, HIV-positives, and patients with autoimmune disorders who have to start an immunosuppressive therapy with anti-TNF-α drugs. On the other hand, a case-by-case evaluation, performed by experts in the public health field, is necessary in order to better understand when to screen and treat some potentially at-risk groups (for instance, migrants from high incidence countries). It is widely accepted that screening has to be performed only in those individuals who want to be treated in case of latent tuberculosis infection diagnosis.[82]

It was proved that treatment of infected individuals with isoniazid for 6–12 months, prescribed at a daily dosage of 5 mg/Kg, reduces the risk of tuberculosis by 60% in a time period longer than 2 years; no differences were found between 6 and 12 months but a higher frequency of hepatic adverse events was recorded with a longer duration.[82]

The effectiveness of this drug for the elimination of mycobacteria, when it is prescribed for 6, 9, or 12 months, is hindered by treatment completion rates ranging from 30 to 64%.[103,104]

Another alternative therapy is a 3-month regimen of isoniazid and rifampicin, whose efficacy and safety profile is comparable to isoniazid prescribed for 6 months.[82]

A recent multi-centre study showed that a weekly combination of rifapentine (900 mg) and isoniazid (900 mg) for 3 months has the same efficacy of isoniazid prescribed for 9 months, but with higher adherence rates.[103]

It is unknown how to manage the contacts of MDR-tuberculosis patients. There is no evidence for a therapy but the only accepted alternative is the active surveillance in the initial years following the close contact.[82]

PREVENTION

Epidemiologic indicators of tuberculosis in high-income countries started to improve following the availability of the anti-tuberculosis drugs after the 1950s' and the implementation of the national tuberculosis programs, along with the social and economic progress.[4,11,12,28,29]

The HIV/AIDS epidemic, the significant migration flows from high-incidence countries, as well as the wrong feeling of a definitive success on infectious diseases owing to the antibiotic therapy were recognized as the main factors responsible for the increase of prevalence and incidence of tuberculosis in developed countries after the 1980s.[4,11,12,28,29,105,106]

Following a dramatic increase of tuberculosis in high- and low-income countries, United Nations declared tuberculosis a public health emergency in 1993 and included the fight against tuberculosis, malaria, and HIV/AIDS among the Millennium Development Goals (MDGs).

The WHO has made tremendous efforts to improve the epidemiological situation of tuberculosid in the last few decades, worldwide.

In 1996, it issued the first global public health strategy called directlt observed treatment short course (DOTS) strategy; after its successful implementation, that strategy was included in another, more comprehensive public health approach 10 years later-the Stop Tuberculosis Strategy, which accounts for the new epidemiological scenario and the emerging public health issues. Both of them were created after interactive discussions among the main governmental and non-governmental stakeholders.[12,13,28,107-112]

The DOTS strategy was focused on the management of the infectious cases in order to interrupt the epidemiological chain of the transmission. It was mainly aimed to diagnose 70% of the sputum smear-positive patients nationwide and to successfully treat 85% of them by 2005. If adequately implemented and scaled-up, it could reduce the tuberculosis notification from 6 to 8%. It is characterized by 5 elements:

- Government dedication to tuberculosis control
- Bacteriological diagnosis through smear microscopy, mostly focused on subjects complaining of tuberculosis symptoms
- Short-course anti-tuberculosis therapy, which has to be standardized and supervised, particularly in the early phase
- Uninterrupted supply of high-quality drugs
- Implementation of a standardized recording and reporting system for the evaluation of treatment outcomes.

The Stop Tuberculosis strategy is characterized by further 6 elements to meet the 2015 MDG targets, that is to halve the prevalence and the mortality due to tuberculosis compared to the figures recorded in 1990 (Table 2). It is focused on the expansion and the national improvement of high-quality DOTS, the issue of tuberculosis/HIV co-infection, MDR-tuberculosis, the improvement of the healthcare systems, the engagement of the care providers, the empowerment of individuals with tuberculosis and of their communities, and promotion of the scientific research. All its elements represent an intentional response to issues and shortcomings detected during the implementation and scale-up of the DOTS strategy-emergence and spread of MDR-tuberculosis, increased incidence of tuberculosis/HIV co-infection, weaknesses

TABLE 2

The World Health Organization Stop Tuberculosis Strategy[109]

- Pursue high-quality DOTS expansion and enhancement
  - Secure political commitment toward tuberculosis, with adequate and continuous financing
  - Ensure early case detection and diagnosis through quality-assured bacteriology
  - Provide standardized treatment with supervision and patient support
  - Ensure effective drug supply and management
  - Monitor and evaluate performance and impact
- Address tuberculosis/HIV co-infection, MDR-tuberculosis, and the needs of poor and vulnerable populations
  - Scale up collaborative tuberculosis/HIV activities
  - Scale up prevention and management of MDR tuberculosis
  - Address the needs of tuberculosis contacts and poor and vulnerable populations
- Contribute to health system strengthening
  - Help improve health policies, human resource development, financing, supplies, service delivery, and information
  - Strengthen infection control in healthcare services, other congregate settings, and households
  - Upgrade laboratory networks and implement the Practical Approach to Lung Health
  - Adapt successful approaches from other fields and sectors and foster action on the social determinants of health
- Engage all care providers
  - Involve all public, voluntary, corporate, and private careproviders through Public-Private Mix approaches
  - Promote use of the ISTC
- Empower people with tuberculosis, and communities through partnership
  - Pursue advocacy, communication, and social mobilization
  - Foster community participation in tuberculosis care
  - Promote use of the Patients' Charter for tuberculosis Care
- Enable and promote research
  - Conduct program-based operational research and introduce new tools into practice
  - Advocate for and participate in research to develop new diagnostics, drugs, and vaccines

DOTS, directly observed treatment, short-course; HIV, human immunodeficiency virus; MDR, multidrug resistant; ISTC, International Standards for Tubuerculosis care.

of the healthcare systems, exclusion of private healthcare systems, unidirectional management of the patients, and few efforts on research on new diagnostics, drugs, and vaccines.

The Stop Tuberculosis strategy is supported by the Global Plan to Stop Tuberculosis (2011–2015), prepared by the Stop Tuberculosis partnership; it was developed in order to discover financial needs, and new political and public health approaches.[112]

Another relevant clinical and public health tool is prepared by the WHO together with numerous stakeholders is the International Standards of Tuberculosis Care (ISTC). It summarizes the standards of care that should be followed by the public and private care-providers while managing suspected or confirmed tuberculosis patients, in order to ensure a high-quality care. In particular, it is focused on early bacteriological diagnosis, accurate prescription of anti-tuberculosis drugs, management of vulnerable groups (for instance, HIV-positives), and recording and reporting of treatment outcomes.[78,79]

Recently, the European Respiratory Society (ERS) and the European Centre for Disease Prevention and Control (ECDC) prepared the European standards to complement the ISTC, that is to adapt them to the epidemiological scenario of the European Union/European economic areas, oriented to the elimination of tuberculosis.[110]

The primary prevention of tuberculosis has not been successful with BCG vaccination. After its introduction in the clinical practice in 1921, several clinical trials evaluated its efficacy.

It consists of a live attenuated strain of *M. bovis* and represents the only registered vaccine for the prevention of tuberculosis. It was proved that it is efficacious in preventing tuberculous meningitis and miliary tuberculosis in children in areas of the world where the disease is endemic. It confers a variable protection against pulmonary tuberculosis, particularly in adolescents and adults.[113-115] Several concerns were raised on its safety in immunocompromised patients, primarily in HIV-positives.[116,117]

It was given 4 billion times until now and is currently prescribed to newborns in high-risk areas as component of the WHO Expanded Program on Immunization.[115,117,118]

Elimination of tuberculosis by 2050 seems unlikely. It is equivalent to an incidence of new sputum smear-positive patients below 1/1 million population.

CONCLUSION

Tuberculosis represents a relevant clinical and public health issue worldwide. However, where the evidence-based WHO public health strategies (i.e., DOTS and Stop Tuberculosis) were implemented and scaled-up, the epidemiological scenario dramatically changed. Unfortunately, numerous geographical areas, particularly in the sub-Saharan Africa, should improve the sustainability of their healthcare systems in order to hinder the spread of tuberculosis, MDR-tuberculosis , and HIV/AIDS. The improvement of the funding system for low-income countries, the sustained political commitment against tuberculosis and HIV/AIDS, the introduction of new healthcare models, as well as the discovery of innovative preventive, therapeutic, and diagnostic means might help in addressing the target of less than 1 new sputum smear-positive case/1 million inhabitants, that is the elimination of tuberculosis. It can be obtained by reducing the incidence and the prevalence of individuals with latent tuberculosis infection, that is the potential source of new tuberculosis cases.[29]

Only a plural, multi-sectorial strategy, adequately funded and supported by the political parties, can eliminate tuberculosis in the near future, following the correct tactics implemented by several countries worldwide.[107,119,120]

REFERENCES

1. Huynh KK, Joshi SA, Brown EJ. A delicate dance: host response to mycobacteria. *Curr Opin Immunol.* 2011;23: 464-72.
2. World Health Organization. Global tuberculosis control 2011. Geneva: WHO. Available from: http://whqlibdoc.who.int/publications/2011/9789241564380_eng.pdf
3. Ahmad S. Pathogenesis, immunology, and diagnosis of latent Mycobacterium tuberculosis infection. *Clin Dev Immunol.* 2011: 2011;814943.
4. Fitzgerald D, Haas DW. Mycobacterium tuberculosis. In: Mandell GL, Bennett JE, Dolin R, eds. Principles and practice of infectious diseases, 6th ed. Philadelphia: Churchill Livingstone; 2005. p. 2852-86.
5. Flynn JL, Chan J, Lin PL. Macrophages and control of granulomatous inflammation in tuberculosis. *Mucosal Immunol.* 2011;4:271-8.
6. Smith I. Mycobacterium tuberculosis pathogenesis and molecular determinants of virulence. *Clin Microbiol Rev.* 2003;16:463-96.
7. Torrelles JB, Schlesinger LS. Diversity in Mycobacterium tuberculosis mannosylated cell wall determinants impacts adaptation to the host. *Tuberculosis (Edinb).* 2010;90:84-93.
8. Mishra AK, Driessen NN, Appelmelk BJ, Besra GS. Lipoarabinomannan and related glycoconjugates: structure, biogenesis and role in Mycobacterium tuberculosis physiology and host-pathogen interaction. *FEMS Microbiol Rev.* 2011;35:1126-57.
9. Karakousis PC, Bishai WR, Dorman SE. Mycobacterium tuberculosis cell envelope lipids and the host immune response. *Cell Microbiol.* 2004;6:105-16.

10. Kaufmann SH, Cole ST, Mizrahi V, Rubin E, Nathan C. Mycobacterium tuberculosis and the host response. *J Exp Med.* 2005;201:1693-7.
11. Rieder H. Epidemiologic basis of tuberculosis control. Paris IUATaLD, 1999.
12. Styblo RMT, public health aspects. Encyclopedia of Human Biology, second edition, volume 8. Academic Press, 1997. pp. 537-558.
13. Raviglione MC. The Global Plan to Stop TB, 2006-2015. *Int J Tuberc Lung Dis.* 2006;10:238-9.
14. Storla DG, Yimer S, Bjune GA. A systematic review of delay in the diagnosis and treatment of tuberculosis. *BMC Public Health.* 2008;8:15.
15. Ngadaya ES, Mfinanga GS, Wandwalo ER, Morkve O. Delay in tuberculosis case detection in Pwani region, Tanzania. A cross sectional study. *BMC Health Serv Res.* 2009;9:196.
16. WHO. WHO policy on TB infection control in health-care facilities, congregate settings and households. Available from: http://whqlibdoc.who.int/publications/2009/9789241598323_eng.pdf
17. Gideon HP, Flynn JL. Latent tuberculosis: what the host "sees"? *Immunol Res.* 2011;50:202-12.
18. Dorhoi A, Reece ST, Kaufmann SH. For better or for worse: the immune response against Mycobacterium tuberculosis balances pathology and protection. *Immunol Rev.* 2011;240:235-51.
19. Kleinnijenhuis J, Oosting M, Joosten LA, Netea MG, Van Crevel R. Innate immune recognition of Mycobacterium tuberculosis. *Clin Dev Immunol.* 2011;2011:405310.
20. Urdahl KB, Shafiani S, Ernst JD. Initiation and regulation of T-cell responses in tuberculosis. *Mucosal Immunol.* 2011;4:288-93.
21. Maglione PJ, Chan J. How B cells shape the immune response against Mycobacterium tuberculosis. *Eur J Immunol.* 2009;39:676-86.
22. Sotgiu G, Ferrara G, Matteelli A, Richardson MD, Centis R, Ruesch-Gerdes S, et al. Epidemiology and clinical management of XDR-TB: a systematic review by TBNET. *Eur Respir J.* 2009;33:871-81.
23. Centers for Disease Control and Prevention (CDC). Emergence of Mycobacterium tuberculosis with extensive resistance to second-line drugs — worldwide 2000-2004. *MMWR Morb Mortal Wkly Rep.* 2006;55:301-5.
24. World Health Organization. Guidelines for the programmatic management of drug-resistant tuberculosis. Geneva, Switzerland, 2008. Available from: http://whqlibdoc.who.int/publications/2008/9789241547581_eng.pdf.
25. World Health Organization. Multidrug and extensively drug-resistant TB (M/XD-TB). 2010 Global report on surveillance and response. Geneva, Switzerland, 2010. Available from: http://whqlibdoc.who.int/publications/2010/9789241599191_eng.pdf.
26. World Health Organization. Extensively drug-resistant tuberculosis (XDR-TB): recommendations for prevention and control. *Wkly Epidemiol Rec.* 2006;81:430-2
27. The Global MDR-TB and XDR-TB response plan 2007-2008. Available from: http://www.who.int/tb/publications/2007/global_response_plan.pdf.
28. Migliori GB, Sotgiu G, Lange C, Centis R. Extensively drug-resistant tuberculosis: back to the future. *Eur Respir J.* 2010;36:475-7.
29. Migliori GB, Loddenkemper R, Blasi F, Raviglione MC. 125 years after Robert Koch's discovery of the tubercle bacillus: the new XDR-TB threat. Is "science" enough to tackle the epidemic? *Eur Respir J.* 2007;29:423-7.
30. Migliori GB, Besozzi G, Girardi E, Kliiman K, Lange C, Toungoussova OS, et al.; SMIRA/TBNET Study Group. Clinical and operational value of the extensively drug-resistant tuberculosis definition. *Eur Respir J.* 2007;30: 623-6.
31. Caminero JA. Multidrug-resistant tuberculosis: epidemiology, risk factors and case finding. *Int J Tuberc Lung Dis.* 2010;14:382-90.
32. Migliori GB, Sotgiu G, Jaramillo E, Mirzayev F, Centis R, Colvin C, et al. Development of a standardised multidrug-resistant/extensively drug-resistant tuberculosis assessment and monitoring tool. *Int J Tuberc Lung Dis.* 2009;13: 1305-8.
33. Migliori GB, Zellweger JP, Abubakar I, Ibraim E, Caminero JA, De Vries G, et al. European union standards for tuberculosis care. *Eur Respir J.* 2012;39:807-19.
34. Migliori GB, Sotgiu G, D'Ambrosio L, Centis R, Lange C, Bothamley G, et al. TB and MDR/XDR-TB in European Union and European Economic Area countries: managed or mismanaged? *Eur Respir J.* 2012;39:619-25.
35. Sotgiu G, Centis R, D'ambrosio L, De Lorenzo S, D'arcy Richardson M, Lange C, et al.; TBNET MDR-TB project. Development of a standardised tool to survey MDR-/XDR-TB case management in Europe. *Eur Respir J.* 2010;36: 208-11.
36. Sotgiu G, D'Ambrosio L, Centis R, Bothamley G, Cirillo DM, De Lorenzo S, et al. TB and M/XDR-TB infection control in European TB reference centres: the Achilles' heel? *Eur Respir J.* 2011;38:1221-3.
37. Orenstein EW, Basu S, Shah NS, Andrews JR, Friedland GH, Moll AP, et al. Treatment outcomes among patients with multidrug-resistant tuberculosis: systematic review and meta-analysis. *Lancet Infect Dis.* 2009;9:153-61.
38. Kim DH, Kim HJ, Park SK, Kong SJ, Kim YS, Kim TH, et al. Treatment outcomes and survival based on drug resistance patterns in multidrug-resistant tuberculosis. *Am J Respir Crit Care Med.* 2010;182:113-9.
39. Chaulk CP, Kazandjian VA. Directly observed therapy for treatment completion of pulmonary tuberculosis: Consensus Statement of the Public Health Tuberculosis Guidelines Panel. *JAMA.* 1998;279:943-8.
40. Johnston JC, Shahidi NC, Sadatsafavi M, Fitzgerald JM. Treatment outcomes of multidrug-resistant tuberculosis: a systematic review and meta-analysis. *PLoS One.* 2009; 4:e6914.
41. Nunn P, Williams B, Floyd K, Dye C, Elzinga G, Raviglione M. Tuberculosis control in the era of HIV. *Nat Rev Immunol.* 2005;5:819-26.
42. Lönnroth K, Jaramillo E, Williams BG, Dye C, Raviglione M. Drivers of tuberculosis epidemics: the role of risk factors and social determinants. *Soc Sci Med.* 2009;68:2240-6.
43. Creswell J, Raviglione M, Ottmani S, Migliori GB, Uplekar M, Blanc L, et al. Tuberculosis and noncommunicable diseases:

neglected links and missed opportunities. *Eur Respir J.* 2011;37:1269-82.

44. Schutz C, Meintjes G, Almajid F, Wilkinson RJ, Pozniak A. Clinical management of tuberculosis and HIV-1 co-infection. *Eur Respir J.* 2010;36:1460-81.
45. Jeon CY, Murray MB. Diabetes mellitus increases the risk of active tuberculosis: a systematic review of 13 observational studies. *PLoS Med.* 2008;5:e152.
46. Stalenhoef JE, Alisjahbana B, Nelwan EJ, van der Ven-Jongekrijg J, Ottenhoff TH, van der Meer JW, et al. The role of interferon-gamma in the increased tuberculosis risk in type 2 diabetes mellitus. *Eur J Clin Microbiol Infect Dis.* 2008;27:97-103.
47. Martens GW, Arikan MC, Lee J, Ren F, Greiner D, Kornfeld H. Tuberculosis susceptibility of diabetic mice. *Am J Respir Cell Mol Biol.* 2007;37:518-24.
48. Shaw JE, Sicree RA, Zimmet PZ. Global estimates of the prevalence of diabetes for 2010 and 2030. *Diabetes Res Clin Pract.* 2010;87:4-14.
49. Harries AD, Billo N, Kapur A. Links between diabetes mellitus and tuberculosis: should we integrate screening and care? *Trans R Soc Trop Med Hyg.* 2009;103:1-2.
50. Dooley KE, Tang T, Golub JE, Dorman SE, Cronin W. Impact of diabetes mellitus on treatment outcomes of patients with active tuberculosis. *Am J Trop Med Hyg.* 2009;80:634-9.
51. Dooley KE, Chaisson RE. Tuberculosis and diabetes mellitus: convergence of two epidemics. *Lancet Infect Dis.* 2009;9:737-46.
52. Lienhardt C, Rodrigues LC. Estimation of the impact of the human immunodeficiency virus infection on tuberculosis: tuberculosis risks re-visited? *Int J Tuberc Lung Dis.* 1997; 1:196-204.
53. Jeon CY, Harries AD, Baker MA, Hart JE, Kapur A, Lönnroth K, et al. Bi-directional screening for tuberculosis and diabetes: a systematic review. *Trop Med Int Health.* 2010;15:1300-14.
54. Hussein MM, Mooij JM, Roujouleh H. Tuberculosis and chronic renal disease. *Semin Dial.* 2003;16:38-44.
55. Woeltje KF, Mathew A, Rothstein M, Seiler S, Fraser VJ. Tuberculosis infection and anergy in hemodialysis patients. *Am J Kidney Dis.* 1998;31:848-52.
56. Rees D, Murray J. Silica, silicosis and tuberculosis. *Int J Tuberc Lung Dis.* 2007;11:474-84.
57. Hnizdo E, Murray J. Risk of pulmonary tuberculosis relative to silicosis and exposure to silica dust in South African gold miners. *Occup Environ Med.* 1998;55:496-502.
58. Barboza CE, Winter DH, Seiscento M, Santos UeP, Terra Filho M. Tuberculosis and silicosis: epidemiology, diagnosis and chemoprophylaxis. *J Bras Pneumol.* 2008; 34:959-66.
59. Solovic I, Sester M, Gomez-Reino JJ, Rieder HL, Ehlers S, Milburn HJ, et al. The risk of tuberculosis related to tumour necrosis factor antagonist therapies: a TBNET consensus statement. *Eur Respir J.* 2010;36:1185-206.
60. Ehlers S. Why does tumor necrosis factor targeted therapy reactivate tuberculosis? *J Rheumatol Suppl.* 2005;74:35-9.
61. Bates MN, Khalakdina A, Pai M, Chang L, Lessa F, Smith KR. Risk of tuberculosis from exposure to tobacco smoke: a systematic review and meta-analysis. *Arch Intern Med.* 2007;167:335-42.
62. Arcavi L, Benowitz NL. Cigarette smoking and infection. *Arch Intern Med.* 2004;164:2206-16.
63. Newton SM, Brent AJ, Anderson S, Whittaker E, Kampmann B. Paediatric tuberculosis. *Lancet Infect Dis.* 2008;8:498-510.
64. Sreeramareddy CT, Ramakrishnareddy N, Shah RK, Baniya R, Swain PK. Clinico-epidemiological profile and diagnostic procedures of pediatric tuberculosis in a tertiary care hospital of western Nepal-a case-series analysis. *BMC Pediatr.* 2010;10:57.
65. Long R, Cowie R. Tuberculosis: 4. Pulmonary disease. *CMAJ.* 1999;160:1344-8.
66. Golden MP, Vikram HR. Extrapulmonary tuberculosis: an overview. *Am Fam Physician.* 2005;72:1761-8.
67. Cruz AT, Starke JR. Clinical manifestations of tuberculosis in children. *Paediatr Respir Rev.* 2007;8:107-17.
68. Myers JN. Miliary, central nervous system, and genito-urinary tuberculosis. *Dis Mon.* 2007;53:22-31.
69. Garg RK, Sharma R, Kar AM, Kushwaha RA, Singh MK, Shukla R, et al. Neurological complications of miliary tuberculosis. *Clin Neurol Neurosurg.* 2010;112:188-92.
70. Garg RK. Tuberculous meningitis. *Acta Neurol Scand.* 2010;122:75-90.
71. Vinnard C, Macgregor RR. Tuberculous meningitis in HIV-infected individuals. *Curr HIV/AIDS Rep.* 2009;6:139-45.
72. Light RW. Update on tuberculous pleural effusion. *Respirology.* 2010;15:451-8.
73. Porcel JM. Tuberculous pleural effusion. *Lung.* 2009;187: 263-70.
74. Cherian A, Thomas SV. Central nervous system tuber-culosis. *Afr Health Sci.* 2011;11:116-27.
75. Schirmer P, Renault CA, Holodniy M. Is spinal tuberculosis contagious? *Int J Infect Dis.* 2010;14:e659-66.
76. Matos MJ, Bacelar MT, Pinto P, Ramos I. Genitourinary tuberculosis. *Eur J Radiol.* 2005;55:181-7.
77. Handa U, Mundi I, Mohan S. Nodal tuberculosis revisited: a review. *J Infect Dev Ctries.* 2012;6:6-12.
78. Tuberculosis Coalition for Technical Assistance. International Standards for Tuberculosis Care (ISTC), second edition. Tuberculosis Coalition for Technical Assistance, The Hague, 2009. Available from : http://www.currytbcenter.ucsf.edu/international/ISTC_Report_2ndEd.pdf.
79. Tuberculosis Coalition for Technical Assistance. International Standards for Tuberculosis Care (ISTC). The Hague: Tuberculosis Coalition for Technical Assistance, 2006. Available from: http://www.who.int/tb/publications/2006/istc_report.pdf.
80. Boehme CC, Nabeta P, Hillemann D, Nicol MP, Shenai S, Krapp F, et al. Rapid molecular detection of tuberculosis and rifampin resistance. *N Engl J Med.* 2010;363:1005-15.
81. World Health Organization. Strategic And Technical Advisory Group For Tuberculosis (STAG-TB). Report of the Tenth Meeting. 2010. Available from: http://www.who.int/tb/advisory_bodies/stag_tb_report_2010.pdf
82. Leung CC, Rieder HL, Lange C, Yew WW. Treatment of latent infection with Mycobacterium tuberculosis: update 2010. *Eur Respir J.* 2011;37:690-711.

83. European Centers of Disease Prevention and Control. Use of interferon-γ release assays in support of TB diagnosis. Stockholm: ECDC;2011. Available from: http://ecdc.europa.eu/en/publications/Publications/1103_GUI_IGRA.pdf
84. Diel R, Goletti D, Ferrara G, Bothamley G, Cirillo D, Kampmann B, et al. Interferon-γ release assays for the diagnosis of latent Mycobacterium tuberculosis infection: a systematic review and meta-analysis. *Eur Respir J.* 2011; 37:88-99.
85. Oxford_Immunotec. T-Spot.TB Package Insert. 2009. Available from: http://www.oxfordimmunotec.com/96-UK.
86. Cellestis. QuantiFERON-TB Gold (In-Tube Method) Package Insert. 2006. Available from: http://www.cellestis.com/IRM/Company/ShowPage.aspx?CPID=1171
87. Sester M, Sotgiu G, Lange C, Giehl C, Girardi E, Migliori GB, et al. Interferon-γ release assays for the diagnosis of active tuberculosis: a systematic review and meta-analysis. *Eur Respir J.* 2011;37:100-11.
88. Jafari C, Thijsen S, Sotgiu G, Goletti D, Domínguez Benítez JA, Losi M, et al.; Tuberculosis Network European Trialsgroup. Bronchoalveolar lavage enzyme-linked immunospot for a rapid diagnosis of tuberculosis: a Tuberculosis Network European Trialsgroup study. *Am J Respir Crit Care Med.* 2009;180:666-73.
89. Jafari C, Kessler P, Sotgiu G, Ernst M, Lange C. Impact of a Mycobacterium tuberculosis-specific interferon-γ release assay in bronchoalveolar lavage fluid for a rapid diagnosis of tuberculosis. *J Intern Med.* 2011;270:254-62.
90. Mitchison DA. The diagnosis and therapy of tuberculosis during the past 100 years. *Am J Respir Crit Care Med.* 2005;171:699-706.
91. World Health Organization. Treatment of Tuberculosis. Guidelines tEWHTscwsospwsoG. REFERENCE NOT COMPLETE
92. Freiden T (editor). Toman's tuberculosis: case detection, treatment and monitoring. 2nd edition. WHO Geneva. 2004. Available from: http://whqlibdoc.who.int/publications/2004/9241546034_1.pdf.
93. Migliori GB, Raviglione MC, Schaberg T, Davies PD, Zellweger JP, Grzemska M, et al. Tuberculosis management in Europe. Task Force of the European Respiratory Society (ERS), the World Health Organisation (WHO) and the International Union against Tuberculosis and Lung Disease (IUATLD) Europe Region. *Eur Respir J.* 1999;14:978-92.
94. National Institute of Clinical Excellence. Tuberculosis: clinical diagnosis and management of tuberculosis and measures for its prevention and control. NICE clinical guideline 117. 2011. Available from: http://www.nice.org.uk/nicemedia/live/13422/53642/53642.pdf
95. Blumberg HM, Burman WJ, Chaisson RE, Daley CL, Etkind SC, Friedman LN, et al.; American Thoracic Society, Centers for Disease Control and Prevention and the Infectious Diseases Society. American Thoracic Society/Centers for Disease Control and Prevention/Infectious Diseases Society of America: treatment of tuberculosis. *Am J Respir Crit Care Med.* 2003;167:603-62.
96. World Health Organization. TB/HIV: a clinical manual, second edition. 2004.
97. Kwara A, Flanigan TP, Carter EJ. Highly active antiretroviral therapy (HAART) in adults with tuberculosis: current status. *Int J Tuberc Lung Dis.* 2005;9:248-57.
98. Burman WJ, Gallicano K, Peloquin C. Therapeutic implications of drug interactions in the treatment of human immunodeficiency virus-related tuberculosis. *Clin Infect Dis.* 1999;28:419-29.
99. Falzon D, Jaramillo E, Schünemann HJ, Arentz M, Bauer M, Bayona J, et al. WHO guidelines for the programmatic management of drug-resistant tuberculosis: 2011 update. *Eur Respir J.* 2011;38:516-28.
101. Mitnick C, Bayona J, Palacios E, Shin S, Furin J, Alcántara F, et al. Community-based therapy for multidrug-resistant tuberculosis in Lima, Peru. *N Engl J Med.* 2003;348:119-28.
102. Kempker RR, Vashakidze S, Solomonia N, Dzidzikashvili N, Blumberg HM. Surgical treatment of drug-resistant tuberculosis. *Lancet Infect Dis.* 2012;12:157-66.
103. World Health Organization. Global Tuberculosis Control: Surveillance, Planning, Financing. WHO Report 2002. Geneva, Switzerland,WHO/CDS/TB/2002.295. Available from: http://library.cphs.chula.ac.th/Ebooks/Annual%20Report/WHO%20Report/WHO%20REPORT%202002.pdf.
104. Sterling TR, Villarino ME, Borisov AS, Shang N, Gordin F, Bliven-Sizemore E, et al.; TB Trials Consortium PREVENT TB Study Team. Three months of rifapentine and isoniazid for latent tuberculosis infection. *N Engl J Med.* 2011;365:2155-66.
105. Horsburgh CR, Goldberg S, Bethel J, Chen S, Colson PW, Hirsch-Moverman Y, et al. Latent TB infection treatment acceptance and completion in the United States and Canada. *Chest.* 2010;137:401-9.
106. Dahle UR, Eldholm V, Winje BA, Mannsåker T, Heldal E. Impact of immigration on the molecular epidemiology of Mycobacterium tuberculosis in a low-incidence country. *Am J Respir Crit Care Med.* 2007;176:930-5.
107. McKenna MT, McCray E, Onorato I. The epidemiology of tuberculosis among foreign-born persons in the United States, 1986 to 1993. *N Engl J Med.* 1995;332:1071-6.
108. Broekmans JF, Migliori GB, Rieder HL, Lees J, Ruutu P, Loddenkemper R, et al.; World Health Organization, International Union Against Tuberculosis and Lung Disease, and Royal Netherlands Tuberculosis Association Working Group. . European framework for tuberculosis control and elimination in countries with a low incidence. Recommendations of the World Health Organization (WHO), International Union Against Tuberculosis and Lung Disease (IUATLD) and Royal Netherlands Tuberculosis Association (KNCV) Working Group. *Eur Respir J.* 2002;19:765-75.
109. Raviglione MC, Uplekar MW. WHO's new Stop TB Strategy. *Lancet.* 2006;367:952-5.
110. Stop TB Partnership and World Health Organization. Global Plan to Stop TB 2006–2015. Geneva, World Health Organization, 2006 (WHO/HTM/STB/2006.35).
111. World Health Organization. Fifty-eighth World Health Assembly: resolutions and decisions. Geneva. 2005. Available from: http://apps.who.int/gb/ebwha/pdf_files/WHA58-REC1/english/A58_2005_REC1-en.pdf

112. World Health Organization. Report on the meeting of the second ad hoc Committee on the TB Epidemic. Recommendations to Stop TB partners. Montreux. 2004. Available from: http://www.stoptb.org/assets/documents/resources/publications/technical/TB-REPORT-24pages.pdf
113. Migliori GB, Sotgiu G, Blasi F, Zumla A, Loddenkemper R, Raviglione MC, et al. Towards the development of EU/EEA Standards for Tuberculosis Care (ESTC). *Eur Respir J.* 2011;38:493-5.
114. Trunz BB, Fine P, Dye C. Effect of BCG vaccination on childhood tuberculous meningitis and miliary tuberculosis worldwide: a meta-analysis and assessment of cost-effectiveness. *Lancet.* 2006;367:1173-80.
115. Sterne JA, Rodrigues LC, Guedes IN. Does the efficacy of BCG decline with time since vaccination? *Int J Tuberc Lung Dis.* 1998;2:200-7.
116. McShane H. Tuberculosis vaccines: beyond bacille Calmette-Guerin. *Philos Trans R Soc Lond B Biol Sci.* 2011;366:2782-9.
117. World Health Organisation. Revised BCG vaccination guidelines for infants at risk for HIV infection. *Wkly Epidemiol Rec.* 2007;82:193-6.
118. Kaufmann SH. Fact and fiction in tuberculosis vaccine research: 10 years later. *Lancet Infect Dis.* 2011; 11:633-40.
119. Zwerling A, Pai M. The BCG world atlas: a new, open-access resource for clinicians and researchers. *Expert Rev Anti Infect Ther.* 2011;9:559-61.
120. Clancy L, Rieder HL, Enarson DA, Spinaci S. Tuberculosis elimination in the countries of Europe and other industrialized countries. *Eur Respir J.* 1991;4:1288-95.

CHAPTER 14

Invasive Fungal Infections in Critically Ill Patients

Stijn I Blot, Koenraad Vandewoude

ABSTRACT

In the past decades, a demographic shift in hospital and intensive care unit (ICU) populations have been taking place with a greater proportion of strongly debilitated patients who are at risk for secondary opportunistic infections such as invasive fungal disease. The utmost important fungal pathogens encountered in ICUs are invasive candidiasis and invasive (pulmonary) aspergillosis. With the exception of candidemia, the diagnosis of invasive fungal infections is problematic. This may lead to a postponed diagnosis and therefore, delayed initiation of antifungal therapy. Despite the availability of potent antifungal agents, mortality associated with invasive fungal infections in critically ill patients remains unacceptably high.

INTRODUCTION

Over the past 3 decades, major advances in healthcare have led to an unwelcome increase in the number of life-threatening infections due to true pathogenic and opportunistic fungi. Invasive candidiasis and invasive aspergillosis are the 2 major manifestations of opportunistic invasive mycoses.[1,2] These infections are being seen in ever increasing numbers, largely because of the increasing size of the population at risk. This population includes recipients of hematopoietic stem cell transplants and solid organ transplants, patients with hematological malignancies, patients infected with human immunodeficiency virus (HIV) developing acquired immunodeficiency syndrome (AIDS), and other persons receiving immunosuppressive treatment. Furthermore, the use of high-grade supportive care in severe and life-threatening diseases, specifically in intensive care units (ICUs), burn patients, and premature neonates, has improved survival but has created a demographic shift in hospital and ICU populations with more debilitated patients at risk for secondary invasive opportunistic infections. These evolutions in medical practice have led to changes in the epidemiology of fungal infections.

The importance of fungi as pathogens in hospitalized patients, in general, and in ICU patients in particular, has increased substantially in the past 3 decades. In the National Nosocomial Infections Surveillance System (NNIS), 1980–1990, the rate of nosocomial fungal infections rose from 2.0 to 3.8 infections/1,000 discharges.[3] In the US, amongst the deaths caused by any infectious disease, those due to mycoses increased from the 10th most common in 1980 to the 7th most common in 1997.[4] The increased incidence of fungal infections has coincided with a decreased mortality from bacterial infections. This is probably the result of better antibiotic therapy, leading to an increased survival of patients who are predisposed to fungal infections, as well as, inappropriate antibiotic therapy disrupting the normal microbial flora on the skin and the mucosal surfaces. The increase in incidence of candidiasis have been most marked during the 1980s,[5,6] but rates appeared to have stabilized in the 1990s.[7] This increasing trend of *Candida* infections over the past decades has been noted in all types of hospitals and wards. The NNIS data showed that between 1980 and 1989, the incidence of primary candidemia increased by 487% in large hospitals and by 219% in smaller hospitals.[5] The overall rate of nosocomial fungal infections increased almost 5-fold over the same period. *Candida* species may account for approximately 8–15% of all nosocomial bloodstream infections albeit that some studies report a much lower incidence of candidemia.[8,9] In the past decades, it has been suggested that in ICUs the incidence of invasive aspergillosis, mainly pulmonary involvement, is on the rise.[10,11] However, diagnosis of invasive aspergillosis is problematic as well, and reliable incidence estimates are scarce as such. As with all opportunistic infections, the case-mix of patients is most probably a major factor influencing the occurrence rate of invasive fungal infections.

A sobering observation in infectious disease medicine and critical care is that invasive fungal infections are often not diagnosed or are diagnosed late in the course of the disease, because diagnostic techniques are less than ideal.[12,13] In a large autopsy study, only 22% of invasive fungal infections were suspected or documented antemortem.[14] Clinicians are often frustrated since the weakness of current clinical, radiological, and mycological diagnostic modalities are nonspecific and insensitive. Thus, it hampers the implementation of the concept of timely appropriate treatment, from which is known that it has a positive impact on outcome in bacterial infections. In spite of the availability of effective azole and polyene antifungals for more than 3 decades and more recently, the development of the new generation triazoles and the echinocandins, fungal infection continues to carry a grim prognosis and is associated with significant morbidity and mortality, thus, representing a growing health-economic burden for modern healthcare systems. A robust management strategy for prophylaxis, diagnosis, and therapy of invasive fungal infections, continues to evade clinicians and mycological experts from developing new noninvasive tools for screening patients at risk and to corroborate diagnosis when clinical argumentation is insufficient in a particular patient.

POSTMORTEM EPIDEMIOLOGICAL EVIDENCE AND TEMPORAL TRENDS

Autopsy data on the incidence of invasive fungal infection provide incontrovertible evidence for the importance of invasive fungal disease in the general population as well as in hospitalized patients.

In a single tertiary care center study, analyzing trends in the postmortem epidemiology of invasive fungal infection between 1978 and 1992, 278 invasive fungal infections were found in a series of 8,214 autopsies (3.38%). Over 12 years, the prevalence of invasive fungal infection rose from 2.2% (1978–1982) and 3.2% (1983–1987) to 5.1% (1998–1992) ($p < 0.001$). This was mainly due to a significant increase in *Aspergillus* infections ($p < 0.001$), whereas the prevalence of *Candida* infections was stable and even showed a declining trend.[14]

The same temporal trend was found in a nationwide Japanese unselected autopsy study, encompassing patients from 1969 to 1994.[15] The frequency of visceral mycoses among the annual total number of autopsy cases increased noticeably from 1.60% in 1969 to a peak of 4.66% in 1990 and 3.17% in 1994. Among them, the incidences of candidiasis and aspergillosis increased the most. After 1990, however, the frequency of visceral mycoses gradually decreased. Until 1989, the predominant causative agent was *Candida* species, followed in order by *Aspergillus* species and *Cryptococcus* species The incidence of invasive candidiasis rose from 0.41% in 1969 to a peak of 1.89% in 1989 and then decreased to 1.12% after 1991. In contrast, the aspergillosis rate rose from 0.39% in 1969 to a peak of 1.55% in 1990 and maintained a constant level of about 1.3% after 1991, surpassing the rate of invasive candidiasis.

Two German studies confirm these findings. In a single center study in a general hospital, the incidence of systemic mycoses was found to be 0.98% in 4,813 necropsies.[16] Whereas candidiasis predominated from 1973 till 1991, a shift towards aspergillosis was noticed in the period of 1992–2001. The invasive candidiasis rate was 0.56%, and the aspergillosis rate was 0.37%. An incidence of 6.6% for invasive candidiasis and of 1.3% for invasive aspergillosis was found in an autopsy study analyzing records between 1994 and 2003.[17] In the setting of tertiary care hospitals, invasive aspergillosis is actually surpassing invasive candidiasis, as the most frequent fungal infection found at autopsy. However, one should consider that most cases clinically classified as 'invasive candidiasis' effectively are candidemia without tissue invasion. This entity of definite fungal infection by *Candida* species may be underestimated in necropsy studies.[18]

DIAGNOSIS OF INVASIVE FUNGAL INFECTION

With the exception of cryptococcal meningitis and candidemia, the diagnosis of invasive fungal infection at an early stage remains difficult. Definite or proven diagnosis still remains on positive histopathological examination. The sampling of body fluids or tissue from protected anatomical sites is often not feasible in critically ill patients. Therefore, diagnosis is often constructed on clinical and radiological data, and an estimation of the probability of acquiring invasive fungal infection based on estimation of host risk factors and epidemiological data. This has led to the concepts of probable and possible fungal disease, which are far more frequent diagnostic categories than proven fungal disease; the latter often being a post-mortem diagnostic finding.

Historically, invasive fungal infection was first recognized problematic in patients with hematological cancer undergoing chemotherapy and in patients receiving allogeneic stem cell transplants; hence, most efforts in optimizing diagnosis and treatment have been directed to this population. However, evidence is accumulating that the groups of patient at risk for developing invasive fungal infection continue to expand. Moreover, the spectrum of *Candida* and *Aspergillus* species infection is wide. Some entities are difficult to characterize, and not always a consensus can be formed definitions in published work.

For immunocompromized patients, an international consensus has been reached by investigators from the Invasive Fungal Infections Co-operative Group (IFICG) of both the European Organization for Research and Treatment of Cancer (EORTC) and the Mycoses Study Group (MSG) of the US National Institute of Allergy and Infectious Diseases (NIAID).[19] The EORTC/MSG developed standard definitions of invasive fungal infections in immunocompromized patients with cancer and in recipients of hematopoietic stem cell transplants. These diagnostic criteria were updated in 2008.[20] According to the revised definitions, invasive fungal disease is categorized in 3 major categories reflecting the diagnostic degree of certainty: proven, probable, and possible invasive fungal disease.[20] A proven diagnosis requires histopathologic evidence of fungal invasion. A diagnosis of probable invasive fungal disease is based on the presence of host factors, clinical features, and positive mycology. Host factors reflect profound immunodeficiency, such as neutropenia or treatment with immunosuppressive agents. Clinical features for invasive fungal disease include medical imaging on computed tomography (CT) scan demonstrating suggestive signs of fungal invasion: dense, well circumscribed lesions, with or without a halo sign, air crescent sign, or cavity. Mycological criteria include either a direct test (cytology, direct microscopy, or culture) on any respiratory tract aspirate, or galactomannan antigen detection on bronchoalveolar lavage (BAL) fluid or serum. A diagnosis of possible invasive fungal disease is reached in the presence of host factors and clinical features, but in the absence of mycological criteria.

These diagnostic criteria proved to be useful in research and practice in severely immunocompromized patients.[21,22] In mechanically ventilated ICU patients, however, diagnosing invasive fungal disease according to this strict classification is problematic due to a number of reasons. First, open lung biopsy might be contraindicated because of coagulation disorders; as such, a diagnosis of proven invasive fungal disease is rare. Second, current definitions of probable or possible invasive fungal disease have been validated only in immunocompromized patients. However, this is a serious drawback as invasive fungal disease may develop in ICU patients without host factors.[23,24] Third, radiological findings in mechanically ventilated patients are nonspecific in the majority of cases[24] in contrast to the very strict definitions of radiological lesions according to the EORTC/MSG criteria.[20] Moreover, these lesions should be documented by computed tomography (CT) scan, which is not always feasible in ICU patients with hemodynamic or respiratory instability. Finally, galactomannan antigen detection on serum is of little value in non-neutropenic patients, as circulating neutrophils are capable of clearing the antigen.

The lack of specific criteria for diagnosing invasive fungal disease in critically ill patients hampers timely initiation of appropriate antifungal therapy and may, as such, compromise the odds of survival.[22,25,26] One of the black boxes in the diagnostic process is the presence of *Aspergillus* species in endotracheal aspirate cultures. This is observed in up to 2% of mechanically ventilated ICU patients.[24,27,28] The relevance of *Aspergillus*-positive endotracheal aspirates was assessed by Vandewoude et al. who proposed a clinical diagnostic algorithm to discriminate *Aspergillus* colonization from invasive pulmonary aspergillosis.[24] The algorithm was derived from the EORTC/MSG definitions and considers an endotracheal aspirate culture to represent invasive pulmonary aspergillosis in the presence of compatible signs, abnormal thoracic medical imaging, and either host factors or BAL fluid positive for *Aspergillus* on direct microscopy and culture (Table 1).

In a cohort of 172 ICU patients with *Aspergillus*-positive endotracheal aspirate cultures, 83 were judged to have invasive pulmonary aspergillosis (48.3%). Histopathology data were available in 26 patients, 19 in the invasive pulmonary aspergillosis group and 9 in the colonization group. In all 26 cases, the diagnosis as based upon the clinical algorithm was confirmed. These data were externally validated in a large multicenter epidemiologic study that included 524 critically ill patients with *Aspergillus*-positive endotracheal aspirates.[29] For semantic clarity, the classification of probable invasive pulmonary aspergillosis in the clinical algorithm was renamed to "putative invasive pulmonary aspergillosis", in order to distinguish from probable invasive pulmonary

TABLE 1

Diagnostic Criteria for Putative Invasive Pulmonary Aspergillosis[24,29]

Putative invasive pulmonary aspergillosis (all 4 criteria must be met)
1. *Aspergillus*-positive lower respiratory tract specimen culture (entry criterion)
2. Compatible signs and symptoms (one of the following)
• Fever refractory to at least 3 days of appropriate antibiotic therapy
• Recrudescent fever after a period of defervescence of at least 48 hours while still on antibiotics and without other apparent cause
• Pleuritic chest pain
• Pleuritic rub
• Dyspnea
• Hemoptysis
• Worsening respiratory insufficiency in spite of appropriate antibiotic therapy and ventilator support
3. Abnormal medical imaging by portable chest X-ray or CT scan of the lungs
4. Either 4a or 4b
4a. Host risk factors (1 of the following conditions)
• Neutropenia (ANC <500/mm^3) preceding or at the time of ICU admission
• Underlying hematological or oncological malignancy treated with cytotoxic agents
• Glucocorticoid treatment (prednisone equivalent >20 mg/day)
• Congenital or acquired immunodeficiency
4b. Semiquantitative *Aspergillus*-positive culture of BAL fluid (+ or ++), without bacterial growth together with a positive cytological smear showing branching hyphae

When ≥1 criterion necessary for a diagnosis of putative invasive pulmonary aspergillosis is not met, the case is classified as *Aspergillus* respiratory tract colonization.

BAL, bronchoalveolar lavage; CT, computed tomography; ANC, absolute neutrophil count; ICU, intensive care unit.

aspergillosis in the EORTC/MSG criteria for invasive fungal disease.

In a subset of 115 pathology-controlled cases ('gold standard') the clinical algorithm reached an area under the receiver operating characteristic curve of 76% [95% confidence interval (CI) 67–85%] while the criteria for probable aspergillosis as defined by the EORTC/MSG only reached an area under curve of 57% (95% CI 46–68%). The positive and negative predictive values were 61% and 92%, respectively. These data stress that in the absence of histopathologic data, the criteria proposed by the EORTC/MSG are of minor value in ICU settings. In the total cohort (n = 524), 79 patients had proven invasive pulmonary aspergillosis (15.1%). According to the EORTC/MSG criteria, 32 patients had probable aspergillosis (6.1%) and 413 patients were not classifiable (78.8%). The algorithm judged 199 patients to have putative aspergillosis (38.0%) and 246 to have *Aspergillus* colonization (46.9%). The algorithm demonstrated favorable operating characteristics to discriminate *Aspergillus* respiratory tract colonization from invasive pulmonary aspergillosis in critically ill patients. In comparison to the EORTC/MSG criteria, this algorithm probably encompasses a greater proportion of the true burden of invasive pulmonary aspergillosis in the ICU.

CLINICAL EPIDEMIOLOGY OF INVASIVE FUNGAL INFECTIONS

Because of the uncertainties in diagnosis, it is difficult to assess the true clinical significance of fungal isolates. As a result, it is troublesome to appreciate the true incidence of invasive candidiasis and invasive aspergillosis. Literature data addressing frequency, diseased pattern, and prognostic data rely on autopsy series, retrospective series, and more recently, prospective series in certain risk groups. By far, the greatest wealth of information exists for nosocomial invasive candidiasis. For invasive aspergillosis, studies have mostly focused on severely immunocompromized and cancer patients. Particularly in non-neutropenic patients, the incidence of invasive aspergillosis is difficult to assess. Data about the incidence of invasive pulmonary aspergillosis in the critically ill are scarce.

INVASIVE CANDIDIASIS AND CANDIDEMIA

Clinical Spectrum and Definitions

The clinical spectrum of diseases related to *Candida* species is wide, and a summary is given in table 2. They can be divided in hematogenous, nonhematogenous, and deep seated infections.

Some entities are difficult to characterize, so in surgical and critically ill patients, there is no uniform consensus in definitions in published work.[30] For practical reasons, it can be considered that invasive candidiasis describes 2 close but distinct entities: candidemia and systemic or disseminated candidiasis.[31] Candidemia refers to the isolation of *Candida* species from the blood. If the patient temporarily presents signs of infection, candidemia is considered proven invasive fungal infection. Candidemia without clinical signs in a neutropenic patient, in the presence of graft vs. host disease or in a patient

TABLE 2
Clinical Spectrum of *Candida* Infections

Hematogenous infections	
• Candidemia	• Osteomyelitis
• Endophthalmitis	• Spondylodiscitis
• Vascular access-related candidemia	• Meningitis
	• Pyelonephritis
• Septic thrombophlebitis	• Pulmonary candidiasis
• Infectious endocarditis	• Hepatosplenic candidiasis
• Arthritis	
Nonhematogenous infections	
• Cutaneous candidiasis	• Vaginitis
• Oropharyngeal candidiasis	
Deep-seated *Candida* species infections	
• Esophageal candidiasis	• Peritonitis
• Cystitis	• Tracheitis, bronchitis

receiving steroids, is considered probable. 'Disseminated candidiasis' refers to conditions where *Candida* invasion is shown from culture or histology results at non-adjacent, normally sterile sites. Such findings confirm hematogenous dissemination, and accordingly, these infections can be categorized as proven. The term invasive candidiasis is sometimes used instead of hematogenous candidiasis, referring to the fact that the development of infection follows host colonization.[32-34] *Candida albicans* is responsible for most infections, but compared to older reports, the share of non-*albicans* species is increasing.[35-38]

Incidence and Temporal Trends

Over the past 3 decades, *Candida* species has become increasingly important as nosocomial pathogens. Since *Candida* species infections are not reportable diseases, published data have been derived from institution-based registries and more recently in multicenter studies, often in predefined patient type groups, such as the critically ill.

Invasive candidiasis was estimated to account for 17% of hospital-acquired infections reported during the European Study on the Prevalence of Nosocomial Infections in Critically Ill Patients (EPIC study).[39] This large multicenter study included 10,038 patients from 1,417 ICUs in 17 European countries in 1992. A criticism to the study concept was that due to imperfection in case definitions, patients categorized as having invasive candidiasis were merely colonized; hence, the point-prevalence estimate of 17% is likely to be an overestimation. In the EPIC II study, comparable data were reported regarding presumed *Candida* infections, hereby, illustrating the ongoing diagnostic fog in these opportunistic infections.[40]

Candidemia represents 10–20% of all invasive candidiasis. This may be considered as the 'tip of the iceberg' of infections by *Candida* species.[3,41,42] In the 80s, a candidemia rate of 0.5% of all medical and surgical discharges was described in a tertiary care center, representing a 20-fold increase as compared to the 70s. Overall mortality in candidemic patients was 57%.[43] In the US, the NNIS program between 1980 and 1989 showed an increase in the proportion of nosocomial infections caused by *Candida* species from 2% in 1980 to approximately, 5% in the period 1986–1989.[44] In an active population-based surveillance for candidemia in 2 North-American metropolitan areas in 1992–1993, the average annual incidence was 8/100,000 population;[6] 19% of patients developed candidemia prior to or on the day of admission.

Subsequently, between 1990 and 1999, the NNIS based registry showed that *Candida* species were responsible for 5–10% of all bloodstream infections[45,46] *Candida* species represented the fourth leading organism, after coagulase-negative staphylococci, *Staphylococcus aureus,* and enterococci.

In a retrospective study on candidemia in a tertiary care hospital in Switzerland between 1989 and 2000, the annual incidence ranged from 0.2 to 0.46/10,000 patient-days. During the study period, a decrease in incidence of candidemia has been noted. The species distribution in patients with candidemia showed that the most commonly identified species were *C. albicans* (66%), followed by *C. glabrata* (17%), and *C. parapsilosis* (6%). In spite of an increase in fluconazole use, the proportion of non-*C. albicans* species remained stable. The overall mortality among patients with candidemia was 44%, with the highest rate in patients over 65 years (52%). Factors independently associated with higher mortality were patient age greater than 65 years, ICU admission, and underlying cancer.

The European Confederation of Medical Mycology (ECMM) prospective, sequential, hospital population-based study through 1997–1999 revealed rates of candidemia ranging from 0.20 to 0.38/1,000 admissions with a 30-day mortality rate of 37.9%.[47] *C. albicans* was identified in 56% of cases. Non-*albicans Candida* species were most frequently isolated from patients with hematological malignancies (65%). With increasing age, an increasing incidence of *C. glabrata* was seen. The 30-day mortality rate was 37.9%. In a series of 294 consecutive candidemia patients between 1989 and 2000 at a large referral center, candidemia incidence ranged from 0.21 to 0.56/10,000 patient days with the highest incidence in 1993 and the lowest in 2000.[48]

Candidemia rates vary according to the characteristics of the population considered and the type of the institution. Rates calculated as incidence-densities (i.e., per 10,000 patient days) better express the risk associated with the case-mix of the population and hence allow some comparisons between studies.[31] The incidence of candidemia reported in observational series range from 2.8 to 22.0 candidemia/10,000 patient-days.[48-50] As already mentioned, case-mix should be considered in the interpretation of such data. Trends over time are also important to consider as indicated in some of the above-mentioned studies.

Although ICUs generally account for only 5% or less of the total admission capacity in acute care hospitals, the majority of patients with invasive candidiasis are diagnosed in those facilities. In a 2-year large-scaled population-based study of nosocomial candidemia in England and Wales, 45.5% of cases occurred in ICUs.[51]

In the EPIC study, 9.3% of bloodstream infections in ICUs were caused by *Candida* species.[39] Voss et al. reported an average incidence of *Candida* bloodstream infections of 5.5/10,000 patients days, ranging from 2.4 (1990) to 7.4/10,000 patient days (1994) with an overall mortality of 58%.[52] In a large Spanish prospective multicenter survey, the incidence of ICU-acquired candidemia was 1/500 admissions.[53] In a 10-year retrospective cohort study (1990–2000) in critically ill medical and surgical patients in France, the mean yearly incidence of candidemia was 2.1/1,000 admissions with *C. albicans* accounting for 55% of all candidemia. The overall mortality was 60.8%.[54] During 1989–1999, a significant decrease in the incidence of hospital-acquired candidemia among ICU patients was noted in US hospitals participating to the NNIS system.[55] More specifically, there was a significant decrease in the incidence of *C. albicans*, whereas the incidence of non-*albicans* species of *Candida* remained stable. Analyzing the bloodstream infections due to non-*albicans* species, there was a significant increase in *C. glabrata* bloodstream infections. This shift was related to the exponentially increased use of fluconazole in ICUs in the past decade.

A prospective hospital-based surveillance of the surgical ICU patients in particular has demonstrated a high incidence of fungal infection. In the National Epidemiology of Mycosis Survey (NEMIS) study concerning patients admitted to surgical ICU in 1993–94, an incidence of even 9.8 *Candida* bloodstream infections/1,000 admissions was observed. In this survey, *Candida* species caused 9.2% of all bloodstream infections diagnosed in surgical ICUs. More than half of these were due to non-*albicans Candida* species.[49]

The second important type of invasive candidiasis is *Candida* peritonitis. In contrast to candidemia, *Candida* peritonitis is more challenging, because of a problematic clinical and microbiological diagnosis. In some reports *Candida* species were the leading or second most frequently isolated pathogens in secondary or tertiary peritonitis.[56-58] On the other hand, in a study of 120 patients with secondary peritonitis, *Candida* species was present in only 12% of the cases, thereby, ranking seventh.[59] Sandven et al. demonstrated *Candida* involvement in 32 of 81 patients with secondary (nonappendicitis) peritonitis (39.5%).[60] After exclusion of cases with community-acquired peritonitis, this percentage increased to 45%. In critically ill patients with secondary or tertiary peritonitis, the significance of *Candida* isolation is controversial.[61] Some studies have found *Candida* species to have only a limited significance,[61,62] while others found it quite relevant.[63] Only in cases with perioperatively documented *Candida* plaques on the peritoneum, or on histology, can a definite diagnosis of *Candida* peritonitis be made. Yet, as soon as *Candida* is cultured from the peritoneum, antifungal therapy is recommended, irrespective of whether this represent colonization or established infection.[64]

Emergence of Non-*Albicans Candida* Species

An increase in the proportion of non-*albicans Candida* strains has been reported in several series, since the late 1980s. In some studies, predominantly in cancer centers, more than half of *Candida* fungemia was due to non-*albicans* isolates. This evolution is in parallel with the widespread introduction of antifungal prophylaxis with triazoles in the 1980s in hemato-oncological patients receiving intensive cytostatic treatment and bone marrow or stem cell transplantation. Antifungal prophylaxis in this patient population is associated with a higher risk of infection with non-*albicans* strains, such as *C. krusei* (with intrinsic resistance to triazoles) or *C. glabrata* (with dose-dependent sensitivity to triazoles).[65,66]

During the 1990s, surveillance programs were established to provide more general epidemiological information on species distribution. These registries show that *C. albicans* remains the most predominant strain in most countries, more in particular in studies in critically ill patients, as well as, in series in which severely immunocompromized patients did not represent a major proportion.[38,67] The long-term effect of fluconazole consumption on distribution of species causing candidemia was investigated in a university hospital during a period of 11 years (1994–2004).[68] Despite long-term exposure to fluconazole, no change in *Candida* ecology was observed. More recently, however, French investigators found a relationship between antifungal drug use in an ICU and changes in drug susceptibility of *Candida* species.[69] The epidemiological shift in species distribution has implications for the guidelines for antifungal management of invasive *Candida* species infections.[34,70] On the individual patient level, prior exposure to fluconazole increases the likelihood of non-albicans *Candida* involvement in case of candidemia.[68,71]

Of particular interest, is the large variation in species distribution in large therapeutic trials (1994–2003), including those evaluating the newer antifungals, in mixed patients populations, as well as non-neutropenic patients with invasive *Candida* infections, showing a progressive decrease of *C. albicans* over time to about half of the isolates. In most of these series, the proportion of *C. krusei* with intrinsic resistance to triazole compounds remains below 5%. Hence, the effect of the ongoing slow shift in species distribution for management of invasive *Candida* infections, in particular in the ICU, may not be exaggerated, since the proportion of strains with high potential or intrinsic resistance to triazole antifungals remains relatively low. This indicates that international therapeutic guidelines should be implemented after careful consideration of the local fungal ecology, exposure to antifungal prophylaxis, patient mix and proportion of immunosuppressed patients.

Pathophysiology of *Candida* Infection

Candida species are normal inhabitants amongst the human endogenous flora. Mucocutaneous surface colonization is rare under normal conditions.[41] Colonization is a prerequisite for the development of invasive infection; it develops as a consequence of *Candida* overgrowth on mucosal or skin surfaces.[72,73] Translocation across a damaged gut barrier is also possible. Exposure to risk factors creates additional opportunities to develop invasion and secondary hematogenous dissemination. Though endogenous colonization is in most cases responsible for the development of invasive disease, nosocomial cross contamination as a result of poor hand hygiene procedures has been described in ICU settings.

Risk Factors for *Candida* Bloodstream Infection

Several retrospective studies have identified multiple risk factors for candidal bloodstream infection.[72,74-79] Most of the risk factors have been repeatedly verified, although others are more controversial. Major risk factors include the use of central venous catheters, total parenteral nutrition (TPN), receipt of multiple antibiotics, extensive surgery and burns, renal failure and hemodialysis, mechanical ventilation, and prior fungal colonization.

The NEMIS evaluated in a prospective way, the risk factors for the acquisition of *Candida* bloodstream infection in surgical ICU patients.[49] The dominant risk factors were prior surgery (relative risk (RR) 7.3), acute renal failure (RR 4.2), and total parenteral nutrition (RR 3.6), with a significant trend toward *Candida* bloodstream infection developing in association with shock, disseminated intravascular coagulation (DIC), and adult respiratory distress syndrome (ARDS). Other important findings included the contributory role of the triple-lumen catheter in surgical patients. Remarkably, in this study, colonization with *Candida* species was not found to be an independent risk factor for *Candida* bloodstream infection. This observation is in contrast to the findings of several previous studies in which colonization was linked to the risk of candidemia.[72,74,77]

Diagnostic Tools

Timely clinical diagnosis of invasive disease caused by *Candida* species remains a challenge for the clinician. Cultures other than blood or obtained from normally sterile sites are nonspecific. Moreover, the mycological cultures may only contribute to diagnosis, late in the course of the infection. Early clinical manifestations of *Candida* infection are nonspecific with the exception of a positive fundoscopic examination. *Candida* endophthalmitis is a rare, but specific finding present in up to 25% of patients in prospective series.[80-82] Diagnosis remains dependent on a high index of suspicion and critical patient assessment and clinical experience.

The finding in a large autopsy study that only 22% of invasive fungal infections were suspected or documented antemortem is sobering.[14] Diagnostic failure or delayed diagnosis and institution of therapy may be a cause of the persisting high mortality, despite the availability of new potent antifungals with less toxicity. In spite of this, serological or molecular techniques to detect *Candida* infections have not been applied in routine clinical practice until now.

Multisite *Candida* Colonization

The relationship between multisite colonization and subsequent development of candidemia has been demonstrated by several investigators.[83-86] Yet, efforts to define a precise cut-off value based on a ratio of cultures positive for *Candida* and the total number of cultures sampled ('colonization index') have been less successful. For example, in a group of 92 medical ICU patients, 36 of whom had a colonization index of 0.5 or more, only 1 patient developed invasive candidiasis.[87] Agvald-Öhman et al. found that 7 of 29 patients with a colonization index of more than 0.5 developed invasive candidiasis, whereas still 3 of 30 patients with an index of less than 0.5 developed systemic *Candida* infection as well.[83] Yet, in logistic regression analysis, the investigators could demonstrate an increased risk for invasive candidiasis in case of increased colonization density in combination with extensive abdominal surgery. The relative weight of distinct body sites being colonized has never been investigated, but it appears that candiduria deserves extra attention as a risk factor for candidemia.[88] Other investigators have also linked the relevance of multisite colonization to other significant risk factors.[89] Therefore, the decision to start presumptive therapy should be based on a broad clinical evaluation instead of multisite *Candida* colonization alone.

Impact of Invasive Candidiasis

The impact of invasive candidiasis on patient outcome has only been established in patients with candidemia. In general, the crude mortality is over 50% and has remained at this level in recent years. The attributable mortality, defined as the proportion of deaths directly related to candidemia, can be determined by a simple comparison of the mortality rates between candidemic and noncandidemic patients in a cohort of consecutive patients. One must be cautious in interpreting these data which are calculated as such, since it is possible to overestimate attributable mortality. Matched cohort studies with strict adjustment for confounding factors are more appropriate. The attributable mortality derived from matched cohort studies range from dramatic proportion (>30%)[50,74] to nonsignificant fractions (5%).[90] High rates of early initiated empiric appropriate antifungal therapy may contribute to better survival.[88,91,92]

Candida peritonitis in critically ill surgical patients carries a very poor prognosis but studies addressing the attributable mortality are lacking. Mortality rates between 52 and 75% have been described.[63,79,93] In a series of 271 patients with peritonitis, Dupont et al.[94] investigated outcome and risk factors for mortality in patients with *Candida* peritonitis. Mortality in patients without *Candida* involvement was 41%, while in the 83 patients with *Candida* peritonitis, ICU mortality was 52%. In a multicenter matched cohort study, Montravers et al. compared 91 patients with *Candida* isolated from the peritoneal cavity with 168 matched control subjects.[63]

Patients eligible for study inclusion were those operated for peritonitis with focus on complex problems, such as perforation, bowel necrosis, and anastomotic leakages.

In nosocomial peritonitis, mortality was significantly higher among patients with *Candida* peritonitis (48% vs. 28%; $p < 0.05$). Additionally, *Candida* peritonitis was identified as an independent predictor of mortality, after adjustment for major confounders, such as source of peritonitis and inappropriate empiric antimicrobial therapy, but not for failure of source control, which is well known as a major factor contributing to unfavorable outcomes.[95]

INVASIVE PULMONARY ASPERGILLUS INFECTIONS

Clinical Spectrum and Definitions

The term 'aspergillosis' refers to several categories of infection: life-threatening acute invasive aspergillosis, chronic necrotizing aspergillosis, aspergilloma or fungus ball, and allergic bronchopulmonary aspergillosis. The lung is the most frequent site of disease. The clinical manifestation and severity of *Aspergillus* disease depend upon the immunologic state of the patient.[96] The 3 principal entities are allergic bronchopulmonary aspergillosis, pulmonary aspergilloma, and invasive aspergillosis.

Depending on the immune status of the patient, it can be speculated that a spectrum of invasive pulmonary aspergillosis exists, from the well-known acute invasive form characteristic for severely immune debilitated patients, over subacute invasive aspergillosis—still with fungal tissue invasion—to chronic cavitary and fibrosing pulmonary and pleural aspergillosis and simple aspergilloma; the latter disease entities with histologic evidence of hyphae in cavities but not in tissues and a chronic inflammation with fibrosis in the tissue surrounding the cavity.[18]

Incidence of Invasive Pulmonary Aspergillosis

Invasive pulmonary aspergillosis mainly affects severely immunocompromized patients, but evidence is emerging that this disease entity is encountered and possibly emerging in other categories of patients without apparent immunodeficiency.[97-102] An important study addressing epidemiology of invasive aspergillosis in an ICU was published by Meersseman et al.[23] The EORTC/MSG diagnostic criteria were applied in this retrospective study. One hundred twenty seven patients out of 1,850 admissions (6.9%), hospitalized between 2000 and 2003 had microbiological or histopathological evidence of *Aspergillus* during their ICU stay. There were 89 cases (70%) without hematological malignancy. These patients were classified as proven invasive aspergillosis (n = 30), probable invasive aspergillosis (n = 37), possible invasive aspergillosis (n = 2), or colonization (n = 20). In these patients, mean Simplified Acute Physiology Score II (SAPS II) was 52 with a predicted mortality of 48%. The observed mortality was 80% (n = 71). Mortality of the proven and the probable invasive aspergillosis was 97% and 87%, respectively. Postmortem examination was done in 46 out of 71 patients, and 27 autopsies (59%) showed hyphal invasion with *Aspergillus*. *Aspergillus* infections occurred in 5 critically ill patients with proven invasive aspergillosis who did not have any predisposing factors according to the currently available definitions.

In an autopsy study of ICU patients, an incidence of invasive aspergillosis of 2.7% of the patients undergoing postmortem examination was found, and COPD was the underlying disease in most of the cases.[103]

The epidemiology of invasive aspergillosis is changing. Invasive disease is increasingly observed in the non-neutropenic phase of hematopoietic stem cell transplantation, and in nonclassic settings, such as critically ill patients in ICUs.[104] These studies imply that invasive disease caused by *Aspergillus* species should be considered in critically ill patients, even in the absence of classic risk factors such as prolonged neutropenia, hematological malignancy, and bone marrow or stem cell transplantation.

Aspergillus Species

The genus comprises about 180 species, of which 33 have been associated with disease in humans. Most infections are caused by *Aspergillus fumigatus, A. flavus, A. terreus,* and *A. niger*, and less commonly, *A. nidulans* can be implicated as a causative pathogen, especially in the setting of chronic, granulomatous disease.[105] Some species, such as *A. terreus*, may exhibit inherent resistance to available antifungal drugs. This species is often resistant to amphotericin B, but still susceptible to the echinocandins and the new-generation triazoles.[106,107]

Pathophysiology of Pulmonary *Aspergillus* Infection

The development of aspergillosis requires the exposure of a susceptible host to a relevant inoculum. The incubation period between exposure and development of the disease is unclear. Invasive aspergillosis most commonly involves the sinopulmonary tract, reflecting inhalation as the principal port of entry. While it is generally accepted that neutrophils and pulmonary macrophages represent the first 2 lines of (innate) host defense against invasive aspergillosis, the recognition of T-cell-mediated immunity is increasing. Specifically pulmonary alveolar macrophages ingest and kill inhaled conidia, while polymorphonuclear neutrophil leucocytes are fungicidal to the hyphal form of *Aspergillus* species. It is likely that neutrophils actively participate in the generation of a subsequent adaptive T-helper cell response, with production of a series of cytokines influencing the inflammatory response and phagocytic activity. In the absence of an adequate neutrophil count and if macrophage function is disturbed, 'escaped' conidia will germinate and form hyphae with the capacity to invade tissue.

There is evidence that acquired dysfunction of neutrophils, monocytes, or macrophages is an important cause of infection in patients with diabetes mellitus, renal or hepatic failure, alcoholism, auto-immune diseases, influenza or HIV infection, burns, and trauma. Distinguishable mechanisms of acquired phagocyte dysfunction include inhibitory effects of metabolic disturbances (e.g., hyperglycemia, uremia), chemical toxins (e.g., ethanol), viral proteins on phagocyte activation, and pathologic activation of phagocytes in the circulation (e.g., after hemodialysis, burns, or cardio-pulmonary bypass). Tissue invasion by *Aspergillus* hyphae may be promoted by temporary dysfunction of phagocytic cells.

In animal models, the protective role of lung surfactant proteins (SP)-A and SP-D and mannose-binding lectin (MBL) in the host defense against invasive aspergillosis was identified. Therapeutic administration of SP-D and MBL proteins in a murine model of pulmonary invasive aspergillosis rescued mice from death. The results suggested that individuals with any structural or functional defects in these innate immune molecules due to genetic variations, or acquired by severe lung disease, might be susceptible to invasive aspergillosis.

Risk Factors for Invasive Pulmonary Aspergillosis

For many years, it has been known that several types of immunosuppression predispose to invasive aspergillosis. Numerically, the most numerous patients are those with prolonged neutropenia and transplant recipients. In addition to neutropenia, corticosteroid treatment is a clear risk factor. Advanced HIV infection, even in the absence of neutropenia or corticosteroid use, may also be predisposing to invasive disease. Patients with chronic granulomatous disease are also at risk for invasive aspergillosis.

As immunosuppressive protocols change and new immunosuppressive agents are made available for patients with autoimmune diseases, it is expected that the traditional risk factors for invasive aspergillosis may also change. Examples of new therapeutic advances are the use of T-cell ablative agents, such as alemtuzumab in solid organ transplantation, and the use of immunomodulatory agents, such as etanercept in rheumatoid arthritis.

In a multicenter hospital-based survey, most *Aspergillus* species culture isolates from nonsterile body sites did not represent disease.[108] However, for high-risk patients, a positive culture result was associated with invasive disease, such as in allogeneic bone marrow transplant recipients (60%), persons with hematologic cancer (50%), and those with signs of neutropenia (60%) or malnutrition (30%). Diagnosis of invasive aspergillosis on the basis of an *Aspergillus* species positive culture of a specimen obtained from a nonsterile body site remained most difficult in the group of patients with an intermediate risk for invasive aspergillosis (10–30%): HIV infection (20%), solid-organ transplantation (20%), corticosteroid use (20%), or an underlying pulmonary disease (10%). It was concluded that in this intermediate risk group with specimens from nonsterile body sites, the clinician must aggressively determine by means of histopathological tests, radiology, and/or serologic tests, the relevance of an *Aspergillus* isolate with regard to disease.

Diagnostic Tools

An accurate diagnosis of invasive aspergillosis is important for several clinical reasons. Early diagnosis is associated with improved patient survival.[22] Deep tissue diagnostic specimens are often difficult to obtain from severely ill patients. Tests with a high negative predictive value may allow expensive and potentially toxic antifungal treatments to be withheld.

Timely diagnosis of invasive aspergillosis, in early stage, remains difficult in immunocompromized patients. In patients with critical illness, the diagnostic process is very difficult, because the symptoms and signs are atypical and the initiation of additional diagnostic examinations is often delayed due to a low index of suspicion—the diagnosis of invasive aspergillosis in apparently immunocompetent patients is often discarded or considered as not plausible.

Although a positive *Aspergillus* species culture in a respiratory tract specimen is neither sensitive, nor specific, it is often the first clue for the diagnosis in critically ill patients.[24,27] Excluding the possibility of contamination during preanalytical phase of a sample, isolation of *Aspergillus* species in the respiratory tract may represent one of the three scenarios:

- Evidence of current disease
- True colonization
- A marker for the future development of disease.

Direct Diagnostic Techniques

In clinical scenarios of high suspicion of opportunistic fungal infections, direct microscopic examination of respiratory samples is of paramount importance. These samples may be obtained either by simple endotracheal aspiration or BAL.[109] Microscopy is an important investigation for several reasons. First, diagnostic yield may be more than for culture alone in infections. The second reason is the rapid turnaround tie of microscopy: results should be available within hours after sampling. Combining microscopy and culture may optimize the diagnostic yield by 15% or more over that of culture alone.[110,111] The use of special stains may increase the sensitivity of microscopy. Within tissue secretions, *Aspergillus* typically appears as slender septate hyphae that exhibit angular dichotomous branching. Demonstration of septate hyphae by direct microscopy is, however, not an unequivocal diagnostic confirmation, because other fungi may have similar appearances.

Culture

A culture yielding *Aspergillus* species in addition to enabling a diagnosis of invasive aspergillosis, may further define therapeutic options via susceptibility testing or the isolation of a species possessing inherent antifungal resistance. The main disadvantage of culture is that it is relatively slow, as the process may take days, is relatively insensitive, and requires specialized expertise for species determination. A positive culture of a tissue sample or sample of a normally sterile site obtained by aseptic technique, establishes the diagnosis of proven invasive diagnosis.

In the absence of such samples, samples obtained from contiguous nonsterile sites, such as the upper or lower respiratory tract, can serve as a surrogate to establish a "putative" diagnosis of invasive pulmonary aspergillosis.[29] It can be assumed that viable hyphal elements are shed into the respiratory tract from infected parenchyma. However, this shedding may appear late in the natural course of the disease, and hence, this can indicate an advanced stage of the disease, less amendable to antifungal treatment. In immunocompromized patients, the overall sensitivity of BAL (combining culture and microscopy), is generally estimated about 50%.[105] The value of this diagnostic technique in nonimmunocompromized patients is a matter of debate and requires further research. However, in the presence of a compatible clinical condition and a radiological picture compatible with pneumonia, the combination of a positive culture and demonstration of septate hyphae in BAL, seems to have a discriminating value. The clinical course in patients fulfilling these criteria is significantly more severe than in other patients with a positive culture, considered colonized.[24]

Serological Techniques

Galactomannan

Galactomannan is a heat-stable hetero-polysaccharide present in the cell wall of most *Aspergillus* and *Penicillium* species[105] The Platelia enzyme-linked immunosorbent assay (ELISA) is available in Europe for more than 15 years and is licensed by the US Food and Drug Administration (FDA). Galactomannan antigen detection either on serum or BAL fluid is now incorporated in the diagnostic criteria for immunocompromized patients.[20]

In terms of analytical specificity on serum, cross reactivity with other filamentous fungi, bacteria, drugs, and cotton swabs have been documented. There have been considerable efforts in establishing the appropriate galactomannan ELISA cut-off to maximize clinical sensitivity of galactomannan ELISA is somewhat variable with a range from 29 to 100%. There are a number of potential reasons for this disparate result. The performance of the assay may differ according to the host group and, therefore, the underlying pathological process. In studies conducted in severely immunocompromized patients, sensitivity has been generally reported in excess of 90%, while in other settings, e.g., chronic granulomatous disease and solid organ transplantation, sensitivity appears to be lower. In a study in critical care patients without proven malignancy, diagnosed with proven or probable aspergillosis, the galactomannan test was twice as positive as in 53% of cases.[23]

An important issue is that galactomannan antigen detection on serum is of little value in non-neutropenic patients as circulating neutrophils are capable of clearing the antigen. Meersseman et al. evaluated the significance of galactomannan detection in BAL fluid in 72 pathology-controlled non-neutropenic ICU patients with an overt risk profile for aspergillosis, as evidenced by thoracic CT scan, underlying and acute conditions.[112] Using a cut-off index of 0.5, the sensitivity and specificity of galactomannan detection in BAL fluid was 88% and 87%, respectively. Therefore, galactomannan antigen detection in the ICU should primarily be advocated on BAL fluid samples instead of on serum.

(1, 3)-β-D-glucan

There has been an emergence of clinical data pertaining to the diagnostic utility of the cell wall component, (1-3)-β-D-glucan in serum.[105] It is present in the cell wall of most fungi; the notable exceptions are *Cryptococcus* species and the zygomycetes. The molecule is ubiquitous in the environment and has been used as a marker of fungal biomass. The presence of (1-3)-β-D-glucan in fungal species other than *Aspergillus* means that its role in establishing a specific diagnosis of invasive aspergillosis is not straightforward. False-positive results have been documented in hemodialysis, cardiopulmonary bypass, treatment with immunoglobulin (IG) preparations, and exposure to glucan containing gauze (e.g., following major surgery). As these factors are very common in ICU patients, it seems that the value of (1-3)-β-D-glucan detection is merely in its high negative predictive value.

Antibodies Directed Toward Aspergillus Species

The demonstration of specific antibody is required to establish the diagnosis of chronic pulmonary aspergillosis.[109] Traditionally, antibody detection has not been considered useful for the diagnosis of acute invasive aspergillosis, following an early study that failed to document antibody formation. Subsequently, antibody has been documented in about one-third of patients with invasive aspergillosis. Furthermore, antibody detection could be useful as a means of establishing a retrospective diagnosis of invasive aspergillosis in profoundly immunocompromized hosts who have undergone immunological reconstitution.

Metabolites

Aspergillus species produce a range of extracellular enzymes as well as primary (e.g., D-mannitol) and secondary metabolites (e.g., gliotoxin), all of which have at least the potential to serve as diagnostic markers for invasive aspergillosis. The detection of metabolites produced by *Aspergillus* species represents an under-researched area at this time in terms of their potential application as noninvasive diagnostic modalities.

Nucleic Acids

As far as the amplification of nucleic acids and diagnosis of invasive aspergillosis is concerned, polymerase chain reaction (PCR) technology has dominated. It can be applied to blood and BAL samples. Specific primers and conditions have been described in various series and will require standardization and validation in reference studies and in multicenter reproducibility assessment as diagnostic tools.

Medical Imaging

Chest CT is an important instrument for the diagnosis of invasive aspergillosis in neutropenic severely immunocompromized patients, even in the absence of evident lesion on a conventional chest X-ray. One or more nodules is the most common finding in early invasive aspergillosis in neutropenic patients and patients after hematological stem cell transplantation.[113] The 'halo sign', a haziness surrounding a nodule or infiltrate, is a characteristic chest CT feature of angio-invasive organisms and is highly suggestive of invasive aspergillosis in patients with prolonged neutropenia.[113] In one study, it was demonstrated that early chest CT in patients with neutropenic fever may lead to earlier diagnosis and initiation of therapy.[114] The same investigators demonstrated that the 'halo sign' was common early in the course of disease but decreased during the first week of treatment, as the frequency of the 'air crescent' sign increased. In spite of a positive clinical response, the volume of the lesions may even increase during the first weeks of therapy; increase in size of pulmonary lesions did not predict a negative response to therapy.[115]

Medical imaging of the thorax in the ICU patients is less pathognomonic due to many confounding factors, such as ventilator-associated pneumonia (VAP), atelectasis, and pleural fluid effusions in ventilated patients. Furthermore, it can be speculated that typical radiological lesions may be less apparent because of the difference in severity and nature of the immune derangements. Typical lesions for invasive aspergillosis, such as the 'halo sign' and the 'air crescent' sign, were only found in 5% in a series of ICU patients.[24] In another study, 'halo sign' was only present in a minority of patients with proven or probable disease, cavitating lesions, or atypical infiltrates with a broad differential diagnosis were present in most patients.[23] This is in agreement with the previous description of the low sensitivity (24%) of the halo and air crescent sign in patients without hematological malignancy as compared with neutropenic patients with hematological malignancy (82%).[116]

HEALTH-ECONOMIC IMPACT OF FUNGAL INFECTION

In a cost-of-illness case-control study, analyzing the average direct medical costs with treating a single episode of care for candidemia, it was shown that average length-of-stay was significantly longer for candidemia patients compared to control patients. A 3:1 matching procedure was done—age, gender, and DRG (diagnosis-related groups). The major cost driver was hospitalization, while use of other medical resources contributed for 11% of the total cost. During the duration of the study, amphotericin B was the drug of choice for treating candidemia.[117]

In a prospective, cohort, observational study, it was shown that patients colonized or infected with *Candida* species, it was demonstrated that *Candida* colonization and infection in critically ill patients is associated with an important economic impact in terms of cost, which increases due to longer stays not only in the ICU but also in the hospital after ICU discharge.[118] Prolonged stay was associated with severity of illness, *Candida* species colonization or infection, infection by other fungi, antifungal therapy, and toxicity associated with this therapy. Compared to noncolonized, noninfected patients, patients with *Candida* species colonization had an extended ICU stay of 6.2 days and an extended hospital stay of 8.6 days. The corresponding figures for *Candida* species infection were 12.7 for ICU stay and 15.5 days for hospital stay.

In the US in 1996, there were an estimated 10,190 aspergillosis-related hospitalizations, based upon an administrative data set of the Healthcare Cost and Utilisation Project; these resulted in 1970 deaths, 176,272 hospital days, and $633.1 million in costs. Although *Aspergillosis*-related hospitalizations accounted for a small percentage of hospitalizations in the US, patients hospitalized with the condition have lengthy hospital stays and high mortality rates.[119] These findings were confirmed in a retrospective analysis of hospital discharge records in Australia.[120] In a large-scale epidemiological study, Tong et al. evaluated the economic impact of aspergillosis in a general hospital population.[121] Aspergillosis was associated with a dramatic economic burden. Overall length of hospitalization was 7.9 vs. 17.7 days and the mean total hospital charge was approximately US $44,000 vs. US $97,000 in non-aspergillosis and aspergillosis patients, respectively. In a matched cohort study of exclusively ICU patients, cases with invasive aspergillosis experienced higher resource utilization in terms of necessity for renal replacement therapy, (43% vs. 21%), prolonged ICU stay (24 days vs. 12 days), and an extended period of ventilator dependency (21 days vs. 9 days).[25] These results are important because in particular extra days in the ICU while being on mechanical ventilation must be considered 'high-cost days'.

The above-mentioned studies examined only direct medical costs. Indirect costs, such as productivity loss by morbidity and mortality were not taken into account. The estimated costs of care may have changed in the last decade because of the use of more expensive antifungal treatments with improved safety and efficacy.

CONCLUSION

Due to a steadily growing population at risk, one might assume an increasing incidence of invasive fungal infections in ICUs. Yet, because of its difficult diagnosis the precise occurrence rate remains unknown. The incidence might differ between units according to the local case-mix. Due to the problematic diagnosis initiation of antifungal therapy is often delayed, thereby being responsible - at least in part - for the detrimental outcomes associated with these infections. Because of the availability of potent antifungal agents, any progress in the field is most likely to be expected from diagnostic tests, allowing a more rapid and unequivocal diagnosis.

REFERENCES

1. Blot S, Vandewoude K. Management of invasive candidiasis in critically ill patients. *Drugs.* 2004;64:2159-75.
2. Kullberg BJ, Oude Lashof AM. Epidemiology of opportunistic invasive mycoses. *Eur J Med Res.* 2002;7:183-91.
3. Beck-Sague C, Jarvis WR. Secular trends in the epidemiology of nosocomial fungal infections in the United States, 1980-1990. National Nosocomial Infections Surveillance System. *J Infect Dis.* 1993;167:1247-51.
4. McNeil MM, Nash SL, Hajjeh RA, Phelan MA, Conn LA, Plikaytis BD, et al. Trends in mortality due to invasive mycotic diseases in the United States, 1980-1997. *Clin Infect Dis.* 2001;33:641-7.
5. Banerjee SN, Emori TG, Culver DH, Gaynes RP, Jarvis WR, Horan T, et al. Secular trends in nosocomial primary bloodstream infections in the United States, 1980-1989. National Nosocomial Infections Surveillance System. *Am J Med.* 1991;91:86S-9S.
6. Kao AS, Brandt ME, Pruitt WR, Conn LA, Perkins BA, Stephens DS, et al. The epidemiology of candidemia in two United States cities: results of a population-based active surveillance. *Clin Infect Dis.* 1999;29:1164-70.
7. Hobson RP. The global epidemiology of invasive *Candida* infections—is the tide turning? *J Hosp Infect.* 2003;55:159-68.
8. Pfaller MA, Diekema DJ, Jones RN, Sader HS, Fluit AC, Hollis RJ, et al. International surveillance of bloodstream infections due to *Candida* species: frequency of occurrence and *in vitro* susceptibilities to fluconazole, ravuconazole, and voriconazole of isolates collected from 1997 through 1999 in the SENTRY antimicrobial surveillance program. *J Clin Microbiol.* 2001;39:3254-9.
9. Sandven P, Bevanger L, Digranes A, Gaustad P, Haukland HH, Steinbakk M. Constant low rate of fungemia in norway, 1991 to 1996. The Norwegian Yeast Study Group. *J Clin Microbiol.* 1998;36:3455-9.
10. Meersseman W, Van Wijngaerden E. Invasive aspergillosis in the ICU: an emerging disease. *Intens Care Med.* 2007; 33:1679-81.
11. Trof RJ, Beishuizen A, Debets-Ossenkopp YJ, Girbes AR, Groeneveld AB. Management of invasive pulmonary aspergillosis in non-neutropenic critically ill patients. *Intensive Care Med.* 2007;33:1694-703.
12. Ostrosky-Zeichner L, Alexander BD, Kett DH, Vazquez J, Pappas PG, Saeki F, et al. Multicenter clinical evaluation of the (1—>3) beta-D-glucan assay as an aid to diagnosis of fungal infections in humans. *Clin Infect Dis.* 2005;41:654-9.
13. Hope WW, Walsh TJ, Denning DW. Laboratory diagnosis of invasive aspergillosis. *Lancet Infect Dis.* 2005;5:609-22.
14. Groll AH, Shah PM, Mentzel C, Schneider M, Just-Nuebling G, Huebner K. Trends in the postmortem epidemiology of invasive fungal infections at a university hospital. *J Infect.* 1996;33:23-32.
15. Yamazaki T, Kume H, Murase S, Yamashita E, Arisawa M. Epidemiology of visceral mycoses: analysis of data in annual of the pathological autopsy cases in Japan. *J Clin Microbiol.* 1999;37:1732-8.
16. Koch S, Hohne FM, Tietz HJ. Incidence of systemic mycoses in autopsy material. *Mycoses.* 2004;47:40-6.
17. Vogeser M, Haas A, Aust D, Ruckdeschel G. Postmortem analysis of invasive aspergillosis in a tertiary care hospital. *Eur J Clin Microbiol Infect Dis.* 1997;16:1-6.
18. Denning DW, Riniotis K, Dobrashian R, Sambatakou H. Chronic cavitary and fibrosing pulmonary and pleural aspergillosis: case series, proposed nomenclature change, and review. *Clin Infect Dis.* 2003;37:S265-80.
19. Ascioglu S, Rex JH, de Pauw B, Bennett JE, Bille J, Crokaert F, et al. Defining opportunistic invasive fungal infections in immunocompromised patients with cancer and hematopoietic stem cell transplants: an international consensus. *Clin Infect Dis.* 2002;34:7-14.
20. De Pauw B, Walsh TJ, Donnelly JP, Stevens DA, Edwards JE, Calandra T, et al.; European Organization for Research and Treatment of Cancer/Invasive Fungal Infections Cooperative Group; National Institute of Allergy and Infectious Diseases Mycoses Study Group (EORTC/MSG) Consensus Group. Revised definitions of invasive fungal disease from the European Organization for Research and Treatment of Cancer/Invasive Fungal Infections Cooperative Group and the National Institute of Allergy and Infectious Diseases Mycoses Study Group (EORTC/MSG) Consensus Group. *Clin Infect Dis.* 2008;46:1813-21.
21. Maertens J, Theunissen K, Verbeken E, Lagrou K, Verhaegen J, Boogaerts M, et al. Prospective clinical evaluation of lower cut-offs for galactomannan detection in adult neutropenic cancer patients and haematological stem cell transplant recipients. *Br J Haematol.* 2004;126:852-60.
22. Nivoix Y, Velten M, Letscher-Bru V, Moghaddam A, Natarajan-Ame S, Fohrer C, et al. Factors associated with overall and attributable mortality in invasive aspergillosis. *Clin Infect Dis.* 2008;47:1176-84.
23. Meersseman W, Vandecasteele SJ, Wilmer A, Verbeken E, Peetermans WE, Van Wijngaerden E. Invasive aspergillosis in critically ill patients without malignancy. *Am J Respir Crit Care Med.* 2004;170:621-5.

24. Vandewoude KH, Blot SI, Depuydt P, Benoit D, Temmerman W, Colardyn F, et al. Clinical relevance of *Aspergillus* isolation from respiratory tract samples in critically ill patients. *Crit Care.* 2006;10:R31.
25. Vandewoude KH, Blot SI, Benoit D, Colardyn F, Vogelaers D. Invasive aspergillosis in critically ill patients: attributable mortality and excesses in length of ICU stay and ventilator dependence. *J Hosp Infect.* 2004;56:269-76.
26. von Eiff M, Roos N, Schulten R, Hesse M, Zuhlsdorf M, van de Loo J. Pulmonary aspergillosis: early diagnosis improves survival. *Respiration.* 1995;62:341-7.
27. Garnacho-Montero J, Amaya-Villar R, Ortiz-Leyba C, Leon C, Alvarez-Lerma F, Nolla-Salas J, et al. Isolation of *Aspergillus* species from the respiratory tract in critically ill patients: risk factors, clinical presentation and outcome. *Crit Care.* 2005;9:R191-9.
28. Vandewoude K, Blot S, Benoit D, Depuydt P, Vogelaers D, Colardyn F. Invasive aspergillosis in critically ill patients: analysis of risk factors for acquisition and mortality. *Acta Clin Belg.* 2004;59:251-7.
29. Blot SI, Taccone FS, Van den Abeele AM, Bulpa P, Meersseman W, Brusselaers N, et al.; AspICU Study Investigators. A Clinical Algorithm to Diagnose Invasive Pulmonary Aspergillosis in Critically Ill Patients. *Am J Respir Crit Care Med.* 2012;186:56-64.
30. Vincent JL, Anaissie E, Bruining H, Demajo W, el-Ebiary M, Haber J, et al. Epidemiology, diagnosis and treatment of systemic *Candida* infection in surgical patients under intensive care. *Intensive Care Med.* 1998;24:206-16.
31. Eggimann P, Garbino J, Pittet D. Epidemiology of *Candida* species infections in critically ill non-immunosuppressed patients. *Lancet Infect Dis.* 2003;3:685-702.
32. Edwards JE Jr, Bodey GP, Bowden RA, Buchner T, de Pauw BE, Filler SG, et al. International Conference for the Development of a Consensus on the Management and Prevention of Severe Candidal Infections. *Clin Infect Dis.* 1997;25:43-59.
33. Buchner T, Fegeler W, Bernhardt H, Brockmeyer N, Duswald KH, Herrmann M, et al. Treatment of severe *Candida* infections in high-risk patients in Germany: consensus formed by a panel of interdisciplinary investigators. *Eur J Clin Microbiol Infect Dis.* 2002;21:337-52.
34. Pappas PG, Rex JH, Sobel JD, Filler SG, Dismukes WE, Walsh TJ, et al. Guidelines for treatment of candidiasis. *Clin Infect Dis.* 2004;38:161-89.
35. Tortorano AM, Dho G, Prigitano A, Breda G, Grancini A, Emmi V, et al. Invasive fungal infections in the intensive care unit: a multicentre, prospective, observational study in Italy (2006-2008). *Mycoses.* 2012;55:73-9.
36. Pfaller MA, Messer SA, Moet GJ, Jones RN, Castanheira M. *Candida* bloodstream infections: comparison of species distribution and resistance to echinocandin and azole antifungal agents in Intensive Care Unit (ICU) and non-ICU settings in the SENTRY Antimicrobial Surveillance Program (2008-2009). *Int J Antimicrob Agents.* 2011;38:65-9.
37. Kett DH, Azoulay E, Echeverria PM, Vincent JL. *Candida* bloodstream infections in intensive care units: analysis of the extended prevalence of infection in intensive care unit study. *Crit Care Med.* 2011;39:665-70.
38. Holley A, Dulhunty J, Blot S, Lipman J, Lobo S, Dancer C, et al. Temporal trends, risk factors and outcomes in albicans and non-albicans candidaemia: an international epidemiological study in four multidisciplinary intensive care units. *Int J Antimicrob Agents.* 2009;33:554. e1-7.
39. Vincent JL, Bihari DJ, Suter PM, Bruining HA, White J, Nicolas-Chanoin MH, et al. The prevalence of nosocomial infection in intensive care units in Europe. Results of the European Prevalence of Infection in Intensive Care (EPIC) Study. EPIC International Advisory Committee. *JAMA.* 1995;274:639-44.
40. Vincent JL, Rello J, Marshall J, Silva E, Anzueto A, Martin CD, et al. International study of the prevalence and outcomes of infection in intensive care units. *JAMA.* 2009;302:2323-9.
41. Jarvis WR. Epidemiology of nosocomial fungal infections, with emphasis on *Candida* species. *Clin Infect Dis.* 1995; 20:1526-30.
42. Pfaller MA. Nosocomial candidiasis: emerging species, reservoirs, and modes of transmission. *Clin Infect Dis.* 1996;22:S89-94.
43. Fraser VJ, Jones M, Dunkel J, Storfer S, Medoff G, Dunagan WC. Candidemia in a tertiary care hospital: epidemiology, risk factors, and predictors of mortality. *Clin Infect Dis.* 1992;15:414-21.
44. Schaberg DR, Culver DH, Gaynes RP. Major trends in the microbial etiology of nosocomial infection. *Am J Med.* 1991;91:72S-5S.
45. Jarvis WR, Martone WJ. Predominant pathogens in hospital infections. *J Antimicrob Chemother.* 1992;29:19-24.
46. Richards MJ, Edwards JR, Culver DH, Gaynes RP. Nosocomial infections in medical intensive care units in the United States. National Nosocomial Infections Surveillance System. *Crit Care Med.* 1999;27:887-92.
47. Tortorano AM, Peman J, Bernhardt H, Klingspor L, Kibbler CC, Faure O, et al. Epidemiology of candidaemia in Europe: results of 28-month European Confederation of Medical Mycology (ECMM) hospital-based surveillance study. *Eur J Clin Microbiol Infect Dis.* 2004;23:317-22.
48. Garbino J, Kolarova L, Rohner P, Lew D, Pichna P, Pittet D. Secular trends of candidemia over 12 years in adult patients at a tertiary care hospital. Medicine (Baltimore). 2002;81:425-33.
49. Blumberg HM, Jarvis WR, Soucie JM, Edwards JE, Patterson JE, Pfaller MA, et al.; National Epidemiology of Mycoses Survey (NEMIS) Study Group. Risk factors for candidal bloodstream infections in surgical intensive care unit patients: the NEMIS prospective multicenter study. The National Epidemiology of Mycosis Survey. *Clin Infect Dis.* 2001;33:177-86.
50. Leleu G, Aegerter P, Guidet B. Systemic candidiasis in intensive care units: a multicenter, matched-cohort study. *J Crit Care.* 2002;17:168-75.
51. Kibbler CC, Seaton S, Barnes RA, Gransden WR, Holliman RE, Johnson EM, et al. Management and outcome of bloodstream infections due to *Candida* species in England and Wales. *J Hosp Infect.* 2003;54:18-24.
52. Voss A, le Noble JL, Verduyn Lunel FM, Foudraine NA, Meis JF. Candidemia in intensive care unit patients: risk factors for mortality. *Infection.* 1997;25:8-11.

53. Nolla-Salas J, Sitges-Serra A, Leon-Gil C, Martinez-Gonzalez J, Leon-Regidor MA, Ibanez-Lucia P, et al. Candidemia in non-neutropenic critically ill patients: analysis of prognostic factors and assessment of systemic antifungal therapy. Study Group of Fungal Infection in the ICU. *Intensive Care Med.* 1997;23:23-30.
54. Charles PE, Doise JM, Quenot JP, Aube H, Dalle F, Chavanet P, et al. Candidemia in critically ill patients: difference of outcome between medical and surgical patients. *Intensive Care Med.* 2003;29:2162-9.
55. Trick WE, Fridkin SK, Edwards JR, Hajjeh RA, Gaynes RP. Secular trend of hospital-acquired candidemia among intensive care unit patients in the United States during 1989-1999. *Clin Infect Dis.* 2002;35:627-30.
56. Nathens AB, Rotstein OD, Marshall JC. Tertiary peritonitis: clinical features of a complex nosocomial infection. *World J Surg.* 1998;22:158-63.
57. Rotstein OD, Pruett TL, Simmons RL. Microbiologic features and treatment of persistent peritonitis in patients in the intensive care unit. *Can J Surg.* 1986;29:247-50.
58. Sawyer RG, Rosenlof LK, Adams RB, May AK, Spengler MD, Pruett TL. Peritonitis into the 1990s: changing pathogens and changing strategies in the critically ill. *Am Surg.* 1992;58:82-7.
59. Sotto A, Lefrant JY, Fabbro-Peray P, Muller L, Tafuri J, Navarro F, et al. Evaluation of antimicrobial therapy management of 120 consecutive patients with secondary peritonitis. *J Antimicrob Chemother.* 2002;50:569-76.
60. Sandven P, Qvist H, Skovlund E, Giercksky KE. Significance of *Candida* recovered from intraoperative specimens in patients with intra-abdominal perforations. *Crit Care Med.* 2002;30:541-7.
61. Rex JH. *Candida* in the peritoneum: passenger or pathogen? *Crit Care Med.* 2006;34:902-3.
62. Peoples JB. *Candida* and perforated peptic ulcers. *Surgery.* 1986;100:758-64.
63. Montravers P, Dupont H, Gauzit R, Veber B, Auboyer C, Blin P, et al. *Candida* as a risk factor for mortality in peritonitis. *Crit Care Med.* 2006;34:646-52.
64. Blot S, De Waele JJ, Vogelaers D. Essentials for selecting antimicrobial therapy for intra-abdominal infections. *Drugs.* 2012;72:e17-32.
65. Wingard JR. Infections due to resistant *Candida* species in patients with cancer who are receiving chemotherapy. *Clin Infect Dis.* 1994;19:S49-53.
66. Wingard JR. Importance of *Candida* species other than C. albicans as pathogens in oncology patients. *Clin Infect Dis.* 1995;20:115-25.
67. Chow JK, Golan Y, Ruthazer R, Karchmer AW, Carmeli Y, Lichtenberg D, et al. Factors associated with candidemia caused by non-albicans *Candida* species versus *Candida albicans* in the intensive care unit. *Clin Infect Dis.* 2008; 46:1206-13.
68. Blot S, Janssens R, Claeys G, Hoste E, Buyle F, De Waele JJ, et al. Effect of fluconazole consumption on long-term trends in candidal ecology. *J Antimicrob Chemother.* 2006; 58:474-7.
69. Fournier P, Schwebel C, Maubon D, Vesin A, Lebeau B, Foroni L, et al. Antifungal use influences *Candida* species distribution and susceptibility in the intensive care unit. *J Antimicrob Chemother.* 2011;66:2880-6.
70. Rex JH, Walsh TJ, Sobel JD, Filler SG, Pappas PG, Dismukes WE, et al. Practice guidelines for the treatment of candidiasis. Infectious Diseases Society of America. *Clin Infect Dis.* 2000;30:662-78.
71. Blot S, Vandewoude K, Hoste E, Poelaert J, Colardyn F. Outcome in critically ill patients with candidal fungaemia: *Candida albicans* vs. *Candida glabrata. J Hosp Infect.* 2001; 47:308-13.
72. Pittet D, Monod M, Suter PM, Frenk E, Auckenthaler R. *Candida* colonization and subsequent infections in critically ill surgical patients. *Ann Surg.* 1994;220:751-8.
73. Petri MG, Konig J, Moecke HP, Gramm HJ, Barkow H, Kujath P, et al. Epidemiology of invasive mycosis in ICU patients: a prospective multicenter study in 435 non-neutropenic patients. Paul-Ehrlich Society for Chemotherapy, Divisions of Mycology and Pneumonia Research. *Intensive Care Med.* 1997;23:317-25.
74. Wey SB, Mori M, Pfaller MA, Woolson RF, Wenzel RP. Risk factors for hospital-acquired candidemia. A matched case-control study. *Arch Intern Med.* 1989;149:2349-53.
75. Eggimann P, Francioli P, Bille J, Schneider R, Wu MM, Chapuis G, et al. Fluconazole prophylaxis prevents intra-abdominal candidiasis in high-risk surgical patients. *Crit Care Med.* 1999;27:1066-72.
76. Borzotta AP, Beardsley K. *Candida* infections in critically ill trauma patients: a retrospective case-control study. *Arch Surg.* 1999;134:657-64.
77. Bross J, Talbot GH, Maislin G, Hurwitz S, Strom BL. Risk factors for nosocomial candidemia: a case-control study in adults without leukemia. *Am J Med.* 1989;87: 614-20.
78. MacDonald L, Baker C, Chenoweth C. Risk factors for candidemia in a children's hospital. *Clin Infect Dis.* 1998; 26:642-5.
79. Calandra T, Bille J, Schneider R, Mosimann F, Francioli P. Clinical significance of *Candida* isolated from peritoneum in surgical patients. *Lancet.* 1989;2:1437-40.
80. Donahue SP. Intraocular candidiasis in patients with candidemia. *Ophthalmology.* 1998;105:759-60.
81. Donahue SP, Greven CM, Zuravleff JJ, Eller AW, Nguyen MH, Peacock JE, Jr., et al. Intraocular candidiasis in patients with candidemia. Clinical implications derived from a prospective multicenter study. *Ophthalmology.* 1994;101:1302-9.
82. Donahue SP, Yu VL. Intraocular candidiasis in candidemic patients. *Eur J Clin Microbiol Infect Dis.* 1997;16:256-7.
83. Agvald-Ohman C, Klingspor L, Hjelmqvist H, Edlund C. Invasive candidiasis in long-term patients at a multidisciplinary intensive care unit: *Candida* colonization index, risk factors, treatment and outcome. *Scand J Infect Dis.* 2008;40:145-53.
84. Desai MH, Herndon DN, Abston S. *Candida* infection in massively burned patients. *J Trauma.* 1987;27:1186-8.
85. Jorda-Marcos R, Alvarez-Lerma F, Jurado M, Palomar M, Nolla-Salas J, Leon MA, et al. Risk factors for candidaemia in critically ill patients: a prospective surveillance study. *Mycoses.* 2007;50:302-10.
86. McKinnon PS, Goff DA, Kern JW, Devlin JW, Barletta JF, Sierawski SJ, et al. Temporal assessment of *Candida* risk

factors in the surgical intensive care unit. *Arch Surg.* 2001;136:1401-8.

87. Charles PE, Dalle F, Aube H, Doise JM, Quenot JP, Aho LS, et al. *Candida* species colonization significance in critically ill medical patients: a prospective study. *Intensive Care Med.* 2005;31:393-400.
88. Blot S, Dimopoulos G, Rello J, Vogelaers D. Is *Candida* really a threat in the ICU? *Curr Opin Crit Care.* 2008;14:600-4.
89. Leon C, Ruiz-Santana S, Saavedra P, Almirante B, Nolla-Salas J, Alvarez-Lerma F, et al. A bedside scoring system ("*Candida* score") for early antifungal treatment in nonneutropenic critically ill patients with *Candida* colonization. *Crit Care Med.* 2006;34:730-7.
90. Blot SI, Vandewoude KH, Hoste EA, Colardyn FA. Effects of nosocomial candidemia on outcomes of critically ill patients. *Am J Med.* 2002 ;113:480-5.
91. Labelle AJ, Micek ST, Roubinian N, Kollef MH. Treatment-related risk factors for hospital mortality in *Candida* bloodstream infections. *Crit Care Med.* 2008;36:2967-72.
92. Morrell M, Fraser VJ, Kollef MH. Delaying the empiric treatment of *Candida* bloodstream infection until positive blood culture results are obtained: a potential risk factor for hospital mortality. *Antimicrob Agents Chemother.* 2005; 49:3640-5.
93. Alden SM, Frank E, Flancbaum L. Abdominal candidiasis in surgical patients. *Am Surg.* 1989;55:45-9.
94. Dupont H, Paugam-Burtz C, Muller-Serieys C, Fierobe L, Chosidow D, Marmuse JP, et al. Predictive factors of mortality due to polymicrobial peritonitis with *Candida* isolation in peritoneal fluid in critically ill patients. *Arch Surg.* 2002;137:1341-6.
95. Blot S, Vandewoude K, De Waele J. *Candida* peritonitis. *Curr Opin Crit Care.* 2007;13:195-9.
96. Denning DW. *Aspergillus* species. In: Mandell GL, Bennett JE, Dolin R, editors. Principles and practice of infectious diseases.5th ed. New York: Churchill Livingstone; 2000. p. 2674-85.
97. Lewis M, Kallenbach J, Ruff P, Zaltzman M, Abramowitz J, Zwi S. Invasive pulmonary aspergillosis complicating influenza A pneumonia in a previously healthy patient. *Chest.* 1985;87:691-3.
98. Pittet D, Huguenin T, Dharan S, Sztajzel-Boissard J, Ducel G, Thorens JB, et al. Unusual cause of lethal pulmonary aspergillosis in patients with chronic obstructive pulmonary disease. *Am J Respir Crit Care Med.* 1996;154:541-4.
99. Bulpa PA, Dive AM, Garrino MG, Delos MA, Gonzalez MR, Evrard PA, et al. Chronic obstructive pulmonary disease patients with invasive pulmonary aspergillosis: benefits of intensive care? *Intensive Care Med.* 2001;27:59-67.
100. Rello J, Esandi ME, Mariscal D, Gallego M, Domingo C, Valles J. Invasive pulmonary aspergillosis in patients with chronic obstructive pulmonary disease: report of eight cases and review. *Clin Infect Dis.* 1998;26:1473-5.
101. Rolando N, Harvey F, Brahm J, Philpott-Howard J, Alexander G, Casewell M, et al. Fungal infection: a common, unrecognised complication of acute liver failure. *J Hepatol.* 1991;12:1-9.
102. Karam GH, Griffin FM, Jr. Invasive pulmonary aspergillosis in nonimmunocompromised, nonneutropenic hosts. *Rev Infect Dis.* 1986;8:357-63.
103. Dimopoulos G, Piagnerelli M, Berre J, Eddafali B, Salmon I, Vincent JL. Disseminated aspergillosis in intensive care unit patients: an autopsy study. *J Chemother.* 2003;15:71-5.
104. Vandewoude KH, Vogelaers D, Blot SI. Aspergillosis in the ICU-the new 21st century problem. *Medical Mycology.* 2006;44:S71-S6.
105. Hope WW, Walsh TJ, Denning DW. Laboratory diagnosis of invasive aspergillosis. *Lancet Infect Dis.* 2005;5:609-22.
106. Iwen PC, Rupp ME, Langnas AN, Reed EC, Hinrichs SH. Invasive pulmonary aspergillosis due to *Aspergillus terreus*: 12-year experience and review of the literature. *Clin Infect Dis.* 1998;26:1092-7.
107. Pfaller MA, Messer SA, Hollis RJ, Jones RN. Antifungal activities of posaconazole, ravuconazole, and voriconazole compared to those of itraconazole and amphotericin B against 239 clinical isolates of *Aspergillus* species and other filamentous fungi: report from SENTRY Antimicrobial Surveillance Program, 2000. *Antimicrob Agents Chemother.* 2002;46:1032-7.
108. Perfect JR, Cox GM, Lee JY, Kauffman CA, de Repentigny L, Chapman SW, et al. The impact of culture isolation of *Aspergillus* species: a hospital-based survey of aspergillosis. *Clin Infect Dis.* 200;33:1824-33.
109. Denning DW, Kibbler CC, Barnes RA. British Society for Medical Mycology proposed standards of care for patients with invasive fungal infections. *Lancet Infect Dis.* 2003;3:230-40.
110. Levy H, Horak DA, Tegtmeier BR, Yokota SB, Forman SJ. The value of bronchoalveolar lavage and bronchial washings in the diagnosis of invasive pulmonary aspergillosis. *Respir Med.* 1992;86:243-8.
111. Fischler DF, Hall GS, Gordon S, Stoler MH, Nunez C. *Aspergillus* in cytology specimens: a review of 45 specimens from 36 patients. *Diagn Cytopathol.* 1997;16:26-30.
112. Meersseman W, Lagrou K, Maertens J, Wilmer A, Hermans G, Vanderschueren S, et al. Galactomannan in bronchoalveolar lavage fluid: a tool for diagnosing aspergillosis in intensive care unit patients. *Am J Respir Crit Care Med.* 2008;177:27-34.
113. Kuhlman JE, Fishman EK, Siegelman SS. Invasive pulmonary aspergillosis in acute leukemia: characteristic findings on CT, the CT halo sign, and the role of CT in early diagnosis. *Radiology.* 1985;157:611-4.
114. Caillot D, Casasnovas O, Bernard A, Couaillier JF, Durand C, Cuisenier B, et al. Improved management of invasive pulmonary aspergillosis in neutropenic patients using early thoracic computed tomographic scan and surgery. *J Clin Oncol.* 1997;15:139-47.
115. Caillot D, Couaillier JF, Bernard A, Casasnovas O, Denning DW, Mannone L, et al. Increasing volume and changing characteristics of invasive pulmonary aspergillosis on sequential thoracic computed tomography scans in patients with neutropenia. *J Clin Oncol.* 2001;19:253-9.
116. Greene RE, Schlamm HT, Stark P, Oestmann JW, Troke P, Patterson TF, et al. Radiological findings in acute invasive pulmonry aspergillosis: utility and reliability of halo sign and air-crescent sign for diagnosis and treatment of invasive pulmonary aspergillosis in high-risk patients. *Clin Microbiol Infect.* 2003;9:O397.

117. Rentz AM, Halpern MT, Bowden R. The impact of candidemia on length of hospital stay, outcome, and overall cost of illness. *Clin Infect Dis*. 1998;27:781-8.
118. Olaechea PM, Palomar M, Leon-Gil C, Alvarez-Lerma F, Jorda R, Nolla-Salas J, et al. Economic impact of *Candida* colonization and *Candida* infection in the critically ill patient. *Eur J Clin Microbiol Infect Dis*. 2004;23:323-30.
119. Dasbach EJ, Davies GM, Teutsch SM. Burden of aspergillosis-related hospitalizations in the United States. *Clin Infect Dis*. 2000;31:1524-8.
120. Slavin M, Fastenau J, Sukarom I, Mavros P, Crowley S, Gerth WC. Burden of hospitalization of patients with *Candida* and *Aspergillus* infections in Australia. *Int J Infect Dis*. 2004;8:111-20.
121. Tong KB, Lau CJ, Murtagh K, Layton AJ, Seifeldin R. The economic impact of aspergillosis: analysis of hospital expenditures across patient subgroups. *Int J Infect Dis*. 2009;13:24-36.

CHAPTER 15

Adjunctive Therapies for Respiratory Infections

Evangelos J Giamarellos-Bourboulis

ABSTRACT

Severe pneumonia is an acute infection of the lower respiratory tract accompanied by at least one organ failure. Cases result from the over-whelming reaction of the host to a pathogen that is entering the lower airways. When severe pneumonia develops, immunoparalysis and pro-coagulant phenomena in the lung predominate. The need to attenuate these phenomena has led to several randomized and non-randomized clinical trials for the evaluation of agents that can modulate the host response to a lung pathogen. Corticosteroids, intravenous immunoglobulin-M, macrolides, and recombinant thrombomodulin have yielded the most promising results and an overview of clinical efficacy is presented here. However, existing clinical evidence is not robust and further clinical trials are required to be conducted to fully define their explicit role for every single patient.

INTRODUCTION

One of the major fights in the history of medicine has been against *Streptococcus pneumoniae*. *S. pneumoniae* is the main cause of community-acquired pneumonia (CAP), which is the sixth leading cause of death in the US and in all developed nations, and mortality ranges between 5 and 36%. The difficulty of the combat of physicians against CAP complicated by pneumococcal bacteremia was shown by Austrian and Gold in their seminal study published in 1964. The authors clearly demonstrated that the physical course of the first 7 days of the disease cannot be changed even with the early start of appropriate antimicrobials. This was a very important finding because it clearly showed for the first time that the outcome of the patients was dependent on the host-bacterial interactions.[1]

The road to death in severe CAP is driven through progression to multiple organ dysfunction syndrome (MODS). Analysis of characteristics of patients with severe CAP enrolled in the recombinant human activated PRotein C Worldwide Evaluation in Severe Sepsis (PROWESS) study showed that 72% of cases were suffering from MODS. The main organ failures in these patients were respiratory failure (87%), cardiovascular failure and shock (66%), acute renal dysfunction (35%), metabolic acidosis (29%), and acute coagulopathy (10%). The main microbial cause of severe CAP in these patients was *S. pneumoniae.*[2]

However, CAP is not the only lower respiratory tract infection that is accompanied by high mortality. Hospital-acquired pneumonia (HAP), although of lower prevalence in the general population than CAP, is a major cause of nosocomial sepsis and death. Ventilator-associated pneumonia (VAP) is the prototype of HAP, and it takes place as a result of mechanical intubation leading to disruption of the physical barriers of the airways. VAP is a sequelae of more than 30% of cases post-intubation and mechanical ventilation; mortality increases up to 70%.[3,4] The pathogens causing VAP are very different than those causing CAP: methicillin-resistant *Staphylococcus aureus* (MRSA) and resistant Gram-negative bacteria predominate.[3,4] The significance of the host-parasite interactions in VAP seem to be equally important, as they are in CAP. A recent study of our group in 213 patients disclosed the significance of single nucleotide polymorphisms (SNPs) at the promoter region of the tumor necrosis factor (TNF) gene as an independent factors for the development of VAP. More precisely, presence of A alleles in at least 1 of the positions -376, -308, and -238 of the TNF promoter was linked with earlier development of VAP after intubation, compared with patients who had only wild-type alleles.[5] It seems that a similar scenario is taking place for patients who suffered lung complications of the recent epidemic of 2009 H1N1 influenza. Obesity, chronic heart failure, allergic bronchial asthma, chronic obstructive pulmonary disease (COPD), and pregnancy were considered important predisposing factors for the development of viral pneumonia during that epidemic. However, it was shown that the frequency of the A allele at the -238 promoter region of TNF was greater than in controls and presence of A alleles at any of the 3 regions of the gene promoter was an independent risk factor for development of viral pneumonia among patients infected by the 2009 H1N1 virus.[6] The last two findings about the importance of SNPs of TNF to predispose to lung infection underscore the importance of the observation stated by Austrian and Gold in 1964, and therefore, other factors apart from administration of the appropriate antimicrobial therapy determine early progression to death after CAP.

The great mortality of CAP and VAP, which seems to be unaltered throughout the last few decades, despite the development of extended-spectrum antimicrobials created the need to better understand the pathogenesis, with special emphasis on how lower respiratory tract infections lead to activation of the immune response and subsequent deterioration of the host. A knowledge of these interactions may create the background for therapeutic intervention, a process known as immunomodulation.[7] The present chapter will try to present an overview of the complex bacterial-host interactions in sepsis with emphasis on the peculiarities of CAP and VAP, and thereafter the broadly-recognized aspects of immunomodulatory interventions will be discussed.

HOST-PATHOGEN INTERACTIONS AND SEVERE LOWER RESPIRATORY TRACT INFECTIONS

Host Immune Response

Sepsis is defined as the systemic inflammatory response syndrome (SIRS) that develops in the field of microbial infections. At the cellular level sepsis is initiated when well-conserved microbial structures, known as pathogen-associated molecular patterns (PAMPs), sensitize the receptors embedded, either on the cell membrane or inside the cell cytoplasm of cells, participating in the innate human defense. These receptors are known as pattern recognition receptors (PRRs). The most broadly recognized PAMPs are endotoxins [lipopolysaccharides (LPS)] of the outer cell membrane of Gram-negative bacteria, muramyl dipeptide (MDP) and lipoteichoic acid (LTA) of Gram-positive cocci, flagellum of Gram-negative bacteria, and CpG motifs of bacterial DNA (Table 1). Common PRRs are Toll-like receptors (TLRs) that are transmembrane receptors, nucleotide-oligomerization domain (NOD)-like receptors (NLRs) that are cytoplasmic receptors and triggering receptors expressed on myeloid cells (TREMs) that are transmembrane receptors. Binding of PAMPs to PRRs of circulating monocytes and tissue macrophages prime, through the sequential activation of a series of adaptor proteins, the activation of transcriptional factors, namely nuclear factor kappa B (NF-κB) and activation protein-1 (AP-1). The end result is the over-whelming production of proinflammatory and anti-inflammatory cytokines. Within the vast context of cytokines, TNF-α, interleukin (IL)-1β, IL-6, IL-8, and interferon-gamma (IFN-γ) are the best described proinflammatory cytokines, whereas IL-10, soluble IL-1 receptor antagonist (IL-1ra), and soluble TNF receptors are the best described anti-inflammatory cytokines. Proinflammatory cytokines try to orchestrate the chemotaxis of neutrophils at the infection site to contain invading microorganisms through increase of vascular permeability and cell migration. Anti-inflammatory cytokines tend to compensate for the excess inflammatory phenomena so that the host is protected. However, sepsis develops as a result of predominance of proinflammatory cytokines (Figure 1).[8]

This innate immune response of the host is in parallel to activating the adaptive immune response. A set of heterodimeric cytokines, namely IL-12/IL-23, are released by monocytes and dendritic cells and they prime the differentiation of Th0 lymphocytes into 4 subsets of functionally distinct cells: Th1 producing IL-2, TNF-α, and IFN-γ, which perpetuate the proinflammatory response; Th2 produces IL-4, IL-5, IL-6, and IL-10, which are anti-inflammatory; Th17 produces IL-17, which is a chemoattractant for neutrophils; and T-regulatory cells (Tregs) that are anti-inflammatory. This transition from the innate to the adaptive host response aims to better coordinate the containment of the infection.[9]

The simplistic description of the immunological phenomena leading to sepsis created the ambition that the development of agents blocking the proinflammatory mediators could substantially decrease sepsis mortality.

TABLE 1

The Most Common Agonists Participating in the Sepsis Process and Their Receptors on Cells of the Innate Host Defense

Agonists	Source	Receptors	Innate immune cell
Endotoxin (lipopolysaccharide)	Gram-negative bacteria	TLR4	Monocytes, macrophages
LOS	*Neisseria meningitidis*	TLR2/4	Monocytes, macrophages
Muramyl dipeptide	Gram-positive cocci	NLRP3	Macrophages
Lipoteichoic acid	Gram-positive cocci	TLR2	Monocytes, macrophages
Flagellin	Gram-negative bacteria	TLR5	Monocytes, macrophages
CpG DNA motifs	Bacteria	TLR9	Monocytes, macrophages
β-D-glucan	*Candida* spp.	Dectin-1	Monocytes, macrophages
ssRNA	Viruses	TLR3	Monocytes, macrophages
HMGB1	Non-histone nucleic human protein	TLR4	Monocytes, macrophages
HSP70	Cell constituent	TLR4	Monocytes, macrophages
Unknown	*Staphylococcus aureus*	TREM-1	Neutrophils
Unknown	*Aspergillus* spp.	TREM-1	Neutrophils
Monosodium urate	Nucleotide metabolite	NLRP3	Macrophages
Mitochondrial DNA	Human nucleic acid	TLR9	Macrophages
Oxygen radicals	Endogenous products	NLRP3	Macrophages

TLR, Toll-like receptor; NLRP, NOD-like receptor; TREM, triggering receptor expressed on myeloid cells; LPS, lipopolysaccharides; LOS, lipo-oligosaccharides; MDP, muramyl dipeptide; LTA, lipoteichoic acid; HMGB1, high mobility group box-1; HSP70, heat shock protein 70.

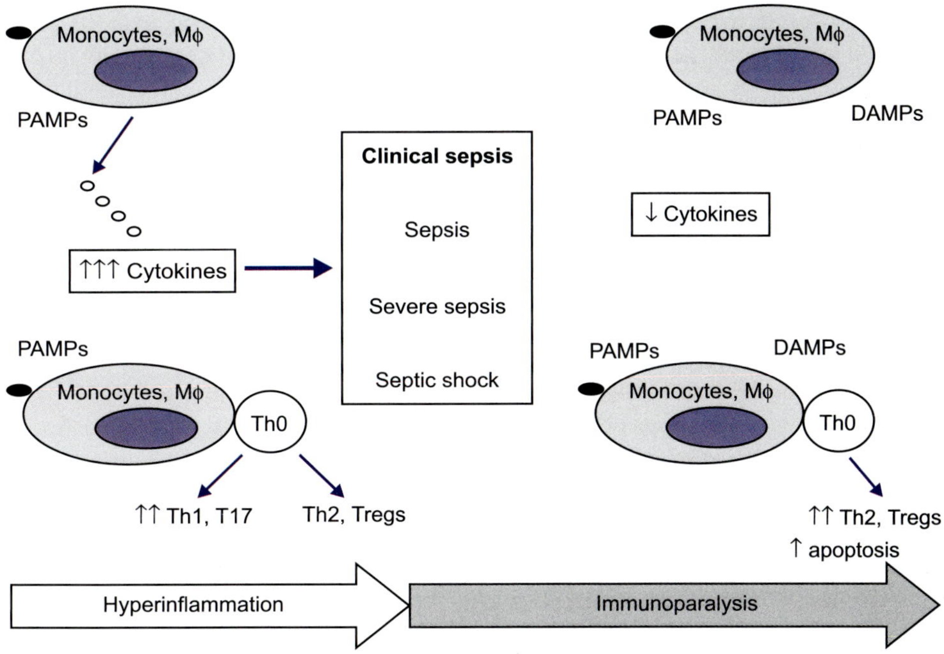

DAMPs, danger-associated molecular patterns; Th, T-helper cells; Tregs, regulatory T cells.

FIGURE 1 Current theory of the immunopathogenesis of sepsis. The complex interaction of pathogen-associated molecular patterns (PAMPs) of invading microorganisms on blood monocytes and tissue macrophages leads to the release of pro- and anti-inflammatory cytokines. Antigen-presentation of PAMPs drives differentiation of Th0 lymphocytes into 4 different functional subsets. Clinical sepsis develops as the results of overwhelming proinflammatory phenomena. At that stage, immunoparalysis predominates with anergy of mononuclear cells, predominance of anti-inflammatory cytokines and lymphocyte apoptosis.

A vast array of mediators, namely antibodies targeting LPS, anti-TNF antibodies, recombinant IL-1ra, and recombinant TNF receptors were tested in both phase II and phase III trials and failed to prolong survival.[10] Attempts to explain failure of these agents led to the understanding that although excess production of pro-inflammatory cytokines leads to sepsis, once clinical signs of severe sepsis develop, the host enters in a complete different immunological phase (Figure 1). This phase is called immunoparalysis and following changes occur during the process:

- Circulating monocytes fail to release cytokines after exposure to PAMPs
- Th2 and Tregs responses predominate over Th1 and Th17 responses
- Antigen presentation through dendritic cells to Th0 lymphocytes fails
- Lymphopenia arises due to generalized apoptosis.[11]

The phenomenon becomes more complex, as it has been recently recognized that endogenous molecules released after tissue destruction during the septic process may stimulate PRRs. These molecules are high mobility group box-1 (HMGB1) and heat-shock protein 70 (HSP70) that sensitize TLR-4; monosodium urate, oxygen radicals, and double-strand DNA that sensitizes NLRs; and mitochondrial DNA that sensitizes TLR-9. These endogenous sensitizers are called danger-associated molecular patterns (DAMPs) or alarmins, and they seem to represent independent sources of activation of the innate host defense.[12]

However, many of the above described elements are nothing but generalizations since it seems that the status of the innate and adaptive immune responses after worsening of the condition of the patient and development of severe sepsis/shock differ in relation with the underlying type of infection. A total of 505 patients were enrolled in a prospective study of 18 study sites, participating in the Hellenic Sepsis Study Group (HSSG). Flow cytometry of circulating mononuclear cells was performed within the first 24 hours from diagnosis. Analysis was focused on the differences between patients with uncomplicated sepsis and patients with severe sepsis/shock, taking into consideration the underlying type of infection. In CAP, a decrease in circulating levels of NK cells, CD4-, CD8-, and of B-lymphocytes were found; in HAP/VAP, the profile was different with apoptosis of NK cells and of NK T cells predominating.[13] Further insight into cytokine responses of patients with VAP showed that the final outcome was greatly dependent on the functional state of circulating monocytes. Monocytes of survivors were able to cause potent release of TNF-α and IL-6 after stimulation with LPS.[14]

Activation of the Coagulation Cascade

A distinct characteristic of the septic response developing in the field of CAP is the excess activation of the coagulation cascade. This takes place either through the direct effect of bacterial PAMPs on alveolar macrophages or through the indirect activation of the coagulation pathways by the cytokine storm. More precisely, tissue factor (TF) is exposed on the cell membranes of monocytes and of endothelial cells during lung infection. This process never occurs under normal conditions. Soluble circulating forms of TF are also found in sepsis. TF forms complexes with activated coagulation factors VII and X, and these TF-VIIa-Xa complexes in conjunction with factor Va stimulate the conversion of prothrombin into thrombin. Thrombin is a proteolytic enzyme, which lyses the amino terminal of protease activator receptors (PAR1, PAR2, PAR3, and PAR4) and renders them susceptible to stimulation by the TF-VIIa-Xa complexes. The PAR-TF-VIIa-Xa interactions prime further generation of proinflammatory cytokines in the lung, leading to the acute respiratory distress syndrome (ARDS). Normally, the action of TF is inhibited by tissue factor pathway inhibitor (TFPI), which is a proteoglycan expressed on the endothelium. It seems that TFPI production is down-regulated in sepsis, which contributes to excess coagulation and inflammation.[15]

These procoagulant phenomena in the lung can be counterbalanced by protein C. This is a zymogen and a natural anticoagulant inhibiting the function of factor Xa. Sensing of excess thrombin leads to the release of thrombomodulin by the endothelial cells. Thrombomodulin binds to thrombin and the thrombin-thrombomodulin complex activates protein C through proteolytic cleavage. Activated protein C also acts on the endothelial PC receptor (EPCR). EPCR is expressed not only on endothelial cells but also on alveolar macrophages. Binding of protein C on EPCR inhibits cytokine production so that activated protein C possesses considerable anti-inflammatory properties.[16] In sepsis, circulating levels of protein C are decreased and this phenomenon is more prominent in the bronchoalveolar lavage (BAL) of patients.[17] Moreover, damage of the endothelium by the excess production of cytokines leads to downregulation of the production of thrombomodulin, thus, priming procoagulant phenomena and enhanced proinflammatory responses.[18]

CLASSIFICATION OF ADJUNCTIVE THERAPIES

Available immunomodulatory therapies targeting the immune response of the host may be divided into the following main categories according to their mechanism of action:

- Modifiers of the immune response: this category comprises of macrolides, intravenously administered immunoglobulins (Ig), and statins
- Inhibitors of the proinflammatory response: this category involves mainly corticosteroids
- Anticoagulants: this category involves recombinant human activated protein C (rhaPC, namely drotrecogin-alpha), recombinant human TFPI (namely tifacogin), and recombinant thrombomodulin (ART-123).

Macrolides

Macrolides are antimicrobial agents with a central lactone ring structure. They possess antimicrobial activity against *S. pneumoniae, S. pyogenes,* viridans streptococci, and atypical pathogens, namely *Chlamydophila pneumoniae, Mycoplasma pneumoniae,* and *Legionella pneumophila.* Their pharmacokinetic profile indicates that they concentrate intracellularly, and makes them a good candidate for the management of infections by atypical intracellular pathogens. The most commonly prescribed drugs of this family are clarithromycin and azithromycin. In the azithromycin molecule, the ketone group at the C3 position of the lactone ring has been replaced by nitrogen allowing for azithromycin to easily accumulate intracellularly.

It was realized that macrolides could modulate the host response when survival of Japanese patients suffering from the fatal disorder, diffuse panbronchiolitis (DPB), was prolonged after addition of erythromycin in the daily treatment regimen. Since this rare disease resembles in pathophysiology with cystic fibrosis (CF), 4 randomized controlled trials (RCTs) were conducted in patients with CF. Results of all the trials indicated that long-term treatment of patients with azithromycin decreased the number of infectious exacerbations and improved lung function, as evidenced by increases of measured forced expiratory volume in the first second (FEV_1) and forced vital capacity (FVC).[19,20]

Two main explanations have been proposed for this non-antimicrobial activity of macrolides: modulation of cytokine production and inhibition of quorum sensing of *Pseudomonas aeruginosa* colonizing the airways. Both, *in vitro* studies and animal studies have shown that macrolides inhibit activation of the transcription factors NF-κB and AP-1, and inhibit production of proinflammatory cytokines by mononuclear cells. Their effect extends well beyond the direct inhibition of cytokine release. They inhibit formation of oxygen radicals and release of metalloproteinases by neutrophils, and they also decrease neutrophils migration. However, a common denominator of CF, DPB, and chronic bronchiectasis is heavy colonization of the airways by mucoid strains of *P. aeruginosa.* These strains communicate with each other and produce a biofilm, allowing firm adherence to the airways by a system of auto-inducer ramnolipid lactones, namely quorum sensing. Macrolides inhibit both the gene expression of *lasI* and *lasR,* respectively, which are involved in the biosynthesis of the 3-C12-homoserine lactone (HSL), and the gene expression of *rhlR* and *rhlI,* which are involved in the biosynthesis of butyryl-C4-HSL.[21] However, a recent trial in patients with CF noncolonized in the airways by *P. aeruginosa* disclosed similar clinical benefit from the chronic intake of azithromycin. This indicates that both mechanisms of action of macrolides are of equal importance in these patients, i.e., attenuation of the inflammatory cascade and inhibition of quorum sensing.[22]

The above described disorders, CF, DPB, and bronchiectasis are chronic inflammatory disorders of the airways. It is, thus, highly questionable whether a family of drugs modulating a chronic inflammatory state may also modulate an acute inflammatory state like CAP. There is extensive bulk of evidence that addition of a macrolide to the treatment regimen of CAP decreases mortality. However, most of the evidence comes from non-randomized studies with great heterogeneity. A summary of findings of these studies is shown in table 2.[23-28] The conclusion of all these studies is that addition of a macrolide to the treatment regimen decreases the mortality of CAP considerably. The most striking finding came from the prospective cohort by Restrepo et al. who studied patients with CAP developing severe sepsis. They showed that addition of a macrolide decreased the hazard ratio (HR) for death even for patients infected by macrolide-resistant *S. pneumoniae* (HR 0.1; $p = 0.005$).[26] However, none of the available studies is double-blind and randomized and designed in the appropriate way to decipher if addition of a macrolide to the treatment regimen may attenuate inflammation and modify the physical course of the disease without acting as an antimicrobial.

To this end, a recent meta-analysis was conducted in all available literature, comprising of 18 observational cohort studies. This meta-analysis included a total of 12,624 patients.[29] Macrolide use was associated with significant lower risk for death in CAP statistically when compared to nonmacrolide use (HR 0.78; $p = 0.010$).

The only way to fully prove the benefit from addition of a macrolide to the physical course of respiratory infections is to study their efficacy in a clinical setting where macrolides cannot act as antimicrobials. To this end, a

TABLE 2

Summary of Observational Studies Indicating the Significance of Treatment with Macrolides for the Outcome of CAP

State	Most common pathogen	Compared regimens	Outcomes
Pneumococcal bacteremia[23]	*S. pneumoniae*	β-lactam (n = 238) β-lactam + macrolide (n = 171)	OR_{death} with macrolides 0.40 (p = 0.03)
CAP[24]	*S. pneumoniae*	β-lactam (n = 270) β-lactam + macrolide (n = 918)	Mortality: β-lactams 13.3% vs. β-lactams + macrolides 6.9% (p = 0.001)
CAP and bacteremia[25]	*S. pneumoniae*	Macrolide combinations (n = 273) All other combinations (n = 1051)	OR_{death} with macrolides 0.61 (p = 0.007) OR_{death} with fluoroquinolones 0.82 (pNS)
Severe sepsis and CAP[26]	*S. pneumoniae*	Macrolide combinations (n = 104) All other combinations (n = 133)	Mortality: macrolide combinations 12.5% vs. 33.8% non-macrolide combinations (p < 0.0001)
Severe CAP[27]	*S. pneumoniae*	Macrolide combinations (n = 46) Fluoroquinolone combinations (n = 54)	Mortality: macrolide combinations 26.1% vs. 46.3% fluoroquinolone combinations HR_{death} 0.48 with macrolides (p = 0.04) HR_{death} 0.44 by severe sepsis with macrolides (p = 0.03)
Out-patients with CAP[28]	NR	Macrolides (n = 1832) Fluoroquinolones (n = 947)	Mortality: macrolides 0.2% vs. fluoroquinolones 3% (p < 0.001)

OR, odds ratio; HR, hazard ratio; NR, not reported; CAP, community-acquired pneumonia.

double-blind, placebo-controlled RCT was conducted in 200 patients suffering from VAP. A hundred patients were blindly assigned to placebo and another 100 patients to clarithromycin. Clarithromycin was administered as single intravenous infusions of 1 g in 1 hour daily for 3 consecutive days. Patients were treated with antimicrobials according to current guidelines. Isolated pathogens from the quantitative tracheobronchial secretions at a density greater than 10^5 cfu/mL were multidrug-resistant isolates of *Acinetobacter baumannii*, *Klebsiella pneumoniae*, and *P. aeruginosa*. Patients were followed-up for 28 days from study enrolment. Primary end-point was sepsis-related mortality. Analysis showed that clarithromycin decreased odds ratio (OR) for death by septic shock and MODS to 3.78 while OR being 19.00 in the placebo arm (p = 0.048). The secondary end-point of the study was the effect on VAP. VAP was resolved considerably earlier in clarithromycin-treated patients (median time to resolution, 10 days) compared with placebo-treated patients (median time to resolution, 15.5 days, p = 0.011 between groups). This was accompanied by a similar effect on the time until weaning from mechanical ventilation. The median time was 22.5 days in the placebo arm, and it was shortened to 16.0 days in the clarithromycin arm (p = 0.049) (Figures 2 and 3).[30]

In parallel with the clinical follow-up of the patients, intense laboratory work-out took place for the first 7 days after allocation to blind treatment in an attempt to decipher the mechanism of action of clarithromycin. Investigation involved:

- Measurements of the ratio of circulating IL-10/TNF-α as an index of the Th2/Th1 balance
- Flow cytometry on freshly isolated monocytes for apoptosis, for expression of TREM-1 and for expression of the costimulatory molecule CD86
- Cytokine stimulation of freshly isolated monocytes.

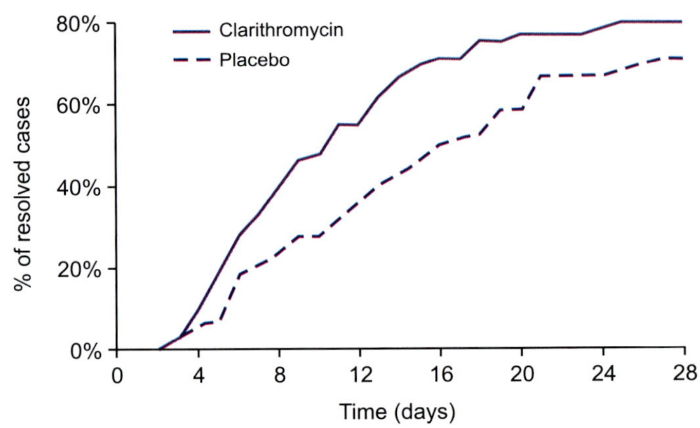

FIGURE 2 Cumulative resolution of ventilator-associated pneumonia (VAP) within 100 patients assigned to placebo and 100 patients treated with a 3-day regimen of clarithromycin. All patients were coadministered antimicrobial therapy according to current guidelines. P between groups: 0.011. *Adapted from* Giamarellos-Bourboulis EJ, Pechere JC, Routsi C, Plachouras D, Kollias S, Raftogiannis M, et al. Effect of clarithromycin in patients with sepsis and ventilator-associated pneumonia. *Clin Infect Dis.* 2008;46:1157-64.

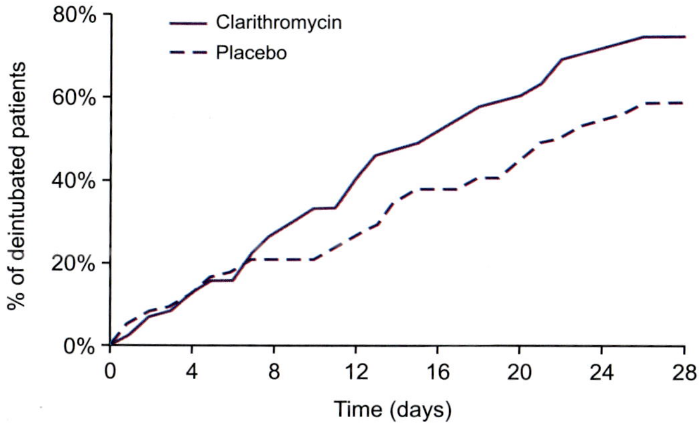

FIGURE 3 Cumulative time to weaning from mechanical ventilation within 100 patients assigned to placebo and 100 patients treated with a 3-day regimen of clarithromycin. All patients were coadministered antimicrobial therapy according to current guidelines. P between groups: 0.049. *Adapted from* Giamarellos-Bourboulis EJ, Pechere JC, Routsi C, Plachouras D, Kollias S, Raftogiannis M, et al. Effect of clarithromycin in patients with sepsis and ventilator-associated pneumonia. *Clin Infect Dis.* 2008;46:1157-64.

No differences were found between the 2 groups over the first 3 days after start of blind treatment. However, significant changes were described in all measured parameters two days after the end of the administration of clarithromycin. More precisely, the ratio of IL-10/TNF-α was decreased, the rate of apoptosis of monocytes was increased, the expression of TREM-1 and of CD86 on circulating monocytes was increased, and *ex vivo* release of TNF-α and of IL-6 from circulating monocytes was increased. These findings were striking among the subset of patients with septic shock and MODS whose risk for death was decreased by clarithromycin treatment. These findings provide a unique characteristic of clarithromycin, as its mechanism of action and benefits in sepsis are the reversal of immunoparalysis evidenced by the correction of the anti-inflammatory/proinflammatory dysregulation, improvement of antigen presentation, and restoration of function of circulating monocytes.[31]

Immunoglobulins

As already described, when the septic patient is developing organ failures, he is in a state of immunoparalysis. At that state, apoptosis of T- and B-lymphocytes predominate, and the patient is not able to produce adequate Ig titers.[32] This is consistent with defective opsonizing capacity of the invading bacteria and defective phagocytosis. To this end, it is thought that intravenous administration of Ig may help contain the infection and prolong survival. Several trials have been conducted in both pediatric and adult populations of patients with severe sepsis and septic shock. A meta-analysis of all 27 conducted RCTs clearly indicated that survival benefit could only be achieved after treatment with intravenous Ig supplemented with IgM. This was translated to 34% reduction of mortality in adults with severe sepsis and 50% reduction of mortality in children with severe sepsis.[33] However, no specific trial has been conducted in patients with CAP.

A novel approach is the development of IgM antibodies targeting specific structures of multidrug-resistant (MDR) bacteria. Panomacumab is a polyclonal IgM antibody targeting isolates of *P. aeruginosa* serotype O11. The drug was tested in one phase IIA open-label, single-arm study in 18 patients with documented acute lung infection by O11-*P. aeruginosa* (15 patients with VAP and 3 patients with HAP). Mean acute physiology and chronic health evaluation II (APACHE II) score of these patients was 17 and overall survival was 82%. The low mortality of patients, taking into consideration the APACHE II score renders this novel approach as a promising method.[34]

Statins

Statins are considered promising anti-inflammatory molecules. They act through inhibition of hydroxy-methylglutaryl-coenzyme A (HMG-CoA) reductase so as to reduce cardiovascular risk for death, and to be considered promising modulators of the immune response of the host. Retrospective meta-analysis of 7 observational cohorts of patients orally treated with statins disclosed borderline protection against the development of severe CAP. However, cohorts enrolled in these meta-analyses presented with great heterogeneity so as to render inconsistent results.[35,36]

Corticosteroids

Corticosteroids are well known anti-inflammatory agents. They attenuate proinflammatory phenomena through inhibition of NF-κB formation and of the subsequent cytokine production. Moreover, through an effect on cellular phospholipase A2, they block biosynthesis of both prostaglandins (PGs) and leukotrienes. However, there is a robust evidence that in patients with septic shock, the hypothalamus-pituitary-adrenal axis is dysregulated leading to relative adrenal insufficiency. The incidence of the phenomenon is high as seen in 60% of studied cases.[37] This relative adrenal insufficiency is defined as any serum cortisol below 10 μg/mL or as any failure of serum cortisol to increase by more than 9 μg/mL from the baseline after stimulation with 250 μg of cosyntropin [synthetic derivative of adrenocorticotropic hormone (ACTH)]. The importance of the phenomenon seems striking for patients with CAP. In CAP, severity is easily assessed by the CURB-65 score taking into consideration the presence of simple clinical signs like confusion, increased serum urea, respiratory rate more than 20 breaths/min, systolic blood pressure less than 90 mmHg, and age more than 65 years. However, an analysis of a multicentric cohort of 984 hospitalized patients with CAP showed that low plasma cortisol was an independent prognostic marker for CAP. Using a cut-off of 795 nmol/L, the investigators demonstrated that even within patients scoring 2 or more values of CURB-65, this cut-off could discriminate nonsurvivors from survivors.[38]

These observations inspired the therapeutic strategy to replace the needs of the patient at septic shock with low dose of hydrocortisone. In their original double-blind RCT, Annane et al.[39] randomized 300 patients with septic shock to the daily intravenous administration of 50 mg of hydrocortisone every 6 hours and 50 μg of fludrocortisone tablets once daily or matched placebo for 7 days. Striking differences were found within the subgroup of patients with relative adrenal insufficiency defined by a positive ACTH test. Stress corticosteroid replacement in these patients significantly reduced the risk for death (HR 0.67, $p = 0.020$) and reduced the time to withdrawal of vasopressors (median time 7 days vs. 10 days in the placebo arm).[39]

The efficacy of stress corticosteroid replacement was debated after the results of the Corticosteroid Therapy of Septic Shock (CORTICUS) study. In this study, 499 patients were blindly assigned to hydrocortisone 50 mg intravenous bolus every 6 hours for 4 days followed by tapering of the dosage and matched placebo. No difference in survival was found between the 2 arms of treatment; however, duration of septic shock was shorter in the hydrocortisone group compared to the placebo group.[40]

A smaller multicenter, double-blind RCT supported a beneficial role of hydrocortisone for the management of severe CAP. However, the treatment regimen was far different than the one used in the study by Annane et al.[39] and in the CORTICUS trial.[40] More precisely, 46 patients were randomized to receive either an intravenous 200 mg loading dose of hydrocortisone followed by a constant 10 mg/hour intravenous infusion for 7 days or matched placebo. At day 8 which was the end of therapy, considerably fewer patients treated with hydrocortisone were still on mechanical ventilation (26% vs. 65% of the placebo arm, $p = 0.008$). Similar findings were reported for the incidence of MODS (35% vs. 70% of the placebo arm, $p = 0.02$).[41]

Although hydrocortisone possesses some anti-inflammatory properties, its anti-inflammatory effect is much lower compared to other corticosteroids. Dexamathasone is the member of this drug family with the major glucocorticosteroid effect and, thus, the greatest anti-inflammatory potency. In a recent study of our group, whole blood was collected from 33 patients with sepsis within the first 24 hours of diagnosis. Whole blood was stimulated with LPS in the absence or presence of serial concentrations of dexamethasone. Results revealed a considerable effect of dexamethasone at added concentrations of 1 and 10 μM to decrease the production of TNF-α, IL-6, IL-8, and IL-10. These dexamethasone concentrations represent maximal achieved serum levels after intravenous administration.[42] In order to demonstrate the significance of these properties of dexamethasone in severe CAP, 304 patients participated in a double-blind RCT: 153 were allocated to placebo treatment and 151 to treatment with dexamethasone. Dexamethasone was administered as 1 bolus loading intravenous dose of 5 mg followed by once daily 5 mg intravenous dose for 3 days. Analysis revealed a significant effect of dexamethasone on the length of hospital stay: median hospital stay was 7.5 days within placebo-treated patients and 6.5 days within dexamethasone-treated patients ($p = 0.048$).[43] A post hoc analysis was conducted, trying to define serum biomarkers that can predict beneficial response to treatment with dexamethasone. Patients were divided into 4 categories:

- Patients with low serum cytokines and low cortisol
- Patients with low serum cytokines and high cortisol
- Patients with high serum cytokines and low cortisol, and
- Patients with high serum cytokines and high cortisol.

A plasma cortisol level below 10 μg/mL was considered "low" and a plasma cortisol level above 10 μg/mL was considered "high". A patient was classified with high serum cytokines as a combination of IL-6 above 92.5 pg/mL, IL-8 above 14.8 pg/mL and monocyte chemotactic protein-1 (MCP-1) above 1154.5 pg/mL. The third combination reflecting patients with high serum cytokines and low cortisol was the best predictor of survival benefit from dexamethasone treatment. More precisely, 42.7% of placebo-treated patients with this combination died as opposed to 0% of dexamethasone-treated patients within this category ($p = 0.020$).[44]

Anticoagulants

The procoagulant phenomena taking place in the lung parenchyma during the sepsis process led to the development of 2 natural human recombinant anticoagulants designing, thus, a novel therapeutic strategy in sepsis with 2 aims: counterbalance the procoagulant phenomena and attenuate hyperinflammation. The first drug of this class was rhaPC (drotrecogin alfa). It was also the first drug in the history of medicine to be approved with the indication of severe sepsis. PROWESS was a phase II, double-blind RCT study enrolling 1890 patients with severe sepsis. The study was prematurely terminated due to the benefit documented within the group of rhaPC-treated patients. Therapy with rhaPC was accompanied by a 19.5% reduction of the relative risk (RR) for death. Based on the results of the PROWESS study showing pronounced treatment benefit for the most severe patients, rhaPC was licensed for patients at severe sepsis with high risk for death. This was defined as APACHE II score more than 25 or as the presence of two or more organ failures.[45] Almost 40% of enrolled patients in the PROWESS study were suffering from severe CAP. Analysis of data coming from these patients showed a statistically significant reduction of the risk for death for patients receiving treatment with rhaPC (HR: 0.81).[2] The treatment arm of PROWESS study was repeated as a single-arm, open-label study using the same inclusion and exclusion criteria as the PROWESS study (ENHANCE US study). This study provided similar survival benefit.[46]

When a double-blind RCT was conducted in patients with APACHE II less than 25, no survival benefit was found.[47] The documented increase in the risk for bleeding in the rhaPC treatment arm led to reconsideration for the usage of rhaPC. A double-blind RCT was conducted in patients with septic shock (PROWESS-SHOCK study). The study failed to provide any treatment benefit. The manufacturer company Eli-Lilly has recently announced the withdrawal of drotrecogin-alfa from the market.

The second drug of this armory was recombinant human TFPI (tifacogin). The drug was administered in 1,754 patients in a large double-blind, phase III RCT of patients at severe sepsis. Almost 50% of the total enrolled population was suffering from CAP. Analysis showed survival benefit from tifacogin treatment only for patients who were not coadministered heparin (mortality 34.6% vs. 42.7% of placebo-treated patients, p = 0.050).[48] These findings prompted the conduct of one phase III RCT in 2,136 patients with severe CAP. The trial failed to show any survival benefit for patients with severe CAP.

ART-123 is already approved in Japan for patients with disseminated intravascular coagulation (DIC). The efficacy of ART123 was tested in a phase III double-blind RCT with sepsis and DIC. The study has been completed after enrolment of 715 patients, but results have not yet been published.

CONCLUSION

The great mortality of severe CAP is based on the complex pathogenesis ending in MODS and putting the life of the patient in danger. Early understanding of the need for adjunctive therapies to the traditional antimicrobials led to the development of drugs that modulated the immune response. However, the present analysis renders evident that most of the developed drugs have failed in terms of efficacy with special emphasis on drotrecogin-alfa and tifacogin (Table 3). The only drugs yielding consistent promising results for effective immunointervention are macrolides. However, even for this class of drugs only one double-blind RCT is available pointing towards improvement of the host upon addition of intravenous clarithromycin in the treatment regimen. It is obvious that there is a long way to go until a novel potent immunomodulator will enter the market for severe CAP. Until then, therapy with macrolides seems to be the most promising alternative.

TABLE 3

Synopsis of Immunomodulatory Therapies for the Management of Severe Community-acquired Pneumonia (CAP) and Existing Clinical Evidence

Drug class	Mechanism of action	Clinical evidence
Macrolides	Reversal of immunoparalysis	↓ Mortality shown in observational studies, 1 RCT: ↓ OR for death by septic shock and MODS; ↑ resolution of VAP
Immunoglobulins-enriched in IgM	↑ Opsonization	↓ Mortality shown in meta-analysis of RCT in sepsis; no data for CAP
Statins		Inconsistent data; no RCT available
Corticosteroids	↓ Adrenal insufficiency; ↓ inflammation	Hydrocortisone replacement reverses septic shock
Anticoagulants	↓ Excess coagulation; ↓ inflammation	Failed clinical development of tifacogin; drotrecogin-alfa was retracted by the manufacturer

IgM, immunoglobulin M; ↓ decrease; ↑ increase; RCT, randomized controlled trial; OR, odds ratio; VAP, ventilator-associated pneumonia.

REFERENCES

1. Austrian R, Gold J. Pneumococcal bacteremia with special references to bacteremic pneumococcal pneumonia. *Ann Intern Med.* 1964;60:759-76.
2. Laterre PF, Garber G, Levy H, Wunderink R, Kinasewitz GT, Sollet JP, et al. Severe community-acquired pneumonia as a cause of severe sepsis: data from the PROWESS study. *Crti Care Med.* 2005;33:952-61.
3. Hunter J, Annadurai S, Rothell M. Diagnosis, management and prevention of ventilator-associated pneumonia in the UK. *Eur J Anaesthesiol.* 2010;24:971-7.
4. Vincent JL. Ventilator-associated pneumonia. *J Hosp Infect.* 2004;57:272-80.
5. Kotsaki A, Raftogiannis M, Routsi C, Baziaka F, Kotanidou A, Antonopoulou A, et al. Genetic polymorphisms within tumour necrosis factor gene promoter region: a role for susceptibility to ventilator-associated pneumonia. *Cytokine.* 2012;59:358-63.
6. Antonopoulou A, Baziaka F, Tsaganos T, Raftogiannis M, Koutoukas P, Spyridaki A, et al. Role of tumor necrosis factor gene single nucleotide polymorphisms in the natural course of 2009 influenza A H1N1 virus infection. *IntJ Infect Dis.* 2012;16:e204-e8.
7. Wunderink RG. Adjunctive therapy in community-acquired pneumonia. *Semin Resp Crit Care Med.* 2009; 30:146-53.
8. Wang H, Ma S. The cytokine storm and factors determining the sequence and severity of organ dysfunction in multiple organ dysfunction syndrome. *Am J Emerg Med.* 2008;26: 711-5.
9. Lyakh L, Trinchieri G, Provezza L, Carra G, Gerosa F. Regulation of interleukin-12/interleukin-23 production and the T-helper 17 response in humans. *Immunol Rev.* 2008;226:112-31.
10. Vincent JL, Sun Q, Dubois MJ. Clinical trials of immunomodulatory therapies in severe sepsis and septic shock. *Clin Infect Dis.* 2003;34:1084-93.
11. Giamarellos-Bourboulis EJ, van de Veerdonk, Mouktaroudi M, Raftogiannis M, Antonopoulou A, Joosten LAB, et al. Inhibition of caspase-1 activation in Gram-negative sepsis and experimental endotoxemia. *Crit Care.* 2011;15:R27.
12. Martinon F, Mayor A, Tschopp J. The inflammasomes: guardians of the body. *Annu Rev Immunol.* 2009;27:229-65.
13. Gogos C, Kotsaki A, Pelekanou A, Giannikopoulos G, Vaki I, Maravitsa P, et al. Early alterations of the innate and adaptive immune statuses is sepsis according to the type of underlying infection. *Crit Care.* 2010;14:R96.
14. Pelekanou A, Tsangaris I, Kotsaki A, Karagianni V, Giamarellou H, Armaganidis A, et al. Decrease of CD4-lymphocytes and apoptosis of CD14-monocytes are characteristic alterations in sepsis caused by ventilator-associated pneumonia: results from an observational study. *Crit Care.* 2009;13:R172.
15. van der Poll T. Tissue factor as an initiator of coagulation and inflammation in the lung. *Crit Care.* 2008;12:S3.
16. Nieuwenhuizen L, de Groot PG, Grutters JC, Biesma DH. A review of pulmonary coagulopathy in acute lung injury, acute respiratory distress syndrome and pneumonia. *Eur J Haematol.* 2009; 82: 413-25.
17. Choi G, Hofstra JJH, Roelofs JJTH, Florquin S, Bresser P, Levi M, et al. Recombinant human activated protein C inhibits local and systemic activation without influencing inflammation during *Pseudomonas aeruginosa* pneumonia in rats. *Crti Care Med.* 2007;35:1362-8.
18. Fournier F. Recombinant human activated protein C in the treatment of severe sepsis: an evidence-based review. *Crit Care Med.* 2004;32:S524-41.
19. Giamarellos-Bourboulis EJ. Macrolides beyond the conventional antimicrobials: a class of potent immuno-modulators. *Int J Antimicrol Agents.* 2008;31:12-20.
20. Cai Y, Chai D, Wang R, Bai N, Liang BB, Liu Y. Effectiveness and safety of macrolides in cystic fibrosis patients: a meta-analysis and systematic review. *J Antimicrob Chemother.* 2011;66:968-78.
21. Corrales-Medina VF, Musher DM. Immunomodulatory agents in the treatment of community-acquired pneumonia: a systematic review. *J Infect.* 2011;63:187-99.
22. Saiman L, Anstead M, Mayer-Hamblett N, Lands LC, Kloster M, Hocevar-Trnka J, et al. Effect of azithromycin on pulmonary function in patients with cystic fibrosis uninfected with *Pseudomonas aeruginosa*: a randomized controlled trial. *JAMA.* 2010;303:1707-15.
23. Martínez JA, Horcajada JP, Almela M, Marco F, Soriano A, Garcia E, et al. Addition of a macrolide to a β-lactam-based empirical antibiotic regimen is associated with lower in-hospital mortality for patients with bacteremic pneumococcal pneumonia. *Clin Infect Dis.* 2003;36:389-95.
24. García Vázquez E, Mensa J, Martínez JA, Marcos MA, Puig J, Ortega M, et al. Lower mortality among patients with community-acquired pneumonia treated with a macrolide plus a beta-lactam agent versus a beta-lactam agent alone. *Eur J Clin Microbiol Infect Dis.* 2005;24:190-5.
25. Metersky ML, Ma A, Houck PM, Bratzler DW. Antibiotics for bacteremic pneumonia: improved outcomes with macrolides but not fluoroquinolones. *Chest.* 2007;131: 466-73.
26. Restrepo MI, Mortensen EM, Waterer GW, Wunderink RG, Coalson JJ, Anzueto A. Impact of macrolide therapy on mortality for patients with severe sepsis due to pneumonia. *Eur Resp J.* 2009;33:153-9.
27. Martin-Loeches I, Lisboa T, Rodriguez A, Patersen A, Putensen C, Annane D, et al. Combination antibiotic therapy with macrolides improves survival in intubated patients with community-acquired pneumonia. *Intensive Care Med.* 2010;36:612-20.
28. Asadi L, Eurich DT, Gamble JM, Minhas-Sandhu JK, Marrie TJ, et al. Guideline adherence and macrolides reduced mortality in outpatients with pneumonia. *Resp Med.* 2012;106:451-8.
29. Asadi L, Sligl WI, Eurich DT, Colmers IN, Tjosvold L, Marrie TJ, et al. Macrolide-based regimens and mortality in hospitalized patients with community-acquired pneumonia: a systemic review and meta-analysis. *Clin. Infect Dis.* 2012;55:371-80.
30. Giamarellos-Bourboulis EJ, Pechère JC, Routsi C, Plachouras D, Kollias S, Raftogiannis M, et al. Effect of clarithromycin in patients with sepsis and ventilator-associated pneumonia. *Clin Infect Dis.* 2008;46:1157-64.

31. Spyridaki A, Raftogiannis M, Antonopoulou A, Tsaganos T, Routsi C, Baziaka F, et al. The effect of clarithromycin in inflammatory markers of patients with ventilator-associated pneumonia and sepsis by Gram-negative bacteria: results from a randomized clinical study. *Antimicrob Agents Chemother.* 2012;56:3819-25.
32. Boomer JS, To K, Chang KC, Takasu O, Osborne DF, Walton AH, Bricker TL, et al. Immunosuppression in patients who die of sepsis and multiple organ failure. *JAMA.* 2011;306: 2594-605.
33. Kreymann KG, de Heer G, Nierhaus A, Kluge S. Use of polyclonal immunoglobulins as adjunctive therapy for sepsis or septic shock. *Crit Care Med.* 2007;35:2677-85.
34. Lu Q, Rouby JJ, Laterre PF, Eggimann P, Dugard A, Giamarellos-Bourboulis EJ, Mercier E, et al. Pharmacokinetics and safety of panobacumab: specific adjunctive immunotherapy in critical patients with nosocomial *Pseudomonas aeruginosa* O11 pneumonia. *J Antimicrob Chemother.* 2011;66:1110-6.
35. Viasus D, Carcia-Vidal C, Gudiol F, Carratalà J. Statins for community-acquired pneumonia: current state of the science. *Eur J Clin Microbiol Infect Dis.* 2010;29:143-52.
36. Kwok CS, Yeong JKY, Turner RM, Cavallazzi R, Singh S, Loke YK. Statins and associated risk of pneumonia a systematic review and meta-analysis of observational studies. *Eur J Clin Pharmacol.* 2012;68:747-55.
37. Annane D, Maxime V, Ibrahim F, Alvarez JC, Abe E, Boudou P. Diagnosis of adrenal insufficiency in severe sepsis and septic shock. *Am J Respir Crit Care Med.* 2006;174:1319-26.
38. Kolditz M, Hoffken G, Martus P, Rohde G, Schutte H, Bals R, et al. Serum cortisol predicts death and critical disease independently of CRB-65 score in community-acquired pneumonia: a prospective observational cohort study. *BMC Infect Dis.* 2012;12:90.
39. Annane D, Sébille V, Charpentier C, Bollaert PE, François B, Korach JM, et al. Effect of treatment with low doses of hydrocortisone and fludrocortisone on mortality in patients with septic shock. *JAMA.* 2002;288:862-71.
40. Sprung CL, Annane D, Keh D, Moreno R, Singer M, Freivogel K, et al. Hydrocortisone therapy for patients with septic shock. *New Engl J Med.* 2008;358:111-24.
41. Confaleroni M, Urbino R, Potena A, Piattella M, Parigi P, Puccio G, et al. Hydrocortisone infusion for severe community-acquired pneumonia. A preliminary randomized study. *Am J Resp Crit Care Med.* 2005;171:242-8.
42. Giamarellos-Bourboulis EJ, Dimopoulou I, Kotanidou A, Livaditi O, Pelekanou A, Tsagarakis S, et al. *Ex-vivo* effect of dexamethasone on cytokine production from whole blood of septic patients: correlation with disease severity. *Cytokine.* 2010;49:89-94.
43. Meijvis SCA, Hardeman H, Remmelts HHF, Heijlingenberg R, Rijkers GT, van Velzen-Blad H, et al. Dexamethasone and length of hospital stay in patients with community-acquired pneumonia: a randomized, double-blind, placebo-controlled trial. *Lancet.* 2011;377:3023-30.
44. Remmelts HHF, Meijvis SCA, Heijligenberg R, Rijkers GT, Oosterheert JJ, Bos WJW, et al. Biomarkers define the clinical response to dexamethasone in community-acquired pneumonia. *J Infect.* 2012;65:25-31.
45. Levi M. Activated protein C in sepsis: a critical review. *Curr Opin Hematol.* 2008;15:481-6.
46. Bernard GR, Margolis BD, Shanies HM, Ely EW, Wheeler AP, Levy H, et al. Extender evaluation of recombinant human activated protein C United States trial (ENHANCE US): a single-arm, phase 3B, multicenter study of drotrecogin alfa (activated) in severe sepsis. *Chest.* 2004;125:2206-16.
47. Toussaint S, Gerlach H. Activated protein C for sepsis. *N Engl J Med.* 2009;361:2646-52.
48. Abraham E, Reinhart K, Opal S, Demeyer I, Doig C, López Rodriguez A, et al. Efficacy and safety of tifacogin (recombinant tissue factor pathway inhibitor) in severe sepsis. *JAMA.* 2003;290:238-47.

CHAPTER 16

Parapneumonic Pleural Effusions

Stavros Anevlavis, Demosthenes Bouros

ABSTRACT

Parapneumonic pleural effusion and pleural empyema can be the complications of pneumonia, bronchiectasis, and lung abscess. Pathophysiologically, they progress from exudate to fibrinopurulent and to empyema phase. There are a number of classifications, ranging from simple classifications (simple, complex, and empyema stage) to more sophisticated [the American College of Chest Physicians classification] and to practical classification (Light et al. 1995 classification). All suspected parapneumonic pleural effusion should undergo thoracocentesis. Imaging by computed tomography and especially by ultrasonography, are useful to correct diagnosis, evaluation, and management. The kind of therapy depends on the classification of the parapneumonic pleural effusion. It cannot be overemphasized that there is a need for rapid evaluation and intervention. Medical treatment embraces antibiotics, tube thoracostomy, and preferably, use of small bore image-guided catheters, fibrinolytics, and in case of failure, medical thoracoscopy or video-assisted thoracic surgery.

INTRODUCTION

Pneumonia, bronchiectasis, and lung abscess can be complicated by parapneumonic pleural effusion and pleural empyema.[1,2]

In the US, about 4 million cases of pneumonia occur annually; 20% of them are being hospitalized, 20% of the hospitalized ones will develop a pleural effusion, 20% will be complicated and will develop an empyema with 20% mortality rate of empyemas. About 1 million patients with pneumonia are hospitalized every year in US, and 20–57% of them develop parapneumonic pleural effusion[3,4] increasing the morbidity and mortality of these patients, despite the advent of potent antibiotics. Empyema is less common, occurring in 5–10% of patients who experience parapneumonic pleural effusion.[5] More frequently, it affects the elderly and debilitated patients with a male to female ratio of 1.8:1. In a review of over 1,300 patients, 70% of parapneumonic pleural effusion cases were due to pneumonia.[5]

Parapneumonic pleural effusion and pleural empyema are characterized by great heterogeneity and it is this heterogeneity that makes it difficult to diagnose and to treat them.[6] Parapneumonic pleural effusions can be small pleural effusions with no complications that can be treated only with antibiotic treatment of the associated pneumonia but sometimes, it can be complicated pleural effusions with many loculations and empyema which can lead to serious complications, such as fibrosis, lung entrapment, inability of the underlying lung to re-expand, and respiratory failure.[7]

DEFINITIONS

An uncomplicated parapneumonic pleural effusion is characterized by its small volume and the absence of loculations. Although there is an ongoing inflammatory process, usually no microbes are cultured. The antibiotic therapy of the underlying pneumonia is usually enough for the treatment of the effusion. A complicated

TABLE 1

Biochemical Characteristics of the Stages of Parapneumonic Pleural Effusions and Empyema

Parameter	Uncomplicated	Undetermined	Complicated
pH	>7.3	7.3–7.1	<7.1
Glucose (mg/dL)	>60	60–40	<40
Lactate dehydrogenase (IU/L)	>500	<1000	>1000

Source: Bouros D, editor. Parapneumonic Pleural Effusions and Empyema. New York: Marcel Dekker; 2010.

parapneumonic pleural effusion is usually the result of the invasion of the infection into the pleural cavity and for its treatment, not only antibiotic therapy is required, but usually, chest tube drainage and in some situations even a surgical intervention is mandatory. The presence of yellow, viscid fluid with putrid smell, full of leukocytes signifies the formation of empyema. An empyema is the collection of pus in the pleural cavity. The pus contains fibrin, destroyed cellular constituents, and microbes either dead or alive. The chemical parameters of the pleural fluid such as the pH are not used in order to define an empyema.[5]

The formation of adhesions composed of fibrin results in the development of a loculated parapneumonic pleural effusion. These adhesions prevent pleural fluid to move freely inside the pleural cavity. When a loculated parapneumonic pleural effusion forms more than one loculus, then it is called multiloculated parapneumonic pleural effusion.[7]

In table 1, the biochemical characteristics of a parapneumonic effusion are shown.

PATHOPHYSIOLOGY AND CLASSIFICATION

The development of a pleural empyema involves a continuous process that starts as an uncomplicated small effusion, without loculations and ends as a pleural empyema characterized by pus, many loculations, and thickened pleural membrane. During the initial hours of development of pneumonia, as a result of the presence of pulmonary pathogens, the pleura react by forming pleural fluid which has the chemical characteristics of an exudate with high levels of leukocytes and increased albumin. Initially, the glucose content of pleural fluid is normal (>60 mg/dL) while the pH is more than 7.30 and the lactic acid dehydrogenase (LDH) concentration and the leucocytes count are low.[7] The increase in the production of interstitial fluid in areas of pneumonia and the increase in the permeability of the pleural capillaries leads to the increase in the production of fluid into the pleura cavity.[8] In order to have a pleural effusion, the quantity of pleural fluid produced must exceed the reabsorption of the fluid by the lymphatics. The reabsorption of the pleural fluid is done through the stomata of the pleural lymphatics. The occlusion of these stomata by fibrin decreases the reabsorption of the pleural fluid.

Mesothelial cells play main role in the inflammatory process that takes place inside the pleural cavity. The mesothelial cells release chemokines and inflammatory cytokines such as interleukin (IL)-1, IL-6, IL-8, monocyte chemotactic protein (MCP)-1, and tumor necrosis factor (TNF)-α, when they are activated by the invasion of bacteria. They also play a role as phagocytes and recruit other inflammatory cells such as polymorphonuclears.[9-11] A chemotactic gradient from the vessels to the pleural cavity is responsible for the movement of the inflammatory cells into the pleural space.[11] When the microbes get into the pleural cavity, the glucose and the pH decrease, LDH in the pleural fluid increases, and it becomes thicker. If proper antibiotic treatment is not instituted in this phase, then the formation of loculi due to the accumulation of fibrin occurs which covers the visceral pleura. It is this fibrin coat that leads to the formation of a trapped lung when the pleural cavity is evacuated from the pleural fluid.

Various classification schemes have been described since 1962 regarding the ways to manage a parapneumonic pleural effusion/pleural empyema.

The first classification was described by Andrews et al. in 1962.[12] The development of a parapneumonic pleural effusion passes through 4 stages:

1. The dry "sicca" pleuritis stage
2. The exudative stage
3. The fibropurulent stage
4. The organization stage.

In the dry "sicca" pleuritis stage, there is a direct extension of the inflammation in the involved area of the pneumonia to the visceral pleura. As a consequence, a local pleuritic reaction is formed. In this stage, the clinician listens to a pleural rub during auscultation and the patient experiences a characteristic chest pain. Chest pain accompanying pneumonia is reported by many patients but the characteristic is that in many cases, there is no pleural fluid.[3,13] In these cases, there is no progression to the next stages of parapneumonic pleural effusion.

In the exudative stage, there is development of a parapneumonic pleural effusion which is small in size; it is exudative with increased neutrophil count but sterile. The ongoing inflammation results in an increase in the production of interstitial fluid and in the permeability of the pleural capillaries leading to an increase in the production of fluid into the pleura cavity.[14] In this stage, usually the pH of the fluid is more than 7.30, glucose levels are above 60 mg/dL, and LDH is more than 500 U/L.[5,7,13,15,16] Antibiotics alone, without the use of chest tube drainage of the pleural space, are enough for the successful treatment of patients in this stage of parapneumonic pleural effusion.

In the fibropurulent stage or bacterial invasion stage, the infection of the pleura occurs which leads to the formation of fibrin which is deposited on both pleural membranes. As a consequence, loculations are formed. As the pneumonia progresses, bacteria invade the pleural cavity. The amount of pleural fluid increases as the endothelial destruction continues. In this stage, there is accumulation of polymorphonuclear cells which are chemo-attracted by IL-8, while the pleural fluid glucose and pH decrease and LDH increases.[17] The ratio of pleural fluid to serum glucose decreases to less than 0.5 with absolute concentration of usually less than 40 mg/dL due to bacterial metabolism.[5,7] The LDH increases by more than 1000 U/L, due to destruction of polymorphonuclear cells. Fibrin and collagen are formed continuously covering both pleural membranes and leading to the formation of loculations making the drainage increasingly difficult. The pleural thickening makes the lung expansion difficult. The deposition of fibrin and collagen and the swelling of the mesothelial cells block the stomata of parietal pleura leading to increase in the volume of the pleural fluid. In this stage, antibiotic therapy alone may result in resolution of the pleural effusion, but usually drainage of the pleural cavity is required later on.[2,18]

In the organization stage or empyema stage, the fibroblasts enter into the pleural cavity and thickening of the pleural membranes occurs with the formation of adhesions leading to single or multiple loculations. The drainage of pleural fluid in this situation is very difficult and usually, the lung cannot be re-expanded. Pus is characterized by high viscosity and contains fibrin, collagen, destroyed cellular constituents, and microbes, either dead or alive. Antibiotic treatment alone is rarely effective in treating empyema. A chest tube drainage is always required in order to have resolution of the empyema. When the empyema drains through the thoracic wall, it is called empyema necessitates and when it drains into the lung it is called bronchopleural fistula. Factors that influence the evolution of an empyema are the type of microbes involved, the immune status of the patient, and the rapidity and effectiveness of the antibiotic treatment.

Many classification schemes have been published which focus on the clinical staging of parapneumonic pleural effusion and empyema.[3,18]

In 1995, Light[18] proposed a classification scheme with its main purpose being to guide the initiation of treatment of a parapneumonic pleural effusion (Table 2). It is a 7 class scheme which classifies the parapneumonic pleural effusion due to characteristics such as: amount

TABLE 2

Classification and Treatment Scheme for Parapneumonic Effusions and Empyema

Class 1 Nonsignificant parapneumonic effusion	• Small: <10 mm thick on decubitus X-ray • Treatment: No thoracentesis indicated
Class 2 Typical parapneumonic effusion	• >10 mm thick • Glucose >40 mg/dL, pH >7.20 • Gram stain and culture negative • Treatment: Antibiotics alone
Class 3 Borderline complicated parapneumonic effusion	• $7.00 < \text{pH} < 7.20$ and/or • Lactate dehydrogenase >1,000 and glucose >40 mg/dL • Gram stain and culture negative • Treatment: Antibiotics plus serial thoracentesis
Class 4 Simple complicated parapneumonic effusion	• pH <7.00 and/or glucose <40 mg/dL and/or • Gram stain or culture positive • Not loculated not frank pus • Treatment: Tube thoracostomy plus antibiotics
Class 5 Complex complicated parapneumonic effusion	• pH <7.00 and/or glucose <40 mg/dL and/or • Gram stain or culture positive • Multiloculated • Treatment: Tube thoracostomy plus thrombolytics (rarely require thoracoscopy or decortication)
Class 6 Simple empyema	• Frank pus present • Single locule or free flowing • Treatment: Tube thoracostomy ± decortication
Class 7 Complex empyema	• Frank pus present • Multiple locules • Tube thoracostomy + thrombolytics • Treatment: Often require thoracoscopy or decortication

Source: Light RW. A new classification of parapneumonic effusions and empyema. *Chest.* 1995;108:299-301.

of pleural fluid, positivity or negativity of Gram's stain and culture of the pleural fluid, pH, glucose, and LDH of the pleural fluid, and loculated or non-loculated parapneumonic pleural effusion. A patient with a parapneumonic pleural effusion is categorized as class 1 (non-significant parapneumonic effusion) if the thickness of the fluid on the decubitus chest radiograph is less than 1 cm. It is recommended not to perform a diagnostic thoracentesis because these effusions are too small to be sampled and almost always resolve after the initiation of the appropriate antimicrobial treatment.[3] A patient has a class 2 parapneumonic effusion if the thickness of the pleural fluid is more than 1 cm on the decubitus film and the pleural fluid glucose level is above 40 mg/dL, pH is above 7.20, LDH level is below 1000 IU/L, and the Gram's stain and culture are negative. Antibiotic therapy alone usually is enough as the therapy of a class 2 parapneumonic effusion. If during the follow-up of the patient, there is an increase in the size of the pleural effusion, then a second thoracentesis must be performed in order to again test the characteristics of the pleural effusion again. A patient has a borderline complicated parapneumonic effusion (class 3) if the pleural fluid pH is between 7.00 and 7.20 or if the pleural fluid LDH is greater than 1000 IU/L and if the pleural fluid glucose is above 40 mg/dL, while the Gram's stain and culture are negative. Antibiotic treatment alone usually is effective in this kind of parapneumonic pleural effusion but in some situations, an interventional method is also required. It is recommended that patients with class 3 parapneumonic effusions and reaccumulation of pleural fluid need to be treated with daily therapeutic thoracenteses. If the pH falls below 7.20, then a chest tube is recommended and if loculations are formed, then the clinician should think about the instillation of intrapleural fibrinolytics. Patients with class 4 (simple complicated parapneumonic pleural effusion) usually will need chest tube placement plus antibiotic therapy while patients with class 5 (complex complicated parapneumonic pleural effusion) require chest tube drainage plus thrombolytics or thoracoscopy if the thrombolytics are ineffective. Patients with class 6 (simple empyema) is proposed to be managed with chest tube placement plus thrombolytics and/or decortication while patients with complex empyema (class 7) usually will need thoracoscopy or decortication.

The American College of Chest Physicians (ACCP) classification scheme for parapneumonic pleural effusion/ pleural empyema,[1] uses characteristics of the pleural effusion in order to classify it into 4 classes determining the risk for poor outcomes. These characteristics are size of the pleural effusion on the chest X-ray, biochemical characteristics of the fluid (pH, glucose, LDH), and results of the Gram stain and cultures (Table 3). Criteria for an effusion to be classified as associated with poor prognosis are: size hemithorax more than 50% on a chest X-ray, presence of loculations, positive culture and/or Gram stain, presence of pus, pH less than 7.20, pleural fluid glucose below 60 mg/dL, or a pleural fluid LDH more than 3 times the upper limit of normal serum levels. ACCP states that patients classified in categories 1 and 2 due to low risk of poor outcomes can be managed with antibiotics alone. For Patients classified in categories

TABLE 3

American College of Chest Physicians Classification of Parapneumonic Effusions

Pleural space anatomy	Pleural fluid bacteriology	Pleural fluid chemistry	Category	Risk of poor outcome	Drainage	Additional fibrinolytic, VATS or surgery required
A0: minimal, free-flowing effusion (<10 mm on lateral decubitus)	AND BX culture and Gram stain results unknown	AND CX pH unknown	1	Very low	No	No
A1: small to moderate free-flowing effusion (<10 mm and <1/2 hemithorax)	AND B0 negative culture and Gram stain	AND C0 pH >7.20	2	Low	No	No
A2: large, free-flowing effusion (≥1/2 hemithorax), loculated effusion, oreffusion with thickened parietal pleura	OR B1 positive culture or Gram stain	OR C1 pH <7.20	3	Moderate	Yes	Yes
	B2 pus		4	High	Yes	Yes

VATS, video-assisted thoracoscopic surgery.

Source: Colice GL, Curtis A, Deslauriers J, Heffner J, Light R, Littenberg B, et al. Medical and surgical treatment of parapneumonic effusions : an evidence-based guideline. *Chest.* 2000;118:1158-71.

TABLE 4

British Thoracic Society Classification Scheme for Parapneumonic Pleural Effusions

Stages	Macroscopic appearance	Pleural fluid characteristics	Comments
Simple parapneumonic	Clear fluid	• pH >7.2 LDH <1000 IU/L • Glucose >2.2 mmol/L • No organisms on culture or Gram stain	• Will usually resolve with antibiotics alone. • Perform chest tube drainage for symptom relief if required
Complicated parapneumonic	Clear fluid or cloudy/turbid	• pH <7.2 • Lactate dehydrogenase >1000 IU/L • Glucose >2.2 mmol/L • May be positive Gram stain/culture	• Requires chest tube drainage
Empyema	Frank pus	• May be positive Gram stain/culture	• Requires chest tube drainage • No additional biochemical tests necessary onpleural fluid (do not measure pH)

Source: Davies CW, Gleeson FV, Davies RJ. BTS guidelines for the management of pleural infection. *Thorax.* 2003;58:ii18-28.

3 and 4, it is recommended to be managed with chest tube drainage in addition to the proper antibiotic therapy.

The simplest classification of parapneumonic pleural effusions has been published in 2003 by the British Thoracic Society (BTS).[8] The macroscopic appearance of the pleural fluid, the biochemical characteristics, and the results of Gram stain and culture are used in order to classify the parapneumonic pleural effusions in 3 categories (Table 4). For the empyema stage (class 3), frank pus is usually drained and there is no need for biochemical testing on it.

A schematic presentation of the classifications of parapneumonic pleural effusions is shown in figure 1.

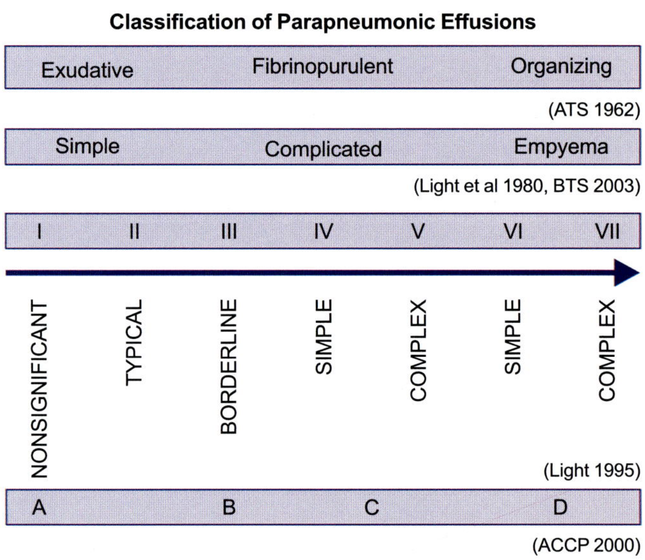

FIGURE 1 Schematic presentation of the classifications of parapneumonic pleural effusions. A figure presenting the different classification schemes from the first by ATS in 1962 to the 2000 one by ACCP.

CLINICAL PRESENTATION

The symptoms of pneumonia involving a parapneumonic pleural effusion or empyema (fever, malaise, cough, dyspnea, and pleuritic type pain) are same as the symptoms of pneumonia without a parapneumonic pleural effusion.[3] Elderly patients may be relatively asymptomatic, presenting only with fatigue or altered mental status, and without pulmonary symptoms. Other factors, such as age, peak temperature, leukocyte count, or number of lobes involved cannot predict the presence of a parapneumonic pleural effusion or differentiate between persons with and without a parapneumonic pleural effusion.[3] Furthermore, the clinical presentation is frequently similar to those for an uncomplicated parapneumonia pleural effusion or a complicated parapneumonia pleural effusion.

Patients with empyema usually represent a neglected pleural infection. Patients who are hospitalized with a parapneumonic pleural effusion and who receive appropriate antibiotic treatment rarely (<2%) develop empyema.[19] In a large study from the UK, patients presented to their physicians 5 days after the onset of pneumonia symptoms with an additional 13-day interval from the time of the initial outpatient visit and admission to the hospital. The admitting physician considered pleural space infection in only 29 (17%) of 119 patients. Delayed thoracentesis in the hospital is also associated with a prolonged hospital stay.[20]

BACTERIOLOGY OF PLEURAL INFECTION

The microbes implicated in the development of pleural infection have changed significantly. There is a difference in the microbes cultured in patients with community acquired and nosocomial parapneumonic pleural effusions.

In patients with community acquired parapneumonic pleural effusions, the microbes most frequently cultured are Gram-positive aerobes.[21] *Streptococcal* species and *S. aureus* account for approximately, 65% of cases.[21-23] Gram-negative organisms, including *Enterobacteriaceae, Escherichia coli,* and *Haemophilus influenzae* are not cultured usually and are found more often in patients with underlying diseases.[24] Anaerobes are cultured in 12–34% of positive pleural fluid cultivations,[19,22,25] while in up to 15%, anaerobes may be the only pathogens found.[4] This high incidence may be due to the indolent nature of these pneumonias. In patients with nosocomial parapneumonic pleural effusion, *S. aureus* is isolated in up to 50% of positive cases.[21] In the rest of the cases, Gram-negative organisms, such as *E. coli, Enterobacter* species, and *Pseudomonas* species are isolated. In patients who are admitted to the intensive care unit (ICU), the rates of Gram-negative aerobes reported are significantly higher.[26,27]

As has been shown in the multicenter intrapleural sepsis trial 1 (MIST1) study by Maskell et al.,[21] which included 434 patients with parapneumonic pleural effusion, streptococcal infection accounted for most of the community-acquired pleural infections. *S. pneumoniae* accounted for 21% of the pleural infections while *S. intermedius* group was responsible for 24% of the parapneumonic pleural effusions. In the hospital-acquired infections, *S. aureus* and enterococci were more frequently cultured. High percentage (25%) attributed to methicillin-resistant *S. aureus* (MRSA). The overall mortality was almost 3 times higher in the patients with hospital-acquired pleural infection as compared to patients who acquired the pleural infection in the community (47% vs. 17%, respectively).

In a large study form Spain that included more than 800 patients with parapneumonic pleural effusion by Falguera et al.,[28] *S. pneumoniae* was cultured in almost 50% of patients with complicated parapneumonic effusion/empyema. Also in this subgroup of patients, anaerobes and Gram-positive cocci were more frequent. In the same study, the investigators proposed 5 factors that could predict the development of complicated parapneumonic pleural effusion/empyema. These factors were: age below 60 years, alcoholism, pleuritic chest pain, tachycardia of more than 100 beats/min, and leukocytosis of more than 15,000/mm^3.

Empyema due to fungi is rare (<1%).[29] In the majority of cases *Candida* species are cultured and are seen mainly in immunosuppressed patients.[30] *Aspergillus* empyema usually occurs as a complication of aspergilloma and chronic necrotizing pulmonary aspergillosis or surgery for lung cancer, tuberculosis, or aspergillosis; it responds to treatment slowly.[31,32]

IMAGING TECHNIQUES

Radiological techniques play an important role in the evaluation and proper management of parapneumonic pleural effusion. Chest X-rays (plain and decubitus) and newer techniques such as ultrasound and contrast-enhanced computed tomography (CT) provide better morphological picture in terms of size and nature of effusion.[2,33]

Chest X-ray

The volume of the pleural fluid, its consistency, the positioning of the patient, and the presence or absence of adhesions plays an important role in the appearance of a parapneumonic pleural effusion on plain chest radiography. When on a chest X-ray there are pulmonary infiltrates accompanied by a pleural effusion, one should always think about a parapneumonic pleural effusion. When there is a suspicion of a pleural effusion, lateral chest X-ray must always be performed, as a pleural effusion may not be seen clearly on a posteroanterior X-ray. Supine radiographs have sensitivity and specificity of about 70% comparing with lateral decubitus films in demonstrating a pleural effusion.[34] The presence of more than 200 mL of pleural fluid usually blunts the lateral costophrenic angle, although in some cases up to 500 mL may be needed in order to have blunting of the costophrenic angle.[35] A meniscus sign is seen in non-loculated pleural effusions in excess of pleural fluid of 500 mL.

Chest Ultrasonography

Ultrasonography may help to detect a pleural effusion in cases where chest X-rays are not helpful. Also, it is widely used to assist a thoracentesis or to insert a thoracic tube. The sensitivity of ultrasonography is higher than that of a chest X-ray (only 5 mL of fluid can be detected).[36-38] Pleural effusions are anechoic and they change their shape during the respiratory cycle of the patient. Ultrasonography has the advantage that it can be performed bedside with a portable machine.[39] Also, the nature of the pleural fluid can be assessed by chest ultrasonography. The appearance of a pleural effusion on ultrasonography can be homogeneously anechoic, complex nonseptated with internal echogenic foci, complex septated, and homogeneously echogenic.[40] Transudative pleural effusions are always anechoic, while

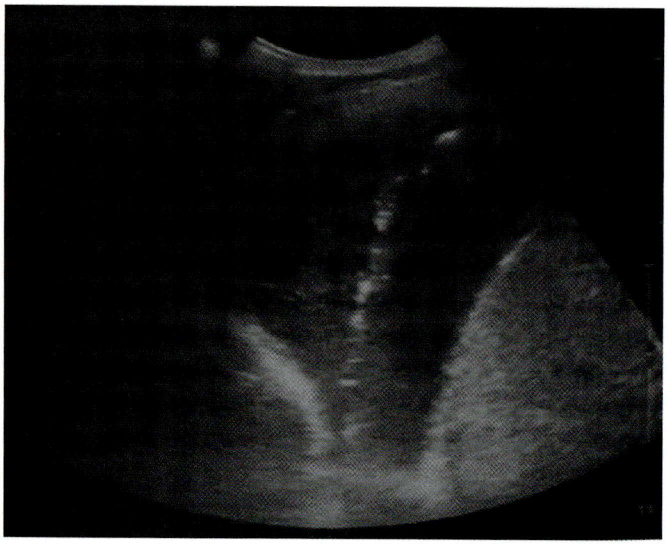

FIGURE 2 A septated pleural effusion. Notice the hyperechoic material (diaphragms and fibrin tissue) in the effusion. (Archive of pneumonology department, University Hospital of Alexandroupolis).

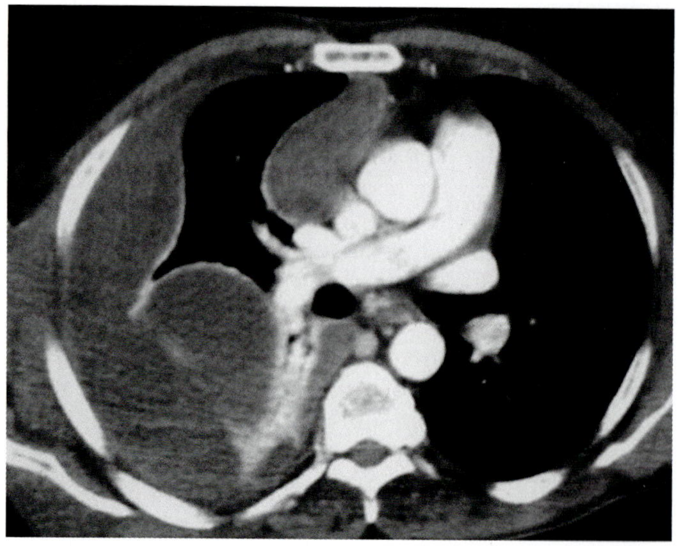

FIGURE 3 Split pleura sign in a loculated pleural effusion. This is a multiloculated right sided parapneumonic effusion. Notice the thickened parietal and visceral pleura (split pleura sign). (Archive of pneumonology department, University Hospital of Alexandroupolis).

exudative ones can be either echogenic or anechoic. Exudative pleural effusions are usually characterized by the presence of septations or by a complex or homogeneously echogenic pattern (Figure 2). Uniformly echogenic collections typically contain blood or debris. In patients who have the clinical picture of infection, the above sign in the chest ultrasonography indicates the presence of pus in almost all the cases.[41] The above characteristics were confirmed in a study by Yang et al.,[40] in which all the exudates were seen as echogenic effusions on chest ultrasonography while empyemas or hemorrhagic pleural effusions had a homogeneously echogenic pattern.

Computed Tomography

Multidetector CT scan offers images of the pleura that help in evaluating and differentiating complex pleural abnormalities.[42] It assists in differentiating pleural from parenchymal abnormalities, discovering pleural fluid loculations in the mediastinal pleura where ultrasound is negative[43] finding the exact place and the volume of the pleural effusion, and providing information for the specific characterization of pleural fluid. Thoracic CT with the use of intravenous contrast medium helps in differentiating between pleural and lung disorders.[44] Thoracic CT has better sensitivity as compared to plain chest X-ray in detecting small pleural effusions.[44] Small pleural effusions form the meniscus sign. Atelectasis of the lung can be seen in large collection of pleural fluid.[45] If we have an accumulation of fluid into the fissures (a finding called pseudotumor), it can be mistaken as pulmonary mass.[46] Pleural effusions, when loculated, have a biconvex morphology, while pulmonary solid lesions distinguish clearly from the effusion.[47,48] The split pleura sign is a clear demarcation of the loculations, due to enhancement of both pleural membranes by the inflammatory process (Figure 3). In 86–100% of empyemas, thickening of the pleural membranes can be seen.[49,50]

Positron Emission Tomography Scan

The use of positron emission tomography (PET) using 2-[18F]-fluoro-2-deoxy-glucose (FDG-PET) in imaging pleural effusions is limited. The uptake differs in situations such as discriminating between pleural infection and malignancy.[51,52]

PLEURAL FLUID ANALYSIS

All suspected parapneumonic pleural effusions should undergo thoracentesis. The pleural fluid should be sent to microbiology lab for Gram's staining and bacterial culture, leukocyte count, and to biochemistry for determination of glucose, LDH, pH, and proteins levels. The pH measurement is done the same way as it is done during the arterial blood pH.[53] Polymorphonuclear leucocytes are the main type of leukocytes found in parapneumonic pleural effusions but there is a variation in the number between simple effusions and empyemas.[15] A lymphocytic exudative pleural effusion is most often tubercular or malignant in origin.

It has been shown clinically[3,15,16] and confirmed by a meta-analysis[54] that a pleural fluid pH below 7.28 strongly suggests that pleural space drainage is necessary for a good outcome. The cutoff point to define a complicated pleural effusion and to consider draining ranged between pH 7.21 and 7.28. A pleural fluid glucose below 40 mg/dL or a ratio of pleural fluid to serum glucose of less than 0.5 and a pleural fluid lactate dehydrogenase (LDH) levels above 1000 IU/L also suggest the need for drainage. In situations other than a parapneumonic pleural effusion, such as a rheumatoid pleural effusion, glucose is also low.

Bacteriological studies must include Gram stain and cultures for anaerobes and aerobes. Delayed thoracocentesis results in prolonged hospitalization.[54,55] If pus is aspirated from the pleural cavity, then the diagnosis of empyema can be made and the patient always requires drainage. The yield of cultures can be improved if the fluid is inoculated in the culture medium bedside.[56]

DIFFERENTIAL DIAGNOSIS

What looks like a parapneumonic pleural effusion is not always the case. Fever, pulmonary consolidations, and a pleural effusion are not only due to pneumonia. Pleural effusions are associated commonly with pulmonary embolism. Twenty-five to fifty percent of cases of pulmonary embolism are complicated with a pleural effusion.[57] The differential diagnosis of a pleural effusion includes diseases such as tuberculosis, systemic lupus erythematosus (SLE), rheumatoid arthritis, sarcoidosis, and drug-induced pleural effusions. The milky appearance of an empyema can be confused sometimes as a chylothorax or pseudochylothorax. The measurement of certain inflammatory biomarkers in the pleural fluid can help in the differential diagnosis of pleural effusions. TNF-α, myeloperoxidase, matrix metalloproteinase-2, IL-8, lipopolysaccharide-binding protein (LBP), matrix metalloproteinase-9, matrix metalloproteinase-8, and C-reactive protein (CRP) have been shown that they can assist in the differential diagnosis of a complicated parapneumonic pleural effusion. Procalcitonin (PCT) levels measured in the pleural fluid have been shown not to be a significant diagnostic tool of pleural infection.[58] In a study by Porcel et al.,[59] the investigators found elevated pleural fluid levels of CRP, soluble triggering receptor expressed on myeloid cells (TREM-1), and LBP in patients with pleural infections, and especially, in cases of complicated parapneumonic pleural effusions.

TREATMENT

The therapeutic options for a parapneumonic pleural effusion depend on the particular stage of the effusion. There must be no delay on the management of an effusion. "The sun should never set on a parapneumonic effusion".[60] A parapneumonic pleural effusion is one of the few clinical situations in which a diagnostic thoracocentesis should be performed. What a clinician should do is to recognize the pathophysiological state and act quickly and appropriately in order to stop the progression of a parapneumonic pleural effusion to empyema. There is no unique therapeutic approach for parapneumonic pleural effusion and empyema.[7,13,57,61]

Uncomplicated parapneumonic effusions resolve with antibiotics alone. Not all complicated parapneumonic effusions have the same response to appropriate antibiotic therapy. Although in some patients therapy with antibiotics only is enough,[43] there are cases that early placement of chest tube drainage speeds clinical recovery and hospital stay.

In 2010, the BTS,[62] published a diagnostic algorithm for the management of patients with pleural effusion. In this algorithm, it is proposed as a first action after the documentation of accumulation of pleural fluid and infection, the start of antibiotics and the diagnostic thoracocentesis. If pus is present, immediately a chest tube is inserted. If no pus is present, the fluid is sent for pH, microbiological investigations, leukocyte count, and staining. If the Gram staining and/or the culture is positive and/or the pH is below 7.2, consider tube thoracotomy. If not, observe the pleural effusion and re-evaluate the patient. If the patient improves after the insertion of the chest tube (5–7 days after the insertion, the fluid and sepsis improve), continue the antibiotic coverage and remove the chest tube. If no improvement is evident, then one has to consider surgical treatment, if the patient is fit for it or less radical surgical techniques, if he is not fit.

Antibiotic Treatment

The initial antibiotic treatment of patients with parapneumonic pleural effusions is generally guided by treatment guidelines for pneumonia. When the results of blood and pleural fluid microbial cultures and antibiotic sensitivities are available, the treatment is altered accordingly. Empirical antibiotic coverage for anaerobes is generally advised, as there is a high incidence of anaerobic infection in empyema and it is difficulty in many clinical laboratories to isolate anaerobes. Antibiotics such as penicillins, cephalosporins, aztreonam, clindamycin, and ciprofloxacin have a good penetrating ability into the pleural cavity.[63] The penetration of intravenous gentamicin is lower in the pus of the empyema as compared to a sterile pleural fluid.[63,64] Choices for community-acquired empyema include intravenous β-lactam-β-lactamase inhibitor with or without macrolide, or alternatively, a newer fluoroquinolone plus cefotaxime or ceftriaxone. In patients with nosocomial parapneumonic pleural effusion coverage for Gram-negative microbes such as third generation cephalosporin plus an aminoglycoside, is necessary. If MRSA infection is probable, vancomycin or linezolid should be prescribed. There are few studies about the use of intrapleural antibiotics with positive results, but there no randomized controlled ones.[23,65]

Repeat Thoracentesis

The presence of clinical factors such as prolonged pneumonia symptoms,[66] comorbid disease,[54] failure to respond to antibiotic therapy, and the presence of anaerobic organisms[4] is suggestive of drainage of the pleural cavity. Chest radiograph findings that are indicative for drainage of the pleural space include an effusion involving more than 50% of the hemithorax,[19] loculations, and an air-fluid level. Stranding or septations noted on an ultrasound suggests the need for pleural space drainage;[67] marked pleural enhancement, pleural thickening, and the split pleura sign noted by chest CT indicate the necessity for pleural space drainage.[68] The split pleura sign clearly demarcates loculations due to enhancement of the pleural membranes by the inflammatory process. Aspiration of pus, an odor characteristic of an anaerobic infection, a positive Gram stain result or a positive culture, pH below 7.20, glucose level below 40 mg/dL, and LDH level above 1000 IU/L, all support the need to drain the pleural space.[3,15,16]

The guidelines published by the ACCP in 2000 recommended drainage of the parapneumonic pleural effusion, when it is stage 3 or 4.[1]

The options for pleural space drainage include repeated thoracocentesis, use of a chest tube, or insertion of a small-bore catheter with the assistance of an imaging technique. There are no randomized controlled studies evaluating the efficacy of daily thoracocentesis. There is big discrepancy between the suggestions of medical and surgical specialties about the best choice of catheter. Usually, large bore (>28 F) chest tubes are placed without radiological assistance. Nowadays, flexible catheters with smaller size (10–14 F) are used frequently. Their introduction is very easy and they produce less discomfort to the patients. The success rate of non-randomized studies of repeated thoracocentesis varies between 24 and 94%, while the mortality rate ranges from 0 to 25%.[23,69] Storm et al.[23] reported a double arm retrospective study of 94 patients with parapneumonic pleural effusion or pleural empyema. One arm included patients that were treated in a medical ward with daily thoracentesis, intravenous antibiotics, and in some of them also with intrapleural antibiotics, and the second arm included patients treated in a surgical department with tube thoracostomy and intravenous antibiotic therapy. The duration of hospital stay was significantly shorter for the patients treated in the medical wards compared to the patients treated in the surgical ward (2.3–5.0 weeks, respectively). Furthermore, pleurocutaneous and bronchopleural fistulas developed more frequently in patients treated by tube drainage than in those treated with the thoracocentesis regimen alone (30 to 10%) and (14 to 4%) for each complication, respectively. In the MIST1 study by Maskel et al.,[70] in the subanalysis, there was no difference in the efficacy of large chest tubes compared with the small bore ones.

Standard chest tubes (size 26–32 F) are often placed without ultrasound or CT guidance by thoracic surgeons for the treatment of complicated parapneumonic pleural effusion and empyema; success rates range from 6 to 76%, with mortality rates of 0–24%.[19,71,72] Drainage failure is a consequence of misplacement of the chest tube, tube malfunction, and loculations. Complications of using standard chest tubes include pain, pneumothorax, hemorrhage, and subcutaneous emphysema.

Small-bore catheters (size 8–14 F), which are more frequently used presently, can be placed under ultrasound or CT guidance. They are used more often in small, without loculations parapneumonic pleural effusions, but they have also been used in empyema with good results. The success rate of these catheters (72–82%) depends on the patients selected, operator's experience, and at which stage the parapneumonic pleural effusion is at the time of insertion.[73-76] Small-bore catheters are better tolerated by the patients while major complications can be avoided. In addition, a small-bore catheter placed with the Seldinger technique, when used for an initial thoracocentesis, can be left in place for continued drainage or removed after complete drainage, if the fluid is nonpurulent and the pH is above 7.30.

Image guided transcutaneous catheter insertion is used increasingly these days as they are more comfortable for pleural drainage. Usually they are inserted by interventional radiologists or pneumonologists with the assistance of ultrasound or CT. Their size is between 8 and 14 F (Malecot or pigtail). Their success rate is increased if they are instituted early in the disease course. The placement of an image guided transcutaneous catheter is indicated for pleural fluid collections that have small amount of fluid and are difficult to access. They are not indicated for empyema. They can also be used for fibrinolytic instillation.

Application of suction (up to -20 cm H_2O) can be employed in order to improve drainage, but there is not enough data from randomized trials to have a consensus on this field.[77,78]

The use of small-bore catheters is proposed in a recent review by Light et al.[79] They have the advantage of easier insertion while the patient experiences less pain having the tube into the pleural cavity. Their insertion should be guided by ultrasound. They are especially good in situations where pleurodesis must be done, as the tube must be left in place for a few days, minimizing the discomfort patient feels. What is needed is a large randomized trial to compare the efficacy and complications of small- and large-bore catheters. Even in situations where the pleural effusion has the consistency of pus, small-bore catheters can be used with success. He suggests the use of large-bore catheters for hemothorax due to the possibility of obstruction due to blood clots.

Intrapleural Fibrinolytics

Intrapleural fibrinolytic therapy was first attempted in 1949.[80] Tillett described the first intrapleural instillation of streptokinase and streptodornase. Fears about systemic side effects and a paucity of controlled clinical trials have unfortunately delayed the use of this method for years. The instillation of streptokinase or urokinase into the pleural cavity proved to be effective and without major complications, it is a choice of treatment in complicated parapneumonic pleural effusions and empyema. Usually after the instillations of fibrinolytics, the need for surgery is minimized.

The dose which is effective varies, but most commonly, 250,000 IU of streptokinase are used and 100,000 IU of urokinase are proven effective. The drug is usually diluted in 100 mL of normal saline and it is instilled in the pleural cavity. The time for which it remains in the pleural cavity varies from 2 to 4 hours. The instillation is 1–2 times/day and duration of treatment is between 3 and 5 days. The effectiveness of the treatment is determined by repeated chest radiographs, ultrasound of the hemithorax, or chest CT scan.

There are numerous case reports and randomized controlled trials (RCTs) reporting the results of using intrapleural instillation of fibrinolytics in pleural infection. It is an effective therapy with no serious complications that increases the drainage of pleural fluid and improves the radiological appearance. Bouros et al. demonstrated that urokinase is a safe intrapleural fibrinolytic.[81] In 20 patients with pleural infection, 50,000 IU of urokinase was instilled and it was proved that urokinase was a safe method of treatment with enhancement of drainage in all patients. The same investigators[82] in a RCT compared the efficacy and safety of streptokinase and urokinase in the treatment of infectious pleural effusions. Fifty consecutive patients were randomized to receive either streptokinase (250,000 IU in 100 mL normal saline) or urokinase (100,000 IU in 100 mL of normal saline) through a chest tube. The investigators were blind to the kind of the fibrinolytic used. The amount of pleural fluid drained was significantly increased after the instillation of fibrinolytics, increasing similarly for both groups of treatment. Most of the patients had clinical improvement with fibrinolytic treatment. The investigators concluded that urokinase is the treatment of choice due to the lower incidence of adverse events and it is only slightly costly. Bouros et al.[83] in another study were able to show that the urokinase effect in empyema was due to the breaking down of the adhesions, and not due to an increase in volume from the instilled urokinase and saline.

Lim and Chin[84] in a controlled, non-randomized trial analyzed the efficacy of 3 different protocols, simple chest tube drainage, adjunctive intrapleural streptokinase, and an aggressive empirical approach incorporating streptokinase and early surgical drainage in patients with parapneumonic pleural effusion and pleural empyema. In 29 patients, tube thoracostomy was performed; in the second group of 23 patients, 250,000 IU streptokinase were instilled intrapleurally on a daily basis, while 17% of the patients underwent surgical intervention. The investigators reported that the average duration of hospitalization and mortality in both streptokinase and early surgical intervention group was significantly lower than with tube drainage alone. The investigators concluded that the combination of intrapleural fibrinolysis with early surgical drainage had an advantage over the other 2 methods of therapy tested, resulting in fewer days of hospitalization and possibly reduces mortality in patients with pleural empyema and high-risk parapneumonic pleural effusions.

Davies et al.,[85] designed a randomized, prospective, control study to test the results of instilling 250,000 IU of streptokinase intrapleurally on a daily basis for 3 consecutive days vs. saline irrigations. Twelve patients were randomized to receive streptokinase and twelve received saline. In the streptokinase group, the daily and the total drainage of pleural fluid was significantly increased. The X-ray improvement was also greater in the streptokinase group than in the saline group. From the saline group, 3 patients were referred for surgery. In the streptokinase group, no patient was referred for surgery. The duration of hospitalization, temperature, and time of normalization of leukocytes was not statistically different between the 2 groups.[85]

Wait et al.[86] reported their experience using intrapleural fibrinolytic instillation and video-assisted thoracoscopic surgery (VATS) in the treatment of parapneumonic pleural effusion. They randomly treated 20 patients either with streptokinase 250,000 IU on a daily basis for 3 consecutive days or the patients underwent VATS. The investigators reported higher success rate of treatment in the VATS group as compared with the patients that received the streptokinase. Also, the in-hospital period of therapy and the number of days of tube thoracostomy were less in the VATS group.[86]

Tuncozgur et al.[87] in a RCT reported a decortication rate of 60% in the placebo (saline) group as compared to 29.1% in the urokinase group—a statistically significant difference. Also, the hospitalization time and the deferverscence time were shorter in the patients in whom fibrinolytic was instilled compared to the patients that received saline and the mean volume of drained fluid during the 5-day treatment period was significantly more in the urokinase patients ($p < 0.001$) as compared to the patients in whom saline was instilled.

In a study by Diacon et al.,[88] the percentage of referral for surgery and the clinical success rate were assessed. This was a RCT that involved 40 patients with pleural empyema. The patients were randomly chosen to receive either fibrinolytic (streptokinase) through a thoracic tube or saline. The clinical success rate in the streptokinase group of patients was almost double (82%) and the rate of referral to surgery was 5 times less in the streptokinase group as compared to the saline group.[88]

Maskell et al.[70] in 2005, reported the results of an UK multicenter, controlled trial of intrapleural instillation of streptokinase in patients with pleural infection. In this study, 454 patients with pleural pus, pleural sepsis with a pH below 7.2, or positive cultures of pleural fluid received on a random basis either streptokinase or placebo. The patients included were older than in most of the other studies (average age 60 years) and had a high prevalence of comorbidities. The primary end point of the study was either the referral for a surgical intervention or the death of a patient at 3 months. The secondary end points included the rate of death and the rate of surgical referral, the duration of in-hospital treatment, and the radiographic appearance. The results were disappointing for the use of streptokinase as an intrapleural fibrinolytic as there were no differences in the end points of the study between the 2 groups of patients. However, there was a lot of criticism for this study.[89-91] Questions were raised about the uniformity of decision-taking across the 52 centers that were included in the study. Also, there was criticism about the use of small bore catheters, without reporting the volume of pleural fluid drained. Because the placebo was shipped to the study centers after the patients were randomized, there were delays in the initiation of the treatment. Finally, the mortality as a primary end-point was criticized, as the patients included were patients over 60 years of age with much comorbidity.

A meta-analysis in 2006 by Tokuda et al.[92] was designed to include all randomized studies that enrolled patients with complicated parapneumonic pleural effusions and empyema and in whom fibrinolytics vs. placebo were used as intrapleural treatment. Primary end points were the reduction in death rate and the rate of surgical referral. The meta-analysis included 575 patients from 5 trials that met the inclusion criteria. The results showed a reduction in death rate which was not significant and the same for the rate of referral for surgical intervention. The investigators suggested that specific groups of patients could be treated with intrapleural fibrinolytics as different trials had different therapeutic results.[92]

Misthos et al.[93] conducted a prospective, randomized trial to examine the effectiveness of intrapleural instillation of fibrinolytics in the treatment of complicated parapneumonic pleural effusions. In one group, patients in whom only chest tube was inserted were included and the other group included patients in whom chest tube was inserted and streptokinase was instilled. They reported tube thoracostomy being successful in 67% of cases, while the streptokinase group had a favorable outcome in 87.7% ($p < 0.05$) with a significant shorter hospitalization. The mortality rate and the rate for surgical referral were significantly lower for the streptokinase group.

In 2008, in a Cochrane library meta-analysis conducted by Cameron et al.,[94] 7 studies and 761 patients were included. The investigators found a significantly reduced rate of surgical referral in all the studies included in the meta-analysis except the one reported by Maskell. In the analysis of the group of patients with multiloculated pleural effusions, they found a positive outcome with the instillation of intrapleural fibrinolytics. Also, the adverse events associated with the instillation of fibrinolytics were not increased.

Other fibrinolytics, like recombinant tissue plasminogen activator (r-TPA) alone or in combination with human recombinant DNase have been shown very effective.

Our group[95] has reported its experience with r-TPA. The study included 20 patients with complicated parapneumonic effusion and pleural empyema. After no improvement with simple chest tube thoracostomy, r-TPA was instilled intrapleurally in a concentration of 25 units diluted in 100 mL of normal saline. The instillation was repeated daily for 5–7 consecutive days. Clinical parameters such as fever and shortness of breath were improved after the therapy with r-TPA. The quantity of pleural fluid increased after the course of r-TPA improving the chest radiography of all the patients.

The overall benefit reported in our trial was 95%. We also documented a decrease in the number of leukocytes and in CRP, suggesting a decrease in the ongoing systemic inflammation. We didn't observe adverse events such as intrapleural or systemic hemorrhage. Also, the prothrombin time and the partial thromboplastin time were not increased, suggesting no systemic effects of the intrapleural instillation of the fibrinolytic.

Light et al.[96] reported their experience with DNase combined with streptokinase (Varidase) in empyema from rabbits. Liquefaction of the thick exudative purulent material was documented by Varidase but not with streptokinase or urokinase monotherapy.

In the effectiveness of the intrapleural instillation of fibrinolytics, is the time of starting the therapy. If after chest tube thoracostomy there is no improvement in the amount of pleural fluid evacuated and the chest X-ray shows no improvement, it is the time to use intrapleural fibrinolytics. The better outcome has been documented with the earlier instillation of the fibrinolytics,[13] measurement of the amount of pleural fluid drained, the number of leukocytes, and monitoring the success of the instillation of fibrinolytics with chest X-rays, ultrasound, or CT is mandatory.

The newer preparations of streptokinase cause fewer allergic reactions compared to the initial use of non-purified preparations. Fever is the most frequent adverse reaction.[13,97,98]

Anaphylactic reactions to urokinase intravenously are rarely reported and are usually mild. There are case reports for only ventricular fibrillation and acute respiratory failure as complications of the intrapleural use of urokinase or streptokinase.[99,100]

We have reported 2 cases[101] of major intrapleural hemorrhage after the instillation of intrapleural r-TPA for complicated parapneumonic pleural effusions. Both of the patients were receiving low molecular weight heparin (one in prophylactic dose and one in therapeutic dose). One of them had to undergo surgical intervention and the other one was conservatively treated.

The intrapleural instillation of fibrinolytic should be used in specific cases. If after 3–5 instillations of a fibrinolytic agent, there is no radiographic improvement and the patient is not getting better, the clinician should consider referring the patient for medical thoracoscopy when it is available or VATS.[102,103] Nowadays, a multicenter, two arms trial comparing the use of intrapleural fibrinolytics vs. medical thoracoscopy in complicated parapneumonic pleural effusions and empyema is scheduled in Europe. Until now, the evidence about the use of intrapleural fibrinolytics suggest that they can be used with good success rates in patients with complicated parapneumonic pleural effusions through large chest tubes and by clinicians, who have an experience with the technique.

Thoracoscopy

Medical thoracoscopy is an endoscopic examination of the pleural space, carried out by a pulmonologist, usually under local anesthesia in the endoscopy room, after induced or spontaneous pneumothorax. It can be performed with entering from 1 or 2 holes.[104-106] Medical thoracoscopy offers aspiration of pus, exploration of the pleural space to identify loculations and adhesions. One can open the loculations and remove the fibrinous membranes, take biopsies, and irrigate the cavity. At the end, a large thoracic tube is placed in order to remove the remaining fluid.

VATS is a mini-invasive technique which is performed in the operating suite under general anaesthesia.[107,108] The 2010 ACCP guidelines,,[62] recommended the usage of VATS in patients at high-risk of unfavorable development (categories 3 and 4). The advantages of VATS over thoracostomy are the less cost, reduced hospital stay, and less pain with fewer complications and success rate between 60% and 100%, that becomes higher if it is used earlier in the course of the disease.[109-111] In a randomized study by Bilgin et al.,[112] 70 patients with pleural empyema were assigned either to VATS or tube thoracostomy alone. In the VATS group, the success rate was 82.8% and in the tube group, the success rate was 62.9%. The duration of hospitalization was statistically shorter in the VATS group (8.3 days compared to 12.8 days, respectively).

In the studies where medical thoracoscopy has been used to treat complicated parapneumonic pleural effusions and empyemas, the success rate was over 73% (73–100%). Emphasis is given to the lower cost compared to VATS and that it can be performed in subjects who are not fit for general anesthesia.[113-115]

When less invasive procedures fail to control pleural sepsis and no re-expansion of the lung is achieved, the decision to proceed to open thoracotomy is taken.[116,117] The decision for a patient to undergo an operation like a decortication depends on the performance status of the patient. When it is done in the acute phase of a parapneumonic pleural effusion, it controls the pleural infection, while a late decortication (>6 months) is aimed to restore chest mechanics by removing a restrictive peel surrounding the lung. The success rate ranges between 87 and 100%, while the mortality rate ranges between 0 and 9%.[7,118,119] A study comparing VATS and thoracotomy shows similar results but with VATS, the hospital stay was shorter and there were advantages in the resolution of the disease and the cosmetic result.[107]

Thoracostomy, a procedure used in debilitated patients, involves rib excision, which produces a stoma allowing the continuous drainage of the pleural space. One or more chest tubes can be inserted through the opening, in order for the pleural cavity to be irrigated daily with a mild antiseptic. A colostomy bag can be used for the drainage collection. The chest tubes can be slowly retracted until complete removal—a process that takes 2–3 months to be completed. A different approach involves packing the empyema cavity with gauze. A more complicated procedure is the Eloesser technique. The time of healing is usually 6 months.[7]

REFERENCES

1. Colice GL, Curtis A, Deslauriers J, Heffner J, Light R, Littenberg B, et al. Medical and surgical treatment of parapneumonic effusions : an evidence-based guideline. *Chest.* 2000;118:1158-71.
2. Hamm H, Light RW. Parapneumonic effusion and empyema. *Eur Respir J.* 1997;10:1150-6.
3. Light RW, Girard WM, Jenkinson SG, George RB. Parapneumonic effusions. A*m J Med.* 1980;69:507-12.
4. Bartlett JG, Finegold SM. Anaerobic infections of the lung and pleural space. *Am Rev Respir Dis.* 1974;110:56-77.
5. Strange C, Sahn SA. The definitions and epidemiology of pleural space infection. *Semin Respir Infect.* 1999;14:3-8.
6. Bouros D, editor. Parapneumonic Pleural Effusions and Empyema. New York: Marcel Dekker; 2010.
7. Light R, editor. Pleural Diseases. Philadelphia, PA:Lippincott and Williams and Wilkins; 2001.
8. Davies CW, Gleeson FV, Davies RJ. BTS guidelines for the management of pleural infection. *Thorax.* 2003;58:ii18-28.
9. Antony VB, Godbey SW, Kunkel SL, Hott JW, Hartman DL, Burdick MD, et al. Recruitment of inflammatory cells to the pleural space. Chemotactic cytokines, IL-8, and monocyte chemotactic peptide-1 in human pleural fluids. *J Immunol.* 1993;151:7216-23.
10. Lin FC, Chen YC, Chen FJ, Chang SC. Cytokines and fibrinolytic enzymes in tuberculous and parapneumonic effusions. *Clin Immunol.* 2005;116:166-73.
11. Mohammed KA, Nasreen N, Hardwick J, Logie CS, Patterson CE, Antony VB. Bacterial induction of pleural mesothelial monolayer barrier dysfunction. *Am J Physiol Lung Cell Mol Physiol.* 2001;281:L119-25.
12. Andrews NC, Parker EF, Shaw RR, Wilson NJ, Webb WR. Management of non tuberculous empyema: a statement of the subcommittee on surgery. *Am Rev Respir Dis* 1962; 85:935-6.
13. Bouros D, Hamm H. Infectious pleural effusions. *Eur Respir Mon.* 2002;22:204-18.
14. Wiener-Kronish JP, Sakuma T, Kudoh I, Pittet JF, Frank D, Dobbs L, et al. Alveolar epithelial injury and pleural empyema in acute P. aeruginosa pneumonia in anesthetized rabbits. *J Appl Physiol.* 1993;75:1661-9.
15. Potts DE, Levin DC, Sahn SA. Pleural fluid pH in parapneumonic effusions. *Chest.* 1976;70:328-31.
16. Potts DE, Taryle DA, Sahn SA. The glucose-pH relationship in parapneumonic effusions. *Arch Intern Med.* 1978;138: 1378-80.
17. Antony VB, Mohammed KA. Pathophysiology of pleural space infections. *Semin Respir Infect.* 1999;14:9-17.
18. Light RW, MacGregor MI, Ball WC, Jr., Luchsinger PC. Diagnostic significance of pleural fluid pH and PCO2. *Chest.* 1973;64:591-6.
19. Ferguson AD, Prescott RJ, Selkon JB, Watson D, Swinburn CR. The clinical course and management of thoracic empyema. *QJM.* 1996;89:285-9.
20. Heffner JE, McDonald J, Barbieri C, Klein J. Management of parapneumonic effusions. An analysis of physician practice patterns. *Arch Surg.* 1995;130:433-8.
21. Maskell NA, Batt S, Hedley EL, Davies CW, Gillespie SH, Davies RJ. The bacteriology of pleural infection by genetic and standard methods and its mortality significance. *Am J Respir Crit Care Med.* 2006;174:817-23.
22. Alfageme I, Munoz F, Pena N, Umbria S. Empyema of the thorax in adults. Etiology, microbiologic findings, and management. *Chest.* 1993;103:839-43.
23. Storm HK, Krasnik M, Bang K, Frimodt-Moller N. Treatment of pleural empyema secondary to pneumonia: thoracocentesis regimen versus tube drainage. *Thorax.* 1992;47:821-4.
24. Chen KY, Hsueh PR, Liaw YS, Yang PC, Luh KT. A 10-year experience with bacteriology of acute thoracic empyema: emphasis on Klebsiella pneumoniae in patients with diabetes mellitus. *Chest.* 2000;117:1685-9.
25. Galea JL, De Souza A, Beggs D, Spyt T. The surgical management of empyema thoracis. *J R Coll Surg Edinb.* 1997;42:15-8.
26. Lin YC, Chen HJ, Liu YH, Shih CM, Hsu WH, Tu CY. A 30-month experience of thoracic empyema in a tertiary hospital: emphasis on differing bacteriology and outcome between the medical intensive care unit (MICU) and medical ward. *South Med J.* 2008;101:484-9.
27. Tu CY, Hsu WH, Hsia TC, Chen HJ, Chiu KL, Hang LW, et al. The changing pathogens of complicated parapneumonic effusions or empyemas in a medical intensive care unit. *Intensive Care Med.* 2006;32:570-6.
28. Falguera M, Carratala J, Bielsa S, Garcia-Vidal C, Ruiz-Gonzalez A, Chica I, et al. Predictive factors, microbiology and outcome of patients with parapneumonic effusion. *Eur Respir J.* 2011;38:1173-9.
29. Rahman NM, Chapman SJ, Davies RJ. The approach to the patient with a parapneumonic effusion. *Clin Chest Med.* 2006;27:253-66.
30. Ko SC, Chen KY, Hsueh PR, Luh KT, Yang PC. Fungal empyema thoracis: an emerging clinical entity. *Chest.* 2000;117:1672-8.
31. Denning DW. Chronic forms of pulmonary aspergillosis. *Clin Microbiol Infect.* 2001;7:25-31.
32. Shiraishi Y, Katsuragi N, Nakajima Y, Hashizume M, Takahashi N, Miyasaka Y. Pneumonectomy for complex aspergilloma: is it still dangerous? *Eur J Cardiothorac Surg.* 2006;29:9-13.
33. Levin DL, Klein JS. Imaging techniques for pleural space infections. *Semin Respir Infect.* 1999;14:31-8.

34. Ruskin JA, Gurney JW, Thorsen MK, Goodman LR. Detection of pleural effusions on supine chest radiographs. *AJR Am J Roentgenol.* 1987;148:681-3.
35. Blackmore CC, Black WC, Dallas RV, Crow HC. Pleural fluid volume estimation: a chest radiograph prediction rule. *Acad Radiol.* 1996;3:103-9.
36. Tayal VS, Nicks BA, Norton HJ. Emergency ultrasound evaluation of symptomatic nontraumatic pleural effusions. *Am J Emerg Med.* 2006;24:782-6.
37. Kocijancic I, Vidmar K, Ivanovi-Herceg Z. Chest sonography versus lateral decubitus radiography in the diagnosis of small pleural effusions. *J Clin Ultrasound.* 2003;31:69-74.
38. Feller-Kopman D. Therapeutic thoracentesis: the role of ultrasound and pleural manometry. *Curr Opin Pulm Med.* 2007;13:312-8.
39. Lichtenstein DA, Menu Y. A bedside ultrasound sign ruling out pneumothorax in the critically ill. Lung sliding. *Chest.* 1995;108:1345-8.
40. Yang PC, Luh KT, Chang DB, Wu HD, Yu CJ, Kuo SH. Value of sonography in determining the nature of pleural effusion: analysis of 320 cases. *AJR Am J Roentgenol.* 1992; 159:29-33.
41. Tu CY, Hsu WH, Hsia TC, Chen HJ, Tsai KD, Hung CW, et al. Pleural effusions in febrile medical ICU patients: chest ultrasound study. *Chest.* 2004;126:1274-80.
42. Ravenel JG, McAdams HP. Multiplanar and three-dimensional imaging of the thorax. *Radiol Clin North Am.* 2003;41:475-89.
43. Strange C, Sahn SA. Management of parapneumonic pleural effusions and empyema. *Infect Dis Clin North Am.* 1991;5:539-59.
44. Evans AL, Gleeson FV. Radiology in pleural disease: state of the art. *Respirology.* 2004;9:300-12.
45. Heffner JE, Klein JS, Hampson C. Diagnostic utility and clinical application of imaging for pleural space infections. *Chest.* 2010;137:467-79.
46. Henschke CI, Davis SD, Romano PM, Yankelevitz DF. Pleural effusions: pathogenesis, radiologic evaluation, and therapy. *J Thorac Imaging.* 1989;4:49-60.
47. Muller NL. Imaging of the pleura. *Radiology.* 1993;186: 297-309.
48. Stark DD, Federle MP, Goodman PC, Podrasky AE, Webb WR. Differentiating lung abscess and empyema: radiography and computed tomography. *AJR Am J Roentgenol.* 1983;141:163-7.
49. Aquino SL, Webb WR, Gushiken BJ. Pleural exudates and transudates: diagnosis with contrast-enhanced CT. *Radiology.* 1994;192:803-8.
50. Waite RJ, Carbonneau RJ, Balikian JP, Umali CB, Pezzella AT, Nash G. Parietal pleural changes in empyema: appearances at CT. *Radiology.* 1990;175:145-50.
51. Duysinx BC, Larock MP, Nguyen D, Corhay JL, Bury T, Hustinx R, et al. 18F-FDG PET imaging in assessing exudative pleural effusions. *Nucl Med Commun.* 2006;27: 971-6.
52. Toaff JS, Metser U, Gottfried M, Gur O, Deeb ME, Lievshitz G, et al. Differentiation between malignant and benign pleural effusion in patients with extra-pleural primary malignancies: assessment with positron emission tomography-computed tomography. *Invest Radiol.* 2005; 40: 204-9.
53. Poe RH, Marin MG, Israel RH, Kallay MC. Utility of pleural fluid analysis in predicting tube thoracostomy/decortication in parapneumonic effusions. *Chest.* 1991;100:963-7.
54. Heffner JE, Brown LK, Barbieri C, DeLeo JM. Pleural fluid chemical analysis in parapneumonic effusions. A meta-analysis. *Am J Respir Crit Care Med.* 1995;151:1700-8.
55. Chu MW, Dewar LR, Burgess JJ, Busse EG. Empyema thoracis: lack of awareness results in a prolonged clinical course. *Can J Surg.* 2001;44:284-8.
56. Runyon BA, Antillon MR, Akriviadis EA, McHutchison JG. Bedside inoculation of blood culture bottles with ascitic fluid is superior to delayed inoculation in the detection of spontaneous bacterial peritonitis. *J Clin Microbiol.* 1990; 28:2811-2.
57. Sahn SA. State of the art. The pleura. *Am Rev Respir Dis.* 1988;138:184-234.
58. Porcel JM. Pleural fluid tests to identify complicated parapneumonic effusions. *Curr Opin Pulm Med.* 2010; 16:357-61.
59. Porcel JM, Vives M, Cao G, Bielsa S, Ruiz-Gonzalez A, Martinez-Iribarren A, et al. Biomarkers of infection for the differential diagnosis of pleural effusions. *Eur Respir J.* 2009;34:1383-9.
60. Sahn SA, Light RW. The sun should never set on a parapneumonic effusion. *Chest.* 1989;95:945-7.
61. Lemmer JH, Botham MJ, Orringer MB. Modern management of adult thoracic empyema. *J Thorac Cardiovasc Surg.* 1985;90:849-55.
62. Davies HE, Davies RJ, Davies CW. Management of pleural infection in adults: British Thoracic Society Pleural Disease Guideline 2010. *Thorax.* 2010;65:ii41-53.
63. Teixeira LR, Sasse SA, Villarino MA, Nguyen T, Mulligan ME, Light RW. Antibiotic levels in empyemic pleural fluid. *Chest.* 2000;117:1734-9.
64. Thys JP, Vanderhoeft P, Herchuelz A, Bergmann P, Yourassowsky E. Penetration of aminoglycosides in uninfected pleural exudates and in pleural empyemas. *Chest.* 1988;93:530-2.
65. Rosenfeldt FL, McGibney D, Braimbridge MV, Watson DA. Comparison between irrigation and conventional treatment for empyema and pneumonectomy space infection. *Thorax.* 1981;36:272-7.
66. Taryle DA, Potts DE, Sahn SA. The incidence and clinical correlates of parapneumonic effusions in pneumococcal pneumonia. *Chest.* 1978;74:170-3.
67. Mayo PH, Doelken P. Pleural ultrasonography. *Clin Chest Med.* 2006;27:215-27.
68. Qureshi NR, Gleeson FV. Imaging of pleural disease. *Clin Chest Med.* 2006;27:193-213.
69. Mandal AK, Thadepalli H. Treatment of spontaneous bacterial empyema thoracis. *J Thorac Cardiovasc Surg.* 1987;94:414-8.
70. Maskell NA, Davies CW, Nunn AJ, Hedley EL, Gleeson FV, Miller R, et al. U.K. Controlled trial of intrapleural streptokinase for pleural infection. *N Engl J Med.* 2005;352: 865-74.
71. Hoover EL, Hsu HK, Webb H, Toporoff B, Minnard E, Cunningham JN. The surgical management of empyema thoracis in substance abuse patients: a 5-year experience. *Ann Thorac Surg.* 1988;46:563-6.

72. Huang HC, Chang HY, Chen CW, Lee CH, Hsiue TR. Predicting factors for outcome of tube thoracostomy in complicated parapneumonic effusion for empyema. *Chest.* 1999;115:751-6.
73. Merriam MA, Cronan JJ, Dorfman GS, Lambiase RE, Haas RA. Radiographically guided percutaneous catheter drainage of pleural fluid collections. *AJR Am J Roentgenol.* 1988;151:1113-6.
74. Silverman SG, Mueller PR, Saini S, Hahn PF, Simeone JF, Forman BH, et al. Thoracic empyema: management with image-guided catheter drainage. *Radiology.* 1988;169:5-9.
75. Shankar S, Gulati M, Kang M, Gupta S, Suri S. Image-guided percutaneous drainage of thoracic empyema: can sonography predict the outcome? *Eur Radiol.* 2000;10: 495-9.
76. Ulmer JL, Choplin RH, Reed JC. Image-guided catheter drainage of the infected pleural space. *J Thorac Imaging.* 1991;6:65-73.
77. Miller KS, Sahn SA. Chest tubes. Indications, technique, management and complications. *Chest.* 1987;91:258-64.
78. Munnell ER. Thoracic drainage. *Ann Thorac Surg.* 1997;63: 1497-502.
79. Light RW. Pleural controversy: optimal chest tube size for drainage. *Respirology.* 2011;16:244-8.
80. Tillett WS, Sherry S. The Effect in Patients of Streptococcal Fibrinolysin (Streptokinase) and Streptococcal Desoxy-ribonuclease on Fibrinous, Purulent, and Sanguinous Pleural Exudations. *J Clin Invest.* 1949;28:173-90.
81. Bouros D, Schiza S, Tzanakis N, Drositis J, Siafakas N. Intrapleural urokinase in the treatment of complicated parapneumonic pleural effusions and empyema. *Eur Respir J.* 1996;9:1656-9.
82. Bouros D, Schiza S, Patsourakis G, Chalkiadakis G, Panagou P, Siafakas NM. Intrapleural streptokinase versus urokinase in the treatment of complicated parapneumonic effusions: a prospective, double-blind study. *Am J Respir Crit Care Med.* 1997;155:291-5.
83. Bouros D, Schiza S, Tzanakis N, Chalkiadakis G, Drositis J, Siafakas N. Intrapleural urokinase versus normal saline in the treatment of complicated parapneumonic effusions and empyema. A randomized, double-blind study. *Am J Respir Crit Care Med.* 1999;159:37-42.
84. Lim TK, Chin NK. Empirical treatment with fibrinolysis and early surgery reduces the duration of hospitalization in pleural sepsis. *Eur Respir J.* 1999;13:514-8.
85. Davies RJ, Traill ZC, Gleeson FV. Randomised controlled trial of intrapleural streptokinase in community acquired pleural infection. *Thorax.* 1997;52:416-21.
86. Wait MA, Sharma S, Hohn J, Dal Nogare A. A randomized trial of empyema therapy. *Chest.* 1997;111:1548-51.
87. Tuncozgur B, Ustunsoy H, Sivrikoz MC, Dikensoy O, Topal M, Sanli M, et al. Intrapleural urokinase in the management of parapneumonic empyema: a randomised controlled trial. *Int J Clin Pract.* 2001;55:658-60.
88. Diacon AH, Theron J, Schuurmans MM, Van de Wal BW, Bolliger CT. Intrapleural streptokinase for empyema and complicated parapneumonic effusions. *Am J Respir Crit Care Med.* 2004;170:49-53.
89. Heffner JE. Multicenter trials of treatment for empyema—after all these years. *N Engl J Med.* 2005;352:926-8.
90. Diacon AH, Koegelenberg CF, Bolliger CT. A trial of intrapleural streptokinase. *N Engl J Med.* 2005;352:2243-5.
91. Bouros D, Antoniou KM, Light RW. Intrapleural streptokinase for pleural infection. *BMJ.* 2006;332:133-4.
92. Tokuda Y, Matsushima D, Stein GH, Miyagi S. Intrapleural fibrinolytic agents for empyema and complicated parapneumonic effusions: a meta-analysis. *Chest.* 2006;129: 783-90.
93. Misthos P, Sepsas E, Konstantinou M, Athanassiadi K, Skottis I, Lioulias A. Early use of intrapleural fibrinolytics in the management of postpneumonic empyema. A prospective study. *Eur J Cardiothorac Surg.* 2005;28:599-603.
94. Cameron R, Davies HR. Intra-pleural fibrinolytic therapy versus conservative management in the treatment of adult parapneumonic effusions and empyema. *Cochrane Database Syst Rev.* 2008;(2):CD002312.
95. Froudarakis ME, Kouliatsis G, Steiropoulos P, Anevlavis S, Pataka A, Popidou M, et al. Recombinant tissue plasminogen activator in the treatment of pleural infections in adults. *Respir Med.* 2008;102:1694-700.
96. Light RW, Nguyen T, Mulligan ME, Sasse SA. The in vitro efficacy of varidase versus streptokinase or urokinase for liquefying thick purulent exudative material from loculated empyema. *Lung.* 2000;178:13-8.
97. Bouros D, Tzouvelekis A, Antoniou KM, Heffner JE. Intrapleural fibrinolytic therapy for pleural infection. *Pulm Pharmacol Ther.* 2007;20:616-26.
98. Bouros D, Schiza S, Siafakas N. Utility of fibrinolytic agents for draining intrapleural infections. *Semin Respir Infect.* 1999;14:39-47.
99. Alfageme I, Vazquez R. Ventricular fibrillation after intrapleural urokinase. *Intensive Care Med.* 1997;23:352.
100. Frye MD, Jarratt M, Sahn SA. Acute hypoxemic respiratory failure following intrapleural thrombolytic therapy for hemothorax. *Chest.* 1994;105:1595-6.
101. Anevlavis S, Archontogeorgis K, Tzouvelekis A, Kouliatsis G, Pozova S, Bougioukas I, et al. Intrapleural r-tPA in Association with Low-Molecular Heparin May Cause Massive Hemothorax Resulting in Hypovolemia. *Respiration.* 2011; 81:513-6.
102. Bouros D, Antoniou KM, Chalkiadakis G, Drositis J, Petrakis I, Siafakas N. The role of video-assisted thoracoscopic surgery in the treatment of parapneumonic empyema after the failure of fibrinolytics. *Surg Endosc.* 2002;16:151-4.
103. Petrakis IE, Kogerakis NE, Drositis IE, Lasithiotakis KG, Bouros D, Chalkiadakis GE. Video-assisted thoracoscopic surgery for thoracic empyema: primarily, or after fibrinolytic therapy failure? *Am J Surg.* 2004;187:471-4.
104. Loddenkemper R. Thoracoscopy—state of the art. *Eur Respir J.* 1998;11:213-21.
105. Mathur PN, Astoul P, Boutin C. Medical thoracoscopy. Technical details. *Clin Chest Med.* 1995;16:479-86.
106. Rodriguez-Panadero F, Janssen JP, Astoul P. Thoracoscopy: general overview and place in the diagnosis and management of pleural effusion. *Eur Respir J.* 2006;28:409-22.
107. Angelillo Mackinlay TA, Lyons GA, Chimondeguy DJ, Piedras MA, Angaramo G, Emery J. VATS debridement

versus thoracotomy in the treatment of loculated postpneumonia empyema. *Ann Thorac Surg.* 1996;61:1626-30.
108. Lawrence DR, Ohri SK, Moxon RE, Townsend ER, Fountain SW. Thoracoscopic debridement of empyema thoracis. *Ann Thorac Surg.* 1997;64:1448-50.
109. Waller DA. Thoracoscopy in management of postpneumonic pleural infections. *Curr Opin Pulm Med.* 2002; 8:323-6.
110. Cassina PC, Hauser M, Hillejan L, Greschuchna D, Stamatis G. Video-assisted thoracoscopy in the treatment of pleural empyema: stage-based management and outcome. *J Thorac Cardiovasc Surg.* 1999;117:234-8.
111. Solaini L, Prusciano F, Bagioni P. Video-assisted thoracic surgery in the treatment of pleural empyema. *Surg Endosc.* 2007;21:280-4.
112. Bilgin M, Akcali Y, Oguzkaya F. Benefits of early aggressive management of empyema thoracis. *ANZ J Surg.* 2006;76: 120-2.
113. Soler M, Wyser C, Bolliger CT, Perruchoud AP. Treatment of early parapneumonic empyema by "medical" thoracoscopy. *Schweiz Med Wochenschr.* 1997;127:1748-53.
114. Colt HG. Thoracoscopy. A prospective study of safety and outcome. *Chest.* 1995;108:324-9.
115. Brutsche MH, Tassi GF, Gyorik S, Gokcimen M, Renard C, Marchetti GP, et al. Treatment of sonographically stratified multiloculated thoracic empyema by medical thoracoscopy. *Chest.* 2005;128:3303-9.
116. Light RW. Parapneumonic effusions and empyema. *Proc Am Thorac Soc.* 2006;3:75-80.
117. Mandal AK, Thadepalli H, Chettipally U. Outcome of primary empyema thoracis: therapeutic and microbiologic aspects. *Ann Thorac Surg.* 1998;66:1782-6.
118. Mayo P. Early thoracotomy and decortication for nontuberculous empyema in adults with and without underlying disease. A twenty-five year review. *Am Surg.* 1985; 51:230-6.
119. Muskett A, Burton NA, Karwande SV, Collins MP. Management of refractory empyema with early decortication. *Am J Surg.* 1988;156:529-32.
120. Light RW. A new classification of parapneumonic effusions and empyema. *Chest.* 1995;108:299-301.

CHAPTER 17

Intensive Care Unit-associated Infections: Pathogenesis, Diagnosis, Management, and Prevention

Timothy L Wiemken, Ruth Carrico, Paula Peyrani, Julio A Ramirez

ABSTRACT

A significant number of hospitalized patients in medical or surgical intensive care units (ICU) require antibiotic therapy for the management of infections. Patients admitted to the medical or surgical ICU without evidence of infection who develop infection while in the ICU are considered to have ICU-associated infections. In this chapter, we will emphasize four of the most common ICU-associated infections, including catheter-associated urinary tract infection, ventilator-associated pneumonia, catheter-associated bloodstream infections, and *Clostridium difficile* infection. The first section will provide an overview of the pathogenesis of each infection, the second section will identify methods to diagnose each of the infections, the third section will summarize the current best practices for the management of each infection, and the fourth and final sections will describe the various methods for the prevention and control of each infection.

INTRODUCTION

A significant number of hospitalized patients in medical or surgical intensive care units (ICUs) require antibiotic therapy for the management of infection. Some of these patients are admitted directly from the community to the ICU for the treatment of serious infection. The most frequent infection for patients requiring admission to the medical ICU is community-acquired pneumonia (CAP) and to the surgical ICU is secondary peritonitis. Patients admitted to the medical or surgical ICU without any evidence of infection and who develop the infection while in the ICU are considered to have ICU-associated infections.

We reviewed data on the use of intravenous antibiotics to treat infection in our hospitalized patients at the Robley Rex Veterans Affairs Medical Center (VAMC) in Louisville, Kentucky to define the most likely sites of infection in patients treated in the medical and surgical ICUs. Using data from over 20,000 courses of intravenous antimicrobial therapy during a 7-year period from our antimicrobial stewardship program at the VAMC, we identified the most frequent sites of infection requiring antibiotic treatment from the community and healthcare settings. Results from these analyses can be found in table 1. Patients in the ICU setting are at a high risk of developing ICU-associated infections. Data from our VAMC showed that the most frequently identified ICU-associated infections requiring intravenous antibiotic therapy include hospital-acquired pneumonias (HAP, 57%) and central line-associated bloodstream infection (CLABSI, 8%) in the medical ICU, and HAP (35%) and peritonitis (11%) in the surgical ICU. We have also recently identified *Clostridium difficile* infection as an emerging ICU-associated infection.

There are multiple reasons that patients in medical and surgical ICUs are at an increased risk for development of ICU-associated infections. Some of these risk factors are well defined in the literature and include the following:

TABLE 1

Most Common Sites of Infection for Patients Treated with Intravenous Antimicrobial Therapy in the Medical and Surgical Intensive Care Units of Robley Rex Veterans Affairs Medical Center, Louisville, Kentucky Between 2002 and 2009

Community-associated infections treated in the ICU setting			ICU-associated infections treated in the ICU setting		
Medical ICU (n = 1868)			*Medical ICU (n = 2486)*		
CAP	n = 870	47%	HAP	n = 1406	57%
Pyelonephritis	n = 144	8%	CLABSI	n = 192	8%
COPD exacerbation	n = 119	6%	Pyelonephritis	n = 86	3%
Surgical ICU (n = 436)			*Surgical ICU (n = 1076)*		
Peritonitis	n = 97	22%	HAP	n = 379	35%
Cholecystitis	n = 66	15%	Peritonitis	n = 113	11%
Soft tissue infection	n = 44	10%	CLABSI	n = 103	10%

ICU, intensive care unit; CAP, community-acquired pneumonia; COPD, chronic obstructive pulmonary disease; HAP, hospital-acquired pneumonia; CLABSI, central-line associated bloodstream infection.

- The increased severity of disease[1]
- High incidence of medical device use, such as central venous catheters
- High burden of antimicrobial therapy and associated collateral damage[3]
- Environmental contamination with microorganisms.[4]

Some novel risk factors include contact with healthcare workers and patient movement. We are currently evaluating the role of the network density between patients and healthcare workers to elucidate the effect of patient-healthcare worker contact on the risk of ICU-associated infection. We are also investigating how patient movement throughout a healthcare facility may affect the risk of ICU-associated infection through environmental contamination, healthcare worker contact, and the inability to sustain or adhere to isolation precautions.[5]

Overall, infections in patients hospitalized in the intensive care unit account for a significant quantity of excess morbidity, mortality, and healthcare costs.[6,7] Therefore, prevention and control of these infections should be of high importance to the healthcare team.

In this chapter, we will focus on the pathogenesis, diagnosis, management, and prevention of four infections commonly seen in the ICU setting:

- Catheter-associated urinary tract infections (CAUTI)
- Ventilator-associated pneumonia (VAP)
- Central line-associated bloodstream (CLABSI)
- *Clostridium difficile* infection (CDI).

A clear understanding of these factors as they relate to the common ICU-associated infections will provide a pathway to reduce the excessive morbidity and mortality in these patients.

CATHETER-ASSOCIATED URINARY TRACT INFECTIONS

Introduction

Urinary tract infections (UTI) are the most common ICU-associated infections.[8] The vast majority of these infections are associated with indwelling urinary catheters and are denoted as CAUTI.[9] Nearly one-fifth of hospitalized patients will have a urinary catheter inserted at some point during their hospitalization,[10] a rate that can be much higher among patients in the ICU.[11] The risk of CAUTI in the general patient population varies but is suggested to range between 3% to 7% per day of urinary catheterization.[8] The duration of catheterization is considered to be the biggest risk factor for acquisition of CAUTIs, with the majority of patients having significant bacterial counts in their urine after 10–20 days of catheterization.[12] Although mortality is low in these patients, the overall morbidity burden is extremely high.[13] Costs for these infections are estimated at approximately USD 3,000/episode.[14] Patients with these infections are at risk for bacteremia and sepsis, which can increase length of stay, risks for other ICU-associated infections, and healthcare costs.[13,15]

Pathogenesis

A depiction of the pathogenesis of CAUTI can be seen in figure 1. The majority of pathogenic bacteria found in the urine originate in the gastrointestinal tract and perineum. These organisms may enter the urinary system through the urethra and reach the urinary bladder, ascend through the ureter to the renal pelvis and parenchyma.[16-18] The majority

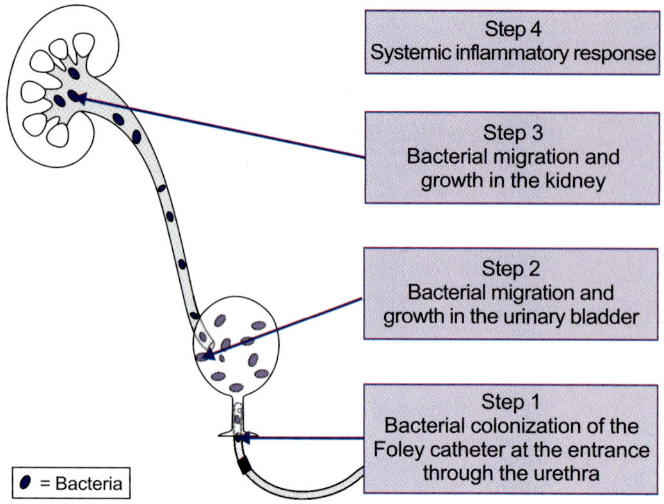

FIGURE 1 Steps in the pathogenesis of catheter-associated urinary tract infections.

of these organisms are introduced extraluminally, through inoculation during catheter insertion.[13] However, they may gain access intraluminally through failure of the closed catheter system or contamination of the collection bag by the hands of healthcare workers.[13,17] For these organisms to cause infection, they must have the appropriate virulence factors, allowing them to attach to the uroepithelium. The most important attachment-related virulence mechanism for organisms causing CAUTI is the ability to produce biofilm.[9] Biofilm is a polysaccharide matrix produced by many bacteria that allows them to attach to various surfaces and also protect them from host immune defenses and antimicrobial agents. The presence of a medical device, such as a urinary catheter, is an opportune site for attachment of bacteria via biofilm. Once the bacteria attach to the catheter and produce biofilm, they are unlikely to be eliminated through any intervention with the exception of removal of the catheter.

Etiology of CAUTI varyies based on the length of catheterization. Common pathogens associated with CAUTI include Enterobacteriaceae, such as *Escherichia coli*, *Klebsiella* species, and *Enterobacter* species. However, in critically ill patients, those with prolonged catheterization, and with prior antimicrobial use, *Psuedomonas aeruginosa*, enterococci, and *Candida* species may be identified.[9] It is important to note that short-term catheterization is associated with single etiology, whereas long-term catheterizations are often polymicrobial.[17,19]

Diagnosis

Clinical diagnosis of CAUTI can often be difficult as patients may present with only fever. Other common symptoms in patients presenting with UTI from the community, such as flank pain or tenderness, may be absent. Therefore, urine culture with a significant amount of microorganisms (typically ≥10^5 colony forming units (cfu)/mL of urine), in conjunction with fever, costovertebral angle pain, or increased white blood cell count is often used as a clinical diagnosis of upper UTI requiring antibiotic therapy. Criteria for diagnosis of CAUTI can be found in table 2. The presence of a urine culture with more than 10^5 cfu without evidence of systemic inflammatory response will diagnose cystitis and asymptomatic or lower UTI.

TABLE 2

Criteria for Clinical Diagnosis of Catheter-associated Urinary Tract Infection

Criteria
• Urine culture with ≥10^5 bacterial colony forming units
Plus at least one of the following:
• Costovertebral angle pain
• Fever (>38°C)
• Leukocytosis

From a surveillance perspective, CAUTIs are defined as outlined by the Centers for Disease Control and Prevention (CDC) and National Healthcare Safety Network (NHSN) definitions for symptomatic UTI or asymptomatic bacteriuria UTI in the presence of a urinary catheter.[20] Although these definitions may not always agree with clinical diagnosis, surveillance definitions are used by infection prevention and control departments to ensure that data are collected in a standardized objective manner. Only through standardized data collection, can outbreaks be detected and appropriate interventions can be instituted.

Management

Although asymptomatic CAUTIs, also called cystitis or lower UTIs in patients with a urinary catheter, are the most common healthcare-associated infections, they should not be treated with antibiotics. Antibiotic therapy is indicated only in patients with symptomatic CAUTI, also called upper UTI or pyelonephritis. The urine Gram's stain and the hospital antibiogram should direct empiric therapy for patients with ICU-associated CAUTIs. If a stratified antibiogram is not available, the results of the Gram's stain should be used to focus therapy. As described previously, patients with short-term catheterization commonly present with Gram-negative rods, such as *E. coli* or *Enterobacter* species. In this case, the CAUTI can be treated empirically with intravenous fluoroquinolones (e.g., ciprofloxacin) or third generation cephalosporins (e.g., ceftriaxone). Due to the likelihood of other etiologic agents, patients with long-term catheterization should be treated with antipseudomonal penicillins (e.g., piperacillin/tazobactam) or cephalosporin (e.g., ceftazidime) in combination with an aminoglycoside (e.g., gentamicin) or an antipseudomonal fluoroquinolone (e.g., ciprofloxacin).

These therapies are directed toward Gram-negative organisms based on the results of the urine Gram's stain. However, if the Gram Stain consistently stain reveals Gram-positive organisms, enterococci or *Staphylococcus aureus* [e.g., methicillin-resistant *S. aureus* (MRSA)] should be considered. For enterococci, patients can be treated with intravenous ampicillin and gentamicin, or vancomycin and gentamicin for penicillin allergic patients. For *S. aureus*, care should be taken to ensure that the seeding of the kidney did not occur from the blood due to an invasive medical device or other extra-urinary source. Intravenous vancomycin can be used for patients with risk factors for MRSA, while nafcillin or cefazolin can be used for patients without risk factors. All patients should be evaluated for clinical stability with the intention to switch the patient from intravenous to oral antimicrobials after stability is reached.

Care must be taken to ensure that the most narrow spectrum antimicrobial agent with activity against the actual etiology of the infection as well as the shortest appropriate length of therapy are instituted to reduce the likelihood of selection for multidrug resistant organisms.

Prevention

The CDC has published guidelines for the prevention of CAUTIs in hospitalized patients.[21] These guidelines are stratified into appropriate use, insertion, and maintenance of the catheter. Recommendations for appropriate usage include minimizing the use and duration of use in all patients, including limiting use for the management of incontinence and for operative patients. Proper techniques for insertion include a focus on hand hygiene prior to manipulation of the urinary catheter, insertion using aseptic technique (e.g., sterile gloves, drape, sponges, antiseptic solutions for skin antisepsis, and lubricant jelly), appropriate anchoring of the device after insertion, and utilization of the smallest bore catheter possible. Appropriate catheter maintenance focuses on the need for a closed drainage system, maintenance of unobstructed urine flow, and use of standard precautions (e.g., hand hygiene and glove use) when manipulating the device. The guidelines do not recommend utilization of complex drainage systems, changing of drainage bags on regular intervals, cleaning the periurethral area while the catheter is in place, or bladder irrigation unless obstruction is anticipated. The guidelines also suggest that changing of the catheter is not recommended. In our experience, we have seen patients developing bacteremia and sepsis after changing the catheter with the same organisms that was present in the urinary bladder. Although the presence of a urinary catheter is strongly associated with the development of a UTI, the use of prophylactic antibiotics may delay the development of a UTI but is associated with it due to antibiotic resistant microorganisms.[22]

VENTILATOR-ASSOCIATED PNEUMONIA

Introduction

VAP is one of the most deadly ICU-associated infections with mortality rates of up to 50%.[23] These infections occur in up to 20% of patients after endotracheal intubation and mechanical ventilation; however, recent advances in prevention are significantly reducing this risk.[24,25] Patients are at a much higher risk for VAP if they have prolonged intubation, paralytic/sedative drugs, advanced age, and enteral feedings.[24] However, many other factors may contribute to a significant proportion of these infections, including supine position and poor oral hygiene.[26] From a healthcare administration standpoint, these infections are increasingly under scrutiny due to their high economic burden on the healthcare facility. One episode of VAP has been estimated to have an attributable cost of between USD 5,000 and 26,000. Furthermore, these patients are estimated to have a 6-fold longer length of hospital stay.[23]

Pathogenesis

A depiction of the pathogenesis of VAP can be seen in figure 2. In healthy individuals, the oropharyngeal space is primarily colonized with Gram-positive organisms. These organisms attach to fibronectin on the surface of the oropharyngeal mucosa.[27] This fibronectin covers Gram-negative bacterial receptor sites on the mucosal cells, preventing colonization by these organisms. However, when patients are hospitalized, they become exposed to a different microflora. If these patients lose their fibronectin, they can become colonized with this new microflora, which includes many multidrug resistant Gram-negative pathogens. Fibronectin may be lost due to the use of antimicrobials, hypotension, hypoxemia, acidosis, or other comorbidities.[28] Due to the varied risks in fibronectin loss in hospitalized patients, each patient

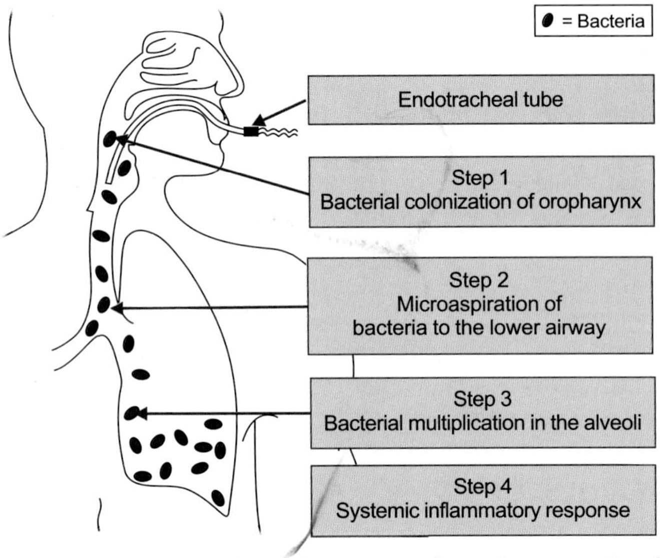

FIGURE 2 Steps in the pathogenesis of ventilator-associated pneumonia.

will have varied changes in the oropharyngeal flora at different times during hospitalization. On top of these factors, oropharyngeal bacteria may produce biofilms and adhere to the endotracheal tube. These bacteria may remain attached to the device until they are aspirated into the alveoli.

Microaspiration is a common event, even in healthy hosts. In fact, up to half of healthy adults may microaspirate during sleep.[29] In intubated patients, subglottic secretions build up around the endotracheal cuff and contain various flora from the patients oropharynx. These secretions may leak around the endotracheal cuff and will be aspirated into the alveolar space. Once present in the alveolar space, these organisms multiply and cause or may cause pneumonia. The host immune defenses prevent a large proportion of pneumonia due to microaspiration through macrophage phagocytosis. These innate immune defenses are responsible for a much lower rate of pneumonia than that of microaspiration. However, if the microorganisms are able to bypass the macrophage, the host will initiate a local and/or systemic inflammatory response.[30] The local immune response includes movement of white blood cells, lymphocytes, and monocytes into the alveoli. This response is primarily mediated by cytokines released from macrophages, including tumor necrosis factor (TNF) and interleukin (IL)-1. Once these cytokines enter the circulation, they will produce a systemic inflammatory response. These immune responses trigger the typical signs and symptoms of pneumonia, including cough, sputum production, tachypnea, pleuritic chest pain, and pulmonary infiltrates. Common bacteria associated with VAP include *P. aeruginosa, S. aureus* (including MRSA), *Klebsiella* species, *Acinetobacter* and *baumannii,* and other Gram-negative rods.[31,32]

Diagnosis

Clinical diagnosis of VAP is performed by a combination of criteria that reflect the local and systemic inflammatory responses to pneumonia in an intubated and ventilated patient. Criteria for this diagnosis can be found in table 3. The first criteria includes the presence of a new and/or progressing pulmonary infiltrate that cannot be explained by another factor, such as pulmonary embolism or congestive heart failure. Various organizations suggest different minimum times that the patient must be on a ventilator to call the pneumonia VAP; but generally, VAP is considered when the pulmonary infiltrate develops 48 hours after intubation. The other clinical criteria used to diagnose VAP include those associated with the local inflammatory response. Microbiological criteria may also be used to diagnose VAP. As bacteria causing VAP will be actively multiplying to significant numbers in the alveolar space, performing quantitative cultures of bronchoalveolar lavage (BAL) increases diagnostic accuracy. Semiquantitative culture of endotracheal aspirates may also be used to identify these bacteria. As BAL may only be performed by a qualified physician, endotracheal aspirates are typically more frequently utilized.

Management

Several risk factors for VAP due to multidrug-resistant organisms have been identified in the literature (Table 4).[32] Patients with VAP without risk factors for multidrug-resistant organisms can be treated empirically with narrow-spectrum antibiotics. On the other hand, patients with risk factors for multidrug-resistant organisms should be treated with broad-spectrum empiric therapy to cover organisms present in a particular ICU. The American

TABLE 3
Criteria for Clinical Diagnosis of Ventilator-associated Pneumonia

Criteria
• New or progressive pulmonary infiltrate
Plus at least one of the following:
• Purulent secretions
• Fever
• Leukocytosis
or
• A bronchoalveolar lavage with ≥10^4 colony forming units/mL

TABLE 4
Risk Factors for Multidrug-resistant Organisms

• Antibiotics within last 30 days prior to diagnosis • Hospitalization for ≥5 days prior to diagnosis • Bronchiectasis (clinical diagnosis) • Known family member with multidrug-resistant organisms • Documented colonization/infection with a multidrug-resistant organism • Hospitalization for ≥2 days within the last 90 days • Residence in a nursing home or extended care facility • Chronic dialysis within the last 30 days • Home infusion therapy (including antibiotics) • Home wound care • Active malignancy (except basal or squamous cell cancer of the skin) • AIDS (clinical diagnosis) • End-stage renal disease (clinical diagnosis) • End-stage liver disease (clinical or histological diagnosis) • End-stage lung disease (e.g., COPD with FEV_1 <30% or O_2 dependent) • Steroids (e.g., predisone >10 mg/day for >7 days) or other immunmodulator • Active chemotherapy within the last 30 days • Active radiotherapy within the last 30 days

AIDS, acquired immunodeficiency syndrome; COPD; chronic obstructive pulmonary disease; FEV_1, forced expiratory volume in 1 second.

Thoracic Society (ATS) guidelines for the management of adults with hospital-acquired, ventilator-associated, and healthcare-associated pneumonia suggest selecting empiric antimicrobial therapy based on whether the patient has late onset VAP (≥5 days) or risk factors for multidrug resistant organisms.[32] If either of these criteria are met, these guidelines suggest using a broad-spectrum therapy for drug resistant pathogens. However, the best method for selection of appropriate empiric therapy should be based on the unit and disease-specific hospital antibiogram. To be useful, the antibiogram should present the number and percentage of organisms identified by body site and unit. We recommend empiric therapy with antibiotics that, according to the local antibiogram, have more than 80% susceptibility to the most likely pathogens.

Once the etiology of the VAP has been identified, the spectrum of therapy should be de-escalated to a more narrow spectrum antimicrobial agent. The goal of this pathogen-directed therapy is to choose the most narrow spectrum antimicrobial that is effective against the pathogen causing the infection. This de-escalation will decrease the risk of "collateral damage", or the disruption of the normal flora, which may predispose the patients to colonization or infection with multidrug-resistant organisms.

Prevention

Mechanisms for the prevention of VAP have been well studied. The most described prevention mechanisms proposed by the Institute for Healthcare Improvement have been combined onto the VAP prevention bundle.[33] This bundle has been shown to reduce the incidence of VAP by more than 45%.[33] The elements of the VAP prevention bundle include:

- Elevation of the head of the patient's bed at 35–40 degrees
- Daily sedation interruptions
- Daily assessment of readiness to wean from the ventilator
- Peptic ulcer disease prophylaxis
- Deep venous thrombosis (DVT) prophylaxis.

Care must be taken with overuse of peptic ulcer disease prophylaxis, as some of these agents have been associated with *C. difficile* infection.[34,35] Other organizations such as the Society for Healthcare Epidemiology of America (SHEA)[24] and the CDC[36] have also issued guidelines for the prevention of VAP and they suggest similar interventions.

CENTRAL LINE-ASSOCIATED BLOODSTREAM INFECTION

Introduction

CLABSIs account for over 10% of all ICU-associated infections in the US.[37] Furthermore, patients with CLABSIs have been documented to have up to 80% increase in all cause, in-hospital mortality compared to hospitalized patients without CLABSIs.[38] Risk factors for CLABSIs include use of catheters with multiple lumens, extended catheterization, femoral catheterization, guidewire catheter exchange, non-sterile catheter insertion, and poor insertion site care.[39] CLABSIs have been estimated to provide USD 6,000–9,000 in excess healthcare costs/infection.[40]

Pathogenesis

A depiction of the pathogenesis of CLABSI can be seen in figure 3. Bacteria causing CLABSI may attach to the catheter intraluminally or extraluminally. The primary mechanism of entry of these bacteria is through colonization on the skin and attachment to the catheter extraluminally. A less likely pathogenesis is intraluminal attachment of bacteria to the catheter via contaminated infusion product.

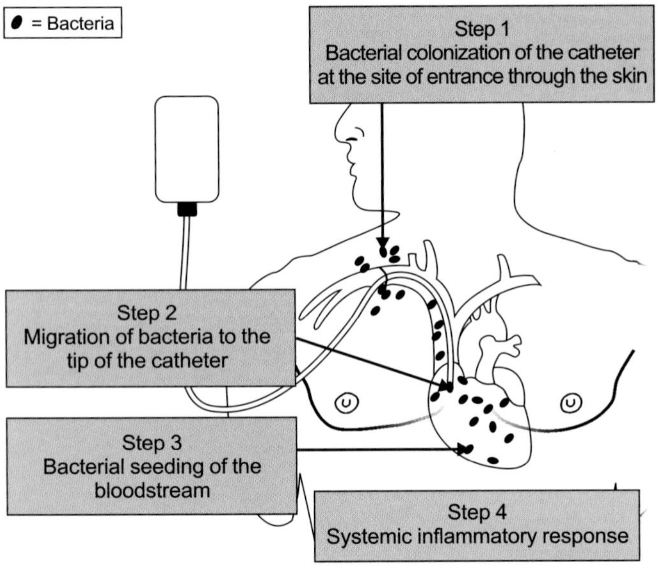

FIGURE 3 Steps in the pathogenesis of catheter-associated bloodstream infections.

From the extraluminal pathogenesis, once the patient is colonized with bacteria near the catheter insertion site, bacteria arrive and attach to the catheter surface. The transfer of these bacteria from the skin to the catheter is most commonly due to the hands of the healthcare worker or patient himself. Once on the surface of the catheter, these bacteria migrate into the inner surface of the catheter and multiply. From the catheter, bacteria may spread locally to the vein causing septic thrombophlebitis. Bacteria may also seed the bloodstream and cause bacteremia. Once bacteria reach the bloodstream, the patient may experience endocarditis, osteomyelitis, or other infections that are due to bacteria entering the bloodstream and seeding other areas of the body.

Diagnosis

CLABSI are often diagnosed clinically in patients with signs and symptoms of infection through bacterial culture from the blood and/or catheter tip if the catheter has been removed. Culturing the tip of the catheter is recommended as part of the diagnostic workup in a patient with suspicion of CLABSI. When central catheters are removed in a patient without clinical suspicion of CLABSI, the tip of the catheter should not be routinely cultured.[2] Criteria for the diagnosis of CLABSI can be found in table 5. Clinically relevant numbers of bacteria are defined as more than 15 cfu on a 5 cm portion of the catheter tip via semiquantitative culture or more than 100 cfu via quantitative broth culture.[2]

One of the challenges for the physician is to define if the organism growing in a blood culture obtained through a catheter has originated from the catheter or is present in the blood as a manifestation of another site of infection (e.g., pneumonia, UTI, etc.). To determine if an organism is originating from the catheter, guidelines recommend drawing one percutaneous blood culture and one culture through the catheter hub at the same time.[2] If the cause of the organism is an infection other than the catheter, the number of organism/mm of blood obtained by a peripheral draw, as well as the one obtained from the catheter will be the same. In these circumstances, the necessary time for the bacteria in the blood culture bottle to reach a level of detection by the microbiology laboratory will be the same. There will be no differential in time to positivity if the infection is not related to the central catheter. On the other hand, if the infection is in the catheter, the blood culture obtained from the central catheter will have a higher concentration of the organisms when compared to the specimen obtained from the peripheral site. Due to higher concentration in the blood culture bottle obtained from the catheter, the time for the organism to reach a level of detection will be significantly reduced. For this, organism that grow from the catheter 2 hours before, the same organism grow from the peripheral site is indicative of CLABSI.[2]

TABLE 5
Criteria for Clinical Diagnosis of Catheter-associated Bloodstream Infection

Criteria
• Culture of the catheter tip with ≥15 colony forming units
or
• Blood culture from the catheter with more than 2 hours differential time to culture positivity in relation to a peripheral blood culture
Plus at least one of the following:
• Fever
• Leukocytosis

Although surveillance definitions may not always agree with clinical diagnosis, they are used by infection prevention and control departments to ensure that data are collected in a standardized, objective manner. Systematic data collection allows for the detection of abnormally high rates and, therefore, do not have to match clinically diagnosed infection. Current surveillance definitions in the US include those proposed by the CDC and NHSN.[20]

Management

After blood cultures are obtained, it is important to begin empiric antimicrobial therapy. It is recommended that empiric therapy should cover the possibility of

MRSA, particularly in institutions where this organism is prevalent.[2] Because of this, vancomycin is often part of the initial empiric therapy for hospitalized patients with suspected CLABSI. Empiric therapy for suspected Gram-negative CLABSIs should be based on the local antibiogram; combination therapy should be used for patients with risk factors for multidrug resistant Gram-negative organisms.[2] Empiric therapy for suspected fungal CLABSIs should include an echinocandin or fluconazole.[2]

Prevention

As is the case with VAP, many prevention mechanisms have been suggested and incorporated into an IHI prevention bundle.[41] The elements of this bundle include five components:

- Hand hygiene
- Maximal barrier precautions upon catheter insertion
- Skin antisepsis prior to insertion with chlorhexidine
- Optimal site selection (avoidance of femoral insertion)
- Daily review of intravenous line necessity with removal of unnecessary lines.

Other strategies that have been suggested include regular full-body bathing with 2% chlorhexidine-impregnated cloths,[42] regular feedback and communication, regarding surveillance process and outcome results, and a focus on staff culture of safety.[43] These evidence-based interventions have been shown to sustain a decrease in CLABSI rates by as much as 60%.[43]

CLOSTRIDIUM DIFFICILE INFECTION

Introduction

C. difficile is an anerobic, spore-forming bacillus that is the most common cause of ICU-associated diarrhea in the US.[44] *C. difficile* infection (CDI) is characterized by diarrhea, though the severity can range from mild to extremely severe. The prototypical CDI consists of watery diarrhea, abdominal distention, increased white blood cell count, and pseudomembranes on the colon. This can progress to fulminant colitis with ileus in a very short period of time. The mortality rate for CDI has been reported to be as high as 80% with very severe CDI.[45] After the initial episode of CDI, it has been estimated that 30% of patients will have a recurrent infection. After one recurrence, this rate may increase to as much as 65% for a subsequent relapse. The cost of one episode of CDI has been estimated to range from USD 2,500–10,000 for uncomplicated cases, with an estimated annual attributable cost to the US in billions of dollars.[45]

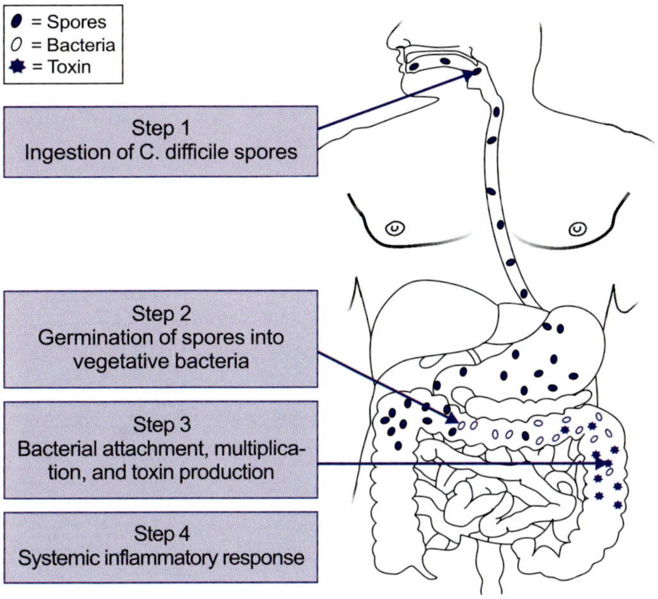

FIGURE 4 Steps in the pathogenesis of *Clostridium difficile* infection.

Pathogenesis

A depiction of the pathogenesis of *C. difficile* infection can be seen in figure 4. *C. difficile* is characterized as a spore-forming bacillus. In the hospital environment, *C. difficile* survives in the form of spores. Colonization of a patient's colon with *C. difficile* spores occurs when the patient comes in contact with the organism in the healthcare environment. This is most likely to occur via contaminated hands of healthcare workers, but may also occur from other mechanisms, such as self-inoculation through fomites or even through foodstuffs.[46,47] Host factors associated with colonization include previous hospitalization, chemotherapy, and lack of antibodies against *C. difficile* toxin B.[44] One of the primary defense mechanisms of the gastrointestinal tract against pathogens is the low pH in the stomach. The use of gastric acid modifying agents allow *C. difficile* spores to bypass the stomach and reach the small bowel.[34] Therefore, the use of these agents may be considered to be another risk factor associated with *C. difficile* colonization.

The next step in the pathogenesis of CDI includes the germination of the *C. difficile* spores into the vegetative form of the organism. It is still unclear as to the mechanisms causing sporulation and germination of this organism; however, various mechanisms have been hypothesized. One of the more common hypotheses includes the importance of bile salts and amino acids, such as taurocholate and glycine in the germination of *C. difficile* spores; however, germination is likely very complex in nature and still poorly understood.[48]

Once vegetative forms of *C. difficile* are present in the gastrointestinal tract, it is necessary to have disruption of the normal gastrointestinal flora for the *C. difficile* to be able to attach and multiply. The most common mechanism for this to occur is through antibiotic use. Even narrow spectrum antimicrobial agents are capable of eradicating many of the normal microorganisms in the gastrointestinal tract and cumulative antibiotic use is significantly associated with CDI.[49]

The final step in the pathogenesis of CDI is the production of toxin by the organism. CDI is a toxin mediated disease and it cannot occur without the toxin. Once germinated, the vegetative form of the organism produces toxins that mediate CDI. The two major toxins of *C. difficile* are toxin A and toxin B; although not all *C. difficile* organisms have the genes necessary to produce these toxins. A new hypervirulent strain of *C. difficile,* NAP-1 or ribotype 027 also produces a binary toxin, although the impact of this toxin on the pathophysiology of the disease is unclear. These toxins inhibit Rho-GTPases, which reduce the integrity of the cell cytoskeleton, leading to death of the intestinal epithelial cells. Once the cells are damaged, they release a number of cytokines and activate neutrophils, which release proinflammatory cytokines. This induces a severe inflammatory response and an increase in intestinal permeability and fluid accumulation within the intestinal lumen, leading to diarrhea.[50] The build-up of neutrophils and dead epithelial cells characterizes the pseudomembrane on the colon of patients with pseudomembranous colitis.

Depending on the amount of toxin produced by the organism, as well as host factors, the patient may have a mild or severe CDI. Severe CDI is characterized by a high white blood cell count (>15,000 cells/μL) or a serum creatinine 1.5 times the patient's normal level. However, some clinicians have suggested more than 20,000 cells/μL as a white blood cell cutoff, while others use scoring systems. One common scoring system provides one point for each of the following criteria:

- Age above 60 years
- Temperature more than 38.3°C
- Serum albumin above 2.5 mg/dL
- Peripheral white blood cell count more than 15,000 cells/μL.

Patients with 2 or more points are considered to have severe disease.

Diagnosis

From a clinical standpoint, CDI is diagnosed when the patient has clinical signs of CDI (diarrhea, abdominal cramps, fever, and leukocytosis), as well as one of the following:

- Laboratory identification of *C. difficile* or *C. difficile* toxin
- Visualization of pseudomembrane on endoscopy.

These criteria can be found in table 6.

TABLE 6

Criteria for Clinical Diagnosis of *Clostridium difficile* Infection

Criteria
• Clinical symptoms of *C. difficile* infection (diarrhea)
Plus one of the following:
• Laboratory identification of *C. difficile* or *C. difficile* toxin
• Visualization of pseudomembranes on endoscopy

Common techniques for laboratory identification include detection of toxins A or B by enzyme immunoassay, detection of toxin activity by cell cytotoxin assay, detection of the genes that encode for toxins A, B or binary toxin by polymerase chain reaction (PCR), and detection of the organism by the glutamate dehydrogenase antigen test, or via anerobic culture. Some investigators suggest using 2-step testing to increase the sensitivity and specificity.[51] These 2-step tests typically include the glutamate dehydrogenase combined with either enzyme immunoassay or PCR. The cell cytotoxin assay is typically considered to be the gold standard test for *C. difficile,* while the glutamate dehydrogenase test has been shown to be equivalent to anerobic culture. Potential issues with the glutamate dehydrogenase test include the detection of *C. difficile* antigen vs. toxin. Detection of the antigen only indicates the presence of the organism and does not differentiate between infection and colonization. Although PCR has become popular recently, it may be less effective at detecting the NAP-1 strain,[53] and there are also concerns regarding its ability to detect organisms causing infection vs. colonization. Without a more clear differentiation between infection and colonization, test results may lead to overtreatment and perpetuation of the CDI cycle.[52]

Management

The most important factor in the management of patients with CDI is to rebuild the normal gastrointestinal flora. This can only be achieved by discontinuing the inciting antimicrobial therapy. However, this is not always possible, so the narrowest spectrum antibiotic in the shortest effective durations should be used. Some studies have suggested the use of prebiotic or probiotic therapy to replenish the normal flora, but results have been conflicting.[53] The lack of effectiveness of probiotics is likely due to the limited range and quantity of bacteria provided in a dose of probiotic. However, recent advances in fecal microbiota transplantation have shown very promising results, with up to 92% of patients resolving CDI after treatment.[54] This may be the only mechanism to truly replenish the entire normal flora in a consistent manner.

Patients may also need to be treated with antimicrobial therapy to resolve the infection. Initial antibiotic therapy for a non-severe CDI typically includes oral metronidazole or oral vancomycin. Cure rates of non-severe CDI have been show to be similar with use of each of these agents. Oral metronidazole has been favored due to the potential risk for vancomycin-resistant enterococcus (VRE) with vancomycin use, as well as the significantly increased costs associated with oral vancomycin.

Approximately, 30% of patients will have recurrent CDI.[45] Initial recurrences are treated in a similar fashion to initial disease although subsequent occurrences may favor use of a pulse tapered oral vancomycin therapy, rifaximin, or fidaxomicin.

Prevention

Prevention of CDI can be difficult due to the spore-forming nature of the organism. Prevention efforts may be fruitful through appropriate hand hygiene, diligent isolation, appropriate environmental disinfection, and antimicrobial stewardship.

It is known that *C. difficile* spores do not respond to alcohol-based hand rubs, and therefore, it has been recommended to use soap and water to physically remove the spores from hands. However, the alcohol based hand rubs will be effective against the vegetative form of the organism. It has also become clear that soap and water is not particularly effective due to the increased ability of *C. difficile* spores to adhere to the human skin. Therefore, interventions that prevent hand contamination, such as universal glove use, has become a favored intervention of late. Appropriate isolation includes use of standard and contact precautions as outlined in the Centers for Disease Control and Prevention isolation guildelines.[55] This includes diligent glove and gown use as well as appropriate hand hygiene.

Since *C. difficile* spores can persist in the environment for a significant period of time, it is important to maintain adequate environmental disinfection protocols.[57] However, the difficulty arises as few disinfectants are effective against *C. difficile* and currently, only hypochlorite and hydrogen peroxide are recommended for disinfection of this organism.[57,58] Antimicrobial stewardship is arguably one of the most important factors in the prevention of CDI. Limiting overuse and misuse of antimicrobials, particularly broad-spectrum antimicrobials, such as carbapenems and fluoroquinolones will limit the collateral damage to the normal gastrointestinal flora of hospitalized patients. Without the disruption of the normal gastrointestinal flora, *C. difficile* will be limited in its ability to germinate, attach to the gastrointestinal epithelia, produce toxin, and cause disease.

CONCLUSION

The last step in the pathogenesis of all ICU-associated infections is the host response with the development of a systemic inflammatory response. This creates a diagnostic challenge for the treating physician, since a patient in the ICU with evidence of fever and leukocytosis may have any of the ICU-associated infections described in this chapter. The initial management requires full clinical evaluation of the patient and appropriate laboratory investigation to define the etiology of infection. Initiation of empiric antibiotic therapy, pending results of the diagnostic work-up is important in ICU patients with evidence of systemic inflammatory response who are clinically unstable. A better understanding of the pathogenesis of ICU-associated infections will facilitate their diagnosis and facilitation appropriate selection of empiric therapy, leading to improved clinical outcomes.

Implementation of prevention bundles in ICU settings are critical for decreasing the incidence of ICU-associated infections. Although 100% prevention of all ICU-associated infections may be an unrealistic achievement for patients in the ICU setting, it should remain the goal for all infection prevention and control programs.

REFERENCES

1. Peyrani P, Allen M, Wiemken TL, Haque NZ, Zervos MJ, Ford KD, et al.; IMPACT-HAP Study Group.. Severity of Disease and Clinical Outcomes in Patients With Hospital-Acquired Pneumonia Due to Methicillin-Resistant Staphylococcus aureus Strains Not Influenced by the Presence of the Panton-Valentine Leukocidin Gene. *Clin Infect Dis*. 2011;53:766-71.
2. Mermel LA, Allon M, Bouza E, Craven DE, Flynn P, O'Grady NP, et al. Clinical practice guidelines for the diagnosis and management of intravascular catheter-related infection: 2009 Update by the Infectious Diseases Society of America. *Clin Infect Dis*. 2009;49:1-45.
3. Paterson DL. "Collateral damage" from cephalosporin or quinolone antibiotic therapy. *Clin Infect Dis*. 2004;38:S341-5.
4. Otter JA, Yezli S, French GL. The role played by contaminated surfaces in the transmission of nosocomial pathogens. *Infect Control Hosp Epidemiol*. 2011;32:687-99.

5. Pallam H, McCurley K, Harting J, Clay J, Muldoon SB, Weimken T, et al. Evaluating the role of the environment in an outbreak investigation of *Acinetobacter baumannii*: application of social network analysis. American Public Health Association. Available from: https://apha.confex.com/apha/138am/webprogram/Paper225261.html. 2010.
6. Fridkin SK, Welbel SF, Weinstein RA. Magnitude and prevention of nosocomial infections in the intensive care unit. *Infect Dis Clin North Am.* 1997;11:479-96.
7. Vincent JL, Rello J, Marshall J, Silva E, Anzueto A, Martin CD, et al.; EPIC II Group of Investigators. International study of the prevalence and outcomes of infection in intensive care units. *JAMA.* 2009;302:2323-9.
8. Lo E, Nicolle L, Classen D, Arias KM, Podgorny K, Anderson DJ, et al. Strategies to prevent catheter-associated urinary tract infections in acute care hospitals. *Infect Control Hosp Epidemiol.* 2008;29:S41-50.
9. Saint S, Chenoweth CE. Biofilms and catheter-associated urinary tract infections. *Infect Dis Clin North Am.* 2003; 17:411-32.
10. Weinstein JW, Mazon D, Pantelick E, Reagan-Cirincione P, Dembry LM, Hierholzer WJ Jr. A decade of prevalence surveys in a tertiary-care center: trends in nosocomial infection rates, device utilization, and patient acuity. *Infect Control Hosp Epidemiol.* 1999;20:543-8.
11. Huang WC, Wann SR, Lin SL, Kunin CM, Kung MH, Lin CH, et al. Catheter-associated urinary tract infections in intensive care units can be reduced by prompting physicians to remove unnecessary catheters. *Infect Control Hosp Epidemiol.* 2004;25:974-8.
12. Riley DK, Classen DC, Stevens LE, Burke JP. A large randomized clinical trial of a silver-impregnated urinary catheter: lack of efficacy and staphylococcal super-infection. *Am J Med.* 1995;98:349-56.
13. Tambyah PA, Maki DG. Catheter-associated urinary tract infection is rarely symptomatic: a prospective study of 1,497 catheterized patients. *Arch Intern Med.* 2000;160:678-82.
14. Saint S. Clinical and economic consequences of nosocomial catheter-related bacteriuria. *Am J Infect Control.* 2000;28: 68-75.
15. Saint S, Kaufman SR, Rogers MA, Baker PD, Boyko EJ, Lipsky BA. Risk factors for nosocomial urinary tract-related bacteremia: a case-control study. *Am J Infect Control.* 2006;34:401-7.
16. Daifuku R, Stamm WE. Association of rectal and urethral colonization with urinary tract infection in patients with indwelling catheters. *JAMA.* 1984;252:2028-30.
17. Stamm WE. Catheter-associated urinary tract infections: epidemiology, pathogenesis, and prevention. *Am J Med.* 1991;91:65S-71S.
18. Tannock GW. The bowel microflora: an important source of urinary tract pathogens. *World J Urol.* 1999;17:339-44.
19. Warren JW, Tenney JH, Hoopes JM, Muncie HL, Anthony WC. A prospective microbiologic study of bacteriuria in patients with chronic indwelling urethral catheters. *J Infect Dis.* 1982;146:719-23.
20. Centers for Disease Control and Prevention. National Healthcare Safety Network (NHSN) Device-associated module. Available from: http://www.cdc.gov/nhsn/psc_da.html. 2012.
21. Gould CV, Umscheid CA, Agarwal RK, Kuntz G, Pegues DA; Healthcare Infection Control Practices Advisory Committee. Guideline for prevention of catheter-associated urinary tract infections 2009. *Infect Control Hosp Epidemiol.* 2010;31:319-26.
22. Hooton TM, Bradley SF, Cardenas DD, Colgan R, Geerlings SE, Rice JC, et al.; Infectious Diseases Society of America. Diagnosis, Prevention, and Treatment of Catheter-Associated Urinary Tract Infection in Adults: 2009 International Clinical Practice Guidelines from the Infectious Diseases Society of America. *Clin Infect Dis.* 2010;50:625-63.
23. Warren DK, Shukla SJ, Olsen MA, Kollef MH, Hollenbeak CS, Cox MJ, et al. Outcome and attributable cost of ventilator-associated pneumonia among intensive care unit patients in a suburban medical center. *Crit Care Med.* 2003;31:1312-7.
24. Coffin SE, Klompas M, Classen D, Arias KM, Podgorny K, Anderson DJ, et al. Strategies to prevent ventilator-associated pneumonia in acute care hospitals. *Infect Control Hosp Epidemiol.* 2008;29:S31-40.
25. Safdar N, Dezfulian C, Collard HR, Saint S. Clinical and economic consequences of ventilator-associated pneumonia: a systematic review. *Crit Care Med.* 2005;33: 2184-93.
26. Kollef MH. The prevention of ventilator-associated pneumonia. *N Engl J Med.* 1999;340:627-34.
27. Woods DE, Straus DC, Johanson WG, Jr., Bass JA. Role of fibronectin in the prevention of adherence of Pseudomonas aeruginosa to buccal cells. *J Infect Dis.* 1981;143:784-90.
28. Ramirez J. Switch therapy in hospitalized patients with serious infections. Pharmacia Corporation; 2002.
29. Huxley EJ, Viroslav J, Gray WR, Pierce AK. Pharyngeal aspiration in normal adults and patients with depressed consciousness. *Am J Med.* 1978;64:564-8.
30. Ramírez P, Ferrer M, Gimeno R, Tormo S, Valencia M, Piñer R, et al. Systemic inflammatory response and increased risk for ventilator-associated pneumonia: a preliminary study. *Crit Care Med.* 2009;37:1691-5.
31. Ibrahim EH, Tracy L, Hill C, Fraser VJ, Kollef MH. The occurrence of ventilator-associated pneumonia in a community hospital: risk factors and clinical outcomes. *Chest.* 2001;120:555-61.
32. American Thoracic Society; Infectious Diseases Society of America. Guidelines for the management of adults with hospital-acquired, ventilator-associated, and healthcare-associated pneumonia. *Am J Respir Crit Care Med.* 2005; 171:388-416.
33. *How-to Guide: Prevent Ventilator-Associated Pneumonia.* Cambridge, MA: Institute for Healthcare Improvement; 2012. Available from: http://www.ihi.org/knowledge/Pages/Tools/HowtoGuidePreventVAP.aspx.
34. Kuehn BM. Reflux drugs linked to C. difficile-related diarrhea. *JAMA.* 2012;307:1014.
35. Kim YG, Graham DY, Jang BI. Proton Pump Inhibitor Use and Recurrent Clostridium difficile-associated Disease: A Case-control Analysis Matched by Propensity Score. *J Clin Gastroenterol.* 2012;46:397-400.
36. Tablan OC, Anderson LJ, Besser R, Bridges C, Hajjeh R; CDC; Healthcare Infection Control Practices Advisory Committee. Guidelines for preventing health-care—

associated pneumonia, 2003: recommendations of CDC and the Healthcare Infection Control Practices Advisory Committee. *MMWR Recomm Rep.* 2004;53:1-36.
37. Klevens RM, Edwards JR, Richards CL Jr, Horan TC, Gaynes RP, Pollock DA, et al. Estimating health care-associated infections and deaths in U.S. hospitals, 2002. *Public Health Rep.* 2007;122:160-6.
38. Siempos, II, Kopterides P, Tsangaris I, Dimopoulou I, Armaganidis AE. Impact of catheter-related bloodstream infections on the mortality of critically ill patients: a meta-analysis. *Crit Care Med.* 2009;37:2283-9.
39. O'Grady NP, Alexander M, Dellinger EP, Gerberding JL, Heard SO, Maki DG, et al.; Healthcare Infection Control Practices Advisory Committee. Guidelines for the prevention of intravascular catheter-related infections. *Infect Control Hosp Epidemiol.* 2002;23:759-69.
40. Saint S, Veenstra DL, Lipsky BA. The clinical and economic consequences of nosocomial central venous catheter-related infection: are antimicrobial catheters useful? *Infect Control Hosp Epidemiol.* 2000;21:375-80.
41. *How-to Guide: Prevent Central Line-Associated Bloodstream Infections.* Cambridge, MA: Institute for Healthcare Improvement; 2012. Available from: http://www.ihi.org/knowledge/Pages/Tools/HowtoGuidePreventCentralLineAssociatedBloodstreamInfection.aspx.
42. Bleasdale SC, Trick WE, Gonzalez IM, Lyles RD, Hayden MK, Weinstein RA. Effectiveness of chlorhexidine bathing to reduce catheter-associated bloodstream infections in medical intensive care unit patients. *Arch Intern Med.* 2007;167:2073-9.
43. Pronovost PJ, Goeschel CA, Colantuoni E, Watson S, Lubomski LH, Berenholtz SM, et al. Sustaining reductions in catheter related bloodstream infections in Michigan intensive care units: observational study. *BMJ.* 2010; 340:c309.
44. Loo VG, Bourgault AM, Poirier L, Lamothe F, Michaud S, Turgeon N, et al. Host and pathogen factors for Clostridium difficile infection and colonization. *N Engl J Med.* 2011;365:1693-703.
45. Dubberke E. Clostridium difficile infection: The scope of the problem. *J Hosp Med.* 2012;7:S1-4.
46. Guerrero DM, Nerandzic MM, Jury LA, Jinno S, Chang S, Donskey CJ. Acquisition of spores on gloved hands after contact with the skin of patients with Clostridium difficile infection and with environmental surfaces in their rooms. *Am J Infect Control.* 2012;40:556-8.
47. Harvey RB, Norman KN, Andrews K, Hume ME, Scanlan CM, Callaway TR, et al. Clostridium difficile in Poultry and Poultry Meat. *Foodborne Pathog Dis.* 2011;8:1321-3
48. Heeg D, Burns DA, Cartman ST, Minton NP. Spores of Clostridium difficile Clinical Isolates Display a Diverse Germination Response to Bile Salts. *PLoS One.* 2012; 7:e32381.
49. Stevens V, Dumyati G, Fine LS, Fisher SG, van Wijngaarden E. Cumulative antibiotic exposures over time and the risk of Clostridium difficile infection. *Clin Infect Dis.* 2011;53:42-8.
50. Carter GP, Rood JI, Lyras D. The role of toxin A and toxin B in the virulence of Clostridium difficile. *Trends Microbiol.* 2012;20:21-9.
51. Clark NS, Doughton MJ, Karas JA, Enoch DA. Two-step algorithm for the detection of Clostridium difficile from stool samples. *J Hosp Infect.* 2011;79:95-6.
52. Kaltsas A, Simon M, Unruh LH, Son C, Wroblewski D, Musser KA, et al. Clinical and laboratory characteristics of Clostridium difficile infection in patients with discordant diagnostic test results. *J Clin Microbiol.* 2012;50:1303-7.
53. Kelly CP, LaMont JT. Clostridium difficile—more difficult than ever. *N Engl J Med.* 2008;359:1932-40.
54. Gough E, Shaikh H, Manges AR. Systematic review of intestinal microbiota transplantation (fecal bacteriotherapy) for recurrent Clostridium difficile infection. *Clin Infect Dis.* 2011;53:994-1002.
55. Siegel JD, Rhinehart E, Jackson M, Chiarello L. 2007 Guideline for Isolation Precautions: Preventing Transmission of Infectious Agents in Health Care Settings. *Am J Infect Control.* 2007;35:S65-164.
56. McFarland LV. What's lurking under the bed? Persistence and predominance of particular Clostridium difficile strains in a hospital and the potential role of environmental contamination. *Infect Control Hosp Epidemiol.* 2002;23: 639-40.
57. Barbut F, Yezli S, Otter JA. Activity in vitro of hydrogen peroxide vapour against Clostridium difficile spores. *J Hosp Infect.* 2012;80:85-7.
58. Mayfield JL, Leet T, Miller J, Mundy LM. Environmental control to reduce transmission of Clostridium difficile. *Clin Infect Dis.* 2000;31:995-1000.

CHAPTER 18

Ventilator-associated Pneumonia

Alejandra López-Giraldo, Rosanel Amaro, Gianluigi L Bassi, Miquel Ferrer, Antoni Torres

ABSTRACT

Ventilator-associated pneumonia (VAP) is an intensive care unit (ICU)—acquired infection that develops in tracheally intubated patients on mechanical ventilation for at least 48 hours. Studies report 5–16 VAP cases/1,000 ventilator days and 20–50% associated mortality, depending on comorbidities, illness severity, pathogens, and quality of antibiotic treatment. Endogenous colonization is pivotal for VAP development. Aerobic Gram-negative pathogens, *Pseudomonas aeruginosa*, and methicillin-resistant *Staphylococcus aureus* (MRSA) are the most common etiologic agents. Preventive strategies, grouped as bundles, have shown efficacy in decreasing VAP incidence and should be implemented in hospital settings. Diagnostic strategies, in the presence of clinical suspicion of nosocomial pneumonia, should include culture of respiratory samples, before starting or changing antibiotics. Etiology and antimicrobial susceptibility of causative VAP microorganisms varies according to the ICU population, duration of hospital stay, and prior antimicrobial therapy. Thus, the choice of empiric treatment should be based on these factors and adjusted or de-escalated following microbiologic results.

INTRODUCTION

Ventilator-associated pneumonia (VAP) is the most common hospital-acquired infection among tracheally intubated and mechanically ventilated patients in the intensive care unit (ICU). In comparison to other ICU-acquired infections, VAP is associated with worse morbidity, mortality, and healthcare costs. Therefore, several preventive strategies are routinely applied to reduce incidence of VAP. Prompt antimicrobial treatment is mandatory following VAP development; nevertheless, there is still lack of consensus on diagnostic approaches. In this chapter, we have described epidemiology, etiology, and risks factors of the disease and have reviewed the evidence on the preventive measures, diagnosis, and treatment of VAP in critically ill and mechanically ventilated patients.

DEFINITION

VAP is a hospital-acquired infection that develops in patients admitted to an ICU, who have been tracheally intubated and have received mechanical ventilation for at least 48 hours.[1,2] Specifically, VAP is defined as an infection of the lung parenchyma caused by pathogens not present or incubating at the time when mechanical ventilation was started.

VAP that occurs during the first 4 days of mechanical ventilation is referred to as early-onset in order to differentiate from late-onset VAP that develops thereafter; the time of onset has important implications on etiology, empirical antimicrobial treatment, and outcomes.[3] Some authors have used a 7 days cutoff.[4] However, it is unknown what is the best cutoff to separate early from late onset pneumonia, since there are no well-designed trials supporting current time limits.

The term VAP is potentially a misnomer, since the endotracheal tube (ETT) plays the most important role in the pathogenesis of VAP. The ETT creates a direct conduit for bacteria to reach lower airways and greatly impairs host defenses. Interestingly, studies have demonstrated that mechanical ventilation could also increase risk of pneumonia.[5-7] Indeed, lungs become highly susceptible to bacterial colonization when injurious ventilatory settings are applied, i.e., with high tidal volumes and low positive end expiratory pressure (PEEP). Therefore, either "ETT-associated pneumonia" or "ventilation-acquired pneumonia" could be better terms to describe pneumonia in tracheally intubated and mechanically ventilated patients. Ventilation-acquired pneumonia would additionally allow physicians and scientists to maintain the current acronym "VAP".[8]

EPIDEMIOLOGY

Incidence

VAP is the most common nosocomial infection in mechanically ventilated patients.[1] The exact incidence of VAP is difficult to establish because of overlapping with lower respiratory tract infections and the difficulties to diagnose it accurately. The incidence density of VAP, expressed as the total number of VAP episodes/1,000 ventilator days, ranges from 5 to 16.[9] VAP prolongs the time on mechanical ventilation and the length of ICU and hospital stay.[10-12]

Incidence rates greatly depend on the type of population studied, presence or absence of risk factors for colonization by multidrug-resistant (MDR) pathogens, and the type and intensity of applied preventive strategies. Additionally, the lack of gold-standard methods to diagnose VAP partly explains why incidence rates vary widely in the literature.

Tracheal intubation and mechanical ventilation are the main risk factors for VAP during the first week of ventilation. Cook et al.[12] estimated that the risk of VAP is 1%/day of mechanical ventilation. They also demonstrated that the risk changes over time, being 3% in the first 5 days on mechanical ventilation, 2% from 5th to 10th day, and 1% for the remaining days. Considering that most of the patients are intubated for less than a week, nearly half of the VAP cases occur during the first days of mechanical ventilation.

Mortality

Hospital mortality rate of patients with VAP is significantly higher than that of patients without VAP. Crude VAP mortality rates range between 20 and 50%, depending on comorbidities, illness severity, pathogens, and quality of antibiotic treatment.[2] Nevertheless, the mortality rates reported in the literature are inconsistent, and thus, the prognostic impact of VAP is debatable.[13] Mortality rates are higher when VAP is associated with bacteremia, especially with *Pseudomonas aeruginosa* or *Acinetobacter* species, medical rather than surgical illness, and treatment with ineffective antibiotic therapy.[1]

The time of VAP onset strongly affects outcomes.[3] Late-onset VAP has the worst prognosis in comparison with early-onset VAP. Typically, late-onset VAP is caused by high-risk microorganisms, and hospital mortality rates can be as high as 65% when VAP is caused by *P. aeruginosa, Acinetobacter* species, or *Stenotrophomonas maltophilia.*

The VAP-predisposition, insult, response, and organ dysfunction (PIRO) score could be useful in daily practice, as it predicts patient's outcome through a simple assessment upon the day of VAP diagnosis. The VAP-PIRO score has proven efficiency in assessing VAP severity and predicting ICU mortality rate.[14] Patients with a score above 2 consistently present worse outcomes.

VAP is associated with higher healthcare costs. Patients who develop VAP remain longer in the ICU and hospital, and the increased level of care and need for additional invasive procedures drastically increases healthcare costs. It has been reported that each case of VAP is associated with additional hospital costs between USD 20,000 and 40,000.[11] These data on the healthcare burden emphasize the need for strong implementation of preventive measures.

PATHOGENESIS

Tracheally intubated patients can be colonized via exogenous and endogenous pathogenic sources. When pathogens gain access to the lower respiratory tract in healthy, nonintubated patients, infection is prevented by several defense mechanisms, such as cough, mucociliary clearance, and cellular and humoral immunity responses to ultimately maintain the sterility of lower respiratory tract. Critically ill patients are already at high risk of infection because of the underlying illness, comorbidities, malnutrition, immunosuppressive treatment, and invasive devices/procedures. However, tracheal intubation is the *conditio sine qua non* (without which it cannot be) for the development of pneumonia, because it facilitates aspiration of oropharyngeal pathogens across its cuff and hinders intrinsic respiratory defenses. Following aspiration and colonization of the airways, the occurrence of VAP primarily depends on the size of the inoculum, patient's functional status, and competency of host defenses.

Role of Tracheal Tube in the Pathogenesis of Ventilator-associated Pneumonia

Pulmonary aspiration of colonized oropharyngeal secretions across the tracheal tube cuff is the main pathogenic mechanism for development of VAP.

The ETT, commonly used in the ICU for long-term mechanically ventilated patients, includes a high-volume low-pressure cuff that was originally designed to control pressure exerted against the tracheal wall and prevent tracheal injury.[15,16] However, the high-volume low-pressure cuff diameter is larger than the tracheal diameter and hence, upon cuff inflation within the trachea, longitudinal folds invariably form along the cuff surface, causing consistent micro and macro aspiration of oropharyngeal secretions.[17]

Pathogens may also grow on the internal surface of the ETT and ultimately, translocate into the lungs. The ETT is commonly made of polyvinyl chloride (PVC) and bacteria easily adhere on its internal surface to form a complex structure called biofilm.[18,19] Bacteria within the biofilm are difficult to eradicate and antibacterial efficacy of the host immune response and antibiotics is largely reduced. During mechanical ventilation, biofilm particles may dislodge into the airways due to inspiratory airflow[17] and invasive medical interventions, such as tracheal aspiration[20] and bronchoscopy.

Sources of Colonization

Tracheally intubated patients can be colonized either exogenously or endogenously. Patients are colonized exogenously by contaminated respiratory equipment, ICU environment, and hands of the ICU staff. Several reports have described ICU outbreaks due to colonized bronchoscopes,[21,22] water supply,[23,24] respiratory equipment,[25,26] humidifiers,[27] ventilator temperature sensors,[28,29] respiratory nebulizers,[30,31] and contaminated environment.[32]

Endogenous colonization is believed to be pivotal for VAP development. It is well acknowledged that in critically ill patients, the oral flora shifts early to a predominance of aerobic Gram-negative pathogens,[33,34] *P. aeruginosa,* and methicillin-resistant *Staphylococcus aureus* (MRSA). Therefore, pulmonary aspiration of oropharyngeal contents increases the risk for airway colonization and infection. There is still controversy regarding the exact sequence of colonization and sources of infection in the pathogenesis of VAP. Early studies by Feldman et al.[35] found that in patients undergoing mechanical ventilation, the oropharynx is the first site to be colonized by pathogens (36 hours), followed by the stomach (36–60 hours), the lower respiratory tract (60–84 hours), and thereafter, the tracheal tube (60–96 hours).

Dental Plaque

ICU patients are at higher risk for dental plaque colonization, due to difficulties in oral hygiene, changes in salivary properties, and change of oral flora by antibiotic therapy. Fourrier et al.[36] found that prolonged ICU stay increases risk for colonization of dental plaque by aerobic pathogens. Moreover, the investigators found that colonization of dental plaque was highly predictive of concurrent or subsequent nosocomial infection.

Stomach

According to the gastropulmonary hypothesis of colonization, the stomach of ICU patients is often colonized by pathogens due to alkalinization of gastric contents by enteral nutrition and stress ulcer prophylaxis. Supine horizontal position and the presence of a nasogastric tube may favor gastroesophageal reflux and translocation of gastric microorganisms into the oropharynx, which are ultimately aspirated across the ETT cuff.[37]

Impairment of Respiratory Defense During Critical Illness and Tracheal Intubation

Anatomical barrier of the larynx structures promptly prevents aspiration of pathogens into the airways. Abduction of the true and false vocal folds allow full closure of the airways; moreover, the airways are additionally protected by the epiglottis that moves over the top of the larynx to divert any fluid or solids from passing into the pyriform sinuses. Following intubation, the tracheal tube completely bypasses these anatomical barriers and creates a direct conduit for bacteria to reach lower airways.

Cough is one of the most efficient mechanisms to prevent further translocation of pathogens that may have gained access into airways. Endotracheal intubation and commonly prescribed sedatives or analgesic, impede efficient coughing.

Mucociliary clearance is the primary innate airway defense mechanism to clear pathogens. Studies in animals have consistently shown that inflation of the ETT cuff within the trachea lowers mucociliary velocity by 37% within an hour and 52% after 2 hours.[38] Clinical studies[39] in critically ill, tracheally intubated patients have confirmed these results and found that mucociliary velocity is highly impaired (0.8–1.4 mm/min); moreover, lower mucociliary clearance has been associated with higher risks for pulmonary complications.

ETIOLOGY AND RISK FACTORS FOR MICROORGANISMS

VAP is caused by several pathogens most commonly found in hospital settings and, in many patients, more than one pathogen may be isolated. *P. aeruginosa, Escherichia coli, Klebsiella pneumoniae*, or *Acinetobacter* species are the most frequent aerobic, Gram-negative pathogens isolated; whereas, *S. aureus* is the predominant Gram-positive pathogen.[1,11,40]

The high rate of polymicrobial infection in VAP has been repeatedly shown. In a study[41] in 124 critically ill patients, 52% had monomicrobial VAP, while 48% presented polymicrobial VAP. In most patients, only 2 bacteria were isolated (34%); however, up to 4 different bacteria coexisted in 6% of the patients. Interestingly, no differences were detected in mortality rate at 30 days between patients with polymicrobial or monomicrobial infection.

Different organisms may be encountered in patients with specific underlying diseases. For instance, patients with chronic obstructive pulmonary disease (COPD) are at an increased risk for *Haemophilus influenzae, Moraxella catarrhalis, P. aeruginosa,* and *Streptococcus pneumoniae* infections.[42] Patients with acute respiratory distress syndrome (ARDS) are at a higher risk for developing VAP caused by *S. aureus, P. aeruginosa,* and *A. baumannii* and often, VAP in these patients is caused by multiple pathogens.[43] Finally, patients with trauma or neurological diseases are at an increased risk for *S. aureus, H. influenzae,* and *S. pneumoniae* infections.[44,45]

It is fundamental to promptly identify MDR pathogens in order to guide the patient regarding an appropriate antibiotic treatment. VAP pathogens that are potentially multidrug-resistant are *P. aeruginosa*, MRSA, *Acinetobacter* species, *S. maltophilia, Burkholderia cepacia,* and extended spectrum β-lactamase (ESBL+) *Klebsiella pneumoniae.* Conversely, *S. pneumoniae, H. influenzae,* methicillin-sensitive *S. aureus,* (MSSA) and antibiotic-sensitive *Enterobacteriaceae* are considered non-MDR pathogens. Patients at risk of being colonized by MDR pathogens are extremely heterogeneous, commonly present several comorbidities, and have received antibiotics prior to and during the course of their hospitalization. The incidence of MDR pathogens is also closely linked to local factors and widely varies from one institution to another.[46] Therefore, clinicians must be aware of the most common microorganisms, associated with both early-onset and late-onset VAP in their own institution to properly administer empiric antimicrobial therapy.

The primary mechanism for VAP development is through aspiration of oropharyngeal contents and the oropharynx is generally colonized by anaerobes. Therefore, the role of anaerobes in the pathogenesis of VAP should be revisited. Importantly, empiric antibiotic therapy active against anaerobic bacteria appears to improve short-term outcomes in patients with VAP.[47]

Fungi are a seldom cause of VAP. *Candida* species and *Aspergillus fumigatus* are the most common isolated fungi, predominately, in immunosuppressed patients. In mechanically ventilated patients, the clinical significance of respiratory tract colonization by *Candida* is controversial. In a retrospective analysis of 639 patients from the Canadian VAP study, 114 patients had *Candida* colonization of the respiratory tract.[48] Interestingly, patients with *Candida* colonization had a significant increase in hospital mortality (34% vs. 21% in patients without *Candida* colonization, p = 0.003). However, it is still unclear whether *Candida* colonization is associated with or responsible for worse outcomes. Moreover, recent reports showed that the isolation of *Candida* species in respiratory samples of ICU patients demonstrates only colonization rather than candidal pneumonia.[49]

It is commonly reported that VAP is infrequently due to viruses; however, it should also be acknowledged that patients with clinical suspicion of VAP are rarely screened for viruses. Daubin et al.[50] studied 139 patients mechanically ventilated for more than 48 hours, of which 28% developed VAP. Although *P. aeruginosa* and MRSA still accounted for most of the VAP cases, herpes simplex virus type 1 was found in 12 cases of VAP and cytomegalovirus (CMV) in 1 case.

DIAGNOSIS

The diagnosis of VAP is very challenging and lacks a gold standard.[51,52] Clinical signs of pneumonia, such as fever, tachycardia, and leukocytosis are too nonspecific to be of diagnostic value for ventilated patients.[2] Moreover, changes of the chest radiograph are often difficult to interpret in patients who originally presented multilobar opacities at admission. Also, chest radiographs may not reveal subtle lung infiltrates that may be detected with computed tomography (CT) scans, particularly in patients with COPD. When infiltrates are evident, it is often difficult to differentiate among cardiogenic and noncardiogenic pulmonary edema, pulmonary contusion, atelectasis, and pneumonia.

In patients with autopsy-proven VAP, no single radiographic sign had a diagnostic accuracy greater than 68% in an early report.[53] The presence of air bronchograms or alveolar opacities in patients without ARDS correlated with pneumonia; however, no such correlation was found for patients with ARDS. Many causes other than pneumonia can explain asymmetrical consolidation in patients with ARDS and marked heterogeneity of radiographic abnormalities has also been reported in patients with uncomplicated ARDS.[54] A clinical study confirmed the presence of lung infection in only 42% of the patients with clinically suspected VAP, with frequent occurrence of multiple infectious and noninfectious processes,[55] indicating a poor correlation between clinical signs and bacteriologic demonstration of VAP.

The lack of accuracy of specific clinical signs of pneumonia led investigators to develop scores to identify respiratory infections. In particular, the clinical pulmonary infection score (CPIS) is based on 6 clinical assessments (temperature, blood leukocyte count, volume and purulence of tracheal secretions, oxygenation, pulmonary radiographic findings, and semiquantitative culture of tracheal aspirate), each of worth between 0 and 2 points (Table 1).[56] The CPIS showed a good correlation with quantitative bacteriology of bronchoalveolar lavage (BAL) samples. Moreover, a value above 6 is a threshold to accurately identify patients with pneumonia. Yet, the value of CPIS still needs to be validated in a large prospective study, especially in patients with bilateral pulmonary infiltrates.

TABLE 1
The Clinical Pulmonary Infection Score

Criteria	0	1	2
Tracheal secretions	Absent	Non-purulent	Abundant and purulent
Chest X-ray infiltrates	None	Diffuse	Localized
Temperature (°C)	≥36.5 and ≤38.4	≥38.5 or ≤38.9	≥39 or ≤36
Leukocytes (per mm^3)	≥4000 and ≤11000	<4000 or >11000	<4000 or >11000 + bands >50% or >500
PaO_2/FiO_2 (mmHg)	>240 or ARDS	—	≤240 no ARDS
Microbiology*	Negative	—	Positive

CPIS is considered positive with a score ≥6.

ARDS, acute respiratory distress syndrome; PaO_2, partial pressure of arterial O_2; FiO_2, fraction of inspired O_2.

Source: Garrouste-Orgeas M, Chevret S, Arlet G, Marie O, Rouveau M, Popoff N, et al. Oropharyngeal or gastric colonization and nosocomial pneumonia in adult intensive care unit patients. A prospective study based on genomic DNA analysis. *Am J Respir Crit Care Med.* 1997;156:1647-55.

Interestingly, following tracheal intubation, the presence of bacteria in the lower airways is not sufficient to diagnose lung infection. Indeed, the tracheobronchial tree and the oropharynx of mechanically ventilated patients are frequently colonized by enteric Gram-negative bacilli.[1,57] Many sampling procedures of respiratory secretions, such as sputum collection, endotracheal aspirates, BAL, and protected specimen brush (PSB) are available. In addition, there are several microbiological techniques, including Gram's staining and intracellular organism count from specimens obtained via BAL. Each diagnostic technique has advantages as well as limitations and provides different diagnostic accuracy.

Qualitative cultures of endotracheal aspirates have a high percentage of false-positive results due to frequent bacterial colonization of the proximal airways in ICU patients. Conversely, quantitative culture techniques of endotracheal aspirates may have an acceptable overall diagnostic accuracy. When patients develop pneumonia, pathogens are present in the lower respiratory tract secretions at concentrations of at least 10^5–10^6 colony forming units (cfu)/mL,[58,59] and contaminants are generally present at less than 10^4 cfu/mL. The current diagnostic threshold proposed for tracheal aspirates is 10^6 cfu/mL. Similarly, PSB collects between 0.001 and 0.01 mL of secretions; therefore the presence of more than 10^3 bacteria in the originally diluted sample (1 mL) actually represents 10^5–10^6 cfu/mL in pulmonary secretions. Finally, 10^4 cfu/mL is considered the cutoff for BAL, which collects 1 mL of secretions in 10–100 mL of effluent.

The importance of a microbiological diagnosis of VAP is aimed not only at determining whether a patient has pneumonia but also for optimizing antimicrobial treatment. To allow narrowing or de-escalation of the initial empiric treatment, antimicrobial susceptibility data should be available as soon as possible. Recently, several alternative techniques to microbial cultures have been developed in order to achieve a more rapid and accurate diagnosis of nosocomial pneumonia. Among the most recent improvements, the direct antibiogram using E-test strips applied directly to respiratory tract samples have proved to be both reliable and effective and can anticipate the availability of antimicrobial susceptibility data by more than 48 hours.[60] Other advances include the clinical application of quantitative polymerase chain reaction (PCR) for direct measurement of microbial genetic material in patient specimens.[61] The mecA gene that confers resistance to methicillin in *S. aureus* can be detected using quantitative PCR, and a study demonstrated that such assessment in mini-BAL samples was able to diagnose MRSA pneumonia rapidly and accurately.[62]

Theoretically, a diagnostic strategy should be sensitive enough to identify the greatest number of patients infected to initiate early adequate empiric antibiotic treatment and provide improvement in outcomes. On the other hand, the strategy must be able to discriminate patients without a true infection and avoid overtreatment with antimicrobial drugs, which may be associated with worse outcomes, due to selection of MDR microorganisms. VAP is clinically suspected when a new or progressive radiographic infiltrate has developed with at least 2 of 3 clinical criteria (fever >38°C, leukocytosis or leucopenia, and purulent secretions). Then, 2 different diagnostic algorithms can be employed to confirm VAP.

The clinical approach recommends treating every patient with suspicion of having a pulmonary infection with new antibiotics, even when the likelihood of infection is low (Figure 1). Antimicrobial therapy is adjusted according to culture results or clinical response. Semiquantitative culture of tracheal aspirates has the advantage that no specialized microbiologic techniques are required, and the sensitivity is high. This clinical strategy provides antimicrobial treatment to the majority of the patients with suspicion of VAP and yields a low rate of false-negatives. In case the tracheal aspirate culture does not demonstrate pathogens and the patient has not received new antibiotics within the previous 72 hours, the diagnosis of pneumonia is unlikely.[63] This strategy is useful in centers where bronchoscopic methods are not always available for sampling the lower respiratory tract. The main drawback of this strategy is that the high sensitivity of semiquantitative cultures of tracheal aspirates leads to overestimation of the incidence of nosocomial pneumonia; hence, unnecessary antimicrobial treatment could be administered.

The bacteriologic strategy is based on the results of quantitative cultures of lower respiratory secretions (Figure 2). Specific threshold cutoffs for each test to discriminate between colonizing microorganisms and those producing infection are used in this strategy. As previously mentioned, the cutoff points used is

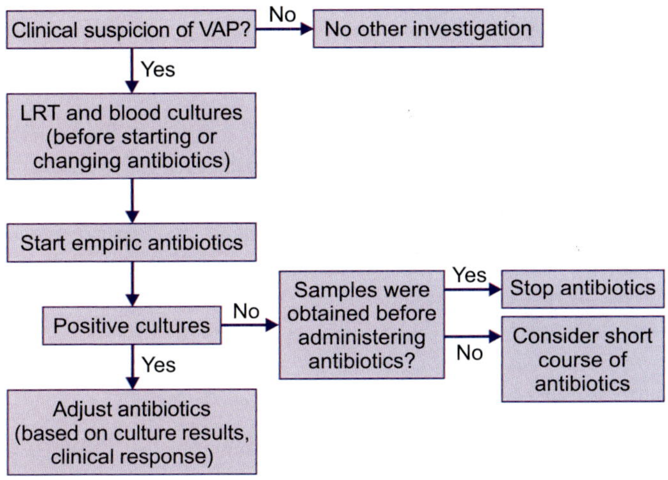

FIGURE 1 Clinical strategy for the empiric treatment of VAP. VAP, ventilator-associated pneumonia; LRT, lower respiratory tract.

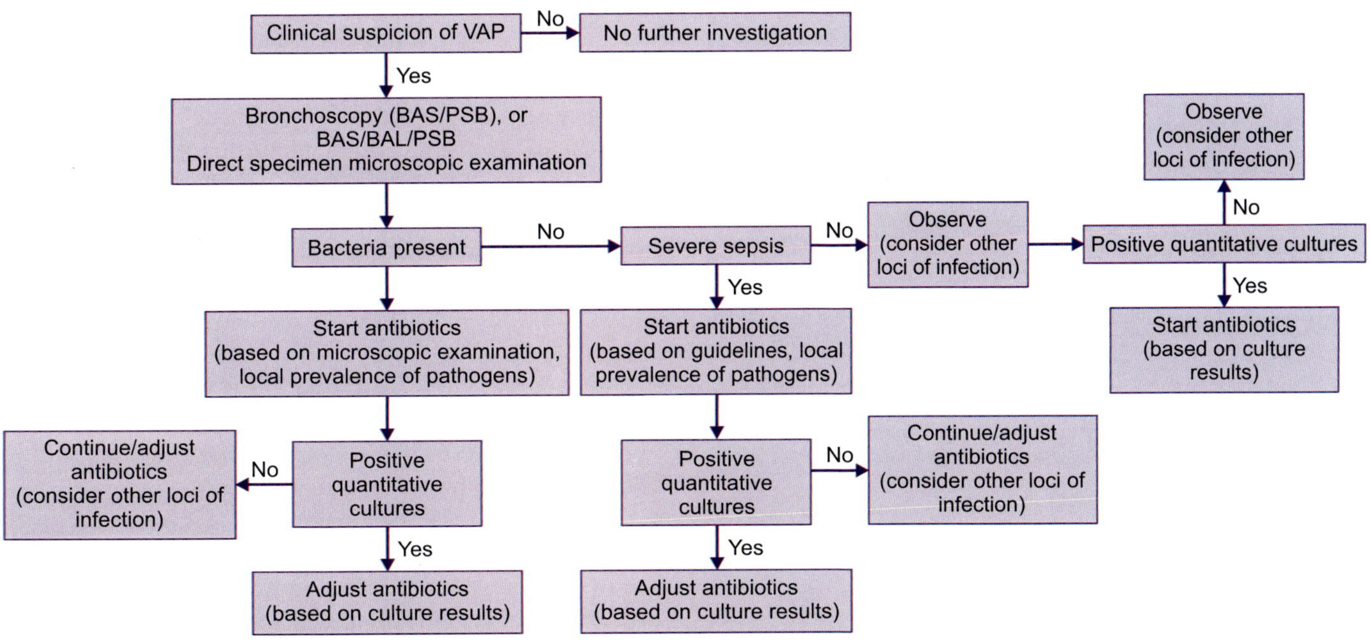

VAP, ventilator-associated pneumonia; BAL, bronchoalveolar lavage; PSB, protected specimen brush; BAS, bronchial aspirate.

FIGURE 2 Bacteriological strategy for the empiric treatment of VAP.

10^6 cfu/mL for bronchial aspirate, 10^4 cfu/mL for BAL, and 10^3 cfu/mL for PSB. Bacteriologic strategy attempts to accurately identify patients with true nosocomial pneumonia in order to treat only infected patients and improve clinical outcomes.[64] Therefore, the strategy reduces risks for overuse of antibiotics, since quantitative cultures yield fewer microorganisms above the threshold in comparison to semiquantitative cultures. Among the disadvantages of the bacteriologic strategy is the possibility of obtaining false-negative results, which lead to delayed antibiotic treatment in a patient with pneumonia. Moreover, results using the microbiology strategy may lack reproducibility, and often no microbiologic information is available at the time of initiation of empiric antibiotic therapy.

Clinical and bacteriologic strategies can be combined into a protocol to improve diagnostic accuracy (Table 2). The protocol begins with clinical suspicion of respiratory infection. The next step is to sample the lower respiratory tract in order to identify the causative microorganism. Sampling should be performed before initiation or change of any antibiotic treatment, even though antibiotic therapy should not be delayed in septic patients. Respiratory tract specimens can be obtained through expectoration, BAS, BAL, or PSB. The latter 2 techniques can be performed through a bronchoscope or blindly. Several other samples should also be collected, as noted in table 2. With clinical suspicion of pneumonia, CPIS should be calculated to improve objective assessment of the clinical parameters (Table 1).

TABLE 2

Diagnostic Protocol to Combine Clinical and Bacteriologic Strategies for the Diagnosis of VAP

- As soon as pneumonia or infection associated with mechanical ventilation is suspected, and before initiating new empiric antibiotic treatment, collect samples as follows:*
  - Expectoration
  - Tracheobronchial aspirate**
  - BAL or mini-BAL**
  - PSB**
- Two blood cultures
- In cases of evidence for parapneumonic effusion, obtain pleural fluid sample
- Obtain *Legionella pneumophila* and *Streptococcus pneumoniae* antigens in urine
- Other lab tests: Complete blood count, serum electrolytes, liver and renal function tests, CRP, PCT, arterial blood gases

VAP, ventilator-associated pneumonia; BAL, bronchoalveolar lavage; PSB, protected specimen brush; CRP, C-reactive protein; PCT, procalcitonin.

*Samples should be sent to the microbiology department, or if not available, maintained in refrigerator at 4°C (only respiratory samples) for a maximum of one hour, for Gram's staining, intracellular organism counting (only in BAL and mini-BAL) and quantitative cultures. The collection of lower respiratory secretion samples should not delay the initiation of empiric treatment in patients with severe sepsis.

**These techniques may be performed by bronchoscopy or blind procedures.

Quantitative cultures are performed with the respiratory secretions obtained by bronchial aspirate, BAL or PSB. The cutoff count to diagnose pneumonia is the following: BAS 10^6 cfu/mL; BAL 10^4 cfu/mL and PSB 10^3 cfu/mL.

TREATMENT

An indiscriminate administration of antibiotics for critically ill patients may contribute to the emergence of multi-resistant pathogens and increase the risk of severe superinfections, ultimately worsening morbidity, mortality, as well as exposing the patient to antibiotic-related adverse effects and higher healthcare costs.[65] Inappropriate therapy is strongly associated with worse survival.[66,67] Several studies showed that inadequate empiric antibiotic treatment, initiated before obtaining the results of cultures from respiratory secretions, was associated with greater hospital mortality rate compared with an antibiotic regimen that provided adequate antimicrobial coverage based on microbiologic culture results.[63,64,68] Nevertheless, the choice of the initial antibiotic treatment is often challenging, due to several factors:

- High frequency of resistant organisms in ICU patients previously treated with antibiotics
- High risks for MDR pathogens in late-onset pneumonia occurring more than 7 days after initiation of mechanical ventilation
- Frequent isolation of multiple organisms from pulmonary secretions when the sampling technique is not specific enough to differentiate colonizing from infecting pathogens.

Once the decision to initiate antimicrobial therapy has been made, the following issues should be considered, in order to achieve the best antimicrobial efficacy and to reduce overuse of antibiotics:

- The most likely etiologic microorganisms
- Choice of the empiric antimicrobials likely to be active against these microorganisms
- The adjustment of therapy following microbiologic results and duration of treatment.

The dynamics of change of oropharyngeal flora during hospital stay can be described as follows:

- Healthy subjects are colonized with normal oropharyngeal flora in which pathogenic microorganisms, such as *S. pneumoniae*, group A streptococci, or meningococci may be transiently found
- Patients with chronic comorbidities or an acute inflammatory process have impairment of normal

immune responses. As a result, *S. aureus* and enterobacteriaceae can colonize the oropharynx

- Patients who have received antibiotic treatment become colonized with resistant pathogens, including ESBL+ enterobacteriaceae, *Enterobacter* species, *P. aeruginosa*, or MRSA
- Patients who have received broad spectrum antibiotics for more than 7 days are often colonized by multi-resistant microorganisms. This leads to emergence of highly-resistant Gram-negative bacilli (*A. baumannii, S. maltophilia, Burkholderia cepacia*) and Gram-positive microorganisms (coagulase-negative *Staphylococcus* and *Enterococcus* species).

Changes in oropharyngeal flora tend to occur progressively so that the presence of microorganisms during one stage often overlaps with the next stage.

Choice of the Empiric Antimicrobials Likely to Be Active Against Causative Microorganisms

The latest guidelines of the America Thoracic Society (ATS)/Infectious Disease Society of America (IDSA) for the management of adult patients with nosocomial pneumonia[1] recommend that the selection of empiric antibiotic therapy for each patient should be based on the timing of onset and presence of risk factors for MDR pathogens. The risk factors for MDR pathogens defined by the ATS/IDSA guidelines are summarized in table 3. An algorithm for the initial management of patients with nosocomial respiratory infection and selection of appropriate antimicrobials is shown in figure 3. The antibiotics recommended by the current ATS/IDSA guidelines are shown in tables 4 and 5. Broad-spectrum empiric antibiotic therapy should be rapidly de-escalated as soon as microbiological data become available in order to limit the emergence of resistance in the hospital.

TABLE 3

Risk Factors for MDR Pathogens Causing Nosocomial Pneumonia

- Antimicrobial therapy in preceding 90 days
- Current hospitalization of 5 days or more
- High frequency of antibiotic resistance in the community or in the specific hospital unit
- Presence of risk factors for HAP:
  - Hospitalization for 2 days or more in the preceding 90 days
  - Residence in a nursing home or extended care facility
  - Home infusion therapy (including antibiotics)
  - Chronic dialysis within 30 days
  - Home wound care
  - Family member with MDR pathogen
- Immunosuppressive disease and/or therapy

MDR, multidrug-resistant; HAP, hospital-acquired pneumonia.

Source: American Thoracic Society; Infectious Diseases Society of America. Guidelines for the management of adults with hospital-acquired, ventilator-associated, and healthcare-associated pneumonia. *Am J Respir Crit Care Med.* 2005;171:388-416.

Antimicrobial Therapy in Special Situations

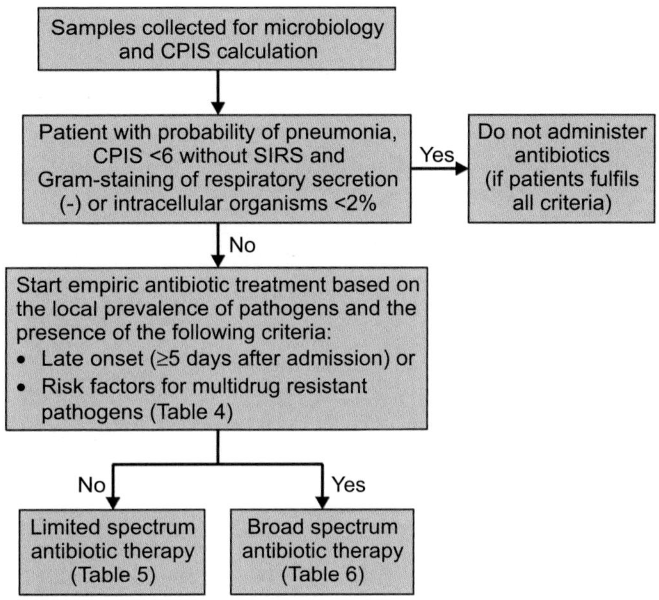

VAP, ventilator-associated pneumonia; CPIS, Clinical Pulmonary Infection Score; SIRS, systemic inflammatory response syndrome; MDR, multidrug resistant.

FIGURE 3 Algorithm for the initial management of patients with VAP and selection of appropriate antimicrobials.

TABLE 4

Initial Empiric Antibiotic Treatment in Nosocomial and VAP of Early-onset in Patients without Risk Factors for Infection by MDR Pathogens

Probable microorganism	Recommended antibiotic
• *Streptococcus pneumoniae*	Ceftriaxone
• *Haemophilus influenzae*	or
• MSSA	Levofloxacin, moxifloxacin
• Enteric Gram-negative bacilli	or
– *Escherichia coli*	Ampicillin/sulbactam
– *Klebsiella pneumoniae*	or
– *Enterobacter* species	Ertapenem
– *Proteus* species	
– *Serratia marcescens*	

VAP, ventilator-associated pneumonia; MDR, multidrug-resistant; MSSA, methicillin-sensitive *Staphylococcus aureus*.

Source: American Thoracic Society; Infectious Diseases Society of America. Guidelines for the management of adults with hospital-acquired, ventilator-associated, and healthcare-associated pneumonia. *Am J Respir Crit Care Med.* 2005;171:388-416.

TABLE 5

Initial Empiric Antibiotic Treatment for Nosocomial and VAP of Late-onset or in Patients with Risk Factors for Infection by MDR Pathogens and Any Degree of Severity

Probable microorganism

Microorganisms mentioned in table 4 plus:

- *Pseudomonas aeruginosa*
- *Klebsiella pneumoniae* (ESBL+)†
- *Acinetobacter* species†
- Other non-fermenting Gram-negative bacteria
- MRSA
- *Legionella pneumophila*‡

Combined antibiotic treatment

- Antipseudomonal cephalosporin (ceftazidime or cefepime)*
  or
- Carbapenem (imipenem, meropenem)*
  or
- β-lactamic/β-lactamase inhibitor (piperacillin-tazobactam)*
  +
- Antipseudomonal fluoroquinolone (ciprofloxacin, levofloxacin)**
  or
- Aminoglycoside** (amikacin)
  ±
- Linezolid or Vancomycin***

VAP, ventilator-associated pneumonia; MDR, multidrug-resistant; ESBL, extended spectrum beta-lactamase; MRSA, methicillin-resistant *Staphylococcus aureus.*

*The choice of β-lactam is made as follows: patients who have not received any antipseudomonal β-lactam within the last 30 days should be administered piperacillin-tazobactam or an antipseudomonal cephalosporin. Patients who have received these drugs should be given empiric therapy with a carbapenem. Patients with infection by ESBL-producing microorganisms should be treated with carbapenem regardless of the results of the antibiogram.

**For combined empiric therapy for MDR Gram-negative bacteria, an antipseudomonal fluoroquinolone should be used in cases of renal failure or concomitant use of vancomycin. In other settings combined empiric therapy is initiated with amikacin and is maintained for a 5-day period.

***Empiric therapy aimed against MRSA is initiated in patients with proven colonization,Ψ previous infection by this microorganism or implementation of mechanical ventilation for more than 6 days. The antibiotic of choice is either vancomycin (except in patients allergic to this medication, creatinine values ≥1.6 mg/dL or in patients presenting signs of empiric treatment failure after 48 hours of antibiotic therapy) or linezolid.

ΨFor epidemiologic surveillance nasal and perineal cultures should be performed on admission and at one-week intervals thereafter while remaining in the ICU.

†If an ESBL+ strain, such as *K. pneumoniae*, or *Acinetobacter* species is suspected, a carbapenem is the first choice.

‡If *L. pneumophila* is suspected, the combination antibiotic regimen should include a macrolide (e.g., azithromycin), or a fluoroquinolone (e.g., ciprofloxacin or levofloxacin) should be used rather than an aminoglycoside.

Source: American Thoracic Society; Infectious Diseases Society of America. Guidelines for the management of adults with hospital-acquired, ventilator-associated, and healthcare-associated pneumonia. *Am J Respir Crit Care Med.* 2005;171:388-416.

The addition of antibiotics with activity against MRSA depends on the local prevalence of MRSA, the presence of risk factors for MRSA, and the severity of infection. In geographic areas with documented presence of community-acquired MRSA (CA-MRSA), severe pneumonia with radiologic images of cavitation, and presence of Gram-positive cocci in respiratory secretions, empiric treatment with linezolid or vancomycin may be appropriate.

Infections by *L. pneumophila* serogroup 1 can be diagnosed by a *Legionella* urinary antigen test. This test should be routinely obtained if the hospital water supply is known to be colonized with *L. pneumophila,* serogroup 1. A fluoroquinolone or a macrolide would be appropriate treatment for *L. pneumophila* infection.

A growing interest in the use of aerosolized antimicrobials to treat VAP has been reported. A recent study showed that nebulization and intravenous infusion of ceftazidime and amikacin provide similar efficiency for treating VAP caused by *P. aeruginosa.*

Modifications of Therapy and Duration of Treatment

After 72 hours, treatment should be adjusted based on the microbiologic results. The initial β-lactam antibiotic should be continued if the microorganism is susceptible to the originally prescribed empiric β-lactam drug. If not, another β-lactam antibiotic, possibly a carbapenem, may be introduced. The empiric antibiotic against MRSA should be discontinued if the presence of this pathogen is not confirmed by cultures. Discontinuation of the fluoroquinolone and, especially, the aminoglycoside should be considered after 3–5 days of treatment. The bactericidal activity of aminoglycosides and fluoroquinolones leads to a rapid reduction in the bacterial load during the initial days of treatment. After this time, monotherapy may be sufficient. This approach would decrease emergence of resistant mutants and minimize nephrotoxicity caused by aminoglycosides.

The majority of infections can be effectively treated with regimens lasting up to 8 days. Four situations may justify prolonged treatment:

- Infection by microorganisms, which may multiply in the cellular cytoplasm, such as *Legionella* species
- The presence of biofilms or prosthetic devices
- The development of tissue necrosis, the formation of abscesses, or infection within a closed cavity, such as empyema
- The persistence of the original infection (such as perforation or endocarditis).

If the clinical course of the pneumonia is favorable, as defined by defervescence, improvement in blood-gas exchanges, and reduction in C-reactive protein (CRP) levels within the first 3–5 days of antimicrobial therapy, treatment may be withdrawn after the completion of 7 days. If the causative microorganism is a nonfermenting Gram-negative bacillus, the treatment can be extended beyond 14 days. In patients with clinical suspicion of ICU-acquired pneumonia who have a CPIS lower than 6 on the third day of treatment, the treatment may be withdrawn.

PREVENTION

Strategies of VAP prevention have focused on avoiding/reducing cross transmission, the likelihood of aspiration across the ETT cuff, and reducing the bacterial load in the oropharynx and gastrointestinal content (Table 6).

TABLE 6

Current Preventive Interventions for VAP

- Implementation, as a bundle, of nosocomial pneumonia preventive strategies that have proven efficacy in reducing morbidity and mortality
- Implementation of educational programs for caregivers and frequent performance feedbacks and compliance assessment
- Strict alcohol-based hand hygiene
- Avoidance of tracheal intubation, use of noninvasice ventilation when appropriate, and daily monitoring of prompt extubation
- Daily vacation from sedation and implementation of weaning protocols
- No ventilatory circuit tube changes unless the circuit is soiled or damaged
- Use of tracheal tube with cuff made of novel materials and shapes
- Use of silver-coated tracheal tube
- Continuous application of low-level of PEEP during tracheal intubation
- Continuous/intermittent aspiration of subglottic secretions
- Internal cuff pressure maintained within the recommended range
- Oral care with antiseptics
- Avoid stress ulcer prophylaxis in very low-risk patients for gastrointestinal bleed and consider use of sucralfate when indicated
- Semi-recumbent patient positioning
- Continuous lateral rotation therapy
- Post-pyloric feeding in patients who have impaired gastric emptying
- Selective digestive decontamination for patients requiring greater than 48 hours of mechanical ventilation

VAP, ventilator-associated pneumonia; PEEP, positive end-expiratory pressure.

The Institute for Healthcare Improvement (IHI) recommends that approaches with proven efficacy for reduction of morbidity and mortality related to infection control should be grouped and implemented together as a bundle because together, they are expected to be more effective than when implemented individually.[69] Designing a preventive bundle is just the first step, and it must be followed by continuous assessment of healthcare personnel compliance and improvements to implement interventions. Several reports[69-71] have found drastic reductions in the incidence of VAP following implementation of VAP-preventive bundles.

General Prophylactic Measures

Maintaining high levels of education among ICU personnel relating to VAP pathophysiology and preventive strategies can be effective in reducing incidence of this complication.[72,73] Respiratory care practitioners and nurses should be the primary recipients of education programs and frequent performance feedback and compliance assessment should be undertaken.[74]

Adherence to simple infection control measures, such as alcohol-based hand disinfection, effectively reduces cross transmission of pathogens and incidence of VAP.[75] The World Health Organization (WHO) has endorsed hand hygiene as the single-most important element of strategies to prevent healthcare-associated infections.[76]

Kollef et al.[77] demonstrated that patient transport outside the ICU was associated with increased risks for VAP. Clinicians and nursing staff should carefully transport intubated patients. In particular, the internal pressure of the ETT cuff should always be kept within the recommended range, particularly when the patient is expected to maintain supine position during diagnostic or therapeutic procedures. Ventilator circuits should be carefully manipulated in order to prevent aspiration of colonized fluids within the circuit.

Daily interruption or decreasing the sedation in order to avoid constant impairment of respiratory defenses, as well as, the avoidance of paralytic agents is highly recommended. It is well acknowledged that prolonged tracheal intubation is associated with VAP. A report by Kress et al.[78] was recently confirmed by Schweickert et al.[79] who studied 128 mechanically ventilated patients randomized to continuous infusions of sedation with or without daily interruption. The authors demonstrated reduction of duration of mechanical ventilation and length of stay in the ICU, when patients were allowed to wake up daily. Results from these clinical trials are challenging standard sedation protocols for intubated patients to reduce length of stay on mechanical ventilation and ultimately, reduce the risks for VAP.

There is an evidence of shorter length of mechanical ventilation, reduced rate of failed extubation, and decreased incidence of VAP when protocol-driven weaning from the ventilator is implemented[80,81] Marelich et al.[80] randomized 385 patients to receive either a protocol-driven weaning procedure or standard care and found that duration of mechanical ventilation was decreased from a median of 124 hours for the control group to 68 hours in the protocol-driven weaning group ($p = 0.0001$). Moreover, a trend towards lower incidence of VAP was found in the treatment group ($p = 0.061$).

Noninvasive Ventilation

Tracheal intubation and mechanical ventilation are the main risk for nosocomial pneumonia and therefore should be avoided whenever possible. Noninvasive ventilation is an attractive alternative for patients with acute exacerbations of COPD or acute hypoxemic respiratory failure, and for some immunosuppressed patients with pulmonary infiltrates and respiratory failure.[82-85] Moreover, noninvasive ventilation can also be used safely in order to facilitate early extubation, especially in hypercapnic patients with COPD.[86] Kohlenberg et al.[87] pooled data of 400 ICUs in Germany, and found mean pneumonia incidence of 1.58 and 5.44 cases/1,000 ventilator days for noninvasive ventilation and invasive mechanical ventilation, respectively. Therefore, when indicated, noninvasive ventilation should be tried in order to avoid tracheal intubation and reduce overall duration of tracheal intubation.

Tracheal Tube Cuff

Several strategies have been applied to improve the design of tracheal tubes and reduce the likelihood of aspiration of pathogen-laden secretions across the cuff. Novel ETT cuffs made of new materials, i.e., polyurethane,[18] silicone, and latex[17,88,89] have been developed and tested in laboratory and clinical trials. Particularly, polyurethane cuff has a thickness of 5–10 μm in comparison to 50 μm of polyvinyl chloride cuffs; hence, upon inflation, smaller folds form and aspiration of secretions above the cuff can be reduced.

The shape of the cuff is an additional factor to prevent pulmonary aspiration.[88,90] In comparison to standard cuffs with cylindrical shape, cuffs designed with a smooth tapering shape allow elimination of folds for a full circumference of the trachea/cuff contact zone, irrespective of the cuff material. Nevertheless, further clinical studies are needed to evaluate efficacy of tapered cuffs.

It is important to maintain the internal pressure of the ETT cuff pressure between 25 and 30 cmH_2O, particularly when no PEEP is applied, in order to prevent either tracheal injury or macroleakage.

Ventilatory settings may play a role in pathogenesis of VAP. In particular, PEEP may decrease the incidence of VAP by counteracting hydrostatic pressure exerted by oropharyngeal secretions above the ETT cuff, hence reducing pulmonary aspiration.[91] A recent report[92] assessed effects of 5–8 cmH_2O of PEEP in normoxemic ventilated patients and showed a significant reduction in VAP.

Tracheal Tubes Coated with Antimicrobial Agents

Coating the ETT with antimicrobial agents, such as silver, is a novel strategy to prevent biofilm formation within its internal surface and, therefore, VAP. The North American Silver-Coated Endotracheal Tube (NASCENT) randomized trial[93] studied 2003 patients expected to require mechanical ventilation for more than 24 hours and randomized them to be intubated with either a silver-coated or a conventional tube. The silver-coated ETT was associated with a lower incidence of microbiologically confirmed VAP with a relative risk (RR) reduction of 35.9%. A retrospective cohort analysis by Afessa B et al.,[94] based on the NASCENT study, showed that the silver-coated ETT was associated with reduced mortality in patients with VAP.

Nevertheless, clinicians should carefully consider benefits and limitations of these new ETTs and properly direct the use of silver coated tubes to patients expected to be ventilated for longer periods of time and with higher associated risk factors for nosocomial pneumonia.

Aspiration of Subglottic Secretions

Aspiration of colonized subglottic secretions, through dedicated ETTs, reduces hydrostatic pressure exerted above the cuff, and potentially prevents macroleakage across the cuff. The latest trial by Lacherade et al.[95] reported a reduction of both early- and late-onset VAP applying intermittent aspiration of subglottic secretions. The investigators included 333 patients randomized to be intubated with either an ETT that allowed drainage of subglottic secretions or a standard ETT. They found an incidence of late-onset VAP in 18.6% of patients in the treatment group vs. 33.0% of the patients in control group ($p = 0.01$). A meta-analysis[96] comprising data from 13 studies and 2442 patients has shown a significant reduction of risk for VAP using these tubes [RR 0.55, 95% confidence interval (CI) 0.46–0.66; $p < .00001$]. The use of subglottic secretion drainage was associated with reduced duration of stay in ICU ($p = 0.03$), decreased duration of mechanical ventilation ($p = 0.03$), and no effect on adverse events or mortality. Nevertheless, the use of these devices has been limited by concerns regarding tracheal mucosal injury and frequent occlusion of the suction port by mucosal blockage or tenuous secretions.[97] Finally, in the above mentioned study by Lacherade, the benefits of intermittent subglottic suction were similar to studies in which continuous aspiration of subglottic secretions was used. Hence, intermittent aspiration (every 4–6 hours) is advisable to avoid potential risks for tracheal injury using continuous aspiration.

Tracheostomy

Tracheostomized patients present the same risks for aspiration of pathogen-laden secretions as do orotracheally intubated patients.[15,98,99] Although early tracheostomy does not reduce risks for VAP, clinicians should consider that it may offer several benefits for mechanically ventilated patients, i.e., improved patient comfort, ability to communicate, capability for oral feeding, less need for sedation and analgesia, and reduced airway resistance in comparison to standard ETTs, which could be extremely important during the weaning period in order to shorten the duration of tracheal intubation.

Ventilator Circuit Management

Results from clinical trials in adults[77,100-106] and meta-analyses[107,108] yield consistent evidence that routine change of the ventilator circuit does not decrease risks and costs for VAP. Therefore, circuits should not be changed, unless the circuit is soiled or damaged. Importantly, the inadvertent flushing of the contaminated condensate into the lower airways should be always avoided by careful emptying ventilator circuits and water traps.[109]

To date, there are no consistent data showing reduction in the incidence of VAP and better outcomes using either heat and moisture exchangers or heated humidifiers. Based on the ongoing controversy, neither humidification strategy can be recommended as a pneumonia prevention tool. However, it is rational to deliver inspiratory gases at body temperature or slightly below and at the highest relative humidity in order to prevent loss of heat and moisture from the airways and more importantly, change in rheologic properties of secretions and impairment of mucociliary clearance.[110] Therefore, the use of heated humidifiers is indicated particularly in patients with hypothermia, prolonged mechanical ventilation, thick secretions, and chronic respiratory disorders.

Body Position

Early studies clearly demonstrated that intubated patients are at a higher risk for gastropulmonary aspiration when placed in the supine position (0°) as compared to a semi-recumbent position (45°).[111,112] Thus, as strongly suggested by the American[1] and European[8] guidelines on nosocomial pneumonia, intubated patients should preferably be kept in the semi-recumbent position (30–45°) rather than supine (0°) to prevent aspiration, especially when receiving enteral feeding.

Stress Ulcer Prophylaxis and Enteral Feeding

Early studies showed that in tracheally intubated patients, gastric pH higher than 4 was consistently associated with gastric colonization. Alkalinization of gastric contents due to drugs for stress ulcer prophylaxis and continuous enteral nutrition were the main risk factors for gastric colonization.

In the ICU, stress ulcer prophylaxis is usually achieved with either sucralfate, histamine type 2 blockers, or proton pump inhibitors. Sucralfate is the only treatment that potentially prevents stress gastrointestinal ulceration without raising gastric pH.

Gastrointestinal bleeding is a serious complication in critically ill patients at high risk for stress ulcers. Therefore, clinicians must weigh the potential benefit of sucralfate (with potentially less VAP and more gastrointestinal bleeding) vs. histamine type 2 blockers/proton pump inhibitors (with potentially more VAP and less gastrointestinal bleeding) and probably, limit stress ulcer prophylaxis to high-risk patients.

Enteral nutrition has been considered a risk factor for the development of VAP, mainly because of increased risks for alkalinization of gastric content, gastroesophageal reflux, and gastropulmonary aspiration. However, its alternative, parenteral nutrition is associated with higher risks for catheter-related infections, complications of line insertion, higher costs, and loss of intestinal villous architecture, which may facilitate enteral microbial translocation. Therefore, the benefits of early nutrition should be balanced with associated increased risks for VAP. Post-pyloric feeding should preferably be indicated in critically ill patients who have impaired gastric emptying.

Modulation of Oropharyngeal and Gastrointestinal Colonization

Extensive efforts have been devoted to modulate oropharyngeal flora of ICU patients and to reduce the risks for aspiration of pathogens. Several antiseptics for oropharyngeal decontamination have been evaluated with overall good results, i.e., chlorhexidine gluconate, iseganan, or povidone iodine. Chlorhexidine is a cationic chlorophenyl bis-biguanide antiseptic that has long been used as an inhibitor of dental plaque formation and gingivitis, and has been the focus of most research among the oropharyngeal antiseptics. The use of oral chlorhexidine to reduce VAP has shown excellent results, particularly in cardiothoracic ICU patients. Results in noncardiac ICU populations are more uncertain.[114,115] Most of the aforementioned studies used chlorhexidine concentrations of 0.12 and 0.2%. However, recent studies in general ICU patients have demonstrated significant reductions in VAP rates when chlorhexidine concentration was increased to 2%.[116,117] Therefore, oral decontamination with chlorhexidine should be routinely used, particularly in cardiothoracic patients. The usefulness of chlorhexidine as VAP preventive strategy in other ICU populations still requires more evidence before putting into general practice, but the use of higher chlorhexidine concentrations has showed promising results.

Selective decontamination of the digestive tract (SDD) has been used as a preventive strategy for nosocomial pneumonia for almost 3 decades.[118] It comprises of a combination of nonabsorbable antibiotics against Gram-negative pathogens (i.e., tobramycin, polymyxin E) and either amphotericin B or nystatin administered into the gastrointestinal tract, in order to prevent oropharyngeal and gastric colonization with aerobic Gram-negative bacilli and *Candida* species, while preserving the anaerobic flora. Some regimens also include a short course of systemic antibiotics (most commonly cefotaxime). Randomized clinical trials (RCTs)[119-121] and meta-analyses[122,123] confirm the results of earlier studies and suggest that selective decontamination of the digestive tract confers protection against pneumonia. Interestingly, selective decontamination of the digestive tract is the only preventive strategies for VAP that has shown reduction of mortality rates.

It is important to acknowledge that prophylactic use of antibiotics to modulate gastrointestinal flora may potentially increase risks for antibiotic resistance, and results from RCTs still remain controversial. Moreover, standard selective decontamination of the digestive tract is aimed at preventing overgrowth of aerobic Gram-negative bacteria, yet it could increase colonization by Gram-positive bacteria, i.e., MRSA and *Enterococcus* species.[120,123] Therefore, during the course of selective decontamination of the digestive tract, it is highly recommended to conduct appropriate surveillance of antibiotic resistance patterns within the ICU and hospital premises.

Several investigators have attempted to modify gastrointestinal and oropharyngeal growth of pathogens through the use of probiotics. Probiotics are viable microorganisms that colonize the host gastrointestinal tract by adhering to the intestinal mucosa and compete with the adhesion of pathogens to epithelial binding sites, thus, creating an unfavorable local milieu for pathogen colonization. In critically ill patients, studies have demonstrated that oral administration of a probiotic *Lactobacillus* preparation delayed respiratory tract colonization with *P. aeruginosa* which resulted in a reduced rate of VAP caused by this pathogen.[124] A meta-analysis of 5 RCTs concluded that probiotic administration was associated with lower incidence of VAP;[125] however, an additional evidence is required before recommending its use in all mechanically ventilated patients.

CONCLUSION

VAP is the most common healthcare-associated infection in the ICU. VAP increases morbidity, mortality, length of stay, and hospital costs. Thus, evidence-based preventive interventions should be implemented in all tracheally intubated patients on mechanical ventilation. VAP diagnosis is challenging and lacks a diagnostic gold-standard, leading to both under-diagnosis and over-diagnosis of the disease. Importantly, a prompt administration of appropriate broad-spectrum antibiotic(s) is mandatory in patients with microbiologic confirmation of VAP.

REFERENCES

1. American Thoracic Society; Infectious Diseases Society of America. Guidelines for the management of adults with hospital-acquired, ventilator-associated, and healthcare-associated pneumonia. *Am J Respir Crit Care Med.* 2005; 171:388-416.
2. Chastre J, Fagon JY. Ventilator-associated pneumonia. *Am J Respir Crit Care Med.* 2002;165:867-903.
3. Langer M, Cigada M, Mandelli M, Mosconi P, Tognoni G. Early onset pneumonia: a multicenter study in intensive care units. *Intensive Care Med.* 1987;13:342-6.
4. Trouillet JL, Chastre J, Vuagnat A, Joly-Guillou ML, Combaux D, Dombret MC, et al. Ventilator-associated pneumonia caused by potentially drug-resistant bacteria. *Am J Respir Crit Care Med.* 1998;157:531-9.
5. Shennib H, Mulder DS, Chiu RC. The effects of pulmonary atelectasis and reexpansion on lung cellular immune defenses. *Arch Surg.* 1984;119;274-7.

6. Nahum A, Hoyt J, Schmitz L, Moody J, Shapiro R, Marini JJ. Effect of mechanical ventilation strategy on dissemination of intratracheally instilled *Escherichia coli* in dogs. *Crit Care Med.* 1997;25:1733-43.
7. Lin CY, Zhang H, Cheng KC, Slutsky AS. Mechanical ventilation may increase susceptibility to the development of bacteremia. *Crit Care Med.* 2003;31:1429-34.
8. Torres A, Ewig S, Lode H, Carlet J; European HAP working group. Defining, treating and preventing hospital acquired pneumonia: European perspective. *Intensive Care Med.* 2009;35:9-29.
9. National Nosocomial Infections Surveillance System. National Nosocomial Infections Surveillance (NNIS) System Report, data summary from January 1992 through June 2004, issued October 2004. *Am J Infect Control.* 2004;32:470-85.
10. Warren DK, Shukla SJ, Olsen MA, Kollef MH, Hollenbeak CS, Cox MJ, et al. Outcome and attributable cost of ventilator-associated pneumonia among intensive care unit patients in a suburban medical center. *Crit Care Med.* 2003;31:1312-7.
11. Rello J, Ollendorf DA, Oster G, Vera-Llonch M, Bellm L, Redman R, et al.; VAP Outcomes Scientific Advisory Group. Epidemiology and outcomes of ventilator-associated pneumonia in a large US database. *Chest.* 2002;122:2115-21.
12. Cook DJ, Walter SD, Cook RJ, Griffith LE, Guyatt GH, Leasa D, et al. Incidence of and risk factors for ventilator-associated pneumonia in critically ill patients. *Ann Intern Med.* 1998;129:433-40.
13. Bekaert M, Timsit JF, Vansteelandt S, Depuydt P, Vésin A, Garrouste-Orgeas M, et al.; Outcomerea Study Group. Attributable mortality of ventilator-associated pneumonia: a reappraisal using causal analysis. *Am J Respir Crit Care Med.* 2011;184:1133-9.
14. Lisboa T, Diaz E, Sa-Borges M, Socias A, Sole-Violan J, Rodríguez A, et al. The ventilator-associated pneumonia PIRO score: a tool for predicting ICU mortality and health-care resources use in ventilator-associated pneumonia. *Chest.* 2008;134:1208-16.
15. Belson TP. Cuff induced tracheal injury in dogs following prolonged intubation. *Laryngoscope.* 1983;93:549-55.
16. Nordin U. The trachea and cuff-induced tracheal injury. An experimental study on causative factors and prevention. *Acta Otolaryngol Suppl.* 1977;345:1-71.
17. Dullenkopf A, Gerber A, Weiss M. Fluid leakage past tracheal tube cuffs: evaluation of the new Microcuff endotracheal tube. *Intensive Care Med.* 2003;29;1849-53.
18. Inglis TJ, Millar MR, Jones JG, Robinson DA. Tracheal tube biofilm as a source of bacterial colonization of the lung. *J Clin Microbiol.* 1989;27:2014-8.
19. Inglis TJ, Lim TM, Ng ML, Tang EK, Hui KP. Structural features of tracheal tube biofilm formed during prolonged mechanical ventilation. *Chest.* 1995;108:1049-52.
20. Ng KS, Kumarasinghe G, Inglis TJ. Dissemination of respiratory secretions during tracheal tube suctioning in an intensive care unit. *Ann Acad Med Singapore.* 1999;28:178-82.
21. Bou R, Aguilar A, Perpiñán J, Ramos P, Peris M, Lorente L, et al. Nosocomial outbreak of Pseudomonas aeruginosa infections related to a flexible bronchoscope. *J Hosp Infect.* 2006;64:129-35.
22. Srinivasan A, Wolfenden LL, Song X, Mackie K, Hartsell TL, Jones HD, et al. An outbreak of *Pseudomonas aeruginosa* infections associated with flexible bronchoscopes. *N Engl J Med.* 2003;348:221-7.
23. Crane LR, Tagle LC, Palutke WA. Outbreak of *Pseudomonas paucimobilis* in an intensive care facility. *JAMA.* 1981;246: 985-7.
24. Eckmanns T, Oppert M, Martin M, Amorosa R, Zuschneid I, Frei U, et al. An outbreak of hospital-acquired *Pseudomonas aeruginosa* infection caused by contaminated bottled water in intensive care units. *Clin Microbiol Infect.* 2008;14:454-8.
25. Lee JK. Two outbreaks of *Burkholderia cepacia* nosocomial infection in a neonatal intensive care unit. *J Paediatr Child Health.* 2008;44:62-6.
26. Kikuchi T, Nagashima G, Taguchi K, Kuraishi H, Nemoto H, Yamanaka M, et al. Contaminated oral intubation equipment associated with an outbreak of carbapenem-resistant *Pseudomonas* in an intensive care unit. *J Hosp Infect.* 2007;65:54-7.
27. Bou R, P Ramos. Outbreak of nosocomial Legionnaires' disease caused by a contaminated oxygen humidifier. *J Hosp Infect.* 2009;71:381-3.
28. Berthelot P, Grattard F, Mahul P, Jospe R, Pozzetto B, Ros A, et al. Ventilator temperature sensors: an unusual source of Pseudomonas cepacia in nosocomial infection. *J Hosp Infect.* 1993.25:33-43.
29. Rogues AM, Maugein J, Allery A, Fleureau C, Boulestreau H, Surcin S, et al. Electronic ventilator temperature sensors as a potential source of respiratory tract colonization with *Stenotrophomonas maltophilia*. *J Hosp Infect.* 2001; 49:289-92.
30. Pegues CF, Pegues DA, Ford DS, Hibberd PL, Carson LA, Raine CM, et al. *Burkholderia cepacia* respiratory tract acquisition: epidemiology and molecular characterization of a large nosocomial outbreak. *Epidemiol Infect.* 1996; 116:309-17.
31. Cobben NA, Drent M, Jonkers M, Wouters EF, Vaneechoutte M, Stobberingh EE. Outbreak of severe *Pseudomonas aeruginosa* respiratory infections due to contaminated nebulizers. *J Hosp Infect.* 1996;33:63-70.
32. Enoch DA, Summers C, Brown NM, Moore L, Gillham MI, Burnstein RM, et al. Investigation and management of an outbreak of multidrug-carbapenem-resistant *Acinetobacter baumannii* in Cambridge, UK. *J Hosp Infect.* 2008; 70:109-18.
33. Johanson WG, Pierce AK, Sanford JP. Changing pharyngeal bacterial flora of hospitalized patients. Emergence of gram-negative bacilli. *N Engl J Med.* 1969;281:1137-40.
34. Johanson WG Jr, Pierce AK, Sanford JP, Thomas GD. Nosocomial respiratory infections with gram-negative bacilli. The significance of colonization of the respiratory tract. *Ann Intern Med.* 1972;77:701-6.
35. Feldman C, Kassel M, Cantrell J, Kaka S, Morar R, Goolam Mahomed A, et al. The presence and sequence of endotracheal tube colonization in patients undergoing mechanical ventilation. *Eur Respir J.* 1999;13:546-51.

36. Fourrier F, Duvivier B, Boutigny H, Roussel-Delvallez M, Chopin C. Colonization of dental plaque: a source of nosocomial infections in intensive care unit patients. *Crit Care Med.* 1998;26:301-8.
37. Safdar N, Crnich CJ, Maki DG. The pathogenesis of ventilator-associated pneumonia: its relevance to developing effective strategies for prevention. *Respir Care.* 2005;50:725-39.
38. Sackner MA, Hirsch J, Epstein S. Effect of cuffed endotracheal tubes on tracheal mucous velocity. *Chest.* 1975; 68:774-7.
39. Konrad F, Schreiber T, Brecht-Kraus D, Georgieff M. Mucociliary transport in ICU patients. *Chest.* 1994;105: 237-41.
40. Kollef MH, Morrow LE, Niederman MS, Leeper KV, Anzueto A, Benz-Scott L, et al. Clinical characteristics and treatment patterns among patients with ventilator-associated pneumonia. *Chest.* 2006;129:1210-8.
41. Combes A, Figliolini C, Trouillet JL, Kassis N, Wolff M, Gibert C, et al. Incidence and outcome of polymicrobial ventilator-associated pneumonia. *Chest.* 2002;121:1618-23.
42. Soler N, Torres A, Ewig S, Gonzalez J, Celis R, El-Ebiary M, et al. Bronchial microbial patterns in severe exacerbations of chronic obstructive pulmonary disease (COPD) requiring mechanical ventilation. *Am J Respir Crit Care Med.* 1998;157:1498-505.
43. Fagon JY, Chastre J. Diagnosis and treatment of nosocomial pneumonia in ALI/ARDS patients. *Eur Respir J Suppl.* 2003;42: 77s-83s.
44. Bronchard R, Albaladejo P, Brezac G, Geffroy A, Seince PF, Morris W, et al. Early onset pneumonia: risk factors and consequences in head trauma patients. *Anesthesiology.* 2004;100:234-9.
45. Sirvent JM, Torres A, Vidaur L, Armengol J, de Batlle J, Bonet A. Tracheal colonisation within 24 h of intubation in patients with head trauma: risk factor for developing early-onset ventilator-associated pneumonia. *Intensive Care Med.* 2000;26:1369-72.
46. Rello J, Sa-Borges M, Correa H, Leal SR, Baraibar J. Variations in etiology of ventilator-associated pneumonia across four treatment sites: implications for antimicrobial prescribing practices. *Am J Respir Crit Care Med.* 1999; 160:608-13.
47. Robert R, Grollier G, Doré P, Hira M, Ferrand E, Fauchère JL. Nosocomial pneumonia with isolation of anaerobic bacteria in ICU patients: therapeutic considerations and outcome. *J Crit Care.* 1999:14:114-9.
48. Delisle MS, Williamson DR, Perreault MM, Albert M, Jiang X, Heyland DK. The clinical significance of *Candida* colonization of respiratory tract secretions in critically ill patients. *J Crit Care.* 2008;23:11-7.
49. Meersseman W, Lagrou K, Spriet I, Maertens J, Verbeken E, Peetermans WE, et al. Significance of the isolation of *Candida* species from airway samples in critically ill patients: a prospective, autopsy study. *Intensive Care Med.* 2009;35:1526-31.
50. Daubin C, Vincent S, Vabret A, du Cheyron D, Parienti JJ, Ramakers M, et al. Nosocomial viral ventilator-associated pneumonia in the intensive care unit: a prospective cohort study. *Intensive Care Med.* 2005;31:1116-22.
51. Niederman MS, Torres A, Summer W. Invasive diagnostic testing is not needed routinely to manage suspected ventilator-associated pneumonia. *Am J Respir Crit Care Med.* 1994;150:565-9.
52. Chastre J, Fagon JY. Invasive diagnostic testing should be routinely used to manage ventilated patients with suspected pneumonia. *Am J Respir Crit Care Med.* 1994; 150:570-4.
53. Wunderink RG, Woldenberg LS, Zeiss J, Day CM, Ciemins J, Lacher DA. The radiologic diagnosis of autopsy-proven ventilator-associated pneumonia. *Chest.* 1992;101:458-63.
54. Meduri GU, Belenchia JM, Estes RJ, Wunderink RG, el Torky M, Leeper KV Jr. Fibroproliferative phase of ARDS. Clinical findings and effects of corticosteroids. *Chest.* 1991;100:943-52.
55. Meduri GU, Mauldin GL, Wunderink RG, Leeper KV Jr, Jones CB, Tolley E, et al. Causes of fever and pulmonary densities in patients with clinical manifestations of ventilator-associated pneumonia. *Chest.* 1994; 106:221-35.
56. Pugin J, Auckenthaler R, Mili N, Janssens JP, Lew PD, Suter PM. Diagnosis of ventilator-associated pneumonia by bacteriologic analysis of bronchoscopic and non-bronchoscopic "blind" bronchoalveolar lavage fluid. *Am Rev Respir Dis.* 1991;143:1121-9.
57. Garrouste-Orgeas M, Chevret S, Arlet G, Marie O, Rouveau M, Popoff N, et al. Oropharyngeal or gastric colonization and nosocomial pneumonia in adult intensive care unit patients. A prospective study based on genomic DNA analysis. *Am J Respir Crit Care Med.* 1997;156:1647-55.
58. Torres A, Martos A, Puig de la Bellacasa J, Ferrer M, el-Ebiary M, González J, Specificity of endotracheal aspiration, protected specimen brush, and bronchoalveolar lavage in mechanically ventilated patients. *Am Rev Respir Dis.* 1993;147:952-7.
59. Jourdain B, Novara A, Joly-Guillou ML, Dombret MC, Calvat S, Trouillet JL, et al. Role of quantitative cultures of endotracheal aspirates in the diagnosis of nosocomial pneumonia. *Am J Respir Crit Care Med.* 1995;152:241-6.
60. Bouza E, Torres MV, Radice C, Cercenado E, de Diego R, Sánchez-Carrillo C, et al. Direct E-test (AB Biodisk) of respiratory samples improves antimicrobial use in ventilator-associated pneumonia. *Clin Infect Dis.* 2007; 44:382-7.
61. Reygaert W. Methicillin-resistant *Staphylococcus aureus* (MRSA): identification and susceptibility testing techniques. *Clin Lab Sci.* 2009:22:120-4.
62. Ost DE, Poch D, Fadel A, Wettimuny S, Ginocchio C, Wang XP. Mini-bronchoalveolar lavage quantitative polymerase chain reaction for diagnosis of methicillin-resistant *Staphylococcus aureus* pneumonia. *Crit Care Med.* 2010; 38:1536-41.
63. Dupont H, Mentec H, Sollet JP, Bleichner G. Impact of appropriateness of initial antibiotic therapy on the outcome of ventilator-associated pneumonia. *Intensive Care Med.* 2001;27:355-62.
64. Sanchez-Nieto JM, Torres A, Garcia-Cordoba F, El-Ebiary M, Carrillo A, Ruiz J, et al. Impact of invasive and

noninvasive quantitative culture sampling on outcome of ventilator-associated pneumonia: a pilot study. *Am J Respir Crit Care Med.* 1998;157:371-6.

65. Kollef MH. Ventilator-associated pneumonia. A multivariate analysis. *JAMA.* 1993;270:1965-70.
66. Celis R, Torres A, Gatell JM, Almela M, Rodríguez-Roisin R, Agustí-Vidal A. Nosocomial pneumonia. A multivariate analysis of risk and prognosis. *Chest.* 1988;93;318-24.
67. Alvarez-Lerma F. Modification of empiric antibiotic treatment in patients with pneumonia acquired in the intensive care unit. ICU-Acquired Pneumonia Study Group. *Intensive Care Med.* 1996;22:387-94.
68. Rello J, Gallego M, Mariscal D, Soñora R, Valles J. The value of routine microbial investigation in ventilator-associated pneumonia. *Am J Respir Crit Care Med.* 1997;156:196-200.
69. Marra AR, Cal RG, Silva CV, Caserta RA, Paes AT, Moura DF Jr, et al. Successful prevention of ventilator-associated pneumonia in an intensive care setting. *Am J Infect Control.* 2009;37:619-25.
70. Al-Tawfiq JA, Abed MS. Decreasing ventilator-associated pneumonia in adult intensive care units using the Institute for Healthcare Improvement bundle. *Am J Infect Control.* 2010;38:552-6.
71. Bird D, Zambuto A, O'Donnell C, Silva J, Korn C, Burke R, et al. Adherence to ventilator-associated pneumonia bundle and incidence of ventilator-associated pneumonia in the surgical intensive care unit. *Arch Surg.* 2010;145: 465-70.
72. Babcock HM, Zack JE, Garrison T, Trovillion E, Jones M, Fraser VJ, et al. An educational intervention to reduce ventilator-associated pneumonia in an integrated health system: a comparison of effects. *Chest.* 2004;125:2224-31.
73. Zack JE, Garrison T, Trovillion E, Clinkscale D, Coopersmith CM, Fraser VJ, et al. Effect of an education program aimed at reducing the occurrence of ventilator-associated pneumonia. *Crit Care Med.* 2002;30:2407-12.
74. Bouadma L, Mourvillier B, Deiler V, Le Corre B, Lolom I, Régnier B, et al. A multifaceted program to prevent ventilator-associated pneumonia: impact on compliance with preventive measures. *Crit Care Med.* 2010;38:789-96.
75. Allegranzi B, D Pittet. Role of hand hygiene in healthcare-associated infection prevention. *J Hosp Infect.* 2009;73: 305-15.
76. Pittet D, Allegranzi B, Boyce J; World Health Organization World Alliance for Patient Safety First Global Patient Safety Challenge Core Group of Experts. The World Health Organization Guidelines on Hand Hygiene in Health Care and their consensus recommendations. *Infect Control Hosp Epidemiol.* 2009;30:611-22.
77. Kollef MH, Von Harz B, Prentice D, Shapiro SD, Silver P, St John R, et al. Patient transport from intensive care increases the risk of developing ventilator-associated pneumonia. *Chest.* 1997;112:765-73.
78. Kress JP, Pohlman AS, O'Connor MF, Hall JB. Daily interruption of sedative infusions in critically ill patients undergoing mechanical ventilation. *N Engl J Med.* 2000; 342:1471-7.
79. Schweickert WD, Gehlbach BK, Pohlman AS, Hall JB, Kress JP. Daily interruption of sedative infusions and complications of critical illness in mechanically ventilated patients. *Crit Care Med.* 2004;32:1272-6.
80. Marelich GP, Murin S, Battistella F, Inciardi J, Vierra T, Roby M. Protocol weaning of mechanical ventilation in medical and surgical patients by respiratory care practitioners and nurses: effect on weaning time and incidence of ventilator-associated pneumonia. *Chest.* 2000;118:459-67.
81. Girard TD, Kress JP, Fuchs BD, Thomason JW, Schweickert WD, Pun BT, et al. Efficacy and safety of a paired sedation and ventilator weaning protocol for mechanically ventilated patients in intensive care (Awakening and Breathing Controlled trial): a randomised controlled trial. *Lancet.* 2008;371:126-34.
82. Brochard L, Mancebo J, Wysocki M, Lofaso F, Conti G, Rauss A, et al. Noninvasive ventilation for acute exacerbations of chronic obstructive pulmonary disease. *N Engl J Med.* 1995;333:817-22.
83. Hilbert G, Gruson D, Vargas F, Valentino R, Gbikpi-Benissan G, Dupon M, et al. Noninvasive ventilation in immunosuppressed patients with pulmonary infiltrates, fever, and acute respiratory failure. *N Engl J Med.* 2001; 344:481-7.
84. Keenan SP. Noninvasive positive pressure ventilation in acute respiratory failure. *JAMA.* 2000;284:2376-8.
85. Nourdine K, Combes P, Carton MJ, Beuret P, Cannamela A, Ducreux JC. Does noninvasive ventilation reduce the ICU nosocomial infection risk? A prospective clinical survey. *Intensive Care Med.* 1999:25:567-73.
86. Burns KE, Adhikari NK, Keenan SP, Meade M. Use of non-invasive ventilation to wean critically ill adults off invasive ventilation: meta-analysis and systematic review. *BMJ.* 2009;338:b1574.
87. Kohlenberg A, Schwab F, Behnke M, Geffers C, Gastmeier P. Pneumonia associated with invasive and noninvasive ventilation: an analysis of the German nosocomial infection surveillance system database. *Intensive Care Med.* 2010;36:971-8.
88. Young PJ, Pakeerathan S, Blunt MC, Subramanya S. A low-volume, low-pressure tracheal tube cuff reduces pulmonary aspiration. *Crit Care Med.* 2006;34:632-9.
89. Young PJ, Blunt MC. Improving the shape and compliance characteristics of a high-volume, low-pressure cuff improves tracheal seal. *Br J Anaesth.* 1999;83:887-9.
90. Dave MH, Frotzler A, Spielmann N, Madjdpour C, Weiss M. Effect of tracheal tube cuff shape on fluid leakage across the cuff: an in vitro study. *Br J Anaesth.* 2010;105: 538-43.
91. Lucangelo U, Zin WA, Antonaglia V, Petrucci L, Viviani M, Buscema G, et al. Effect of positive expiratory pressure and type of tracheal cuff on the incidence of aspiration in mechanically ventilated patients in an intensive care unit. *Crit Care Med.* 2008;36:409-13.
92. Manzano F, Fernández-Mondéjar E, Colmenero M, Poyatos ME, Rivera R, Machado J, et al. Positive-end expiratory pressure reduces incidence of ventilator-associated pneumonia in nonhypoxemic patients. *Crit Care Med.* 2008;36:2225-31.

93. Kollef MH, Afessa B, Anzueto A, Veremakis C, Kerr KM, Margolis BD, et al.; NASCENT Investigation Group Silver-coated endotracheal tubes and incidence of ventilator-associated pneumonia: the NASCENT randomized trial. *JAMA*. 2008;300:805-13.
94. Afessa B, Shorr AF, Anzueto AR, Craven DE, Schinner R, Kollef MH. Association between a silver-coated endotracheal tube and reduced mortality in patients with ventilator-associated pneumonia. *Chest.* 2010;137:1015-21.
95. Lacherade JC, De Jonghe B, Guezennec P, Debbat K, Hayon J, Monsel A, et al. Intermittent subglottic secretion drainage and ventilator-associated pneumonia: a multicenter trial. *Am J Respir Crit Care Med.* 2010;182: 910-7.
96. Muscedere J, Rewa O, McKechnie K, Jiang X, Laporta D, Heyland DK. Subglottic secretion drainage for the prevention of ventilator-associated pneumonia: a systematic review and meta-analysis. *Crit Care Med.* 2011;39: 1985-91.
97. Dragoumanis CK, Vretzakis GI, Papaioannou VE, Didilis VN, Vogiatzaki TD, Pneumatikos IA. Investigating the failure to aspirate subglottic secretions with the Evac endotracheal tube. *Anesth Analg.* 2007;105:1083-5, table of contents.
98. Elpern EH, Scott MG, Petro L, Ries MH. Pulmonary aspiration in mechanically ventilated patients with tracheostomies. *Chest.* 1994;105:563-6.
99. Leder SB. Incidence and type of aspiration in acute care patients requiring mechanical ventilation via a new tracheotomy. *Chest.* 2002;122:1721-6.
100. Dreyfuss D, Djedaini K, Weber P, Brun P, Lanore JJ, Rahmani J, et al. Prospective study of nosocomial pneumonia and of patient and circuit colonization during mechanical ventilation with circuit changes every 48 hours versus no change. *Am Rev Respir Dis.* 1991;143:738-43.
101. Fink JB, Krause SA, Barrett L, Schaaff D, Alex CG. Extending ventilator circuit change interval beyond 2 days reduces the likelihood of ventilator-associated pneumonia. *Chest.* 1998;113:405-11.
102. Han JN, Liu YP, Ma S, Zhu YJ, Sui SH, Chen XJ, et al. Effects of decreasing the frequency of ventilator circuit changes to every 7 days on the rate of ventilator-associated pneumonia in a Beijing hospital. *Respir Care.* 2001;46:891-6.
103. Hess D, Burns E, Romagnoli D, Kacmarek RM. Weekly ventilator circuit changes. A strategy to reduce costs without affecting pneumonia rates. *Anesthesiology.* 1995; 82:903-11.
104. Kotilainen HR, Keroack MA. Cost analysis and clinical impact of weekly ventilator circuit changes in patients in intensive care unit. *Am J Infect Control.* 1997;25:117-20.
105. Kollef MH, Prentice D, Shapiro SD, Fraser VJ, Silver P, Trovillion E, et al. Mechanical ventilation with or without daily changes of in-line suction catheters. *Am J Respir Crit Care Med.* 1997;156:466-72.
106. Long MN, Wickstrom G, Grimes A, Benton CF, Belcher B, Stamm AM. Prospective, randomized study of ventilator-associated pneumonia in patients with one versus three ventilator circuit changes per week. *Infect Control Hosp Epidemiol.* 1996;17:14-9.
107. Stamm AM. Ventilator-associated pneumonia and frequency of circuit changes. *Am J Infect Control.* 1998;26:71-3.
108. Han J, Liu Y. Effect of ventilator circuit changes on ventilator-associated pneumonia: a systematic review and meta-analysis. *Respir Care.* 2010;55:467-74.
109. Cook D, De Jonghe B, Brochard L, Brun-Buisson C. Influence of airway management on ventilator-associated pneumonia: evidence from randomized trials. *JAMA.* 1998;279:781-7.
110. Hirsch JA, Tokayer JL, Robinson MJ, Sackner MA. Effects of dry air and subsequent humidification on tracheal mucous velocity in dogs. *J Appl Physiol.* 1975;39:242-6.
111. Torres A, Serra-Batlles J, Ros E, Piera C, Puig de la Bellacasa J, Cobos A, et al. Pulmonary aspiration of gastric contents in patients receiving mechanical ventilation: the effect of body position. *Ann Intern Med.* 1992;116:540-3.
112. Orozco-Levi M, Torres A, Ferrer M, Piera C, el-Ebiary M, de la Bellacasa JP, et al. Semirecumbent position protects from pulmonary aspiration but not completely from gastroesophageal reflux in mechanically ventilated patients. *Am J Respir Crit Care Med.* 1995;152:1387-90.
113. Donowitz LG, Page MC, Mileur BL, Guenthner SH. Alteration of normal gastric flora in critical care patients receiving antacid and cimetidine therapy. *Infect Control.* 1986;7:23-6.
114. Pineda LA, Saliba RG, El Solh AA. Effect of oral decontamination with chlorhexidine on the incidence of nosocomial pneumonia: a meta-analysis. *Crit Care.* 2006;10:R35.
115. Chan EY, Ruest A, Meade MO, Cook DJ. Oral decontamination for prevention of pneumonia in mechanically ventilated adults: systematic review and meta-analysis. *BMJ.* 2007;334:889.
116. Tantipong H, Morkchareonpong C, Jaiyindee S, Thamlikitkul V. Randomized controlled trial and meta-analysis of oral decontamination with 2% chlorhexidine solution for the prevention of ventilator-associated pneumonia. *Infect Control Hosp Epidemiol.* 2008;29:131-6.
117. Koeman M, van der Ven AJ, Hak E, Joore HC, Kaasjager K, de Smet AG, et al. Oral decontamination with chlorhexidine reduces the incidence of ventilator-associated pneumonia. *Am J Respir Crit Care Med.* 2006;173:1348-55.
118. Stoutenbeek CP, van Saene HK, Miranda DR, Zandstra DF. The effect of selective decontamination of the digestive tract on colonisation and infection rate in multiple trauma patients. *Intensive Care Med.* 1984;10:185-92.
119. de Jonge E, Schultz MJ, Spanjaard L, Bossuyt PM, Vroom MB, Dankert J, et al. Effects of selective decontamination of digestive tract on mortality and acquisition of resistant bacteria in intensive care: a randomised controlled trial. *Lancet.* 2003;362:1011-6.
120. de Smet AM, Kluytmans JA, Cooper BS, Mascini EM, Benus RF, van der Werf TS, et al. Decontamination of the digestive tract and oropharynx in ICU patients. *N Engl J Med.* 2009;360:20-31.
121. Krueger WA, Lenhart FP, Neeser G, Ruckdeschel G, Schreckhase H, Eissner HJ, et al. Influence of combined intravenous and topical antibiotic prophylaxis on the incidence of infections, organ dysfunctions, and mortality in critically ill surgical patients: a prospective,

stratified, randomized, double-blind, placebo-controlled clinical trial. *Am J Respir Crit Care Med.* 2002;166: 1029-37.

122. Liberati A, D'Amico R, Pifferi S, Torri V, Brazzi L, Parmelli E. Antibiotic prophylaxis to reduce respiratory tract infections and mortality in adults receiving intensive care. *Cochrane Database Syst Rev.* 2009;(4): CD000022.
123. D'Amico R, Pifferi S, Leonetti C, Torri V, Tinazzi A, Liberati A. Effectiveness of antibiotic prophylaxis in critically ill adult patients: systematic review of randomised controlled trials. *BMJ.* 1998;316:1275-85.
124. Morrow LE, Kollef MH, Casale TB. Probiotic prophylaxis of ventilator-associated pneumonia: a blinded, randomized, controlled trial. *Am J Respir Crit Care Med.* 2010;182: 1058-64.
125. Siempos II, Ntaidou TK, Falagas ME. Impact of the administration of probiotics on the incidence of ventilator-associated pneumonia: a meta-analysis of randomized controlled trials. *Crit Care Med.* 2010;38:954-62.

CHAPTER 19

Diagnosis and Management of Hospital-acquired Pneumonia Due to Methicillin-resistant *Staphylococcus aureus*

Carolina de La Cuesta, Juan M del Rio, Daniel H Kett

ABSTRACT

Hospital-acquired methicillin resistant *Staphylococcus aureus* (MRSA) pneumonia continues to be associated with increased resource utilization, morbidity, and mortality. Clinicians face the difficult decision as to select the most appropriate antibiotic for patients with MRSA pneumonias. Vancomycin continues to have clinical utility and guidelines recommend dosing vancomycin to a target trough levels between 15 and 20 mg/L. However, due to the relatively poor penetration of vancomycin into the lungs and rising minimum inhibitory concentrations (MICs) in many geographical areas, there are concerns as to vancomycin's effectiveness in MRSA pneumonia. In a randomized controlled trial (RCT) of patients with MRSA pneumonia, linezolid demonstrated improved clinical efficacy compared to vancomycin; however, survival was not improved. Identifying patients who would benefit from linezolid over vancomycin as initial anti-MRSA therapy requires further study. Based on the current literature, other antibiotics with MRSA activity have a more limited role and are not generally used as initial therapy. Combination therapy also requires additional study.

INTRODUCTION

Hospital-acquired pneumonia (HAP), ventilator-associated pneumonia (VAP), and healthcare-associated pneumonia are among the most common nosocomial infections. Despite advances in antimicrobial therapy and the use of better supportive care modalities, these remain important causes of morbidity and mortality in patients receiving intensive care. The increase in morbidity and mortality associated with nosocomial infections, including pneumonias, are partly due to increasing antibiotic resistance.[1,2] The American Thoracic Society (ATS) and the Infectious Diseases Society of America (IDSA) published an updated guideline for the management of healthcare-associated pneumonia, HAP, and VAP in 2005 which emphasized early, appropriate antibiotics in adequate doses.[3] As methicillin-resistant *Staphylococcus aureus* (MRSA) accounts for a large percentage of healthcare-associated pneumonia, HAP, and VAP cases,[4-7] these guidelines recommend that patients with risk factors for infection with multidrug-resistant (MDR) pathogens should receive broad-spectrum empiric therapy with activity against gram-negative pathogens and an antibiotic with activity against MRSA.[3]

The guidelines recommend that vancomycin should be dosed to achieve target trough levels of 15–20 mg/L.[3] The same vancomycin troughs are also recommended for serious infections due to *S. aureus* and MRSA (including pneumonia) in a consensus review of therapeutic monitoring of vancomycin by the American Society of Health-System Pharmacists (ASHP), Society of Infectious Diseases Pharmacists (SIDP), and the IDSA[8] and in the recently published IDSA Clinical Practice Guidelines for the treatment of MRSA infections.[3,9-11]

The choice of antimicrobial therapy for pneumonia patients should be based on the clinical characteristics of the individual patient, the local prevalence of *S. aureus,* and its resistance profile. Antibiotics with activity against MRSA are summarized in table 1. Multiple studies in patients with MRSA pneumonia evaluating alternative antibiotics to vancomycin have been completed (Table 2). Based on these studies, only vancomycin and linezolid are approved by the US Food and Drug Administration (FDA) for the treatment of nosocomial pneumonia due to MRSA. Additionally, quinupristin/dalfopristin has approval for patients with pneumonia in Europe. Other antibiotics have clinical activity against MRSA and have been studied in either patients with pneumonia or other serious infections due to MRSA. Given the importance of determining the appropriate initial therapy in these seriously ill pneumonia patients and the debate surrounding the appropriate empiric antibiotics, we review the current diagnostic strategies and antibiotic therapy available to treat patients with hospital-acquired MRSA (HA-MRSA) pneumonia.

DIAGNOSIS OF PNEUMONIA

Clinical suspicion of pneumonia involves patients with a new or progressive infiltrates on chest radiograph and at least 2 of the following: new or increased cough or sputum production, fever, hypothermia, leukocytosis, left shift, leukopenia, or deterioration of pulmonary function. However, the diagnostic accuracy of clinical criteria is low.[12] Therefore, patients suspected to have nosocomial pneumonia should have a comprehensive medical history and undergo a thorough physical examination. This approach helps to identify other areas of potential infection and in pneumonia patients, to estimate its severity. A detailed history can also assist in identifying risks factors for MDR pathogens such as MRSA.[1,13,14]

Chest X-rays can provide the degree of anatomic involvement, as well as assessment of complications such as pleural effusions, cavitation, and/or necrotizing lesions. Preferably, the chest X-ray includes both posterior, anterior, and lateral views. Portable anteroposterior chest imaging offers less information and should be reserved for patients on mechanical ventilation or who have other positional limitations.[3] While in patients suspected to have pneumonia, a thoracic computed tomography (CT) scan may offer advantages and improve the diagnostic yield,[15] its role in the routine diagnosis of pneumonia in the intensive care unit (ICU) population requires further studies.

Arterial oxygen saturation should also be assessed. In less severely ill patients, pulse oximetry may be sufficient. In patients with suspected respiratory or metabolic abnormalities, such as the critically ill, arterial blood gas analysis is generally preferred. Arterial blood gas analysis also allows clinicians to determine the arterial oxygen tension to fractional inspiratory oxygen ratio (PaO_2/FiO_2), establish the degree of alveolar to arterial oxygen gradient, and better assessment of the appropriate oxygen supplementation and/or the need for mechanical ventilation. Other laboratory data such as blood cells count and metabolic panel may help determine the pneumonia severity by identifying if other organ involvement exists.[16,17] Guidelines recommend that blood cultures should be collected to identify a possible extrapulmonary source of infection.[3] When chest radiology suggests that an effusion is present, a diagnostic thoracentesis should be considered. This allows differentiation between parapneumonic and complicated effusion such as an empyema.

The clinical pulmonary infection score (CPIS) has been used as clinical criteria for decision-making regarding antibiotic therapy in patients with suspected pneumonia.[18] Using a modified CPIS score (Table 3) in patients with a low clinical suspicion of pneumonia (CPIS <6) at time of diagnosis and again on day 3, may allow for early discontinuation of antibiotics without any negative impact on outcomes.[19]

Microbiologic Identification

The microbiological evaluation of patients with HAP includes qualitative and quantitative culture of respiratory secretions. Sputum is generally considered a poor diagnostic specimen, in part because it can be contaminated by upper respiratory flora and may not come from the infected area. Methods to collect lower respiratory samples and protect them from contamination include bronchoscopy-directed methods and non-bronchoscopic 'blind' techniques. Many studies have compared qualitative and quantitative microbiological results on lower respiratory specimens obtained by different sampling methods. The conclusions remain contentious and are beyond the scope of this review.

The diagnostic approach for suspected nosocomial pneumonia has been best studied in patients with VAP. Using quantitative cultures derived from bronchoscopic lavage fluid, compared to a clinical management strategy, investigators found a reduction in antibiotic usage and a trend towards improved survival favoring the invasive technique.[20] However, other studies comparing therapy based on quantitative culture results to therapy guided by non-quantitative cultures of endotracheal aspirates did not find differences in hospital mortality, length of stay, or duration of mechanical ventilation.[21-23] Cost, feasibility, and safety considerations seem to favor endotracheal

TABLE 1
Summary of MRSA Antibiotics

Drug name	Mechanism of action	Mechanism of resistance	Dose	Major side effects	Indications	Note
Vancomycin	Bactericidal; inhibits cell wall and RNA synthesis	High level vancomycin resistance is rare, and is acquired via plasmid (from enterococci). Has been reported in US, India, and Iran	15 mg/kg IV every 12 hours (with therapeutic drug monitoring and drug adjustment)	Renal impairment, infusion reactions, IgA bullous dermatitis	FDA approved for infections due to MRSA, including HAP	Remains gold standard agent for empiric treatment of MRSA infections in hospitalized patients
Linezolid	Bactericidal against *Streptococcus* spp., bacteriostatic against *Staphylococcal* and *Enterococci* species. Binds to 50S ribosomal subunit inhibiting protein synthesis	Results from G257GT mutation in drug target site, acquired via plasmid. Resistant isolates reported in 2008 where secondary to acquisition of a chloramphenicol-florfenicol resistant gene which mediates methylation. This affects binding and is thought to have been acquired from CONS	600 mg IV or PO every 12 hours	Thrombocytopenia, optic and peripheral neuropathy, gastro-intestinal side effects	FDA approved for infections due to MRSA, including HAP	Initial studies showed non inferiority to vancomycin. A recent randomized clinical trial in nosocomial pneumonia due to MRSA noted improved clinical and microbiological success of linezolid over vancomycin. Linezolid may also inhibits *S. aureus* toxin production
Teicoplanin	Bactericidal glycopeptide, which inhibits cell wall synthesis. Produced by fermentation of *Actinoplanes teicomyceticus*	High-level resistance is achieved by replacing the C-terminal D-alanyl-D-alanine of the nascent peptidoglycan with D-alanyl–D-lactate or D-alanyl–D-serine, thus reducing the affinities of glycopeptides for cell wall targets. Reorganization of the cell wall is directed by the expression of the van gene clusters	400 mg (6 mg/kg) IV every 12 hours for 3 doses and then 400 mg daily. IM formulation is also available	Hearing and vestibular disturbances, exanthema, erythema, pruritus, fever bronchospasm or anaphylactic reactions. Elevated creatinine, liver enzymes, nausea, vomiting, eosinophilia, thrombocytopenia, leukopenia	Potentially serious Gram-positive infections, including those which cannot be treated with other antimicrobial drugs	Clinical trials compared to linezolid have show equivalent clinical or microbiologic success
Telavancin	Bactericidal lipoglicopeptide. Membrane depolarization and peptidoglycan synthesis inhibitor	*In vitro* it has displayed low potential for selection of resistance among MRSA and VRE. Acquisition of Van gene from enterococci may affect its action but not to the extent as in vancomycin	10 mg/kg IV every 24 hours	Taste disturbances, contraindicated in pregnancy, nephrotoxicity, QT prolongation, infusion reaction-red man syndrome	Approved in US and Canada for complicated SSSI	Not inferior to vancomycin in patients with HAP or VAP, higher cure rates if vancomycin MIC >1 mg/L

Continued

Table 1 *continued*

Drug name	Mechanism of action	Mechanism of resistance	Dose	Major side effects	Indications	Note
Quinupristin/ dalfopristin	Bacteriostatic for *Enterococci faecium*, bactericidal for *Staphyloccocus*. Binds to 50S subunit inhibiting early phase (dalfopristin), and late phase (quinupristin) of protein synthesis	Modification of the target	7.5 mg/kg IV every 12 hours	Arthralgias and myalgias, gastro-intestinal side effects, hyperbilirubinemia, increase LDH	Indicated for nosocomial pneumonia in Europe but not in the US, due to a non-significantly lower clinical efficacy than vancomycin	—
Tigecycline	Bacteriostatic glycylcycline, binds to 30S subunit inhibiting protein synthesis	Tigecycline is not affected by the two major tetracycline-resistance mechanisms, ribosomal protection and efflux. Not affected either by target-site modifications, macrolide efflux pumps or enzyme target changes. In multidrug-resistant Gram-negative organism resistance has been associated with efflux pumps	100 mg IV once, then 50 mg IV every 12 hours	Gastrointestinal effects	FDA approved in US for intraabdominal infections, SSSI and CAP. Approved in Europe for intraabdominal infections and complicated SSSI	Some *in vitro* activity against VRE. In patients with VAP, tigecycline was found to have a decresed clinical response and increased mortality compared to imipenem
Ceftaroline	5th generation bactericidal cephalosporin; inhibits mucopeptide synthesis	Efflux pumps and membrane permeability changes	600 mg IV every 12 hours	Gastrointestinal effects, increased liver function test, rash, hypokalemia	FDA approved in for acute bacterial SSSI (including MRSA) and CAP (not MRSA)	Not approved for HAP or VAP. Not yet approved for use in Europe
Rifampin	Inhibits DNA dependent RNA polymerase	Mutation in target DNA dependent RNA polymerase	300 mg PO twice daily	Orange body fluids, gastrointestinal side effects, increase liver enzymes, drug interactions, and flu-like symptoms with interruption of therapy	For synergistic effect, penetrates biofilm and it is active against non-dividing bacteria	Small randomized trial in South Korea has suggested that rifampin added to vancomycin 1 g every IV Q day, may provide benefit patients with confirmed MRSA HAP

Continued

Table 1 *continued*

Drug name	Mechanism of action	Mechanism of resistance	Dose	Major side effects	Indications	Note
Daptomycin	Bactericidal lipopeptide; binds to and depolarizes bacterial membrane, causing inhibition of protein, DNA and RNA synthesis (cyclic lipopeptide)	Not clear, likely change in surface membrane charge	4 mg/kg/day IV in SSSI without bacteremia and right side endocarditis. 6 mg/kg/day IV complicated SSSI and rapid progressing, sepsis, VISA and OM and 8 mg/kg/day IV for VRE	Gastrointestinal effects	Approved for complicated SSSI, right sided endocarditis and bacteremia in adults	Not effective or approved for pneumonia due to drug inactivation by lung surfactant
Clindamicyn	Binds to 50S ribosomal subunit inhibiting protein synthesis	Modification of ribosomal target site	600–2700 mg IV/IM/PO divided every 6–12 hours	*Clostridium difficile* associated diarrhea, thrombocytopenia	Uncomplicated skin abscess caused by CA-MRSA	Drug of choice for lung abscess, may inhibits *S. aureus* toxin production
TMP/SMX	TMP: folate antagonist selectively inhibits dihydrofolate reductase. SMX: bacteriostatic, competitively inhibits bacterial or fungal dihydropteroate synthetase, preventing PABA conversion to folic acid and inhibiting growth	Mutation in enzyme involved in folic acid synthesis, preventing drug binding	TMP/SMX dose is generally 160/800 mg IV/PO every 12 hours	Nephrotoxicity, gastrointestinal effects, hypersensitivity reaction	Uncomplicated skin abscess caused by CA-MRSA	No prospective clinical trials in nosocomial pneumonia patients due to MRSA

FDA, Food and Drug Administration; MRSA, *methicillin-resistant Staphylocuccus aureus*; HAP, hospital-acquired pneumonia; CONS, coagulase negative *S. aureus*; SSSI; Skin and Skin Structure Infection; VRE; Vancomycin-resistant *Enterococcus*; VAP, ventilator-associated pneumonia; LDH, lactate dehydrogenase; CAP, community-acquired pneumonia; VISA, vancomycin intermediate/resistant *Staphylococcus aureus*; CA-MRSA, community-acquired MRSA; TMP/SMX, Trimethoprim/sulfamethoxazole; PABA, para-aminobenzoic acid; IV, intravenous.

TABLE 2
Summary of Clinical Trials in MRSA Pneumonia

Reference	Intervention	Type of study	Population/subjects	Results
Rubenstein, et al. 2001[88]	Linezolid vs. Vancomycin	Prospective, double blinded, multicenter, RCT	Gram-positive HAP/VAP N = 396	Clinical response 66.4% vs. 68.1%; CI -14.9–11.3; p = 0.79
				Bacteriologic response 67.9% vs. 71.8%; CI -22.8–15; p = 0.69
				Eradication rates for MRSA 65.2% and 77.8%
				Mortality rates 17.7% vs. 25.4%; p = 0.06
Wunderink, et al. 2003[89]	Linezolid vs. Vancomycin	Prospective, double blinded, multicenter, RCT	Gram-positive HAP/VAP N = 623	Clinical response 67.9% vs. 64.9%; CI -7.1–13
				Bacteriologic response 61.8% vs. 53.2%; CI -6.8–24
				Eradication rates for MRSA 63.2% vs. 43.5%
				Mortality rates 19.9% vs. 20.2%
Wunderink, et al. 2003[90]	Linezolid vs. Vancomycin	Retrospective analysis of data from two prospective, RCT, double-blind studies	Gram-positive HAP/VAP N = 1019	Clinical response for *S. aureus* 51.5% vs. 43.4%; p = 0.18
				Clinical response for MRSA 59% vs. 35.5%; p < 0.01
				Survival rates for the MRSA subset 80.0% vs. 63.5%; p = 0.03
Kollef, et al. 2004[91]	Linezolid vs. Vancomycin	Retrospective analysis of data from two prospective, RCT, double-blind studies	Gram-positive HAP/VAP N = 544	Clinical response MRSA 62.2% vs. 21.1%; CI -16.8–12.8; p = 0.001
				Eradication rates for MRSA 60.5% and 22.9%
				Survival rates for the MRSA subset 84.1% vs. 61.7%; p = 0.02
Wunderink, et al. 2012[109]	Linezolid vs. Vancomycin	RCT, double-blinded, 2 parallel studies	Gram-positive HAP N = 1225 (MRSA pts N = 448)	Clinical response 57.6% vs. 46.6%; CI 0.5–21.6; p = 0.042
				Microbiologic response at end of study 58.1% vs. 47.1%
				Mortality rate 60-day 15.7% vs. 17.0%
Cepeda, et al. 2004[95]	Linezolid vs. Teicoplanin	Double blind, double dummy, prospective, randomized study	Gram-positive infections N = 204 HAP, N = 50	Clinical response HAP 83.3% vs. 82.8% CI –0.215–0.226; p = 1.00
				Microbiologic response HAP 83.3% vs. 68.2%; CI –0.135–0.438; p = 0.44
				Overall mortality rate18% vs. 24.5%; p = 0.3
Wilcox, et al. 2004[94]	Linezolid vs. Teicoplanin	Randomized, controlled, open-label, multicenter study	Gram-positive infections N = 430 HAP, N = 116	Clinical response HAP 96.2% vs. 92.9%
				Overall microbiologic response *S. aureus* 75.8% vs. 65.5%; p = 0.218
				Overall mortality rate 6.8% vs. 8.2%
Tascini, et al. 2009[93]	Linezolid vs. Teicoplanin	Comparative, retrospective study	Gram-positive HAP N = 169 (included skin, pneumonia, others)	Clinical response 83.9% vs. 69.2%; p = 0.002
				Mortality rate 9.8% for both groups
Freire, et al. 2010[101]	Tigecycline vs. Imipenem/ cilastin	Multicenter, RCT, double-blind study	HAP/VAP and non VAP N = 945 (MRSA N = 57)	Clinical response MRSA (Non VAP) 47.1% vs. 73.7%; CI -16.8–12.8
				Clinical response MRSA (VAP) 40% and 81.8%
				Mortality rate in the VAP groups 19.1 % and 12.5%
Rubenstein, et al. 2011[97]	Telavancin vs. Vancomycin	RCT, double-blinded, 2 parallel studies	Gram-positive HAP N = 1503 MRSA N = 290	Clinical response 82.4% vs. 80.7%
				Mortality rate 21.5% vs. 16.6%
Fagon, et al. 2000[20]	Quinupristin/ dalfopristin vs. Vancomycin	Prospective, open label, multicenter, RCT	Gram-positive HAP/VAP N = 298	Clinical response 56.3% vs. 58.3%; CI -16.8–12.8
				Bacteriologic response 54.2% vs. 53.7%; CI -16.1–17
				Overall equivalent by pathogen clinical success rates for *S. pneumoniae*, *S. aureus*, and MRSA
				Mortality rates 25.3% vs. 21.6%; p = 0.45

Continued

Table 2 *continued*

Reference	Intervention	Type of study	Population/subjects	Results
Jung YJ, et al. 2010[106]	Vancomycin/ Rifampin vs. Vancomycin	Prospective, randomized open label study	Gram-positive HAP N = 183	Clinical response in MRSA subjects 53.7% vs. 31.0%; p = 0.47
				Microbiologic response eradication rate did not differ between groups p = 0.472
				ICU mortality rates at day 28:22% vs. 38.1%; p = 0.151 at day 60:26.8% vs. 50%; p = 0.042

HAP, hospital-acquired pneumonia; VAP, ventilator-associated pneumonia; RCT, randomized controlled trial; CI, confidence interval; MRSA, methicillin-resistant *Staphylococcus aureus*; ICU, intensive care unit.

TABLE 3

Modified Clinical Pulmonary Infection Score[23]

Criteria		Points
Temperature (°F)	*Temperature (°C)*	
≥97.7 and ≤101.1	≥36.5 and ≤38.4	0
≥101.3 and ≤102	≥38.5 and ≤38.9	1
≥102.2 and ≤96.8	≥39 and ≤36	2
Blood leukocytes (mm^3)		
≥4,000 and ≤11,000		0
<4,000 or >11,000		1
Band forms ≥50%		1
Tracheal secretions		
Absence of tracheal secretions		0
Presence of nonpurulent tracheal secretions		1
Presence of purulent tracheal secretions		2
Oxygenation: (PaO_2/FiO_2 mmHg)		
>240 or ARDS (ARDS defined as PaO_2/FiO_2 ≥200, pulmonary arterial wedge pressure ≤18 mmHg, and acute bilateral infiltrates)		0
≤240 and no ARDS		1
Pulmonary radiography		
No infiltrate		0
Diffuse (or patchy) infiltrate		1
Localized infiltrate		2
Progression of pulmonary infiltrate		
No radiographic progression		0
Radiographic progression (after CHF and ARDS are excluded)		2
Culture of tracheal aspirate		
Pathogenic bacteria' cultured in rare or light quantity or no growth		0
Pathogenic bacteria cultured in moderate or heavy quantity		1
Same pathogenic bacteria seen on Gram stain		1

ARDS, acute respiratory distress syndrome; PaO_2/FiO_2, ratio of partial pressure of arterial O_2 to the fraction of inspired O_2; CHF, congestive heart failure.

aspirates which are simple and safe to obtain. In patients with suspected pneumonia, a quantitative or semi-quantitative lower respiratory tract culture should be obtained prior to the administration and/or adjustment of antibiotics.[21,23-26]

In comparison with quantitative cultures, the microscopic evaluation of bronchoalveolar lavage (BAL) specimens may be useful in ventilated patients with suspected pneumonia. Investigators have found that the presence of intracellular organisms within the inflammatory cells of lavage fluid may be a rapid and specific test for the diagnosis of pneumonia.[24,25] Alternatively, Kirtland et al., found that no clinical criteria, or combination of clinical criteria could be correlated with the presence or absence of histologic pneumonia. However, a lavage fluid analysis with less than 50% neutrophils had a 100% negative predictive value for histologic evidence of pneumonia.[12]

Innovative techniques, such as the use of polymerase chain reaction (PCR) for molecular identification of MRSA has been shown to be efficacious for detection of nasal colonization and bloodstream infections.[26] Specific molecular assays for rapid MRSA detection in respiratory tract specimens are being developed. Other possibilities for diagnostic approach include PCR analysis of pleural fluid for differentiation of MRSA and *Streptococcus pneumoniae*.[27] Further studies are needed to demonstrate the accuracy and cost-effectiveness of these newer methods in the diagnosis of pneumonia.

INCIDENCE AND EPIDEMIOLOGY

MRSA was seen within a few years after the introduction of methicillin in 1959. Since that time, MRSA has increased in prevalence worldwide as both a nosocomial and more recently, a community-acquired pathogen.[28] MRSA remains one of the principal resistant pathogens causing complicated skin and skin-structure infections (cSSSI) and serious hospital-acquired infections including bacteremias and nosocomial pneumonias.[29]

Currently, in the US, more than 60% of *S. aureus* infections in the ICUs are caused by methicillin resistant strain.[30] In both hospitalized patients and the critically ill, the presence of MRSA, compared with methicillin sensitive *S. aureus* (MSSA) infections, is independently associated with and increased length of stay—a significantly greater likelihood of hospital death.[29-32]

Hospital-acquired pneumonia is associated with increased rates of morbidity, mortality, healthcare expenses, and resources consumption.[33] Mortality related directly to HAP has been estimated between 33 and 55%;[34] although more recent studies debate the attributable mortality associated with VAP.[35,36] Determinants of prognosis in patients with nosocomial pneumonia include the effectiveness of antibiotic treatment administered (active against the causative organism), sufficient antibiotic concentration in the site of infection (adequate treatment), and timely prescription. There is a consistent finding that early and appropriate antimicrobial therapy can reduce mortality in patient with HAP.[35,37-41] In a recent study of patients with septic shock, of which a large percentage were pneumonia patients, inappropriate initial antimicrobial therapy was associated with a 5-fold reduction in survival.[3,42] In numerous pneumonia studies, *S. aureus* has been one of the microorganisms commonly associated with inappropriate treatment, again in these patients.[37-40]

RESISTANCE AND VIRULENCE

MRSA is a major cause of hospital-acquired infections that are becoming increasingly difficult to treat because of the emerging resistance to many current antibiotic classes. Methicillin resistance in *S. aure*us results from acquisition of the *mecA* gene located within the mobile element known as staphylococcal cassette chromosome mec *(SCCmec)*. HA-MRSA infections are generally caused by MDR strains that possess *SCCmec* types I, II, and III, whereas community-acquired MRSA (CA-MRSA) carries *SCCmec* IV, V, or VII. *SCCmec* type IV clone exhibiting the USA300 pulse-field electrophoresis profile predominates in the US.[43]

Staphylococcus aureus can express multiple virulence factors, including adhesins (fibronectin binding protein and protein A) that mediate binding to host cells, enzymes (proteins and lipases), toxins [alfa-hemolysins (αHL) and Panton-valentine leukocidin (PVL)], soluble modulins, and capsular polysaccharides. Expressions of virulent factors are controlled by the accessory gene regulator (agr) system, which varies between strains. PVL is a bicomponent pore-forming exotoxin produced by 2–3% of clinical *S. aureus* isolates[42] and is secreted by strains of MRSA that are generally associated with community outbreaks.[44]

In the US, the primary MRSA circulating clone in the community corresponds to the USA300 and PVL is thought to be related to both the virulence and poor clinical outcomes associated with these infections. Antibiotic susceptibility patterns also do not necessarily predict whether the isolate is a PVL-producing strain or not.[45] In addition, PVL production varies significantly among different clinical isolates,[7] suggesting other factors affect the phenotype and therefore, the need for ICU care. Although debate continues regarding whether the PVL toxin is the most important virulence factor or not,[46,47] presence of PVL appears to be a marker for the more virulent strains.

The CA-MRSA strains in the US most closely associated with community outbreaks, USA300 and USA400, often contain the PVL genes and are associated with skin and soft tissue infections (SSTIs).[48] Community-acquired pneumonia (CAP) has been reported in addition to the more common soft tissue infections with these strains. Gillet et al.[49] found that the overall mortality in patients with CAP with PVL-producing strains of *S. aureus* was 56%.[49,50]

In the US, 300 strains of MRSA are being identified in the hospital setting[45,51,52] which may make the traditional classification of MRSA as community-acquired vs. hospital-acquired less important in the future. To date, in patients with HAP or VAP due to MRSA, the severity of disease and clinical outcomes are not influenced by the presence of the PVL gene, possibly due to the lack of expression of the exotoxin.[51] These authors hypothesize that in contrast to CAP, where the initiation of treatment is often delayed, the initiation of antibiotics in patients with HAP or VAP often occurs within 24 hours from development of pneumonia signs or symptoms. Early institution of therapy in nosocomial MRSA pneumonia may be an important factor in reducing the capability of MRSA to produce PVL exotoxin.[53]

Overall, clinical assessments, bacteriologic surveillance, and other diagnostic tools increase the sensitivity for diagnosing HAP, with the goal of providing timely, adequate antimicrobial therapy and avoid both over- and undertreatment of these serious infections. Daily assessment of the antibiotic need, including when to start, escalate, deescalate, or discontinue antibiotics needs to be a part of the clinical decision-making in the management of HAP.

TREATMENT

Guidelines for the treatment of nosocomial pneumonia recommend an initial empiric therapy, either vancomycin or linezolid, in hospitals with a high prevalence MRSA or in nosocomial pneumonia due to *S. aureus*.[3] Other agents used to treat MRSA, such as teicoplanin and televancin have more limited regional availability. Additionally, multiple other antibiotics have activity against MRSA but have not been well studied in patients with pneumonia (Table 1).

The choice of antimicrobial therapy for pneumonia patients should be based on the clinical characteristics of the individual patients, the local prevalence of *S. aureus*, and its resistance profile. Currently only vancomycin and linezolid[3] are approved by the US FDA for the treatment of nosocomial pneumonia due to MRSA. Additionally, quinupristin/dalfopristin have approval for patients with pneumonia in Europe.[20]

Vancomycin

As vancomycin has been available for over 50 years, clinicians are familiar with its use.[39,54] Vancomycin has been the cornerstone of therapy for serious MRSA infections and its usage has increased dramatically worldwide since the mid-1980.[55] Recent guidelines have supported weight based prescription of vancomycin, with the recommended dose of 15–20 mg/kg intravenously every 8–12 hours in patients with normal renal function. The recommended targeted trough levels are between 15–20 mg/L.[8] This dosing strategy is aimed toward achieving an area under the curve (AUC)/minimal inhibitory concentration (MIC) ratio of at least 400. Even with the recently increased dosage of vancomycin, the acquisition cost is significantly lower than the newer, branded anti-MRSA agents.

Vancomycin is a hydrophilic molecule with a slow bactericidal mechanism against MRSA that inhibits cell-wall formation.[56] As a hydrophilic drug, vancomycin levels are affected by the patient's volume of distribution, frequently abnormal in ICU population. Also, due to its hydrophilic property, vancomycin penetrates poorly into the lung parenchyma[57] with the drug's level in the alveoli and endothelial lining fluid being only a fraction of its concentration in the blood.[57-60] Therefore, even with the current vancomycin dosing regimens, it may be difficult to achieve adequate tissue concentrations, especially, when the MIC to vancomycin is increased.

The lower vancomycin local concentration has been suggested as a potential reason for treatment failure.[57] Attempts to increase vancomycin doses to increase local concentrations has not resulted in improvement of vancomycin efficacy and may be associated with increased toxicity.[61,62] Vancomycin use is associated with nephrotoxicity, especially, when administered with other nephrotoxic agents such as aminoglycosides[10,63,64] or when used at higher than conventional doses (1 g every 12 hours).[64,65] Vancomycin trough levels above 15 mg/L[66] and high dosages (> 4 g/day) are independently associated with risk of nephrotoxicity.[67] Additionally, there appears to be an exposure-response relationship between initial vancomycin trough levels and occurrence and mean time to nephrotoxicity.[66]

Geographical variation in *S. aureus* susceptibility to vancomycin has been reported. Many centers have noted progressive increases in the MIC90 of Staphylococcal species to vancomycin,[68-72] while other investigators have failed to confirm this finding.[73-75] The inconsistent findings related to vancomycin MIC creep may arise from differences in susceptibility testing methods, including how the isolates were stored prior to testing.[76,77]

In a cohort of 158 patients with HA-MRSA pneumonia, Haque et al., demonstrated an association between increasing vancomycin MICs and mortality, even in patients with vancomycin MICs generally considered within the susceptible range.[78] Additionally, prior vancomycin exposure has been found to be an independent predictor of treatment failure.[79] Therefore, in pneumonia patients with prior vancomycin exposure or in areas where MRSA is known to have higher average MICs to vancomycin, antibiotic selection should be based on the patient's clinical condition and the associated risk of failure. When appropriate, alternative therapies should be considered.

Linezolid

Linezolid is a synthetic oxazolidione with bacteriostatic action against MRSA. Linezolid binds to 50s ribosomal subunit inhibiting protein synthesis via a different pathway than other commonly prescribed antibiotics. This mechanism of action makes the development of cross-linked resistance less likely. Linezolid resistance was initially reported to occur most commonly as a result of a G2576T mutation in the drug target site. This mutation has appeared only sporadically and is usually mediated by the presence of mutation in 1 or more alleles of the target 23s rRNA gene. An outbreak of MRSA infections resistant to linezolid occurred due to clonal isolates with the chloramphenicol/florfenicol resistant gene—a gene responsible for the methylation of the 23S rRNA subunit.[80] This gene is thought to have been transmitted horizontally via plasmid from coagulase negative staphylococci.[81] *Staphylococcus aureus* isolates with linezolid-chloramphenicol/florfenicol resistant gene mediated gene resistance have recently been reported in the US.[81] Despite the sporadic outbreaks of linezolid resistance being reported,[82] after a decade of use, approximately 99% of the *S. aureus* are sensitive to linezolid.[80]

The pharmacokinetics of linezolid appears to be less affected in critically ill pneumonia patients. The lung concentration of linezolid, as measured from alveolar epithelium, is approximately, 4 times that of the plasma concentration.[83] Dosing of linezolid is 600 mg every 12 hours and can be administered either intravenously or preorally. The goal of dosing should be to obtain an AUC/MIC between 80 and 120.[84,85] A recent retrospective study in patients with documented or suspected MRSA infections found the standard dosing of linezolid failure to reach the target pharmacokinetic goals in 30% of patients. An additional 12% of patients had overexposure to linezolid, partly associated with concomitant use of omeprazole, amlodipine, or amiodarone.[86] The clinical impact of not achieving these pharmacokinetic goals is still to be determined and to date, measurement of linezolid levels is not commonly performed.

Major side effects associated with linezolid includes dose- and time-dependent thrombocytopenia. Therefore, patients receiving prolonged administration of linezolid should undergo serial complete blood cell count monitoring. Other less frequent, but serious side effects include lactic acidosis, possible serotonin syndrome, and neuropathy.[87]

Clinical Trials of Linezolid in Pneumonia

Linezolid has been studied in multiple populations associated with MRSA pneumonia. Most studies used vancomycin as the comparator, with the most recent trial using weight-based dosing of vancomycin. In 2001, Rubenstein et al.[88] reported the results of a prospective, randomized trial in patients with nosocomial pneumonia, in which 203 patients received intravenous linezolid 600 mg twice daily and 193 patients received vancomycin 1 g intravenously twice daily. Patients in both arms received aztreonam for Gram-negative coverage. In evaluated patients, clinical cure rates [71 (66.4%) of 107 for linezolid vs. 62 (68.1%) of 91 for vancomycin, p = 0.79] and microbiological success rates [36 (67.9%) of 53 for linezolid vs. 28 (71.8%) of 39 for vancomycin, p = 0.69) were similar between treatment groups. Additionally, the eradication rates of MRSA and safety evaluations were similar between treatment groups. In 2003, Wunderink et al.[89] reported the results of another prospective, randomized trial of linezolid and vancomycin, with the use of aztreonam for Gram-negative coverage. A total of 623 patients were enrolled, with 321 in the linezolid group and 302 in the vancomycin group. Again, in evaluated patients, there were no significant differences between the linezolid and vancomycin groups in clinical cure rates [114 of 168 (67.9%) for linezolid and 111 of 171 [64.9%1) for vancomycin] or microbiologic success rates [47 of 76 (61.8%) for linezolid and 42 of 79 (53.2%) for vancomycin].

Based on the data collected in both prospective trials, Wunderink et al.[90] performed a retrospective analysis in the patients with documented *S. aureus* pneumonia. Of the combined 1,019 patients enrolled, 339 patients had *S. aureus* pneumonia, with 160 of these being methicillin resistant. In the MRSA subset, patients receiving linezolid compared to vancomycin had improved clinical cure rates [59.0% (36 of 61 patients) vs. 35.5% (22 of 62 patients), p < 0.01)] and survival [80.0% (60 of 75 patients) vs. 63.5% (54 of 85 patients) p = 0.03]. Kollef et al.[91] performed an additional retrospective analysis of this database. In the 544 patients with suspected VAP, including 264 patients with documented Gram-positive VAP and 91 patients with VAP due to MRSA, the clinical cure rates and survival favored linezolid over vancomycin. Comparing linezolid to vancomycin in the MRSA VAP patients, the clinical cure rate was 62.2% vs. 21.2%. (p = 0.001) and survival was 84.1% vs. 61.7% (p = 0.02), respectively.

While retrospective analysis suggested that in pneumonia due to MRSA, linezolid had improved clinical outcomes and survival compared to vancomycin, a recent meta-analysis of prospective randomized trials that tested linezolid vs. glycopepetides (vancomycin or teicoplanin) did not demonstrate clinical superiority of linezolid for the treatment of nosocomial pneumonia even in the cohort of patients with pneumonia due to MRSA.[92]

Recently, the results from a randomized, prospective, double-blind, controlled, multicenter trial study was undertaken to assess efficacy and safety of linezolid, compared with a weight-based vancomycin regimen, for treatment of MRSA nosocomial pneumonia has been published. Study patients received either intravenous linezolid (600 mg every 12 hours) or vancomycin (15 mg/kg every 12 hours). Vancomycin dose was adjusted on the basis of trough levels. Of the 1225 pneumonia patients randomized, 448 had documented MRSA. The primary end point was clinical success at end of study in evaluable per-protocol patients (n = 348 patients). For the primary endpoint, 95 of 165 (57.6%) linezolid-treated patients achieved clinical success compared with 81 of 174 (46.6%) vancomycin-treated patients [95% confidence interval (CI) 0.5–21.6%; p = 0.042). Additionally, in this population 58.1% of linezolid-treated patients had microbiologic success (eradication or presumed eradication), compared with 47.1% of vancomycin treated patients at the end of study (95% CI 0.4–21.5%). Similar differences in outcomes were noted at other study endpoint. Despite the improved clinical success and microbiologic eradication, the 60 day mortality was similar (15.7% in linezolid-treated patients and 17.0% in vancomycin-treated patients).

Teicoplanin

Teicoplanin is a glycopeptide, which inhibits cell wall synthesis and has similar concerns to other glycopeptides related to its poor penetration into the lung parenchyma, nephrotoxicity, and mechanism of development of resistance. In seriously ill pneumonia patients, intravenous teicoplanin is generally prescribed as 400 mg (6 mg/kg) intravenously every 12 hours for three doses and then, 400 mg daily. Intramuscular formulation is also available. Teicoplanin is not available in the US.

In a retrospective, single center study comparing teicoplanin to linezolid in Gram-positive infections including pneumonia, patients treated with teicoplanin were found to have a lower clinical success and longer hospital stay than those receiving linezolid.[93] In a prospective study in patients with suspected or proven Gram-positive infection, clinical cure rates in the linezolid-treated patient were superior to teicoplanin (95.5% vs. 87.6%, p = 0.005).[94] However, in the subset of pneumonia patients, clinical cure rates were not statistically different (96.2% vs. 92.9%, respectively).[94] In a population of critically ill patients with Gram-positive infections, including those with pneumonia, teicoplanin and linezolid had similar efficacy and safety.[95]

Telavancin

Telavancin is a bactericidal lipoglycopeptide, with bactericidal effects against Gram-positive bacteria including MRSA. It is approved in the US for the treatment of cSSSI.[96]

Two double-blind studies comparing telavancin vs. vancomycin for HAP due to Gram-positive infections have been performed. In the combined trials, over 1500 patients were in the all-treated population and the cure rates between televancin and vancomycin were similar (58.9% vs. 59.5%; 95% CI 0.56–4.3%). While treatment with telavancin achieved higher cure rates in patients with monomicrobial *S. aureus* infection and comparable cure rates in patients with MRSA infection, in patients with mixed Gram-positive or Gram-negative infections, cure rates were higher in the vancomycin group. Mortality was similar in the telavancin-treated and vancomycin-treated groups (20.0% vs. 18.6%; 95% CI 12.6–5.3%). In a subgroup analysis of patient with MRSA pneumonia in which isolates had a vancomycin MIC of more than 1 μg/L or greater, there was an improved clinical response in patients receiving telavancin (87.1% vs. 74.3% clinical response; p = 0.03).[97] Renal dysfunction was more common in patients receiving telavancin than in those receiving vancomycin (16% vs. 10%), but this difference was not statistical.

While the primary end point of the studies was met, indicating that the clinical response in the treatment of HAP due to Gram-positive pathogens telavancin is non-inferior to vancomycin, televancin is not currently approved by the FDA for use in HAP. Due to the possible increased risk of nephrotoxicity in the patients receiving telavancin, there is limited approval of televancin in Europe for the treatment of HAP and VAP. In Europe, telavancin is approved for treatment in patients with pneumonia known or suspected to be caused by MRSA in situations where other alternatives are not suitable.[98] Indications for cSSSI in Europe has been withdrawn.

Quinupristin/Dalfopristin

Quinupristin/dalfopristin is a semisynthetic parenteral streptogramin consisting of 2 components that produce a synergistic, *in vitro* effect against a wide spectrum of Gram-positive pathogens including MRSA. The 2 major components are quinupristin (30%), a group B streptogramin and dalfopristin (70%), a group A streptogramin. Streptogramins are members of the macrolide-lincosamide-streptogramin group of antibiotics due to the similar mechanism of action which includes inhibition of bacterial protein synthesis. Quinupristin/dalfopristin has a good safety profile and it is effective in the treatment of infections due to MRSA. Quinupristin/dalfopristin is indicated for the treatment of nosocomial pneumonia in Europe but not in the US, reportedly due to the non-statistically significant but lower clinical efficacy than vancomycin in nosocomial pneumonia due to MRSA.

A prospective, randomized, open-label, multicenter, clinical trial of intravenous quinupristin/dalfopristin vs. vancomycin in the treatment of nosocomial pneumonia caused by Gram-positive pathogens enrolled 298 patients. In the bacteriologically evaluable population, therapy was clinically successful (cure or improvement) in 49 (56.3%) of patients receiving quinupristin/dalfopristin and 49 (58.3%) patients receiving vancomycin [difference, –2.0% (95% CI –16.8–12.8%)]. The number of MRSA cases was relatively small, but the clinical success rates were comparable between quinupristin/dalfopristin and vancomycin groups (6/20 vs. 8/18, respectively). Equivalent clinical success rates were also observed in the all-treated population.[99]

Tigecycline

Tigecycline is the first commercially available member of the glycylcyclines class of antibiotics. It is a bacteriostatic antimicrobial that binds to the 30S ribosomal subunit inhibiting protein synthesis. Tigecycline is approved in the US for treatment of adults with cSSSI, complicated intra-abdominal infections, and CAP[100] and in Europe for cSSSI and intra-abdominal infections.[100] In a clinical trial of 945 patients with nosocomial pneumonia, the clinical response of the patients treated with tigecycline was lower (67%) in comparison to the group treated with imipenem (78%). In the case of MRSA pneumonia, vancomycin was added to the patients treated with imipenem.[101] These results may be due to a low concentration of tigecycline in the epithelial lining fluid; hence, a higher dose of the drug might improve the clinical results.[102]

Ceftaroline and Ceftobiprole

Cephalosporin antibiotics with activity against MRSA, such as ceftaroline and ceftobiprole, have recently been developed. They are 5th generation cephalosporins which inhibit cell wall mucopeptide synthesis.

Ceftaroline, the active component of the pro-drug ceftaroline fosamil, is a 5th generation cephalosporin that is approved in the US for acute bacterial SSSI and CAP[103] and yet not approved in Europe. It has been shown to be non-inferior than vancomycin plus aztreonam in SSSI, and to ceftriaxone in CAP. At present, there is no data available in case of nosocomial pneumonia.[104]

In a randomized phase III trial comparing ceftobiprole to ceftazidime combined with linezolid in nosocomial pneumonia patients, the primary endpoint of clinical success met its non-inferiority criteria. However, in the subgroup of patients with VAP,[105] significantly lower cure rates were observed in ceftobiprole-treated patients.

Rifampin

Rifampin inhibits RNA dependent DNA polymerase and has bactericidal effects against most Gram-positive organisms including MRSA. Rifampin distributes well to the body and achieves a good concentration in various organs and body fluids. Resistant strains are observed rapidly when used as a single agent due to a mutation in the DNA dependent RNA polymerase. It has been used in combination with other agents that are active against *S. aureus* to treat staphylococcal infections.

In a small, randomized prospective study in patients with nosocomial pneumonia, rifampin has been used in combination with vancomycin Results suggested that vancomycin plus rifampin may be more effective than vancomycin alone in clinical cure and mortality in the treatment of nosocomial MRSA pneumonia.[106] However, microbiological eradication was unchanged. Further studies are needed to determine the potential benefit of adding rifampin to others antibiotic therapy for patients with MRSA pneumonia.

Daptomycin

Daptomycin is a cyclic lipopeptide derived from the fermentation of *Streptomyces roseosporus*. It binds to bacterial membranes causing a rapid depolarization of the membrane potential, which inhibits DNA, RNA, and protein synthesis. The mechanism of resistance is not fully understood and to date, there are no known transferable bacterial elements that confer resistance to daptomycin. This agent is approved in Europe for the treatment of complicated SSSIs, right-sided endocarditis, and *S. aureus* bacteremia in adults.[107] Animal data (mice, rats, and sheep) indicate that the penetration of daptomycin into BAL epithelial lining fluid was low with a ratio of 0.02 (or 2% of penetration relative to serum).[108] Daptomycin is not effective or approved for pneumonia due to its inactivation by lung surfactant.

CONCLUSION

Methicillin-resistant Staphylococcus aureus pneumonia continues to be associated with increased morbidity, mortality, and utilization of healthcare resources. Currently, there are multiple options for the treatment of patients with MRSA pneumonias. Vancomycin has over 50 years of clinical experience and continues to have clinical utility; however, concerns have been raised as to its effectiveness in pneumonia patients due to its relative poor penetration into the lungs and rising MICs in many geographical areas. When prescribed for MRSA pneumonia, vancomycin should be dosed to achieve target through levels of 15–20 mg/L.[9] Linezolid is an alternative to vancomycin in patients with MRSA pneumonia. In a recent randomized controlled trial (RCT) in patients with pneumonia due to MRSA, linezolid compared to vancomycin demonstrated improved clinical efficacy.[109] However, survival was not improved. Therefore, further studies and clinical experience are required to identify patients who would benefit from linezolid over vancomycin as initial anti-MRSA therapy. Potential populations include patients in areas with high rates of increased vancomycin MICs (>1 mg/mL), with prior vancomycin exposure, and/or in more severally ill patients such as those in the ICU or with VAP, or. Based on the current literature, other antibiotics such as teicoplanin, telavancin, tigecycline, quinupristin/dalfopristin and the cephalosporins with MRSA activity have a more limited role and should not generally be used as initial therapy. Combination therapy, with rifampin and vancomycin is promising but also requires additional study.[110]

REFERENCES

1. Fridkin SK, Steward CD, Edwards JR, Pryor ER, McGowan JE Jr, Archibald LK, et al. Surveillance of antimicrobial use and antimicrobial resistance in United States hospitals: project ICARE phase 2. Project Intensive Care Antimicrobial Resistance Epidemiology (ICARE) hospitals. *Clin Infect Dis.* 1999;29:245-52.
2. Pinner RW, Teutsch SM, Simonsen L, Klug LA, Graber JM, Clarke MJ, et al. Trends in infectious diseases mortality in the United States. *JAMA.* 1996;275:189-93.
3. American Thoracic Society; Infectious Diseases Society of America. Guidelines for the management of adults with hospital-acquired, ventilator-associated, and healthcare-associated pneumonia. *Am J Respir Crit Care Med.* 2005; 171:388-416.
4. Rubinstein E, Kollef MH, Nathwani D. Pneumonia caused by methicillin-resistant *Staphylococcus aureus. Clin Infect Dis.* 2008;46:S378-85.
5. Kollef MH, Shorr A, Tabak YP, Gupta V, Liu LZ, Johannes RS. Epidemiology and outcomes of health-care-associated pneumonia: results from a large US database of culture-positive pneumonia.[Erratum appears in Chest. 2006 Mar;129(3):831]. *Chest.* 2005;128:3854-62.
6. Micek ST, Kollef KE, Reichley RM, Roubinian N, Kollef MH. Health care-associated pneumonia and community-acquired pneumonia: a single-center experience. *Antimicrob Agents Chemother.* 2007;51:3568-73.
7. Kawasaki S, Aoki N, Kikuchi H, Nakayama H, Saito N, Shimada H, et al. Clinical and microbiological evaluation of hemodialysis-associated pneumonia (HDAP): should HDAP be included in healthcare-associated pneumonia? *J Infect Chemother.* 2011;17:640-5.
8. Rybak M, Lomaestro B, Rotschafer JC, Moellering R Jr, Craig W, Billeter M, et al. Therapeutic monitoring of vancomycin in adult patients: a consensus review of the American Society of Health-System Pharmacists, the Infectious Diseases Society of America, and the Society of Infectious Diseases Pharmacists. *Am J Health Syst Pharm.* 2009;66:82-98.
9. Liu C, Bayer A, Cosgrove SE, Daum RS, Fridkin SK, Gorwitz RJ, et al. Clinical practice guidelines by the Infectious Diseases Society of America for the treatment of methicillin-resistant *Staphylococcus aureus* infections in adults and children. *Clin Infect Dis.* 2011;52:e18-55.
10. Rybak MJ, Lomaestro BM, Rotschafer JC, Moellering RC Jr, Craig WA, Billeter M, et al. Therapeutic monitoring of vancomycin in adults summary of consensus recommendations from the American Society of Health-System Pharmacists, the Infectious Diseases Society of America, and the Society of Infectious Diseases Pharmacists. *Pharmacotherapy.* 2009;29:1275-9.
11. Liu C, Bayer A, Cosgrove SE, Daum RS, Fridkin SK, Gorwitz RJ, et al. Clinical practice guidelines by the infectious diseases society of america for the treatment of methicillin-resistant Staphylococcus aureus infections in adults and children: executive summary. *Clin Infect Dis.* 2011;52:285-92.
12. Kirtland SH, Corley DE, Winterbauer RH, Springmeyer SC, Casey KR, Hampson NB, et al. The diagnosis of ventilator-associated pneumonia: a comparison of histologic, microbiologic, and clinical criteria. *Chest.* 1997;112:445-57.
13. Chastre J, Fagon JY. Ventilator-associated pneumonia. *Am J Respir Crit Care Med.* 2002;165:867-903.
14. Richards MJ, Edwards JR, Culver DH, Gaynes RP. Nosocomial infections in medical intensive care units in the United States. National Nosocomial Infections Surveillance System. *Crit Care Med.* 1999;27:887-92.
15. Hayden GE, Wrenn KW. Chest radiograph vs. computed tomography scan in the evaluation for pneumonia. *J Emerg Med.* 2009;36:266-70.
16. Delclaux C, Roupie E, Blot F, Brochard L, Lemaire F, Brun-Buisson C. Lower respiratory tract colonization and infection during severe acute respiratory distress syndrome: incidence and diagnosis. *Am J Respir Crit Care Med.* 1997;156:1092-8.
17. Markowicz P, Wolff M, Djedaini K, Cohen Y, Chastre J, Delclaux C, et al. Multicenter prospective study of ventilator-associated pneumonia during acute respiratory distress syndrome. Incidence, prognosis, and risk factors. ARDS Study Group. *Am J Respir Crit Care Med.* 2000;161: 1942-8.
18. Pugin J, Auckenthaler R, Mili N, Janssens JP, Lew PD, Suter PM. Diagnosis of ventilator-associated pneumonia by bacteriologic analysis of bronchoscopic and non-bronchoscopic "blind" bronchoalveolar lavage fluid. *Am Rev Respir Dis.* 1991;143:1121-9.
19. Singh N, Rogers P, Atwood CW, Wagener MM, Yu VL. Short-course empiric antibiotic therapy for patients with pulmonary infiltrates in the intensive care unit. A proposed solution for indiscriminate antibiotic prescription. *Am J Respir Crit Care Med.* 2000;162:505-11.
20. Fagon JY, Chastre J, Wolff M, Gervais C, Parer-Aubas S, Stéphan F, et al. Invasive and noninvasive strategies for management of suspected ventilator-associated pneumonia. A randomized trial. *Ann Intern Med.* 2000;132: 621-30.
21. Sanchez-Nieto JM, Torres A, Garcia-Cordoba F, El-Ebiary M, Carrillo A, Ruiz J, et al. Impact of invasive and non-invasive quantitative culture sampling on outcome of ventilator-associated pneumonia: a pilot study.[Erratum appears in *Am J Respir Crit Care Med.* 1998;157:1005]. *Am J Respir Crit Care Med.* 1998;157:371-6.
22. Canadian Critical Care Trials Group. A randomized trial of diagnostic techniques for ventilator-associated pneumonia. *N Engl J Med.* 2006;355:2619-30.
23. Sole Violan J, Fernandez JA, Benitez AB, Cardenosa Cendrero JA, Rodriguez de Castro F. Impact of quantitative invasive diagnostic techniques in the management and outcome of mechanically ventilated patients with suspected pneumonia. *Crit Care Med.* 2000;28:2737-41.

24. Sirvent JM, Vidaur L, Gonzalez S, Castro P, de Batlle J, Castro A, et al. Microscopic examination of intracellular organisms in protected bronchoalveolar mini-lavage fluid for the diagnosis of ventilator-associated pneumonia. *Chest.* 2003;123:518-23.
25. Timsit JF, Cheval C, Gachot B, Bruneel F, Wolff M, Carlet J, et al. Usefulness of a strategy based on bronchoscopy with direct examination of bronchoalveolar lavage fluids in the initial antibiotic therapy of suspected ventilator-associated pneumonia. *Intensive Care Med.* 2001;27:640-7.
26. Carroll KC. Rapid diagnostics for methicillin-resistant Staphylococcus aureus: current status. *Mol Diagn Ther.* 2008;12:15-24.
27. Utine GE, Pinar A, Ozcelik U, Sener B, Yalcin E, Dogru D, et al. Pleural fluid PCR method for detection of *Staphylococcus aureus, Streptococcus pneumoniae* and *Haemophilus influenzae* in pediatric parapneumonic effusions. *Respiration.* 2008;75:437-42.
28. Enright MC, Robinson DA, Randle G, Feil EJ, Grundmann H, Spratt BG. The evolutionary history of methicillin-resistant *Staphylococcus aureus* (MRSA). *Proc Natl Acad Sci U S A.* 2002;99:7687-92.
29. de Kraker ME, Wolkewitz M, Davey PG, Koller W, Berger J, Nagler J, et al.; BURDEN Study Group. Clinical impact of antimicrobial resistance in European hospitals: excess mortality and length of hospital stay related to methicillin-resistant *Staphylococcus aureus* bloodstream infections. [Erratum appears in *Antimicrob Agents Chemother.* 2011; 55:3646 Note: multiple author names added]. *Antimicrob Agents Chemother.* 2011;55:1598-605.
30. Klein E, Smith DL, Laxminarayan R. Hospitalizations and deaths caused by methicillin-resistant Staphylococcus aureus, United States, 1999-2005. *Emerg Infect Dis.* 2007;13: 1840-6.
31. Hanberger H, Walther S, Leone M, Barie PS, Rello J, Lipman J, et al. Increased mortality associated with methicillin-resistant *Staphylococcus aureus* (MRSA) infection in the intensive care unit: results from the EPIC II study. *Int J Antimicrob Agents.* 2011;38:331-5.
32. Athanassa Z, Siempos II, Falagas ME. Impact of methicillin resistance on mortality in *Staphylococcus aureus* VAP: a systematic review. *Eur Respir J.* 2008;31:625-32.
33. Craven DE, Steger KA, Barber TW. Preventing nosocomial pneumonia: state of the art and perspectives for the 1990s. *Am J Med.* 1991;91:44S-53S.
34. Heyland DK, Cook DJ, Griffith L, Keenan SP, Brun-Buisson C. The attributable morbidity and mortality of ventilator-associated pneumonia in the critically ill patient. The Canadian Critical Trials Group. *Am J Respir Crit Care Med.* 1999;159:1249-56.
35. Dupont H, Mentec H, Sollet JP, Bleichner G. Impact of appropriateness of initial antibiotic therapy on the outcome of ventilator-associated pneumonia. *Intensive Care Med.* 2001;27:355-62.
36. Bekaert M, Timsit JF, Vansteelandt S, Depuydt P, Vesin A, Garrouste-Orgeas M, et al. Attributable mortality of ventilator-associated pneumonia: a reappraisal using causal analysis. *Am J Respir Crit Care Med.* 2011;184:1133-9.
37. Rello J, Rue M, Jubert P, Muses G, Sonora R, Valles J, et al. Survival in patients with nosocomial pneumonia: impact of the severity of illness and the etiologic agent. *Crit Care Med.* 1997;25:1862-7.
38. Luna CM, Vujacich P, Niederman MS, Vay C, Gherardi C, Matera J, et al. Impact of BAL data on the therapy and outcome of ventilator-associated pneumonia. *Chest.* 1997; 111:676-85.
39. Kollef MH. Antimicrobial therapy of ventilator-associated pneumonia: how to select an appropriate drug regimen. *Chest.* 1999;115:8-11.
40. Alvarez-Lerma F. Modification of empiric antibiotic treatment in patients with pneumonia acquired in the intensive care unit. ICU-Acquired Pneumonia Study Group. *Intensive Care Med.* 1996;22:387-94.
41. Ruiz M, Torres A, Ewig S, Marcos MA, Alcon A, Lledo R, et al. Noninvasive versus invasive microbial investigation in ventilator-associated pneumonia: evaluation of outcome. *Am J Respir Crit Care Med.* 2000;162:119-25.
42. Kumar A, Zarychanski R, Light B, Parrillo J, Maki D, Simon D, et al.; Cooperative Antimicrobial Therapy of Septic Shock (CATSS) Database Research Group. Early combination antibiotic therapy yields improved survival compared with monotherapy in septic shock: a propensity-matched analysis. *Crit Care Med.* 2010;38:1773-85.
43. David MZ, Daum RS. Community-associated methicillin-resistant *Staphylococcus aureus*: epidemiology and clinical consequences of an emerging epidemic. *Clin Microbiol Rev.* 2010;23:616-87.
44. Vandenesch F, Naimi T, Enright MC, Lina G, Nimmo GR, Heffernan H, et al. Community-acquired methicillin-resistant *Staphylococcus aureus* carrying Panton-Valentine leukocidin genes: worldwide emergence. *Emerg Infect Dis.* 2003;9:978-84.
45. Popovich KJ, Weinstein RA, Hota B. Are community-associated methicillin-resistant *Staphylococcus aureus* (MRSA) strains replacing traditional nosocomial MRSA strains? *Clin Infect Dis.* 2008;46:787-94.
46. Bubeck Wardenburg J, Bae T, Otto M, Deleo FR, Schneewind O. Poring over pores: alpha-hemolysin and Panton-Valentine leukocidin in *Staphylococcus aureus* pneumonia. *Nat Med.* 2007;13:1405-6.
47. Labandeira-Rey M, Couzon F, Boisset S, Brown EL, Bes M, Benito Y, et al. *Staphylococcus aureus* Panton-Valentine leukocidin causes necrotizing pneumonia. *Science.* 2007; 315:1130-3.
48. Deresinski S. Methicillin-resistant *Staphylococcus aureus*: an evolutionary, epidemiologic, and therapeutic odyssey. *Clin Infect Dis.* 2005;40:562-73.
49. Gillet Y, Issartel B, Vanhems P, Fournet J-C, Lina G, Bes M, et al. Association between *Staphylococcus aureus* strains carrying gene for Panton-Valentine leukocidin and highly lethal necrotising pneumonia in young immunocompetent patients. *Lancet.* 2002;359:753-9.
50. Gillet Y, Vanhems P, Lina G, Bes M, Vandenesch F, Floret D, et al. Factors predicting mortality in necrotizing community-acquired pneumonia caused by *Staphylococcus aureus* containing Panton-Valentine leukocidin. *Clin Infect Dis.* 2007;45:315-21.
51. Peyrani P, Allen M, Wiemken TL, Haque NZ, Zervos MJ, Ford KD, et al. Severity of disease and clinical outcomes in patients with hospital-acquired pneumonia due to

methicillin-resistant *Staphylococcus aureus* strains not influenced by the presence of the Panton-Valentine Leukocidin gene. *Clin Infect Dis.* 2011;53:766-71.
52. Maree CL, Daum RS, Boyle-Vavra S, Matayoshi K, Miller LG. Community-associated methicillin-resistant *Staphylococcus aureus* isolates causing healthcare-associated infections. *Emerg Infect Dis.* 2007;13:236-42.
53. Hamilton SM, Bryant AE, Carroll KC, Lockary V, Ma Y, McIndoo E, et al. In vitro production of panton-valentine leukocidin among strains of methicillin-resistant *Staphylococcus aureus* causing diverse infections. *Clin Infect Dis.* 2007;45:1550-8.
54. Kollef MH. Vancomycin for methicillin-resistant *Staphylococcus aureus* pneumonia: the good, the bad, and the ugly. *Crit Care Med.* 2012;40:330-2.
55. Sakoulas G, Moellering RC Jr. Increasing antibiotic resistance among methicillin resistant *Staphylococci aureus* strains. *Clin Infect Dis.* 2008;46:S360-7.
56. Hospira. Vancomycin Package Insert (2008). Available from: http://www.4legpharma.com/Product%20Inserts/Hospira/Vancomycin_10gBUlkPack_10-2008.pdf.
57. Scheetz MH, Wunderink RG, Postelnick MJ, Noskin GA. Potential impact of vancomycin pulmonary distribution on treatment outcomes in patients with methicillin-resistant *Staphylococcus aureus* pneumonia. *Pharmacotherapy.* 2006;26:539-50.
58. Cruciani M, Gatti G, Lazzarini L, Furlan G, Broccali G, Malena M, et al. Penetration of vancomycin into human lung tissue. J *Antimicrob Chemother.* 1996;38:865-9.
59. Lamer C, de Beco V, Soler P, Calvat S, Fagon JY, Dombret MC, et al. Analysis of vancomycin entry into pulmonary lining fluid by bronchoalveolar lavage in critically ill patients. *Antimicrob Agents Chemother.* 1993;37:281-6.
60. Georges H, Leroy O, Alfandari S, Guery B, Roussel-Delvallez M, Dhennain C, et al. Pulmonary disposition of vancomycin in critically ill patients. *Eur J Clin Microbiol Infect Dis.* 1997;16:385-8.
61. Hidayat LK, Hsu DI, Quist R, Shriner KA, Wong-Beringer A. High-dose vancomycin therapy for methicillin-resistant *Staphylococcus aureus* infections: efficacy and toxicity. *Arch Intern Med.* 2006;166:2138-44.
62. Jeffres MN, Isakow W, Doherty JA, McKinnon PS, Ritchie DJ, Micek ST, et al. Predictors of mortality for methicillin-resistant *Staphylococcus aureus* health-care-associated pneumonia: specific evaluation of vancomycin pharmacokinetic indices. *Chest.* 2006;130:947-55.
63. Rybak MJ, Lomaestro BM, Rotschafer JC, Moellering RC, Craig WA, Billeter M, et al. Vancomycin therapeutic guidelines: a summary of consensus recommendations from the infectious diseases Society of America, the American Society of Health-System Pharmacists, and the Society of Infectious Diseases Pharmacists.[Erratum appears in *Clin Infect Dis.* 2009;49:1465]. *Clin Infect Dis.* 2009;49:325-7.
64. Sorrell TC, Collignon PJ. A prospective study of adverse reactions associated with vancomycin therapy. *J Antimicrob Chemother.*1985;16:235-41.
65. Cantu TG, Yamanaka-Yuen NA, Lietman PS. Serum vancomycin concentrations: reappraisal of their clinical value. *Clin Infect Dis.* 1994;18:533-43.
66. Cano EL, Haque NZ, Welch VL, Cely CM, Peyrani P, Scerpella EG, et al. Incidence of nephrotoxicity and association with vancomycin use in intensive care unit patients with pneumonia: retrospective analysis of the IMPACT-HAP Database. *Clin Ther.* 2012;34:149-57.
67. Lodise TP, Miller CD, Graves J, Evans A, Graffunder E, Helmecke M, et al. Predictors of high vancomycin MIC values among patients with methicillin-resistant *Staphylococcus aureus* bacteraemia. *J Antimicrob Chemother.* 2008; 62:1138-41.
68. Awad SS, Elhabash SI, Lee L, Farrow B, Berger DH. Increasing incidence of methicillin-resistant *Staphylococcus aureus* skin and soft-tissue infections: reconsideration of empiric antimicrobial therapy. *Am J Surg.* 2007;194: 606-10.
69. Rhee KY, Gardiner DF, Charles M. Decreasing in vitro susceptibility of clinical *Staphylococcus aureus* isolates to vancomycin at the New York Hospital: quantitative testing redux. *Clin Infect Dis.* 2005;40:1705-6.
70. Wang G, Hindler JF, Ward KW, Bruckner DA. Increased vancomycin MICs for *Staphylococcus aureus* clinical isolates from a university hospital during a 5-year period. *J Clin Microbiol.* 2006;44:3883-6.
71. Dhand A, Sakoulas G. Reduced vancomycin susceptibility among clinical *Staphylococcus aureus* isolates ('the MIC Creep'): implications for therapy. *F1000 Med Rep.* 2012;4:4.
72. Ho PL, Lo PY, Chow KH, Lau EH, Lai EL, Cheng VC, et al. Vancomycin MIC creep in MRSA isolates from 1997 to 2008 in a healthcare region in Hong Kong. J Infect. 2010;6:140-5.
73. Sader HS, Fey PD, Limaye AP, Madinger N, Pankey G, Rahal J, et al. Evaluation of vancomycin and daptomycin potency trends (MIC creep) against methicillin-resistant *Staphylococcus aureus* isolates collected in nine U.S. medical centers from 2002 to 2006.[Erratum appears in *Antimicrob Agents Chemother.* 2010;54:1383 Note: Fish, Douglas N [corrected to Madinger, Nancy]]. *Antimicrob Agents Chemother.* 2009;53:4127-32.
74. Ahlstrand E, Svensson K, Persson L, Tidefelt U, Soderquist B. Glycopeptide resistance in coagulase-negative staphylococci isolated in blood cultures from patients with hematological malignancies during three decades. *Eur J Clin Microbiol Infect Dis.* 2011;30:1349-54.
75. Gasch O, Ayats J, Angeles Dominguez M, Tubau F, Linares J, Pena C, et al. Epidemiology of methicillin-resistant *staphylococcus aureus* (MRSA) bloodstream infection: secular trends over 19 years at a university hospital. *Medicine (Baltimore).* 2011;90:319-27.
76. Edwards B, Milne K, Lawes T, Cook I, Robb A, Gould IM. Is vancomycin MIC "creep" method dependent? Analysis of methicillin-resistant *Staphylococcus aureus* susceptibility trends in blood isolates from North East Scotland from 2006 to 2010. *J Clin Microbiol.* 2012;50:318-25.
77. van Hal SJ, Barbagiannakos T, Jones M, Wehrhahn MC, Mercer J, Chen D, et al. Methicillin-resistant *Staphylococcus aureus* vancomycin susceptibility testing: methodology correlations, temporal trends and clonal patterns. *J Antimicrob Chemother.* 2011;66:2284-7.
78. Haque NZ, Zuniga LC, Peyrani P, Reyes K, Lamerato L, Moore CL, et al. Relationship of vancomycin minimum

inhibitory concentration to mortality in patients with methicillin-resistant *Staphylococcus aureus* hospital-acquired, ventilator-associated, or health-care-associated pneumonia. *Chest.* 2010;138:1356-62.

79. Kullar R, Leonard SN, Davis SL, Delgado G Jr., Pogue JM, Wahby KA, et al. Validation of the effectiveness of a vancomycin nomogram in achieving target trough concentrations of 15-20 mg/L suggested by the vancomycin consensus guidelines. *Pharmacotherapy.* 2011;31:441-8.
80. Jones RN, Fritsche TR, Sader HS, Ross JE. LEADER surveillance program results for 2006: an activity and spectrum analysis of linezolid using clinical isolates from the United States (50 medical centers). *Diagn Microbiol Infect Dis.* 2007;59:309-17.
81. Morales G, Picazo JJ, Baos E, Candel FJ, Arribi A, Pelaez B, et al. Resistance to linezolid is mediated by the cfr gene in the first report of an outbreak of linezolid-resistant Staphylococcus aureus. *Clin Infect Dis.* 2010;50:821-5.
82. Sánchez García M, De la Torre MA, Morales G, Peláez B, Tolón MJ, Domingo S, et al. Clinical outbreak of linezolid-resistant Staphylococcus aureus in an intensive care unit. *JAMA.* 2010;303:2260-4.
83. Conte JE Jr., Golden JA, Kipps J, Zurlinden E. Intrapulmonary pharmacokinetics of linezolid. *Antimicrob Agents Chemother.* 2002;46:1475-80.
84. Jones RN, Fritsche TR, Sader HS, Ross JE. Zyvox Annual Appraisal of Potency and Spectrum Program Results for 2006: an activity and spectrum analysis of linezolid using clinical isolates from 16 countries. *Diagn Microbiol Infect Dis.* 2007;59:199-209.
85. Pea F, Viale P. Pharmacodynamics of antibiotics to treat multidrug-resistant Gram-positive hospital infections. *Expert Rev Anti Infect Ther.* 2007;5:255-70.
86. Pea F, Furlanut M, Cojutti P, Cristini F, Zamparini E, Franceschi L, et al. Therapeutic drug monitoring of linezolid a retrospective monocentric analysis. . *Antimicrob Agents Chemother.* 2010;54:4605-10.
87. Zyvox. 2012; Available from: http://labeling.pfizer.com/ShowLabeling.aspx?id=649.
88. Rubinstein E, Cammarata S, Oliphant T, Wunderink R, Linezolid Nosocomial Pneumonia Study G. Linezolid (PNU-100766) versus vancomycin in the treatment of hospitalized patients with nosocomial pneumonia: a randomized, double-blind, multicenter study. *Clin Infect Dis.* 2001;32:402-12.
89. Wunderink RG, Cammarata SK, Oliphant TH, Kollef MH; Linezolid Nosocomial Pneumonia Study Group. Continuation of a randomized, double-blind, multicenter study of linezolid versus vancomycin in the treatment of patients with nosocomial pneumonia. *Clin Ther.* 2003;25: 980-92.
90. Wunderink RG, Rello J, Cammarata SK, Croos-Dabrera RV, Kollef MH. Linezolid vs vancomycin: analysis of two double-blind studies of patients with methicillin-resistant *Staphylococcus aureus* nosocomial pneumonia. *Chest.* 2003;124:1789-97.
91. Kollef MH, Rello J, Cammarata SK, Croos-Dabrera RV, Wunderink RG. Clinical cure and survival in Gram-positive ventilator-associated pneumonia: retrospective analysis of two double-blind studies comparing linezolid with vancomycin. *Intensive Care Med.* 2004;30:388-94.
92. Kalil AC, Murthy MH, Hermsen ED, Neto FK, Sun J, Rupp ME. Linezolid versus vancomycin or teicoplanin for nosocomial pneumonia: a systematic review and meta-analysis. *Crit Care Med.* 2010;38:1802-8.
93. Tascini C, Gemignani G, Doria R, Biancofiore G, Urbani L, Mosca C, et al. Linezolid treatment for gram-positive infections: a retrospective comparison with teicoplanin. *J Chemother.* 2009;21:311-6.
94. Wilcox M, Nathwani D, Dryden M. Linezolid compared with teicoplanin for the treatment of suspected or proven Gram-positive infections. *J Antimicrob Chemother.* 2004; 53:335-44.
95. Cepeda JA, Whitehouse T, Cooper B, Hails J, Jones K, Kwaku F, et al. Linezolid versus teicoplanin in the treatment of Gram-positive infections in the critically ill: a randomized, double-blind, multicentre study. *J Antimicrob Chemother.* 2004;53:345-55.
96. Stryjewski ME, Graham DR, Wilson SE, O'Riordan W, Young D, Lentnek A, et al. Telavancin versus vancomycin for the treatment of complicated skin and skin-structure infections caused by gram-positive organisms. *Clin Infect Dis.* 2008;46:1683-93.
97. Rubinstein E, Corey GR, Stryjewski ME, Kanafani ZA. Telavancin for the treatment of serious gram-positive infections, including hospital acquired pneumonia. *Expert Opin Pharmacother.* 2011;12:2737-50.
98. Committee for Medicinal Product for Human Use (CHMO). Summary of opinion (initial authorization): Vibativ-Telavancin. European Medicines Agency. Available from: http://www.ema.europa.eu/docs/en_GB/document_library/Summary_of_opinion_-_Initial_authorisation/human/001240/WC500106519.pdf
99. Fagon J, Patrick H, Haas DW, Torres A, Gibert C, Cheadle WG, et al. Treatment of gram-positive nosocomial pneumonia. Prospective randomized comparison of quinupristin/dalfopristin versus vancomycin. Nosocomial Pneumonia Group.[Erratum appears in *Am J Respir Crit Care Med.* 2001;163:1759-60]. *Am J Respir Crit Care Med.* 2000;161:753-62.
100. TYGACIL® (tigecycline) FOR INJECTION for intravenous use. 2010; Available from: http://www.accessdata.fda.gov/drugsatfda_docs/label/2010/021821s021lbl.pdf?utm_source=fdaSearch&utm_medium=website&utm_term=tigecycline package insert&utm_content=9.
101. Freire AT, Melnyk V, Kim MJ, Datsenko O, Dzyublik O, Glumcher F, et al. Comparison of tigecycline with imipenem/cilastatin for the treatment of hospital-acquired pneumonia. *Diagn Microbiol Infect Dis.* 2010;68:140-51.
102. Burkhardt O, Rauch K, Kaever V, Hadem J, Kielstein JT, Welte T. Tigecycline possibly underdosed for the treatment of pneumonia: a pharmacokinetic viewpoint. *Int J Antimicrob Agents.* 2009;34:101-2.
103. Forest. Teflaro. 2010; Available from: http://www.accessdata.fda.gov/drugsatfda_docs/label/2010/200327s000lbl.pdf.
104. Saravolatz LD, Stein GE, Johnson LB. Ceftaroline: a novel cephalosporin with activity against methicillin-resistant *Staphylococcus aureus*. *Clin Infect Dis.* 2011;52:1156-63.
105. Noel GJ, Strauss RS, Shah A, Bagchi P. Ceftobiprole versus ceftazidime combined with linezolid for treatment of patients with nosocomial pneumonia. Program and

abstracts of the 48th Annual Interscience Conference on Antimicrobial Agents and Chemotherapy. Washington, DC; 2008. Abstract K-486.
106. Jung YJ, Koh Y, Hong S-B, Chung JW, Ho Choi S, Kim NJ, et al. Effect of vancomycin plus rifampicin in the treatment of nosocomial methicillin-resistant *Staphylococcus aureus* pneumonia. *Crit Care Med.* 2010;38:175-80.
107. Pharmaceuticals C. Daptomycin. 2010; Available from: http://www.cubicin.com/pdf/PrescribingInformation.pdf.
108. Steenbergen JN, Alder J, Thorne GM, Tally FP. Daptomycin: a lipopolipeptide antibiotic for the treatment of serious Gram positive infections. *J Antimicrob Chemother.* 2005; 55:283-8.
109. Wunderink RG, Niederman MS, Kollef MH, Shorr AF, Kunkel MJ, Baruch A, et al. Linezolid in methicillin-resistant *Staphylococcus aureus* nosocomial pneumonia: a randomized, controlled study. *Clin Infect Dis.* 2012;54: 621-9.
110. Beltrametti F, Consolandi A, Carrano L, Bagatin F, Rossi R, Leoni L, et al. Resistance to glycopeptide antibiotics in the teicoplanin producer is mediated by van gene homologue expression directing the synthesis of a modified cell wall peptidoglycan. *Antimicrob Agents Chemother.* 2007;51: 1135-41.

CHAPTER 20

Management of Multidrug-resistant Pathogens

Helen Giamarellou

ABSTRACT

Nosocomial infections caused by multidrug resistant and extensively drug resistant Gram-negative pathogens represent a major therapeutic problem worldwide. The so-called ESKAPE microorganisms, from the initials of the most frequently isolated MDR bacteria, i.e., *Enterococcus faecium, Staphylococcus aureus, Klebsiella pneumoniae, Acinetobacter baumannii, Pseudomonas aeruginosa,* and *Enterobacter species*, emphasize the "eskape" effect of antibacterial agents. Particularly *K. pneumoniae* strains producing carbapebemases reach mortality rates exceeding 35%, mainly because of the lack of active antimicrobials. The last resort antibiotics are colistin, tigecycline, and fosfomycin which particularly in combination with an aminoglycoside or with each other, have shown promising *in vivo* efficacy in the critically ill host. However, due to their increased use, resistance is rapidly mounting. Unfortunately, new therapeutic options, like plazomycin and the extended spectrum β-lactamases/carbapenem inhibitors are still under development in ongoing clinical trials. In the meantime, the clinician should react by applying antibiotic stewardship and strict infection control programs.

INTRODUCTION

Infections caused by multidrug-resistant (MDR) bacteria present nowadays daily challenges to physicians and their patients all over the world and especially in the nosocomial setting.[1,2] During the last decade, the efforts to combat MDR microorganisms mainly focused on Gram-positive bacteria and drug companies have developed several novel antimicrobial agents to fight them. Unfortunately, the growing problem of multidrug resistance in Gram-negative bacteria was not paralleled with similar efforts. As a result, there are now a growing number of reports on infections caused by Gram-negative microorganisms for which no adequate therapeutic options exist. Thus return to the "Preantibiotic Era" has become a reality and a nightmare in many parts of the world. Therefore, the World Health Organization has identified antimicrobial resistance as one of the three most important problems for human health. In 2008 this phenomenon has been characterized with the word "ESKAPE", from the initials of the most frequent MDR microorganisms, i.e., *Enterococcus faecium, Staphylococcus aureus, Klebsiella pneumoniae, Acinetobacter baumannii, Pseudomonas aeruginosa* and *Enterobacter spp.*, emphasizing that they "eskape" the effect of antibacterial agents.[3] It should be clarified that microorganisms are characterized as MDR (i.e., acquired nonsusceptibility to at least one agent in three or more antimicrobial classes), extensively drug resistant-extensively drug-resistant (XDR) (i.e., resistant to all but one or two antibiotics, colistin or/and tigecycline) or pandrug-resistant-PDR (i.e., resistant to all available classes).[4]

It is well-known that critically ill patients, because of frequent exposure to antibiotics are prone to colonization and subsequent infections by MDR pathogens. On the other hand, the latter hosts frequently intubated and mechanically ventilated, whereas disrupted skin and mucosal barriers, as well as the use of invasive devices render them vulnerable to serious infections, for which the available antibiotics could be almost nil. Even more in the critically ill intubated patients pharmacokinetics/pharmacodynamics (PK/PDs) of antibiotics are prone to major alterations hindering successful therapy while leading to resistant development.[5,6]

The main mechanism of resistance in Gram-negative bacteria is the production of extended spectrum β-lactamases (ESBL).[1,5] As of January 10, 2012 more than 950 (http://www.lahey.org/studies/) different plasmid-mediated ESBLs have been described conferring resistance to penicillins and most cephalosporins including the third generation and cefepime, whereas AmpC enzymes, upregulation of efflux pumps, altered penicillin binding proteins, as well as changes in membrane porins result in non-ESBL-resistant phenotypes.[5] In Europe ESBL-producing *Escherichia coli*, which is the most predominant among infections caused by ESBL-producing strains, prevailed from 1.8% to 19.2% in blood stream infections from 28 European countries in 2009.[7-9] The other major reservoir of ESBL genes in hospitalized patients is *Klebsiella pneumoniae* which varies from 0% to 70% in bloodstream infections (BSI) associated also with nosocomial outbreaks.[10-13].

Probably the extensive use of carbapenems for treating infections caused by ESBL producing bacteria, triggered Gram-negative microorganisms to the production of carbapenemases. Until January 10, 2012, more than 126 carbapenemases, i.e., enzymes capable to hydrolyze carbapenems, have been described (http://www.lahey.org/studies/). The most prevalent ones belong to: (1) group B (metallo-beta-lactamases) in which VIM, *integral membrane protein* (IMP) and *New Delhi-Metallo* (NDM) enzymes are classified, (2) group A (serine β-lactamases) in which *Klebsiella pneumoniae* carbapenemase (KPC) enzymes represent along with NDM the predominant worldwide enzymes,[1,5] and (3) group D in which OXA-48 is the commonest carbapenemase. The most recently detected carbapenemase is NDM, with steeply increasing reports of infections or fecal carriage in Europe, related to transfer of patients from endemic countries, like hospitals in India and Pakistan. It is of interest that blaNDM-1 harboring bacteria were obtained from seepage water samples, as well as from public tap water samples in New Delhi, indicating its spread also through the oral-fecal route.[14-20].

The first KPC was isolated in 1996 from *K. pneumoniae* in USA.[21] As of 2011 notable numbers of outbreaks have been described in Israel and USA, whereas due to the fact that plasmids carrying KPC genes are extremely mobile, KPC have been also demonstrated in other species of *Enterobacteriaceae*, like *E. coli* and *Enterobacter* species.[22-25] Carbepenemases are most prevalent in Greece with resistance rates to carbapenems in *K. pneumoniae* ICU blood isolates reaching 80% in 2011.[26-29] Unfortunately, the number of reported outbreaks in other European countries is also rapidly cumulating since transfer of patients or even carriers across borders facilitate the dissemination of KPC-producing *K. pneumoniae* in worldwide. In general, bacteremias with carbapenemase-producing *K. pneumoniae* (CPKP) carry a mortality rate ranging from 22% to 75%.[2] However, it should be pointed out that estimation of the excess risk of dying or the attributable length of stay, because of the coexistence of many confounding factors, is difficult.[5]

According to the available multicenter surveillance studies, among 33 European countries participating in the European Antimicrobial Resistance Surveillance System (EARS Net) in 2007, six countries reported carbapenem resistance rates of more than 25% among *P. aeruginosa* isolates.[1] On the other hand, the proportion of carbapenem resistant *A. baumannii* strains has been reported as high as 85% in bloodstream isolates from ICU patients in Greece and 48% in clinical isolates from hospitalized patients in Spain and Turkey.[1,30] It should be pointed out that besides their ability to hydrolyze carbapenems, carbapenemase producing Gram-negatives often confer resistance to other major classes of antibiotics, such as aminoglycosides, cephalosporins, and quinolones limiting even more the antibiotic armamentarium.

At a large international meeting organized by Biomerieux in France last year, the prophetic title given was: "Ready for a world without antibiotics?"[31] At least the title was a question and not an affirmative statement. The limited treatment options for the clinician are the revival of colistin and fosfomycin, as well as an improved tetracycline, tigecycline, compounds, that are active both *in vitro* and *in vivo* against several MDR and XDR microorganisms.[32-34] However, their active life is dependent on their prudent use by the clinicians and particularly the intensivist.

COLISTIN

Polymyxins are an old class of cyclic polypeptide antibiotics that was discovered in 1947 from *Bacillus polymyxa*.[32,35,36] They consist of polymyxins A-E, of which only polymyxin B and polymyxin E (colistin) are currently in the market. Colistin is available in two forms: colistin sulfate (tablets or syrup for bowel decontamination and powder for topical use) and colistin methanesulfonate (colistimethate sodium; CMS) for parenteral use. In the USA, as well as in Brazil, polymyxin B sulfate is also used parenterally.[37]

The mode of action of colistin is the bacterial cell membrane, where the polycationic peptide ring interacts with the lipid A of the lipopolysaccharide, allowing penetration through the outer membrane by displacing Ca^{2+} and Mg^{2+}.[35,38] Colistin is inherently active *in vitro* against *Enterobacteriaceae* (*E. coli, Klebsiella* spp., *Enterobacter* spp., *Citrobacter* spp., *Salmonella* spp., and *Shigella* spp.), *Haemophilus influenzae, Legionella pneumophila, P. aeruginosa, Acinetobacter* spp., *Stenotrophomonas maltophilia,* and *Aeromonas* spp. including most of the XDR strains,[39] whereas *Proteus* and *Providencia* spp. are inherently resistant.[40] Heteroresistance to colistin in MDR *A. baumannii* strains as well as *K. pneumoniae*[41] has been attributed to potentially suboptimal dosing regimens.[40] Resistance to colistin is based on alterations at the outer membrane of the cell, such as reduction in cell envelope Mg^{2+} and Ca^{2+} contents, lipid alteration, and substitution of protein OprH for magnesium.[38] Since 2005, the Clinical Laboratory Standards Institute (CLSI) established minimum inhibitory concentration (MIC) breakpoints of less than or equal to 2mg/L for *P. aeruginosa* (susceptibility [S] ≤2 mg/L, resistance [R] ≥8 mg/L) and *Acinetobacter* spp. (S ≤ 2mg/L, R ≥4 mg/L), whereas the European breakpoints published by the European Committee on Antimicrobial Susceptibility Testing (EUCAST) [S ≤2 mg/L, R ≥4 mg/L] include only the *Enterobacteriaceae*.[42,43] In terms of disk susceptibility testing, CLSI recommends susceptibility breakpoints only for *P. aeruginosa* (10 µg colistin disk; R ≤10 mm, S ≥11 mm). It should be clarified that the formulation of colistin that must be used in susceptibility tests is colistin sulfate and not CMS.

In vitro interactions of colistin led to synergistic results with rifampicin and meropenem against *A. baumannii* and *P. aeruginosa* including *K. pneumoniae* KPC (+) strains.[35,44-46] However, in the latter combination, strains exhibiting an MIC to colistin more than or equal to 16 µg/mL, proved to be antagonistic against *K. pneumoniae* isolates. Colistin exhibits concentration-dependent bacterial killing activity with rapid bactericidal activity and a significant postantibiotic effect against Gram-negative organisms.[47] Pharmacodynamically, the unbound area under the concentration-time curve (fAUC)/MIC ratio is the parameter best associated with its efficacy.[48]

It should be emphasized that CMS is a prodrug of colistin which is slowly released *in vivo* to active colistin and inactive CMS. It should be also made clear that 2.4 mg of CMS contains 1 mg colistin base, and that pure colistin base has a potency of 30,000 IU/mg whereas CMS is only 12,500 IU/mg.[32,33,35] Because of the lack of accurate PK/PD information in non-CF patients, the optimal dosage of colistin is unclear. CMS in patients with normal renal function is usually given in the USA at a dose of 2.5–5.0 mg/kg per day (31,200–62,500 IU/kg) intravenously in 2–4 equal doses.[49,50] In the UK, CMS is given at a dose of 4–6 mg/kg/day (50,000–75.000 IU/kg) in three divided doses for adults and children with bodyweight of less than or equal to 60 kg and at a dose of 80–160 mg (1–2 million IU) every 8 hours for body weight more than 60 kg.[49,50] However, it should be pointed out that older pharmacokinetic data were based on microbiological assays and should be considered as inaccurate, because of instability of CMS in aqueous media. Most kinetic information was derived from cystic fibrosis (CF) patients, whether it is not known if data from those patients can be extrapolated to the critically ill individuals since in CF patients several antibiotics display shorter half-lives.[51] On the other hand, colistin kinetics in the various body compartments requires further exploration in well-designed studies.

Despite the existing information on colistin serum kinetics, the knowledge of the appropriate dosage of colistin was still an unknown issue, until recently when colistin was investigated in 18 critically ill ICU patients.[52] After applying a novel rapid chromatography-tandem mass spectrometry method the half-life of CMS disposition was estimated 2.3 hours, whereas for colistin it was 14.4 hours with Cmax of 0.60 µg/mL after the first dose of 3 million IU, and 2.3 µg/mL following repeated administration of 3 million IU every 8 hours.[53] The latter results indicated that colistin concentrations in blood remain below the MIC sensitivity breakpoint (2 µg/mL) after the first few doses of the currently used regimen. Therefore, a loading dose of 9 million IU followed by a maintenance dose of 4.5 million IU every 12 hours has been suggested by the authors, resulting in the same average steady state concentration of colistin as with the current dosing schedule, but this being achieved much faster. The latter finding is of particular importance for the critically ill patients in whom appropriate and adequate antimicrobial therapy within the first hour of severe sepsis and septic shock is essential.[54] Colistin and CMS pharmacokinetic parameters derived from the pre-reported 18 critically ill patients are described in table 1.

After applying the same methodology, the same group of investigators evaluated CMS and colistin kinetics, following a 6 million IU loading dose in 10 critically ill patients with normal renal function and infections caused by MDR Gram-negatives aiming also to explore the bacteria kill following different dosing regimens by predictions using a pharmacokinetic-pharmacodynamic model developed from an in vitro study on *Pseudomonas aeruginosa*.[55] For CMS, a two-compartment model best

TABLE 1

Pharmacokinetic parameters of colistin methanesulfonate and colistin in critically ill patients[28,35]

Parameter	CMS (RSE%)	Colistin (RSE%)
t½ (hour)	2.3	14.4
C_{max} predicted (µg/mL)	NA	NA
First dose	NA	0.60
Steady state	NA	2.3
CL (L/hour)	13.7 (10)	9.09 (19)
Vd (L)	28.9 (22)	189 (12)

CL, total body clearance; C_{max}, maximum concentration; NA, not available; RSE, relative standard error; t½, half-life; Vd, volume of distribution

described the pharmacokinetics, and the half-lives of the two phases were estimated to 0.026 hours and 2.2 hours, respectively. For colistin, a one-compartment model was sufficient and the estimated half-life was 18.5 hours. The predictions suggested that the time to 3 log bacterial kill was reduced to half for a 6 million IU loading dose compared to the dose of 3 million IU.

Recently, a new pharmacokinetic approach was published regarding the appropriate therapeutic dosing of colistin in various patients category including renal insufficiently.[56] According to the latter study when targeting peak blood levels of 2 µg/mL (the break-point of susceptibility) in all patient category, a loading dose should be given, which is calculated after dividing body weight by 7.5 (not to exceed 10 million IU), whereas the maintenance dose follows after 24 hours. Maintenance dose is found after dividing creatinine clearance by 10, adding 2 and administering it into 2–3 doses per day. In hemodialysis 1 million IU is given every 12 hours with another 30% of the daily dose to be given post-hemodialysis. It is interesting that in patients on continuous hemofiltration a very high 12 million IU dose (in two or three daily doses) was suggested. In the above schedule (1) between real and ideal body weight the ideal should be chosen and (2) for daily doses above 10 million IU special attention to renal function should be given.

From 2003 to 2007, 175 non-CF patients who were mostly suffering from pneumonia were given intravenous polymyxin B therapeutically for infections due to MDR Gram-negative bacteria with clinical response rates ranging from 47.3% to 95% and mortality rates from 20% to 48%.[35,37] However, all studies were retrospective and polymyxin B was usually given in combination with other antibacterials, obscuring the precise evaluation of the results. From 1999 until August 2005, in seven retrospective studies involving almost 300 non-CF patients, among whom most represented ICU patients with ventilator-associated pneumonia (VAP), intravenous CMS was given at a dose of 1–3 million IU every 8 hours for 12–22 days.[57-63] In almost all patients, at a rate close to 50%, either MDR *P. aeruginosa* or MDR *A. baumannii* were isolated in relevant cultures. Irrespective of the susceptibility patterns of the isolated pathogens, as a rule, CMS was given in combination mostly with imipenem. Clinical cure rates ranged between 57% and 73%, with mortality rates of 20–61.9% indicating the diversity of the included patients. It should be pointed out that clinical efficacy in nosocomial pneumonia exceeding 50% was comparable to previously reported rates of outcome with piperacillin/tazobactam, imipenem/cilastatin and ciprofloxacin. However, all reported studies shared similar drawbacks, i.e., (1) absence of a control group, (2) retrospective design, (3) variable dosing and duration of therapy, (4) simultaneous administration of other antibiotics (mostly imipenem) in 70–100% of cases, (5) no monitoring of resistance development during and at the end of therapy, (6) a wide range of nephrotoxicity of 8–37%, which, however, due to the retrospective character of the studies cannot be attributed exclusively to colistin, and (7) lack of PK/PDs issues which were almost unexplored.

After 2006, two retrospective but monotherapy studies with CMS were published.[64,65] In the first study, no difference in mortality rates (51.6% vs. 45.1%) was observed between 31 patients with VAP caused by isolates susceptible only to colistin who were treated with CMS and 30 patients with VAP caused by carbapenem-susceptible strains who were treated with a carbapenem as monotherapy.[64] It was concluded that VAP episodes with XDR pathogens susceptible only to colistin (including mainly *A. baumannii* and *P. aeruginosa*) can be treated effectively using CMS, whereas the carbapenem-resistance pattern of pathogens should be suspected in patients with previous VAP or prior antibacterial use for more than 10 days preceding the current VAP episode. In the largest retrospective matched case-control study thus far to assess the efficacy of monotherapy with CMS, the latter was compared with imipenem in VAP caused by isolates susceptible only to colistin (n = 60) or carbapenem susceptible strains (n = 60) of *A. baumannii* (51.6% vs. 61.7%) or *P. aeruginosa* (48.4% vs. 38.3%).[65] A favorable clinical response was observed in 75% of patients in each group without any difference in the time to resolution of infectious parameters.

However, in a third study, in which 200 patients were given colistin as monotherapy, clinical response and infection-related mortality did not differ from the control group.[66] Even more, the authors reported that colistin was associated with a higher mortality rate with fever prolongation, as well as longer hospital stay and statistically significant increase in the incidence of superinfections with *Proteus* spp. However, due to the nonrandomized study design, it seems that patients with fewer therapy options received colistin, whereas initiation of colistin was delayed. On the other hand, in a Greek retrospective analysis of 258 MDR and XDR *P. aeruginosa* and *A. baumannii* infections, monotherapy results with colistin were exactly the same with the results obtained when colistin was combined with meropenem (83% vs. 83%), but monotherapy was superior when compared with colistin given with other antibiotics, an observation attributed to the low number of patients included, as well as to the retrospective character of the study.[67]

The clinical relevance of a high loading dose of 9 million IU of CMS to be followed by 4.5 million IU every 12 hours, as suggested by Plachouras et al.[51] was recently prospectively evaluated in 28 critically ill patients with severe sepsis or septic shock suffering from BSI (64.3%) and VAP (35.7%) caused by A. *baumannii* (46.4%), *K. pneumoniae* (46.4%), and *P. aeruginosa* (7.2%).[68] The isolated strains were either susceptible only to colistin or also to gentamicin (8 strains). CMS was given as monotherapy in 14 patients, whereas in the remaining 14 in combination with gentamicin or carbapenems. Clinical cure was observed in 23 (82.1%) cases. Acute kidney injury developed during five treatment courses (17.8%), but did not require renal replacement therapy, and subsided within 10 days from CMS discontinuation. No correlation was found between serum creatinine variation (baseline-peak) and daily and cumulative doses of CMS, and between serum creatinine variation (baseline-peak) and duration of CMS treatment. The authors concluded that in severe infections caused by colistin-sensitive Gram-negative bacteria, the high-dose extended interval CMS regimen has a high efficacy, without significant renal toxicity.

Adjunctive inhalation therapy has been suggested in case of VAP in the effort to improve therapeutic results.[69] Korbila et al.[70] in a retrospective cohort study reported on 78 patients with VAP, who received IV plus inhaled CMS at an average daily dose of 2.1 ± 0.9 million IU, in comparison to 43 patients in whom only the IV route was used. In bronchial secretion cultures *A. baumannii* predominated in 76% to be followed by *P. aeruginosa* in 18%. Cure rates mounted 79.5% versus 60.5% (p = 0.025) with no difference in toxicity or death rate. However, the necessity of the application of a special mesh-vibrating nebulizer in order CMS to reach the alveoli, a method not used in the latter study, should be pointed out. On the contrary, in a recent matched case control study adjunctive inhalation therapy in 43 patients with VAP was not found of any additional benefit when compared to another group of 43 patients, who served as the control.[71] As in the Korbila study,[70] *A. baumannii* was the predominant pathogen.

Recently, a retrospective, 1:1 matched case-control study of aerosolized colistin (AS) plus IV colistin vs IV colistin alone in 208 ICU patients with VAP caused by colistin only susceptible *A. baumannii, P. aeruginosa,* or *K. pneumoniae* has been reported. The AS-IV colistin cohort had a higher clinical cure rate (69.2% vs. 54.8%, p = 0.03) and required fewer days of mecnanical ventilation after VAP onset (8 days vs. 12 days, p = 0.001), with eradication of pathogens more common in the AS-IV colistin group (63.4% vs. 50%, p = 0.08). The obtained results suggest that AS colistin might be a beneficial adjunct to IV colistin in the management of VAP caused by XDR Gram-negatives.[72] On the other hand, the efficacy of inhaled monotherapy with CMS with the exception of cystic fibrosis is probably indicated only in case of bronchiectasis and ventilation assosiated trecheobronchitis (VAT).[73,74]

Of particular interest are the successful results of intraventricular or intrathecal colistin in *A. baumannii* meningitis complicating neurosurgery. A review of the available literature regarding intraventricular or intrathecal administration of colistin in MDR and XDR *A. baumannii* ventriculitis/meningitis identified a total of 83 episodes in 81 patients.[75] The median dose of local colistin was 125,000 IU (10 mg) with a range of 20,000 IU (1.6 mg) to 500,000 IU (40 mg) in adults, whilst a dose of 2.000 IU/kg (0.16 mg/kg) up to 125,000 IU (10 mg) was used in the pediatric population. The median duration of treatment was 18.5 days, whilst the median time to achieve sterilization of cerebrospinal fluid was 4 days. The rate of successful outcome was 89%, and toxicity related to treatment mainly manifested as reversible chemical ventriculitis/meningitis, was observed in nine cases (11%).

The influence of immunosuppression on the activity of colistin has been evaluated retrospectively on 95 cancer patients diagnosed with infections caused by MDR *P. aeruginosa.*[76] Between January 2001 and 2004, 31 patients were treated with either colistin (colistin group) or 64 with at least one active antipseudomonal agent (a β-lactam antibiotic or a quinolone) as the control group. The overall clinical response rates were 52% in the colistin group and 31% in the control group (p = 0.055). Multiple logistic regression analysis showed that patients treated with colistin were 2.9 times more likely than those in the control group to experience a clinical response to therapy (p = 0.026), whereas neutropenia in 14 versus 24 patients without, did not influence the results.

Colistin therapy in critically ill patients with chronic renal failure (CRF) was evaluated in a recent prospective case-control study of 94 patients admitted to medical

ICUs.[77] All patients were suffering from infections caused by XDR *A. baumannii* or *P. aeruginosa* and received CMS 2–3 million IU every 8 hours or 2 million IU every 24 or 48 hours in case of CRF. Bacteriological cure was observed in 87% of patients with CRF and in 95% of patients without CRF ($p = 0.890$), whereas mortality in patients with CRF did not differ when compared to that in patients in the control group. It is of interest that simultaneous nephrotoxic agents and total defined daily dose of colistin did not influence the incidence of nephrotoxicity. It was concluded that in critically ill patients with CRF, colistin therapy, although used at a reduced dosage, was as effective as in patients without CRF. However, Plachouras et al.[52] as well as Garonzik et al.[56] recommended dosage schedules that differ significantly compared to those used by Turkoglu et al.[77] indicating the necessity of further studies in the field of CRF.

With the exception of children with CF or burns, safety and efficacy issues of colistin use in pediatric patients are rare in the literature, whereas the optimal dosage schedule has not yet been determined. In a recent retrospective Greek report, 13 patients without CF or burns (22 days to 14 years) received 19 courses of CMS for treating pneumonia, central nervous system infection, bacteremia, or complicated soft tissue infection.[78] MDR *A. baumannii, Enterobacter cloacae, K. pneumoniae,* and *P. aeruginosa* were the isolated pathogens. Colistin daily dose ranged between 40,000 IU/kg and 225,000 IU/kg and duration of therapy from 1 day to 133 days. Sixteen of nineteen courses were successfully treated with only two of the three deaths being infection-related. Because other antibiotics active against the isolated pathogens were given simultaneously in 17 infection episodes, the real efficacy of colistin was difficult to be evaluated. However, its safety, with the exception of one patient who expressed increased serum creatinine associated also with gentamicin co-administration, was satisfactory.

It is well known that polymyxins possess endotoxin-binding capacity. Therefore, hemoperfusion with polymyxin B bound to polystyrene fibers has been studied.[79,80] This intervention is commonly used in Japan in the treatment of sepsis and has shown a significant reduction in all-cause mortality. RCTs are, therefore, required to establish the safety and effects of polymyxin B hemoperfusion in sepsis.

The most common and important adverse effects of colistin are nephrotoxicity and neurotoxicity.[32,35,81] In contrast to older information, recent data indicate that nephrotoxicity in ICU patients after CMS administration ranges from 0% to 53%, but the applied criteria tend to overestimate the incidence of kidney injury. Safety data from 19 courses of prolonged intravenous CMS administration (mean duration 43.4 days and mean daily dose 4.4 million IU) showed that the median creatinine value increased only by 0.25 mg/dL, which returned close to baseline at the end of therapy.[82] Despite the already reported findings in Turkoglu et al. study,[77] nephrotoxicity in other studies independently predicted fewer cures of infection and increased mortality, whereas total cumulative colistin dose was associated with kidney damage, suggesting that shortening of treatment duration could decrease the incidence of nephrotoxicity, which however, was reversible in most patients.[81,83] The reported discrepancies and the wide range in nephrotoxicity rates should be attributed to the following reasons: (1) improvement in supportive care offered to seriously ill patients, (2) the effort to avoid simultaneous administration of other nephrotoxic drugs, (3) the different formulations of colistin which lack sulfate impurities, and (4) the applied definitions of nephrotoxicity, which differ in the reported studies.[35] Recently in a rat model, it was observed that ascorbic acid, a chain-breaking antioxidant and free radical scavenger, protects against the nephrotoxicity and apoptosis caused by colistin affecting also its pharmacokinetics.[84]

The incidence of neurotoxicity in earlier studies of colistin reached approximately 7%.[82,85] Facial paresthesias, dizziness, weakness, vertigo, visual disturbances, confusion, ataxia, and neuromuscular blockade leading to respiratory failure and apnea have been reported. Unfortunately, only one study included prospective electrophysiological testing among 12 colistin recipients with evidence of neuromuscular junction blockade, whereas findings consistent with critical polyneuropathy were seen in six of the tested patients.[82,85] Intraventricular high-dose administration may also cause convulsions. However, it seems that both neurotoxicity and nephrotoxicity are dose dependent and reversible.[50] Bronchoconstriction has been also reported with aerosolized CMS, which is an adverse effect that can be controlled by the inhalation of ß-adrenoceptor agonists before CMS administration.[86]

Unfortunately, as early as 2007, the excessive use of colistin led to the emergence of colonization with colistin-resistant *K. pneumoniae* strains, mounting to 30%, as well as superinfections with *Proteus* and *Serratia* spp., strains inherently resistant to colistin in patients receiving CMS for more than 12 days.[87-89] On the other hand, the emergence of *K. pneumoniae* strains producing KPC enzymes, rendering them XDR with the exception to colistin, resulted in excessive empirical use of colistin. This led to a cluster of multiclonal XDR *Klebsiella* strains implicated in bacteremias, VAP and soft tissue infections, mostly in patients who had prolonged administration of colistin (median 27 days).[89] In case of outbreaks horizontal transmission of XDR *Klebsiella* strains through caregivers' hands was also proved by repetitive extragenic palindromic-polymerase chain reaction.[87] The analysis of risk factors after a Greek ICU outbreak with PDR *P. aeruginosa* causing VAP revealed that the sole independent predictors were the administration of colistin for more than or equal to 13 days or the combined use of colistin with a carbapenem for more than 20 days.[90] The outbreak resolved after a reduction in the days of therapy with colistin plus reinforcement of infection control measures. Additionally, in a recent matched case-control study, the use of colistin for more than 14 days was determined in the multivariable model, as the only independent risk factor ($p = 0.002$) related to resistance development of *K. pneumoniae*, *A. baumannii* and *P. aeruginosa* to colistin.[91]

To rescue colistin and while awaiting culture results it seems that physicians in the current nosocomial XDR status should consider empirical therapy with colistin whenever confronting: (1) severe nosocomial sepsis/or septic shock in settings with XDR prevalence, (2) in serious nosocomial infections, whenever risk factors for XDR gram-negatives are present, i.e., preceded VAP episodes, preceded therapy with a carbapenem or superinfection while treated with a carbapenem, preceded ICU hospitalization, known colonization with XDR strains. Not to be forgotten that after culture results, colistin in case of alternative antibiotics should be de-escalated.

TIGECYCLINE

Tigecycline is a newer semisynthetic glycylcycline that represents a modified minocycline.[35] It was approved in 2005 by the FDA and in 2006 by the European Medicines Agency (EMA) for the treatment of complicated skin and skin structure infections and complicated intra-abdominal infections in adults.[92] Additionally, in March 2009, the FDA-approved tigecycline for treating community-acquired pneumonia (CAP) caused by *Streptococcus pneumoniae*, including cases with concurrent bacteremia, *H. influenzae*, and *L. pneumophila*.[93] However, the EMA has raised concerns about the evidence available from clinical studies in patients with CAP and the manufacturing company has withdrawn the application for this indication in the European market.[94]

Tigecycline overcomes many well-known mechanisms of resistance that inactivate older tetracyclines, as the active efflux and the ribosomal protection mechanism.[95] By definition it is a static drug; however, a possible bactericidal activity has been demonstrated requiring further exploration.[96] Tigecycline is active *in vitro* against a wide range of aerobic and anaerobic bacteria, including methicillin-resistant *S. aureus*, methicillin-resistant *S. epidermidis*, *S. pneumoniae* (penicillin-intermediate and -resistant included), vancomycin-resistant *Enterococcus faecium* and several anaerobic species (including *Bacteroides fragilis*), as well as *Enterobacteriaceae*, *S maltophilia* and *Acinetobacter* spp. A high percent of MDR *A. baumannii* strains, ESBL producing *Enterobacteriaceae*, and carbapenemase producing *K. pneumoniae* are also susceptible.[97-100] The breakpoints of susceptibility of tigecycline against *Enterobacteriaceae* are less than or equal to 2 μg/mL, whereas for *Acinetobacter baumannii* they should be probably increased to less than or equal to 4 μg/mL.[101]

Unfortunately, tigecycline is inherently vulnerable to the chromosomal-encoded multidrug efflux pumps of *Pseudomonas* spp., *Proteus* spp., *Providencia* spp., and *Morganella morganii*.[102] The question of potential *in vitro* synergy between tigecycline and other antimicrobials had an indifferent response in the majority of combinations but very rare antagonism.[35] A bactericidal synergistic effect of tigecycline plus amikacin against *A. baumannii* and *Proteus vulgaris*, and of tigecycline plus colistin against MBL- and ESBL-producing *K. pneumoniae* has been described.[103] Tigecycline is not currently approved for infections caused by MDR *A. baumannii*; however, off-label use in that indication is increasing globally because of the appealing in vitro spectrum of tigecycline and the lack of other active antimicrobial agents against XDR strains.

Tigecycline is available as an intravenous formulation and is administered at a 50 mg dose as a 1-hour infusion every 12 hours, after an initial loading dose of 100 mg.[104] After a dose of 50 mg, tigecycline exhibits linear pharmacokinetics, C_{max} of 0.62 ± 0.09 mg/mL, and a half-life of 37 ± 12 hours with protein binding capacity at 78% have been reported.[105,106] The drug does not affect the cytochrome P450 enzyme family and is primarily excreted in the bile.[105,106] Kinetics are not changed in severe renal failure or hemodialysis; however, a 50% reduction of the maintenance dose is recommended in severe hepatic insufficiency.[105,107] Tigecycline concentrations have been calculated in the epithelial lining fluid (ELF) and alveolar cells, which are considered as the most appropriate indicators for evaluating the extracellular and intracellular "drug-pathogen" interaction, respectively.[108] Tigecycline concentrations in ELF were found very low (0.02 ± 0.01 mg/L), whereas a very low ELF: plasma concentration ratio indicated a suboptimal penetration into the extracellular lung compartment probably insufficient to eradicate Gram-negative extracellular bacteria, such as

TABLE 2

Main Plasma Pharmacokinetic Parameters of Tigecycline in Humans[35,105,106]

Plasma parameter	Pharmacological studies		Efficacy studies
	100 mg	50 mg	50 mg
C_{max} (µg/mL)			
30-min infusion	1.15 ± 0.32	0.87 ± 0.23	0.80 ± 0.46
60-min infusion	0.90 ± 0.27	0.63 ± 0.10	0.49 ± 0.28
C_{min} (µg/mL)	NA	0.13 ± 0.08	0.16 ± 0.09
CL (L/hour)	21.8 ± 8.9	23.8 ± 7.8	19.9 ± 8.1
t½ (hour)	27.1 ± 14.3	42.4 ± 35.3	NA
AUC^{24} (mg hour/L)	NA	4.70 ± 1.70	5.85 ± 2.48
AUC∞ (mg hour/L)	5.19 ± 1.86	NA	NA
Fraction unbound (%)	13-29	13-20	NA
Vd (L)	568 ± 244	639 ± 307	NA

AUC, area under the concentration-time curve to time t; CL, total body clearance; Cmax, maximum concentration; C_{min}, minimum concentration; NA, not available; t½, half-life; Vd, volume of distribution

TABLE 3

Pharmacokinetic Parameters of Tigecycline in Various Body Tissues[35,106,107]

Body tissue	Number of subjects	Concentration after single 100 mg IV dose	
		4 hour	12 hour
Bile (µg/mL)	24	309 ± 420	148 ± 155
Gall bladder (mg/kg)	24	6.6 ± 6.6	7.3 ± 7.9
Colon (mg/kg)	24	0.55 ± 0.34	1.3 ± 2.4
Lung (mg/kg)	14	0.76 ± 0.67	0.38 ± 0.26
Bone (mg/mL)	25	0.07 ± 0.04	0.12 ± 0.13
Synovial fluid (µg/kg)	25	0.12 ± 0.06	0.09 ± 0.05
Cerebrospinal fluid (µg/mL)	17	0.015 ± 0.003	0.025 ± 0.005

IV, intravenous

K. pneumoniae. The main pharmacokinetic parameters of tigecycline in plasma and various body tissues are described in tables 2 and 3.

From January 2007 until April 2009, nine studies related to MDR Gram-negative infections were published or became available online.[109-117] Most of the studies were retrospective and noncomparative, with low numbers of monotherapies; therefore, the elucidation of the true role of tigecycline in the outcomes is difficult. In order to bypass some of these methodological problems, a retrospective study in three tertiary Greek hospitals was performed.[116] Forty-five adult patients (35 in the ICU) met strictly defined criteria for infections with MDR Gram-negative pathogens and were subsequently analyzed. They received tigecycline at standard dose for 28 *A. baumannii* and 23 *K. pneumoniae* infections with an MDR or XDR profile: 21 VAP and healthcare-associated pneumonia (HCAP), 10 BSI and 14 surgical infections. Tigecycline was administered either as monotherapy (22 patients) or as presumed active monotherapy (23 patients). In the latter group, all co-administered antimicrobials were resistant *in vitro* against the targeted pathogen. Successful clinical response rates of 90.5% and 80% were recorded for VAP/HCAP and BSI, respectively, with an overall successful clinical response of 80%. A similar successful clinical response of 85% was also observed in 20 patients in septic shock. Regarding microbiological response, 13 episodes of superinfections and breakthrough infections were observed in 10 patients with pathogens inherently resistant to tigecycline (i.e., *Proteus* spp., *Providencia* spp., *P. aeruginosa*, etc.). Unfortunately, the decreased susceptibility of tigecycline in *A. baumannii* complex and several Enterobacteriaceae, has been ascribed to the overexpression of various efflux pumps.[35,118]

In particular, in a prospective, double blind, randomized trial, tigecycline at the conventional dose in comparison to imipenem was given in 511 patients with HAP/VAP. In the final evaluation, tigecycline did not reach "noninferiority" compared to imipenem.[119] The latter result was mainly attributed to 140 patients with VAP mostly caused by *A. baumannii*, in whom cure rates reached only to 57% versus 94.7% with imipenem, leading to a negative approval by the FDA. A plausible explanation for the reported failures in patients with VAP, and not in HAP patients, could be attributed to the lower drug exposure due to physiological changes that occur in patients with VAP. Even more the low tigecycline levels in serum (≤0.6 μg/mL) after the conventional therapeutic schedule (50 mg, IV 12 hourly) is a matter of concern, because of the reported breakthrough bacteremias whenever the MICs exceeded the C_{max}, as well as for reaching the pharmaceutical target only with tigecycline MICs of less than or equal to 0.25 μg/mL.[120] Therefore, studies with higher tigecycline doses (i.e., 150–200 mg 12 hourly) to reach the target attainment with MICs 0.5-1 μg/mL are urgently required. Subsequently, the results of a recent study where tigecycline was prescribed at two high-dosage regimens (150 mg followed by 75 mg every 12 hours in 23 patients or 200 mg followed by 100 mg every 12 hours in 20 patients) versus imipenem at a dose of 1 g every 8 hours in 24 patients for treating HAP, despite the rather low numbers of recruited patients are of importance.[121] On the other hand, the *in vivo* validity of combinations, either with a carbapenem or with colistin or with an aminoglycoside, deserve further exploitation.[122]

In a recent review, the effectiveness of tigecycline in 77 severe infections caused by *K. pneumoniae* producing carbapenemases, the results of which were derived from 34 already published studies, revealed failure rates with tigecycline monotherapy mounting 46%, whereas in case of co-administration with colistin or an aminoglycoside or meropenem (when the MIC of meropenem was ≤4 μg/mL), relevant rates were 15% and 0%, depicting at least the necessity of combinations with active *in vitro* antibiotics, whenever tigecycline is given for XDR *K. pneumoniae* infection.[123]

Safety analysis of the phase II studies revealed a significant number of patients reporting mild to moderate gastrointestinal adverse events, including nausea (24.4–34.5%), vomiting (19.2%), and diarrhea (8.5%), whereas few cases with pancreatitis have been reported.[124-126] The possibility of GI adverse events, including decreased fibrinogen levels (Giamarellou H unpublished data) as well as the warning regarding increased mortality, is of concern. The FDA in a pooled analysis of 13 clinical trials reported an increased mortality risk associated with the use of tigecycline compared to that of other drugs used to treat a variety of serious infections, but not at a statistically significant level.[127] In a recent meta-analysis of 14 randomized trials, comprising about 7,400 patients, treatment success was lower with tigecycline compared with control antibiotic agents, but the difference was not statistically significant.[128] Adverse events were more frequent in the tigecycline groups than in the control groups, whereas all-cause mortality was higher in the tigecycline group than in the comparator groups, but the difference was not statistically significant. Therefore, it seems that monotherapy may be used as effectively and safely as the comparison therapy for complicated skin and skin-structure infection, complicated intra-abdominal infections, CAP, and infections caused by methicillin-resistant *Staphylococcus aureus* (MRSA)/vancomycin-resistant enterococci (VRE). However, because of the higher risk of mortality, adverse events, and emergence of resistant isolates, prudence with the clinical use of tigecycline monotherapy is required. Particularly for carbapenemase producing *K. pneumoniae* strains the combination with another active *in vitro* antibiotic like colistin; gentamicin or even meropenem (whenever the MIC is ≤8 μg/mL) is indicated.[123] On the other hand, the lack of activity of tigecycline against *P. aeruginosa* mandates the addition of an antipseudomonal antibiotic in the case of empirical therapy in the critically ill patient. Even more, according to the recent World Society of Emergency Surgery (WSES) consensus conference guidelines of 2011, in hospital acquired intra-abdominal infections in both non-critically and critically ill patients, tigecycline is recommended to be administered empirically in combination with piperacillin in order to cover the gap of *P. aeruginosa*.[127]

FOSFOMYCIN

Fosfomycin is an antibiotic of the 70s that inhibits bacterial cell wall biosynthesis by inactivating the enzyme pyruvyl transferase, which is required for the synthesis of the bacterial cell wall peptidoglycan.[130,131] As fosfomycin tromethamine, a soluble salt of fosfomycin is licensed in several parts of the world as single-dose oral therapy for uncomplicated urinary tract infections (UTIs) in women caused by *E. coli* and *Enterococcus faecalis*. The available formulation for IV administration is fosfomycin disodium. It is bactericidal against a broad spectrum of Gram-positive and Gram-negative bacteria including MRSA, the group of *Enterobacteriaceae* and *P. aeruginosa* possessing a low potential for cross resistance with other classes of antibiotics. It is also active in vitro against carbapenem-resistant *P. aeruginosa* and *K. pneumonia*.[132,133] However, *Acinetobacter* spp. is inherently resistant to fosfomycin. In a Greek study, the *in vitro* susceptibility of XDR Enterobacteriaceae reached 91.8%, whereas among KPC (+) *K. pneumoniae* 93% were found susceptible with MIC_{90} of 64 μg/mL.[132] Because of the lack of a universal breakpoint, the threshold of 64 μg/mL is considered by many investigators as the upper limit of susceptibility. Regarding *in vitro* interactions of fosfomycin with other antimicrobial agents, combinations were never antagonistic whereas synergy with imipenem or meropenem was found in 30–78% of KPC (+) *K. pneumoniae* strains and 70% of *P. aeruginosa*.[134] With the use of colistin and tigecycline, 35% synergistic results were observed *in vitro* against *K. pneumoniae* KPC (+) strains.[134]

Fosfomycin at a therapeutic dose of 6–8 g every 6–8 hours IV exhibits a T½ of 2.4–4.1 hours with peak serum blood levels of 105–120 μg/mL post 4 g IV dose and 260–442 μg/mL post 8 g IV dose.[131] Advantageous kinetics into various body compartments have been described, including the CSF where levels of 38–62 μg/mL were detected, whereas in case of co-administration of an aminoglycoside, fosfomycin was found protective against aminoglycoside-induced nephrotoxicity.[135]

Clinical data with fosfomycin for MDR infections are very scarce. In a recently published review of the 64 existing, mostly retrospective fosfomycin studies, among 1,529 patients with non-MDR pathogens, 81.1% were successfully treated with a dose of 2–24 g IV daily for a great variety of infections.[136] The major pathogens were *P. aeruginosa, S. aureus, Enterobacter* spp., and *Klebsiella* spp. Fosfomycin was not given as monotherapy but in combination with aminoglycosides, cephalosporins, or penicillins. In a recent French report, the efficacy of parenteral fosfomycin at a dose mostly of 4 g IV every 8 hours, especially against MDR and XDR bacterial infections was analyzed in 116 patients in a prospective cohort study.[137] The main indications for use were osteomyelitis, lung infection, urinary tract infection, and bacteremia. The bacteria most frequently involved were *P. aeruginosa* and methicillin-resistant *S. aureus*. MDR microorganisms were isolated in 71.5% of cases, especially MDR *P. aeruginosa* (n = 28), among which 24 strains were XDR. Critical situations were common, with 44.0% of hospitalizations occurring in an ICU and 22.4% presenting with septic shock. The overall outcome was favorable in 76.8% of cases. However, fosfomycin was given in combination with other antibiotics hindering the real evaluation of the drug.

Clinical experience in XDR pathogens with the exception of anecdotal cases is limited to a recently published multicentre, observational and prospective case series study performed in 11 Greek ICUs.[138] All consecutive fosfomycin-treated patients suffering from XDR or PDR fosfomycin-susceptible, microbiologically documented infections were recorded. Bacteremia and ventilator-associated pneumonia were the main infections. Carbapenemase-producing *K. pneumoniae* and *P. aeruginosa* were isolated in 41 and 17 cases, respectively. All isolates exhibited an XDR or PDR profile, being fosfomycin-susceptible by microbiological definition. Fosfomycin was administered intravenously at a median dose of 24 g/day for a median of 14 days, mainly in combination with colistin or tigecycline. Clinical outcome at day 14 was successful in 54.2% of patients, whilst failure, indeterminate outcome and superinfection were documented in 33.3%, 6.3% and 6.3%, respectively. All-cause mortality at day 28 was 37.5%. Bacterial eradication was observed in 56.3% of cases. The main adverse event was reversible hypokalaemia, as also reported in other studies.[139] Resistance development during therapy, which has been a matter of concern in previous studies occurred only in 3 cases.[140] Authors concluded that the necessity of combination with other antibiotics requires further investigation.

β-LACTAMS

The Inhibitors

Since the last 15 years, the spread of ESBLs and particularly of CTX-M enzymes in Enterobacteriaceae has become a serious public health problem worldwide. ESBL-producing *Escherichia coli* (ESBL-EC) are now a frequent cause of infection both in the community and in healthcare centers. Carbapenems, which are not affected by ESBLs, are considered the drugs of choice for treating severe infections caused by ESBL producers. Therefore, clinicians are increasingly forced to consider the use of carbapenems as empiric or definitive therapy in moderate to severe community-onset and nosocomial infections whenever an ESBL-producing organism is suspected or demonstrated. This might lead to an increase in the consumption of carbapenems, a particularly worrisome event in a scenario where carbapenemase-producing organisms are also spreading. Thus, alternatives to carbapenems for the treatment of ESBL producers are urgently needed. ESBLs are inhibited by β-lactamase inhibitors. Although hyper production of β-lactamases or additional resistance mechanisms may hamper the activity of these compounds, β-lactam/β-lactam inhibitor (BLBLI) combinations, such as amoxicillin clavulanate or piperacillin-tazobactam (PTZ) remain active against a considerable proportion of ESBL-producing enterobacteria, particularly *E. coli*, in many areas of the world. In this context, a study was recently published aiming in the post hoc analysis of patients with BSI due to ESBL-EC using data from six published prospective cohorts.[133] Mortality and length of hospital stay in patients treated with an active BLBLI (amoxicillin-clavulanic acid at a dose of 1.2 g 8 hourly IV and PTZ at a high dose of 4.5 g 6 hourly IV) or a carbapenem, were compared in two cohorts: the empirical therapy cohort (ETC) and the definitive therapy cohort (DTC) including 103 and 174 patients, respectively. At day

30 for those treated with BLBLI versus carbapenems, mortality was 9.7% versus 19.4% for the ETC and 9.3% versus 16.7% for the DTC, respectively (P >0.2, log-rank test). No association of increased mortality was observed between either empirical therapy with BLBLI or definitive therapy. However, physicians should be careful since in case of production of ESBL, in order to administer PTZ, the MIC of the isolated pathogen, should be less than or equal to 8 μg/mL for the PK/PD target to be attained (time above the MIC >50%) and, therefore, the highest dose should be prescribed. On the other hand, the reported series concerned mostly secondary bacteremias of urinary or biliary tract origin without any clinical experience in the respiratory tract rendering the extrapolation of the results difficult in case of lung infections.

Sulbactam, a β-lactamase plasmid-mediated inhibitor, active by itself in vitro against MDR A. baumannii strains, is available in the market only in combination with ampicillin at a ratio of 2:1 given in serious infections at a dose of 3 g 6 hourly IV.[35] In vivo, in combination with ampicillin, it was given at a high dose (18-24 g) in 161 patients derived from six separate studies, several of whom were suffering from VAP caused by Acinetobacter.[35] A successful therapeutic result was obtained in 46%-88%. However, controlled prospective well designed studies are required in order sulbacram to obtain a definitive place in the antimicrobial armamentarium against MDR/XDR microorganisms.

Temocillin

Temocillin, a 6-α-methoxy derivative of ticarcillin, is currently approved for treatment of infections due to members of the *Enterobacteriaceae* in Belgium and the United Kingdom.[142] It is stable against hydrolysis by most β-lactamases, including ESBLs and AmpC-type, *in vitro* studies reporting MICs at which 90% of bacteria are inhibited, between 16 μg/mL and 32 μg/mL.[143] Temocillin was also found active *in vitro* against *K. pneumoniae KPC (+)* strains at an MIC of 16 μg/mL inhibiting 40% and at 32 μg/mL 90% of the strains.[144] The British Society for Antimicrobial Chemotherapy has determined temocillin susceptibilities at less than 8 μg/mL and less than or equal to 32 μg/mL for systemic and urinary tract infections, respectively.[142] One gram of temocillin is known to achieve a peak serum concentration of approximately 160 μg/mL with serum binding of 85% and a half-life of 4–5 hours. The recommended dose in UTIs is 500 mg IV every 12 hours obtaining a urinary concentration approximately 500 μg/mL. Despite its activity against MDR pathogens and its safety profile, it is unexplained why temocillin market still remains so limited.

Cephalosporins

Existing clinical studies concerning the impact of therapy with third-generation cephalosporins or cefepime in infections caused by ESBL-producing Enterobacteriaceae, are retrospective, nonrandomized, and have been carried out with a small number of patients and low-dosage schedules that lack PK/PD correlations with clinical efficacy.[145] Rates of clinical failure and mortality are higher than those in studies with non-ESBL-producing Enterobacteriaceae. Therefore, in settings with a high prevalence of ESBL-producing Enterobacteriaceae, empirical therapy with advanced third generation cephalosporins or even cefepime should be avoided.[145]

Carbapenems

It is well-recognized that carbapenems either as imipenem, meropenem, or doripenem or even ertapenem (which is inherently inactive against *P. aeruginosa* and *A. baumannii* strains) represent the last resort antibiotics for MDR Gram-negative pathogens. Unfortunately, several carbapenemases numbering 126 enzymes have been reported until January 10, 2012 with capacity to hydrolyze carbapenems and almost all cephalosporins and the inhibitors as well.[1,2,14-20,30,34] The most frequently isolated and most important carbapenems are:[1,5,14-30] (1) the IMP-type enzymes, first detected in Japan in the late 1980s in *P. aeruginosa* strains; (2) the VIM-type enzymes, first discovered in Verona in the late 1990s and since then reported worldwide, detected in *P. aeruginosa* strains and Enterobacteriaceae; (3) the KPC enzymes, first isolated from a *K. pneumoniae* strain in 1996 in the state of New York, subsequently spread to different species of Enterobacteriaceae and isolated mostly in Israel, Greece, and the Southern European countries; (4) the NDM-type enzymes, the latest addition to carbapenems characterized by their propensity for intercontinental dissemination, a fact of great concern. NDM-1 was first detected in a strain of *K. pneumoniae* isolated in 2008 in a patient returning to Sweden from India, where NDM-1 is widespread in Enterobacteriaceae, subsequently spread from travelers to India and Pakistan to UK and almost to the five continents; and (5) the OXA-48 and OXA-181 type enzymes mostly detected in *A. baumannii* and mainly reported from Turkey.

Initially, it was considered that therapeutic administration of a carbapenem in case of production of a carbapenemase was prohibited. However, it was well-recognized that both VIM and KPC producing *K. pneumoniae* can exhibit low MICs to carbapenems with a range of 0.12–32 μg/mL, 28–79% possessing MICs less than or equal to 4 μg/mL.[123,146] On the other hand, the new EUCAST breakpoints at least for meropenem and imipenem are equal to 2 μg/mL with resistant strains indicated by MICs more than or equal to 8 μg/mL.[147] Therefore, the question whether or not a carbapenem can be safely administered in similar situations required investigation. In a Greek prospective observational study in a total of 162 consecutive patients with *K. pneumoniae* bacteremia,[148] the mortality rates for patients infected with VIM-positive strains possessing an MIC less than or equal to 4 μg/mL were categorized as follows: (1) combination therapy with two active drugs (one of which was meropenem); 8.3%; (2) therapy with one active *in vitro* drug; 27%; and (3) inappropriate definitive therapy; 27.8%. Therefore, it was concluded that carbapenem monotherapy (imipenem, meropenem, doripenem) for strains with MIC more than 4 μg/mL should be prohibited, whereas for strains with low MICs (≤4 μg/mL) is better to be avoided, at least as monotherapy.

In a recent literature review, including 34 studies compiled from MEDLINE, 297 patients infected with CPKP strains and suffering mostly from bacteremia and VAP were studied.[117] According to the administered therapeutic regimen, seven groups of patients were recognized: (1) Regimen A (36 patients); combination therapy with two active drugs one of which was a carbapenem with MIC less than or equal to 4 μg/mL; (2) Regimen B (62 patients); combination therapy with two active drugs not including a carbapenem; (3) Regimen C (21 patients); monotherapy with an aminoglycoside; (4) Regimen D (36 patients); monotherapy with a carbapenem (MIC ≤4 μg/mL); (5) Regimen E (14 patients); monotherapy with tigecycline; (6) Regimen F (72 patients); monotherapy with colistin; and (7) Regimen G (56 patients); inappropriate therapy. Failure rates were 8.3%, 29%, 24%, 25%, 35.7%, 47.2%, and 54% for the seven regimens, respectively. Regarding statistical analysis, the following results were obtained: A versus B p = 0.02, A versus E p = 0.03, A versus F p = 0.0001, A versus G p = less than 0.0001, G versus B p = 0.014, G versus C p = 0.04, G versus D p= 0.03, G versus E p= NS, G versus F p= NS. From the reported results it is evident that carbapenems, at least in case of bacteremia or VAP, could be a reasonable treatment option against carbapenemase producing *K. pneumoniae*, provided that: (1) the carbapenem MIC for the infecting organism is less than or equal to 4 μg/mL (or even 8 μg/mL); (2) carbapenem is given in combination with another active *in vitro* compound, i.e., colistin, tigecycline or an aminoglycoside; (3) in case of carbapenem MIC more than 8 μg/mL the combination of two active *in vitro* antibiotics excluding carbapenems, might be superior of any active monotherapy; and (4) the carbapenem should be given in high dose and prolonged infusions (3 hours for meropenem, 4 hours for doripenem), based on the fact that the efficacy of the carbapenems depends on the time that blood levels are sustained above the MIC (T >MIC = 40–50%). On the other hand, in an effort to exploit PK/PDs of doripenem, it has been observed that a dose of 1 g as a 4 hour infusion every 8 hour reaches the target for strains with MICs as high as 8 μg/mL restoring, therefore, its activity against isolates with decreased susceptibility or even resistant to doripenem. In agreement with the latter findings are the results of a recent retrospective cohort study in which the overall 28 day crude mortality rate of 41 patients with KPC-producing *K. pneumoniae* bacteremia was 30.9%.[149] In the multivariate analysis, definitive therapy with a comparison regimen was independently associated with survival (p = 0.02), the 28-day mortality rate being 13.3% in the combination therapy group compared with 57.8% in the monotherapy group (p = 0.01). The most commonly used combinations were colistin/polymyxin B or tigecycline combined with a carbapenem. Therefore, the obtained results in KPC-producing *K. pneumoniae* were in agreement with those of the latter review[120] indicating the necessity of combination therapy even with three active *in vitro* antibiotics, preferentially including a carbapenem when susceptibility data allow it (MIC ≤4 μg/mL).[150]

All newer carbapenem, like doripenem, biapenem, panipenem/betamipron, tebipenem, and tomopenem are not active against MDR strains resistant to the older ones.[151] However, it should be pointed out that doripenem, the most recently FDA-approved carbapenem, although exhibiting an antimicrobial spectrum similar to meropenem against Gram-negative pathogens, it possesses two- to fourfold lower MICs against *P. aeruginosa* compared with meropenem.[152] Another potential advantage of doripenem, over the other carbapenems, is its lower propensity for the selection of resistance *in vitro*. Interestingly, doripenem retains activity against *Pseudomonas* strains displaying poring mutations (OprD-mediated resistance) to imipenem.[35] Therefore, it might be an option against strains with isolated resistance to imipenem. Preliminary data indicate that PK/PD applications, by means of prolonged 4-hour infusion supported by the relative stability of the infusate in ambient conditions, may help in the treatment of *K. pneumoniae* KPC (+) strains with borderline MICs, thus overcoming low-level resistance.[153] Exploiting PK/PD evidence, in a large, phase III study of 531 patients with VAP, a 4-hour intravenous infusion of doripenem (500 mg every 8 hours) was effective and therapeutically noninferior to imipenem/cilastatin, exhibiting clinical cure rates of 68.3% versus 64.2% for imipenem.[154] It was of importance that in patients infected with *P. aeruginosa*, doripenem cured 80.0% whereas imipenem/cilastatin only 42.9% (pNS), with microbiological eradiation in 65.0% and 37.5% of patient, respectively.[154]

All other new carbapenems in preclinical phase, are advantageous *in vitro* only because of their enhanced activity against the Gram-positives including MRSA and VRE strains. Even ceftaroline which is already in the USA market, as well as ceftobiprole, the so-called fifth generation cephalosporins, possess activity against MRSA, but they offer no advantage against Gram-negatives.[151]

Recently, the Bulik and Nicolau revolutionary successful approach of the combination of two carbapenems (DC) was applied for the first time in three patients.[155,156] The regimen included the administration of ertapenem, based on its increased affinity for KPC carbapenemases, hindering subsequently doripenem or meropenem degradation in the environment of the targeted CPKP strains. Patients suffered from pandrug-resistant KPC-2 *K. pneumoniae* bacteremia (2) and urinary tract infection (1). Two of them were septic with high MICs to all carbapenems (MIC >32 µg/mL) as well as to all available antibiotics. All responded successfully to the administration of 1 g ertapenem, 1 hour infusion, given every 24 hours, to be followed by 2 g meropenem every 8 hours in 3 hours infusion, without relapse at the follow-up.

Other Therapeutic Options

Plazomicin (ACHN-490), a neoglycoside derivative of sisomicin that evades all plasmid-mediated aminoglycoside-modifying enzymes is also active *in vitro* against ESBLs, MBL, KPC, and OXA-48 carbapenemase producing Enterobacteriaceae.[147] However, it is not active against 16S rRNA methylase positive strains an enzyme spread in several parts of the world. In a multinational Phase II study in patients with cUTIs and acute pyelonephritis, satisfactory clinical response was observed without evidence of nephro- or ototoxicity.[158]

Among new β-lactamase inhibitors in ongoing studies, avibactam (NXL-104), including ESBL, OXA-48, AmpC and KPC enzymes, in combination with ceftazidime plus metronidazole versus imipenem is currently evaluated in UTIs, whereas MK7655, another inhibitor active against KPC and AmpC enzymes in cIAI.[151,159]

The clinician should also not forget to test in vitro the possibility of MDR or even XDR strains to be susceptible to chloramphenicol or to trimethoprim-sulfamethoxazole or even nitrofurantoin in the case of lower UTIs.[160]

CONCLUSION

Facing the critical shortage of new antibiotics in development against MDR-XDR bacteria, it is time for medical personnel to react now. There is no doubt that reducing the consequences of antibiotic resistance requires a multifact approach including rational use of all existing antibacterial agents appropriate selection, high dosage and reduced length of therapy, as well as application of de-escalation.[161] On the other hand, the control of the spread of resistant microorganisms in the hospital setting by the strict application of infection control measures and particularly of "hand hygiene" and "cohorting" of colonized or infected patients with XDR or PDR microorganisms, are the cornerstones of nosocomial infection prevention, as well as of reduction of resistance rates in nasty bugs.[162,163]

REFERENCES

1. Souli M, Galani I, Giamarellou H. Emergence of extensively drug-resistant and pandrug-resistant gram-negative bacilli in Europe. *Euro Surveill.* 2008;13.pii:19045.
2. Souli M, Galani I, Antoniadou A, et al. An outbreak of infection due to beta-Lactamase Klebsiella pneumoniae carbapenemase 2-producing *K. pneumoniae* in a Greek University Hospital: molecular characterization, epidemiology, and outcomes. *Clin Infect Dis.* 2010;50:364-73.
3. Boucher HW, Talbot GH, Bradley JS. Bad bugs, no drugs: no ESKAPE! An update from the Infectious Diseases Society of America. *Clin Infect Dis.* 2009;48:1-12.
4. Magiorakos AP, Srinivasan A, Carey RB, et al. Multidrug-resistant, extensively drug-resistant and pandrug-resistant bacteria: an international expert proposal for interim standard definitions for acquired resistance. *Clin Microbiol Infect.* 2012;18:268-81.
5. van Duijn PJ, Dautzenberg MJ, Oostdijk EA. Recent trends in antibiotic resistance in European ICUs. *Curr Opin Crit Care.* 2011;17:658-65.
6. Lambert ML, Suetens C, Savey A, et al. Clinical outcomes of health-care-associated infections and antimicrobial resistance in patients admitted to European intensive-care units: a cohort study. *Lancet Infect Dis.* 2011;11:30-8.
7. Meyer E, Schwab F, Schroeren-Boersch B, et al. Dramatic increase of third-generation cephalosporin-resistant E. coli in German intensive care units: secular trends in antibiotic drug use and bacterial resistance, 2001 to 2008. *Crit Care.* 2010;14:R113.
8. Vincent JL, Rello J, Marshall J, et al. International study of the prevalence and outcomes of infection in intensive care units. *JAMA.* 2009;302:2323-9.

9. European Centre for Disease Prevention and Control. Annual Epidemiological Report on Communicable Diseases in Europe 2010. Stockholm: ECDC; 2010.
10. Dumpis U, Iversen A, Balode A, et al. Outbreak of CTX-M-15-producing Klebsiella pneumoniae of sequence type 199 in a Latvian teaching hospital. *APMIS.* 2010;118:713-6.
11. Nielsen JB, Skov MN, Jørgensen RL, et al. Identification of CTX-M15-, SHV-28-producing Klebsiella pneumoniae ST15 as an epidemic clone in the Copenhagen area using a semi-automated Rep-PCR typing assay. *Eur J Clin Microbiol Infect Dis.* 2011;30:773-8.
12. Ruiz E, Rojo-Bezares B, Sáenz Y, et al, et al. Outbreak caused by a multi-resistant Klebsiella pneumoniae strain of new sequence type ST341 carrying new genetic environments of aac(6')-Ib-cr and qnrS1 genes in a neonatal intensive care unit in Spain. *Int J Med Microbiol.* 2010;300:464-9.
13. Vranic-Ladavac M, Bosnjak Z, Beader N, et al. Clonal spread of CTX-M-15-producing Klebsiella pneumoniae in a Croatian hospital. *J Med Microbiol.* 2010;59:1069-78.
14. Cornaglia G, Giamarellou H, Rossolini GM. Metallo-β-lactamases: a last frontier for β-lactams? *Lancet Infect Dis.* 2011;11:381-93.
15. Kumarasamy KK, Toleman MA, Walsh TR, et al. Emergence of a new antibiotic resistance mechanism in India, Pakistan, and the UK: a molecular, biological, and epidemiological study. *Lancet Infect Dis.* 2010;10:597-602.
16. Sidjabat H, Nimmo GR, Walsh TR, et al. Carbapenem resistance in Klebsiella pneumoniae due to the New Delhi Metallo-β-lactamase. *Clin Infect Dis.* 2011;52:481-4.
17. Walsh TR, Weeks J, Livermore DM, et al. Dissemination of NDM-1 positive bacteria in the New Delhi environment and its implications for human health: an environmental point prevalence study. *Lancet Infect Dis.* 2011;11:355-62.
18. Struelens MJ, Monnet DL, Magiorakos AP, et al. New Delhi metallo-beta-lactamase 1-producing Enterobacteriaceae: emergence and response in Europe. *Euro Surveill.* 2010;15. pii: 19716.
19. Deshpande P, Shetty A, Kapadia F, et al. New Delhi metallo 1: have carbapenems met their doom? *Clin Infect Dis.* 2010;51:1222.
20. Hammerum AM, Toleman MA, Hansen F, et al. Global spread of New Delhi metallo-β-lactamase 1. *Lancet Infect Dis.* 2010;10:829-30.
21. Yigit H, Queenan AM, Anderson GJ, et al. Novel carbapenem-hydrolyzing beta-lactamase, KPC-1, from a carbapenem-resistant strain of Klebsiella pneumoniae. *Antimicrob Agents Chemother.* 2001;45:1151-61.
22. Grundmann H, Livermore DM, Giske CG, et al. Carbapenem-non-susceptible Enterobacteriaceae in Europe: conclusions from a meeting of national experts. *Euro Surveill.* 2010;15. pii:19711.
23. Kassis-Chikhani N, Decré D, Ichai P, et al. Outbreak of Klebsiella pneumoniae producing KPC-2 and SHV-12 in a French hospital. *J Antimicrob Chemother.* 2010;65:1539-40.
24. Naas T, Nordmann P, Vedel G, et al. Plasmid-mediated carbapenem-hydrolyzing beta-lactamase KPC in a Klebsiella pneumoniae isolate from France. *Antimicrob Agents Chemother.* 2005;49:4423-4.
25. Petrella S, Ziental-Gelus N, Mayer C, et al. Genetic and structural insights into the dissemination potential of the extremely broad-spectrum class A beta-lactamase KPC-2 identified in an Escherichia coli strain and an Enterobacter cloacae strain isolated from the same patient in France. *Antimicrob Agents Chemother.* 2008;52:3725-36.
26. Hellenic Center for Infectious Disease Control, Ministry of Health (KEEL), National School of Public Health (NSPH). (2011). Greek System for the Surveillance of Antimicrobial Resistance. [online] Available from: www.mednet.gr/whonet. [Accessed January, 2014].
27. Cuzon G, Naas T, Demachy MC, et al. Plasmid-mediated carbapenem-hydrolyzing beta-lactamase KPC-2 in Klebsiella pneumoniae isolate from Greece. *Antimicrob Agents Chemother.* 2008;52:796-7.
28. Tsakris A, Kristo I, Poulou A, et al. First occurrence of KPC-2-possessing Klebsiella pneumoniae in a Greek hospital and recommendation for detection with boronic acid disc tests. *J Antimicrob Chemother.* 2008;62:1257-60.
29. Vatopoulos A. High rates of metallo-beta-lactamase-producing Klebsiella pneumoniae in Greece--a review of the current evidence. *Euro Surveill.* 2008;13.pii: 8023.
30. Giamarellou H, Antoniadou A, Kanellakopoulou K. Acinetobacter baumannii: a universal threat to public health? *Int J Antimicrob Agents.* 2008;32:106-19.
31. Carlet J, Mainardi JL. Antibacterial agents: back to the future? Can we live with only colistin, co-trimoxazole and fosfomycin? *Clin Microbiol Infect.* 2012;18:1-3.
32. Giamarellou H. Multidrug resistance in Gram-negative bacteria that produce extended-spectrum beta-lactamases (ESBLs). *Clin Microbiol Infect.* 2005;11:1-16.
33. Giamarellou H. Multidrug-resistant Gram-negative bacteria: how to treat and for how long. *Int J Antimicrob Agents.* 2010;36:S50-4.
34. Hanberger H, Giske CG, Giamarellou H. When and how to cover for resistant gram-negative bacilli in severe sepsis and septic shock. *Curr Infect Dis Rep.* 2011;13:416-25.
35. Giamarellou H, Poulakou G. Multidrug-resistant Gram-negative infections: what are the treatment options? *Drugs.* 2009;69:1879-901.
36. Li J, Nation RL. Old polymyxins are back: is resistance close? *Clin Infect Dis.* 2006;4:663-4.
37. Kwa A, Kasiakou SK, Tam VH, et al. Polymyxin B: similarities to and differences from colistin (polymyxin E). *Expert Rev Anti Infect Ther.* 2007;5:811-21.
38. Moore RA, Chan L, Hancock RE. Evidence for two distinct mechanisms of resistance to polymyxin B in Pseudomonas aeruginosa. *Antimicrob Agents Chemother.* 1984;26:539-45.
39. Gales AC, Jones RN, Sader HS. Global assessment of the antimicrobial activity of polymyxin B against 54 731 clinical isolates of Gram-negative bacilli: report from the SENTRY antimicrobial surveillance programme (2001-2004). *Clin Microbiol Infect.* 2006;12:315-21.
40. Li J, Rayner CR, Nation RL, et al. Heteroresistance to colistin in multidrug-resistant Acinetobacter baumannii. *Antimicrob Agents Chemother.* 2006;50:2946-50.
41. Meletis G, Tzampaz E, Sianou E, et al. Colistin heteroresistance in carbapenemase-producing Klebsiella pneumoniae. *J Antimicrob Chemother.* 2011;66:946-7.
42. Clinical Laboratory Standards Institute. Performance standards for antimicrobial susceptibility testing. 16th International Supplement M-100-S15. Wayne (PA): CLSI, 2005.
43. European Committee on Antimicrobial Susceptibility Test. (2008) Miscellaneous antimicrobials: EUCAST clinical MIC breakpoints 2008-06-19 (v 2.3). [online]. Available from:

www.srga.org/eucastwt/MICTAB/MICmiscellaneous.html. [Accessed August, 2009].

44. Giamarellos-Bourboulis EJ, Sambatakou H, Galani I, et al. In vitro interaction of colistin and rifampin on multidrug-resistant Pseudomonas aeruginosa. *J Chemother.* 2003;15:235-8.
45. Souli M, Rekatsina PD, Chryssouli Z, et al. Does the activity of the combination of imipenem and colistin in vitro exceed the problem of resistance in metallo-beta-lactamase-producing Klebsiella pneumoniae isolates? *Antimicrob Agents Chemother.* 2009;53:2133-5.
46. Giamarellos-Bourboulis EJ, Xirouchaki E, Giamarellou H. Interactions of colistin and rifampin on multidrug-resistant Acinetobacter baumannii. *Diagn Microbiol Infect Dis.* 2001;40:117-20.
47. Li J, Turnidge J, Milne R, et al. In vitro pharmacodynamic properties of colistin and colistin methanesulfonate against Pseudomonas aeruginosa isolates from patients with cystic fibrosis. *Antimicrob Agents Chemother.* 2001;45: 781-5.
48. Bergen PJ, Li J, Nation RL, et al. Comparison of once-, twice- and thrice-daily dosing of colistin on antibacterial effect and emergence of resistance: studies with Pseudomonas aeruginosa in an in vitro pharmacodynamic model. *J Antimicrob Chemother.* 2008;61:636-42.
49. Lim LM, Ly N, Anderson D, et al. Resurgence of colistin: a review of resistance, toxicity, pharmacodynamics, and dosing. *Pharmacotherapy.* 2010;30:1279-91.
50. Giamarellou H. Treatment options for multidrug-resistant bacteria. *Expert Rev Anti Infect Ther.* 2006;4:601-18.
51. de Groot R, Smith AL. Antibiotic pharmacokinetics in cystic fibrosis. Differences and clinical significance. *Clin Pharmacokinet.* 1987;13:228-53.
52. Plachouras D, Karvanen M, Friberg LE, et al. Population pharmacokinetic analysis of colistin methanesulfonate and colistin after intravenous administration in critically ill patients with infections caused by gram-negative bacteria. *Antimicrob Agents Chemother.* 2009;53:3430-6.
53. Jansson B, Karvanen M, Cars O, et al. Quantitative analysis of colistin A and colistin B in plasma and culture medium using a simple precipitation step followed by LC/MS/MS. *J Pharm Biomed Anal.* 2009;49:760-7.
54. Kumar A, Roberts D, Wood KE, et al. Duration of hypotension before initiation of effective antimicrobial therapy is the critical determinant of survival in human septic shock. *Crit Care Med.* 2006;34:1589-96.
55. Mohamed AF, Karaiskos I, Plachouras D, et al. Application of a loading dose of colistin methanesulphonate (CMS) in critically ill patients: population pharmacokinetics, protein binding and prediction of bacterial kill. *Antimicrob Agents Chemother.* 2012;56:4241-9.
56. Garonzik SM, Li J, Thamlikitkul V, et al. Population pharmacokinetics of colistin methanesulfonate and formed colistin in critically ill patients from a multicenter study provide dosing suggestions for various categories of patients. *Antimicrob Agents Chemother.* 2011;55:3284-94.
57. Levin AS, Barone AA, Penço J, et al. Intravenous colistin as therapy for nosocomial infections caused by multidrug-resistant Pseudomonas aeruginosa and Acinetobacter baumannii. *Clin Infect Dis.* 1999;28:1008-11.
58. Linden PK, Kusne S, Coley K, et al. Use of parenteral colistin for the treatment of serious infection due to antimicrobial-resistant Pseudomonas aeruginosa. *Clin Infect Dis.* 2003;37: e154-60.
59. Markou N, Apostolakos H, Koumoudiou C, et al. Intravenous colistin in the treatment of sepsis from multiresistant Gram-negative bacilli in critically ill patients. *Crit Care.* 2003;7:R78-83.
60. Michalopoulos AS, Tsiodras S, Rellos K, et al. Colistin treatment in patients with ICU-acquired infections caused by multiresistant Gram-negative bacteria: the renaissance of an old antibiotic. *Clin Microbiol Infect.* 2005;11:115-21.
61. Kasiakou SK, Michalopoulos A, Soteriades ES, et al. Combination therapy with intravenous colistin for management of infections due to multidrug-resistant Gram-negative bacteria in patients without cystic fibrosis. *Antimicrob Agents Chemother.* 2005;49:3136-46.
62. Garnacho-Montero J, Ortiz-Leyba C, Jiménez-Jiménez FJ, et al. Treatment of multidrug-resistant Acinetobacter baumannii ventilator-associated pneumonia (VAP) with intravenous colistin: a comparison with imipenem-susceptible VAP. *Clin Infect Dis.* 2003;36:1111-8.
63. Reina R, Estenssoro E, Sáenz G, et al. Safety and efficacy of colistin in Acinetobacter and Pseudomonas infections: a prospective cohort study. *Intensive Care Med.* 2005;31:1058-65.
64. Rios FG, Luna CM, Maskin B, et al. Ventilator-associated pneumonia due to colistin susceptible-only microorganisms. *Eur Respir J.* 2007;30:307-13.
65. Kallel H, Hergafi L, Bahloul M, et al. Safety and efficacy of colistin compared with imipenem in the treatment of ventilator-associated pneumonia: a matched case-control study. *Intensive Care Med.* 2007;33:1162-7.
66. Paul M, Bishara J, Levcovich A, et al. Effectiveness and safety of colistin: prospective comparative cohort study. *J Antimicrob Chemother.* 2010;65:1019-27.
67. Falagas ME, Rafailidis PI, Ioannidou E, et al. Colistin therapy for microbiologically documented multidrug-resistant Gram-negative bacterial infections: a retrospective cohort study of 258 patients. *Int J Antimicrob Agents.* 2010;35:194-9.
68. Dalfino L, Puntillo F, Mosca A, et al. High dose, extended-interval colistin administration in critically ill patients: Is this the right dosing strategy? a preliminary study. *Clin Infect Dis.* 2012;54:1720-6.
69. Michalopoulos A, Papadakis E. Inhaled anti-infective agents: emphasis on colistin. *Infection.* 2010;38:81-8.
70. Korbila IP, Michalopoulos A, Rafailidis PI, et al. Inhaled colistin as adjunctive therapy to intravenous colistin for the treatment of microbiologically documented ventilator-associated pneumonia: a comparative cohort study. *Clin Microbiol Infect.* 2010;16:1230-6.
71. Kofteridis DP, Alexopoulou C, Valachis A, et al. Aerosolized plus intravenous colistin versus intravenous colistin alone for the treatment of ventilator-associated pneumonia: a matched case-control study. *Clin Infect Dis.* 2010;51:1238-44.
72. Tumbarello M, De Pascale G, Trecarichi EM, et al. Effect of aerosolized colistin as adjunctive treatment on the outcomes of microbiologically documented ventilator-associated pneumonia caused by colistin-only susceptible gram-negative bacteria. *Chest.* 2013;144:1768-75.
73. Rubin BK. Aerosolized antibiotics for non-cystic fibrosis bronchiectasis. *J Aerosol Med Pulm Drug Deliv.* 2008;21:71-6.
74. Athanassa ZE, Markantonis SL, Fousteri MZ, et al. Pharmacokinetics of inhaled colistimethate sodium (CMS) in mechanically ventilated critically ill patients. *Intensive Care Med.* 2012;38:1779-86.

75. Cascio A, Conti A, Sinardi L, et al. Post-neurosurgical multidrug-resistant Acinetobacter baumannii meningitis successfully treated with intrathecal colistin. A new case and a systematic review of the literature. *Int J Infect Dis.* 2010;14:e572-9.
76. Hachem RY, Chemaly RF, Ahmar CA, et al. Colistin is effective in treatment of infections caused by multidrug-resistant Pseudomonas aeruginosa in cancer patients. *Antimicrob Agents Chemother.* 2007;51:1905-11.
77. Turkoglu M, Dizbay M, Ciftçi A, et al. Colistin therapy in critically ill patients with chronic renal failure and its effect on development of renal dysfunction. *Int J Antimicrob Agents.* 2012;39:142-5.
78. Iosifidis E, Antachopoulos C, Ioannidou M, et al. Colistin administration to pediatric and neonatal patients. *Eur J Pediatr.* 2010;169:867-74.
79. Cruz DN, Perazella MA, Bellomo R, et al. Effectiveness of polymyxin B-immobilized fiber column in sepsis: a systematic review. *Crit Care.* 2007;11:R47.
80. Cruz DN, Antonelli M, Fumagalli R, et al. Early use of polymyxin B hemoperfusion in abdominal septic shock: the EUPHAS randomized controlled trial. *JAMA.* 2009; 301:2445-52.
81. Spapen H, Jacobs R, Van Gorp V, et al. Renal and neurological side effects of colistin in critically ill patients. *Ann Intensive Care.* 2011;1:14.
82. Falagas ME, Rizos M, Bliziotis IA, et al. Toxicity after prolonged (more than four weeks) administration of intravenous colistin. *BMC Infect Dis.* 2005;5:1.
83. Yahav D, Farbman L, Leibovici L, et al. Colistin: new lessons on an old antibiotic. *Clin Microbiol Infect.* 2012;18:18-29.
84. Yousef JM, Chen G, Hill PA, et al. Ascorbic acid protects against the nephrotoxicity and apoptosis caused by colistin and affects its pharmacokinetics. *J Antimicrob Chemother.* 2012;67:452-9.
85. Bosso JA, Liptak CA, Seilheimer DK, et al. Toxicity of colistin in cystic fibrosis patients. *DICP.* 1991;25:1168-70.
86. Falagas ME, Kasiakou SK. Colistin: the revival of polymyxins for the management of multidrug-resistant gram-negative bacterial infections. *Clin Infect Dis.* 2005;40:1333-41.
87. Antoniadou A, Kontopidou F, Poulakou G, et al. Colistin-resistant isolates of Klebsiella pneumoniae emerging in intensive care unit patients: first report of a multiclonal cluster. *J Antimicrob Chemother.* 2007;59:786-90.
88. Marchaim D, Chopra T, Pogue JM, et al. Outbreak of colistin-resistant, carbapenem-resistant Klebsiella pneumoniae in metropolitan Detroit, Michigan. *Antimicrob Agents Chemother.* 2011;55:593-9.
89. Kontopidou F, Plachouras D, Papadomichelakis E, et al. Colonization and infection by colistin-resistant Gram-negative bacteria in a cohort of critically ill patients. *Clin Microbiol Infect.* 2011;17:E9-E11.
90. Mentzelopoulos SD, Pratikaki M, Platsouka E, et al. Prolonged use of carbapenems and colistin predisposes to ventilator-associated pneumonia by pandrug-resistant Pseudomonas aeruginosa. *Intensive Care Med.* 2007;33: 1524-32.
91. Matthaiou DK, Michalopoulos A, Rafailidis PI, et al. Risk factors associated with the isolation of colistin-resistant gram-negative bacteria: a matched case-control study. *Crit Care Med.* 2008;36:807-11.
92. Kasbekar N. Tigecycline: a new glycylcycline antimicrobial agent. *Am J Health Syst Pharm.* 2006;63:1235-43.
93. Department of Health and Human Services. (2009). Letter to Wyeth Pharmaceuticals, Inc. [online]. Available from: www.accessdata.fda.gov/drugsatfda_docs/appletter/2009/021821s013,021821s017,021821s018ltr.pdf. [Accessed January, 2014].
94. European Medicines Agency. (2009). Questions and answers on the withdrawal of the application for a change to the marketing authorization for tygacil. Doc. Ref. EMEA/245771/2008. [online]. Available from www. emea.europa.eu/humandocs/PDFs/EPAR/tygacil/24577108en.pdf. [Accessed January, 2014].
95. Noskin GA. Tigecycline: a new glycylcycline for treatment of serious infections. *Clin Infect Dis.* 2005;41:S303-14.
96. Petersen PJ, Jones CH, Bradford PA. In vitro antibacterial activities of tigecycline and comparative agents by time-kill kinetic studies in fresh Mueller-Hinton broth. *Diagn Microbiol Infect Dis.* 2007;59:347-9.
97. Bouchillon SK, Iredell JR, Barkham T, et al. Comparative in vitro activity of tigecycline and other antimicrobials against Gram-negative and Gram-positive organisms collected from the Asia-Pacific Rim as part of the Tigecycline Evaluation and Surveillance Trial (TEST). *Int J Antimicrob Agents.* 2009;33:130-6.
98. Castanheira M, Sader HS, Deshpande LM, et al. Anti-microbial activities of tigecycline and other broad-spectrum antimicrobials tested against serine carbapenemase-and metallo-beta-lactamase-producing Enterobacteriaceae: report from the SENTRY Antimicrobial Surveillance Program. *Antimicrob Agents Chemother.* 2008;52:570-3.
99. Souli M, Kontopidou FV, Koratzanis E, et al. In vitro activity of tigecycline against multiple-drug-resistant, including pan-resistant, gram-negative and gram-positive clinical isolates from Greek hospitals. *Antimicrob Agents Chemother.* 2006;50:3166-9.
100. Kelesidis T, Karageorgopoulos DE, Kelesidis I, et al. Tigecycline for the treatment of multidrug-resistant Enterobacteriaceae: a systematic review of the evidence from microbiological and clinical studies. *J Antimicrob Chemother.* 2008;62:895-904.
101. Jones RN, Ferraro MJ, Reller LB, et al. Multicenter studies of tigecycline disk diffusion susceptibility results for Acinetobacter spp. *J Clin Microbiol.* 2007;45:227-30.
102. Dean CR, Visalli MA, Projan SJ, et al. Efflux-mediated resistance to tigecycline (GAR-936) in Pseudomonas aeruginosa PAO1. *Antimicrob Agents Chemother.* 2003;47: 972-8.
103. Vouillamoz J, Moreillon P, Giddey M, et al. In vitro activities of tigecycline combined with other antimicrobials against multiresistant gram-positive and gram-negative pathogens. *J Antimicrob Chemother.* 2008;61:371-4.
104. Tygacil® [package insert]. Philadelphia (PA): Wyeth Pharmaceuticals Inc.; 2005.
105. Meagher AK, Ambrose PG, Grasela TH, et al. Pharmacokinetic/pharmacodynamic profile for tigecycline-a new glycylcycline antimicrobial agent. *Diagn Microbiol Infect Dis.* 2005;52:165-71.
106. MacGowan AP. Tigecycline pharmacokinetic/pharmacodynamic update. *J Antimicrob Chemother.* 2008;62:i11-6.
107. Giamarellou H, Poulakou G. Pharmacokinetic and pharmacodynamic evaluation of tigecycline. *Expert Opin Drug Metab Toxicol.* 2011;7:1459-70.

108. Conte JE, Golden JA, Kelly MG, et al. Steady-state serum and intrapulmonary pharmacokinetics and pharmacodynamics of tigecycline. *Int J Antimicrob Agents.* 2005;25: 523-9.
109. Schafer JJ, Goff DA, Stevenson KB, et al. Early experience with tigecycline for ventilator-associated pneumonia and bacteremia caused by multidrug-resistant Acinetobacter baumannii. *Pharmacotherapy.* 2007;27:980-7.
110. Anthony KB, Fishman NO, Linkin DR, et al. Clinical and microbiological outcomes of serious infections with multidrug-resistant gram-negative organisms treated with tigecycline. *Clin Infect Dis.* 2008;46:567-70.
111. Swoboda S, Ober M, Hainer C, et al. Tigecycline for the treatment of patients with severe sepsis or septic shock: a drug use evaluation in a surgical intensive care unit. *Antimicrob Chemother.* 2008;61:729-33.
112. Vasilev K, Reshedko G, Orasan R, et al. A Phase 3, open-label, non-comparative study of tigecycline in the treatment of patients with selected serious infections due to resistant Gram-negative organisms including Enterobacter species, Acinetobacter baumannii and Klebsiella pneumoniae. *J Antimicrob Chemother.* 2008;62:i29-40.
113. Gallagher JC, Rouse HM. Tigecycline for the treatment of Acinetobacter infections: a case series. *Ann Pharmacother.* 2008;42:1188-94.
114. Curcio D, Fernández F, Vergara J, et al. Late onset ventilator-associated pneumonia due to multidrug-resistant Acinetobacter spp.: experience with tigecycline. *J Chemother.* 2009;21:58-62.
115. Gordon NC, Wareham DW. A review of clinical and microbiological outcomes following treatment of infections involving multidrug-resistant Acinetobacter baumannii with tigecycline. *J Antimicrob Chemother.* 2009;63:775-80.
116. Poulakou G, Kontopidou FV, Paramythiotou E, et al. Tigecycline in the treatment of infections from multi-drug resistant gram-negative pathogens. *J Infect.* 2009;58:273-84.
117. Maltezou HC, Giakkoupi P, Maragos A, et al. Outbreak of infections due to KPC-2-producing Klebsiella pneumoniae in a hospital in Crete (Greece). *J Infect.* 2009;58:213-9.
118. Ruzin A, Keeney D, Bradford PA. AdeABC multidrug efflux pump is associated with decreased susceptibility to tigecycline in Acinetobacter calcoaceticus-Acinetobacter baumannii complex. *J Antimicrob Chemother.* 2007;59: 1001-4.
119. Freire AT, Melnyk V, Kim MJ, et al. Comparison of tigecycline with imipenem/cilastatin for the treatment of hospital-acquired pneumonia. *Diagn Microbiol Infect Dis.* 2010;68:140-51.
120. Peleg AY, Potoski BA, Rea R, et al. Acinetobacter baumannii bloodstream infection while receiving tigecycline: a cautionary report. *J Antimicrob Chemother.* 2007;59:128-31.
121. Ramirez J, Dartois N, Gandjini H, et al. Randomized phase 2 trial to evaluate the clinical efficacy of two high-dosage tigecycline regimens versus imipenem-cilastatin for treatment of hospital-acquired pneumonia. *Antimicrob Agents and Chemother.* 2013;57:1756-62.
122. Kontopidou F, Giamarellou H, Katerelos P, et al. Infections caused by carbapenem-resistant Klebsiella pneumoniae among patients in intensive care units in Greece: a multi-centre study on clinical outcome and therapeutic options. *Clin Microb and Infect.* 2014;20:O117-23.
123. Tzouvelekis LS, Markogiannakis A, Psichogiou M, et al. Carbapenemases in Klebsiella pneumoniae and other Enterobacteriaceae: an evolving crisis of global dimensions. *Clin Microbiol Rev.* 2012;25:682-707.
124. Scaglione F. Comment on: Efficacy and safety of tigecycline: a systematic review and meta-analysis. *J Antimicrob Chemother.* 2011;66:2892-3.
125. Cai Y, Wang R, Liang B, et al. Systematic review and meta-analysis of the effectiveness and safety of tigecycline for treatment of infectious disease. *Antimicrob Agents Chemother.* 2011;55:1162-72.
126. Yahav D, Lador A, Paul M, et al. Efficacy and safety of tigecycline: a systematic review and meta-analysis. *J Antimicrob Chemother.* 2011;66:1963-71.
127. US Food and Drug Administration. (2010). FDA Drug Safety Communication: Increased risk of death with Tygacil (tigecycline) compared to other antibiotics used to treat similar infections (Sept 1, 2010). [online]. Available from: www.fda.gov/Drugs/DrugSafety/ucm224370.htm. [Accessed January, 2014].
128. Tasina E, Haidich AB, Kokkali S, et al. Efficacy and safety of tigecycline for the treatment of infectious diseases: a meta-analysis. *Lancet Infect Dis.* 2011;11:834-44.
129. Sartelli M, Viale P, Koike K, et al. WSES consensus conference: Guidelines for first-line management of intra-abdominal infections. *World J Emerg Surg.* 2011;6:2.
130. Raz R. Fosfomycin: an old-new antibiotic. *Clin Microbiol Infect.* 2012;18:4-7.
131. Popovic M, Steinort D, Pillai S, et al. Fosfomycin: an old, new friend? *Eur J Clin Microbiol Infect Dis.* 2010;29:127-42.
132. Falagas ME, Maraki S, Karageorgopoulos DE, et al. Antimicrobial susceptibility of multidrug-resistant (MDR) and extensively drug-resistant (XDR) Enterobacteriaceae isolates to fosfomycin. *Int J Antimicrob Agents.* 2010;35: 240-3.
133. Endimiani A, Patel G, Hujer KM, et al. In vitro activity of fosfomycin against blaKPC-containing Klebsiella pneumoniae isolates, including those nonsusceptible to tigecycline and/or colistin. *Antimicrob Agents Chemother.* 2010;54:526-9.
134. Souli M, Galani I, Boukovalas S, et al. In vitro interactions of antimicrobial combinations with fosfomycin against KPC-2-producing Klebsiella pneumoniae and protection of resistance development. *Antimicrob Agents Chemother.* 2011;55:2395-7.
135. Pfausler B, Spiss H, Dittrich P, et al. Concentrations of fosfomycin in the cerebrospinal fluid of neurointensive care patients with ventriculostomy-associated ventriculitis. *J Antimicrob Chemother.* 2004;53:848-52.
136. Falagas ME, Giannopoulou KP, Kokolakis GN, et al. Fosfomycin: use beyond urinary tract and gastrointestinal infections. *Clin Infect Dis.* 2008;46:1069-77.
137. Dinh A, Salomon J, Bru JP, et al. Fosfomycin: efficacy against infections caused by multidrug-resistant bacteria. *Scand J Infect Dis.* 2012;44:182-9.
138. Pontikis K, Karaiskos I, Bastani S, et al. Outcomes of critically ill intensive care unit patients treated with fosfomycin for infections due to pandrug-resistant and extensively drug-resistant carbapenemase-producing Gram-negative bacteria. *Int J Antimicrob Agents.* 2014;43: 52-9.

139. Florent A, Chichmanian RM, Cua E, et al. Adverse events associated with intravenous fosfomycin. *Int J Antimicrob Agents.* 2011;37:82-3.
140. Karageorgopoulos DE, Wang R, Yu XH, et al. Fosfomycin: evaluation of the published evidence on the emergence of antimicrobial resistance in Gram-negative pathogens. *J Antimicrob Chemother.* 2012;67:255-68.
141. Rodríguez-Baño J, Navarro MD, Retamar P, et al. Extended-Spectrum Beta-Lactamases–Red Española de Investigación en Patología Infecciosa/Grupo de Estudio de Infección Hospitalaria Group. β-Lactam/β-lactam inhibitor combinations for the treatment of bacteremia due to extended-spectrum β-lactamase-producing Escherichia coli: a post hoc analysis of prospective cohorts. *Clin Infect Dis.* 2012;54:167-74.
142. Adams-Haduch JM, Potoski BA, Sidjabat HE, et al. Activity of temocillin against KPC-producing Klebsiella pneumoniae and Escherichia coli. *Antimicrob Agents Chemother.* 2009;53:2700-1.
143. Rodriguez-Villalobos H, Malaviolle V, Frankard J, et al. In vitro activity of temocillin against extended spectrum beta-lactamase-producing Escherichia coli. *J Antimicrob Chemother.* 2006;57:771-4.
144. Naesens R, Ursi JP, Van Schaeren J, et al. In vitro activity of tigecycline against multidrug-resistant Enterobacteriaceae isolates from a Belgian hospital. *Eur J Clin Microbiol Infect Dis.* 2009;28:381-4.
145. Giamarellou H. beta-Lactams without a suicide inhibitor. *Clin Microbiol Infect.* 2008;14:194-7.
146. Daikos GL, Markogiannakis A. Carbapenemase-producing Klebsiella pneumoniae: (when) might we still consider treating with carbapenems? *Clin Microbiol Infect.* 2011;17: 1135-41.
147. European Committee on Antimicrobial Susceptibility Testing. (2012). Clinical breakpoints-bacteria (v 2.0) valid from 2012-01-01. [online]. Available from www.eucast.org/clinical_breakpoints. [Accessed January, 2014].
148. Daikos GL, Petrikkos P, Psichogiou M, et al. Prospective observational study of the impact of VIM-1 metallo-beta-lactamase on the outcome of patients with Klebsiella pneumoniae bloodstream infections. *Antimicrob Agents Chemother.* 2009;53:1868-73.
149. Qureshi ZA, Paterson DL, Potoski BA, et al. Treatment outcome of bacteremia due to KPC-producing Klebsiella pneumoniae: superiority of combination antimicrobial regimens. *Antimicrob Agents Chemother.* 2012;56:2108-13.
150. Tumbarello M, Viale P, Viscoli C, et al. Predictors of mortality in bloodstream infections caused by Klebsiella pneumoniae carbapenemase-producing K. pneumoniae: importance of combination therapy. *Clin Infect Dis.* 2012;55:943-50.
151. Bassetti M, Ginocchio F, Giacobbe DR, et al. Development of antibiotics for Gram-negatives: where now? *Clin Investig.* 2011;1:211-27.
152. Castanheira M, Jones RN, Livermore DM. Antimicrobial activities of doripenem and other carbapenems against Pseudomonas aeruginosa, other nonfermentative bacilli, and Aeromonas spp. *Diagn Microbiol Infect Dis.* 2009;63: 426-33.
153. Ikawa K, Morikawa N, Uehara S, et al. Pharmacokinetic-pharmacodynamic target attainment analysis of doripenem in infected patients. *Int J Antimicrob Agents.* 2009; 33:276-9.
154. Chastre J, Wunderink R, Prokocimer P, et al. Efficacy and safety of intravenous infusion of doripenem versus imipenem in ventilator-associated pneumonia: a multicenter, randomized study. *Crit Care Med.* 2008;36: 1089-96.
155. Crandon JL, Bulik CC, Nicolau DP. In vivo efficacy of 1- and 2-gram human simulated prolonged infusions of doripenem against Pseudomonas aeruginosa. *Antimicrob Agents Chemother.* 2009;53:4352-6.
156. Giamarellou H, Galani L, Baziaka F, et al. Effectiveness of a double-carbapenem regimen for infections in humans due to carbapenemase-producing pandrug-resistant Klebsiella pneumoniae. *Antimicrob Agents Chemother.* 2013;57:2388-90.
157. Endimiani A, Hujer KM, Hujer AM, et al. ACHN-490, a neoglycoside with potent in vitro activity against multidrug-resistant Klebsiella pneumoniae isolates. *Antimicrob Agents Chemother.* 2009;53:4504-7.
158. Galani I. Plazomicin. *Drugs of the future.* 2014;39:25-35.
159. Lucasti C, Popescu I, Ramesh MK, et al. Comparative study of the efficacy and safety of ceftazidime/avibactam plus metronidazole versus meropenem in the treatment of complicated intra-abdominal infections in hospitalized adults: results of a randomized, double-blind, Phase II trial. *J Antimicrob Chemother.* 2013;68:1183-92.
160. Livermore DM, Warner M, Mushtaq S, et al. What remains against carbapenem-resistant Enterobacteriaceae? Evaluation of chloramphenicol, ciprofloxacin, colistin, fosfomycin, minocycline, nitrofurantoin, temocillin and tigecycline. *Int J Antimicrob Agents.* 2011;37:415-9.
161. Pakyz AL, Oinonen M, Polk RE. Relationship of carbapenem restriction in 22 university teaching hospitals to carbapenem use and carbapenem-resistant Pseudomonas aeruginosa. *Antimicrob Agents Chemother.* 2009;53:1983-6.
162. Carmeli Y, Akova M, Cornaglia G, et al. Controlling the spread of carbapenemase-producing Gram-negatives: therapeutic approach and infection control. *Clin Microbiol Infect.* 2010;16:102-11.
163. Schwaber MJ, Lev B, Israeli A, et al. Containment of a country-wide outbreak of carbapenem-resistant Klebsiella pneumoniae in Israeli hospitals via a nationally implemented intervention. *Clin Infect Dis.* 2011;52: 848-55.

CHAPTER 21

Using PK/PD Properties of Antibiotics in the Treatment of Respiratory Infections

Francesco Scaglione

ABSTRACT

Anti-infective pharmacodynamic investigation is a critical tool for development of optimal dosing strategies and for establishment of definitions of clinically relevant drug resistance. The efficacy of an antimicrobial agent is dependent on its pharmacokinetic and pharmacodynamic properties. Classically, the pharmacokinetic describes the absorption, distribution, metabolism, and excretion, as well as the magnitude of the dosing regimen. The pharmacodynamics profile is a function of the concentrations achieved in tissues, body fluids, and the infection site relative to the *in vitro* microbiological activity of a given agent. The pharmacokinetic and pharmacodynamics profiles can be different for the various antimicrobial agents, an understanding of these characteristics for each agent is crucial in determining effective antibiotic dosing regimens. Some classes of antibiotics, such as the β-lactams or flucytosine antifungal, are characterized by time-dependent bactericidal activity, which means that free-drug concentrations higher than the minimum inhibitory concentration (MIC) for an adequate percentage of time in a dosing interval (%T > MIC) must be maintained for efficacy. Other drugs, such as the aminoglycosides, fluoroquinolones, or amphotericin B, exhibit concentration-dependent bactericidal activity, which requires an adequate maximum concentration/MIC ratio or area under the concentration-time curve/MIC ratio for efficacy.

In this chapter, we described the essential pharmacological aspects of the different antimicrobial agents drugs, including their pharmacokinetics/pharmacodynamic principles, with a focus on the respiratory tract infections.

INTRODUCTION

Pharmacokinetic/pharmacodynamic (PK/PD) characterization of antimicrobial agents has allowed a better understanding of why a particular dosing regimen achieves clinical success or failure. Antimicrobial dosing regimens historically have been based on the premise that serum concentrations must be higher than the minimum inhibitory concentration (MIC) of the antimicrobial against the pathogen. However, the relationship between serum concentrations and bacterial eradication has only recently been clearly defined. Although the MIC is an important measure of antimicrobial activity, it does not take into account patient-, drug-, and pathogen-related factors that influence the outcome of antimicrobial therapy. Increasing pathogen resistance and documented treatment failures, particularly in respiratory tract infections, indicate a need to use dosing strategies with available agents to maximize antimicrobial effectiveness and limit the spread of resistance. Using techniques first pioneered by Eagle et al., and further developed by Craig and co-workers, dose selection has become a much more sophisticated process over previous empirical methods. *In vitro* and *in vivo* experiments are used to define a relationship between drug concentration (PK) and effect (PD) and allow for a clear target to be identified so that efficacy is achieved in the clinical setting.

TABLE 1

Definitions of Pharmacokinetic Parameters

Parameter	Description
Bioavailability	Proportion of drug absorbed into the systemic circulation after administration. Drugs administered intravenously are usually 100% bioavailable (some are given as prodrugs); other dosage forms may be less bioavailable
C_{max}	Peak serum concentration of drug achieved following administration of a single dose
T_{max}	Time to reach peak serum concentration
Vd	Volume of distribution. A relative measure of the distribution of the drug throughout the body. Vd > 4 L indicates drug is distributed outside the plasma
AUC	Area under the serum concentration-time curve
t½	Elimination half-life. Time required for serum concentration of drug to be reduced by 50%. Also referred to as bt½ to differentiate it from at½, which designates the distribution t½ of a drug
Cl	A measurement of the excretion ability from the body. When referring to the function of the kidney, clearance is considered to be the amount of liquid filtered out of the blood that gets processed by the kidneys or the amount of blood cleaned per time because it has the units of a volumetric flow rate [volume/time]
T > MIC	Amount of time that the serum concentration is above the minimum inhibitory concentration required for bactericidal/static effects. Applicable to antimicrobials only

It is now understood that to achieve bacteriologic and clinical success, sufficient concentrations of antimicrobial at the site of infection must be maintained for an adequate period of time. These dynamics are determined by combining drug PK/PD data with MIC data. Different classes of antimicrobials have different patterns of bactericidal action based on PK and PD characteristics, and these patterns influence antimicrobial efficacy. PK/PD characteristics of an antimicrobial need to be integrated with MIC data to guide dosing strategies and predict bacteriologic and clinical outcomes. This approach not only improves antimicrobial efficacy but also serves to limit development of further pathogen resistance.

Principles of Pharmacokinetics and Pharmacodynamics

Pharmacokinetics describes the absorption, distribution, metabolism, and elimination characteristics of a drug in the human body (Table 1). PK parameters that have been shown to correlate with antimicrobial efficacy are area under the serum-concentration-time profile [area under the curve (AUC)], peak serum concentration (C_{max}), amount of time that the serum concentration of drug is above the MIC (T > MIC), the serum half-life, and penetration of drug into tissues.

Pharmacodynamics refers to the actions the drug exerts in the body, including therapeutic effects. Drug PD correlates for antimicrobial therapy are MIC and duration of bactericidal effects, including persistent antibiotic effects [post-antibiotic effects (PAE)], rate of killing, and rate of development of resistant mutants. Some antimicrobials continue to have bactericidal effects even after the antimicrobial has been cleared from the infection site. These PAEs are observed *in vivo* with inhibitors of protein and nucleic acid synthesis with Gram-negative bacilli and Gram-positive cocci and with β-lactams against *Staphylococcus aureus*, but not with β-lactams against Gram-negative bacilli or streptococci.

Thus, β-lactams that exhibit time-dependent killing usually have minimal or short PAEs, which are therefore of negligible value in contributing to additional antimicrobial efficacy. Antimicrobials that inhibit protein and nucleic acid synthesis can be thought of as having a substantial PAE. A long PAE prevents regrowth after antimicrobial concentrations fall below the MIC.

Antimicrobials exhibiting PAEs may be administered less frequently than would be predicted based on elimination half-life (t½). Thus, PAEs have a major impact on dosing. An understanding of these concepts has led to improved dosing regimens for current antibiotics as well as the establishment of appropriate dosing regimens for new antibiotics. This has improved patient care.

The PK/PD indices typically used for antimicrobials include the time the free drug concentration remains above the MIC (fT > MIC) expressed as a percent of the dosing interval, the ratio of the maximum concentration and MIC (Cmax/MIC), and the ratio of the 24-hour area under the concentration-time curve and MIC (AUC0-24/MIC).

The inter-relationships between these parameters are illustrated in figure 1 and reported in table 2.

The PK/PD parameters that best correlate with efficacy for the various classes of antimicrobials are shown in table 3.

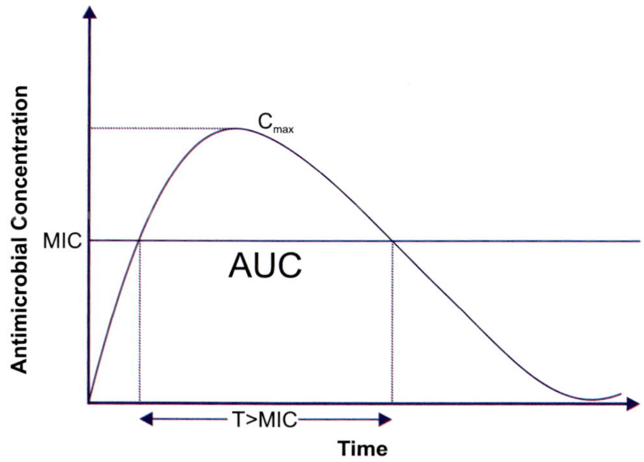

AUC, area under the serum concentration-time curve; C_{max}, maximum plasma concentration; MIC, minimal inhibitory concentration (*in vitro*).

FIGURE 1 PK/PD Correlation of antimicrobials. T more than MIC = time the concentration exceeds the minimum inhibitory concentration.

The index that best correlates with a particular antibiotic depends on several factors. One of these factors is the pattern of microbial kill exhibited by the drug, which is frequently referred to as either time-dependent killing or concentration-dependent killing. Antibiotics that display time-dependent killing typically reach a maximum effect at a concentration ca. 4 × MIC. Once this maximum effect is reached, increasing the concentration does not increase the rate of bacterial death, as shown for ticarcillin in figure 2. Antibiotics that display concentration-dependent killing produce an increasing effect as the concentration increases, as shown for tobramycin and ciprofloxacin in figure 2.

However, categorizing an agent's antimicrobial activity as time- or concentration-dependent is not always obvious, as shown in figure 3 where profiles for concentrations more than 4 × MIC appear similar for all compounds.[7]

TABLE 2
Pharmacokinetics/Pharmacodynamics Indices

Indices	Definition	Dimensions
MIC	Minimum inhibitory concentration. Note: Any calculation or expression of the MIC should include a description of the method by which the MIC was determined	Concentration (e.g., mg/L or mg/mL)
f	Prefix indicating that the pharmacokinetic parameter values or PK/PD index values used are unbound (free) fractions of the drug	Not applicable
AUC/MIC	The area under the concentration-time curve over 24 hours in steady-state divided by the MIC If a subscript indicating another time-period is not present, the AUC is assumed to be the 24 hour value at steady-state For unbound fraction of the drug, use *f*AUC/MIC	No dimensions
Peak/MIC (C_{max}/MIC) (ratio)	The peak level divided by the MIC For unbound fraction of the drug, use *f*Peak/MIC or *f* C_{max}/MIC	No dimensions
Time > MIC (to be written as T > MIC)	The cumulative percentage of a 24 hour period that the drug concentration exceeds the MIC at steady state Pharmacokinetic conditions Note: If the period is other than 24 hour, this should be stated explicitly For unbound fraction of the drug, use *f*T > MIC	%
In vitro PAE	It is defined as the period of suppression of bacterial growth after short exposure of organisms to an antimicrobial Note: The PAE using bacterial counts as a parameter is calculated by PAE = T C where T is the time required for the bacterial counts of the exposed cultures to increase one $\log_{10}$ above the counts observed immediately after washing/ dilution and C is the corresponding time required for the counts of the untreated cultures	Time (e.g., hours)
In vivo PAE	The difference in time for the number of bacteria in a tissue of treated animals versus controls to increase 1 $\log_{10}$ over values when drug concentrations in serum or the infection site fall below the MIC. The *in vivo* PAE thus includes the effects of sub-MIC concentrations	Time (e.g., hours)

PAE, post-antibiotic effects; AUC, area under curve; MIC, minimum inhibitory concentration; PK, pharmacokinetic; PD, pharmacodynamics.

TABLE 3

Antimicrobial Agents Classified by Pharmacokinetic/Pharmacodynamic Pattern

Drug class	Pharmacodynamic class	Magnitude
β-lactams	Time-dependent	T > MIC: 40–50% 80–100% in critically ill or immunocompromised patients
Macrolides	Time-dependent (with moderate to prolonged persistent effect)	AUC/MIC = 25–35
Fluoroquinolones	Concentration-dependent (with prolonged persistent effect)	AUC/MIC = 25–35 (*S. pneumoniae*) >100 (Gram-negatives)
Aminoglycosides	Concentration-dependent (with prolonged persistent effect)	C_{max}/MIC > 10
Tigecycline	Time dependent (with prolonged persistent effect)	AUC/MIC 18 (cSSSIs) and 7 (cIAIs)
Linezolid	Time dependent (with prolonged persistent effect)	AUC0-24/MIC 48 (pneumococci) 83 (staphylococci), >100 critically ill
Vancomycin	Time dependent	AUC0-24/MIC ≥400
Amphotericin B	Concentration dependent	C_{max}/MIC >40
Triazoles	Time dependent	AUC0-24/MIC ≥25 (fluconazole)
Echinocandins	Concentration dependent	C_{max}/MIC 10 (plasma); AUC/MIC 250 (tissue)

MIC, minimum inhibitory concentration; AUC, area under curve; cSSSIs, complicated skin and skin-structure infections; CIAIs, complicated intra-abdominal infections.

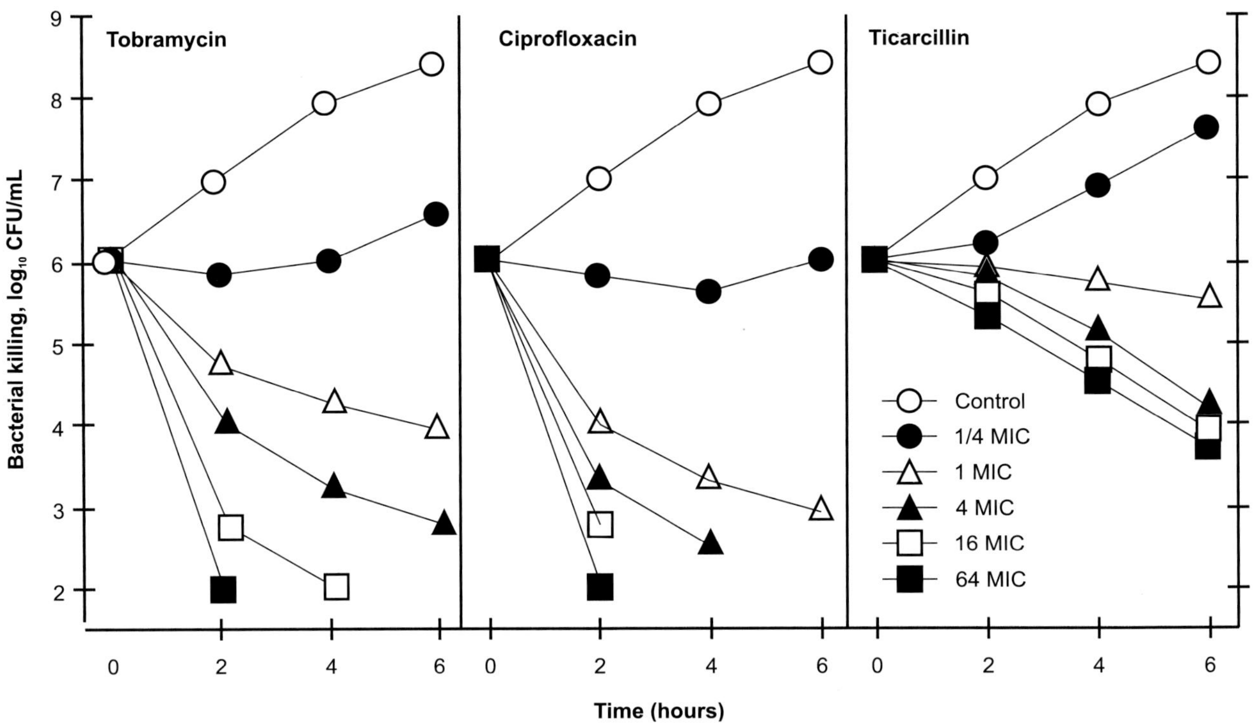

MIC, minimum inhibitory concentration; CFU, colony-forming units.

FIGURE 2 Time-kill curves with *Pseudomonas aeruginosa* ATCC 27853, showing tobramycin and ciprofloxacin as having concentration-dependent kill kinetics and ticarcillin as having time-dependent kill kinetics. *Source:* Craig WA, Ebert SC. Killing and regrowth of bacteria in vitro: a review. *Scand J Infect Dis Suppl.* 1990;74:63-70.

Concentration-dependent antibiotics usually correlate efficacy with exposure and the MIC, i.e., the C_{max}/MIC or the AUC0-24/MIC.

The efficacy of time-dependent antimicrobials usually depends on fT more than MIC as a percentage of the dosing interval. However, time-dependent

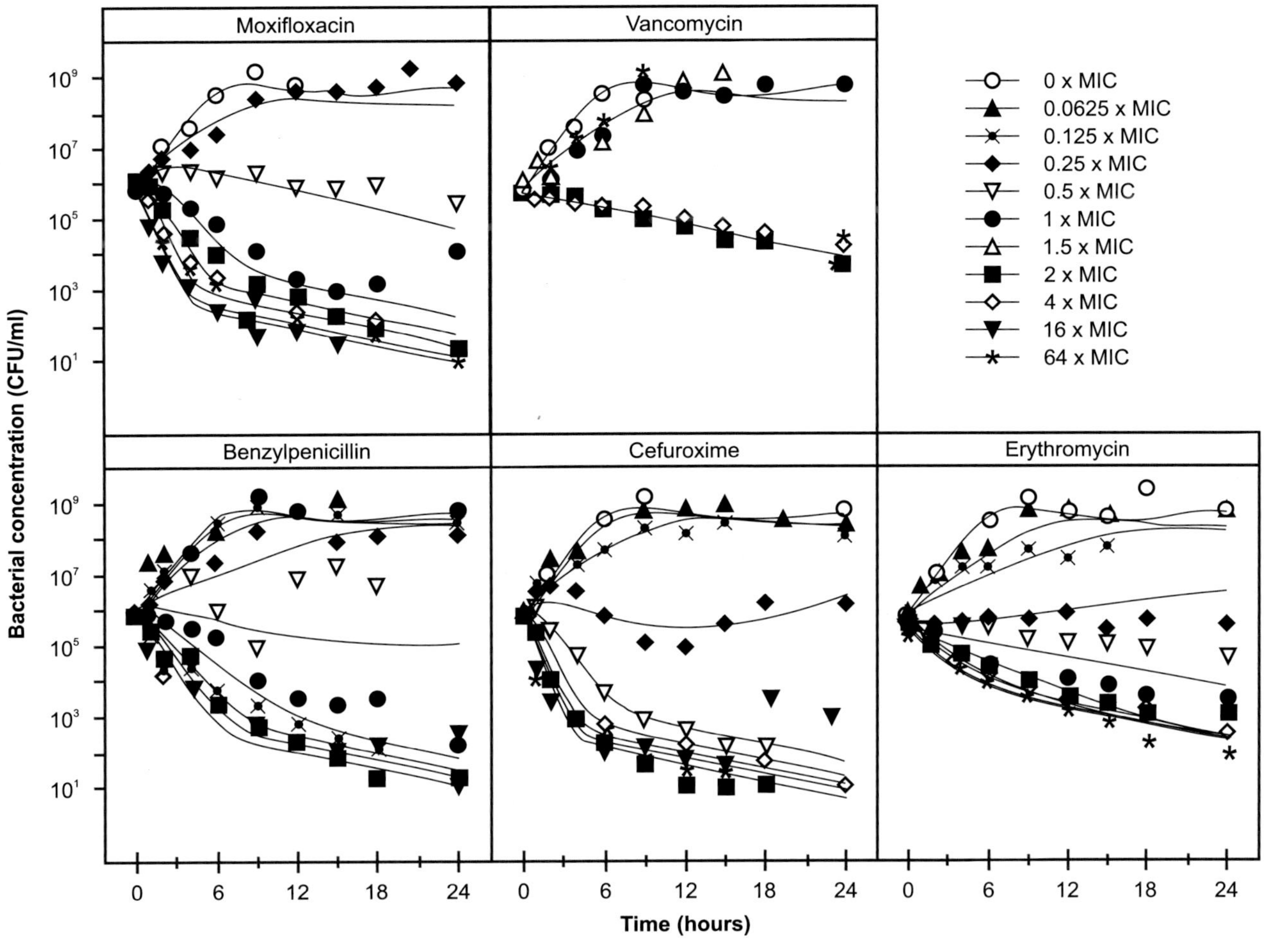

MIC, minimum inhibitory concentration; CFU, colony-forming units.

FIGURE 3 Time-kill curves for *S. pyogenes* showing that there is little difference in the kill kinetics among several antibiotics. The glycopeptide vancomycin displays different time-dependent kill kinetics compared with the other antibiotics presented. *Source:* Nielsen EI, Viberg A, Lowdin E, Cars O, Karlsson MO, Sandstrom M. Semimechanistic pharmacokinetic/pharmacodynamic model for assessment of activity of antibacterial agents from time-kill curve experiments. *Antimicrob Agents Chemother.* 2007;51: 128-36.

antibiotics that display a prolonged PAE, i.e., the persistence of activity after removal of the drug or after concentrations drop below the MIC,[8,9] often correlate well with the AUC0-24/MIC. Although the mechanisms of the PAE have been speculated, the PAE appears to depend on the drug, the pathogen, and the infection model. However, the term PAE is used collectively to explain residual effects of complex PK and PD processes that are not well-defined.

Other factors that influence the significance of PK/PD indices for predicting clinical efficacy that are often overlooked include protein binding and tissue distribution.[7] It is important to consider that only free concentrations should be taken into account in these indices as only free drug has the ability to exhibit a pharmacological effect. Similarly, it follows that the most relevant concentration for antibiotic efficacy would be the concentration within the interstitial space fluid (ISF) of target tissues, as most infections are located outside the plasma or serum where drug concentrations are commonly monitored.

The PK/PD relationship of various antimicrobial classes will be discussed in the next paragraphs.

β-*Lactams*

β-lactam antibiotics, which include the penicillins, cephalosporins, carbapenems, and monobactams, work by binding to penicillin-binding proteins, so inhibiting cell wall synthesis.

This mechanism of action is consistent with time-dependent killing. The efficacy of β-lactams correlate generally well with fT more than MIC. The time needed for the concentration to remain above the MIC is slightly different but consistent within subclass as long as only free concentrations are considered owing to the fact that protein binding can vary greatly between compounds, e.g., 2% for meropenem and ca. 90% for ertapenem.

The fT more than MIC needed for bactericidal effects in Gram-negative bacteria is ca. 40–50% for carbapenems, 50–70% for penicillins, and 70–80% for cephalosporins. For Gram-positive bacteria, the fT more than MIC needed for maximum effect is ca. 25–45% for carbapenems, 35–50% for penicillins, and 40–50% for cephalosporins.[12] It can be seen that the carbapenems display efficacy with a lower fT more than MIC, mainly because this subclass displays the fastest rate of kill.[3]

Aminoglycosides

The PK and PD of the aminoglycosides are well-characterized and appear to be consistent throughout the class. The mechanism of action of this class produces the inhibition protein synthesis by binding to the 30S ribosomal subunit and this class displays a concentration-dependent killing pattern and a relative long PAE, as is the case for the aminoglycosides. With these PD characteristics, the efficacy of aminoglycosides in clinical studies correlates with a C_{max}/MIC ratio that should exceed 10[13] or an AUC0-24/MIC ratio between 80 and 100 for maximum effects in animal models of infection.

Allowing a larger less frequent dose and subsequent larger C_{max}, better efficacy may be achieved due to prevention of the development of resistant mutants, the mechanism of antibacterial uptake and other PAE mechanisms. Once daily dose appear the best dosing regimen for aminoglycosides, but more data are needed to show a statistically better clinical outcome with a once daily dosing regimen.

Fluoroquinolones

The fluoroquinolones inhibiting type II topoisomerases, also called DNA gyrase, and topoisomerase IV prevent DNA replication and may also affect bacterial membranes. The fluoroquinolones display concentration-dependent killing and both the AUC0-24/MIC and Cmax/MIC ratios are correlated with efficacy. However, the high target C_{max}/MIC ratio may aid in the prevention of resistance development.[14] In Gram-negative respiratory infections, an AUC0-24/MIC ratio of 125 (free ~75) and an AUC0-24/MIC of more than or equal to 87 (free ~62) was found to be efficacious for ciprofloxacin[15] and levofloxacin,[16] respectively. For Gram-positive pathogens, such as *Streptococcus pneumoniae*, the breakpoints appear to be lower. In patients with community-acquired pneumonia or acute exacerbation of chronic bronchitis who received either levofloxacin or gatifloxacin, a free AUC0-24/MIC ratio above 33.7 provided complete efficacy.[17] A C_{max}/MIC ratio of 12.2 was also found to predict efficacy for levofloxacin in a clinical study.[16]

The magnitude of the plasma-based PK/PD indices that correlate with efficacy are in good agreement among this class. The magnitudes of these targets are also similar to the aminoglycosides when comparing free AUC0-24/MIC. However, the fluoroquinolones distribute more extensively into tissue, with free tissue/free plasma ratios of ca. 0.9 to more than 2. Therefore, it is somewhat surprising that the magnitude of these indices associated with efficacy is not lower and this may be due to the higher killing rate of aminoglycosides compared to fluoroquinolones.

Oxazolidinone

Linezolid is the only approved oxazolidinone for clinical use. The mechanism of action of this class is inhibition of protein synthesis at the initiation stage by binding to the 50S subunit of the bacterial ribosome. The efficacy of linezolid, although this antibiotic displays time-dependent kill kinetics, best correlates with the AUC0-24/MIC ratio. The AUC0-24/MIC ratio required for a bacteriostatic effect with linezolid was 48 for pneumococci and 83 for staphylococci in the neutropenic murine thigh infection model.[18] In critically ill patients with bacteremia, an AUC0-24/MIC of more than or equal to 105 and a time above MIC of 82% was associated with a faster time to bacterial eradication.[19]

Tetracyclines and Glycylcycline

The mechanism of action of this antibiotic class is inhibition of protein synthesis by binding to the 30S subunit of the bacterial ribosome. The tetracyclines display a time-dependent killing pattern and exhibit a considerable PAE, particularly with tigecycline.[20] The best PK/PD index correlating with efficacy is the AUC0-24/MIC. However, time above the MIC for free drug levels versus effect also had a high correlation coefficient. In clinical trials with patients with complicated skin and skin-structure infections or complicated intra-abdominal infections, the AUC/MIC ratios of 17.9 and 6.96, respectively, produced a better outcome.

The PAE of this class of antibiotic may be the result of extensive tissue distribution resulting in higher active concentrations at the site of action. Tigecycline, is the most extensively distributed compound in this class, with a volume of distribution (Vd) of 7–10 L/kg.[21] The high Vd reflects that free concentrations in the ISF could be significantly higher than in plasma. This theory is supported by the low PK/PD target values calculated for tigecycline from clinical trials.

Macrolides, Ketolides, and Azalides

The mechanism of action involves reversible binding to the 50S ribosomal subunit and prevention of protein synthesis. Although this type of mechanism usually results in a bactericidal agent, the macrolides can display bacteriostatic or bactericidal killing depending on the pathogen. Overall, this class mainly displays time-dependent killing.[22] A residual antimicrobial effect or PAE is observed for the macrolides; however, no single PK/PD parameter appears to correlate with efficacy for all members in this class, and all three target parameters have been suggested. This is likely due to several factors, including differences in kill kinetics and large differences in PK properties.[23]

Animal models of infection suggest that the AUC/MIC ratio based on free drug AUC values that correlate with efficacy against *S. pneumoniae* for most macrolides, azalides is 25–35.

This relative low PK/PD targeted index depends probably from the high tissue concentration of these antibiotics. These antibiotics accumulate intracellularly, especially azithromycin and telithromycin, with an ion trapping mechanisms. Moreover, the macrolides may be carried to the infection site by white blood cells resulting in a lower magnitude of the appropriate PK/PD index for efficacy.

Glycopeptides

Glycopeptides inhibit cell wall synthesis inhibiting peptidoglycan synthesis by forming hydrogen bonds with bacterial cell wall intermediate peptide. They display time-dependent killing *in vitro*. However, dalbavancin has been shown to display bactericidal concentration-dependent activity *in vitro*. The neutropenic mouse thigh infection model revealed the AUC/MIC to be predictive of efficacy with vancomycin against *S. aureus*. In a clinical study involving patients with *S. aureus* lower respiratory tract infection receiving vancomycin, an AUC0-24/MIC ratio of more than or equal to 400 resulted in a significantly better clinical outcome and bacteriological response.[24] A magnitude of 400 appears high compared with other antibiotics, however, this value is in better agreement when free tissue concentrations are considered. This compound displays a variable protein binding, ca. 10–80%, and penetration into the ISF may be less than free plasma concentrations.[25]

Teicoplanin is a glycopeptide with similar efficacy of vancomycin, approved for the treatment of lower respiratory tract infections, including those caused by MRSA, in some parts of Europe but not in the USA.

Teicoplanin is generally considered to have a favorable safety profile compared with vancomycin, with lower risk of nephrotoxicity and reactions resulting from histamine release (such as red man syndrome). PK/PD profile of teicoplanin is not well-established but similarly to vancomycin AUC/MIC ratio should correlate with efficacy.

Antifungal Pharmacodynamics

Extensive experimental and clinical antifungal PD studies have been undertaken relative to invasive candidiasis. Fewer investigations have addressed these questions for fungi that produce primary fungal pneumonia. However, thus far the observations from study of fungi, such as *Aspergillus* species have been quite similar to those with *Candida* species.

Although PK/PD parameters of antifungals are identified primarily in animal models, are often remarkably consistent for infections in humans. In spite of these limitations, results from preclinical PK/PD studies have already proven useful as a guide for establishing human dosing regimens and susceptibility breakpoints for resistant, or less common fungal pathogens.[26] Current knowledge concerning the magnitude of PK/PD parameters and antifungal efficacy for *Candida* and *Aspergillus* infections is summarized below according to the class of antifungal.

Polyene Pharmacodynamics

Despite the drug's toxicity, amphotericin B (AMB) remains an important treatment option for life threatening mycoses because of the drug's broad spectrum of activity and low potential for cross-resistance with other antifungals. AMB binds to ergosterol in the fungal cell membrane causing depolarization and increased permeability resulting in rapid cell death. AMB is an amphiphilic molecule, virtually insoluble in water, capable of forming salts only in basic or acidic environments. The drug was traditionally prepared as a micellar suspension with the bile salt deoxycholate (D-AMB). After many years of clinical use in this form, actually the drug is available complexed with phospholipid ribbons (Amphotericin B lipid complex) or cholesterol disks (amphotericin B cholesterol dispersion), or incorporated into unilamellar liposomes (L-AMB).

Amphotericin B formulations display *in vitro* and *in vivo* concentration-dependent fungicidal activity with a prolonged post-antifungal effect (PAFE) against *Candida* species, *Cryptococcus neoformans*, and *Aspergillus* species. The activity is maximized once peak (C_{max}) plasma drug concentrations surpass the MIC of the infecting pathogen by fourfold to tenfold and aspergillosis.[27,28]

However, only a small and saturable portion of AMB is microbiologically active in tissue, irrespective of the total tissue accumulation or concurrent plasma concentrations of the drug.[26] In respiratory infections in humans, the PK/PD values correlating with efficacy are comparable with those obtained in acute experimental infections. In a subset of patients for whom detailed PK and MIC data were available, patients with a plasma L-AMB C_{max}/MIC ratio exceeding 40 were more likely to achieve a complete versus partial clinical response.[29] For most adults, standard dosages of L-AMB (3–5 mg/kg) should surpass a C_{max}/MIC of 40 unless the pathogen has an AMB MIC of 2 mg/mL or greater.[27]

Triazole Pharmacodynamics

The triazole antifungals are a class of synthetic compounds that target fungal cytochrome P450-dependent enzyme lanosterol 14-a-demethylase inhibiting the fungal cell ergosterol biosynthesis.

Both *in vitro* and *in vivo* PD studies have been performed with all of the available triazole antifungals against *Candida* species. A prolonged concentration-dependent PAFE is observed *in vivo*.[30] AUC/MIC is the PK/PD parameter that best correlates with triazole activity against *Candida* species. Most studies have reported that the plasma AUC/MIC ratio, when corrected for protein binding, must surpass 25 for triazoles to be effective, or expressed more simply, concentrations of the triazoles must average at roughly 1 x MIC during the 24-hour dosing interval (1 x MIC x 24 hours = AUC/MIC of 24).[25]

Although fewer PK/PD studies have been completed for filamentous fungi, preclinical and clinical experience with itraconazole, voriconazole, and posaconazole have found that a trough plasma concentration of roughly 500–1,500 ng/mL is required for efficacy in either the prevention or treatment of aspergillosis.[31] Because of the significant patient-to-patient PK variability of the lipophilic, mould-active triazoles, plasma drug concentration monitoring has been proposed as an approach to individualize drug dosing, particularly in patients with poor oral intake, complex medication regimens, or changing hepatic, dysfunction.[32]

Echinocandin Pharmacodynamics

Echinocandins have become a preferred treatment option for invasive candidiasis because of their novel mechanism of action and excellent safety profile, and are proposed to be used in combination with polyenes or triazoles for refractory aspergillosis. Echinocandins inhibit the synthesis of 1,3-b-D-glucan, a key structural polysaccharide in the cell wall of *Candida* and *Aspergillus* species. The three currently available echinocandins caspofungin, micafungin, and anidulafungin are similar in terms of their spectrum of activity and PK with some differences in metabolism. The echinocandins exhibit concentration-dependent killing with a prolonged PAFE against *Candida* species.[25] In the experimental animal models of candidiasis and aspergillosis, echinocandin activity is optimized when plasma C_{max}/MIC ratio approaches 10 or the tissue 24-hour area under the curve to MIC ratio (AUC/MIC) exceeds 250.[33]

PHARMACOKINETICS/PHARMACODYNAMICS CONSIDERATION ON VENTILATOR-ASSOCIATED PNEUMONIA

The institution of mechanical ventilation affects cardiac output and hepatic blood flow. It increases intrathoracic pressure, which compresses the ventricles, decreases venous return, and decreases ventricular filling, leading to a reduction in cardiac output and consequently a decrease in hepatic and kidney blood flow. Theses ventilation-induced reductions in liver and kidney blood flow may be expected to decrease clearance of drugs. Many other factors can affect drug PK in patients with ventilator-associated pneumonia (VAP). These include age, organ dysfunction, drug interactions, and other therapeutic interventions, e.g., hemodynamically active drugs and continuous renal replacement therapies.[12]

Moreover, variations in extracellular fluid content and/or in renal or liver function are probably the most relevant and frequent pathophysiological mechanisms affecting drug disposition in critically ill patients. Several pathophysiological conditions may cause an increase in the Vd, such that an increase in dosage should be considered. Hypoalbuminemia, a common condition in critically ill patients, may contribute to fluid extravasation and antimicrobial dilution by reducing plasma oncotic pressure, whereas the increase in the free fraction of drugs may increase their Vd. Moreover, renally excreted, highly albumin-bound antimicrobials (e.g., teicoplanin, ceftriaxone and ertapenem) are more extensively distributed, but also more rapidly eliminated. Hemodynamically active drugs (e.g., dopamine, dobutamine, and furosemide) can modify renal blood flow and thereby glomerular filtration, tubular secretion rates, and renal clearance.

In this context, renally excreted hydrophilic antimicrobials (e.g., β-lactams, aminoglycosides, and glycopeptides) and moderately lipophilic antimicrobials (e.g., ciprofloxacin, gatifloxacin, and levofloxacin) are at higher risk of presenting substantial daily fluctuations in plasma concentration, which may require repeated dosage adjustment. Hydrophilic antimicrobials exhibit distribution limited mainly to the extracellular space; consequently their plasma and interstitial concentrations may drop dramatically if substantial fluid extravasation to the interstitial space occurs. In all the pathophysiological situations described above, higher dosages for most hydrophilic antimicrobials should be considered to ensure therapeutic concentrations. By contrast, for lipophilic antimicrobials presenting a larger Vd, the dilution of interstitial fluids is less relevant.

Therapeutic drug monitoring can be of great value in patients with VAP, helping to optimize drug exposure in the individual patient. Clinical practice has demonstrated its positive effect on both clinical outcome and cost of hospitalization.

CONCLUSION

Inappropriate dosing of antimicrobials in community-acquired as well as in hospital-acquired reproductive tract infections is a major cause of concern as it increases the risk of clinical failure and is a major risk factor for the development and spread of bacterial resistance. *In vitro* susceptibility data alone were the most important parameters on which was based a rational choice of antimicrobial treatment. Advances in our understanding of PK/PD now enable us to predict antimicrobial efficacy; the choice of the antimicrobial and its administration at the right dose and at right interval between doses optimize antibacterial therapy, the risk of failure is minimized and the high eradication rates should decrease the risk of emergence of resistance and its subsequent spread.

REFERENCES

1. Eagle H, Fleischman R, Levy M. 'Continuous' vs. 'discontinuous' therapy with penicillin; the effect of the interval between injections on therapeutic efficacy. *N Engl J Med.* 1953;248(12):481-8.
2. Eagle H, Fleischman R, Musselman AD. The bactericidal action of penicillin in vivo: the participation of the host, and the slow recovery of the surviving organisms. *Ann Intern Med.* 1950;33(3):544-71.
3. Craig WA. Pharmacokinetic/pharmacodynamic parameters: rationale for antibacterial dosing of mice and men. *Clin Infect Dis.* 1998;26(1):1-10.
4. Ambrose PG, Bhavnani SM, Rubino CM, et al. Pharmacokinetics–pharmacodynamics of antimicrobial therapy: it's not just for mice anymore. *Clin Infect Dis.* 2007;44(1):79-86.
5. Vogelman B, Gudmundsson S, Leggett J, et al. Correlation of antimicrobial pharmacokinetic parameters with therapeutic efficacy in an animal model. *J Infect Dis.* 1988;158(4):831-47.
6. Craig WA. Interrelationship between pharmacokinetics and pharmacodynamics in determining dosage regimens for broad-spectrum cephalosporins. *Diagn Microbiol Infect Dis.* 1995;22(1-2):89-96.
7. Barbour A, Scaglione F, Derendorf H. Class-dependent relevance of tissue distribution in the interpretation of anti-infective pharmacokinetic/pharmacodynamic indices. *Int J Antimicrob Agents.* 2010;35(5):431-8.
8. Bundtzen RW, Gerber AU, Cohn DL, et al. Postantibiotic suppression of bacterial growth. *Rev Infect Dis.* 1981;3(1):28-37.
9. Craig WA. Post-antibiotic effects in experimental infection models: relationship to in-vitro phenomena and to treatment of infections in man. *J Antimicrob Chemother.* 1993;31(Suppl. D):149-58.
10. Schmidt S, Rock K, Sahre M, et al. Effect of protein binding on the pharmacological activity of highly bound antibiotics. *Antimicrob Agents Chemother.* 2008;52(11):3994-4000.
11. Burgess DS, Frei CR. Comparison of lactam regimens for the treatment of Gram-negative pulmonary infections in the intensive care unit based on pharmacokinetics/pharmacodynamics. *J Antimicrob Chemother.* 2005;56(5):893-8.
12. Scaglione F, Paraboni L. Pharmacokinetics/pharmacodynamics of antibacterials in the Intensive Care Unit: setting appropriate dosing regimens. *Int J Antimicrob Agents.* 2008;32(4):294-301.
13. Kashuba AD, Nafziger AN, Drusano GL, et al. Optimizing aminoglycoside therapy for nosocomial pneumonia caused by Gram-negative bacteria. *Antimicrob Agents Chemother.* 1999;43(3):623-9.
14. Preston SL, Drusano GL, Berman AL, et al. Pharmacodynamics of levofloxacin: a new paradigm for early clinical trials. *JAMA.* 1998;279(2):125-9.
15. Forrest A, Nix DE, Ballow CH, et al. Pharmacodynamics of intravenous ciprofloxacin in seriously ill patients. *Antimicrob Agents Chemother.* 1993;37(5):1073-81.
16. Drusano GL, Preston SL, Fowler C, et al. Relationship between fluoroquinolone area under the curve: minimum inhibitory concentration ratio and the probability of eradication of the infecting pathogen, in patients with nosocomial pneumonia. *J Infect Dis.* 2004;189(9):1590-7.
17. Ambrose PG, Grasela DM, Grasela TH, et al. Pharmacodynamics of fluoroquinolones against Streptococcus pneumoniae in patients with community-acquired respiratory tract infections. *Antimicrob Agents Chemother.* 2001;45:2793-7.
18. Andes D, van Ogtrop ML, Peng J, et al. In vivo pharmacodynamics of a new oxazolidinone (linezolid). *Antimicrob Agents Chemother.* 2002;46(11):3484-9.
19. Rayner CR, Forrest A, Meagher AK, et al. Clinical pharmacodynamics of linezolid in seriously ill patients treated in

a compassionate use programme. *Clin Pharmacokinet.* 2003;42(15):1411-23.
20. van Ogtrop ML, Andes D, Stamstad TJ, et al. In vivo pharmacodynamic activities of two glycylcyclines (GAR-936 and WAY 152,288) against various Gram-positive and Gram-negative bacteria. *Antimicrob Agents Chemother.* 2000;44(4):943-9.
21. Conte JE, Golden JA, Kelly MG, et al. Steady-state serum and intrapulmonary pharmacokinetics and pharmacodynamics of tigecycline. *Int J Antimicrob Agents.* 2005;25(6):523-9.
22. Andes D, Anon J, Jacobs MR, et al. Application of pharmacokinetics and pharmacodynamics to antimicrobial therapy of respiratory tract infections. *Clin Lab Med.* 2004;24(2):477-502.
23. Jain R, Danziger LH. The macrolide antibiotics: a pharmacokinetic and pharmacodynamic overview. *Curr Pharm Des.* 2004;10(25):3045-53.
24. Moise-Broder PA, Forrest A, Birmingham MC, et al. Pharmacodynamics of vancomycin and other antimicrobials in patients with Staphylococcus aureus lower respiratory tract infections. *Clin Pharmacokinet.* 2004;43(13):925-42.
25. Skhirtladze K, Hutschala D, Fleck T, et al. Impaired target site penetration of vancomycin in diabetic patients following cardiac surgery. *Antimicrob Agents Chemother.* 2006;50(4):1372-5.
26. Andes D. Pharmacokinetics and pharmacodynamics of antifungals. *Infect Dis Clin North Am.* 2006;20(3):679-97.
27. Andes D, Safdar N, Marchillo K, et al. Pharmacokinetic pharmacodynamic comparison of amphotericin B (AMB) and two lipid-associated AMB preparations, liposomal AMB and AMB lipid complex, in murine candidiasis models. *Antimicrob Agents Chemother.* 2006;50:674-84.
28. Wiederhold NP, Tam VH, Chi J, et al. Pharmacodynamic activity of amphotericin B deoxycholate is associated with peak plasma concentrations in a neutropenic murine model of invasive pulmonary aspergillosis. *Antimicrob Agents Chemother.* 2006;50:469-73.
29. Hong Y, Shaw PJ, Nath CE, et al. Population pharmacokinetics of liposomal amphotericin B in pediatric patients with malignant diseases. *Antimicrob Agents Chemother.* 2006;50(3):935-42.
30. Andes D. In vivo pharmacodynamics of antifungal drugs in treatment of candidiasis. *Antimicrob Agents Chemother.* 2003;47(4):1179-86.
31. Denning DW, Ribaud P, Milpied N, et al. Efficacy and safety of voriconazole in the treatment of acute invasive aspergillosis. *Clin Infect Dis.* 2002;34(5):563-71.
32. Trifilio S, Pennick G, Pi J, et al. Monitoring plasma voriconazole levels may be necessary to avoid subtherapeutic levels in hematopoietic stem cell transplant recipients. *Cancer.* 2007;109(8):1532-5.
33. Louie A, Deziel M, Liu W, et al. Pharmacodynamics of caspofungin in a murine model of systemic candidiasis: importance of persistence of caspofungin in tissues to understanding drug activity. *Antimicrob Agents Chemother.* 2005;49(12):5058-68.
34. Scaglione F, Esposito S, Leone S, et al. Feedback dose alteration significantly affects probability of pathogen eradication in nosocomial pneumonia. *Eur Respir J.* 2009; 34(2):394-400.
35. Mouton JW, Dudley MN, Cars O, et al. Standardization of pharmacokinetic/pharmacodynamic (PK/PD) terminology for anti-infective drugs: an update. *J Antimicrob Chemother.* 2005;55(5):601-7.

CHAPTER 22

Scores for the Assessment of Pneumonia Severity and Outcome

Benjamin Klapdor, Santiago Ewig

ABSTRACT

The assessment of severity of community-acquired pneumonia (CAP) is a major criterion for the decision of where to treat the patient and determines the amount of diagnostic workup and the selection of empiric antimicrobial treatment.

Several severity scores have been developed and evaluated, including the pneumonia severity index (PSI) as well as the confusion, urea levels, respiratory rate, blood pressure, and age more than 65 years (CURB-65) score and its modifications. PSI is equivalent to CURB-65 or the CRB-65 (confusion, respiratory rate, blood pressure, and age more than 65 years) scores in hospitalized patients. PSI has the advantage that it can identify low-risk patients, while the CURB-65/CRB-65 identify high-risk patients. CRB-65 is superior in terms of simplicity, whereas CURB-65 requires the determination of urea. PSI is obviously overtly complex in the ambulatory settings. Limitations include lacking impact analyses in different settings and possibly, worse predictive power in younger as well as elderly patients residing in nursing homes.

Similarly, several predictive score to identify severe CAP requiring intensive care unit (ICU) admission have been evaluated, including the modified American Thoracic Society (ATS) rule, the Infectious Disease Society of America (IDSA)/ATS rule, the SMART-COP rule, the España rule and the risk of early admission (REA)-ICU index. All the scores provide reasonable operative characteristics. However, predictive tools perform within a wide range in different settings. Furthermore, none seems to be truly superior in a clinically relevant manner.

Few investigations have assessed severity rules for hospital-acquired pneumonia (HAP). Rules such as the predisposition, insult, response, and organ dysfunction (PIRO) score and the IBMP score still await validation.

Altogether, severity scores are meant as an adjunct to clinical judgment and in case of doubt, such judgment should always overrule classification according to predictive tools.

COMMUNITY-ACQUIRED PNEUMONIA

General Population

The assessment of severity is a key step in the management of patients with community-acquired pneumonia (CAP)[1] and is recommended by all authoritative guidelines for the management of adult patients with CAP.[2-5] It is a major criterion to decide where to treat the patient and determines the amount of diagnostic work-up and selection of empiric antimicrobial treatment. Thus, it has a major impact in terms of outcome and costs.[1] The last decades have seen a major effort in derivation and validating scores that might be used for the initial assessment of severity of CAP. No doubt, major advances have been made in the understanding of factors determining severity and the advantages and limitations of predictive tools for assessing CAP severity.

Pneumonia Severity Index

Pneumonia Severity Index (PSI) is a prediction rule for 30-day mortality of patients with CAP. It was developed by Fine et al. in 1997.[6] Its primary goal was to identify patients at low-risk who might be treated safely as outpatients.

According to the PSI, patients are classified in 5 risk classes (I–V) including patients with low-risk (I–III), intermediate-risk (IV), and high-risk (V). PSI risk class is assessed in 2 steps. The first step includes the assessment of the criteria age (threshold >50 years), the presence of 5 comorbidities (history of neoplastic disease, congestive heart failure, cerebrovascular disease, renal disease, and liver diseases), and 5 vital sign abnormalities (altered mental status, pulse ≥125/min, respiratory rate ≥30/min, systolic blood pressure <90 mmHg, and temperature <35°C or ≥40°C) on initial physical examination (Tables 1 and 2). If the patient meets none of these criteria, risk class will be determined as I. If the patient meets at least 1 of these criteria, the patient will be assigned to risk classes II–V according to step 2.

This includes the calculation of a score according to the 11 parameters of step 1, and additionally, 2 demographic factors (male sex and nursing home residence) and 7 laboratory and radiographic findings [arterial pH <7.35, blood urea nitrogen ≥30 mg/dL (11 mmol/L), sodium <130 mmol/L, hematocrit <30%, partial pressure of arterial oxygen (PaO_2) <60 mmHg, and pleural effusion] (Table 3). Patients are assigned to risk class II with a score of 70 or less, risk class III with a score of 71–90, risk class IV with a score of 91–130, and risk class V with

TABLE 1

Step One of Pneumonia Severity Index: Identifying Patients in Risk Class I

Age >50 years	Yes/No
History of coexisting conditions	
Neoplastic disease	Yes/No
Congestive heart failure	Yes/No
Cerebrovascular disease	Yes/No
Renal disease	Yes/No
Liver disease	Yes/No
Abnormalities on physical examination	
Altered mental status	Yes/No
Pulse ≥125/minute	Yes/No
Respiratory rate ≥30/minute	Yes/No
Systolic blood pressure <90 mmHg	Yes/No
Temperature <35°C or ≥40°C	Yes/No

If all "No" assign patient to risk class I.
If any "Yes" assign patient to risk class II–V according to step 2.

TABLE 2

Pneumonia Severity Index: Definitions

- **Neoplastic disease:** Any cancer except basal or squamous cell cancer of the skin that was active at the time of presentation or diagnosed within 1 year of presentation
- **Liver disease:** Clinical or histologic diagnosis of cirrhosis or another form of chronic liver disease, such as chronic active hepatitis
- **Congestive heart failure:** Systolic or diastolic ventricular dysfunction documented by history, physical examination and chest radiograph, echocardiogram, multiple-gated acquisition scan, or left ventriculography
- **Cerebrovascular disease:** Clinical diagnosis of stroke or transient ischemic attack or stroke documented by MRI or CT scan
- **Renal disease:** History of chronic renal disease or abnormal blood urea nitrogen and creatinine concentrations documented in the medical record
- **Altered mental status:** Disorientation with respect to person, place, or time that is not known to be chronic, stupor, or coma

MRI, magnetic resonance imaging; CT, computed tomography.

TABLE 3

Step Two of Pneumonia Severity Index: Scoring System for Assignment to Risk Classes II–V

Demographic factor	
Age	
Men	Age (year)
Women	Age (year) −10
Nursing home resident	+10
Coexisting illness	
Neoplastic disease	+30
Liver disease	+20
Congestive heart failure	+10
Cerebrovascular disease	+10
Renal disease	+10
Physical examination findings	
Altered mental status	+20
Respiratory rate ≥30/min	+20
Systolic blood pressure <90 mmHg	+20
Temperature <35°C or ≥40°C	+15
Pulse ≥125/min	+10
Laboratory and radiographic findings	
Arterial pH <7.35	+30
Blood urea nitrogen ≥30 mg/dL (11 mmol/L)	+20
Sodium <130 mmol/L	+20
Glucose ≥250 mg/dL (14 mmol/L)	+10
Hematocrit <30%	+10
Partial pressure of arterial oxygen <60 mmHg	+10
Pleural effusion	+10

TABLE 4

Pneumonia Severity Index: Risk Class-specific Mortality Rates

Risk class	Score	Risk level	30-day mortality (%)
I	—	Low	0.1–0.4
II	≤70	—	0.6–0.7
III	71–90	—	0.9–2.8
IV	91–130	Intermediate	8.2–9.3
V	>130	High	27.9–31.1

scores of more than 130. In the derivation and validation cohorts mortality rates of risk classes I–V were 0.1–0.4%, 0.6–0.7%, 0.9–2.8%, 8.2–9.3%, and 27.9–31.1%, respectively (Table 4).[6]

CURB and Its Modifications

In the classical study by the British Thoracic Society (BTS) from 1987, 4 criteria were identified as predictors of in-hospital death: respiratory rate, blood pressure, blood urea nitrogen, and confusion.[7] Originally, these 4 criteria were included in 3 predictive rules, including three criteria each (the third rule included oxygenation and white blood cell or lymphocyte count). Neill et al. presented the predictive power of a modified BTS rule, including all 4 criteria mentioned above.[8] In a study that followed, Lim et al. investigated the predictive power of CURB (confusion, urea, respiratory rate, and blood pressure) and its modifications CURB-65 and CRB-65.[9] CURB resulted in inferior predictions of death, whereas CURB-65 performed among the 3 scores. Since urea is not readily available in the ambulatory setting, CRB-65 was primarily thought as a simplification of CURB-65 with inferior but acceptable performance.

CURB-65

According to the CURB-65 score, patients can be categorized in 3 risk classes.[9] Parameters included are new onset pneumonia-associated mental confusion (mental test score ≤8[10] or disorientation in person, place or time), urea levels above 7 mmol/L, respiratory rate of more than 30/min, hypotension with systolic blood pressure less than 90 mmHg or diastolic blood pressure less than 60 mmHg, and age above 65 years (Table 5). One point is given for each parameter present at first presentation, which results in CURB-65 scores of 0–5. Mortality increases with score points. The derivation and validation study showed 30-day mortality for patients with 0–1, 2, and 3–5 points of 1.5%, 9.2%, and 22%, respectively (Table 6).[9]

TABLE 5

CURB-65 Score

- **C**onfusion*
- **U**rea >7 mmol/L
- **R**espiratory rate ≥30/min
- **B**lood pressure (systolic <90 mmHg or diastolic ≤60 mmHg)
- Age ≥**65** years

*Mental test score ≤8[10] or disorientation in person, place, or time.

TABLE 6

CURB-65: Risk Classes

CURB-65	Risk class	30-day mortality (%)
0–1	Low	1.5
2	Intermediate	9.2
3 or more	High	22

TABLE 7

CRB-65 Score

- **C**onfusion*
- **R**espiratory rate ≥30/min
- **B**lood pressure (systolic <90 mmHg or diastolic ≤60 mmHg)
- Age ≥**65** years

*Mental test score ≤8[10] or disorientation in person, place, or time.

TABLE 8

CRB-65: Risk Classes

CRB-65	Risk class	30-day mortality (%)
0	Low	1.2
1–2	Intermediate	8.2
3–4	High	31

CRB-65

CRB-65 is a simplified modification of the CURB-65 omitting urea. Only parameters of clinical assessment are included and a laboratory measurement is not needed (Table 7). One point is given for each parameter present at first presentation, which results in CRB-65 scores of 0–4. The original derivation and validation study showed 30-day mortality for patients with 0, 1–2, and 3–4 points of 1.2%, 8.2%, and 31%, respectively (Table 8).[9]

Other Scores

Generic Scores

Barlow et al.[11] used 2 generic scores, the systemic inflammatory response syndrome (SIRS),[12] and the standardized early warning score (SEWS)[11] to assess CAP severity. For SEWS severe CAP was diagnosed at a score of more than 4. For SIRS, severe CAP was diagnosed at the presence of at least 2 criteria (temperature <36°C or >38°C, pulse >90/min, respiratory rate >20/min and leucocyte count <4,000 or >12,000 cells/mm^3) and hypotension (defined as a systolic blood pressure <90 mmHg) and/or organ hypoperfusion [defined as new onset confusion mental state questionnaire (MSQ ≤8/10 or a 2 point drop)] (Table 9). Both, SIRS and SEWS showed less predictive power than CURB-65.[11]

PIRO Score for Community-acquired Pneumonia

The predisposition, insult, response, and organ dysfunction (PIRO) score for CAP is based on the PIRO concept.[13-17] The PIRO concept reflects a multidimensional concept of severity based on 4 dimensions judged to be critical for the resulting severity of pneumonia. The score was developed by Rello et al. in order to stratify patients with CAP who were admitted to an intensive care unit (ICU) into different 28-day mortality risk groups.[18] For every condition of predisposition (comorbidities, age >70 years), insult (bacteremia, multilobar opacities in chest radiograph), response (shock, severe hypoxemia), and organ dysfunction [acute renal failure, acute respiratory distress syndrome (ARDS)], 1 point is given, which leads to scores of 0–8 points (Tables 10 and 11). Patients with 0–2 points were classified as low-risk, 3 points mild-risk, 4 points high-risk, and 5–8 points very high-risk patients with a 28-day mortality ranging from 3.6 to 76.3% (Table 12). The PIRO score also predicts length of stay in the ICU and requirement of mechanical ventilation.[18]

CORB

Confusion oxygen saturation, respiratory rate, and blood pressure (CORB) score, a modification of CURB,

TABLE 9

Generic Scores

SIRS	≥2 of the following criteria: temperature <36°C or >38°C, pulse >90/min, respiratory rate >20/min, and leucocyte count <4 or >12 cells/mm^3
Severe CAP	SIRS plus hypotension and/or organ hypoperfusion
SEWS	Complex scoring system based on respiratory rate, SaO_2, temperature, blood pressure, heart rate, neurological response, and urine output*

SIRS, systemic inflammatory response syndrome; SEWS, standardized early warning score; CAP, community-acquired pneumonia; SaO_2, percentage of available hemoglobin saturated with oxygen.

SEWS chart: http://www.healthcareimprovementscotland.org/previous_resources/benchmarking_report/emergency_medical_admissions_s.aspx

TABLE 10

PIRO Score for CAP

Predisposition	Comorbidities (COPD or immunocompromised)	1 Point
	>70 years	1 Point
Insult	Bacteremia	1 Point
	Multilobar opacities in chest radiograph	1 Point
Response	Shock	1 Point
	Severe hypoxemia	1 Point
Organ dysfunction	Acute renal failure	1 Point
	Acute respiratory distress syndrome	1 Point
	Score range	0–8 Points

CAP, community-acquired pneumonia; COPD, chronic obstructive pulmonary disease.

TABLE 11

PIRO Score for CAP: Definitions

- **Immunocompromised:** Primary immunodeficiency of immunodeficiency secondary to radiation treatment, use of cytotoxic drugs or steroids (>20 mg of prednisolone or the equivalent/day for >2 weeks) or AIDS or malignancy
- **Shock:** Need for vasopressors for >4 hours after adequate fluid replacement
- **Severe hypoxemia:** PaO_2/F_IO_2 ratio <300 mmHg requiring mechanical ventilation
- **Acute renal failure:** Total urine output of <80 mL in 4 hours

PaO_2/F_IO_2, ratio of partial pressure of arterial oxygen to the fraction of inspired oxygen; CAP, community-acquired pneumonia; AIDS, acquired immunodeficiency syndrome.

TABLE 12

Risk According to PIRO Score for CAP

Score	Risk level	28-day mortality (%)
0–2	Low	3.6
3	Mild	13.0
4	High	43.0
5–8	Very high	76.3

CAP, community-acquired pneumonia.

was described by Buising et al. in 2007.[19] This score replaces urea by oxygen saturation below 90% (Table 13). It is a simple tool to predict in-hospital death and/or requirement for ventilatory or inotropic support in the emergency department. Patients with a score of 2 or more are identified as having severe CAP.[19]

A-DROP

Another variation of CURB is age, dehydration, respiratory failure, orientation disturbance, and blood pressure

TABLE 13

CORB Score

- **C**onfusion (new onset, or worsening of preexisting state)
- **O**xygen saturation ≤90% (on any F_IO_2)
- **R**espiratory rate ≥30/min
- **B**lood pressure (systolic <90 mmHg or diastolic ≤60 mmHg)

(A-DROP) score, which was described by Shindo et al. in 2008 and predicts 30-day mortality (Table 14).[20] Every parameter present at first presentation has a value of 1 point. The investigators suggested patients with 0–1 points for outpatient treatment, 2–3 points for hospitalization, and 4–5 for ICU treatment (Table 15).[20]

Critical Appraisal

Developing a prognostic model is a 3-stage process, including derivation (creating the rule), validation (applying the rule to new populations of patients to confirm its accuracy), and impact analysis (applying the rule and determining the impact on clinical outcomes).[21] Although many validation studies have been conducted, studies, including impact analysis are rare. In addition to these processes, practical issues are also important, particularly in the ambulatory setting.

Validation of Predictive Tools for the Assessment of Community-acquired Pneumonia Severity

PSI and CURB-65/CRB-65 are the most extensively evaluated tools for the initial assessment of severity of CAP. Numerous studies were conducted to validate these scores with a total of more than 80,000 patients for PSI and more than 15,000/390,000 patients for CURB-65/CRB-65, respectively.[22] Other scores, like systolic blood pressure, multilobar involvement as in chest X-ray, albumin, respiratory rate tachycardia, confusion, lower oxygen, and pH (SMART-COP) score, PIRO score for CAP, CORB, and A-DROP are only validated in relatively small cohorts and, thus, need further investigation, including head-to-head comparison with the PSI and CURB-65/CRB-65 scores prior to be introduced in clinical practice.

TABLE 14

A-DROP Score

- **A**ge (male ≥70 years, female ≥75 years)
- **D**ehydration (blood urea nitrogen ≥210 mg/L)
- **R**espiratory failure (SaO_2 ≤90% or PaO_2 ≤60 mmHg)
- **O**rientation disturbance (confusion)
- **P**ressure (diastolic blood pressure ≤60 mmHg or systolic <90 mmHg)

SaO_2, percentage of available hemoglobin saturated with oxygen; PaO_2, partial pressure of arterial oxygen.

TABLE 15

A-DROP: Risk Classes

Score	Risk class	Proposed treatment setting
0–1	Low	Outpatient treatment
2–3	Intermediate	Hospitalization
4–5	High	ICU treatment

ICU, intensive care unit.

A study performed by Aujesky et al. compared the PSI and CURB-65 score and found a slight but significantly higher predictive accuracy with the PSI.[23] Additionally, PSI identified more patients at low risk. Moreover, Ananda-Rajah et al. found that in contrast to PSI, CURB-65 was neither sensitive nor specific for predicting mortality in CAP patients.[24]

In contrast, Capelastegui et al. did not find any differences in the predictive powers of PSI, CURB-65, and CRB-65.[25] The findings of Man et al. also support that these tools are equivalent in predicting the 30-day mortality.[26] In 2009, Ewig et al. found CRB-65 a powerful tool for the assessment of CAP severity in a cohort of 388,406 in-patients, confirming its potential to predict in-hospital mortality in a 3 class manner [mortality in low-risk group (CRB-65 0) 2–3%, 13% moderate-risk (CRB-65 1–2), and 34% high risk (CRB-65 3–4)].[27] In contrast, although CRB-65 is particularly recommended for community use,[9] only 1 study validated this score in a primary care setting.[28] In this study, CRB-65 performed well despite a low overall mortality rate.

In 2010, 2 meta-analyses compared the performance of PSI and CURB-65/CRB-65. Chalmers et al.[22] included 40 studies and found PSI slightly superior in identifying low-risk patients and CURB-65/CRB-65 in identifying high-risk patients. However, significant differences in overall test performance among these 3 scores were not found. Loke et al.[29] included 23 studies and found PSI more sensitive and less specific than CURB-65/CRB-65 and vice versa, which is consistent with the findings of Chalmers et al.

Most recent data from the German mandatory quality assurance program of hospitalized patients with CAP including more than 600,000 patient data sets evaluating different age thresholds within the CRB-65 indicate that an age of 50 years is an optimal threshold in terms of predictive power for patients of age below 65 years [area under curve (AUC) 0.73], with good identification of low-risk patients (CRB-50 risk class I: 1.3% deaths, negative predictive value 98.7%). However, in patients aged ≥65 years, AUC of CRB-65 is lower (0.64). Even worse, in patients aged more than 65 years residing in nursing homes, predictive power is low (AUC 0.61) and mortality already reaches 18% in the lowest CRB-80 risk class (Ewig et al. data in review).

Some data are available for biomarkers as predictors of death. In 1 study, midregional pro-atrial natriuretic peptide (MR-proANP) and C-terminal proarginine-vasopressin (CT-proAVP) are useful new biomarkers for the risk stratification of CAP patients. They are significantly lower in CAP survivors and correlate with the severity of the disease measured by CRB-65 score.[30] In a more recent study, ANP was more accurate than C-reactive protein (CRP) and procalcitonin (PCT) to predict appropriate admission.[31]

Since biomarkers, such as PCT and midregional pro-adrenomedullin (MR-proADM) have been shown to be of considerable prognostic value, the incorporation of biomarkers into severity rules might be appealing. Adding CRP levels to PSI, CURB-65 and CRB-65 scales improves the 30-day mortality prediction.[32] PCT levels on admission predicted severity and outcome of CAP with a similar prognostic accuracy as the CRB-65 score.[33] Moreover, PCT levels provided independent identification of patients at low risk of death within CRB-65 risk classes. In a study to follow, MR-proADM was an independent and strong predictor of short- and long-term mortality, superior to CRB-65; moreover, the combination of CRB-65 and MR-proADM performed best.[34] However, these promising results lack prospective validation in larger and independent cohorts.

Impact Analysis of Predictive Tools in the Community

PSI was prospectively validated as a tool to guide site of treatment decisions.[35] Renaud et al. compared outpatient treatment rates in hospitals that used the PSI with hospitals that did not use the PSI for the assessment of CAP severity. They found higher outpatient treatment rates in hospitals that used PSI without compromising the patients' safety.[36] Such studies have not been conducted for CURB-65/CRB-65.[35]

Practical Issues in the Use of Predictive Tools

The PSI comprises 20 parameters and requires several laboratory tests. This makes it considerably complex and impractical for routine use, especially in a community setting. In contrast, the main advantage of CURB-65/CRB-65 is its simplicity.[35] CURB-65 includes only physical examination findings and one laboratory test and for the assessment of CRB-65, no technical investigation is needed at all. In several studies, CURB-65 and CRB-65 were shown to perform equally well.[11,22,26,28,37-39] Chalmers et al. showed that a simplified CRB-65 score containing systolic blood pressure below 90 mmHg alone performed equally well to standard CRB-65 score and CURB-65 score for the prediction of 30-day mortality.[39] The simplified CRB-65 score was also equivalent for prediction of mechanical ventilation and/or inotropic support to standard CRB-65 and CURB-65.

A CRB-65 of 1 implies increased risk. According to this, hospitalization would have to be considered for all patients with CAP above the age of 65 years, which seems inadequate.[35] Bont et al. showed in a study of elderly outpatients that age should not be the only criterion for hospitalization.[28] The investigators suggested that in view of overall low mortality rates in primary care, new studies should focus on less severe outcomes.

Advantages and Limitations of Predictive Tools

To sum up, the available literature suggests that:

- PSI is equivalent to CURB-65/CRB-65 in hospitalized patients, with advantages for the PSI to identify low risk and for the CURB-65/CRB-65 to identify high-risk patients
- CRB-65 is superior in terms of simplicity, whereas CURB-65 is in need of the determination of urea and PSI obviously being over complex in the ambulatory setting
- On the other hand, whereas the use of PSI was proven to reduce hospital admissions of low-risk patients without compromising safety, no impact analysis of CURB-65/CRB-65 is available
- Only 1 study has assessed the use of CRB-65 in outpatients
- Most recent data indicate that CRB-65 is not a useful predictive tool in elderly patients residing in nursing homes.

Another criticism that has frequently been raised, is that all predictive tools including age as criterion for severity may be particularly vulnerable to bias in younger patients. This bias might be of most concern when applying the PSI, which implies a high bearing of age.[1]

Thus, all 3 tools are imperfect. In the meta-analysis by Chalmers et al., only PSI achieved a negative likelihood ratio below 0.1 and none achieved a positive likelihood ratio above 10.[22] The investigators also noticed that the performance of scores varied significantly between different studies in different healthcare systems. Thus, it seems necessary to consider local recalibration of the score if the population of patients to which the score is being applied is significantly different from the original derivation population. Disappointingly, the most recent data evaluating different age thresholds clearly shows that CRB-65 is not suitable for patients with nursing home-acquired pneumonia, and overall, it is less useful in the elderly (Ewig et al. in press).

Evidently, PSI and CURB-65/CRB-65 are clearly not suitable for predicting need for ICU treatment.[22,40,41] Scores for this purpose are discussed separately. It may be due to the reason that many patients ultimately dying with CAP are not suitable for ICU admission because of advanced aged and disabling comorbidities.

Despite important limitations, the predictive tools presented are clearly useful for the initial evaluation of patients presenting with CAP and as a consequence, have been introduced in all authoritative guidelines of the management of this condition. While the Infectious Disease Society of America (IDSA)/American Thoracic Society (ATS) guidelines[4] recommend the use of the PSI, the European[5] (and German[2]) guidelines opted for the use of CRB-65, mainly because of its splendid simplicity. In fact, the potential of age and 3 clinical criteria to predict death from CAP without any need for more elaborate criteria is impressive. The British guidelines[3] recommend the use of CURB-65 for patients presenting to the hospital and CRB-65 for the outpatient setting. All guidelines unanimously point out the limitations of these tools and strongly advice to use these tools as an adjunct to clinical judgment. It is important to bear in mind that even patients at low risk may be the candidates for observation in an intermediate care unit or even, ICU admission. This may be particularly true for younger patients.

In case of doubt, clinical judgment should always overrule classification according to predictive tools; however, the reasons for doubt should be expressively documented. Finally, the many potential reasons for hospitalization other than only severity should always be remembered.

Severe Community-acquired Pneumonia

In view of the limited predictive power of PSI and CURB-65 to predict ICU admission, scores for the prediction of severe CAP requiring ICU admission have been evaluated.

Modified American Thoracic Society Rule

The first rule was presented by the ATS guidelines in 1993.[42] ICU admissions should be considered in the presence of 1 or more of criteria identified as predictive for in-hospital death. However, a validation study by Ewig et al. could show that these criteria had a sensitivity of 98% sensitive but a limited specificity of only 32%. Therefore, a prediction rule with patients admitted to a respiratory ICU used as reference was derived.[43] This rule [presence of 2 or 3 "minor criteria" (systolic blood pressure <90 mmHg, multilobar involvement, PaO_2/F_IO_2 <250 mmHg) or one of 2 "major criteria" (requirement of mechanical ventilation, presence of septic shock)] (Table 16), later addressed as modified ATS rule, had a sensitivity of 78%, specificity of 94%, positive predictive value of 75%, and negative predictive value of 95%. This rule was included in the ATS guidelines from 2001.[44]

Infectious Disease Society of America/ American Thoracic Society Rule

The 2007 guidelines for the management of CAP in adults of the IDSA and the ATS proposed the IDSA/ATS rule,[4] which is a revision of the modified ATS rule. It includes 9 "minor criteria" (respiratory rate ≥30/min, PaO_2/F_IO_2 ratio <250 mmHg, multilobar infiltrates, confusion/disorientation, uremia (blood urea nitrogen level ≥20 mg/dL), leukopenia (WBC count, <4,000 cells/mm³), thrombocytopenia (platelet count, <100,000 cells/mm³), hypothermia (core temperature, <36°C), and hypotension requiring aggressive fluid resuscitation) instead of the 3 "minor criteria" of the modified ATS rule (Table 17). ICU treatment was recommended in the presence of at least 3 "minor criteria" or 1 "major criterion".[4]

SMART-COP

SMART-COP is a tool that predicts the need for intensive respiratory or vasopressor support in CAP patients that has been described by Charles et al. in 2008.[41] Scores are calculated according to 3 "major criteria" [systolic blood

TABLE 16
Modified ATS Rule

Modified ATS Rule
Major criteria
• Need for mechanical ventilation
• Septic shock
Minor criteria
• Systolic blood pressure <90 mmHg
• Multilobar infiltrates
• PaO_2/F_IO_2 ratio <250 mmHg
Severe CAP
• Presence of ≥1 major criteria or ≥2 minor criteria

ATS, American Thoracic Society; CAP, community-acquired pneumonia; PaO_2/F_IO_2, ratio of partial pressure of arterial oxygen to the fraction of inspired oxygen.

TABLE 17
IDSA/ATS Rule

Major criteria
• Need for mechanical ventilation
• Septic shock
Minor criteria
• Respiratory rate ≥30/min
• PaO_2/F_IO_2 ratio <250 mmHg
• Multilobar infiltrates
• Confusion/disorientation
• Uremia (blood urea nitrogen level ≥20 mg/dL)
• Leukopenia (WBC count <4,000 cells/mm^3)
• Thrombocytopenia (platelet count <100,000 cells/mm^3)
• Hypothermia (core temperature <36°C)
• Hypotension requiring aggressive fluid resuscitation
Severe CAP
• Presence of ≥1 major criteria or ≥3 minor criteria

IDSA, Infectious Disease Society of America; ATS; American Thoracic Society; CAP community-acquired pneumonia; PaO_2/F_IO_2, ratio of partial pressure of arterial oxygen to the fraction of inspired oxygen; WBC, white blood cell.

TABLE 18
SMART-COP Score

Criteria			Score
Systolic blood pressure <90 mmHg			2 points
Multilobar chest X-ray involvement			1 point
Albumin <3.5 g/dL			1 point
Respiratory rate			
Age	≤50 years	>50 years	1 point
Respiratory rate	≥25/min	≥30/min	
Tachycardia ≥125 beats/min			1 point
Confusion (new onset)			1 point
Oxygen low			
Age	≤50 years	>50 years	
PaO_2	<70 mmHg	<60 mmHg	2 points
or SaO_2	≤93%	≤90%	
or PaO_2/F_IO_2	<333 mmHg	<250 mmHg	
P Arterial pH <7.35			2 points

PaO_2, partial pressure of arterial oxygen; SaO_2, percentage of available hemoglobin saturated with oxygen; PaO_2/F_IO_2, ratio of partial pressure of arterial oxygen to the fraction of inspired oxygen.

pressure <90 mmHg, low oxygen levels (age adjusted cutoffs as given in Table 18), and arterial pH <7.35] and 4 "minor criteria" (multilobar chest X-ray involvement, albumin <3.5 g/dL, respiratory rate (age adjusted cutoffs as given in Table 18), tachycardia ≥125 beats/min and new onset confusion). "Major criteria" count 2 points and "minor criteria" count 1 point (Table 18). Corresponding to the calculated points, patients are assigned to 4 risk classes from low- to very high-risk of needing intensive respiratory or vasopressor support (Table 19).[41]

For a primary care setting, in which laboratory measurement is not available, SMRT-CO, a modified version omitting albumin, oxygen level and arterial pH measurement, was suggested (Table 20).[41]

A SMART-COP score of more than 3 points identified 92% of patients who received intensive respiratory or vasopressor support, including 84% of patients who did not need immediate admission to the ICU. In comparison, a SMRT-CO score of more than 2 points identified 90.1% of these patients. An increasing SMART-COP score was associated with an increased rate of receipt of intensive respiratory or vasopressor support and a higher mortality.[41]

España Rule

The España rule is a clinical prediction rule for identifying patients with severe CAP in the emergency department.[45] España et al. derived this prediction rule using a combined reference including 3 parameters: mechanical ventilation, septic shock, and mortality. The variables of the score were also grouped in 6 "minor criteria" (confusion, urea ≥30 mg/dL, respiratory rate >30/min, multilobar bilateral infiltrates, PaO_2 <54 mmHg or PaO_2/F_IO_2 <250, mmHg and age ≥80 years) and 2 "major criteria" (arterial pH <7.35 or systolic blood pressure <90 mmHg) (Table 21). Severe CAP was defined in the presence

TABLE 19
Risk of Needing IRVS According to SMART-COP Score

Score	Risk level	Need of IRVS
0–2	Low	—
3–4	Moderate	1 in 8
5–6	High	1 in 3
≥7	Very high	2 in 3

IRVS, intensive respiratory and vasopressor support.

TABLE 20
Risk of Needing IRVS According to SMRT-CO Score

Score	Risk level	Need of IRVS
0	Very low	—
1	Low	1 in 20
2	Moderate	1 in 10
3	High	1 in 6
≥4	Very high	1 in 3

IRVS, intensive respiratory and vasopressor support.

TABLE 21

España Rule

Major criteria
• Arterial pH <7.30
• Systolic pressure <90 mmHg
Minor criteria
• Confusion
• Urea >30 mg/dL
• Respiratory rate >30/min
• X-Ray multilobar/bilateral
• PaO_2 <54 mmHg or PaO_2/F_IO_2 <250 mmHg
• Age ≥80 years
Severe CAP
• Presence of ≥1 major criteria or ≥2 minor criteria

PaO_2, partial pressure of arterial oxygen; PaO_2/F_IO_2, ratio of partial pressure of arterial oxygen to the fraction of inspired oxygen; CAP, community-acquired pneumonia.

of at least 1 "major criterion" or 2 "minor criteria". In the validation group, this rule was 84% sensitive, 60% specific, with a positive predictive value of 22%, and a negative predictive value of 97%. In fact, these operative characteristics were not superior to the modified ATS score (AUC 0.72 vs. 0.71).[45]

Risk of Early Admission to Intensive Care Unit Index

A further prediction rule for ICU admission focused on patients presenting with no obvious reason for immediate ICU admission (not requiring immediate respiratory or circulatory support) on days 1–3 of emergency department.[46] The Risk of Early Admission to ICU index (REA-ICU index) included 11 criteria independently associated with ICU admission: male gender, age less than 80 years, comorbid conditions, respiratory rate of more than 30 breaths/min, heart rate of more than 125 beats/min, multilobar infiltrate or pleural effusion, white blood cell count less than 3 or more than 20 × 10^9/L, hypoxemia (oxygen saturation <90% or PaO_2 <60 mmHg), blood urea nitrogen above 11 mmol/L, pH below 7.35, and sodium below 130 mmol/L (Table 22). The REA-ICU index stratified patients into 4 risk classes with a risk of ICU admission on days 1–3 ranging from 0.7 to 31%. The AUC was 0.81 [95% confidence interval (CI) 0.78–0.83] in the overall population.[46]

Validation Studies of Predictive Rules for Severe Community-acquired Pneumonia

A validation study of the modified ATS rule in the same setting achieved comparable prediction for the admission

TABLE 22

REA-ICU Index Criteria

Criteria	Score
Male gender	1 point
Age <80 years	1 point
≥1 comorbid condition	1 point
Respiratory rate ≥30 breaths/min	1 point
Heart rate ≥125 beats/min	1 point
Multilobar infiltrates or pleural effusion	1 point
White blood cell count <3 or ≥20 × 10^9/L	1 point
Hypoxemia (oxygen saturation <90% or PaO_2 <60 mmHg)	1 point
Blood urea nitrogen <11 mmol/L	1 point
Arterial pH <7.35	1 point
Sodium <130 mmol/L	1 point

REA-ICU, risk of early admission to intensive care unit; PaO_2, partial pressure of arterial oxygen.

to the ICU.[47] However, 2 validation studies from the US[48,49] and 1 from Australia[40] revealed much more variable predictions. The only consistent finding across all studies was a high-negative predictive value.

The operative characteristics of the IDSA/ATS rule in a validation cohort were comparable to the modified ATS rule.[50] Similarly, in a Greek study limited to patients with pneumococcal CAP, the performance of the 2007 IDSA/ATS criteria was not superior to the 2001 modified ATS rule in predicting ICU admission.[51]

Evidently, "major criteria" are self-evident and less helpful for the clinicians. Therefore, the focus has shifted to the predictive potential of the 9 "minor criteria" listed in the 2007 IDSA/ATS guideline update. Two studies have evaluated these "minor criteria", using ICU admission as reference for severe CAP. Using 4 rather than 3 "minor criteria" improved the positive predictive value from 54 to 81%, with a stable negative predictive value of 94–92%.[52] Similarly, Phua et al. found positive and negative predictive values of the "minor criteria" of 52.9% and 92.3%, respectively, for ICU admission.[53]

In a validation study of the España rule in the same setting, these criteria had a comparable AUC of 0.75.[54]

Chalmers et al. presented a validation study of predictive rules for severe CAP applying perhaps, the best methodology.[55] Two references for severe CAP at admission were used; ICU admission as decided by the attending physicians and the need for ventilatory support and vasopressor use; in addition, the prediction of mortality was evaluated. The validation was restricted to patients with "minor criteria", thereby, excluding patients with an immediate need for mechanical ventilation and/or vasopressor support. Patients with treatment limitations (i.e., no indication for ICU) were excluded. The resulting study population was fundamentally different from those in previous studies. Of 1723 initially eligible patients, 98 were excluded because of the presence of "major criteria" and 563 because of treatment restrictions. These numbers confirm the high percentage of patients with evident severe CAP at admission (32% of patients meeting criteria of severe CAP according to IDSA/ATS guidelines) and the magnitude of patient numbers with CAP as terminal event (33% of the total population) in such validation studies. As a consequence, patient age was very low (mean 63 years, no patient older than 74 years), comorbidity was exceedingly low (44% of patients without any comorbidity), and mortality resulted much lower than in other studies (4.5% overall, 16% of patients meeting criteria for severe CAP according to IDSA/ATS guidelines). In this population, the IDSA/ATS criteria achieved the highest and statistically superior predictions compared to several predictive rules, including ATS 2001 criteria, España rule, and SMART-COP rule. Interestingly, there were only minimal differences in predictions of severe CAP using either ICU admission or the requirement for mechanical ventilation or vasopressor support (MV/VS) as reference. All rules failed to achieve a positive and negative likelihood ratio of more than 10 and less than 1, respectively, thought to indicate confident clinical predictions.[56]

Role of biomarkers in addition to severity scoring was investigated by Ramírez et al.[57] PCT, CRP, tumor necrosis factor (TNF)-α, and interleukin (IL)-6 levels all were higher in ICU-admitted patients; however, the IDSA/ATS "minor severity criteria" predicted better ICU admission. Inflammatory biomarkers identified patients needing ICU, including those with delayed ICU admission. Patients with severe CAP, "minor criteria" and low levels of PCT were identified as a group that may be safely admitted to wards.[57]

Critical Appraisal

All the scores presented provided reasonable operative characteristics. However, predictive tools were performed within a wide range in different settings. Furthermore, none seems to be truly superior in a clinically relevant manner.

Several methodological issues deserve consideration for an appropriate interpretation of predictive tools for severe CAP. The reference "admission to the ICU" is determined by local admission policies limiting external validity. Thus, it is observed that the rules derived from treatment setting, perform formidably well when validated in the same setting but perform less favorably when used in a difference set up. Changing clinical practices also affect the performance of predictive rules. Such changes include the emergence of intermediate care units in the late 90s in many hospitals, some even as specialized respiratory units and non-invasive ventilation as a standardized care for respiratory failure, occasionally delivered even in the respiratory ward. Such settings of intensified care outside the ICU challenge the use of "admission to the ICU" as a reference to define severe pneumonia. Patients who formerly would have been admitted at the ICU may now be treated in non-ICU settings (at the cost of specificity of severity criteria). On the other hand, patients without severe respiratory or hemodynamic compromise might nevertheless be subject to monitoring in the initial phase of management (at the cost of sensitivity of severity criteria).[58]

The alternative suggested by España et al. relies on the 3 most severe outcomes of CAP including mechanical ventilation, septic shock, and mortality as reference outcome. This approach, however, remains questionable. First, this reference obviously excludes important and frequent presentations of severe CAP, e.g., acute respiratory failure not requiring mechanical ventilation and severe sepsis. Second, factors not related to mortality, such as comorbidity, delayed timing, and inadequacy of treatment, and complications—each might predict such outcome. Finally, this approach suffers from an obvious circular reasoning. The 2 major criteria, mechanical ventilation and septic shock, are deconstructed into predictive variables, which finally are presented as predicting the 2 major criteria.[58,59]

In contrast, the SMART-COP approach leaves behind the treatment setting as reference and defines independent critical endpoints. Unfortunately, predictions of severe CAP in external settings were not superior to previous ones. This finding might be explained by two reasons. First, IRVS might not be an unequivocally objective reference since the decision to start ventilatory support remains to some extent on clinical judgment. Second, hidden treatment restrictions in face of elderly, highly comorbid, and disabled patients may preclude intensive respiratory or vasopressor support; although the rule may predict its application.[58]

Overall, criteria to define severe CAP seem very similar across all approaches (except the PIRO approach). In fact, all criteria relate to 3 categories, i.e., acute respiratory failure, severe sepsis/septic shock, and radiographic spread. An important difference between various criteria is whether they are present at admission or during follow-up.

It is perhaps astonishing that simple criteria may reflect highly complex pathophysiological processes. Nevertheless, tachypnea or the PaO_2/F_IO_2 can reflect acute respiratory failure, and hypotension as well as pneumonia-related mental confusion can reflect severe sepsis. The addition of more criteria reflecting acute respiratory failure and/or severe sepsis and septic shock does not improve the performance of a severity rule. Obviously, due to the limited prevalence of each criterion reflecting severe sepsis, adding more criteria result in higher thresholds at the cost of sensitivity of the rule. Therefore, the inflation of the modified ATS rule as presented in the most recent update of the IDSA/ATS guidelines does not generate a relevant increase in predictive power.[58]

The inclusion of "major criteria" is subjected to criticism. In fact, "major criteria" are self-evident since they predict severe CAP in patients who have already received treatment for the most severe complications of CAP. "Major criteria" might remain useful for purposes of patient classification in studies. "Minor criteria", however, are less sensitive and the increase in the number of criteria does not overcome this problem. Accordingly, rules that do not include "major criteria" (España and the SMART-COP rules) have a limited sensitivity.[58]

The evolution of pneumonia severity is not sufficiently reflected by any predictive rule. An attempt to account for this was made in the modified ATS rule, classifying criteria as being present at admission or during follow-up. However, only "major criteria" were provided as evolutionary criteria. Thus, patients developing severe CAP after admission but not requiring mechanical ventilation and/or without septic shock remain unidentified.

Evidently, patients at risk of developing severe CAP during the course of the illness are particularly important to identify since they may be subject to preventive measures even outside ICU. In fact, the chance to improve outcomes of such patients might be regarded considerably higher than for patients with septic shock.[58]

Practical Issues

Scores for severe CAP might appear to be rigid tools of limited sensitivity, possibly inferior to a pathophysiologically informed and alert clinical assessment.[60]

In order to use predictive tools adequately, it is mandatory to understand what severe CAP is. Pneumonia may be addressed as severe either as a consequence of alveolar infectious inflammation resulting in serious ventilation-perfusion-mismatches, reaching a dead space ventilation up to 50%, as well as shunt up to 20%, i.e., acute respiratory failure,[61] or by the SIRS together with severe hypoperfusion and multiorgan failure, i.e., severe sepsis and/or septic shock. Another reason for severe pneumonia may be pneumonia-related and non-pneumonia-related complications.

Severity assessment should identify patients in need of any type of what may be addressed as "intensified treatment", i.e., monitoring of vital signs and oxygenation, independently from the need for ICU or even intermediate care admission. Basically, "intensified treatment" comprises the monitoring of respiratory rate, oximetry, heart rate, and blood pressure. Patients with acute respiratory failure may then receive oxygen supplementation and/or noninvasive ventilator support and in those with hypotension should receive early goal directed treatment, at least aggressive fluid resuscitation. From this point of view, the only patients with an absolute indication for admission to the ICU are those meeting "major criteria".[58]

Since rules for severe pneumonia basically represent an aid to recognize acute respiratory failure and severe sepsis/septic shock, all criteria reflecting acute respiratory failure and hemodynamic compromise may be used to assess severity by the clinician. However, predictive scores remain an aid to clinical judgment and must not be used independently from such judgment. Scores falling shortly below the defined thresholds may nonetheless reflect transition to severe CAP, particularly in younger patients who might compensate acute respiratory failure much more effectively.[58]

Pneumonia severity is not a static event but a dynamic process that mirrors the inflammatory response. The initial 24–48 hours after first presentation are the most vulnerable to pneumonia progression and ultimately, lethal outcomes.[46] Some data suggest that a delayed transfer to the ICU may adversely affect the outcome.[62,63] Therefore, a continuous re-evaluation for the development of acute respiratory failure, hypotension, as well as the presence of pneumonia-related complications and decompensated comorbidities is mandatory.[58]

Another important challenge in some very elderly and severely disabled patients may be to consider treatment restrictions, such as withholding ICU admission.[58]

Today, the modified ATS rule, IDSA/ATS rule, or the SMART-COP rule can be regarded as equally predictive to identify severe pneumonia. The first rule has the advantage of perfect simplicity. The exact role of biomarkers within such rules has not yet been settled. However, rules remain an aid to a sensible clinical assessment. Such assessment requires knowledge about the key features behind severity of pneumonia, i.e., acute respiratory failure, hypotension, and organ failure, as well as possible pneumonia-related complications and decompensated (mainly cardiovascular) comorbidities.[58]

HOSPITAL-ACQUIRED PNEUMONIA

Compared to CAP, the role of severity assessment in hospital-acquired pneumonia (HAP) is far less prominent, since HAP is less common in the non-ventilated patients than in the ventilated patients and most cases with HAP occur in the ICU or intermediate care units. Thus, predictive tools for in-hospital mortality are designed primarily for prognostic purposes, which may get relevant in patient stratification within study protocols. Any predictive tool will have to be compared to the generic APACHE II score,[64] although SAPS II[65] was also shown to be a predictor of severity and outcome.[66]

VAP-PIRO Score

The VAP-PIRO score was developed in 2008 by Lisboa et al. to assess severity and stratify mortality risk of patients with VAP.[67] It is based on the PIRO concept.[13-17] One point is given for predisposition (comorbidities: COPD, immunocompromised, congestive heart failure, chronic renal failure, chronic hepatopathy), insult (bacteremia), response (systolic BP <90 mmHg or need for vasopressor drugs), and organ failure (ARDS) resulting in scores from 0 to 4 (Table 23). The risk is low for patients with scores of 0–1, high with scores of 2, and very high with scores of 3–4 points (Table 24). The best cutoff to predict ICU mortality was more than 2 points with a sensitivity of 79.8% and specificity of 73.4%.[67]

The VAP PIRO score was validated in only 1 recent study. It was not better than APACHE II and VAP APACHE II and not a good predictor of ICU and 28-day mortality. Further studies are needed to validate this score.[68]

IBMP-10 Score

The IBMP-10-prediction rule was derived in 2 steps. First, univariate analysis identified variables predictive of death. Second, from the group of variables with *P* values below 0.1, a group of 5 variables was selected; the 5 variables needed to be easily obtainable and to represent a combination of criteria in different dimensions, including the patient's history, physical examination findings, laboratory values, and manifestations noted by chest radiography. The resulting IBMP-10 score assigned 1 point to each of the following variables:

- The presence of **i**mmunodeficiency
- **B**lood pressure below 90 mmHg (systolic) or below 60 mmHg (diastolic)
- **M**ultilobar infiltrates noted on a chest radiograph
- **P**latelet count below 100,000/mm^3
- Duration of hospitalization before the onset of VAP of more than **10** days (Tables 25 and 26).[69]

In the derivation study, the IBMP-10 score had higher sensitivity, specificity, and AUC to predict mortality, compared with the APACHE II scoring system; the AUC was 0.743 for the APACHE II score and 0.824 for the IBMP-10 score ($p < 0.001$).[69]

Unfortunately, in the first validation study, the IBMP-10 score was less reliable than the APACHE II score in predicting 14-day mortality in this independent population of VAP patients.[70]

TABLE 23
VAP-PIRO Score

Predisposition	Comorbidities*
Insult	Bacteraemia
Response	Systolic blood pressure <90 mmHg#
Organ failure	ARDS

*COPD, Immunocompromised, chronic heart failure, chronic renal failure, chronic hepatopathy
#or need of vasopressor drugs to maintain blood pressure.
VAP, ventilator-associated pneumonia; COPD, chronic obstructive pulmonary disease; ARDS, acute respiratory distress syndrome.

TABLE 24
Risk According to VAP-PIRO Score

Score	Risk level	ICU mortality (%)
0–1	Low	13.9
2	High	52.9
3–4	Very high	79.5

VAP, ventilator-associated pneumonia; ICU, intensive care unit.

TABLE 25
IBMP-10 Score

- **I**mmunodeficiency
- **B**lood pressure <90 mmHg (systolic) or <60 mmHg (diastolic)
- **M**ultilobar infiltrates noted on a chest radiograph
- **P**latelet count <100,000/mm^3
- Duration of hospitalization before the onset of VAP >**10** days

VAP, ventilator-associated pneumonia.

TABLE 26
Mortality According to IBMP-10 Score

Score	Mortality* (%)
0	2
1	9
2	24
3	50
4	67

*All-cause during the 14-day study period.

These results indicate that much more investigation will be needed to achieve a predictive tool for HAP with sufficient external validity.

REFERENCES

1. Ewig S, Welte T. CRB-65 for the assessment of pneumonia severity: who could ask for more? *Thorax.* 2008;63: 665-6.
2. Höffken G, Lorenz J, Kern W, Welte T, Bauer T, Dalhoff K, et al.; Paul-Ehrlich-Gesellschaft für Chemotherapie; Deutschen Gesellschaft für Pneumologie und Beatmungsmedizin; Deutschen Gesellschaft für Infektiologie und vom Kompetenznetzwerk CAPNETZ. Epidemiology, diagnosis, antimicrobial therapy and management of community-acquired pneumonia and lower respiratory tract infections in adults. Guidelines of the Paul-Ehrlich-Society for Chemotherapy, the German Respiratory Society, the German Society for Infectiology and the Competence Network CAPNETZ Germany. *Pneumologie.* 2009;63:e1-68.
3. Lim WS, Baudouin SV, George RC, Hill AT, Jamieson C, Le Jeune I, et al.; Pneumonia Guidelines Committee of the BTS Standards of Care Committee. BTS guidelines for the management of community acquired pneumonia in adults: update 2009. *Thorax.* 2009;64:iii1-55.
4. Mandell LA, Wunderink RG, Anzueto A, Bartlett JG, Campbell GD, Dean NC, et al. Infectious Diseases Society of America/American Thoracic Society consensus guidelines on the management of community-acquired pneumonia in adults. *Clin Infect Dis.* 2007;44:S27-72.
5. Woodhead M, Blasi F, Ewig S, Garau J, Huchon G, Ieven M, et al. Guidelines for the management of adult lower respiratory tract infections—full version. *Clin Microbiol Infect.* 2011;17:E1-59.
6. Fine MJ, Auble TE, Yealy DM, Hanusa BH, Weissfeld LA, Singer DE, et al. A prediction rule to identify low-risk patients with community-acquired pneumonia. *N Engl J Med.* 1997;336:243-50.
7. Community-acquired pneumonia in adults in British hospitals in 1982-1983: a survey of aetiology, mortality, prognostic factors and outcome. The British Thoracic Society and the Public Health Laboratory Service. *Q J Med.* 1987;62:195-220.
8. Neill AM, Martin IR, Weir R, Anderson R, Chereshsky A, Epton MJ, et al. Community acquired pneumonia: aetiology and usefulness of severity criteria on admission. *Thorax.* 1996;51:1010-6.
9. Lim WS, van der Eerden MM, Laing R, Boersma WG, Karalus N, Town GI, et al. Defining community acquired pneumonia severity on presentation to hospital: an international derivation and validation study. *Thorax.* 2003;58:377-82.
10. Qureshi KN, Hodkinson HM. Evaluation of a ten-question mental test in the institutionalized elderly. *Age Ageing.* 1974;3:152-7.
11. Barlow G, Nathwani D, Davey P. The CURB65 pneumonia severity score outperforms generic sepsis and early warning scores in predicting mortality in community-acquired pneumonia. *Thorax.* 2007;62:253-9.
12. American College of Chest Physicians/Society of Critical Care Medicine Consensus Conference: definitions for sepsis and organ failure and guidelines for the use of innovative therapies in sepsis. *Crit Care Med.* 1992;20:864-74.
13. Levy MM, Fink MP, Marshall JC, Abraham E, Angus D, Cook D, et al. 2001 SCCM/ESICM/ACCP/ATS/SIS International Sepsis Definitions Conference. *Crit Care Med.* 2003;31:1250-6.
14. Angus DC, Burgner D, Wunderink R, Mira J-P, Gerlach H, Wiedermann CJ, et al. The PIRO concept: P is for predisposition. *Crit Care.* 2003;7:248-51.
15. Vincent J-L, Opal S, Torres A, Bonten M, Cohen J, Wunderink R. The PIRO concept: I is for infection. *Crit Care.* 2003;7:252-5.
16. Gerlach H, Dhainaut J-F, Harbarth S, Reinhart K, Marshall JC, Levy M. The PIRO concept: R is for response. *Crit Care.* 2003;7:256-9.
17. Vincent J-L, Wendon J, Groeneveld J, Marshall JC, Streat S, Carlet J. The PIRO concept: O is for organ dysfunction. *Crit Care.* 2003;7:260-4.
18. Rello J, Rodriguez A, Lisboa T, Gallego M, Lujan M, Wunderink R. PIRO score for community-acquired pneumonia: a new prediction rule for assessment of severity in intensive care unit patients with community-acquired pneumonia. *Crit Care Med.* 2009;37:456-62.
19. Buising KL, Thursky KA, Black JF, MacGregor L, Street AC, Kennedy MP, et al. Identifying severe community-acquired pneumonia in the emergency department: a simple clinical prediction tool. *Emerg Med Australas.* 2007; 19:418-26.
20. Shindo Y, Sato S, Maruyama E, Ohashi T, Ogawa M, Imaizumi K, et al. Comparison of severity scoring systems A-DROP and CURB-65 for community-acquired pneumonia. *Respirology.* 2008;13:731-5.
21. McGinn TG, Guyatt GH, Wyer PC, Naylor CD, Stiell IG, Richardson WS. Users' guides to the medical literature: XXII: how to use articles about clinical decision rules. Evidence-Based Medicine Working Group. *JAMA.* 2000; 284:79-84.
22. Chalmers JD, Singanayagam A, Akram AR, Mandal P, Short PM, Choudhury G, et al. Severity assessment tools for predicting mortality in hospitalised patients with community-acquired pneumonia. Systematic review and meta-analysis. *Thorax.* 2010;65:878-83.
23. Aujesky D, Auble TE, Yealy DM, Stone RA, Obrosky DS, Meehan TP, et al. Prospective comparison of three validated prediction rules for prognosis in community-acquired pneumonia. *Am J Med.* 2005;118:384-92.
24. Ananda-Rajah MR, Charles PGP, Melvani S, Burrell LL, Johnson PDR, Grayson ML. Comparing the pneumonia severity index with CURB-65 in patients admitted with community acquired pneumonia. *Scand J Infect Dis.* 2008; 40:293-300.
25. Capelastegui A, España PP, Quintana JM, Areitio I, Gorordo I, Egurrola M, et al. Validation of a predictive rule for the management of community-acquired pneumonia. *Eur Respir J.* 2006;27:151-7.
26. Man SY, Lee N, Ip M, Antonio GE, Chau SSL, Mak P, et al. Prospective comparison of three predictive rules for assessing severity of community-acquired pneumonia in Hong Kong. *Thorax.* 2007;62:348-53.

27. Ewig S, Birkner N, Strauss R, Schaefer E, Pauletzki J, Bischoff H, et al. New perspectives on community-acquired pneumonia in 388, 406 patients. Results from a nationwide mandatory performance measurement programme in healthcare quality. *Thorax.* 2009;64:1062-9.
28. Bont J, Hak E, Hoes AW, Macfarlane JT, Verheij TJM. Predicting death in elderly patients with community-acquired pneumonia: a prospective validation study reevaluating the CRB-65 severity assessment tool. *Arch Intern Med.* 2008;168:1465-8.
29. Loke YK, Kwok CS, Niruban A, Myint PK. Value of severity scales in predicting mortality from community-acquired pneumonia: systematic review and meta-analysis. *Thorax.* 2010;65:884-90.
30. Krüger S, Ewig S, Kunde J, Hartmann O, Suttorp N, Welte T. Pro-atrial natriuretic peptide and pro-vasopressin for predicting short-term and long-term survival in community-acquired pneumonia: results from the German Competence Network CAPNETZ. *Thorax.* 2010; 65:208-14.
31. Claessens Y-E, Mathevon T, Kierzek G, Grabar S, Jegou D, Batard E, et al. Accuracy of C-reactive protein, procalcitonin, and mid-regional pro-atrial natriuretic peptide to guide site of care of community-acquired pneumonia. *Intensive Care Med.* 2010;36:799-809.
32. Menéndez R, Martínez R, Reyes S, Mensa J, Filella X, Marcos MA, et al. Biomarkers improve mortality prediction by prognostic scales in community-acquired pneumonia. *Thorax.* 2009;64:587-91.
33. Krüger S, Ewig S, Marre R, Papassotiriou J, Richter K, von Baum H, et al. Procalcitonin predicts patients at low risk of death from community-acquired pneumonia across all CRB-65 classes. *Eur Respir J.* 2008;31:349-55.
34. Krüger S, Ewig S, Giersdorf S, Hartmann O, Suttorp N, Welte T. Cardiovascular and inflammatory biomarkers to predict short- and long-term survival in community-acquired pneumonia: Results from the German Competence Network, CAPNETZ. *Am J Respir Crit Care Med.* 2010;182:1426-34.
35. Ewig S, Torres A. Severity scores for CAP. Much workload for the next bias. *Thorax.* 2010;65:853-5.
36. Renaud B, Coma E, Labarere J, Hayon J, Roy P-M, Boureaux H, et al. Routine use of the Pneumonia Severity Index for guiding the site-of-treatment decision of patients with pneumonia in the emergency department: a multicenter, prospective, observational, controlled cohort study. *Clin Infect Dis.* 2007;44:41-9.
37. Singanayagam A, Chalmers JD, Hill AT. Severity assessment in community-acquired pneumonia: a review. *QJM.* 2009;102:379-88.
38. Bauer TT, Ewig S, Marre R, Suttorp N, Welte T. CRB-65 predicts death from community-acquired pneumonia. *J Intern Med.* 2006;260:93-101.
39. Chalmers JD, Singanayagam A, Hill AT. Systolic blood pressure is superior to other haemodynamic predictors of outcome in community acquired pneumonia. *Thorax.* 2008;63:698-702.
40. Buising KL, Thursky KA, Black JF, MacGregor L, Street AC, Kennedy MP, et al. A prospective comparison of severity scores for identifying patients with severe community acquired pneumonia: reconsidering what is meant by severe pneumonia. *Thorax.* 2006;61:419-24.
41. Charles PGP, Wolfe R, Whitby M, Fine MJ, Fuller AJ, Stirling R, et al. SMART-COP: a tool for predicting the need for intensive respiratory or vasopressor support in community-acquired pneumonia. *Clin Infect Dis.* 2008; 47:375-84.
42. Niederman MS, Bass JB Jr, Campbell GD, Fein AM, Grossman RF, Mandell LA, et al. Guidelines for the initial management of adults with community-acquired pneumonia: diagnosis, assessment of severity, and initial antimicrobial therapy. American Thoracic Society. Medical Section of the American Lung Association. *Am Rev Respir Dis.* 1993;148:1418-26.
43. Ewig S, Ruiz M, Mensa J, Marcos MA, Martinez JA, Arancibia F, et al. Severe community-acquired pneumonia. Assessment of severity criteria. *Am J Respir Crit Care Med.* 1998;158:1102-8.
44. Niederman MS, Mandell LA, Anzueto A, Bass JB, Broughton WA, Campbell GD, et al. Guidelines for the management of adults with community-acquired pneumonia. Diagnosis, assessment of severity, antimicrobial therapy, and prevention. *Am J Respir Crit Care Med.* 2001;163:1730-54.
45. España PP, Capelastegui A, Gorordo I, Esteban C, Oribe M, Ortega M, et al. Development and validation of a clinical prediction rule for severe community-acquired pneumonia. *Am J Respir Crit Care Med.* 2006;174:1249-56.
46. Renaud B, Labarère J, Coma E, Santin A, Hayon J, Gurgui M, et al. Risk stratification of early admission to the intensive care unit of patients with no major criteria of severe community-acquired pneumonia: development of an international prediction rule. *Crit Care.* 2009;13:R54.
47. Ewig S, de Roux A, Bauer T, García E, Mensa J, Niederman M, et al. Validation of predictive rules and indices of severity for community acquired pneumonia. *Thorax.* 2004;59:421-7.
48. Angus DC, Marrie TJ, Obrosky DS, Clermont G, Dremsizov TT, Coley C, et al. Severe community-acquired pneumonia: use of intensive care services and evaluation of American and British Thoracic Society Diagnostic criteria. *Am J Respir Crit Care Med.* 2002;166:717-23.
49. Riley PD, Aronsky D, Dean NC. Validation of the 2001 American Thoracic Society criteria for severe community-acquired pneumonia. *Crit Care Med.* 2004;32:2398-402.
50. Liapikou A, Ferrer M, Polverino E, Balasso V, Esperatti M, Piñer R, et al. Severe community-acquired pneumonia: validation of the Infectious Diseases Society of America/American Thoracic Society guidelines to predict an intensive care unit admission. *Clin Infect Dis.* 2009;48: 377-85.
51. Kontou P, Kuti JL, Nicolau DP. Validation of the Infectious Diseases Society of America/American Thoracic Society criteria to predict severe community-acquired pneumonia caused by *Streptococcus pneumoniae. Am J Emerg Med.* 2009;27:968-74.
52. Brown SM, Jones BE, Jephson AR, Dean NC. Validation of the Infectious Disease Society of America/American Thoracic Society 2007 guidelines for severe community-acquired pneumonia. *Crit Care Med.* 2009;37:3010-6.

53. Phua J, See KC, Chan YH, Widjaja LS, Aung NW, Ngerng WJ, et al. Validation and clinical implications of the IDSA/ATS minor criteria for severe community-acquired pneumonia. *Thorax*. 2009;64:598-603.
54. España PP, Capelastegui A, Quintana JM, Bilbao A, Diez R, Pascual S, et al. Validation and comparison of SCAP as a predictive score for identifying low-risk patients in community-acquired pneumonia. *J Infect*. 2010;60: 106-13.
55. Chalmers JD, Taylor JK, Mandal P, Choudhury G, Singanayagam A, Akram AR, et al. Validation of the Infectious Diseases Society of America/American Thoratic Society minor criteria for intensive care unit admission in community-acquired pneumonia patients without major criteria or contraindications to intensive care unit care. *Clin Infect Dis*. 2011;53:503-11.
56. Ewig S. Gains and limitations of predictive rules for severe community-acquired pneumonia. *Clin Infect Dis*. 2011;53:512-4.
57. Ramírez P, Ferrer M, Martí V, Reyes S, Martínez R, Menéndez R, et al. Inflammatory biomarkers and prediction for intensive care unit admission in severe community-acquired pneumonia. *Crit Care Med*. 2011;39:2211-7.
58. Ewig S, Woodhead M, Torres A. Towards a sensible comprehension of severe community-acquired pneumonia. *Intensive Care Med*. 2011;37:214-23.
59. Ewig S. Against misleading predictions for severe community-acquired pneumonia. Am J *Respir Crit Care Med*. 2007;175:289-90.
60. Vincent J-L, Opal SM, Marshall JC. Ten reasons why we should NOT use severity scores as entry criteria for clinical trials or in our treatment decisions. *Crit Care Med*. 2010;38:283-7.
61. Gea J, Roca J, Torres A, Agustí AG, Wagner PD, Rodriguez-Roisin R. Mechanisms of abnormal gas exchange in patients with pneumonia. *Anesthesiology*. 1991;75:782-9.
62. Renaud B, Santin A, Coma E, Camus N, Van Pelt D, Hayon J, et al. Association between timing of intensive care unit admission and outcomes for emergency department patients with community-acquired pneumonia. *Crit Care Med*. 2009;37:2867-74.
63. Renaud B, Brun-Buisson C, Santin A, Coma E, Noyez C, Fine MJ, et al. Outcomes of Early, Late, and No Admission to the Intensive Care Unit for Patients Hospitalized with Community-acquired Pneumonia. *Acad Emerg Med*. 2012;19:294-303.
64. Knaus WA, Draper EA, Wagner DP, Zimmerman JE. APACHE II: a severity of disease classification system. *Crit Care Med*. 1985;13:818-29.
65. Le Gall JR, Lemeshow S, Saulnier F. A new Simplified Acute Physiology Score (SAPS II) based on a European/ North American multicenter study. *JAMA*. 1993;270: 2957-63.
66. Froon AH, Bonten MJ, Gaillard CA, Greve JW, Dentener MA, de Leeuw PW, et al. Prediction of clinical severity and outcome of ventilator-associated pneumonia. Comparison of simplified acute physiology score with systemic inflammatory mediators. *Am J Respir Crit Care Med*. 1998;158:1026-31.
67. Lisboa T, Diaz E, Sa-Borges M, Socias A, Sole-Violan J, Rodríguez A, et al. The ventilator-associated pneumonia PIRO score: a tool for predicting ICU mortality and health-care resources use in ventilator-associated pneumonia. *Chest*. 2008;134:1208-16.
68. Furtado GH, Wiskirchen DE, Kuti JL, Nicolau DP. Performance of the PIRO score for predicting mortality in patients with ventilator-associated pneumonia. *Anaesth Intensive Care*. 2012;40:285-91.
69. Mirsaeidi M, Peyrani P, Ramirez JA. Predicting mortality in patients with ventilator-associated pneumonia: The APACHE II score versus the new IBMP-10 score. *Clin Infect Dis*. 2009;49:72-7.
70. Wiskirchen DE, Kuti JL, Nicolau DP. Acute physiology and chronic health evaluation II score is a better predictor of mortality than IBMP-10 in patients with ventilator-associated pneumonia. *Surg Infect (Larchmt)*. 2011;12:385-90.

CHAPTER 23

Biomarkers in the Diagnosis and Treatment of Respiratory Infections

Dimitrios K Matthaiou, Irene D Karampela, Apostolos D Armaganidis, George Dimopoulos

ABSTRACT

Delays in diagnosing and administering appropriate empirical treatment can make the difference between life and death in patients with respiratory tract infections. Hence, methods have been developed including rapid tests that detect pathogen-specific molecules and can be done even at the bedside and biomarkers. Biomarkers are measurable biological parameters that participate in pathophysiological processes and may indirectly help in diagnosing a probable pathology, predicting its course and, in some cases, even contribute to the duration of treatment. Each one of them may help in different aspects of disease management including differential diagnosis, predictor of severity or mortality, etc. However, one should keep in mind that none of them can be separately used safely. Biomarkers are tools that should always be used in conjunction with each other and with clinical signs and imaging findings to ensure maximal efficacy and have an impact on the patient's course.

INTRODUCTION

When a patient presents with clinical signs and symptoms suggestive of an infection of the respiratory tract, the golden rule in diagnosing it, as any other infection, is the isolation of the responsible pathogen. However, the isolation, if possible, is cumbersome and time consuming. Often, delays in diagnosing and administering appropriate empirical treatment make the difference between life and death.

Hence, other methods have been developed including rapid tests that detect pathogen-specific molecules and can be done even at the bedside and biomarkers. The latter are measurable biological parameters, such as enzymes, hormones and other substances or even phenotypes, that participate in pathophysiological processes and may indirectly help in diagnosing a probable pathology, predicting its course, and, in some cases, even contribute to the duration of treatment.

In order for such a method to be useful, it should have high sensitivity and high specificity. Sensitivity is defined as the proportion of individuals who have the pathology in question and test positive for it. Specificity is defined as the proportion of individuals who do not have the pathology in question and test negative for it. In other words, the higher sensitivity a method has, the fewer false negative results it will yield, and the higher specificity it has, the fewer false positive results it will yield.

An alternative methodology of assessing the diagnostic value of a biomarker is the measurement of the area under the curve (AUC) of a receiver operating characteristic (ROC) curve. It is a measure of diagnostic accuracy and a combination in a way of the aforementioned methodologies. It may take values from 0 to 1. The greater the value it takes, the higher the diagnostic accuracy of the biomarker.

This chapter concentrates on the use and impact of novel biomarkers in diagnosis, prognosis and treatment of respiratory tract infections, including procalcitonin (PCT), proadrenomedullin (Pro-ADM), neopterin, presepsin and soluble triggering receptor expressed on myeloid cells-1 (sTREM-1).

PROCALCITONIN

Procalcitonin is a precursor peptide consisting 116 peptides. It includes calcitonin, catacalcin, and the N-terminal end. In healthy subjects, it is produced by thyroid C (parafollicular) cells. However, extrathyroidal production may also happen in various noninfectious conditions, such as cancer, acute pancreatitis, and acute myocardial infarction, but also during infection. In case of infection, it is mainly produced by neuroendocrine lung cells and monocytes. The physiological role of its increased production is not fully understood.

In healthy adults, PCT is detected in traces. However, it normally increases during the first days of life in full-term neonates.[1] Factors inducing PCT production include exotoxins, TNF-α, and other cytokines. PCT is rapidly produced after the onset of infection.[2,3] All the amounts of PCT that are produced in thyroid cells are cleaved to calcitonin. However, PCT that is produced extrathyroidally is directly released in the bloodstream without cleavage. Although renal insufficiency may slightly prolong the half-life of PCT, renal elimination does not constitute a major elimination mechanism. Thus, PCT serum concentration depends mainly on its production rate.[4,5] PCT may be detected in serum, but is also traceable in other body fluids including pleural fluid and bronchoalveolar lavage. Although steroids were found to modify the levels of other biomarkers, no such influence has been reported.[6]

Procalcitonin is measured by quantitative or semi-quantitative techniques; the latter being used as point-of-care test with inferior performance compared to quantitative laboratory tests. The first laboratory-based test used was a "sandwich" immunoluminometric assay known as LUMI test. Subsequently, LIA test was developed. Kryptor test is the most recent evolution of LIA test using time resolved amplified cryptate emission (TRACE) technology and yield more rapid and sensitive results. Other newly developed assays based on the same principle include ADVIA and VIDAS.

Procalcitonin serum concentration in healthy individuals is lower than 0.1 ng/mL. PCT levels of up to 0.25 ng/mL are considered to denote low likelihood of infection, while levels more than 0.25 ng/mL possibly indicate a bacterial infection. PCT greater than 0.5 ng/mL is considered to indicate high probability of bacterial infection, which requires antibiotic treatment.[7]

Procalcitonin role in the prognosis and diagnosis of respiratory infections has been widely studied. Regarding community-acquired pneumonia (CAP), PCT was found to have high diagnostic accuracy of up to 0.88[8] and to be a good predictor of mortality with an AUC ranging from 0.60 to 0.82 depending on the day of measurement.[9-11] PCT levels are not only significantly higher in CAP nonsurvivors than in CAP survivors[12] but also increase with severity of CAP with an AUC of 0.69.[8,13] Furthermore, increased PCT levels on admission were independently associated with higher risk of treatment failure.[14] Regarding other clinical scores, PCT was strongly correlated with various scores including PSI, CURB-65 and A-DROP,[10] and in combination with the former two may contribute in adverse event prediction.[11] However, PCT fails to differentiate between CAP due to typical and atypical bacteria.[13]

In patients with ventilator-associated pneumonia, PCT has a high discriminative capacity yielding and AUC of 0.83, which in combination with CPIS may reach 0.96. The optimal cut-off for PCT-CPIS combination of more than 3 ng/mL and more than 6 points, respectively, has a sensitivity of 67% and a specificity of 100%, thus excluding false-positive diagnoses of VAP under these cut-offs.[15] Furthermore, decreasing PCT concentration is a strong predictor of survival in such patients.[16,17]

In patients with COPD, PCT levels were significantly higher in patients with pneumonia or bacterial exacerbation than in patients with exacerbations of different origin.[18,19] However, there is no difference after the patients return to stable state.[20] To discriminate between patients with mixed bacterial-viral infection and patients with viral infection alone, PCT yielded an AUC 0.70.[19] It has been suggested that a PCT cut-off level of 0.1 ng/mL may be more appropriate than 0.25 ng/mL to predict the probability of bacterial infection in severe COPD patients with pneumonia.[21] It should also be noted that PCT concentration was found to be independently associated with increased risk for ICU mortality.[22]

Procalcitonin contribution has also been studied in the management of patients with H1N1 influenza. PCT concentrations were significantly lower in patients with pneumonia caused by H1N1 influenza alone than in patients with mixed bacterial and viral pneumonia.[23,24] Similarly, patients with pneumonia due to H1N1 pneumonia had significantly lower PCT levels compared to patients with acute bacterial CAP. In both patient groups, PCT decreased with time but remained significantly lower in patients with H1N1 pneumonia.[25] The optimal cut-off to differentiate bacterial from viral etiology of pneumonia ranged from 0.35 ng/mL to 1.5 ng/mL. Likewise, sensitivity and specificity for each of the cut-offs varied greatly.[23,24,26,27] Similarly, the AUC ranged from 0.78 to 0.88.[24,27]

In children with pneumonia, the optimal cut-off to differentiate bacterial from viral etiology was suggested to be 2 ng/mL. Sensitivity and specificity ranged from 50% to 62.7% and 80% to 96%, respectively.[28] The AUC for PCT to differentiate viral and bacterial infections was 0.93.[29] However, it should be noted that, in malaria-endemic areas, the presence of malaria parasites may hamper this differentiation.[30]

In patients with tuberculosis, PCT levels are low but increase significantly with increasing severity of tuberculosis and may predict mortality risk.[31] PCT levels are significantly higher in patients with CAP compared to patients with tuberculosis. The AUC for PCT to differentiate between CAP and tuberculosis was 0.87. Tuberculosis patients with PCT higher than 0.5 ng/mL had significantly shorter survival than those with less than 0.5 ng/mL.[32,33] It should also be noted that in case of pleurisy this cut-off of PCT in pleural fluid does not allow the safe diagnosis of tuberculous compared to nontuberculous origin.[34] In patients, HIV (to whom atypical presentation of respiratory infections may confound diagnosis) and PCT levels are also significantly higher in patients with CAP compared to patients with tuberculosis.[35] The optimal cut-off to distinguish CAP from tuberculosis in such patients was suggested to be 3 ng/mL. Sensitivity and specificity were both 82%.[36]

Measurement of PCT concentration was found to be a useful tool for monitoring the efficacy of antibiotic treatment of respiratory infections and guiding the duration of antibiotic administration. Several studies have been performed in various settings including primary care, medical wards and ICU. In pooled analyses of studies with relevant data, PCT-guided therapy in patients with respiratory tract infections was found to significantly reduce antibiotic exposure without an increase in mortality, treatment failure, ICU admission and length of stay.[37,38] Regarding the effect on cost containment in a study considering a scenario of 6-day PCT measurement and a 2-day shortening of antibiotic administration, a mean daily reduction in antibiotic costs of Can$148.26 (ranging between Can$59.30 and Can$296.52) was estimated.[39]

Key Points

- PCT is useful in distinguishing bacterial from viral pneumonia
- PCT greater than 0.5 ng/mL is considered to indicate high probability of bacterial infection, which requires antibiotic treatment
- PCT increases along with increasing severity of CAP
- PCT is a good predictor of mortality
- PCT-guided therapy in patients with respiratory tract infections may reduce antibiotic exposure and cost of care without an increase in mortality and treatment failure.

PROADRENOMEDULLIN

Adrenomedullin (ADM), which was isolated in 1993 from pheochromocytoma, belongs to the calcitonin peptide family and originates from a member of the CALC gene family, namely CALC-V gene.[40]

It is a strong endogenous vasodilator and has numerous other effects on various organs including the heart, the kidney, the brain and pituitary, and the uterus and ovary. ADM plays a role in cell growth and apoptosis, as well as in sepsis.[41] It is also considered to have bactericidal properties.[42]

The hypotensive effect of ADM is considered to be caused by a combination of two separate mechanisms. The first is the result of the direct effect of ADM on smooth muscle cells and cause the increase of intracellular cAMP, probably by inactivating the myosin light chain kinase. The second mechanism is the result of ADM effect on vascular endothelial cells and causes the increase of concentration of calcium ions. Subsequently, nitric oxide (NO) synthase is activated and NO is released resulting in smooth muscle cells relaxation.[43]

Adrenomedullin is highly upregulated during the hyperdynamic phase of sepsis.[44,45] It reduces vascular hyperpermeability and down-regulates the inflammatory response.[46,47] These effects are considered to contribute in improving survival. However, later on during the hypodynamic phase of sepsis, vascular responsiveness is greatly reduced.[48]

It is ubiquitously found throughout body tissues along with the other derivatives of the precursor peptide. However, the highest amounts are found in pheochromocytoma and the adrenal medulla. Significant amounts may be found in the heart, lungs and kidneys.[41,49] It may be detected in plasma, urine, cerebrospinal fluid, amniotic fluid and sweat. Its concentration in urine is six times higher than that of plasma. ADM levels may be increased in various conditions including cardiovascular, renal, respiratory and endocrine disorders. Also, its concentrations elevate in hepatic cirrhosis, cancer and sepsis.

Knowing the ADM levels may be useful in monitoring sepsis. However, ADM measurement is very cumbersome due to technical difficulties and its rapid clearance from the circulation.[41,50] Pro-ADM is a peptide generated from

ADM precursor along with ADM and other molecules. It is a mid-regional fragment of the original 185 aminoacid-long peptide spanning from aminoacids 45 to 92. It is more stable than ADM, it is metabolically inactive and it is produced in directly correlated amounts with ADM. Thus, it is preferred to be measured in septic patients instead of ADM.

Proadrenomedullin is measured by a sandwich immunoluminometric assay. Its mean plasma concentration in healthy individuals varies from 0.33 nmol/L to 0.46 nmol/L.[51-53] It is not known how pro-ADM is cleared from the body. It has been suggested that it is cleared by renal secretion, as it was found to be associated with cystatin C. Other factors found to positively correlate with pro-ADM levels were age, obesity and lipid profile.[53] It should be noted that steroid pretreatment was found to inhibit pro-ADM in a dose-dependent manner.[54]

Proadrenomedullin has been evaluated in the diagnosis of patients with lower respiratory tract infections (LRTIs) including CAP and COPD.

In table 1, there is a summary of studies assessing pro-ADM in patients with CAP. Pro-ADM levels were significantly higher than those of healthy individuals and the baseline median varied from 1.0 nmol/L to 2.4 nmol/L. Pro-ADM median levels in survivors varied from 0.59 nmol/L to 1.7 nmol/L, while in nonsurvivors from 1.44 nmol/L to 5.0 nmol/L, a statistically significant increase. It should also be noted that pro-ADM levels increased with increasing severity of CAP. Suberviola et al.[55] found pro-ADM concentration to be higher in patients with renal failure, although not significantly, while a significant correlation with creatinine was suggested by Christ-Crain et al.[56] Although pro-ADM concentration seems to be accurate as a prognostic tool for CAP, its value is not modified by different possible CAP etiologies.[57] Furthermore, pro-ADM levels were significantly higher in patients with multilobar pneumonia compared to patients with unilateral pneumonia.[56] High peak levels of pro-ADM during initial hospitalization were also associated with higher risk of long-term mortality.[58]

To predict short-term mortality, the AUC for pro-ADM varied from 0.72 to 0.86. When it was combined with clinical scores, including CURB-65 and PSI, the AUC was further increased.[55,56,59-62] Pro-ADM was better correlated to PSI than other scores and biomarkers.

However, the optimal cut-off to predict short-term mortality exhibited great variability between studies ranging from 0.96 nmol/L to 4.86 nmol/L. Likewise, sensitivity and specificity for each of the cut-offs varied greatly. Under this context, setting cut-offs to predict mortality may be futile. Focus should rather be put on the utilization of pro-ADM as a predictor of CAP severity.

In patients with COPD exacerbations, pro-ADM admission levels were significantly associated with mortality as well as correlated with length of hospital stay. It should be noted that no significant correlation was found between pro-ADM concentration and COPD severity. Pro-ADM levels were significantly high in nonsurvivors compared to survivors [1.07 (0.95-2.8) nmol/L and 0.82 (0.58-1.22) nmol/L, respectively]. Similar differences were also found between long-term nonsurvivors and survivors. The optimal cut-off to predict 2-year mortality was 0.77 nmol/L. Sensitivity and specificity were 81% and 53%, respectively.[63]

Currently, there are no studies focusing on optimizing treatment duration with pro-ADM-based algorithms. Its importance lies in using pro-ADM as a diagnostic and prognostic tool.

TABLE 1

Summary of Studies Assessing Proadrenomedullin in Patients with Community-acquired Pneumonia

Study (Ref.)	Baseline median (range) (nmol/L)	Survivors median (range) (nmol/L)	Nonsurvivors median (range) (nmol/L)	AUC	Sensitivity (cut-off in nmol/L)	Specificity (cut-off in nmol/L)
Christ-Crain[56]	1.1 (0.6–1.9)	1.0 (0.6–1.6)	2.1 (1.5–3.0)	0.76	80% (1.8)	72% (1.8)
Huang[59]	1.0 (0.7–1.5)	0.9 (0.7–1.4)	1.6 (1.1–2.8)	0.76	68% (1.3) 46% (1.8)	73% (1.3) 86% (1.8)
Krueger[60]	NR	0.59 (0.43–0.94)	1.44 (0.99–2.36)	0.85	77.8% (0.96)	76.3% (0.96)
Albrich[62]	1.2 (0.8–1.9)	NR	NR	0.76	NR	NR
Suberviola[55]	2.4 (1.4–5.6)	1.7 (1.3–3.1)	5.0 (1.9–10.1)	0.72	53% (4.86)	84% (4.86)
Bello[57]	NR	0.86 (0.59–1.91)	2.34 (1.19–4.23)	0.86	92% (1.07)	67.5% (1.07)
Schuetz[61]	1.1 (0.9–1.3)	NR	NR	0.76	NR	NR

AUC, area under the ROC curve; NR, not reported.

Key Points

- Pro-ADM levels increase with increasing severity of CAP
- Pro-ADM cannot be used for the discrimination of CAP etiology
- Pro-ADM is inhibited by steroid pretreatment in a dose-dependent manner
- Pro-ADM is a better predictor of CAP and COPD severity than of mortality.

NEOPTERIN

Neopterin is a pyrazino-(2,3-d-)-pyrimidine molecule and belongs to the chemical group of pteridines, namely aromatic pteridines. It is the catabolic result of guanosine triphosphate (GTP) cleavage by GTP-cyclohydrolase I, along with 7,8-dihydroneopterin.[64] Its production is stimulated by interferon-gamma (INF-γ), which is released by T-lymphocytes and especially the Th-1-type ones. In primates, it is synthetized almost exclusively in monocytes and macrophages,[65] although it may be also detectable in microglial cells of the central nervous system.[66]

Neopterin is an indirect marker of macrophage activation and the subsequent synthesis of free radicals. However, since both neopterin and reactive oxygen metabolites production is regulated by INF-γ stimulation, a correlation between neopterin levels and the amount of oxidative stress has been established. Neopterin has a dual role of noncompetitive inhibition of xanthine oxidase, which is an enzyme generating free oxygen radicals, and that of enhancing the effect of H_2O_2, HOCl, chloramine and other reactive substances.[67] However, it is not clear which of these roles predominates in vivo. Neopterin's counterpart, dihydroneopterin, acts as free radical scavenger. Thus, its biosynthesis acts as a regulator of the immune response generated by activated macrophages and the measurement of its levels can be of clinical value in conditions associated with cell-mediated immunity.

Neopterin can be measured by various methods including ELISA, radioimmunoassay (RIA) and high-performance liquid chromatography (HPLC). It may be detected in various body fluids including in serum, urine, pleuritic fluid, cerebrospinal fluid, ascetic fluid, pancreatic juice, bronchoalveolar lavage (BAL) fluid and synovial fluid.[67-69]

Neopterin levels in blood may be influenced by age. The mean value is about 6 nmol/L until adulthood, lowers down to 5 nmol/L till the 8th decade of life and then rises sharply to a mean of 8.5 nmol/L. These variations are associated with renal function. As individuals get older and renal function compromises, neopterin accumulates. Likewise, the same phenomenon may happen in patients with renal insufficiency.[69] At this point, it should be noted that the renal clearance of creatinine and neopterin is similar. Thus, neopterin/creatinine ratio is used as a formula to overcome the problem of neopterin accumulation due to a possible renal insufficiency. Contrary to that, steroids may cause a decrease in neopterin concentration. Hence, measurements should be done before the commencement of steroid treatment.[70]

Increased concentrations may be detected in various conditions including infectious diseases, cancer, autoimmune diseases, cardiovascular disease and allograft rejection. Regarding infectious diseases, neopterin levels increase when cell-mediated immunity is activated, namely in infections caused by intracellular bacteria and viruses. Such infections include tuberculosis, HIV, hepatitis B and C, CMV and EBV infections, dengue fever, measles, influenza, malaria, melioidosis, borreliosis, leprosy and schistosomiasis.

In patients with LRTIs, neopterin levels could contribute in discriminating between viral or bacterial etiology of such infections. In a comparison of neopterin concentrations in patients with viral LRTIs, mostly by influenza, with those of patients with bacterial LRTIs, the former group had a twofold higher increase of neopterin levels compared to the latter. Compared to healthy controls, the increase was fivefold. The median values were 30.5, 18.7 and 5.8 nmol/L, respectively. When a cut-off value of at least 15 nmol/L for neopterin was used to diagnose a viral LRTI against a bacterial LRTI or healthy subject, the sensitivity and specificity were 86.7% and 69.5%, respectively. The AUC for using neopterin to distinguish between viral from bacterial LRTI was 0.832. When neopterin was used in combination with CRP and CRPxPCT the AUCs were 0.857 and 0.856, respectively.[71]

In patients with COPD, no difference was found in neopterin levels between different clinical states including stability, exacerbations and pneumonia. However, neopterin was increased and its mean values were 17.1 ng/mL, 17.4 ng/mL and 22.3 ng/mL, respectively. Additionally, neopterin levels were significantly increased during COPD exacerbations when the culture result was normal flora or negative, indicating a possible viral etiology. It should be noted that neopterin also increased 1 month after the exacerbation during the recovery phase. It was independently associated with 2-year survival and significantly correlated with the time to next exacerbation.[72] Regarding other nonviral respiratory infections, neopterin levels were found to be significantly increased in patients with Legionellosis, and *Pneumocystis jirovecii* pneumonia.[73]

Neopterin levels were also assessed in patients with influenza. The mean concentration was 18.8±11.9 nmol/L and it was significantly increased in comparison with healthy controls.[74] In patients with severe acute respiratory syndrome (SARS), neopterin mean concentration was 34.2±20 nmol/L. Neopterin increased from the first day, reached its peak on day 3, remained high for 8 days and fell below 10 nmol/L after 11 days of the onset of symptoms. It may be explained by the activation of the cellular immune system due to viral replication and cytolysis. After seroconversion and attenuation of viral replication occurs, neopterin concentration decreases to normal. It should also be noted that higher levels were associated with longer fever period. Thus, neopterin levels could be used as an indicator of SARS severity.[75]

In patients with tuberculosis, neopterin was measured in blood, urine, BAL and pleural fluid in several studies. In table 2, there is a summary of such studies, reporting neopterin concentrations in various body fluids. Neopterin mean values in serum varied from 20.6 nmol/L to 69.5 nmol/L.[76-81] Neopterin mean values in urine, pleural and BAL fluid varied from 718.5 µmol/mol to 759.2 µmol/mol creatinine,[77,78] 39 nmol/L to 42 nmol/L,[77,81] and 33.36 nmol/L to 88.6 nmol/L,[78,80] respectively. All studies comparing neopterin levels in patients with tuberculosis compared to other groups including patients with cancer, other diseases or healthy individuals, the former had significantly higher levels.[77,78,80,81] It should be noted that serum levels were roughly equal to pleural fluid levels. BAL fluid neopterin levels were suggested to indicate the degree of disease activity in patients with tuberculosis.[80]

Measurement of neopterin concentration may be a useful tool for monitoring the efficacy of treatment and the compliance of patients with tuberculosis. In HIV-negative patients with active pulmonary tuberculosis receiving treatment for 6 months, neopterin levels decreased from a mean pretreatment value of 69.5 nmol/L to 12.9 nmol/L at the end of treatment.[76] Likewise, in HIV-positive patients with tuberculosis, neopterin levels decreased from a mean pretreatment value of 39.9 nmol/L to almost normal range at the end of treatment.[79] A possible explanation of the marginally increased values of neopterin at the end of anti-tuberculosis treatment may be the presence of scant amounts of antigens which continue to trigger a limited cell-mediated immune response and the subsequent low neopterin release.

Key Points

- Neopterin is of clinical value in conditions associated with cell-mediated immunity
- Neopterin increases in infections caused by intracellular bacteria and viruses
- Neopterin is useful in distinguishing between bacterial and viral etiology of LRTIs
- Neopterin is useful for monitoring the efficacy of treatment and the compliance of patients with tuberculosis.

PRESEPSIN

Cluster of Differentiation 14 (CD14) is a gene encoding a protein taking part in the innate immune response. This protein is mostly expressed in macrophages and monocytes. Its role lies mainly in mediating bacterial phagocytosis by inducing cytokine secretion. The induction of cytokine secretion takes place after the ligation of CD14 with bacterial lipopolysaccharide (LPS). LPS cannot directly bind to CD14. This is done with the help of LPS binding protein (LBP). Then the LPS-LBP compound binds to CD14 and subsequently to Toll-Like Receptor 4 (TLR-4) to stimulate the immune response.[82]

CD14 is integrated into the cellular membrane. However, it may be also found in a soluble form. Soluble CD14 is produced in two ways. It may either be released by monocytes or cut-off from the membrane. In both cases, it lacks the glycosylphosphatidylinositol moiety, by which it is integrated into the membrane. CD14 in its soluble form is also called presepsin and has an increasing role in diagnosing sepsis.[83]

TABLE 2

Studies Reporting Neopterin Concentrations in Various Body Fluids of Patients with Tuberculosis

Study (Ref)	Serum mean ± SD (nmol/L)	Urine mean ± SD (µmol/mol creatinine)	Pleural mean ± SD (nmol/L)	BAL fluid mean ± SD (nmol/L)	Assay
Turgut[76]	69.5 ± 29.4	NR	NR	NR	ELISA
Tozkoparan[77]	38.3 ± 14.2	759.2 ± 622.7	39 ± 14.2	NR	HPLC
Yuksekol[78]	20.6 ± 12.1	718.5 ± 594.4	NR	33.3 ± 18.6	HPLC
Immanuel[79]	39.9 (range 32.1–47.7)	NR	NR	NR	HPLC
Mohamed[80]	61.3 ± 29.4	NR	NR	88.6 ± 27.4	RIA
Baganha[81]	41.3 ± 25	NR	42 ± 23	NR	RIA

SD, standard deviation; BAL, bronchoalveolar lavage; NR, not reported; HPLC, high-performance liquid chromatography; RIA, radioimmunoassay.

Presepsin, as well as its integrated counterpart, may bind with high affinity with the LPS. Thus, it may have a dual role in generating the immune response. First, it may facilitate the response of cells that lack the integrated CD14 protein by helping in binding the LPS to TLR-4. Its high affinity for LPS and its high quantities during inflammation may detain a compelling response by competing with membrane CD14 for LPS.[84] However, when its concentration increases over a certain threshold it may have a pathogenic role in sepsis.[85]

Presepsin mean serum levels in healthy individuals vary depending on the method used, which may be either ELISA or a rapid method using chemiluminescence enzyme immunoassay. With ELISA, mean serum levels in healthy individuals are about 3 ng/mL in adults and 7 ng/mL in children.[86,87] With rapid testing, mean serum levels in healthy individuals are 160 pg/mL.[88] Presepsin increases in various conditions both infectious and noninfectious including sepsis, AIDS, systemic lupus erythematosus, severe burns, malaria and acute respiratory distress syndrome.[89,90]

Several studies were conducted regarding the variations of presepsin levels and its role in the pathogenicity of diseases. In vitro, presepsin was suggested to be upregulated by LPS stimulation. The initial effect of LPS stimulation started after 6–15 hours. Except LPS, other bacterial wall components were found to have a similar effect.[91] Comparable findings regarding presepsin increase during the first hours after sepsis onset *in vivo* are reported elsewhere.[90]

In animal studies, it was suggested that *Streptococcus pneumoniae* specifically uses presepsin in the bronchoalveolar compartment to cause invasive disease by a TLR-independent mechanism.[92] Also, it was found that presepsin in cerebrospinal fluid may have an important role in the pathogenesis of bacterial meningitis. Its concentration increases after induction by bacterial constituents and contributes, in turn, in a markedly increased local cytokine response.[93]

In human studies, presepsin was found to be increased in smokers and patients with COPD. However, the increase was considered more of an inhibitory mechanism to prevent an overwhelming inflammatory response.[84] It was also found to reach high concentrations in the lungs of patients with ARDS. More specifically, presepsin levels in the bronchoalveolar lavage fluid were found to be strongly related to total protein, and polymorphonuclear neutrophil concentration, suggesting a contribution of presepsin to lung inflammation in ARDS.[94] In Japanese children, *CD14-550 C/T* was associated with RSV bronchiolitis. This finding suggests that the varying roles of presepsin in the pathogenicity of diseases may be determined by different genetic factors.[95]

Presepsin has been evaluated in the diagnosis of several conditions. In table 3, there is a summary of studies assessing presepsin either alone or in comparison with other biomarkers in sepsis and various diseases. In terms of the AUC for presepsin compared to other biomarkers, it varied from 0.817 to 0.998. It scored better than other biomarkers including PCT, IL-6 and others. Sensitivity varied from 80.1% to 87.8% and specificity varied from 81% to 81.4%. However, the cut-off values, which were used, varied considerably.

A common outcome among different studies was that presepsin levels were significantly higher in patients with sepsis compared to healthy individuals, non-septic patients or patients with other conditions, including SIRS.[96-98] Regarding pediatric patients, presepsin

TABLE 3

Summary of Studies Assessing Presepsin in Sepsis and Various Diseases

Study (Ref)	Setting	AUC	Mean ± SD (median)	Sensitivity (cut-off)	Specificity (cut-off)	Assay
Endo[96]	Sepsis	0.908	(1579 pg/mL)	87.8% (600 pg/mL)	81.4% (600 pg/mL)	Pathfast
Shozushima[98]	Sepsis	0.845	817.9 ± 572.7 pg/mL	80.1% (415 pg/mL)	81% (415 pg/mL)	Pathfast
Marcos[83]	Pneumonia in children	0.998	(1433 ng/mL)	93.6% (8444 ng/mL)	100% (8444 ng/mL)	ELISA
Yaegashi[90]	Sepsis	0.817	(220.7 ng/mL)	—	—	ELISA
Okamura[97]	Sepsis	—	2363 ± 2161 pg/mL	—	—	Pathfast
Burgmann[99]	Gram (+) sepsis	—	4.86 ± 0.36 μg/mL	—	—	ELISA
Landmann[100]	Gram (-) septic shock	—	(3.23 μg/mL)	—	—	ELISA Western blot

AUC, area under the ROC curve; SD: standard deviation.

concentration was significantly higher in children with pneumonia compared to children with cystic fibrosis, and asthma.[83] Patients with severe sepsis were reported to have presepsin levels up to 1992.9±1509.2, which were more than double that of patients with sepsis.[98] An interesting finding was that in patients with Gram (-) sepsis presepsin levels were significantly higher at the day of diagnosis compared to other groups. Also, as time progressed presepsin levels of patients with Gram (+) sepsis who did not survive were significantly higher than of those who survived.[99] A similar finding was suggested in patients with Gram (-) septic shock, whose presepsin levels had a prognostic value.[100] It should be noted that fluctuations in the presepsin concentrations correlated positively with the clinical diagnosis of sepsis and the success of therapy, respectively.[90]

Currently, there are no studies focusing on optimizing treatment duration with presepsin-based algorithms. Its importance lies in using presepsin as a diagnostic tool.

Key Points

- Presepsin is useful as a biomarker in the diagnosis of sepsis
- Presepsin levels may have a prognostic value for sepsis
- Presepsin levels in patients with Gram (-) sepsis are significantly higher at the day of diagnosis compared to other groups of patients
- Presepsin may also increase in noninfectious conditions.

sTREM-1

Triggering receptor expressed on myeloid cells-1 belongs to the immunoglobulin superfamily and is expressed on the surface of immune cells, like neutrophils, monocytes and macrophages. TREM-1 is an activating receptor signaling pathways in amplifying the inflammatory response. It is expressed on phagocytes after exposure to infectious agents. It has been intensely investigated during the past few years for its role in innate immunity and inflammatory response to bacterial infection.

Activation of TREM-1 by an agonistic TREM-1 antibody results in an increase in cytokine and chemokine secretion. Treatment of monocytes with the same antibody results in increased expression of molecules related to antigen presentation and T-cell activation. Although its natural ligand is unknown, Toll-like receptor agonists stimulate TREM-1 upregulation and function. TREM-1 blockade attenuates inflammation and may decrease bacterial sepsis mortality. Altered TREM-1 expression on neutrophils after exposure to bacterial products is a factor of susceptibility to bacterial infection.[101]

The soluble form of TREM-1 (sTREM-1) is released from activated phagocytes and can be found in plasma, urine, cerebrospinal fluid, alveolar lining fluid and pleural fluid. Since infectious agents stimulate expression of TREM-1 and release of sTREM-1, it may serve as a more direct marker of infection than CRP and PCT. Data on the diagnostic value of sTREM-1 are contradicting. A recent meta-analysis showed that plasma sTREM-1 had a moderate diagnostic performance in differentiating sepsis from SIRS, with a sensitivity of 79% and a specificity of 80% (AUC=0.87), thus making it insufficient as a single marker for the diagnosis of sepsis.[102] There are also recent reports of elevated plasma sTREM-1 in noninfectious inflammatory diseases like trauma, pancreatitis, heart surgery and cardiac arrest,[103] which are in agreement with the moderate specificity of sTREM-1 as a biomarker for sepsis. However, sTREM-1 kinetics in sepsis may have predictive value. A prospective study in critically ill patients with sepsis, severe sepsis or septic shock found that an elevated baseline sTREM-1 level was an independent protective factor, while a progressive decline of plasma sTREM-1 concentration correlated with a favorable outcome.[104] Recent studies confirm these findings, reporting that sTREM-1 levels reflect the severity of sepsis more accurately than those of CRP and PCT and are more sensitive for dynamic evaluations of sepsis prognosis[105-107] In a recent study, urine sTREM-1 was investigated for its possible diagnostic value for sepsis. The investigators reported that urine sTREM-1 is more sensitive than WBC, serum CRP and serum PCT for the early diagnosis of sepsis, as well as for dynamic assessments of severity and prognosis and it might also serve as an early index of acute kidney injury in sepsis patients.[108]

The value of sTREM-1 has also been investigated in the diagnosis of local infections. sTREM-1 determination in bronchoalveolar lavage fluid correctly classified pulmonary versus nonpulmonary origin of sepsis in 93% of patients in a medical intensive care unit. Even when PCT concentration remained low, sTREM-1 assessment allowed for the detection of sepsis due to ventilator-associated pneumonia in 50% of cases.[109] sTREM-1 in pleural fluid has been shown to have a good diagnostic accuracy for bacterial pleural effusions.[110,111] sTREM-1 determination in fine needle aspiration fluid in patients with severe acute pancreatitis might help in diagnosing infected necrosis according to a recent study.[112]

As sTREM-1 comprise a promising field of investigation in the diagnosis and treatment of severe sepsis and chronic inflammation, till date none of the proposed biomarkers had sufficient sensitivity and specificity to diagnose sepsis over SIRS in critically ill patients, but rather a combination of several biomarkers should be used for improved diagnostic accuracy.[113]

Key Points

- sTREM-1 in combination with other markers may help in diagnosing sepsis
- sTREM-1 kinetics in sepsis may have predictive value
- Elevated baseline sTREM-1 levels may be a protective factor, while a progressive decline of plasma sTREM-1 concentration correlate with a favorable outcome in patients with sepsis.

CONCLUSION

Novel biomarkers may prove to be a useful arrow in the clinician's quiver in the diagnosis and treatment of respiratory infections. Each one of them may help in different aspects of disease management including differential diagnosis, predictor of severity or mortality, etc. However, one should keep in mind that none of them can be separately used safely. Biomarkers are tools that should always be used in conjunction with each other and with clinical signs and imaging findings to ensure maximal efficacy and have an impact on the patient's course.

REFERENCES

1. Oczenski W, Fitzgerald RD, Schwarz S. Procalcitonin: a new parameter for the diagnosis of bacterial infection in the peri-operative period. *Eur J Anaesthesiol.* 1998;15(2):202-9.
2. Dandona P, Nix D, Wilson MF, et al. Procalcitonin increase after endotoxin injection in normal subjects. *JClinEndocrinol Metab.* 1994;79(6):1605-8.
3. Nijsten MW, Olinga P, The TH, et al. Procalcitonin behaves as a fast responding acute phase protein in vivo and in vitro. *Crit Care Med.* 2000;28(2):458-61.
4. Maruna P, Nedelnikova K, Gurlich R. Physiology and genetics of procalcitonin. *Physiol Res.* 2000;49(Suppl 1):S57-61.
5. Meisner M, Lohs T, Huettemann E, et al. The plasma elimination rate and urinary secretion of procalcitonin in patients with normal and impaired renal function. *Eur J Anaesthesiol.* 2001;18(2):79-87.
6. Perren A, Cerutti B, Lepori M, et al. Influence of steroids on procalcitonin and C-reactive protein in patients with COPD and community-acquired pneumonia. *Infection.* 2008;36(2):163-6.
7. Schuetz P, Albrich W, Christ-Crain M, et al. Procalcitonin for guidance of antibiotic therapy. *Expert Rev Anti Infect Ther.* 2010;8(5):575-87.
8. Muller B, Harbarth S, Stolz D, et al. Diagnostic and prognostic accuracy of clinical and laboratory parameters in community-acquired pneumonia. *BMC Infect Dis.* 2007;7:10.
9. Horie M, Ugajin M, Suzuki M, et al. Diagnostic and prognostic value of procalcitonin in community-acquired pneumonia. *The Am J Med Sci.* 2012;343(1):30-5.
10. Kasamatsu Y, Yamaguchi T, Kawaguchi T, et al. Usefulness of a semi-quantitative procalcitonin test and the A-DROP Japanese prognostic scale for predicting mortality among adults hospitalized with community-acquired pneumonia. *Respirology.* 2012;17(2):330-6.
11. Schuetz P, Suter-Widmer I, Chaudri A, et al. Prognostic value of procalcitonin in community-acquired pneumonia. *Eur Respir J.* 2011;37(2):384-92.
12. Park JH, Wee JH, Choi SP, et al. The value of procalcitonin level in community-acquired pneumonia in the ED. *Am J Emerg Med.* 2012;30(7):1248-54.
13. Kruger S, Ewig S, Papassotiriou J, et al. Inflammatory parameters predict etiologic patterns but do not allow for individual prediction of etiology in patients with CAP: results from the German competence network CAPNETZ. *Respir Res.* 2009;10:65.
14. Menendez R, Cavalcanti M, Reyes S, et al. Markers of treatment failure in hospitalised community acquired pneumonia. *Thorax.* 2008;63(5):447-52.
15. Ramirez P, Garcia MA, Ferrer M, et al. Sequential measurements of procalcitonin levels in diagnosing ventilator-associated pneumonia. *Eur Respir J.* 2008;31(2):356-62.
16. Luyt CE, Guerin V, Combes A, et al. Procalcitonin kinetics as a prognostic marker of ventilator-associated pneumonia. *Am J Respir Crit Care Med.* 2005;171(1):48-53.
17. Seligman R, Meisner M, Lisboa TC, et al. Decreases in procalcitonin and C-reactive protein are strong predictors of survival in ventilator-associated pneumonia. *Crit Care.* 2006;10(5):R125.
18. Bafadhel M, Clark TW, Reid C, et al. Procalcitonin and C-reactive protein in hospitalized adult patients with community-acquired pneumonia or exacerbation of asthma or COPD. *Chest.* 2011;139(6):1410-8.
19. Falsey AR, Becker KL, Swinburne AJ, et al. Utility of serum procalcitonin values in patients with acute exacerbations of chronic obstructive pulmonary disease: a cautionary note. *Int J Chron Obstruct Pulmon Dis.* 2012;7:127-35.
20. Chang C, Yao WZ, Chen YH, et al. The changes and clinical implications of serum procalcitonin in acute exacerbations of chronic obstructive pulmonary disease. *Zhonghua Jie He He Hu Xi Za Zhi.* 2006;29(7):444-7.
21. Daubin C, Parienti JJ, Fradin S, et al. Procalcitonin levels and bacterial aetiology among COPD patients admitted to the ICU with severe pneumonia: a prospective cohort study. *BMC Infect Dis.* 2009;9:157.
22. Rammaert B, Verdier N, Cavestri B, et al. Procalcitonin as a prognostic factor in severe acute exacerbation of chronic obstructive pulmonary disease. *Respirology.* 2009;14(7):969-74.
23. Ahn S, Kim WY, Kim SH, et al. Role of procalcitonin and C-reactive protein in differentiation of mixed bacterial infection from 2009 H1N1 viral pneumonia. *Influenza Other Respir Viruses.* 2011;5(6):398-403.
24. Song JY, Cheong HJ, Heo JY, et al. Clinical, laboratory and radiologic characteristics of 2009 pandemic influenza A/H1N1 pneumonia: primary influenza pneumonia versus concomitant/secondary bacterial pneumonia. *Influenza Other Respir Viruses.* 2011;5(6):e535-43.
25. Piacentini E, Sanchez B, Arauzo V, et al. Procalcitonin levels are lower in intensive care unit patients with

H1N1 influenza A virus pneumonia than in those with community-acquired bacterial pneumonia. A pilot study. *J Crit Care.* 2011;26(2):201-5.

26. Cuquemelle E, Soulis F, Villers D, et al. Can procalcitonin help identify associated bacterial infection in patients with severe influenza pneumonia? A multicentre study. *Intensive Care Med.* 2011;37(5):796-800.
27. Ingram PR, Inglis T, Moxon D, et al. Procalcitonin and C-reactive protein in severe 2009 H1N1 influenza infection. *Intensive Car Med.* 2010;36(3):528-32.
28. Toikka P, Irjala K, Juven T, et al. Serum procalcitonin, C-reactive protein and interleukin-6 for distinguishing bacterial and viral pneumonia in children. *Pediatr Infect Dis J.* 2000;19(7):598-602.
29. Moulin F, Raymond J, Lorrot M, et al. Procalcitonin in children admitted to hospital with community acquired pneumonia. *Arch Dis Child.* 2001;84(4):332-6.
30. Diez-Padrisa N, Bassat Q, Machevo S, et al. Procalcitonin and C-reactive protein for invasive bacterial pneumonia diagnosis among children in Mozambique, a malaria-endemic area. *PLoS One.* 2010;5(10):e13226.
31. Rasmussen TA, Sogaard OS, Camara C, et al. Serum procalcitonin in pulmonary tuberculosis. *Int J Tuberc Lung Dis.* 2011;15(2):251-6.
32. Kang YA, Kwon SY, Yoon HI, et al. Role of C-reactive protein and procalcitonin in differentiation of tuberculosis from bacterial community acquired pneumonia. *Korean J Intern Med.* 2009;24(4):337-42.
33. Ugajin M, Miwa S, Shirai M, et al. Usefulness of serum procalcitonin levels in pulmonary tuberculosis. *Eur Respir J.* 2011;37(2):371-5.
34. Cakir E, Deniz O, Ozcan O, et al. Pleural fluid and serum procalcitonin as diagnostic tools in tuberculous pleurisy. *Clin Biochem.* 2005;38(3):234-8.
35. Nyamande K, Lalloo UG. Serum procalcitonin distinguishes CAP due to bacteria, mycobacterium tuberculosis and PJP. *Int J Tuberc Dis.* 2006;10(5):510-5.
36. Schleicher GK, Herbert V, Brink A, et al. Procalcitonin and C-reactive protein levels in HIV-positive subjects with tuberculosis and pneumonia. *Eur Respir J.* 2005;25(4):688-92.
37. Li H, Luo YF, Blackwell TS, et al. Meta-analysis and systematic review of procalcitonin-guided therapy in respiratory tract infections. *Antimicrob Agents Chemother.* 2011;55(12):5900-6.
38. Schuetz P, Briel M, Christ-Crain M, et al. Procalcitonin to guide initiation and duration of antibiotic treatment in acute respiratory infections: an individual patient data meta-analysis. *Clin Infect Dis.* 2012;55(5):651-62.
39. Heyland DK, Johnson AP, Reynolds SC, et al. Procalcitonin for reduced antibiotic exposure in the critical care setting: a systematic review and an economic evaluation. *Crit Care Med.* 2011;39(7):1792-9.
40. Christ-Crain M, Müller B. Biomarkers in respiratory tract infections: diagnostic guides to antibiotic prescription, prognostic markers and mediators. *Eur Respir J.* 2007;30(3):556-73.
41. Eto T. A review of the biological properties and clinical implications of adrenomedullin and proadrenomedullin N-terminal 20 peptide (PAMP), hypotensive and vasodilating peptides. *Peptides.* 2001;22(11):1693-711.
42. Marutsuka K, Nawa Y, Asada Y, et al. Adrenomedullin and proadrenomudullin N-terminal 20 peptide (PAMP) are present in human colonic epithelia and exert an antimicrobial effect. *Exp Physiol.* 2001;86(5):543-5.
43. Shimekake Y, Nagata K, Ohta S, et al. Adrenomedullin stimulates two signal transduction pathways, cAMP accumulation and Ca2+ mobilization, in bovine aortic endothelial cells. *J Biol Chem.* 1995;270(9):4412-7.
44. Wang P, Ba ZF, Cioffi WG, et al. The pivotal role of adrenomedullin in producing hyperdynamic circulation during the early stage of sepsis. *Arch Surg.* 1998;133(12):1298-304.
45. Wang P, Zhou M, Ba ZF, et al. Up-regulation of a novel potent vasodilatory peptide adrenomedullin during polymicrobial sepsis. *Shock.* 1998;10(2):118-22.
46. Gonzalez-Rey E, Chorny A, Varela N, et al. Urocortin and adrenomedullin prevent lethal endotoxemia by down-regulating the inflammatory response. *Am J Pathol.* 2006;168(6):1921-30.
47. Temmesfeld-Wollbruck B, Brell B, David I, et al. Adrenomedullin reduces vascular hyperpermeability and improves survival in rat septic shock. *Intensive Care Med.* 2007;33(4):703-10.
48. Wang P, Yoo P, Zhou M, et al. Reduction in vascular responsiveness to adrenomedullin during sepsis. *J Surg Rese.* 1999;85(1):59-65.
49. Marutsuka K, Hatakeyama K, Sato Y, et al. Immunohistological localization and possible functions of adrenomedullin. *Hypertens Res.* 2003;26(Suppl):S33-40.
50. Hinson JP, Kapas S, Smith DM. Adrenomedullin, a multifunctional regulatory peptide. *Endocr Rev.* 2000;21(2):138-67.
51. Caruhel P, Mazier C, Kunde J, et al. Homogeneous time-resolved fluoroimmunoassay for the measurement of midregional proadrenomedullin in plasma on the fully automated system B.R.A.H.M.S KRYPTOR. *Clinical Biochem.* 2009;42(7-8):725-8.
52. Morgenthaler NG, Struck J, Alonso C, et al. Measurement of midregional proadrenomedullin in plasma with an immunoluminometric assay. *Clin Chem.* 2005;51(10):1823-9.
53. Smith JG, Newton-Cheh C, Hedblad B, et al. Distribution and correlates of midregional proadrenomedullin in the general population. *Clin Chem.* 2009;55(8):1593-5.
54. de Kruif MD, Lemaire LC, Giebelen IA, et al. The influence of corticosteroids on the release of novel biomarkers in human endotoxemia. *Intensive Care Med.* 2008;34(3):518-22.
55. Suberviola B, Castellanos-Ortega A, Llorca J, et al. Prognostic value of proadrenomedullin in severe sepsis and septic shock patients with community-acquired pneumonia. *Swiss Med Wkly.* 2012;142:w13542.
56. Christ-Crain M, Morgenthaler NG, Stolz D, et al. Pro-adrenomedullin to predict severity and outcome in community-acquired pneumonia [ISRCTN04176397]. *Crit Care.* 2006;10(3):R96.
57. Bello S, Lasierra AB, Minchole E, et al. Prognostic power of proadrenomedullin in community-acquired pneumonia is independent of aetiology. *Eur Respir J.* 2012;39(5):1144-55.
58. Guertler C, Wirz B, Christ-Crain M, et al. Inflammatory responses predict long-term mortality risk in community-acquired pneumonia. *Eur Respir J.* 2011;37(6):1439-46.

59. Huang DT, Angus DC, Kellum JA, et al. Midregional proadrenomedullin as a prognostic tool in community-acquired pneumonia. *Chest.* 2009;136(3):823-31.
60. Kruger S, Ewig S, Giersdorf S, et al. Cardiovascular and inflammatory biomarkers to predict short- and long-term survival in community-acquired pneumonia: results from the German Competence Network, CAPNETZ. *Am J Respir Crit Care Med.* 2010;182(11):1426-34.
61. Schuetz P, Wolbers M, Christ-Crain M, et al. Prohormones for prediction of adverse medical outcome in community-acquired pneumonia and lower respiratory tract infections. *Crit Care.* 2010;14(3):R106.
62. Albrich WC, Dusemund F, Ruegger K, et al. Enhancement of CURB65 score with proadrenomedullin (CURB65-A) for outcome prediction in lower respiratory tract infections: derivation of a clinical algorithm. *BMC Infect Dis.* 2011;11:112.
63. Stolz D, Christ-Crain M, Morgenthaler NG, et al. Plasma pro-adrenomedullin but not plasma pro-endothelin predicts survival in exacerbations of COPD. *Chest.* 2008;134(2):263-72.
64. Werner ER, Werner-Felmayer G, Fuchs D, et al. Tetrahydrobiopterin biosynthetic activities in human macrophages, fibroblasts, THP-1, and T 24 cells. GTP-cyclohydrolase I is stimulated by interferon-gamma, and 6-pyruvoyl tetrahydropterin synthase and sepiapterin reductase are constitutively present. *J Biol Chem.* 1990; 265(6):3189-92.
65. Huber C, Batchelor JR, Fuchs D, et al. Immune response-associated production of neopterin. Release from macrophages primarily under control of interferon-gamma. *J Exp Med.* 1984;160(1):310-6.
66. Millner MM, Franthal W, Thalhammer GH, et al. Neopterin concentrations in cerebrospinal fluid and serum as an aid in differentiating central nervous system and peripheral infections in children. *Clinical Chem.* 1998;44(1):161-7.
67. Berdowska A, Zwirska-Korczala K. Neopterin measurement in clinical diagnosis. *J Clin Pharm Ther.* 2001; 26(5): 319-29.
68. Hagberg L, Dotevall L, Norkrans G, et al. Cerebrospinal fluid neopterin concentrations in central nervous system infection. *J Infect Dis.* 1993;168(5):1285-8.
69. Werner ER, Bichler A, Daxenbichler G, et al. Determination of neopterin in serum and urine. *Clin Chem.* 1987;33(1): 62-6.
70. Oda K, Arai T, Nagase M. Increased serum and urinary neopterin in nephrotic syndrome indicate cell-mediated immune dysfunction. *Am J Kidney Dis.* 1999;34(4):611-7.
71. Ip M, Rainer TH, Lee N, et al. Value of serum procalcitonin, neopterin, and C-reactive protein in differentiating bacterial from viral etiologies in patients presenting with lower respiratory tract infections. *Diagn Microbiol Infect Dis.* 2007;59(2):131-6.
72. Lacoma A, Prat C, Andreo F, et al. Value of procalcitonin, C-reactive protein, and neopterin in exacerbations of chronic obstructive pulmonary disease. *Int J Chron Obstruct Pulmon Dis.* 2011;6:157-69.
73. Prat C, Dominguez J, Andreo F, et al. Procalcitonin and neopterin correlation with aetiology and severity of pneumonia. *J Infect.* 2006;52(3):169-77.
74. Chan CP, Choi JW, Cao KY, et al. Detection of serum neopterin for early assessment of dengue virus infection. *J Infect.* 2006;53(3):152-8.
75. Zheng B, Cao KY, Chan CP, et al. Serum neopterin for early assessment of severity of severe acute respiratory syndrome. *Clin Immunol.* 2005;116(1):18-26.
76. Turgut T, Akbulut H, Deveci F, et al. Serum interleukin-2 and neopterin levels as useful markers for treatment of active pulmonary tuberculosis. *Tohoku J Exp Med.* 2006;209(4):321-8.
77. Tozkoparan E, Deniz O, Cakir E, et al. The diagnostic values of serum, pleural fluid and urine neopterin measurements in tuberculous pleurisy. *Int J Tuberc Lung Dis.* 2005;9(9):1040-5.
78. Yuksekol I, Ozkan M, Akgul O, et al. Urinary neopterin measurement as a non-invasive diagnostic method in pulmonary tuberculosis. *Int J Tuberc Lung Dis.* 2003;7(8):771-6.
79. Immanuel C, Rajeswari R, Rahman F, et al. Serial evaluation of serum neopterin in HIV seronegative patients treated for tuberculosis. *Int J Tuberc Lung Dis.* 2001;5(2):185-90.
80. Mohamed KH, Mobasher AA, Yousef AR, et al. BAL neopterin: a novel marker for cell-mediated immunity in patients with pulmonary tuberculosis and lung cancer. *Chest.* 2001;119(3):776-80.
81. Baganha MF, Mota-Pinto A, Pego MA, et al. Neopterin in tuberculous and neoplastic pleural fluids. *Lung.* 1992;170(3):155-61.
82. Hailman E, Vasselon T, Kelley M, et al. Stimulation of macrophages and neutrophils by complexes of lipopolysaccharide and soluble CD14. *J Immunol.* 1996;156(11): 4384-90.
83. Marcos V, Latzin P, Hector A, et al. Expression, regulation and clinical significance of soluble and membrane CD14 receptors in pediatric inflammatory lung diseases. *Respir Res.* 2010;11:32.
84. Regueiro V, Campos MA, Morey P, et al. Lipopolysaccharide-binding protein and CD14 are increased in the bronchoalveolar lavage fluid of smokers. *Eur Respir J.* 2009;33(2):273-81.
85. Landmann R, Reber AM, Sansano S, et al. Function of soluble CD14 in serum from patients with septic shock. *J Infect Dis.* 1996;173(3):661-8.
86. Sack U, Burkhardt U, Borte M, et al. Age-dependent levels of select immunological mediators in sera of healthy children. *Clin Diagn Lab Immunol.* 1998;5(1):28-32.
87. Grunwald U, Kruger C, Westermann J, et al. An enzyme-linked immunosorbent assay for the quantification of solubilized CD14 in biological fluids. *J Immunol Methods.* 1992;155(2):225-32.
88. Spanuth E, Wilhelm J, Loppnow H, et al. Diagnostic and Prognostic Value of Presepsin (Soluble CD14 Subtype) in Emergency Patients with Early Sepsis Using the New Assay PATHFAST Presepsin. IFCC World Lab/EuroMedLab Proceedings; 2011.
89. Wenisch C, Wenisch H, Parschalk B, et al. Elevated levels of soluble CD14 in serum of patients with acute Plasmodium falciparum malaria. *Clin Exp Immunol.* 1996;105(1):74-8.
90. Yaegashi Y, Shirakawa K, Sato N, et al. Evaluation of a newly identified soluble CD14 subtype as a marker for sepsis. *J Infect Chemother.* 2005;11(5):234-8.

91. Landmann R, Knopf HP, Link S, et al. Human monocyte CD14 is upregulated by lipopolysaccharide. *Infect Immun.* 1996;64(5):1762-9.
92. Dessing MC, Knapp S, Florquin S, et al. CD14 facilitates invasive respiratory tract infection by Streptococcus pneumoniae. *Am J Respir Crit Care Med.* 2007;175(6):604-11.
93. Cauwels A, Frei K, Sansano S,et al. The origin and function of soluble CD14 in experimental bacterial meningitis. *J Immunol.* 1999;162(8):4762-72.
94. Martin TR, Rubenfeld GD, Ruzinski JT, et al. Relationship between soluble CD14, lipopolysaccharide binding protein, and the alveolar inflammatory response in patients with acute respiratory distress syndrome. *Am J Respir Crit Care Med.* 1997;155(3):937-44.
95. Inoue Y, Shimojo N, Suzuki Y, et al. CD14-550 C/T, which is related to the serum level of soluble CD14, is associated with the development of respiratory syncytial virus bronchiolitis in the Japanese population. *J Infect Dis.* 2007;195(11):1618-24.
96. Endo S, Suzuki Y, Takahashi G, et al. Usefulness of presepsin in the diagnosis of sepsis in a multicenter prospective study. *J Infect Chemother.* 2012;18(6):891-7.
97. Okamura Y, Yokoi H. Development of a point-of-care assay system for measurement of presepsin (sCD14-ST). *Clin Chim Acta.* 2011;412(23-24):2157-61.
98. Shozushima T, Takahashi G, Matsumoto N, et al. Usefulness of presepsin (sCD14-ST) measurements as a marker for the diagnosis and severity of sepsis that satisfied diagnostic criteria of systemic inflammatory response syndrome. *J Infect Chemother.* 2011;17(6):764-9.
99. Burgmann H, Winkler S, Locker GJ, et al. Increased serum concentration of soluble CD14 is a prognostic marker in gram-positive sepsis. *Clin Immunol Immunopatholo.* 1996;80(3 Pt 1):307-10.
100. Landmann R, Zimmerli W, Sansano S, et al. Increased circulating soluble CD14 is associated with high mortality in gram-negative septic shock. *J Infect Dis.* 1995;171(3):639-44.
101. Sharif O, Knapp S. From expression to signaling: roles of TREM-1 and TREM-2 in innate immunity and bacterial infection. *Immunobiology.* 2008;213(9-10):701-13.
102. Wu Y, Wang F, Fan X, et al. Accuracy of plasma sTREM-1 for sepsis diagnosis in systemic inflammatory patients: a systematic review and meta-analysis. *Crit Care.* 2012;16(6):R229.
103. Adib-Conquy M, Monchi M, Goulenok C, et al. Increased plasma levels of soluble triggering receptor expressed on myeloid cells 1 and procalcitonin after cardiac surgery and cardiac arrest without infection. *Shock.* 2007;28(4):406-10.
104. Gibot S, Cravoisy A, Kolopp-Sarda MN, et al. Time-course of sTREM (soluble triggering receptor expressed on myeloid cells)-1, procalcitonin, and C-reactive protein plasma concentrations during sepsis. *Crit Care Med.* 2005;33(4):792-6.
105. Li L, Zhu Z, Chen J, et al. Diagnostic value of soluble triggering receptor expressed on myeloid cells-1 in critically ill, postoperative patients with suspected sepsis. *Am J Med Sci.* 2013;345(3):178-84.
106. Su L, Han B, Liu C, et al. Value of soluble TREM-1, procalcitonin, and C-reactive protein serum levels as biomarkers for detecting bacteremia among sepsis patients with new fever in intensive care units: a prospective cohort study. *BMC Infect Dis.* 2012;12:157.
107. Zhang J, She D, Feng D, et al. Dynamic changes of serum soluble triggering receptor expressed on myeloid cells-1 (sTREM-1) reflect sepsis severity and can predict prognosis: a prospective study. *BMC Infect Dis.* 2011;11:53.
108. Su LX, Feng L, Zhang J, et al. Diagnostic value of urine sTREM-1 for sepsis and relevant acute kidney injuries: a prospective study. *Crit Care.* 2011;15(5):R250.
109. Gibot S, Cravoisy A, Dupays R, et al. Combined measurement of procalcitonin and soluble TREM-1 in the diagnosis of nosocomial sepsis. *Scand J Infect Dis.* 2007;39(6-7):604-8.
110. Porcel JM, Vives M, Cao G, et al. Biomarkers of infection for the differential diagnosis of pleural effusions. *Eur Respir J.* 2009;34(6):1383-9.
111. Summah H, Tao LL, Zhu YG, et al. Pleural fluid soluble triggering receptor expressed on myeloid cells-1 as a marker of bacterial infection: a meta-analysis. *BMC Infect Dis.* 2011;11:280.
112. Lu Z, Liu Y, Dong YH, et al. Soluble triggering receptor expressed on myeloid cells in severe acute pancreatitis: a biological marker of infected necrosis. *Intensive Care Med.* 2012;38(1):69-75.
113. Gibot S, Bene MC, Noel R, et al. Combination biomarkers to diagnose sepsis in the critically ill patient. *Am J Respir Crit Care Med.* 2012;186(1):65-71.

CHAPTER 24

Vaccine-preventable Respiratory Infections

Gernot GU Rohde

ABSTRACT

Prevention is one of the cornerstones of management of respiratory infections, and vaccines play the most important role in this respect. Currently, there are vaccines available for the prevention of seasonal and pandemic influenza and pneumococcal disease. For seasonal influenza, there are 2 different types of vaccine available, the trivalent, injectable inactivated vaccine (TIV) and the live-attenuated (LAIV) nasal spray flu vaccine. Different formulations of the TIV are available for all ages, whereas the LAIV is approved for use in healthy people of 2–49 years of age, who are not pregnant. These vaccines have a good safety profile and are effective but their efficacy ranges between 30 and 60%. For the prevention of pneumococcal disease, a 23-valent polysaccharide (PPV) vaccine and newer conjugated vaccines are available. Efficacy of PPV against invasive pneumococcal disease ranges between 50 and 70%. PPV seems to be not efficacious against pneumococcal pneumonia in small children or elderly patients. The new conjugated vaccines promise to provide better protection.

INTRODUCTION

Prevention is a cornerstone of management of respiratory infections, and vaccines play the most important role in this respect. Currently, there are vaccines available for the prevention of seasonal and pandemic influenza and pneumococcal disease. We have an experience of more than half a decade with respiratory vaccines and the current pandemics have re-emphasized their importance.

INFLUENZA

Influenza Viruses

Influenza viruses are single-stranded RNA viruses with a segmented genome,[1] belonging to the family of *Orthomyxoviruses*. Segmentation of the genome allows exchange of gene fragments during simultaneous infection of host cells of different species. This phenomenon is called "antigenic shift" and is responsible for the emergence of new serotypes against which there is no or insufficient specific immunity in the population.[2] Depending on the virulence of newly emerged serotypes, epidemics or even pandemics may occur. Such pandemics were observed in 1890, 1900, 1918–19, 1957, 1968, and recently, in 2009 (H1N1).[3] Spontaneous mutations in the viral surface proteins, hemagglutinin, and neuraminidase, are responsible for the so-called "antigenic drift". In case they result in changes of the viral amino acid structure, preexisting antibodies might not or insufficiently be able to bind viral particles.[4] This phenomenon is responsible for the annual flu waves observed worldwide.

Epidemiology

The World Health Organization (WHO) estimated that every year 3–5 million cases of severe infection occur worldwide in high-income countries resulting in additional mortality in the range of 250,000–500,000. Risk groups for the development of serious complications include persons above 65 years of age, persons with chronic medical conditions, persons with conditions that compromise respiratory function or ability to handle secretions, residents of long-term-care facilities, pregnant women, children/adolescents receiving chronic aspirin therapy, and children between 6 months to 5 years of age.[5]

The Vaccines

Seasonal Vaccines

In light of the frequent variations in circulating influenza strains, the composition of the seasonal influenza vaccine has to be adapted to the strains of virus identified, as those likely to be the circulating strains for that particular influenza season.[2] For seasonal influenza, there are 2 different types of vaccine available.

The first one is the trivalent, inactivated vaccine (TIV), which is injected into the muscle of the upper arm or thigh. This trivalent vaccine usually contains an influenza B virus, influenza A (H1N1) virus, and influenza A (H3N2) virus strains. There are different preparations of these vaccines containing either the entire whole inactivated virus (whole virus vaccines), virus particles that have been disrupted by detergents or solvents (split vaccines), or vaccines that only contain purified hemagglutinin and neuraminidase (subunit vaccines).[6]

According to Centers of Disease Control and Prevention (CDC), this so-called "flu shot" is approved for use in subjects older than 6 months, including healthy people and people with chronic medical conditions.[7] There are 3 different formulations of this vaccine:

- The regular flu shot approved for children aged 6 months and older
- The high-dose flu shot approved for subjects, 65 years and older, and
- The intradermal flu shot approved for subjects, 18–64 years of age.

The indication for the regular flu shot has recently changed. Since the beginning of 2010, the Advisory Committee on Immunization Practices (ACIP) has issued the recommendation to vaccinate all persons aged 6 months or older. This so-called "universal vaccination" aims at expanding protection against flu to more people.

The high-dose flu shot contains 4 times the amount of antigen contained in regular flu shots in order to create a stronger immune response in elderly people (approved for people 65 and older).

The intradermal flu vaccine is injected into the skin instead of the muscle. This allows for use of a much smaller needle than the regular flu shot, and it requires fewer antigens to be as effective as the regular flu shot. This vaccine was licensed by the US Food and Drug Administration (FDA) for use in the US for the 2011–2012 flu season and is at the moment approved for people between 18 and 64 years of age.

The second one is the nasal spray flu vaccine, which is a live-attenuated influenza vaccine (LAIV).[8] This type of vaccine was introduced with the idea that a stronger immune response can be obtained in comparison to inactivated vaccines. A meta-analysis of 9 randomized controlled trials indicated that efficacy of LAIVs was significantly higher that TIVs in children.[9]

Live-attenuated vaccines contain viable viral particles with diminished virulence.

It is only approved for use in healthy individuals between 2 and 49 years of age, who are not pregnant. This range can be explained by concerns over wheezing and excess hospitalizations in children younger than 2 years resulting from the pivotal licensure trials.[10] Moreover, a *post hoc* analysis of a critical study showed no efficacy for subjects aged 50–64 years.[11] Due to the fact that this is a LAIV, transmission of the vaccine strains to other persons by close contact is an issue, and it has been observed in approximately 2% of cases.[12] Recent research shows that LAIVs has higher efficacy mainly in young children aged 6 months to 7 years compared to TIV.[13] It is still unclear how these findings will translate into recommendations.

Pandemic Vaccines

After the seasonal flu vaccines, pandemic flu vaccines have been developed.[14] In response to the outbreak of the bird flu in 2004–2005, an H5N1 vaccine was approved by the FDA. This monovalent vaccine contains the A/Vietnam/1203/2004 influenza strain and is not commercially available but has been stockpiled by the Federal Government to be used in the event of a pandemic.[2,14]

Five years later, another pandemic influenza outbreak was recognized. A novel H1N1 strain emerged and a monovalent vaccine using the A/California/07/2009 (H1N1) strain was manufactured within a very short time period. It was approved by the FDA and WHO for prevention of novel H1N1 as an inactivated, adjuvant injectable vaccine, and also as a live-attenuated intranasal formulation.[14,15]

Efficacy

Vaccination is considered to be the most effective strategy to control influenza. This is for 2 reasons: first, the efficacy of antivirals to combat influenza is still low and second, vaccination becomes particularly important when a new subtype or distantly related strain of virus enters the human population causing a worldwide epidemic or pandemic. Depending upon the virulence of the emerging virus, a lack of preexisting immunity could lead to overwhelming morbidity and mortality.[14] In the northern hemisphere, flu vaccination should be performed yearly in October and November. In the southern hemisphere, influenza strains to be included into vaccine are selected in February.[16] The development of an adequate antibody response needs 2 weeks.[17] Protection against infection with vaccine strains is in general good in healthy persons below the age of 60 years and ranges between 70 and 100%.[18] However, a recent Cochrane analysis revealed that effects on outcomes, such as workdays lost and reduction of influenza symptoms were moderate.[19] It was found that in the situation of vaccine matching the viral circulating strain and high circulation, 4% of unvaccinated people compared to 1% of vaccinated people developed influenza symptoms.[19] The corresponding figures for poor vaccine matching were 2% and 1%, respectively.[19] It is estimated that efficacy of flu vaccination is lower in elderly patients, probably due to a phenomenon called "immunosenescence". This refers to the fact that the capacity of the immune system decreases with age. There is a paucity of clinical trials investigating efficacy and effectiveness in the elderly.[20] There seems to be an effect on influenza symptoms but reports on other outcomes, such as reduction of complications like hospital admission or pneumonia, are scarce.[20] In general, efficacy is estimated to range between 30 and 60% among the elderly or young children.[18] However, there are some promising results from more recent studies indicating positive effects on hospitalization rates and mortality.[21,22] Nevertheless, a recent meta-analysis concluded that evidence for protection in adults aged 65 years or older is lacking.[13] Clinical studies are underway to evaluate the efficacy of high-dose vaccines, intradermal vaccines, and adjuvanted vaccines in these populations. Initial results seem to be encouraging.[23] Estimations of the health impact and cost-effectiveness of adjuvantes influenza vaccines have demonstrated that use of these vaccines in older adults and young children would result in clinical benefits and would be economically attractive.[24]

In specific patients groups, such as patients with chronic obstructive pulmonary disease (COPD), a significant reduction in the total number of exacerbations could be demonstrated.[25] Moreover there are reports on the reduction of all-cause mortality in COPD patients.[26] There are a limited number of studies investigating the effects of flu vaccination on asthma exacerbations and there seems to be less effect on this outcome.[27]

Further research is needed to develop more effective seasonal influenza vaccines that provide long-lasting immunity, especially in persons at high-risk of complications, such as elderly patients and patients with immunodeficiency. Another important aspect is to obtain broad protection against strains that differ in their antigen structure from vaccine viruses because selection of optimal vaccine strains remains difficult.[3,28]

Safety

Inactivated influenza vaccines have a favorable safety profile. The most common adverse events include a painful arm and redness at the injection site. Systemic symptoms, such as fever or malaise are less commonly reported.[29]

There has been a concern that flu vaccination could be associated with Guillain-Barré syndrome. A series of large cohort studies showed convincingly that there is no increase in the incidence of Guillain-Barré syndrome after flu vaccination. A recent study from the CDC on vaccination against pandemic flu demonstrated absence of increased risk for Guillain-Barré syndrome.[30] In contrast, there seems to be a protective effect.[31] This is conceivable because influenza-like illnesses themselves seem to be relevant triggering events for GBS.[32]

As far as LAIVs are concerned, the most common adverse events are nasal congestion, headache, myalgias, or fever.[29] Moreover, an increased risk of wheezing in some young children has been reported, and the vaccine is not recommended for children younger than 2 years and between the age of 2 and 4 years with a history of recurrent wheezing or reactive airways disease.[8]

PNEUMOCOCCAL VACCINES

Pneumococci

Streptococcus pneumoniae, often referred to as *Pneumococcus*, is a Gram-positive lancet-shaped bacterium, often presents as pairs (diplococci). The bacterium possesses a capsule composed of polysaccharide that completely envelops the pneumococcal cell.[33] Differences within this polysaccharide structure determine the serotypes, of which 91 different serotypes are known at present. Only a small subset of these serotypes causes the majority of pneumococcal disease worldwide.[34]

Colonization of mucosal surfaces in the upper respiratory tract is considered to be an important step in the pathogenesis of infective disease and has been demonstrated in approximately 40% of the population.[35] Colonization is especially prevalent in children.[36]

Epidemiology

According to WHO, about 14.5 million episodes of serious pneumococcal disease occurred in children aged between 1 and 59 months. On the other side of the age spectrum, more than 500,000 cases of pneumococcal disease were reported in adults above 50 years of age in the US.[37] The CDC reports that data from community-based studies indicate that the overall annual incidence of pneumococcal bacteremia in the US is estimated to be 15–30 cases/100,000 population. Again, this rate is higher for children below 2 years of age (160 cases/100,000 population) and for persons above 65 years of age (50–83 cases/100,000 population).[38]

Polysaccharide Vaccines

The first pneumococcal vaccines were polysaccharide vaccines. The first tetravalent vaccine was introduced as early as 1945 but was not used widely due to emergence of penicillin antibiotics at the same time.[39] Pneumococcal vaccine development was resumed in the late 1960s, because it became clear that penicillin was not able to cure all pneumococcal diseases, and first resistant strain were identified.

In 1977, a pneumococcal polysaccharide vaccine covering 14 serotypes was licenced in the US.[40] Six years later, in 1983, the still available 23-valent polysaccharide vaccine (PPV23) was introduced covering the following capsular polysaccharide antigen serotypes: 1, 2, 3, 4, 5, 6B, 7F, 8, 9N, 9V, 10A, 11A, 12F, 14, 15B, 17F, 18C, 19A, 19F, 20, 22F, 23F, and 33F.[41] They are considered to be responsible for about 95% of invasive pneumococcal infections. The introduction of this vaccine clearly was a step forward. The effectiveness ranges from 50 to 70% prevention of invasive pneumococcal disease (IPD) in elderly persons for vaccine-strains.[42] However, efficacy against all-cause pneumonia could not be convincingly demonstrated.[43] Moreover, children below 2 years of age are not sufficiently protected, because of lack of immunogenicity. A further limitation is the lack of effect on nasopharyngeal pneumococcal carriage.

Possible explanations for these limitations can be found in the immunology of polysaccharide vaccines. Common polysaccharide vaccines induce a B-cell mediated immune response leading to production of protective antibodies by plasma cells. Plasma cells live for up to 4 years only and cannot be boosted. The short life span of plasma cells probably is 1 of the reasons for the so-called hyporesponsiveness observed after revaccination.[42]

Lack of efficacy in children and elderly persons, failure to efficiently prevent pneumococcal pneumonia, waning immunity with age, and comorbidities, as well as the limited duration of protection (2–5 years) associated with the inability to elicit a memory immune response, led to the development of new pneumococcal vaccines.[44]

Conjugated Vaccines

Conjugated pneumococcal vaccines consist of serotype-specific polysaccharide that is chemically linked (conjugated) to a protein carrier; for example diphtheria toxoid, tetanus toxoid, or non-typable *Haemophilus influenzae* proteins. This conjugated vaccine is then able to elicit T-cell-dependent responses and induce immunologic memory in addition to the induction of antibodies by plasma cells. In 2000, the first conjugated pneumococcal vaccine was introduced, covering 7 serotypes (PCV7: 4, 6B, 9V, 14, 18C, 19F, and 23F). In 2009, PCV9 was licensed covering two additional serotypes (1 and 5) and Synflorix, a 10-serotypes conjugate vaccine covering serotypes 1, 4, 5, 6B, 7F, 9V, 14, 18C, 19F, and 23F.

In 2010, PCV13[45] was licensed that contains 4 additional serotypes compared to PCV10 (3, 6A, 7F, and 19A). PCV13 was licensed on the basis of noninferiority trials compared to PCV7 and was shown to be at least as safe and effective.[46] It replaced PCV7 in the childhood immunization schedules of the US and UK in 2010.[47]

Conjugate vaccines have demonstrated efficacy not only against invasive pneumococcal disease but also against other pneumococcal infections, such as pneumonia and acute otitis media,[48] which significantly broadened the indications.

Efficacy

The first efficacy studies were performed in the US with PCV7 and showed 97.4% efficacy against IPD caused by vaccine serotypes and 89.1% against all strains.[49] Further post-marketing trials confirmed the marked effects on IPD.[44] In the year 2000, PCV7 was introduced into national immunization schemes of various countries.[44] In addition to the effects in children and adults on IPD, administration of PCV7 also resulted in a significant reduction of nonbacteremic pneumonia, otitis media, the need for tympanic tubes, and the number of cases of otorrhea and of various antimicrobial resistant strains in children below 5 years of age.[44] Interestingly, the rate of pneumococcal infections also declined in unvaccinated children above 5 years of age and adults including individuals older than 65 years of age (herd effect).[50]

Choice of serotypes included in pneumococcal vaccines is based on the epidemiology of these sero types and their clinical relevance. Successful implementation of vaccination strategies using highly efficacious vaccines might lead to replacement of vaccine strains by nonvaccine strains. Serotype replacement after the introduction of PCV7 has been widely studied. It has been recently shown that PCV7 serotypes have been nearly completely replaced by other strains, with the relatively virulent 19A being the most common serotype.[51] This strain is now included in the 13-valent conjugated vaccine. Further surveillance is necessary in order to identify the most relevant serotypes and to possibly adapt vaccination strategies and vaccines.

Current Recommendations

The current recommendation of the ACIP is to use PCV13 as a 4-dose series at ages 2, 4, 6, and 12–15 months. For children who have underlying medical conditions, a supplemental PCV13 dose is recommended at 71 months. Children aged 2–18 years with underlying medical conditions should also receive PPV23 after completing all recommended doses of PCV13.[52] Further guidance for children, who started with PCV7 or received PPV23 can also be found in these recommendations.[52]

Currently, the CDC recommends to use PPV23 for prevention of pneumococcal disease in:[53]

- All adults of 65 years of age and older
- Anyone between 2 and 64 years of age, who has a long-term health problem, such as heart disease, lung disease, sickle cell disease, diabetes, alcoholism, cirrhosis, leakage of cerebrospinal fluid, or cochlear implant
- Anyone between 2 and 64 years of age, who has a disease or condition that lowers the body's resistance to infection, such as Hodgkin's disease, lymphoma or leukemia, renal failure, multiple myeloma, nephrotic syndrome, human immunodeficiency virus (HIV) infection or acquired immunodeficiency syndrome (AIDS), damaged spleen or no spleen, and organ transplant
- Anyone between 2 and 64 years of age, who is taking a drug or treatment that lowers the body's resistance to infection, such as long-term steroids, certain cancer drugs, radiation therapy
- Any adult between 19 and 64 years of age, who is a smoker or has asthma
- Residents of nursing homes or long-term care facilities.

Safety

Based on almost 30 years of clinical experience, PPV23 is generally considered safe.[54] Mild transient local side effects are relatively common after administration, but moderate systemic reactions and more severe local reactions are rare.[55]

A systematic review of the safety of conjugated pneumococcal vaccines found that PCV7 may result in more local reactions and fever when compared to certain other vaccines.[56] These adverse effects were mild and self-limiting. There are conflicting reports about increased risk of adverse effects in patients with asthma.[56] Coadministration with other childhood vaccines seems to be well tolerated and safe.[57]

CONCLUSION

In general, the currently available respiratory vaccines can be considered to be safe, effective, and efficacious. The indication for influenza vaccination has recently changed to a universal vaccination of all persons aged 6 months or older in the US. Future research will show what effects this policy will have on the burden of influenza in this country. The integration of influenza into the childhood vaccination program solves 1 important problem, namely that of vaccine uptake, which has been demonstrated to be generally low.

Pneumococcal vaccination has been included into the childhood vaccination schedule only some years ago with the advent of conjugated vaccines. This introduction resulted in an impressive reduction of pneumococcal diseases not only in children but also in the general population.

These concepts point to the future of respiratory vaccines, which lies in the further development of highly immunogenic and safe vaccines and the implementation into established vaccination programmes or schedules.

REFERENCES

1. Knipe DM, Howley PM, Griffin DE, Lamb RA, Martin MA, Roizman B, et al. editors. Fields Virology. Philadelphia, PA:Lippincott Williams & Wilkins;2001.
2. Rohde G. Influenza A. Prevention and Treatment. *Hot Topics in Respir Med.* 2010;5:23-9.
3. LaRussa P. Pandemic novel 2009 H1N1 influenza: what have we learned? *Semin Respir Crit Care Med.* 2011;32: 393-9.
4. Rohde GG. Influenza: Clinical symptoms, diagnostics and therapy. *Internist (Berl).* 2011;52:1047-52.
5. Center for Disease Control and Prevention. Key Facts about Influenza (Flu) & Flu Vaccine. Available from: http://www.cdc.gov/flu/keyfacts.htm. March 2012.

6. Dormitzer PR, Galli G, Castellino F, Golding H, Khurana S, Del Giudice G, et al. Influenza vaccine immunology. *Immunol Rev*. 2011;239:167-77.
7. Center for Disease Control and Prevention. Key Facts About Seasonal Flu Vaccine. Available from: http://www.cdc.gov/flu/protect/keyfacts.htm. July 2012.
8. Belshe RB, Edwards KM, Vesikari T, Black SV, Walker RE, Hultquist M, et al. Live Attenuated versus Inactivated Influenza Vaccine in Infants and Young Children. *N Engl J Med*. 2007;356:685-96.
9. Rhorer J, Ambrose CS, Dickinson S, Hamilton H, Oleka NA, Malinoski FJ, et al. Efficacy of live attenuated influenza vaccine in children: A meta-analysis of nine randomized clinical trials. *Vaccine*. 2009;27:1101-10.
10. Belshe RB, Ambrose CS, Yi T. Safety and efficacy of live attenuated influenza vaccine in children 2-7 years of age. *Vaccine*. 2008;26:D10-6.
11. Ambrose CS, Luke C, Coelingh K. Current status of live attenuated influenza vaccine in the United States for seasonal and pandemic influenza. *Influenza Other Respi Viruses*. 2008;2:193-202.
12. Block SL, Yogev R, Hayden FG, Ambrose CS, Zeng W, Walker RE. Shedding and immunogenicity of live attenuated influenza vaccine virus in subjects 5-49 years of age. *Vaccine*. 2008;26:4940-6.
13. Osterholm MT, Kelley NS, Sommer A, Belongia EA. Efficacy and effectiveness of influenza vaccines: a systematic review and meta-analysis. *Lancet Infect Dis*. 2012;12:36-44.
14. Rockman S, Brown L. Pre-pandemic and pandemic influenza vaccines. *Hum Vaccin*. 2010;6:792-801.
15. Use of influenza A (H1N1) 2009 monovalent vaccine: recommendations of the Advisory Committee on Immunization Practices (ACIP), 2009. *MMWR Recomm Rep*. 2009;58:1-8.
16. World Health Organization. Recommended composition of influenza virus vaccines for use in the 2012 southern hemisphere influenza season. Available from: http://www.who.int/influenza/vaccines/virus/recommendations/2011_09_recommendation.pdf. October 2011.
17. Ellebedy AH, Webby RJ. Influenza vaccines. *Vaccine*. 2009; 27:D65-8.
18. Clark NM, Lynch JP 3rd. Influenza: epidemiology, clinical features, therapy, and prevention. *Semin Respir Crit Care Med*. 2011;32:373-92.
19. Jefferson T, Di Pietrantonj C, Rivetti A, Bawazeer GA, Al-Ansary LA, Ferroni E. Vaccines for preventing influenza in healthy adults. *Cochrane Database Syst Rev*. 2010;7:CD001269.
20. Jefferson T, Di Pietrantonj C, Al-Ansary LA, Ferroni E, Thorning S, Thomas RE. Vaccines for preventing influenza in the elderly. *Cochrane Database Syst Rev*. 2010;(2): CD004876.
21. Tessmer A, Welte T, Schmidt-Ott R, Eberle S, Barten G, Suttorp N, et al. Influenza vaccination is associated with reduced severity of community-acquired pneumonia. *Eur Respir J*. 2011;38:147-53.
22. Groenwold RH, Hoes AW, Hak E. Impact of influenza vaccination on mortality risk among the elderly. *Eur Respir J*. 2009;34:56-62.
23. Parodi V, de Florentiis D, Martini M, Ansaldi F. Inactivated influenza vaccines: recent progress and implications for the elderly. *Drugs Aging*. 2011;28:93-106.
24. Fisman DN, Tuite AR. Estimation of the health impact and cost-effectiveness of influenza vaccination with enhanced effectiveness in Canada. *PLoS One*. 2011;6:e27420.
25. Poole P, Chacko E, Wood-Baker R, Cates C. Influenza vaccine for patients with chronic obstructive pulmonary disease. *Cochrane Database Syst Rev*. 2006;(1):CD002733.
26. Schembri S, Morant S, Winter JH, MacDonald TM. Influenza but not pneumococcal vaccination protects against all-cause mortality in patients with COPD. *Thorax*. 2009;64:567-72.
27. Cates CJ, Jefferson TO, Rowe BH. Vaccines for preventing influenza in people with asthma. *Cochrane Database Syst Rev*. 2008;(2):CD000364.
28. Schultz-Cherry S, Jones JC. Influenza vaccines: the good, the bad, and the eggs. *Adv Virus Res*. 2010;77:63-84.
29. Fiore AE, Bridges CB, Cox NJ. Seasonal influenza vaccines. *Curr Top Microbiol Immunol*. 2009;333:43-82.
30. Centers for Disease Control and Prevention (CDC). Safety of influenza A (H1N1) 2009 monovalent vaccines - United States, October 1-November 24, 2009. *MMWR Morb Mortal Wkly Rep*. 2009;58:1351-6.
31. Pesek R, Lockey R. Vaccination of adults with asthma and COPD. *Allergy*. 2011;66:25-31.
32. Lehmann HC, Hartung HP, Kieseier BC, Hughes RA. Guillain-Barre syndrome after exposure to influenza virus. *Lancet Infect Dis*. 2010;10:643-51.
33. Todar K. Todar's Online Textbook of Bacteriology 2012. Available from: http://www.textbookofbacteriology.net.
34. Bogaert D, De Groot R, Hermans PW. Streptococcus pneumoniae colonisation: the key to pneumococcal disease. *Lancet Infect Dis*. 2004;4:144-54.
35. Kadioglu A, Weiser JN, Paton JC, Andrew PW. The role of *Streptococcus pneumoniae* virulence factors in host respiratory colonization and disease. *Nat Rev Microbiol*. 2008;6:288-301.
36. Loda FA, Collier AM, Glezen WP, Strangert K, Clyde WA Jr, Denny FW. Occurrence of Diplococcus pneumoniae in the upper respiratory tract of children. *J Pediatr*. 1975;87: 1087-93.
37. Weycker D, Strutton D, Edelsberg J, Sato R, Jackson LA. Clinical and economic burden of pneumococcal disease in older US adults. *Vaccine*. 2010;28:4955-60.
38. Prevention of pneumococcal disease: recommendations of the Advisory Committee on Immunization Practices (ACIP). *MMWR Recomm Rep*. 1997;46:1-24.
39. Finch R. Is pneumococcal infection a preventable disease? *J Infect*. 1988;17:95-8.
40. Ho CF, Lin TY. Pneumococcal vaccines. *Chang Gung Med J*. 2005;28:765-72.
41. Kyaw MH, Clarke S, Edwards GF, Jones IG, Campbell H. Serotypes/groups distribution and antimicrobial resistance of invasive pneumococcal isolates: implications for vaccine strategies. *Epidemiol Infect*. 2000;125:561-72.
42. Artz AS, Ershler WB, Longo DL. Pneumococcal vaccination and revaccination of older adults. *Clin Microbiol Rev*. 2003; 16:308-18.

43. Moberley SA, Holden J, Tatham DP, Andrews RM. Vaccines for preventing pneumococcal infection in adults. *Cochrane Database Syst Rev.* 2008;(1):CD000422.
44. Arguedas A, Soley C, Abdelnour A. Prevenar experience. *Vaccine.* 2011;29:C26-34.
45. Paradiso PR. Advances in pneumococcal disease prevention: 13-valent pneumococcal conjugate vaccine for infants and children. *Clin Infect Dis.* 2011;52:1241-7.
46. Jefferies JM, Macdonald E, Faust SN, Clarke SC. 13-valent pneumococcal conjugate vaccine (PCV13). *Hum Vaccin.* 2011;7:1012-8.
47. Centers for Disease Control and Prevention (CDC). Invasive pneumococcal disease and 13-valent pneumococcal conjugate vaccine (PCV13) coverage among children aged </=59 months—selected U.S. regions, 2010—2011. *MMWR Morb Mortal Wkly Rep.* 2011;60:1477-81.
48. Klugman KP, Madhi SA, Huebner RE, Kohberger R, Mbelle N, Pierce N. A trial of a 9-valent pneumococcal conjugate vaccine in children with and those without HIV infection. *N Engl J Med.* 2003;349:1341-8.
49. Black S, Shinefield H, Fireman B, Lewis E, Ray P, Hansen JR, et al. Efficacy, safety and immunogenicity of heptavalent pneumococcal conjugate vaccine in children. Northern California Kaiser Permanente Vaccine Study Center Group. *Pediatr Infect Dis J.* 2000;19:187-95.
50. Miller E, Andrews NJ, Waight PA, Slack MP, George RC. Herd immunity and serotype replacement 4 years after seven-valent pneumococcal conjugate vaccination in England and Wales: an observational cohort study. *Lancet Infect Dis.* 2011;11:760-8.
51. Wroe PC, Lee GM, Finkelstein JA, Pelton SI, Hanage WP, Lipsitch M, et al. Pneumococcal Carriage and Antibiotic Resistance in Young Children Before 13-valent Conjugate Vaccine. *Pediatr Infect Dis J.* 2012;31:249-54.
52. Nuorti JP, Whitney CG. Prevention of pneumococcal disease among infants and children - use of 13-valent pneumococcal conjugate vaccine and 23-valent pneumococcal polysaccharide vaccine - recommendations of the Advisory Committee on Immunization Practices (ACIP). *MMWR Recomm Rep.* 2010;59:1-18.
53. Centers for Disease Control and Prevention (CDC); Advisory Committee on Immunization Practices. Updated recommendations for prevention of invasive pneumococcal disease among adults using the 23-valent pneumococcal polysaccharide vaccine (PPSV23). *MMWR Morb Mortal Wkly Rep.* 2010;59:1102-6.
54. European Centre for Disease Prevention and Control. Use of pneumococcal polysaccharide vaccine for subjects over 65 years of age during an inter-pandemic period. Technical Report. Stockholm, 2007.
55. Ortqvist A. Pneumococcal vaccination: current and future issues. *Eur Respir J.* 2001;18:184-95.
56. Destefano F, Pfeifer D, Nohynek H. Safety profile of pneumococcal conjugate vaccines: systematic review of pre- and post-licensure data. *Bull World Health Organ.* 2008;86:373-80.
57. Oosterhuis-Kafeja F, Beutels P, Van Damme P. Immunogenicity, efficacy, safety and effectiveness of pneumococcal conjugate vaccines (1998-2006). *Vaccine.* 2007;25:2194-212.

CHAPTER 25

Pulmonary Endothelium in Sepsis and Infections

Ioanna Nikitopoulou, Nikolaos A Maniatis, Anastasia Kotanidou, Stylianos E Orfanos

ABSTRACT

Endothelial cells possess major metabolic properties, with the endothelial barrier maintenance being a key regulator of fluid and macromolecule exchange, thus preserving lung and whole body homeostasis. Since endothelium forms the inner cellular lining of blood and lymphatic vessels and covers a large surface area widely distributed in all tissues, it constitutes a major target of human bacterial pathogens. During an inflammatory reaction, the endothelial surface is exposed to infectious agent-derived products, as pathogenic bacteria can produce numerous molecules in order to alter their uptake by endothelial cells, disseminate in tissues, and manipulate host immune responses.

In this chapter, we present an overview of the interactions that pathogens establish with the endothelium, triggering inflammatory responses and promoting invasion and even disruption of the endothelial barrier. Novel aspects of endothelial dysfunction induced by infectious agents are discussed, as well as the different strategies that pathogenic bacteria have evolved to damage the endothelium. Finally, examples of specific pathologies induced by microorganisms affecting the pulmonary endothelium, as well as endothelia of extrapulmonary tissues, will be thoroughly analyzed.

INTRODUCTION

The lung's primary function as a gas-exchanging organ depends on the existence of an elaborate network of blood vessels, which, by forming a low-resistance circuit with a large contact surface to alveolar airspaces, facilitates oxygenation of the entire cardiac output at rest and during exercise. This precisely tuned system is frequently involved in infectious processes by regulating adhesion of immune cells and diapedesis into the underlying tissue, a necessary step in order for the immune system's innate and acquired response to unfold. In some cases, the pulmonary circulation serves as a portal of entry for pathogens and, relatively infrequently, it becomes the primary target. Vascular injury may be incurred during the host's confrontation with pathogens which, when severe, can lead to significant organ dysfunction. This manifests itself most commonly as pulmonary edema due to increased vascular permeability to plasma fluid, a complication known as acute lung injury (ALI) or, in advanced instances, the acute respiratory distress syndrome (ARDS). Moreover, remodeling of pulmonary vessels in response to certain infections may lead to pulmonary arterial hypertension (PAH), mostly in high-prevalence areas. In the following pages we will give a brief overview of basic principles of endothelial biology and physiology and describe how these are perturbed in the setting of various infections.

BASIC FUNCTIONS

The vascular endothelium lines the inner surface of blood vessels, establishing a multifunctional, semipermeable cellular barrier at the blood-tissue interface.[1]

Developmentally, endothelium arises from mesoderm via the differentiation of hemangioblasts and/or angioblasts. However, other cell lineages may transdifferentiate into endothelial cells and vice versa.[2] Endothelial cells are highly metabolically active and play important roles in many physiological functions, including regulation of pulmonary and systemic vascular resistance, proliferation control of vascular smooth muscle cells and fibrocytes, innate and adaptive immunity. Endothelial cell phenotypes are differentially regulated in space and time, giving rise to the phenomenon of structural and functional heterogeneity.[3]

Leukocyte trafficking and hemostasis constitute further important functions of the endothelium. Passage of leukocytes from blood to underlying tissue involves a multistep adhesion operation, which includes initial attachment, rolling, arrest (i.e., firm adhesion) and transmigration.[1] Platelet aggregation and adhesion are prevented or attenuated by secretion of nitric oxide (NO) and prostacyclin, which help to maintain blood in a fluid state; conversely, clotting may be facilitated on the endothelial surface, in order to repair a breach in the integrity of the vascular wall.

The regulated transport of water, solutes and macromolecules in "continuous" endothelia (as found in pulmonary, coronary skeletal muscle and brain vascular beds), depends on tight control of endothelial permeability properties and generally occurs via paracellular and transcellular pathways.[4] The passage of water and solutes is limited by the endothelial barrier, comprising multiple inter-endothelial connections (tight and adherens junctions), while macromolecules with molecular radii greater than 3 nm are preferentially carried by vesicular shuttling systems, as shown for albumin.[5] Paracellular permeability is regulated by a complex interplay of cellular adhesive forces balanced against barrier-disruptive forces generated by actinomyosin molecular motors. The restrictive properties of the pulmonary endothelial barrier to the passage of macromolecules[2] are primarily due to closed interendothelial junctions (IEJs) and integrin-extracellular matrix (ECM) associations.

LUNG ENDOTHELIUM IN DISEASE

Endothelial alterations in the setting of infection comprise the loss of vascular integrity, increased expression of leukocyte adhesion molecules, a change in phenotype from anti- to prothrombotic, cytokine production and upregulation of HLA molecules.[3,4] The first stage of activation is endothelial cell stimulation or type 1 activation, which does not require *de novo* protein synthesis or gene upregulation. Endothelial cells retract from each other, express P-selectin leading to increased neutrophil adhesion, and release von Willebrand factor which regulates platelet adherence to the subendothelium. Type 2 activation requires upregulation of mRNA expression and *de novo* protein synthesis, particularly of cytokines and adhesion molecules. The endothelium produces vascular cell adhesion molecule-1 (VCAM-1), intercellular adhesion molecules (ICAM-1 and ICAM-2) and E-selectin, promoting the binding of leukocytes (Figure 1). This adhesion process is associated with increased expression of endotoxin/cytokine inducible genes, which are involved in determining vasomotor tone, particularly those encoding for the production of NO, endothelins (ETs) and cyclooxygenase products.

Pulmonary edema due to increased endothelial permeability is the hallmark of ALI/ARDS.[5] Vasoactive mediators, including thrombin, bradykinin, histamine, vascular endothelial growth factor (VEGF), and others act via cell-surface receptors to disrupt the organization of IEJs and integrin-ECM complexes, thereby opening the junctional barrier.[6] The resulting intercellular gap formation allows leakage of plasma water and proteins into the interstitium. When filtered fluid exceeds lymphatic clearance capacity, alveolar flooding ensues and gas exchange is impeded. In sepsis-induced ALI, the pulmonary endothelium demonstrates increased permeability and promotes leukocyte transmigration.[7] Characteristically, alveolar spaces from patients with ALI/ARDS are lined with an amorphous material known as hyaline membrane, felt to represent fibrin deposits and attesting to the aforementioned breakdown of endothelial integrity in addition to activation of coagulation.[8]

Pulmonary arterial hypertension is probably the hallmark disease related to chronic pulmonary vasculopathy and endotheliopathy. PAH is associated with hypertrophy and hyperplasia of smooth muscle cells in small precapillary pulmonary arteries. Recent evidence suggests that early PAH is associated with increased endothelial apoptosis, whereas more advanced pulmonary hypertension is characterized by reduced endothelial apoptosis and formation of plexiform lesions.[9] Plexiform lesions result from excess endothelial cell proliferation in parallel with neovessel formation. The endothelial cells lining the plexiform lesions and the sites of angiogenesis seem to be phenotypically distinct, suggesting differential angiogenic activity within the plexiform lesion.[10] Pulmonary endothelial dysfunction is a key pathophysiological component of PAH, includes critical disruptions of the endothelial paracrine properties, and may also favor pulmonary intravascular clotting by altering the production of anticoagulant factors.[11]

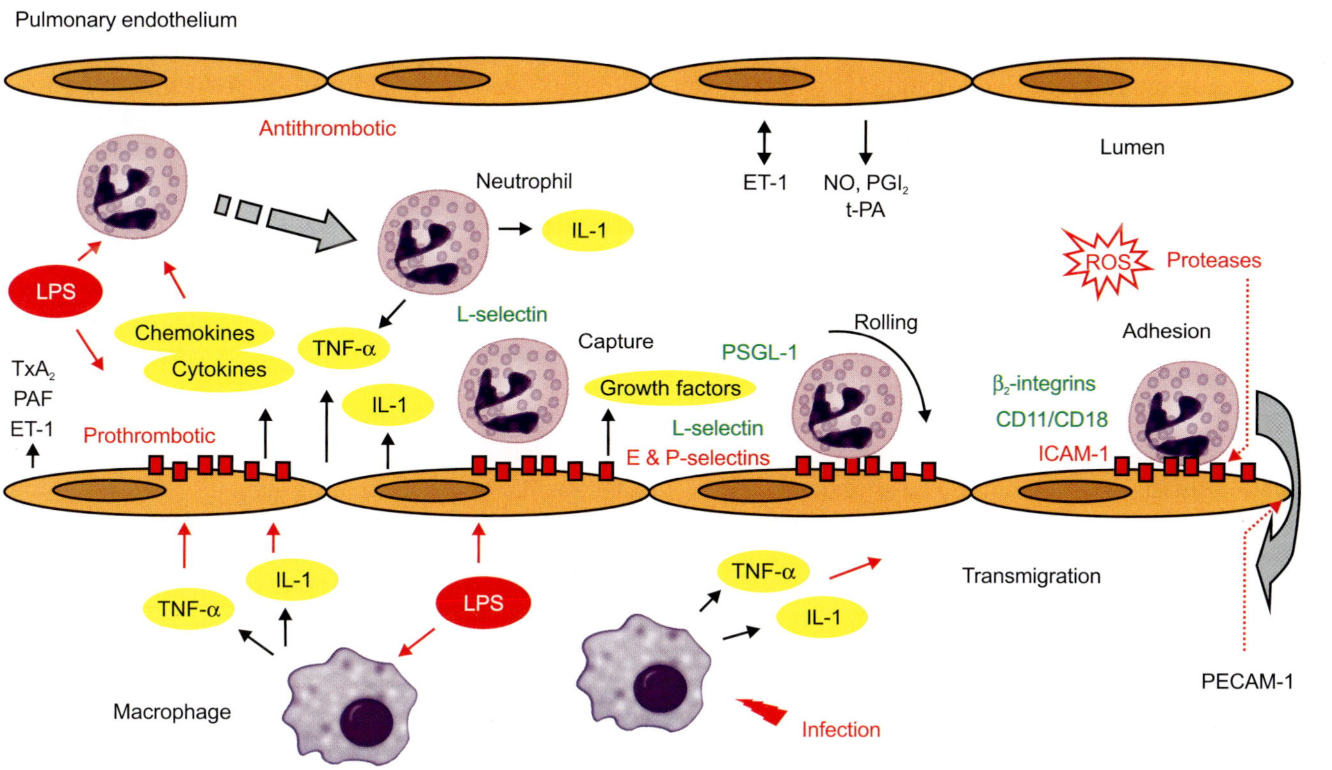

LPS, lipopolysaccharide; TNF-α, tumor necrosis factor-α; IL-1 interleukin-1; NO, nitric oxide; ET-1, endothelin-1; PGI_2, prostacyclin; TxA2, thromboxane A2; PAF, platelet-activating factor; t-PA, tissue plasminogen activator; ROS, reactive oxygen species; PSGL-1, P-selectin glycoprotein-1; ICAM-1, intercellular adhesion molecule-1; PECAM-1, platelet-endothelial cell adhesion molecule-1. adhesion molecules; Red arrows, action; black arrows, synthesis (and uptake for ET-1); dotted arrows, location.

FIGURE 1 Major endothelial functional properties in the normal lung and mechanisms of pulmonary endothelial injury induced by infection. Neutrophil adhesion to endothelial cells is a multistage process, essential for successful neutrophil migration and extravasation. The initial phase, neutrophil capture and rolling, is mediated by cell adhesion molecules of the selectin family. The second phase is firm neutrophil adhesion and requires ICAM-1 expression on endothelial cells, which is augmented by inflammatory mediators such as tumor necrosis factor-α and IL-1. Neutrophil transmigration is the third phase of the adhesion cascade and depends on the presence of a chemotactic gradient and the platelet-endothelial cell adhesion molecule 1 (PECAM-1) expressed on endothelial cell junctions. *Source:* Orfanos SE, Mavrommati I, Korovesi I,et al. Pulmonary endothelium in acute lung injury: from basic science to the critically ill. *Intensive Care Medicine.* 2004;30(9):1702-14.

An attractive hypothesis about the stimulus preceding the vasoconstrictive/vasoproliferative events is that endothelial injury leads to apoptosis of inactive cells, destabilization of the pulmonary vascular intima, preferably at branching points, and uncontrolled proliferation of endothelial cells. Most of the physiological consequences of PAH would then emanate from the resultant narrowing of the pulmonary vessels.

Changes in EC phenotype have been linked to abnormalities in bone morphogenetic proteins (BMPs) and VEGF signaling.[12] Recently BMPs were shown to render cultured endothelial cells more resistant to apoptotic stimuli,[13] and mutations in the BMP receptor gene accompanied by a decrease in the alveolar density of BMP receptor expression in patients with heritable PAH have been the first genetic abnormalities reported in PAH.[14]

Endothelial Responses to Pathogens

Since blood vessels are widely distributed in all tissues, they constitute a preferred interface for systemic dissemination of human bacterial pathogens. Dysfunction or disruption of the endothelial barrier provides a highly effective means for bacteria to spread into tissues, leading to major pathologies.

Pathogenic bacteria can produce numerous molecules in order to adhere to the endothelium and damage it.[15] Firm bacterial adhesion to endothelial cells and triggering of endothelial membrane reorganization are probably general requisites to resist the shear stress exerted by the blood flow, enabling colonization and the development of severe cardiovascular and metastatic infections.[16] In addition, bacteria can subvert cell membrane organization and receptor signaling to persist at the surface or translocate through endothelial barriers.[17]

Finally, pathogenic bacteria have evolved mechanisms in order to avoid or promote their uptake by endothelial cells, disseminate in tissues and manipulate host innate and adaptive immune responses.

Sepsis is the immediate consequence of bacterial access and multiplication in the bloodstream: sepsis is the systemic inflammatory response to infection from invasive pathogens that is clinically manifested by two or more of (1) fever or hypothermia, (2) rapid heart rate, (3) increased respiratory rate or hypocapnia, and (4) leukocytosis or leukopenia, or presence of immature (band) forms more than 10% of circulating leukocytes.[18] Severe sepsis is accompanied by organ dysfunctions, while septic shock, which is associated with compromised circulation, is the most common cause of death among hospitalized patients in noncoronary intensive-care units. More specifically, a related meta-analysis reported an overall mortality rate of 49.7%, although these rates increase in patients of higher illness severity (52% in patients with severe sepsis, and 82% in patients with septic shock).[19]

Although best studied in response to lipopolysaccharide (LPS) from Gram-negative bacteria, the septic syndrome can also be triggered by Gram-positive bacterial, fungal or viral infections. LPS is a major constituent of the Gram-negative bacterial cell wall essential for the integrity of the bacterial cell.[20] The portion of LPS that causes shock is the innermost and most highly conserved phosphoglycolipid, lipid A, known as bacterial endotoxin. Multicellular organisms have evolved proteins specialized for the recognition of LPS. These proteins are found both on the surface of phagocytic cells and as soluble proteins in the blood.[21] LPS is removed by (1) macrophages through scavenger receptors that are highly expressed in the liver and are thus positioned to remove LPS from portal blood draining the intestines, and (2) by neutrophils through the primary granule protein, bactericidal permeability increasing (BPI) protein, which is toxic to Gram-negative bacteria. The homologous LPS-binding protein transfers LPS to membrane-bound or soluble CD14, enabling interactions with Toll-like receptors (TLRs) on the phagocyte membrane. In mice and humans the LPS receptor includes CD14, an LPS-interacting moiety, TLR4, the signal transducing element, and MD-2, a small extracellular protein tightly bound to TLR4.

Endotoxins are recognized primarily by the complex formed by MD2 (also known as ly96), TLR4 and CD14.[20] Polymorphism in human TLR4 modulates the efficiency of recognition of various types of endotoxin and the extent of the inflammatory response. Individuals with a less responsive TLR4 have a higher incidence of infections by Gram-negative bacteria and of septic shock.[22]

Toll-like receptors are involved in the septic shock syndrome. The physiological function of signaling through phagocyte TLRs is to induce the release of the cytokines tumor necrosis factor-alpha (TNF-α), interleukin (IL)-1, IL-6, IL-8 and IL-12 and trigger the inflammatory response, which is critical to containing bacterial infection in the tissues.[23] However, if infection disseminates in the blood, the widespread activation of phagocytes in the bloodstream is catastrophic. Cytokine production in the bloodstream results in widespread endothelial cell activation, with expression of adhesion molecules, activation of the coagulation cascade and the production of chemokines and cytokines by the endothelial cells themselves, with consequent amplification of the inflammatory cascade. The adhesion of circulating neutrophils on the endothelium and their activation result in both oxidative and elastase-mediated damage, resulting in the loss of vascular integrity and failure to maintain adequate blood pressure. TNF-α and IL-1 also depress myocardial function directly. Refractory shock, with leakage of edema fluid, and the failure of organs with large capillary beds, such as the lung and kidney, leads to death.

Molecular Pathways in Sepsis

Recognition of pathogen-associated molecular patterns (PAMPs) by the extracellular domains of the TLRs on both endothelial and immune cells has as a result the expression of proinflammatory mediators, after initiation of signal transduction pathways that lead to the activation of mitogen-activated protein (MAP) kinases, such as p38 and Jun amino-terminal kinase (Jnk) proteins, as well as nuclear factor-κB (NF-κB).[24]

All TLRs use a common adaptor protein, MyD88, that when associated with a TLR, recruits members of the IL-1 receptor– associated kinase family through death domain and activates TNF-receptor-associated factor 6 (TRAF6). Biochemical evidence indicates that TRAF6 activates a MAP kinase called transforming growth factor β-activated kinase (TAK-1). Activated TAK-1 phosphorylates kinases upstream of p38 MAPKs and JNK and can also activate the IκBα kinase complex (IKK), which consists of the kinases IKKα and IKKβ and the scaffolding protein IKKγ (NEMO).

The phosphorylation of IκBα leads to its degradation, the release of NF-κB, and the activation of NF-κB-dependent genes (Figure 2).

Rho GTPases are proved to be crucial regulators of the expression of inflammatory genes, due to their ability to activate Jnk proteins, p38 and NF-κB downstream of TLRs. Rho GTPases can be targets for both Gram-negative and Gram-positive pathogenic bacteria,[25] and

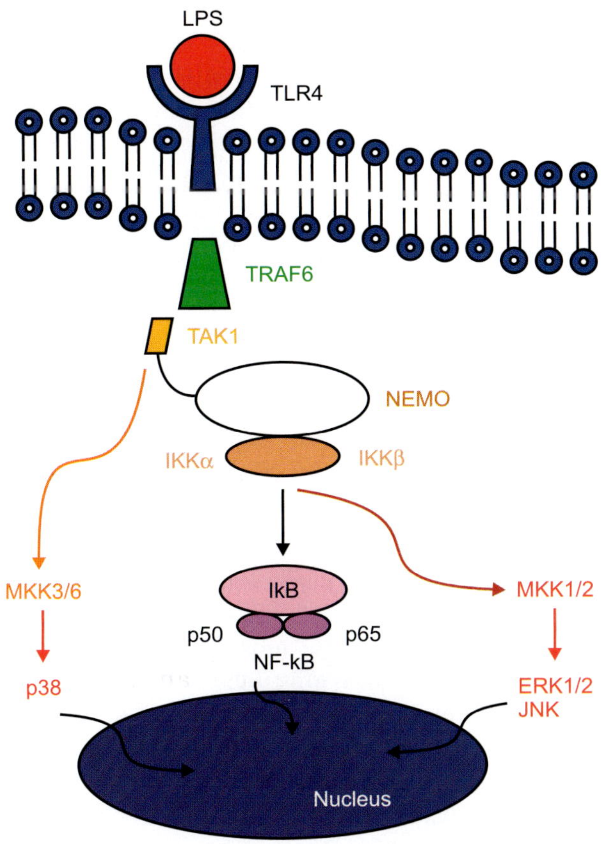

TLR, toll-like receptors; LPS, lipopolysaccharide; TRAF6, tumor necrosis factor-receptor-associated factor 6; TAK1, transforming growth factor β-activated kinase 1; IKK, IκBα kinase complex; MAP, mitogen-activated protein.

FIGURE 2 The TLR4-mediated signaling pathway. Upon LPS recognition, TLR4 recruits its downstream adaptor TRAF6, and TAK1 activation is induced. Activated TAK1 phosphorylates the IKK complex, consisting of IKKα, IKKβ, and NEMO (IKKγ). Phosphorylation of IκB leads to degradation of its proteins and subsequent translocation of NF-κB. Apart from the IKK complex, MAP kinase pathways are activated, thereby inducing transcription factor activation.

the production of inflammatory mediators in endothelial cells is the result of Rho protein activation by bacterial virulence factors. The response to direct activation of Rho proteins by the cytotoxic necrotizing factor 1 toxin of the pathogen *Escherichia coli* is an example.[26] To date, septic shock is basically induced by endotoxin and superantigen proteins that are produced by various Gram-positive cocci as well as by Gram-negative bacteria.

ENDOTHELIUM AND INFECTIONS

Specific Interactions of Microorganisms with the Endothelium

The endothelial surface is exposed to pathogens, pathogen-derived products and agents of the activated host defense during an inflammatory reaction. The endothelium is not only specifically targeted by infective agents like Rickettsia or Bartonella; it is involved in virtually most acute inflammatory responses.[27] As analyzed, pathogens attack the endothelium by a wide variety of strategies, including activation of receptor-mediated pathways, release of toxins or intracellular replication and chronic parasitism (Figure 3). Intracellular colonization of endothelial cells and spreading through an intracellular route require specific virulence strategies aimed at escaping intracellular destruction by lysosomes.[28] For instance, obligate intracellular bacteria that target the endothelium, such as Rickettsia spp., have evolved strategies to limit their lysosomal degradation on entry into the host cell by modulating membrane trafficking or triggering the rupture of the phagosomal membrane.[29,30]

All the aforementioned pathophysiological events affect the endothelial phenotype, resulting in endothelial barrier dysfunction, increased leukocyte-endothelial interaction, mediator release, and procoagulant activity.

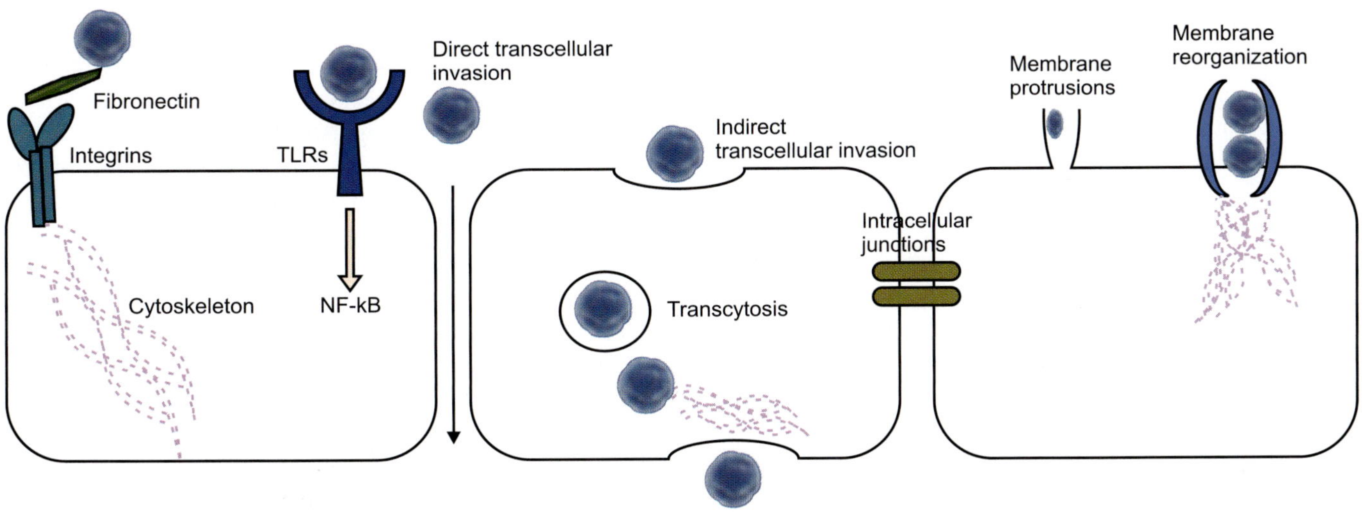

FIGURE 3 Pathogenic bacterial mechanisms for targeting the endothelium.

Moreover, endothelial responses retroact on the invading pathogen as well as on host defense pathways resulting in a complex and dynamic interaction. The endothelium proceeds with great effort against the pathogen, thus it could be supported that endothelial activation contributes considerably to inflammation and the resulting clinical characteristics.

In this chapter, microorganisms directly targeting the pulmonary endothelium will be presented, as well as some infectious agents that intensely affect the vascular endothelium although the lung is not their primary target.

Pathogenic bacteria have developed several mechanisms to promote their adherence to the endothelium and some host features are also recruited. Membrane-anchored fibronectin-binding protein A helps *S. aureus* to form adhesion-like attachment sites and move at the surface of endothelial cells. TLRs on endothelial cells recognize PAMPs on the bacterial surface and a defense pathway is initiated. Bacteria can penetrate endothelial cells by direct transcellular invasion through macroapertures, while massive membrane reorganizations can also take place, as for *Bartonella henselae*. Membrane protrusions induced by *Neisseria meningitides* allow the bacterium to resist blood flow forces and to destabilize cellular junctions.

Staphylococcus aureus

Staphylococcus aureus, a facultative anaerobic Gram-positive coccus that can be potentially harmful in humans, is in many cases the leading cause of endovascular bacterial infections, including infective endocarditis, thrombophlebitis, or vascular graft infection. For most pathogenic events of staphylococcal disease, contact of the bacterium with the host tissue is needed.

Staphylococcus aureus expresses a number of bacterial cell wall-anchored proteins, which mediate bacterial adherence to host cells and ECM components.[31] Among these, adhesins, which recognize fibronectin and fibrinogen, are the most prominent. Adhesins possess a conserved signal essential for their incorporation into the cell wall by sortase. This sorting signal comprises a conserved motif which is cleaved by sortase and covalently links the adhesins to bacterial wall peptidoglycan. More than 20 members of this family of cell wall-anchored proteins have been identified in the *S. aureus* genome. Staphylococcal invasion of endothelial cells is achieved by binding of bacterial adhesins to host cell adhesion receptors. Bacteria-associated adhesive glycoproteins, in particular fibronectin, are recognized by endothelial cells via integrins. The process involves binding of adhesins to receptors of the integrin β1 family on the host cell plasma membrane.

An exception to *S. aureus* contact with the host tissue is toxin-mediated disease. Various clinical isolates of S. aureus directly cross the endothelial barrier by producing the exotoxin epidermal-cell differentiation inhibitor (EDIN).[32] EDIN factors enter cells by macropinocytosis and can inactivate the GTPase RhoA by catalyzing its ADP-ribosylation at Asp-41.[25] RhoA and Rho-associated protein kinase inhibition result in complete disruption of the cell's actin cytoskeleton and formation of transcellular tunnels, named macroapertures.[33] The inactivation of RhoA and the formation of macroapertures do not alter the organization of adherens junctions. Strikingly, macroapertures are highly dynamic, opening and closing in minutes.

Aspergillus Fumigatus

Invasive aspergillosis can cause significant mortality and is characterized by vascular invasion and thrombosis. *Aspergillus fumigatus* is the most common Aspergillus species causing invasive infections. Numerous conidia are released into the atmosphere, and due to their small size they deposit in pulmonary alveoli after they are inhaled. Once the conidia reach the alveoli, they produce hyphae that invade the pulmonary parenchyma and have a marked tropism for blood vessels. Thus, a key finding in invasive aspergillosis is angioinvasion, which subsequently leads to thrombosis.[34]

During angioinvasion, *Aspergillus fumigatus* hyphae interact with the vascular endothelium. Once the hyphae have entered the bloodstream, they must adhere to and penetrate the endothelial cell lining of the blood vessels to invade the deep tissues of the target organs. It is shown that pathogenesis of invasive aspergillosis involves interactions of *Aspergillus fumigatus* conidia and hyphae with endothelial cells,[35] as both forms of the organism induce endothelial cell microfilament rearrangement and subsequent endocytosis. The internalized organisms injure the endothelial cells and stimulate them to express tissue factor (or thromboplastin or CD142*36*), providing a potential mechanism for the vascular invasion and thrombosis during invasive aspergillosis.

Bartonella henselae

Bartonella spp. have been recognized as causative agents of several human diseases, including bacillary angiomatosis, cat-scratch disease, chronic bacteremia, chronic lymphadenopathy, meningoencephalitis, stellar retinitis, myelitis, granulomatous hepatitis, endocarditis, osteomyelitis, and peliosis hepatis. As a facultative intracellular bacterium, Bartonella interacts closely with its host cells. The Bartonella-endothelial cell interaction is not restricted to angiogenesis stimulation.[37] Invasion of endothelial cells was described for *B. quintana*,[38] *B. henselae*,[39] and *B. bacilliformis*,[40] and a proinflammatory activation of endothelial cells was postulated, which is thought to be a result of receptor ligand interactions between the activated endothelium and circulating neutrophils.[41]

The bacterial ligands that may be involved in adherence may include bundle-forming pili and several outer-membrane proteins. The endothelial receptors involved in Bartonella adhesion may include ICAM-1, which has been shown to be enriched especially at the tips of the protrusions of the endothelial membrane. Interestingly, ICAM-1 and E-selectin expression is upregulated via NF-κB translocation, induced by *B. henselae*.[39]

Endothelial cells are invaded by two mechanisms: (1) endocytosis of bacteria and (2) the engulfment of clustered bacteria by a unique host cell structure called the invasome. Invasion is associated with cytoskeletal rearrangements, themselves induced by Bartonella via Rho GTPase signaling.[42]

Specifically, *B. henselae* factors can induce vasoproliferative lesions in the skin and internal organs of immunocompromised patients as well as cat scratch disease in immunocompetent individuals. *B. henselae* adhesion to human cells is promoted by Bartonella adhesin (badA), the structure of which has been recently resolved.[43] BadA mediates the binding of *B. henselae* to ECM proteins and to endothelial cells, possibly through β1 integrins. Colonization and invasion of the endothelium, which occurs following a specific sequence of host-microorganism interactions, is a crucial event in the pathogenicity of this bacterium. *B. henselae* enters human endothelial cells *in vitro* by two alternative routes: either by an endocytic uptake of individual bacteria, giving rise to Bartonella-containing vacuoles,[44] or by the formation of membrane waves, which form large protrusions that surround bacterial aggregates and eventually promote their internalization.

Hantaviruses

Hantaviruses cause two potentially lethal diseases, Hantavirus pulmonary syndrome (HPS) and hemorrhagic fever with renal syndrome (HFRS); both diseases result in defects in vascular permeability and platelet function.[45,46] The HPS-associated viruses are members of the genus Hantavirus, family Bunyaviridae. Hantaviruses have a worldwide distribution and are broadly split into the New World Hantaviruses, which include those causing HPS, and the Old World Hantaviruses, which are associated with HFRS. Pathogenic new world Hantaviruses infect the lung microvascular endothelium, resulting in microvascular leakage, the hallmark of HPS. The severe phase of the disease develops with the onset of the pulmonary edema, hypotension and shock.[47] Recognition of PAMPs by host cells leads to activation of innate immune responses such as the type I interferons (IFNs) and of proinflammatory cytokines responsible initially for restriction of viral replication and spread. Innate immunity is considered the first line of defense of the host to RNA virus infections. The subsequently activated adaptive immune responses contribute to virus elimination.[48] The basis of lung vascular leakage during Hantavirus infection, and ultimately HPS, is not well-understood. The progression to HPS is likely a multifactorial process with contributions directly from the virus replication and indirectly from the immune response induced by the virus. An immune-mediated basis of disease is supported by studies demonstrating that Hantavirus infection is associated with endothelial cell and leukocyte activation and release of proinflammatory lymphokines, thus affecting endothelial integrity.[49,50] Infection of monocytes, macrophages and T cells results in production of inflammatory mediators, including IFN-γ, IL-1a, IL-6 and TNF-α, which have been detected at high levels in HPS patients.[51] By demonstrating a direct virus effect on vascular endothelium, recent studies have cast some doubts on the established paradigm that HPS is solely an immune-modulated disease. These studies are based on: (1) the virus receptor usage, (2) the fact that pathogenic Hantaviruses can sensitize the endothelium and cause vascular hyperpermeability in response to exogenously added VEGF,[52] and (3) that Hantavirus replication alone can cause loss of the integrity of the endothelial cell barrier.[53]

Bacillus anthracis

Bacillus anthracis, the causative agent of anthrax, is a Gram-positive, spore-forming, rod-shaped bacterium, with a width of 1–1.2 μm and a length of 3–5 μm. It is known to synthesize a protein capsule (D-glutamate) and forms a calmodulin-dependent adenyl cyclase exotoxin known as edema factor (EF). Its oval spores are located centrally in a nonswollen sporangium, and they are highly resistant to extreme temperatures, low-nutrient environments, and harsh chemical treatments.[54]

Lethal toxin (LeTx) and edema toxin (ETx) production are key events to the virulent effects of this lethal bacterium. These are binary-type toxins comprising a protective antigen necessary for their cellular uptake, and either lethal or EFs.[55] LeTx is composed of protective antigen and lethal factor, while ETx is made up of protective antigen and EF.

Primary cellular receptors for protective antigen have been identified and the processing of the completed toxins clarified. Consistent with the ability of LeTx to inhibit MAP kinase function, it is indicated that it may also suppress the inflammatory response. Moreover, evidence suggests that direct effect of LeTx on endothelial cell function could contribute to shock.[56] Despite that, LeTx can also be immunosuppressive[57] by inhibiting cytokines of the innate immune response and impairing neutrophil chemotaxis. Therapies under development which target several steps in the cellular uptake and function of these two toxins have been effective in both *in vitro* and *in vivo* systems. A future research goal could be to study the combination of these agents with conventional treatments.

Rickettsiae

Rickettsiae, a diverse group of intracellular Gram-negative bacteria, invade and infect the vasculature, causing endothelial dysfunction[58] and the subsequent clinical characteristics of the spotted fever and typhus groups of diseases. *Rickettsia rickettsii* and *Rickettsia conorii* represent the etiologic agents for Rocky Mountain spotted fever and boutonneuse fever, respectively. These diseases are transmitted from ticks to humans and are characterized by widespread infection of the vascular endothelium, microvascular injury, and vasculitis. The clinical features of rickettsial diseases correspond to damage of the main target cells, i.e., the endothelial cells, particularly those in the lungs and brain. Because of experimental limitations imposed by the obligate intracellular nature of the organism, little is known about specific virulence determinants utilized by Rickettsia spp. Insight into the virulence of *R. rickettsii*, was achieved with the discovery that it promotes direct cell-to-cell spread through an intracellular actin-based motility (ABM) system.[59] Bacteria move forward through the cytoplasm into tips of membranous protrusions by stimulating host cell actin polymerization. Pseudopodia can be subsequently engulfed by neighboring cells, while escape from the double membrane vacuole allows infection of the new cytoplasm.[60] The ability of spotted fever group rickettsiae to spread via ABM within the endothelium, by directly passing from one cell to another, allows evasion of the host humoral immune response, minimizes exposure to antibiotics, and maintains rickettsiae within their required intracellular area.

Neisseria meningitidis

Interactions of *Neisseria meningitidis* with human endothelia rank among the best characterized examples of complex molecular signaling pathways being hijacked by a bacterial pathogen to allow it to adhere to the endothelial cell surface, elicit its uptake into nonphagocytic cells and translocate through paracellular pathways (cell junctions) and transcellular pathways (transcytosis). *N. meningitidis* is a Gram-negative bacterium which, due to its tendency to interact with endothelial cells, can be responsible for severe sepsis. In particular, interaction with brain capillaries can also trigger cerebrospinal meningitis,[17] as bacterial crossing of the blood-brain barrier initiates an inflammatory response in the subarachnoidal space. Systemic bacteria are exposed to drag forces generated by the bloodstream, thus the transiently slowed blood flow found in the cerebral microcirculation can be responsible for the preferential attachment of *N. meningitidis* to cerebral vessels and, therefore, for the brain tropism of this pathogen.

Plasmodium falciparum

The most severe clinical complications of malaria caused by the protozoan parasite *Plasmodium falciparum* are cerebral malaria and noncardiogenic pulmonary edema.[61] Pulmonary complications include a prolonged impairment of gas transfer, due to increased pulmonary capillary permeability causing ALI,[62] or the most severe ARDS. The latter is a major prognostic determinant in both African and Western adults and is associated with a high fatality rate of 60–70% in the absence of ventilatory support.[63] In either clinical presentation, increased vascular permeability is a major component of the pathologic process.

The onset of ARDS commonly occurs a few days after the start of treatment, when parasitemia and systemic proinflammatory cytokines have decreased significantly or the infection has cleared. The etiology of the protracted pulmonary complication of severe falciparum malaria is currently unclear. It has been postulated that endothelial cell injury could occur as a result of a persistent local inflammatory response. Recently it was demonstrated that parasite products can directly alter the integrity of endothelial junctional complexes and may thus contribute to the pulmonary pathologic processes in severe falciparum malaria.[64] Disruption of junctional proteins was dependent on the activity of Src-family kinases, which have been widely implicated in the negative regulation of endothelial barrier function.

Schistosoma

Schistosomiasis is the most common cause of PAH worldwide, imposing a significant medical and epidemiologic challenge in the pulmonary hypertension field especially in the developing world.[65]

The sexual cycle of Schistosoma occurs in vertebrates, where the female worms produce thousands of eggs, that are eliminated by the urine (in the case of *Schistosoma haematobium*) and feces (in the cases of *S. mansoni* and *S. japonicum*) into the water. Under favorable environmental conditions, eggs release ciliated larvae, called miracidia, that swim and penetrate the specific snail intermediate hosts where they undergo transformation into sporocytes.

Portal hypertension precedes PAH in schistosomiasis and facilitates shunting from the portal system to systemic circulation, allowing the passage of schistosome eggs from the liver to the lungs. Acute cutaneous infection causes inflammation at the site of parasite penetration followed by a subacute immune complex-mediated hypersensitivity response as the parasite migrates through the lungs. Chronic *schistosomiasis infection* induces a granulomatous inflammation around ova deposited in the tissue. In particular, *Schistosoma mansoni* migrates to the portal venous system and causes periportal fibrosis in a subset of individuals that appears to be the precursor of chronic pulmonary disease.

The pulmonary histopathology of schistosomiasis-associated PAH is particular and specific, with a characteristic dark pigment widely detected nearby the vascular lesions. Although the cause of this pigment is still unknown, it probably indicates debris left from the parasite or remaining material of the host response.[66] The schistosomiasis-associated pathology is more likely caused by the severe granulomatous inflammation and following fibrosis induced by parasite eggs that become trapped in host organs. The primary response, a type 1 helper T cell (Th1)-mediated phenomenon, is caused by migrating parasites in the circulatory system, and involves a characteristic production of IL-1,[67] IL-12,[68] IFN-γ,[69] TGF-β, and TNF-α. The secondary response, a Th2 response, is caused by schistosome eggs and egg-derived antigens. The secretion of IL-4, IL-5, IL-10, and IL-13 is the result of the passage from Th1 to Th2 response.

The direct effects of Schistosoma infection on the pulmonary vasculature have not been yet thoroughly studied. Recently, cytokines were correlated with pulmonary remodeling, as some of them were increased in parallel with vascular changes and plexiform lesion formation. Furthermore, another report showed a positive correlation between the lung egg burden and the number of muscularized small peripheral vessels.[70]

Medications such as the anthelmintic PZQ and the antimalarial artemether are used to treat schistosomiasis infection,[71] whereas the medical treatment of schistosomiasis-associated PAH has not been well-studied. Phosphodiesterase inhibitors may be of benefit in patients with schistosomiasis-associated PAH.[72]

Human Immunodeficiency Virus

In human immunodeficiency virus (HIV) infected patients vascular complications have emerged as a significant source of morbidity and mortality.[73] These vascular complications include myocardial and pericardial tumors, cardiomyopathy, peripheral vasculitis, ischemic heart disease, and pulmonary hypertension.[74] Thus, HIV-related PAH is one of the long-term complications of HIV infection that has become increasingly apparent in recent years.

Pulmonary arterial hypertension can complicate the course of HIV infection regardless of the route of HIV transmission, the stage of HIV infection, and the degree of immunosuppression. The clinical presentation and underlying pathology of PAH associated with HIV infection are similar to those encountered in other forms of PAH, although there are data suggesting a greater inflammatory component in the HIV-related form.[75]

Human immunodeficiency virus-related PAH is rare and the pathobiological mechanism leading to its development remains unclear. The prevalence of PAH was estimated to be approximately 0.5% in HIV-infected patients in a study before the highly active antiretroviral therapy era.[76] This rate is 25-fold higher than the prevalence of PAH in the general population.[77]

Histologically, HIV-infected patients do not differ from uninfected counterparts with PAH; 80% of HIV-infected patients also exhibit the concentric laminar intimal fibrosis, medial hypertrophy and plexiform lesions that are hallmarks of PAH. Additional landmarks include augmented expression of smooth muscle cell/fibroblast growth factors such as platelet-derived growth factor (PDGF).

Monocytes and macrophages are known to migrate through the endothelium to ensure immune surveillance and replenishment of myeloid cells. A study indicated that HIV affects the dynamics of the endothelial cell microenvironment, as HIV-infected macrophages are capable of migration through the endothelium but not re-entry into the bloodstream, suggesting that the presence of "trapped" macrophages in tissues may result in defective monocyte/macrophage-mediated immune responses.[78] There is no evidence that HIV infects the pulmonary vascular endothelium, but HIV proteins are known to be noxious to endothelial cells; viral proteins and their interactions with molecular partners in the infected host are strong candidates for cause-effect relationships, because they may promote apoptosis, growth and proliferation.[79]

A paradigm of an HIV protein implicated in the pathology of PAH is the envelope surface glycoprotein-120 (gp-120), which helps HIV to attach and fuse through the host cell membrane. Cell-free HIV-1 gp-120, which has been detected in the blood and cerebrospinal fluid of HIV patients, stimulates proinflammatory cytokine production from monocytes/macrophages, increases the secretion of endothelin-1, and induces apoptosis of human lung endothelial cells.[80]

The HIV protein Tat (transactivator of transcription) also activates endothelial cells, and has angiogenic properties. Postmortem studies in HIV patients with cardiomyopathy showed that HIV infection was restricted to inflammatory cells, while no virus was found in endothelial cells or cardiomyocytes. Extended observations in vitro demonstrated that the HIV proteins gp-120 and Tat generated proapoptotic signals that induced apoptosis in adjacent cardiomyocytes.[81]

CONCLUSION

Scientific evidence supports the important role of endothelial cells in innate immunity and defense. During infection, endothelial cells orchestrate basic functions such as immune cell migration toward pathogens and damaged tissue healing. Cellular microbiology combined with genetics, biophysics, epidemiology and imaging approaches, has been extremely helpful in revealing key molecular steps involved in endothelium infection by bacteria and other microorganisms.

The interplay between pathogens and the host cell membrane or cell-cell junctions is characterized by high complexity, including the pathogen effect on host gene expression. Microorganisms have evolved various strategies to pass through the endothelial layer by disrupting and destroying the host microenvironment. Better understanding of host-pathogen interactions will hopefully allow the development of effective countermeasures that could interfere with the initial steps of these processes, in an effort to achieve early disease control.

Note: In this chapter, the terms acute lung injury (ALI) and acute respiratory distress syndrome (ARDS) are used, to express the ALI/ARDS pathological continuum. The term ALI is not in use anymore and the lung injury syndrome is now characterized as mild, moderate and severe ARDS.[82] We chose to maintain the old terminology since it is used in the related references.

REFERENCES

1. Orfanos SE, Mavrommati I, Korovesi I,et al. Pulmonary endothelium in acute lung injury: from basic science to the critically ill. *Intensive Care Medicine.* 2004;30(9): 1702-14.
2. Lampugnani MG, Resnati M, Dejana E, et al. The role of integrins in the maintenance of endothelial monolayer integrity. *The Journal of Cell Biology.* 1991;112(3): 479-90.
3. Wort SJ, Evans TW. The role of the endothelium in modulating vascular control in sepsis and related conditions. *British Medical Bulletin.* 1999;55(1):30-48.
4. Aird WC. Phenotypic heterogeneity of the endothelium: II. Representative vascular beds. *Circulation Research.* 2007; 100(2):174-90.
5. Maniatis NA, Kotanidou A, Catravas JD, et al. Endothelial pathomechanisms in acute lung injury. *Vascular Pharmacology.* 2008;49(4-6):119-33.
6. Fein A, Grossman RF, Jones JG, et al. The value of edema fluid protein measurement in patients with pulmonary edema. *The American Journal of Medicine.* 1979;67(1):32-8.
7. Andonegui G, Bonder CS, Green F, et al. Endothelium-derived Toll-like receptor-4 is the key molecule in LPS-induced neutrophil sequestration into lungs. *The Journal of Clinical Investigation.* 2003;111(7):1011-20.
8. Bachofen H, Bachofen M, Weibel ER. Ultrastructural aspects of pulmonary edema. *Journal of Thoracic Imaging.* 1988;3(3):1-7.
9. Michelakis ED. Spatio-temporal diversity of apoptosis within the vascular wall in pulmonary arterial hypertension: heterogeneous BMP signaling may have therapeutic implications. *Circulation Research.* 2006;98(2): 172-5.
10. Cool CD, Stewart JS, Werahera P, et al. Three-dimensional reconstruction of pulmonary arteries in plexiform pulmonary hypertension using cell-specific markers. Evidence for a dynamic and heterogeneous process of pulmonary endothelial cell growth. *The American Journal of Pathology.* 1999;155(2):411-9.
11. Budhiraja R, Tuder RM, Hassoun PM. Endothelial dysfunction in pulmonary hypertension. *Circulation.* 2004; 109(2):159-65.
12. Voelkel NF, Vandivier RW, Tuder RM. Vascular endothelial growth factor in the lung. *American Journal of Physiology.* 2006;290(2):L209-21.
13. Teichert-Kuliszewska K, Kutryk MJ, Kuliszewski MA, et al. Bone morphogenetic protein receptor-2 signaling promotes pulmonary arterial endothelial cell survival: implications for loss-of-function mutations in the pathogenesis of pulmonary hypertension. *Circulation Research.* 2006;98(2):209-17.
14. Atkinson C, Stewart S, Upton PD, et al. Primary pulmonary hypertension is associated with reduced pulmonary vascular expression of type II bone morphogenetic protein receptor. *Circulation.* 2002;105(14):1672-8.
15. Lemichez E, Lecuit M, Nassif X, et al. Breaking the wall: targeting of the endothelium by pathogenic bacteria. *Nature Reviews Microbiology.* 2010;8(2):93-104.
16. Mairey E, Genovesio A, Donnadieu E, et al. Cerebral microcirculation shear stress levels determine Neisseria meningitidis attachment sites along the blood-brain barrier. *The Journal of Experimental Medicine.* 2006;203(8):1939-50.

17. Kim KS. Mechanisms of microbial traversal of the blood-brain barrier. *Nature Reviews.* 2008;6(8):625-34.
18. American College of Chest Physicians/Society of Critical Care Medicine Consensus Conference: definitions for sepsis and organ failure and guidelines for the use of innovative therapies in sepsis. *Critical Care Medicine.* 1992;20(6):864-74.
19. Angus DC, Wax RS. Epidemiology of sepsis: an update. *Critical Care Medicine.* 2001;29(7 Suppl):S109-16.
20. Miller SI, Ernst RK, Bader MW. LPS, TLR4 and infectious disease diversity. *Nature Reviews.* 2005;3(1):36-46.
21. Fraser JD, Proft T. The bacterial superantigen and superantigen-like proteins. *Immunological Reviews.* 2008;225:226-43.
22. Lorenz E, Mira JP, Frees KL, et al. Relevance of mutations in the TLR4 receptor in patients with gram-negative septic shock. *Archives of Internal Medicine.* 2002;162(9):1028-32.
23. Takeda K, Kaisho T, Akira S. Toll-like receptors. *Annual Review of Immunology.* 2003;21:335-76.
24. Brodsky IE, Medzhitov R. Targeting of immune signalling networks by bacterial pathogens. *Nature Cell Biology.* 2009; 11(5):521-6.
25. Boquet P, Lemichez E. Bacterial virulence factors targeting Rho GTPases: parasitism or symbiosis? *Trends in Cell Biology.* 2003;13(5):238-46.
26. Munro P, Flatau G, Doye A, et al. Activation and proteasomal degradation of rho GTPases by cytotoxic necrotizing factor-1 elicit a controlled inflammatory response. *The Journal of Biological Chemistry.* 2004;279(34):35849-57.
27. Hippenstiel S, Suttorp N. Interaction of pathogens with the endothelium. *Thrombosis and Haemostasis.* 2003;89(1): 18-24.
28. Tuomanen E. Entry of pathogens into the central nervous system. *FEMS Microbiology Reviews.* 1996;18(4):289-99.
29. Finlay BB, Cossart P. Exploitation of mammalian host cell functions by bacterial pathogens. *Science (New York, NY).* 1997;276(5313):718-25.
30. Walker DH, Ismail N. Emerging and re-emerging rickettsioses: endothelial cell infection and early disease events. *Nature Reviews.* 2008;6(5):375-86.
31. Chavakis T, Wiechmann K, Preissner KT, et al. Staphylococcus aureus interactions with the endothelium: the role of bacterial "secretable expanded repertoire adhesive molecules" (SERAM) in disturbing host defense systems. *Thrombosis and Haemostasis.* 2005;94(2):278-85.
32. Czech A, Yamaguchi T, Bader L, et al. Prevalence of Rho-inactivating epidermal cell differentiation inhibitor toxins in clinical Staphylococcus aureus isolates. *The Journal of Infectious Diseases.* 2001;184(6):785-8.
33. Boyer L, Doye A, Rolando M, et al. Induction of transient macroapertures in endothelial cells through RhoA inhibition by Staphylococcus aureus factors. *The Journal of Cell Biology.* 2006;173(5):809-19.
34. Fraser RS. Pulmonary aspergillosis: pathologic and pathogenetic features. *Pathology Annual.* 1993;28 Pt 1:231-77.
35. Lopes Bezerra LM, Filler SG. Interactions of Aspergillus fumigatus with endothelial cells: internalization, injury, and stimulation of tissue factor activity. *Blood.* 2004; 103(6):2143-9.
36. Doshi SN, Marmur JD. Evolving role of tissue factor and its pathway inhibitor. *Critical Care Medicine.* 2002;30(5 Suppl): S241-50.
37. Greub G, Raoult D. Bartonella: new explanations for old diseases. *Journal of Medical Microbiology.* 2002;51(11):915-23.
38. Brouqui P, Raoult D. Bartonella quintana invades and multiplies within endothelial cells in vitro and in vivo and forms intracellular blebs. *Research in Microbiology.* 1996;147(9):719-31.
39. Dehio C, Meyer M, Berger J, et al. Interaction of Bartonella henselae with endothelial cells results in bacterial aggregation on the cell surface and the subsequent engulfment and internalisation of the bacterial aggregate by a unique structure, the invasome. *Journal of Cell Science.* 1997;110 (Pt 18):2141-54.
40. Blumwald E, Fortin MG, Rea PA, et al. Presence of Host-Plasma Membrane Type H-ATPase in the Membrane Envelope Enclosing the Bacteroids in Soybean Root Nodules. *Plant Physiology.* 1985;78(4):665-72.
41. Dehio C. Bartonella interactions with endothelial cells and erythrocytes. *Trends in Microbiology.* 2001;9(6):279-85.
42. Verma A, Davis GE, Ihler GM. Formation of stress fibres in human endothelial cells infected with Bartonella bacilliformis is associated with altered morphology, impaired migration and defects in cell morphogenesis. *Cellular Microbiology.* 2001;3(3):169-80.
43. Kaiser PO, Riess T, Wagner CL, et al. The head of Bartonella adhesin A is crucial for host cell interaction of Bartonella henselae. *Cellular Microbiology.* 2008;10(11):2223-34.
44. Kyme PA, Haas A, Schaller M, et al. Unusual trafficking pattern of Bartonella henselae -containing vacuoles in macrophages and endothelial cells. *Cellular Microbiology.* 2005;7(7):1019-34.
45. Macneil A, Nichol ST, Spiropoulou CF. Hantavirus pulmonary syndrome. *Virus Research.* 2011;162(1-2):138-47.
46. Mackow ER, Gavrilovskaya IN. Cellular receptors and hantavirus pathogenesis. *Current Topics in Microbiology and Immunology.* 2001;256:91-115.
47. Khan AS, Khabbaz RF, Armstrong LR, et al. Hantavirus pulmonary syndrome: the first 100 US cases. *The Journal of Infectious Diseases.* 1996;173(6):1297-303.
48. Garcia-Sastre A, Biron CA. Type 1 interferons and the virus-host relationship: a lesson in detente. *Science (New York, NY).* 2006;312(5775):879-82.
49. Marsac D, Garcia S, Fournet A, et al. Infection of human monocyte-derived dendritic cells by ANDES Hantavirus enhances pro-inflammatory state, the secretion of active MMP-9 and indirectly enhances endothelial permeability. *Virology Journal.* 2011;8:223.
50. Zaki SR, Greer PW, Coffield LM, et al. Hantavirus pulmonary syndrome. Pathogenesis of an emerging infectious disease. *The American Journal of Pathology.* 1995;146(3):552-79.
51. Mori M, Rothman AL, Kurane I, et al. High levels of cytokine-producing cells in the lung tissues of patients with fatal hantavirus pulmonary syndrome. *The Journal of Infectious Diseases.* 1999;179(2):295-302.
52. Gavrilovskaya IN, Gorbunova EE, Mackow NA, et al. Hantaviruses direct endothelial cell permeability by sensitizing cells to the vascular permeability factor VEGF, while angiopoietin 1 and sphingosine 1-phosphate inhibit

hantavirus-directed permeability. *Journal of Virology.* 2008;82(12):5797-806.
53. Shrivastava-Ranjan P, Rollin PE, Spiropoulou CF. Andes virus disrupts the endothelial cell barrier by induction of vascular endothelial growth factor and downregulation of VE-cadherin. *Journal of virology.* 2010;84(21):11227-34.
54. Li Y, Sherer K, Cui X, et al. New insights into the pathogenesis and treatment of anthrax toxin-induced shock. *Expert Opinion on Biological Therapy.* 2007;7(6):843-54.
55. Sherer K, Li Y, Cui X, et al. Lethal and edema toxins in the pathogenesis of Bacillus anthracis septic shock: implications for therapy. *American Journal of Respiratory and Critical Care Medicine.* 2007;175(3):211-21.
56. Warfel JM, Steele AD, D'Agnillo F. Anthrax lethal toxin induces endothelial barrier dysfunction. *The American Journal of Pathology.* 2005;166(6):1871-81.
57. Stearns-Kurosawa DJ, Lupu F, Taylor FB, et al. Sepsis and pathophysiology of anthrax in a nonhuman primate model. *The American Journal of Pathology.* 2006;169(2):433-44.
58. Walker DH, Valbuena GA, Olano JP. Pathogenic mechanisms of diseases caused by Rickettsia. *Annals of the New York Academy of Sciences.* 2003;990:1-11.
59. Heinzen RA, Hayes SF, Peacock MG, et al. Directional actin polymerization associated with spotted fever group Rickettsia infection of Vero cells. *Infection and Immunity.* 1993;61(5):1926-35.
60. Tilney LG, Portnoy DA. Actin filaments and the growth, movement, and spread of the intracellular bacterial parasite, Listeria monocytogenes. *The Journal of Cell Biology.* 1989; 109(4 Pt 1):1597-608.
61. White NJ, Ho M. The pathophysiology of malaria. *Advances in Parasitology.* 1992;31:83-173.
62. Taylor WR, Canon V, White NJ. Pulmonary manifestations of malaria: recognition and management. *Treatments in Respiratory Medicine.* 2006;5(6):419-28.
63. Bruneel F, Hocqueloux L, Alberti C, et al. The clinical spectrum of severe imported falciparum malaria in the intensive care unit: report of 188 cases in adults. *American Journal of Respiratory and Critical Care Medicine.* 2003; 167(5):684-9.
64. Gillrie MR, Krishnegowda G, Lee K, et al. Src-family kinase dependent disruption of endothelial barrier function by Plasmodium falciparum merozoite proteins. *Blood.* 2007; 110(9):3426-35.
65. Graham BB, Bandeira AP, Morrell NW, et al. Schistosomiasis-associated pulmonary hypertension: pulmonary vascular disease: the global perspective. *Chest.* 2010;137(6 Suppl):20S-9S.
66. Kolosionek E, Graham BB, Tuder RM, et al. Pulmonary vascular disease associated with parasitic infection--the role of schistosomiasis. *Clin Microbiol Infect.* 2010;17(1):15-24.
67. He YX, Chen L, Ramaswamy K. Schistosoma mansoni, S. haematobium, and S. japonicum: early events associated with penetration and migration of schistosomula through human skin. *Experimental Parasitology.* 2002;102(2):99-108.
68. Pearce EJ, Cheever A, Leonard S, et al. Schistosoma mansoni in IL-4-deficient mice. *International Immunology.* 1996;8(4):435-44.
69. Dessein A, Kouriba B, Eboumbou C, et al. Interleukin-13 in the skin and interferon-gamma in the liver are key players in immune protection in human schistosomiasis. *Immunological Reviews.* 2004;201:180-90.
70. Crosby A, Jones FM, Southwood M, et al. Pulmonary vascular remodeling correlates with lung eggs and cytokines in murine schistosomiasis. American Journal of *Respiratory and Critical Care Medicine.* 2010;181(3):279-88.
71. Aragon AD, Imani RA, Blackburn VR, et al. Towards an understanding of the mechanism of action of praziquantel. *Molecular and Biochemical Parasitology.* 2009;164(1): 57-65.
72. Correa Rde A, Moreira MV, Saraiva JM, et al. Treatment of schistosomiasis-associated pulmonary hypertension. *J Bras Pneumol.* 2011;37(2):272-6.
73. Cicalini S, Almodovar S, Grilli E, et al. Pulmonary hypertension and human immunodeficiency virus infection: epidemiology, pathogenesis, and clinical approach. *Clin Microbiol Infect.* 2011;17(1):25-33.
74. Monsuez JJ, Charniot JC, Escaut L, et al. HIV-associated vascular diseases: structural and functional changes, clinical implications. *International Journal of Cardiology.* 2009;133(3):293-306.
75. Janda S, Quon BS, Swiston J. HIV and pulmonary arterial hypertension: a systematic review. *HIV Medicine.* 2010; 11(10):620-34.
76. Opravil M, Pechere M, Speich R, et al. HIV-associated primary pulmonary hypertension. A case control study. Swiss HIV Cohort Study. *American Journal of Respiratory and Critical Care Medicine.* 1997;155(3):990-5.
77. Petitpretz P, Brenot F, Azarian R, et al. Pulmonary hypertension in patients with human immunodeficiency virus infection. Comparison with primary pulmonary hypertension. *Circulation.* 1994;89(6):2722-7.
78. Westhorpe CL, Zhou J, Webster NL, et al. Effects of HIV-1 infection in vitro on transendothelial migration by monocytes and monocyte-derived macrophages. J*ournal of Leukocyte Biology.* 2009;85(6):1027-35.
79. Mette SA, Palevsky HI, Pietra GG, et al. Primary pulmonary hypertension in association with human immunodeficiency virus infection. A possible viral etiology for some forms of hypertensive pulmonary arteriopathy. *The American Review of Respiratory Disease.* 1992;145(5):1196-200.
80. Kanmogne GD, Kennedy RC, Grammas P. Analysis of human lung endothelial cells for susceptibility to HIV type 1 infection, coreceptor expression, and cytotoxicity of gp120 protein. *AIDS Research and Human Retroviruses.* 2001;17(1):45-53.
81. Fiala M, Popik W, Qiao JH, et al. HIV-1 induces cardiomyopathyby cardiomyocyte invasion and gp120, Tat, and cytokine apoptotic signaling. *Cardiovascular Toxicology.* 2004;4(2):97-107.
82. Ranieri VM, Rubenfeld GD, Thompson BT, et al. Acute respiratory distress syndrome: the Berlin definition. *JAMA* 2012;307:2526-33.

CHAPTER 26

Bioterrorism and Respiratory Infections

Petros Kopterides, Nikitas Nikitas, Dimitrios K Matthaiou, Apostolos D Armaganidis, George Dimopoulos

ABSTRACT

The terrorist attacks on the US on September 11, 2001 and the subsequent anthrax attacks later that months, reminded the scientific community as well as the public of the world's dire vulnerability to asymmetric threats, especially biological warfare. The lung represents an attractive target site for biologic agents due to continunous exposure to the atmosphere and its wide absorptive surface area. In this chapter, we describe the key features of the multitude of pathogens that may be weaponized to attack the respiratory system, the clinical syndromes they cause, and how they might be used in biowarfare. Finally, we discuss the appropriate means to reach a specific diagnosis and the currently recommended, therapeutic and logistic responses to their potential use.

INTRODUCTION

Bioterrorism can be defined as the use of pathogens (e.g., bacteria, viruses) or their biologic products (e.g., toxins) for the sake of war or terrorism. These agents may potentially cause acute illness or death to humans, animals and plants.[1] The *Working Group for Civilian Biodefense* has specified the key features that characterize the elements of biologic agents that make them particularly effective as weapons: high associated morbidity/mortality, raised potential for person-to-person spread due to highly infectious capacity, lack of rapidly available diagnostic tests for their detection, and/or universally effective vaccines for their prevention, great potential to cause anxiety and fear to a great mass of population, environmental stability, widespread availability, and feasibility of production, modification and development.[2]

The use of microbial pathogens as potential war agents dates from the ancient times. Among the most frequently cited are the poisoning of water supplies in the sixth century *BC.* with the fungus *Claviceps purpurea* (rye ergot) by the Assyrians, the hurling of the dead bodies of *plague* victims over the walls of the city of Kaffa by the Tartar army in 1346, and the efforts by the British to spread *smallpox* via contaminated blankets to the native American population loyal to the French in 1767. Although the use of chemical weapons in wartime took place in the not-too-distant past, the tragic events of September 11, 2001 dramatically changed the mindset of the international community regarding both our vulnerability to bioterrorists' attacks and the seriousness and intent of governments to protect their citizens against future attacks.[3]

Agents of bioterrorism can be used in their naturally occurring forms or they can be modified in order to result in maximal impact. A number of laboratory approaches, generally implemented to process the microbes or their toxins in a manner that would ensure a devastating effect of a release, fall under the general term of *"weaponization"*. Among the most commonly used approaches are: (1) the genetic modification of microbes for the purposes of antimicrobial resistance or evasion by the immune system, (2) the creation of fine-particle aerosols, (3) the chemical treatment to stabilize and prolong infectivity and

(4) the alteration of host range through changes in surface proteins. The most striking example of weaponization is that of *anthrax* by means of production of vast amounts of spores in an aerosolized form for prolonged periods of time.[4]

The *United States (US) Centers for Disease Control (CDC) and Prevention* has identified a number of potential biological threats and has classified them into three categories A, B, and C, based on their overall potential to cause harm (Table 1).

High-priority agents include organisms that can be easily disseminated or transmitted from person-to-person, cause high mortality, create social disruption and, therefore, require special action for public health preparedness. The highest priority agents (*Category A*) include *anthrax* and *smallpox*. These agents are of particular concern because they can be grown easily in large quantities and are sturdy organisms, resistant to destruction. They are also particularly well-suited to airborne dissemination. *Category B* agents include those that are moderately easy to spread and generally cause less morbidity and mortality than *Category A*, but may require enhanced diagnostic capacity or surveillance techniques. Examples include *Q fever* and *brucellosis*. *Category C* agents include emerging infectious diseases threats that could be quite easily engineered for mass dissemination, either because of ready availability or ease of production and transport. These are usually agents of significant potential morbidity and/or mortality. Examples include *Nipah* virus, *Hantavirus*, *severe acute respiratory syndrome (SARS) coronavirus*, pandemic *influenza* virus (H5N1) and multidrug-resistant *tuberculosis*.

Even though the *CDC* classification scheme groups the various biological agents together on the basis of their potential to cause damage and irrespective of their microbiology profile, we herein chose to present the viral and bacterial agents in two separate sections, in order to make it easier for the reader to follow the data.

VIRAL AGENTS

Hemorrhagic Fever Viruses

Hemorrhagic fever viruses (HFVs) comprise a particular group of viral agents, causing a discrete clinical syndrome manifested by acute onset of fever and severe bleeding diathesis and generally termed as *viral hemorrhagic fever*

TABLE 1

Centers for Disease Control Classification of Bioterrorism Agents

Category A	Category B	Category C
Anthrax (*Bacillus anthracis*)	Brucellosis (*Brucella* species)	Nipah virus
Botulism (*Clostridium botulinum* toxin)	Epsilon toxin of *Clostridium perfringens*	Hantavirus
Plague (*Yersinia pestis*)	Food safety threats (e.g., *Salmonella* species, *Escherichia coli* O157:H7, *Shigella*)	SARS coronavirus
Smallpox (*Variola major*)	Glanders (*Burkholderia mallei*)	Pandemic influenza viruses
Tularemia (*Francisella tularensis*)	Melioidosis (*Burkholderia pseudomallei*)	
Viral hemorrhagic fevers [filoviruses (e.g., Ebola) and arenaviruses (e.g., Lassa)]	Psittacosis (*Chlamydophila psittaci*)	
	Q fever (*Coxiella burnetii*)	
	Ricin toxin from *Ricinus communis*	
	Staphylococcal enterotoxin B	
	Typhus fever (Rickettsia prowazekii)	
	Viral encephalitis [alpha viruses (e.g. Venezuelan equine encephalitis)]	
	Water safety threats (e.g., *Vibrio cholerae*, *Cryptosporidium parvum*)	

SARS, severe acute respiratory syndrome

(*VHF*). Many viruses have been identified as potential causes of *VHF* and are classified into four discrete families: *Filoviridae, Arenaviridae, Bunyaviridae,* and *Flaviviridae.*[5]

The incidence of *VHF* is clearly associated firstly with the geographic distribution and emergence of the respective *HFVs* (mainly in parts of Africa, Asia, Middle East and South America), secondly with the local variable complex biological and ecological systems and finally with the respective climate and seasonal conditions or alterations. With the exception of *Yellow fever* and *Dengue fever* viruses, most of the *HFVs* are characterized by a human-independent zoonotic cycle. During their typical life-cycle, *HFVs* are transferred to humans from their respective animal or arthropod reservoirs via specific biological carriers, such as mosquitoes and ticks, or through contaminated animal feces or urine. The recently recognized natural reservoirs of *Ebola* virus are the bats species of *Hypsignathus monstrosus, Epomops franqueti,* and *Myonycteris torquata,*[6] whereas the respective reservoirs of *Marburg* virus are the bats species of *Rousettus aegyptiacus.*[7] Unlike the *Rift Valley fever* and *Flaviviridae*-related infections, human-to-human transmission can be augmented by close contact. The airborne transmission is also a possibility. Sexually-transmitted infection has been reported for *Filoviridae* and *Arenaviridae*-related infections. In addition, a pattern of nosocomial spread of infection has been reported for *Crimean-Congo hemorrhagic fever,* as well as *Ebola* and *Marburg VHFs.* It is widely accepted that most of the *HFVs* can be transmitted among humans through aerosols. Even though this pattern of transmission is not the most frequent, it concerns the predominant human-to-human transmission pattern during an epidemic.[8] Moreover, aerosol transmission cases have been reported among laboratory workers including all *HFV* families.

Most of *HFVs* have been extensively studied and weaponized in the *US* and the former *Union of Soviet Socialist Republics* (*USSR*).[8] *Yellow fever* virus has been weaponized by North Korea, whereas a Japanese terrorist group has tried unsuccessfully to acquire and use *Ebola* virus. As the majority of *HFVs* may be easily transmitted through aerosols, they can infect laboratory animals. Moreover, they are associated with high morbidity and mortality, since there are no effective vaccines or medications for prevention or treatment of the resultant infections, respectively. Thus, *HFVs* constitute potential biological threats to be used for warfare or biological terrorist attacks.[9]

Hemorrhagic fever viruses potentially associated with biowarfare or bioterrorism are *Hantavirus, Ebola* and *Marburg* viruses (*Filoviridae*), *Lassa fever, Machupo, Junin, Guanarito* and *Sabia* viruses (*Arenaviridae*), *Rift Valley fever* virus (*Bunyaviridae*) and *Yellow fever* virus, *Omsk hemorrhagic fever* virus, and *Kyasanur Forest disease* virus (*Flaviviridae*). Most of these *HFVs* have been already modified to be used as biological weapons. On the contrary, there have been no reports of similar weaponization approaches for *Dengue fever* virus and *Crimean-Congo hemorrhagic fever* virus. Main reasons for the aforementioned lack of relative approaches may be the inability of aerosol transmission or the mild clinical disease manifestations (although, rarely, more severe disease may be associated with infection by specific serotypes).

All members of the *HFVs* group are small lipid-coated RNA viruses, which are clinically associated with similar hemorrhagic syndromes. The usual incubation period of *HFVs*-related syndromes varies between 1 day and 21 days. The clinical syndrome can be complicated by severe bleeding diathesis, acute respiratory and renal failure, depending to an extent to the respective responsible viral agent. All *HFVs* may cause microangiopathic vascular and capillary leak syndromes.[10] The severity of *HVFs* syndromes varies from a relatively mild to a fatal fulminant multiorgan disease. However, most of the infected patients manifest a nonspecific systemic febrile illness without predominant organ involvement.[10]

Flaviviridae Ebola and *Marburg* are endemic in sub-Saharan Africa. *Ebola* virus was named from the so-called river in Democratic Republic of the Congo, where it was first isolated in 1976. Among the four discrete viral strains already recognized, three have been linked to human infection. Natural local disease epidemics in various Africa states are further expanded by the poor hygiene conditions in almost all public hospitals. Eight known large-scale epidemics of *Ebola* virus have been reported since 1970s in various African states (three in Sudan in 1976, 1979 and 2004, two in Democratic Republic of the Congo in 1976 and 1995, one in Uganda in 2000-2001 and two in Congo and Gabon in both 2002-2003 and 2007).[10] Most of the 1,200 reported cases—resulting in almost 900 deaths—have been attributed to direct close contact with infected individuals. *Marburg* virus took its name from the German city where it was first isolated and identified in 1967.[11] The original infectious carriers were green monkeys sent from Uganda for testing. Seven, out of 31, infected humans finally succumbed.[11] Afterward, most of the reported cases mainly concerned laboratory workers who had handled previously infected African green monkeys during experiments,[11] whereas a small number of cases have been reported from East and South Africa.[10]

After initial human infection, both *Ebola* and *Marburg* viruses can be transmitted through close personal contact with blood and body fluids of previously infected individuals.

As a result, healthcare personnel are extremely vulnerable to infection as it is shown by a recent epidemic in Uganda in 2000, where 64% of healthcare workers were infected.[12] Airborne transmission does not seem to constitute the predominant way of human-to-human transmission. Both viruses cause similar clinical illness to infected individuals, sharing similar symptoms and laboratory derangements. After a short mean incubation period of 6 days (2–21 days for *Ebola* and 3–10 days for *Marburg* virus, respectively), patients experience nonspecific systemic symptoms, like high fever and chills, malaise and anorexia, headache and myalgias, pharyngitis and diffuse erythematous rash, as well as, gastrointestinal symptoms: abdominal pain, nausea, vomiting and diarrhea.[13] Three days following the onset of febrile illness, hemorrhagic manifestations become apparent as diffuse purpuric or petechial rash, conjunctival hemorrhages, gum bleeding, upper gastrointestinal bleeding, etc. Hemorrhagic manifestations are present in 20% of patients and the predominant site of involvement is the gastrointestinal tract. Main causes of death are hemorrhagic shock or multiorgan dysfunction syndrome. Risk of human-to-human transmission is highest during the end-stage of the disease rather than during the incubation period, when it is almost negligible.[13] *Ebola* virus can be continually isolated from the semen of infected individuals during a prolonged convalescent period. Natural occurring *Ebola* virus infection cases result in 72% mortality rates, whereas the respective rates for *Marburg* virus are approximately 23%.[14] All infected individuals should be hospitalized in isolated wards and all necessary provisional measures should be taken by the healthcare personnel to minimize the risk of transmission among them (e.g. by using protective clothing, gloves and glasses in every contact with the patient).

Six, out of the twenty, isolated *Arenaviridae* members constitute potential human pathogens and five of those can be the cause of *VHF* syndrome: *Junin, Guanarito, Machupo, Sabia* and *Lassa*. The lymphocytic choriomeningitis virus is associated only with neurological manifestations.

Lassa fever remains endemic in western African territories with an annual incidence of 100,000–300,000 documented infections that result in approximately 5,000 deaths. The *New World Arenaviridae* are the main cause of hemorrhagic fever in South America, especially in a restricted rural province of Argentina (*Junin*), in savanna of Bolivia Beni province (*Machupo*), in Venezuelan valleys (*Guanarito*), and in Brazil (*Sabia*).[15] Each responsible virus is associated with a respective rodent species which serves as the animal reservoir for the virus without developing clinical disease. Human infection is mainly caused by the exposure to aerosolized animal secretions (e.g., urine) through inhalation, oral consumption of infected provisions and direct contact with skin.[10] These types of hemorrhagic fevers may be transmitted from human-to-human in the hospital or domestic setting. In the latter cases, the direct contact with contaminated secretions is regarded as a more frequent pattern of transmission than aerosol exposure.[10] After a mean incubation period of 10–14 days, most patients remain asymptomatic or develop a mild flu-like syndrome. Overt disease onset is usually mild, characterized by low-grade fever and fatigue, lasting for a period of 2–4 days. In more severe disease presentation, generalized weakness, retro-orbital headache, arthralgias, myalgias, pharyngitis, nonproductive cough and conjunctivitis ensue.[10] Abdominal pain, facial edema, conjunctival hemorrhages, gastrointestinal bleeding, hematuria, encephalitis, capillary leak syndrome and shock constitute manifestations of fulminant and often fatal disease presentation. Severe acute hepatitis with respective striking transaminases' elevation can occur in *Lassa fever* cases. Additionally, in *Lassa fever* cases, pulmonary manifestations may be severe, with acute respiratory distress syndrome (*ARDS*) constituting a frequent complication. Severe bleeding diathesis and neurologic symptoms like delusion, confusion, encephalopathy, convulsions and coma are more frequent with *New World Arenaviridae* than *Lassa fever* virus. Similarly, leucopenia, lymphopenia and thrombocytopenia are more frequent in the former than in the latter group.

Diffuse bleeding diathesis may be initiated 5 days after fever onset and can be further complicated by dehydration, intravascular volume depletion, severe bleeding from multiple sites or internal organs, and shock. The mortality rates in such *Lassa fever* cases approximate 15–20%; whereas the total mortality rates for all *HFVs* are much lower (1–2%). Mortality rates are highest among pregnant patients (16%), usually accompanied by fetal death as well. Both *Junin* and *Machupo* viruses show high mortality rates, varying between 10% and 16%.

Rift Valley fever is endemic in southern and eastern African and sub-Saharan African territories as well as in Madagascar. It is prevalent in domestic animals (cows, sheep, goats, and camels), whereas sporadic cases have been reported in humans. *Bunyaviridae* are usually transmitted via mosquitoes of *Aedes* genus. However, close contact with blood or other fluids of infected animals may also contribute to the infection of human individuals. Aerosol transmission has been reported in cases of laboratory workers who have been infected while handling viral cultures. Incubation period is usually short (2–6 days). The febrile phase of the acute illness may be further divided in two distinct periods: the first period usually lasts 4 days and is usually followed by a nonfebrile interval of a few days duration. After that, the second febrile period of 2–4 days duration typically ensues. Although most clinical cases follow a mild course, severe cases characterized by hemorrhagic encephalitis and retinopathy, may occur.[10] The hemorrhagic manifestations are usually fully developed within the first 2–4 days from disease onset, in less than 1% of patients, while convalescent period rapidly ensues, within 2–7 days from disease onset. Mortality rates in cases of *Rift Valley fever* are approximately 1%, mainly attributed to severe hemorrhagic manifestations.[10]

Crimean-Congo hemorrhagic fever is endemic in Africa, Europe and Asia, with reported endemic outbreaks in South Africa, Kosovo, Albania, Iran and Pakistan, in 2001. It is a tick-borne disease, characterized by high mortality rates in humans. Nosocomial outbreaks have been also reported among laboratory personnel. While many domestic and wild animals can be infected by the virus, humans may be infected, either by direct contact with contaminated animal blood or tissues or by a tick bite. The incubation period lasts 1–3 days and the disease onset is acute, manifested by fever, myalgias, light-headedness, and cervical spinal pain, headache accompanied by photophobia, abdominal pain, vomiting and diarrhea. Agitation and aggressive behavior typically ensue, followed by somnolence and depression at later stages of the illness. Frequently observed clinical signs are tachycardia, lymphadenopathy, hepatomegaly associated with mild hepatitis and diffuse petechial rash with mucosal involvement. Hemorrhagic manifestations include upper gastrointestinal bleeding with melena, gross hematuria, gingival bleeding and epistaxis. Acute respiratory failure, as part of multiorgan failure, may develop later than the fifth day of overt clinical illness. Therapy is usually limited to supportive measures, although ribavirin has also been tried without significant clinical benefit. Thus, mortality rates are high (30%).

Yellow fever is an acute illness, typically transmitted via mosquitoes, sharing many common clinical manifestations with other *HFVs*. However, severe hepatic involvement constitutes a more common and cardinal clinical feature of Y*ellow fever* compared to other *HFVs*. Following an incubation period of 3–6 days, a rapid onset of fever, generalized discomfort, weakness, headache, nausea and vomiting typically ensue. Those nonspecific systemic symptoms usually predominate for 3 days, followed by a spontaneous remission of clinical symptoms in the next 24 hours. Then, jaundice, oliguria, hemodynamic instability and bleeding may manifest.[10] Severe forms of *Yellow fever* are characterized by a high mortality rate of 50%. Similar to *Yellow fever*, both *Omsk hemorrhagic fever* and *Kyasanur Forest disease* are caused by *Flaviviridae*, which are mainly transmitted to humans via tick bites and, less frequently, through aerosolized particles.

Infection with *HFVs* should be suspected in any patient who presents with acute severe hemorrhagic manifestations, especially after a recent travel in endemic regions of the disease, or in periods of bioterrorist threats and attacks.[9] Except in cases of *Lassa fever*, thrombocytopenia and leucopenia are common laboratory features of *VHFs*. However, thrombocytopenia is not severe enough to solely account for the hemorrhagic symptoms and signs. Other common laboratory features are proteinuria and elevation of liver enzymes. Jaundice mainly develops in *Yellow fever* and *Rift Valley fever* cases,[8] whereas disseminated intravascular coagulation (*DIC*), although reported in many cases of *VHFs*, cannot be considered as typical for any of the distinct syndromes.

Diagnostic methods involved in *VHFs* are the isolation of the virus and detection of specific antibodies (including *IgM* subtype); using enzyme-linked immunosorbent assays (*ELISA*). Reverse-transcription polymerase chain reaction (*RT-PCR*) may also be used for the detection of viral genome in biologic fluids and tissues. Handling of studied samples and viral cultures should be restricted in highly specialized laboratories, where maximum security precautions can be maintained.[8]

Ribavirin, a nucleoside analogue, has been proposed as a potential antiviral agent in the treatment or prevention of *Arenaviridae* and *Bunyaviridae* infections.[16] It has already been used in the treatment of hepatitis C and respiratory syncytial virus as well as *Crimean-Congo hemorrhagic fever* virus, *Hantavirus* and *Arenaviridae* (*Lassa* and *New World* viruses) infections. Ribavirin should be administered intravenously (*iv*), within 6 days of the disease onset, according to the following formula: a loading dose of 30 *mg/kg*, followed by 60 *mg/kg* divided in four daily doses for 4 days and then 24 *mg/kg* in three daily doses for the rest 6 days. Intravenous hyperimmune globulin, administered within 8 days of the disease onset, could be effective in the treatment of *Junin* virus infection. Interferon-alpha has shown a protective effect when tested in animal models of *Rift Valley fever* infection and is generally limited to the very early stages of the infection. The combination of ribavirin and interferon-alpha may be associated with a more protective effect, although not enough supportive evidence for human infection is available.[17]

When a patient presents with symptoms compatible to *VHFs*, he/she must be isolated and supportive treatment must be administered as soon as possible along with ribavirin, where indicated. This approach must be continued until the diagnosis of *VHFs* can be confirmed or ruled out. Although nowadays a number of potentially efficient vaccines are under various clinical trials, none of those is licensed to be used for the prevention of *VHFs*. *Yellow fever* is the only *VHF* for which an efficient vaccine is licensed.[16] Recently, it has been reported that a single dose of live-attenuated stomatitis virus vaccine, molecularly modified to express a glycoprotein of *Ebola* virus, has effectively prevented the development of fatal clinical syndrome after the exposure of rodents and monkeys to the virus.[18] Additionally, an effective and safe vaccine against *Ebola* virus has already been tried in a small patient cohort (20 patients) in a phase I study.[19]

In conclusion, although not enough evidence is available, it can be assumed that many of the *HFVs* (*Ebola, Marburg, Lassa, New World Arenaviridae, Rift Valley fever, Yellow fever, Omsk hemorrhagic fever, Kyasanur Forest disease*) can be considered as potential bioterrorist threats. Most of those have been extensively studied, modified and weaponized in many countries. A possible spread of *HFVs* in aerosolized form could result into severe morbidity and mortality, provided that neither effective preventive vaccination nor effective treatment regimens exist against them.

Smallpox (*Variola*)

Variola virus has been recognized as the causative agent of *smallpox*, a highly infectious disease characterized by fever, rash and a high associated mortality rate. According to the *World Health Organization* (*WHO*), the disease was eradicated globally in 1979 through a program that included widespread immunization.[20] The last known case in the world, in September 1978, resulted from a laboratory accident in Birmingham, England. Although there have been no reported cases since, continued interest in this virus remains because of the concern regarding its use as a potential agent of bioterrorism.[21,22]

Typically the disease occurs in two main clinical forms: *variola major*, which is a serious illness with a high mortality rate of 30–50%, and *variola minor*, which is a milder infection with a substantially lower mortality rate of less than 1%.[23] The two forms are caused by different strains of *variola* virus. Respiratory viral shedding and infectivity is highest at the beginning of the rash.[24] However, transmission is not widespread and is usually confined to unimmunized persons sharing living quarters. Among unvaccinated family members, approximately 58% contracted *smallpox* compared with 4% in vaccines. The severity of the illness, which usually confines the patient to bed and restricts contact, may contribute to the relatively low attack rate. Because of long incubation times, transmission intervals are 2–3 weeks apart; thus, emerging cases of *smallpox* would appear in a community over many months.

Variola virus is an orthopoxvirus of the *Poxviridae* family. It is a large (200–400 *nm*) *DNA* virus that lacks icosahedral symmetry. The virus consists of an outer membrane, two lateral bodies, and a dumbbell-shaped core that contains a single molecule of double-stranded *DNA*.[25] The entire 186,000 base-pair genome has been sequenced[26] and the majority of the genes are found to be closely related to the genes of *vaccinia* virus, the virus used to vaccinate against *smallpox*.[27] While *variola minor* strains have high sequence similarity to *variola major* strains, it is believed that changes in differential gene expression may explain the differences in virulence. However, because of their high sequence similarity, it is difficult to distinguish *variola minor* from *variola major* in the laboratory. Newer diagnostic tests, under development, may differentiate the two strains of virus.[28]

Human-to-human transmission of *smallpox* virus is generally mediated by the expectoration of upper airway secretions.[23,29] Inhaled secretions, containing the virus, enter the respiratory tract where viruses are multiplied locally and then spread to regional lymph nodes via circulating macrophages.[24] Multiplication within lymph nodes leads to a primary viremia with dissemination of virus to lymphoid organs. Viral amplification within lymphoid organs leads to a secondary viremia, which is associated with the onset of symptoms and the characteristic *smallpox* rash. Virus can be isolated from the oropharynx, skin lesions, bone marrow, spleen, liver, and kidneys. The virus is localized within small dermal blood vessels, produces endothelial swelling and infection of epidermal cells and results in characteristic vesicles in skin and mucous membranes. Extension of infection into the corium and sebaceous glands produces the "pockmarks" or scars which, upon healing, are the hallmarks of prior *smallpox* infection.

The most vulnerable individuals against *smallpox* are infants, the elderly, and the immunosuppressed individuals, particularly those with T-cell deficits. Milder forms are observed in patients with a history of previous immunization. *Variola major* is classified into five clinical categories, each associated with a different level of severity of disease: ordinary type, modified type, flat type, hemorrhagic type and *variola* sine eruption. All of those forms have a characteristic rash, except for *variola* sine eruption.

In ordinary type *smallpox*, the incubation period ranges from 7 days to 19 days.[24] A pre-eruptive phase, lasting 2–4 days, is characterized by the sudden onset of high fever, severe headache, backache, and malaise. Vomiting and diarrhea may also occur.[23] The associated rash may be either confluent, present on face and forearms, or semi-confluent, present on the face with discrete rash elsewhere, or discrete rash on all involved areas with normal skin between pustules. Clinical outcome for ordinary type smallpox is closely linked to the type of the accompanying rash. Mortality rates are approximately 62% for confluent infection, 37% for semi-confluent and 9% for discrete rash.[23] Death usually results from coagulopathy, hypotension and multiorgan failure.[30]

The eruptive phase is characterized by lesions on the mucous membranes, followed approximately 24 hours later by the cutaneous rash. Intraoral lesions first appear as papules, followed by vesicles on the tongue and palate. The spread of the exanthema is centrifugal, involving initially the face, followed by proximal extremities, the trunk and the distal extremities.[31] The exanthema typically begins as small macules ("herald spots") on the face. Macules evolve to papules by day two of the rash, vesicles by days four to five, and pustules by day seven. Fever occasionally recurs during the pustular phase.[32] Crusts develop by day 14 and heal with residual depigmentation.

The modified form of *smallpox* is similar to ordinary disease, except that the phases of the rash develop more rapidly and pustular lesions are smaller.[23] Flat type is characterized by pustules which remain flat and are usually confluent or semi-confluent occurs mainly in children and is often fatal. The hemorrhagic form of disease, in which skin lesions and mucous membranes become hemorrhagic, is the rarest form. Profound prostration, heart failure, diffuse bleeding, and bone marrow suppression commonly result in a fatal outcome within 3–4 days. Pregnant women are predisposed to this type of *smallpox*.[24] *Variola* sine eruptions occur among vaccinated individuals or in partially immune patients who have been previously infected. Typically, these patients have fever but no rash.[23]

The most important potential complications of *smallpox* include secondary bacterial skin infections, keratitis and corneal ulcerations leading to blindness, viral arthritis, osteomyelitis, bacterial pneumonia, orchitis and encephalitis.[23,29] Nonspecific laboratory findings, including granulocytopenia, thrombocytopenia, and lymphocytosis are common during the prodromal and early rash phase. Leukocytosis often occurs when vesicles become pustular. DIC is often seen in patients with hemorrhagic *smallpox*.[23]

With the worldwide eradication of *smallpox*, routine vaccination with *vaccinia* virus is no longer performed. However, after the *anthrax* bioterrorism attack in 2001, the *US* government tried to improve preparedness for the intentional or accidental release of *variola* virus. Initially, this began with attempts to vaccinate a large number of potential first-responders and healthcare workers.[33,34] There has also been funding for the development and production of a modern-day *smallpox* vaccine as well as the development of antipoxvirus therapeutics.

Identification of a case of smallpox should be a public health emergency. Thus, any use of the smallpox vaccine, in the setting of suspected smallpox bioterrorism, should be done only after direct consultation with state and local health officials, along with the CDC. The Advisory Committee on Immunization Practices has published recommendations for smallpox vaccination in routine nonemergency and emergency settings,33,35 which can be found at: www.cdc.gov/mmwr/preview/mmwrhtml/rr5010a1.htm and www.cdc.gov/mmwr/preview/mmwrhtml/rr5207a1.htm.

Vaccination with *vaccinia* virus is carried out as a scarification; an infectious dose is placed on a bifurcated sterile needle and gently penetrated several times into the epidermis of the deltoid region of the arm. Two to five days after primary vaccination, a papule forms and becomes a vesicle 2–3 days later. The vesicle reaches a maximum size by day 8–10. A scab forms within 2 weeks leaving behind a scar when healing is complete. Mild fever and localized lymphadenopathy are often present during the first 2 weeks after vaccination. With the worldwide eradication of *smallpox* and the suspension of *vaccinia* virus as a routine vaccine, there is a growing population that is susceptible to *smallpox*. Concerns have been raised that *variola* virus might be used as a biological warfare agent.[32] Contraindications against *smallpox* vaccination include: patients with immunodeficiencies, individuals with a history of eczema or other exfoliative skin condition and pregnant women.[36]

Category C Biological Threats

Viruses that are grouped in *category C* of biological threats can be considered as emerging potential bioterrorism agents, which either have been recently molecularly modified in the laboratory in order to meet the characteristics of such an agent, or carry this potential when are still in their natural form. Examples of viruses meeting those criteria are *avian influenza H5N1* virus, *Nipah* and *SARS coronavirus*, respectively.

Highly pathogenic *avian H5N1 influenza* virus now appears to be endemic among bird and poultry populations in Eurasia.[37] Sporadic transmission to humans raises concern that the H5N1 virus may mutate or combine with genetic material from co-infecting human *influenza* viruses to generate a novel strain, capable of sustained human-to-human transmission with pandemic potential. In fact, *WHO* has described the potential threat from H5N1 as a "public health crisis".

The first association of *avian influenza H5N1* with clinical respiratory disease occurred in Hong Kong in 1997, when 18 human cases were noted during a poultry outbreak of highly pathogenic H5N1 *influenza* in live-bird markets.[38,39] This outbreak was associated with a high mortality rate (33%), a high incidence of pneumonia (61%) and a high rate of intensive care (51%).

Human *influenza* is transmitted by inhalation of infectious droplets and droplet nuclei, by direct contact, and possibly by indirect (fomite) contact. For human *influenza* A (H5N1) infections, bird-to-human is the predominant route of transmission, whereas limited, nonsustained human-to-human transmission has also rarely been reported.

Researchers in the *US* and the Netherlands reported recently the creation of recombinant H5N1 *influenza* viruses that are transmissible in ferrets, an excellent model for human *influenza* infections.[40] In the fall of 2011, a *US* government advisory panel, the *National Science Advisory Board for Biosecurity*, asked the journals *Science* and *Nature,* which were considering publishing these data, to withhold details that would allow replication of the experiments because of concerns about this information being used for bioterrorism. This intervention spurred much debate.[41-43] A group of experts that met at the *WHO* in February 2012 recommended that the full results of these studies be published, though a moratorium on publication has been temporarily extended until details are worked out.

Both H5 and H7 subtypes possess the ability to evolve into highly pathogenic virus strains. The more recent circulating H5 viruses appear to be more pathogenic in mammals and birds than the earlier H5 viruses, a feature that may precede emergence of reassorted H5 strains with pandemic potential.[44,45]

Following exposure to infected poultry, the incubation period for human H5N1 infection is 7 days or less.[46] Respiratory illness is the most common manifestation, but patients with solely gastrointestinal or central nervous system involvement have also been described. Common presenting features are fever (75%), cough (89%), dyspnea (81%), bilateral pulmonary infiltrates (72%), lymphopenia (73%), and increased aminotransferases [aspartate aminotransferase (AST), 69%; alanine aminotransferase (ALT), 61%]. Diarrhea and mucosal bleeding at presentation are more common among patients who die. The risk of death is highest among individuals younger than 16 years of age.

Respiratory symptoms may be accompanied by gastrointestinal symptoms, headache, myalgias, sore throat, rhinorrhea or, uncommonly, conjunctivitis or bleeding gums.[38,46] Diarrhea is a prominent presenting symptom, along with respiratory distress, in several case series.[38,47] Complications include multiorgan failure with renal dysfunction and cardiac compromise, pulmonary hemorrhage, pneumothorax and pancytopenia.[48] Most deaths have been related to respiratory failure. Patients with severe disease often have leukopenia, neutropenia, lymphopenia, and thrombocytopenia on hospital admission.[49,50] Other laboratory abnormalities include elevated levels of aminotransferases, lactate dehydrogenase (LDH), creatine kinase, and hypoalbuminemia. Radiographic findings of H5N1 avian *influenza* include diffuse, multifocal, or patchy infiltrates, interstitial infiltrates and segmental or lobular consolidation. Progression to respiratory failure is typically associated with diffuse bilateral ground-glass infiltrates.

The diagnosis of H5N1 avian *influenza* can be made by viral culture in appropriate biocontainment or *PCR* assay for H5N1 *RNA* or immunofluorescence test for antigen with the use of monoclonal antibody against H5 or a fourfold rise in H5-specific antibody in paired serum samples. When suspecting highly pathogenic avian *influenza,* specimens must be handled and processed using appropriate biosafety precautions. Therefore, clinicians must alert their laboratory personnel of any clinical suspicion of avian *influenza,* so that the samples will be processed in the appropriate facility.[51] Specimens should be collected and shipped immediately to the appropriate level 3 testing laboratory.

The threat of an avian *influenza* pandemic has prompted global preparedness plans. A national surveillance system for avian *influenza* in Thailand led to a decrease in the median time from procurement of samples to results of testing from 17 days to 18 days. In the event of a pandemic, or in a bioterrorist attack, the presence of such programs should help in the containment of disease.

Nipah Virus

The primary animal reservoirs of the virus are bats of the genus *Pteropus*.[52] *Nipah* virus-infected pigs have clinical disease, manifested by neurologic and respiratory symptoms.[53] The mode of transmission between pigs is probably through direct contact with infected fluid such as urine, saliva, pharyngeal, and bronchial secretions. Other domestic animals such as cats and dogs have also been shown to have a positive serology for *Nipah* virus.[54]

Human infection occurs through direct contact with respiratory secretions and urine from infected pigs.[55] Another mode of transmission is occupational contact, including abattoir workers and pork sellers.[56] There is also evidence that *Nipah* virus may be transmitted from human-to-human.[57]

Among patients with *Nipah* virus infection who have a well-defined exposure to another infected patient, the median incubation period is 9 days (range, 6–11 days)[58] *Nipah* virus causes primarily an encephalitic syndrome with a high mortality rate ranging between 40% and 70%.[54] The initial presentation includes nonspecific systemic symptoms such as sudden onset of fever, headache, myalgias, nausea and vomiting. Meningismus is seen in approximately one-third of patients. However, marked nuchal rigidity and photophobia are uncommon. In approximately 60% of patients, the disease progresses rapidly, with deterioration in consciousness leading to coma within 5–7 days. Generalized seizures occur in approximately 20% of patients. Other neurologic findings associated with *Nipah* encephalitis include segmental myoclonus, cerebellar dysfunction, tremors and areflexia. Brainstem involvement, characterized by pinpoint, nonreactive pupils, abnormal doll's eye reflex, tachycardia and hypertension, occurs in the more severe cases and portends a poorer prognosis.[54] A smaller number of patients may present with atypical pneumonia and diffuse interstitial lung infiltrates.[58]

The laboratory abnormalities in *Nipah* encephalitis are nonspecific. Abnormalities of the cerebrospinal fluid (*CSF*) are observed in the majority of cases. Most have an increased cell count (range: 10–800 cells/mL), with lymphocyte predominance, and an elevated protein concentration (range: 50–250 mg/dL). The *CSF* glucose concentration is normal and red blood cells are not usually present.

Virus isolation is not routinely done since *Nipah* virus is classified as a biosafety level-4 agent. Therefore, other methods, such as serology or *PCR*, are employed. Supportive care is the mainstay of treatment, including intensive care monitoring. Mechanical ventilation for airway protection should be initiated with the onset of neurologic deterioration. Ribavirin has also been given empirically, without solid evidence of clinical effectiveness.[54]

SARS Coronavirus

According to *WHO*, a case of SARS is notifiable if it occurs in an individual with laboratory confirmation of infection who either meets the clinical case definition or has worked in a laboratory with live *SARS coronavirus* or with clinical specimens infected with *SARS coronavirus*.[59]

The clinical case definition includes: history of fever or documented fever and one or more symptoms of lower respiratory tract illness (i.e., cough and shortness of breath) and radiographic evidence of lung infiltrates consistent with pneumonia or *ARDS* or autopsy findings consistent with the pathology of pneumonia or *ARDS* without an identifiable cause and no alternative diagnosis fully explaining the illness.

Based upon the clusters of cases in Hong Kong and Canada, *SARS coronavirus* could clearly spread from person-to-person and could be acquired from face-to-face contact, suggesting droplet spread.[60-62] There has also been speculation that other modes of spread, such as fecal-oral or airborne might be possible. Transmission to healthcare workers has been a common feature of most *SARS* outbreaks, emphasizing the need for strict hygiene measures when such cases are handled in healthcare settings. A possible contributing factor is that peak viral shedding in respiratory secretions, as determined by *PCR*, occurs 6–11 days following the onset of illness, at a time of severe respiratory symptoms.[63] This late viral excretion peak is an unusual feature of *SARS*, when compared with other respiratory viral infections.

The incubation period for *SARS* is usually 2–7 days.[64] The prodrome phase is often prolonged, lasting for 3–7 days and is characterized by fever (>38°C) malaise, headache, and myalgias.[65] Most patients have no upper respiratory symptoms during this stage. At the end of this prodrome, the respiratory phase typically begins with a nonproductive cough. Dyspnea may follow and may progress to respiratory failure, with progressive pulmonary infiltrates on chest X-ray, necessitating mechanical ventilation. Other less common symptoms are diarrhea (20%) and chest pain or pleurisy (22%). Most common laboratory abnormalities are lymphopenia (66%) and elevated LDH (46%) and ALT (44%).[66] Thrombocytopenia is present in 30% while a high LDH level is usually associated with a poor outcome.[67]

Chest X-ray patterns range from normal to diffuse interstitial infiltrates characteristic of *ARDS*.[68] Computed tomographic (*CT*) scanning may show parenchymal abnormalities in patients with apparently normal chest X-rays. Infiltrates are usually ground-glass in character and peripheral in location.

When *SARS* is suspected, specimens for *PCR* testing should be obtained from at least two sites, such as the respiratory tract, stool, and serum or plasma. *PCR* testing should be performed as early in the illness as possible and, if symptoms progress or persist, repeat 5–7 days later. Acute and convalescent serum should also be collected for serologic testing.

The control of *SARS* through the rigorous application of barrier methods represents one of the landmark accomplishments of infectious diseases epidemiology and public health coordination. One of the characteristics of the infection, namely the low contagiousness of patients during the prodrome, probably may contribute to the success of control efforts, since patients could, in the outbreak situation, be identified and placed on isolation before they become infectious to contacts. Quarantine of patients, use of masks, gloves and gowns by the healthcare personnel, and closure of schools, hospitals, and clubs, probably all may effectively contribute to containment of the outbreak.[69,70]

BACTERIAL AGENTS

Bacillus anthracis

History

The biological agent most probable to be used in future bioterrorist attacks is *Bacillus anthracis* (*BA*). In a 1970 *WHO* report,[71] it was estimated that if 50 *kg* of *BA* spores were released by an airplane as aerosol 2 *km* away of an urban center with a population of 500,000, there would be approximately 95,000 deaths. In fact, *BA* spores were sent to several places across the *US* right after the attacks of September 11, 2001. There were 22 confirmed or possible *anthrax* (A) infections; among them, 11 cases represented pulmonary infections and five were fatal. In an accidental leakage of *BA* spores from a biological weapons industry located in *Sverdlovsk*, a Russian city with a population of 1,200,000, there were 42 confirmed deaths in a 50 *km* radius.[72,73]

Microbiology

Bacillus anthracis is an anaerobic, nonmotile, *Gram (+)* bacillus with a centrally positioned spore. The chains of the pathogenic microbial forms usually have a capsule. *BA* grown in blood agar in 18–24 hours. Several biochemical tests may help in discriminating from other species members. *BA* spores grow in *Petri* dishes, in soil, in dead animal tissues, but not in the blood and tissues of infected animals. They are resistant to most antiseptics, drying and boiling for 10 minutes. They need to be boiled at 120°C for at least 15 minutes to be inactivated. They can survive in arid conditions for years.[74]

Epidemiology: Clinical Manifestations

There are three clinical entities of *anthrax*:[75] (1) cutaneous A which is the most common, (2) gastrointestinal A which is caused by the consumption of infected meat and, (3) respiratory A which is caused by inhalation of spores. Until the recent outbreaks in the *US* and former *USSR*, respiratory A occurred sporadically, mainly in individuals with occupational exposure to infected animals. Regarding its pathogenicity, it seems that *BA* spores that lie in particles of 2–5 μm in diameter may be deposited on the alveoli and phagocytized by alveolar macrophages. Those spores that evade phagocytosis are transported via the lymphatic system to the hilar and mediastinal lymph nodes, where new bacilli are formed and toxins are produced. The latter eventually enter the circulation and lead to multiorgan failure or even death. According to animal studies, a dose of 2,500–55,000 *BA* spores may cause the death of half of the exposed population.[76]

Historically, respiratory A is a biphasic disease. During the first phase, which lasts approximately 4 days, there may be myalgias, fatigue, nonproductive cough, retrosternal pain and fever. A temporary improvement may be seen after the first days. The second phase, which lasts 24 hours and may often, be fatal, presents with acute respiratory distress. Swelling of the lymph nodes may cause tracheal compression with wheezing. Central nervous system involvement may present with meningism, drowsiness, and/or coma in half of the cases. The most recent data, regarding the clinical manifestation of respiratory A, come from the *US* outbreak in 2001. All patients had fever with chills and malaise, dyspnea, thoracic pain, cough, nausea and headache. The majority of patients had hypoxemia and elevated transaminases; the median *WBC* count was 9,800/*mL*. All chest X-rays were pathological; the commonest findings were mediastinal dilatation (70%), infiltrates (70%) and pleural effusions (80%).[77] There were similar findings in the thoracic *CT*.

During its first phase, diagnosis of respiratory A is difficult. Symptoms are mild and quite similar to those of common cold. Hupert et al[78] concluded that fever and cough could not discriminate A from other diseases, after retrospectively studying the clinical characteristics of 28 respiratory A cases (from 1920 to 2001), of 2,762 *influenza* cases and of 1,932 cases with noninfluenza viral infection. On the contrary, the presence of neurological symptoms (apart from headache), dyspnea, nausea or vomiting, and auscultatory findings increased the probability for *anthrax* infection. Rhinorrhea and quinsy increased the probability for viral infection. Blood culture is a very sensitive method and becomes positive in 6–24 hours. Sputum cultures rarely lead to the correct diagnosis. Nasal swabs may be used for the commencement of antibiotic therapy but not to rule out infection.

In conclusion, the presence of several patients with fever and respiratory failure who eventually die should raise suspicion of a respiratory *anthrax* outbreak, especially if there are accompanying imaging findings of mediastinal dilatation (due to mediastinal lymphadenopathy), pleural effusions, and isolation of *Gram (+)* bacilli in blood or CSF.

Prevention

There are no data supporting human-to-human transmission but a person's clothing and body may be contaminated with *anthrax* spores.[72,76] The usual measures for the prevention of microbe dissemination are suggested for all types of *anthrax* infections. However, the use of special breathing masks is not necessary. There is no need of vaccination of individuals close to the patient, unless there is an indication of exposure to the same source of anthrax. The usual disinfectants, such as hypochlorite salt, are effective in cleaning surfaces that are infected with *anthrax*.[79]

The *FDA* has approved a vaccine under the brand name *BioThrax* to be administered in five-dose series followed by annual boosters to maintain immunity. Recent simulation studies suggest that post-attack prophylactic vaccination and antibiotic therapy is the most effective and least expensive strategy. However, strategies to reduce deaths from such an attack are cost-effective, only if large exposures are certain. In such cases, a faster response is more beneficial than enhanced surveillance.[80,81]

Treatment

Given the rapid clinical course of respiratory *anthrax*, early administration of antibiotic treatment is of paramount importance. *BA* is highly sensitive to penicillin, amoxicillin, chloramphenicol, doxycycline, erythromycin, streptomycin, and ciprofloxacin. It is resistant to third-generation cephalosporins, cotrimoxazole, and aztreonam.[82] After the attacks in 2001, *CDC* issued guidelines suggesting combination treatment with 2 or 3 antibiotics.[83] According to these guidelines, the first-line treatment for adult patients includes the *iv* administration of ciprofloxacin 400 *mg* or doxycycline 100 *mg q12h* in combination with 1–2 antibiotics that demonstrate *in vitro* activity, such as rifampicin, vancomycin, ampicillin, penicillin, imipenem, clindamycin and clarithromycin. Very recently, *FDA* approved the use of levofloxacin to treat patients with pneumonic plague in the event of a bioterrorist attack.[84] Penicillin and ampicillin should not be administered as monotherapy due to the possibility of beta-lactamase induction. Furthermore, if there is a suspicion of meningeal involvement, doxycycline's low penetration of the blood-brain barrier should be kept in mind. The total duration of antibiotic treatment, initially *iv* and subsequently per os, should be 2 months due to the probability of spores remaining in the organism after the initial exposure.

Francisella tularensis

History

Francisella tularensis has long been recognized as a possible biological weapon. For example, it was studied by the Japanese army in Manchuria between 1932 and 1945, during the 50's and the 60's by the *US* army and the former *USSR*. In 1969, a special *WHO* committee estimated that the dissemination of 50 *kg* of *F. tularensis* in the form of aerosol, over an area with a population of 500,000, would cause 250,000 severe infections and 19,000 deaths.

Microbiology

Tularemia (T) is caused by *F tularensis*, a *Gram (-)* microbe, which grows intracellularly, like *Mycobacteria, Brucella, Legionella* and *Listeria*. It cannot be readily differentiated from other bacteria through conventional diagnostic techniques. Due to the recent advances in molecular methods, laboratory tests based on *PCR* may lead to its rapid and reliable identification. *F. tularensis* includes two main subspecies, *Francisella tularensis ssp. tularensis* (*Jellison* type A) and *Francisella tularensis ssp. holarctica* (*Jellison* type B). Type A is found in North America and is the main subspecies in the continent while type B is widely spread at the northern hemisphere and is the only subspecies found in Europe.

Epidemiology: Clinical Manifestations

The natural reservoir of *F. tularensis* is not known. Although type A outbreaks are associated with increased prevalence among *Lagomorpha* and *Rodentia*, these animals do not seem to be able to "maintain" the bacteria between the outbreaks, because they either do not seem to survive the infection or become immune to it. However, the bacterium may survive in water and mud for months and is transmitted from rabbits to humans through ticks and/or direct contact with infected animals.

Before the emergence of effective antibiotics, mortality due to type A was reported to be as high as 5–10%. The infectious dose for humans is very low: 10 bacteria in subcutaneous inoculation or 25 in aerosol.[85] However, human-to-human transmission has not been described. Type B is also associated with rodents and hares and is transmitted to human through direct contact with animals, aerogenous exposure, infected food or water and tick bites. Type B is less harmful than type A and not lethal to humans. However, it may cause severe disease and, in case of delayed antibiotic management, the clinical course may be long and complicated.

Tularemia is endemic in most northern hemisphere countries. In America, it is reported in Canada, *US* and Mexico. Seasonal distribution in *US* presents a peak from November to February, which is associated with hunting, and a second one during the summer, which is associated with the exposure to tick bites. T is widely found in Eurasia (mainly in the former *USSR* and Scandinavia). Recently (1999–2000), 327 T cases were reported in postwar Kosovo and were attributed to the degradation of public health services and to the infection of food and water supplies by rodents.[86]

Tularemia's clinical form depends on the point of entry. Ulceroglandular form is caused by tick bites in the *US* and in areas of central Europe[87] and by mosquitoes in northern Europe.[88] Hunters may get infected through abrasions after direct contact with infected animals. Oculoglandular form is probably caused by aerogenous exposure or inoculation through the patient's fingers. Oropharyngeal form is associated with the consumption of infected food and water. Pneumonic T is caused by inhalation of a bacterium-containing aerosol. Although it is rarer than ulceroglandular form, it tends to cause outbreaks.

Tularemia's incubation period usually lasts 3–5 days, but it may vary from 1 day to 21 days. Disease onset may be acute, with high fever, chills, malaise, nausea and headache. The duration of fever may vary from days to several weeks. Dry cough may be often present, even without pneumonia. Disease severity may vary according to the causative T type. In type A infection, the patient's clinical course may be complicated with septic shock. Mortality of type A T is 1–2%. Although pneumonic T classically presents with pneumonia symptoms, it may also present without severe respiratory symptoms. Type A pneumonic T is mostly associated with mortality. The patient presents with fever with chills, dyspnea, cough, thoracic pain and severe sweating. Cough may be productive and the patient can look highly "toxic". In 50% of the cases there is relative bradycardia. In some cases, erythema nodosum or multiforme may appear. Radiological findings vary. Hilar lymphadenopathy is a remarkable but nonspecific finding. It should be noted that T may cause various manifestations like septicemia, meningitis, endocarditis and hepatic or renal failure.[89,90]

Routine blood tests do not yield specific results. Median *WBC* count is 10,500/*mL*, with mild lymphocytosis. There is a mild elevation of transaminases.[91] The bacterium is rarely isolated in blood or sputum cultures. Thus, the microbiological diagnosis depends on serological methods. It should be noted, that there is a probability of cross-reaction with *Brucella* or *Yersinia* and that the presence of *IgM* antibodies against *F. tularensis* does not indicate recent infection.[85] Furthermore, serological diagnosis needs at least 14 days to be finalized. Thus, the clinician must administer empirical treatment under the appropriate circumstances.

Prevention

Vaccination with live attenuated bacteria may confer at least partial protection against pneumonic T. Vaccination is not recommended for post-exposure prophylaxis, unless it is administered to laboratory staff. Prophylactic antibiotic therapy of individuals in close contact with infected patients as well as isolation of patients is not recommended.[92] Hospitals should take routine measures. No special procedures, regarding clothes disinfection, are necessary.

Treatment

Tularemia treatment is based on intramuscular (*im*) aminoglycoside administration (*im* streptomycin 1 *g q12h* as first-line treatment and *im* or *iv* gentamicin 5 *mg/kg q24h* as alternative treatment because it is bactericidal and is associated with low recurrence rates. Tetracyclines are bacteriostatic antibiotics and are associated with relatively high recurrence rates, so they should be used in milder type B *tularemia* infections. It should be noted, that macrolides, co-trimoxazole and beta-lactams[93] are not reliable antibiotics against T. Thus, the usual combination of a macrolide with a third-generation cephalosporin, which is empirically used for the treatment of community-acquired pneumonia, is not effective against pneumonic T. Quinolones may be used as an alternative, especially for type B infections,[94] but more data are warranted.

Yersinia pestis

History

The plague of Justinian (541-542 AD) is the first known *plague* pandemic. It is considered to have started in Egypt. At its peak, the *plague* killed 10,000 people daily and annihilated 40% of Constantinople's population. The second great *plague* pandemic, also known as *Black Plague*, started in 1346 and finally killed 20–30 million people in Europe, or one-third of its total population.[95] The third pandemic started in China in 1855 and finally killed over 12 million people.[96] During the Second World War, a secret branch of the Japanese army reportedly spread infected fleas in inhabited Chinese regions, thus causing *plague* outbreaks. In 1970, the *WHO* reported that if 50 *kg* of the bacterium were disseminated as aerosol over a city with a population of

500,000, at least 150,000 inhabitants would be infected with pneumonic plague and this would cause 36,000 deaths. In the former *USSR*, relevant projects using plague as a potential biological weapon were more advanced than those of the *US*.

Microbiology

Yersinia pestis is a nonmotile, *Gram (-)* bacillus belonging to the *Enterobacteriaceae*. It needs around 48 hours to form its colonies, but because they are smaller from those of other members of *Enterobacteriaceae*, they may not be noticed at first.[96]

Epidemiology: Clinical Manifestations

Human *plague* usually presents in its bubonic form after a bite by an infected flea. The migration of the flea population to humans precedes the death of a large number of rats, which constitutes its natural reservoir. Although most patients who get infected this way develop bubonic *plague*, some of the patients may also develop pneumonic *plague* and transmit it through droplets.[97] *Plague* is an enzootic disease of rats, squirrels, dogs and rodents in every inhabited continent except Oceania. During the last 50 years, there is an annual mean incidence of 1,700 cases worldwide. Although pneumonic *plague* is rare, outbreaks have been reported. A lesson from an epidemic in Manchuria in 1910-11 was that low temperature, increased humidity, and overcrowding in confined spaces helped in the spread of the disease.

The pathogenesis and clinical manifestations of *plague* after a biological strike are different from naturally occurring disease. The inhaled bacilli of *Y. pestis* are the causative agents of primary pneumonic *plague*. The time from exposure to emergence of the first symptoms is 2–4 days.[98] The first signs of the disease are fever with cough, which usually is productive with watery and bloody/purulent expectoration and dyspnea. Gastrointestinal symptoms are prominent, including nausea, emesis, abdominal pain and diarrhea. The following stages of primary pneumonic SARS, severe acute respiratory syndrome *plague* are similar with those of any other rapidly progressing pneumonia. In contrast to secondary pneumonic *plague*, primary disease is not usually accompanied with lymphadenopathy. Radiological findings may vary, but bilateral pulmonary infiltrates are very common. As a result of multiorgan failure, laboratory findings include leukocytosis, coagulation disorders, transaminases and urea elevation. The time from exposure to death is reported to be 2–4 days in most epidemics.

Taking into account the rarity of *plague* and the probability the first cases to be the precursor to an outbreak, clinical or laboratory suspicion should lead to mobilization of the appropriate resources. Unfortunately, no surveillance and early warning systems against aerosol containing *plague* bacilli are available. The first indication of a probable bioterrorist attack would be an outbreak of severe pneumonia and septicemia. A sudden increase in previously healthy patients with fever, cough, dyspnea and thoracic pain, whose disease has a deadly outcome, should raise the suspicion of pneumonic *plague* or respiratory *anthrax*.[99] The presence of hemoptysis is in favor of *plague*.

There is no widely available rapid diagnostic test for *plague*. Sputum or blood may reveal *Gram (-)* bacilli. Rarely, when a lymph node is palpable in pneumonic *plague*, it may be aspired and stained. Sputum, blood and lymph node cultures usually get positive in 24–48 hours.

Prevention

From the very moment that pneumonic *plague* is suspected or diagnosed, every individual with fever or cough in the supposed area of exposure should immediately receive appropriate prophylactic antibiotic treatment. Treatment delays until the confirmation of diagnosis reduce survival. Asymptomatic individuals that came in close contact with patients who have not completed pneumonic *plague* treatment should receive prophylactic treatment for 7 days and be vigilant for the emergence of fever or cough. Contact with a patient in a distance less than 2 *m* is considered as close contact.[99]

According to the experience gained from large epidemics of pneumonic *plague* of the previous century, the use of disposable surgical masks, as well as gowns, gloves and eye protection, for the prevention of the disease transmission is recommended.[100,101] The patients must be isolated during the first 48 hours of antibiotic therapy and until clinical improvement. If the patients are too many to be separately isolated, they may remain in the same room as long as they receive appropriate antibiotic treatment and wear surgical masks. Hospital rooms and fomites should be disinfected and burial of the deceased should be done following standardized protocols. Procedures that may form aerosols should be avoided.

There are no data indicating that *plague* bacilli are a threat for the population after the initial aerosol is dissolved. In contrast to *B. anthracis*, there is no form of spores in *Y. pestis* life cycle. Also, *Y. pestis* is very sensitive to the effect of direct sunlight and heat and does not survive away from the host. Thus, disinfection of areas that were exposed to plague aerosol is not necessary.

Treatment

The treatment of choice for *plague* is the *im* administration of streptomycin 1 *g q12h* and *im* or *iv* administration of gentamicin 5 *mg/kg q24h*. Alternatively, gentamicin may be administered *im* or *iv* with a loading dose of 2 *mg/kg* and then 1.7 *mg/kg q8h*. Other choices include doxycycline 100 *mg iv q12h* or 200 *mg iv q24h*, ciprofloxacin 400 *mg iv q12h* and chloramphenicol 25 *mg/kg iv q6h*. Inappropriate antibiotic therapy includes aztreonam, ceftazidime, cefazolin, and rifampicin. In case of an outbreak, parenteral treatment with aminoglycosides is recommended. In case of an epidemic, when parenteral administration may not be possible, oral treatment with doxycycline or ciprofloxacin is recommended. Patients with pneumonic *plague* may experience *ARDS, DIC*, septic shock and multiorgan failure. Thus, apart from antibiotic treatment, an admission to the intensive care unit may become necessary.

Coxiella burnetii

Microbiology

Coxiella burnetii is a *Gram (-)* coccobacillus, member of the family *Rickettsiaceae*. An important feature is its potential of antigenic variation due to the partial lipopolysaccharide (*LPS*) loss. When isolated from humans or animals, *C. burnetii* expresses phase I antigens and it is very virulent whereas, after reculturing, *LPS* modification leads to a phase II antigenic shift and the creation of a less virulent form. This phenomenon is important for the serological discrimination between acute and chronic *Q fever*.[102]

Epidemiology—Clinical Manifestations

Q fever is a zoonosis caused by *Coxiella burnetii*, a rickettsial species found worldwide except New Zealand.[103,104] Cattle, sheep, goats, domestic animals (cats, dogs), wild rodents, birds and ticks are the main reservoirs of the microbe. In contrast to other rickettsioses, ticks are not considered to be transmitters of the disease to humans, but they are the natural reservoir of *C. burnetii* and the reason of disease transmission to animals. Humans may be infected by consuming infected food or water or by inhaling *C. burnetii* that is contained in aerosols of infected tissues. Direct contact with infected animals or other types of infected material has been associated with the disease spread. In European outbreaks caused by aerosol inhalation, a mean of 4–150 patients per country per year is reported.[105] Human-to-human transmission is extremely rare,[106] although cases of sexual transmission or transmission after contact with an infected pregnant woman or even after blood transfusion or bone marrow transplantation have been described. People with the highest risk for *Q fever* are those coming in contact with potentially infected animals.

The interest in using *Q fever* as a potential biological weapon comes from the fact that an aerosol of the agent may infect humans. The infectious dose of *Q fever* is 1–10.[107] *Q. burnetii* is resistant to heat, drying and common disinfectants and may survive in the environment for long periods in the form of spores. Another potential route of transmission could be through a sabotage of the food supply chain. All available data show that this agent has never been used as a biological weapon. It is considered rather unlikely to be used as such, because it has a long incubation period, it causes low mortality and many infections are subclinical. In cases of deliberate release of *Q. burnetii*, the clinical picture would be similar with the naturally occurring disease.

An epidemiological indication that may raise suspicion of a *Q fever* attack would be the onset of a febrile disease outbreak in an urban environment, with a peak of cases indicating exposure to a common source without secondary transmission. If 50 *kg* of *C. burnetii* are released near a city with a population of 500,000, it is estimated that there will be 150 deaths, 125,000 inhabitants will stop their everyday activity,[108] and almost 9,000 will develop endocarditis in the following months.[109] Livestock could also be a target. Causing outbreaks at livestock could raise concerns due to the fear of consuming infected meat.

The clinical manifestation of *Q fever* varies widely. It may be asymptomatic or acute, accompanied by pneumonia or hepatitis, or chronic, that usually emerges as endocarditis. Acute disease develops in 50% of infected patients. Incubation period usually lasts 2–3 weeks, but may vary from 9 days to 39 days, depending on the initial inoculum. A self-limiting febrile disease is probably the commonest form of *Q fever* and may be confused with an acute viral infection. Most of the signs and symptoms are nonspecific. The disease onset is often abrupt with high fever, chills, sweating, severe retrobulbar headache, malaise, myalgias, confusion, drowsiness, nausea, emesis, diarrhea, abdominal pain, nonproductive cough, quinsy and thoracic pain. Almost 50% of those patients will develop pneumonia, which may present as an atypical or a fulminant pneumonia or more often as a febrile disease without prominent respiratory symptoms.[110,111] Chest X-rays may reveal no findings (10%) or present nonsegmental or segmental subpleural infiltrates, nodular opacities, pleural effusions, atelectasias and, rarely, hilar lymphadenopathy.[112] Differential diagnosis includes other pneumonias caused by *Legionella pneumophila, Mycoplasma pneumoniae, Chlamydophila psittaci,* and *Chlamydophila pneumoniae.* Acute or chronic granulomatous hepatitis is common.[113] Other disease manifestations include meningoencephalitis, aseptic meningitis, myelitis, optic neuritis, peripheral neuropathy, pericarditis, maculopapular or purpuric rash, hemolytic anemia, thyroiditis, erythema nodosum, pancreatitis, etc. During pregnancy, although most of the cases are asymptomatic, there is a danger of endometrial death. Laboratory tests show mild leukocytosis (30%), thrombocytopenia (25%) and elevated levels of transaminases and alkaline phosphatase (70%). Chronic *Q fever* persists for more than 6 months and may develop even 1 year following the initial infection.

Q fever diagnosis depends on serological tests. Indirect immunofluorescence remains the test of choice. *IgM* and *IgG* antibodies recognizing phase II antigens can be detected 2–3 weeks after infection. The presence of *IgG* antibodies recognizing phase I antigens in a titer higher than 1:800 indicates chronic infection.[114] Antibodies against both antigenic phases persist for months or year after the initial infection. The effort of isolating the microbe in various types of cultures is usually negative. *DNA* amplification with *PCR* is a specific and sensitive diagnostic technique. *C. burnetii* may also be detected in recently fixed tissue using *ELISA* or monoclonal antibodies.[114]

Prevention

In case of biological strike, two different approaches may be followed; either everybody should receive antibiotics to prevent complications or only severely ill patients should be treated.[115] Chemoprophylaxis with tetracycline 500 *mg q6h* or doxycycline 100 *mg q12h* for 5–7 days is effective if it commences 8–12 hours after exposure. Inactivated vaccine is recommended to individuals with increased occupational risk of exposure to *C. burnetii.* It is not available for the general population and is not recommended as post-exposure prophylaxis.

Standardized prophylactic procedures are recommended for the hospital staff that comes in contact with patients with *Q fever*. Mask and gloves should be used during obstetric procedures to prevent direct contact and contact with droplets. Leakage of potentially infected material should be disinfected with hypochlorite salt 0.05% and peroxide 5%. Hazardous biological waste should be sterilized. Infected equipment may be disinfected with disinfectants, sterilization or boiling for 10 minutes. However, spores may be resistant to regular disinfection, diluted bleach, ultraviolet radiation, heat, and drying, osmotic and oxidative stress.

Treatment

Most cases of *Q fever* are asymptomatic and spontaneously recover. However, antibiotic treatment may shorten the duration of the disease and lower the risk of complications, such as endocarditis. Without treatment, mortality rate is 1%. Doxycycline is the treatment of choice (100 *mg iv* or *per os q12h* for 14 days).[115] Fluoroquinolones have shown good results. In patients with chronic infection, mortality rates are 30–60% and the antibiotic treatment should include combinations of doxycycline with fluoroquinolone or rifampicin or co-trimoxazole for at least 4 years or doxycycline and hydroxychloroquine for 1.5–3 years. Is should be noted that hydroxychloroquine alkalifies the phagolysosome, thus enhancing doxycycline activity.

Burkholderia mallei

History

The sole report of *Burkholderia mallei* as a biological agent was during the First World War, when it was used by the Germans against livestock, especially horses, of the allies. Animals in the *US* east coast, Romania, Norway, Spain, Argentina and the Russian Eastern Front were infected. Research on *B. mallei* use as a biological weapon was conducted by the Japanese Unit 731 and the *US* army during the Second World War and by the *US* and *USSR* army post-war.[116,117]

Microbiology

B. mallei, the causative agent of *glanders*, is a *Gram (-)* nonmotile, oxidase-positive, obligate mammalian bacterium.[118] It is closely related to *Burkholderia pseudomallei*, as it was demonstrated by special molecular identification techniques. Its extracellular polysaccharide capsule is an important virulence determinant.[119] Although it may not persist in the environment, it was found in the immediate surroundings, e.g. stables, of its equine host for limited period of time up to 6 weeks.

Epidemiology—Clinical Manifestations

The natural reservoir of *B. mallei* includes members of the *Equidae*, namely horses, donkeys and mules. However, other animals, including dogs and cats, and humans may also be infected. It is endemic in Africa, South America and Asia, especially Middle East, and it is recognized as an occupational risk for workers coming in contact with horses, such as veterinarians, butchers, and horse handlers.

Transmission may occur by direct contact with infected animals, their meat and their discharges and secretions. Infection may happen by inoculation through skin lesions, through mucosal surfaces and through inhalation of infected aerosols, which is the most possible route in case of a terrorist attack. Humans may develop the following forms: cutaneous, septicemic, upper respiratory and pulmonary *glanders*. The incubation period may vary from a couple of days to several months. There are reports of latent focus reactivation after many years of the initial infection.

Glanders emerges with fever, chills and malaise. When the upper respiratory tract is infected, there may be ulcers of the nasal and buccopharyngeal mucosa with subsequent mucopurulent discharge. In the pulmonary form, necrosis of the tracheobronchial tree may occur. Furthermore, there may be cervical or mediastinal lymphadenopathy and pustular skin lesions, which may resemble *smallpox*.[119] Bilateral bronchopneumonia, pulmonary infiltrates, and cavitating lesions may be found during chest radiography. Regarding laboratory findings, there may be a mild leukocytosis, if any, and transaminases' elevation, which may signify hepatic infection. *B. mallei* may be isolated from blood, sputum, urine and skin lesion cultures. However, it may readily be misidentified as *B. pseudomallei* or as a *Pseudomonas* species.

Prevention

There is no vaccine to prevent disease in humans. The most important step in preventing a potential outbreak is the control of the disease in the livestock. In case of human infection, there should be isolation of the infected individuals. Due to the high infectiveness of equine secretions, laboratory staff should be very cautious when handling suspicious specimens.[120,121]

Treatment

Data regarding treatment of *glanders* are scarce. As far as we know, *B. mallei* have a similar susceptibility profile with *B. pseudomallei*. It is resistant to penicillin, ampicillin, and first- and second-generation cephalosporins. It is susceptible to gentamicin, clarithromycin, azithromycin, doxycycline, imipenem, co-trimoxazole, and ceftazidime. Treatment of choice consists of ceftazidime or meropenem or imipenem in combination with co-trimoxazole for 10–14 days. Also, a combination of imipenem with doxycycline has been used.[121] To avoid reactivation eradication therapy of minimum 3 months with co-trimoxazole combined with doxycycline is suggested.

Burkholderia pseudomallei

History

Burkholderia pseudomallei, the etiological agent of *melioidosis*, are closely related to *B. mallei*. Its potential as a biological agent has been studied by both the *US* and the *USSR* during the Second World War and the post-war era. However, it has never been used for biological warfare and has never been weaponized.[122]

Microbiology

B. pseudomallei is a *Gram (-)*, oxidase (+) bacterium, with many similarities to *B. mallei*, of which it is considered to be a precursor. However, it is motile and may bear polar flagella. It persists in soil and water and may be readily found in endemic areas, but it does not form spores.

Epidemiology—Clinical Manifestations

B. pseudomallei is found on the soil and surface water. It is considered endemic in countries of Southeastern Asia, which constituted former Indochina, and Northern Australia. Hence, animals that come in contact with contaminated soil and water, including cats, sheep, horses and goats, may be infected. However, some species, including cattle, buffalos and crocodiles, seem to have developed some kind of resistance.[123]

Transmission may occur by various routes, the most common of which is percutaneous inoculation through skin lesions. Other routes include inhalation of infective aerosols, especially during extreme weather conditions like monsoons, ingestion or even sexual transmission. In all types of transmission, except inhalation, pneumonia comes as a result of hematogenous spread. *B. pseudomallei* is recognized as an occupational risk in rice paddy farmers. However, the most important risk factors for developing severe *melioidosis* are diabetes mellitus, renal disease, thalassemia, and cystic fibrosis. The incubation period may vary from 1 day to 3 weeks.[124]

Clinically, *melioidosis* may occur in four forms: localized infection, bloodstream infection, pulmonary infection and disseminated infection. Pulmonary infection is the result of the hematogenous spread of the initial suppurative skin infection. It may emerge with high fever, dyspnea, prostration, pleurisy, and productive cough with purulent excretions or even hemoptysis.[125] However, it should be noted that the clinical picture may vary from mild pneumonia to fulminant infection with high mortality of up to 90%.

There are no radiological findings that may safely establish the diagnosis and differentiate it from other causes of pneumonia. Chest radiography may reveal segmental or lobar consolidations, infiltrates, and cavitations. However, lung abscesses, pleural effusions and mediastinal lymphadenopathy are rare.[126]

B. pseudomallei may be isolated from blood and sputum cultures and from throat, skin lesion and rectal swabs. Commercially available culture media or Ashdown's media may be used. However, misidentification as *Pseudomonas* species is not uncommon. Serological tests, including indirect hemagglutination test and *ELISA*, may be useful, but mostly in cases of tourists. Locals have high titers of positive antibodies due to the high rates of previous infection, which limit the diagnostic accuracy of the aforementioned tests. Even if serological tests yield positive results, a positive culture is needed to confirm the diagnosis.

Prevention

There is no vaccine against *B. pseudomallei*. As human-to-human and laboratory spread are rare, patient isolation is not deemed necessary. Standard laboratory practices and disinfection are considered as adequate measures.[118] In special cases, post-exposure prophylaxis with doxycycline, cotrimoxazole or amoxicillin/clavulanate could be administered.[127] Due to the environmental abundance of *B. pseudomallei*, prevention measures should be concentrated on the minimization of exposure to wet soil and water in endemic areas. Protective gloves and footwear are recommended.

Treatment

Like *B. mallei, B. pseudomallei* is resistant to ampicillin, penicillin, first and second generation cephalosporins, but also to aminoglycosides including gentamicin, tobramycin and streptomycin. Ceftazidime is the treatment of choice, which is administered for a minimum of 10–14 days. An open randomized trial of 161 patients comparing the combination of chloramphenicol/doxycycline/trimethoprim/sulfamethoxazole with ceftazidime showed that patients treated with ceftazidime had 50% lower mortality.[128] Imipenem was found to be as effective as ceftazidime. Although amoxicillin/clavulanate was effective as initial therapy, it failed as eradication therapy. Co-trimoxazole may be added to the aforementioned agents for initial therapy. The eradication regimen should last at least for 3 months and usually includes a combination of co-trimoxazole and doxycycline.

Chlamydophila psittaci

History

The etiological agent of *psittacosis* (parrot fever) was discovered over a hundred years ago. In 1930, there was an outbreak caused by Amazon parrots, which were exported from Argentina to various parts of the world, infecting roughly 800 people worldwide. Twenty years ago, an outbreak was reported in Philadelphia without any associated fatalities.[129] Both *US* and the former *USSR* conducted research on *C. psittaci* as a potential biological agent but none of them weaponized it.

Microbiology

C. psittaci is a *Gram (-)*, obligatory intracellular bacterium. It has five serovars (A to E), all of which have been identified as the cause of human disease.[130,131] As other members of the *Chlamydiaceae, C. psittaci* is not able to metabolically sustain itself and, therefore, it uses *ATP* from the host cell. Thus, it may persist in the environment for only a couple of days in the form of infected bird secretions and for 3 weeks in straw. It is not resistant to heat, dryness and disinfectants.

Epidemiology—Clinical Manifestations

The natural reservoirs of *C. psittaci* are various types of birds, but it may also infect animals and humans. It has been recognized as occupational hazard for pet shop employees, poultry workers, veterinarians, and slaughterhouse workers. It is not considered endemic in some specific region. However, small outbreaks may occur in places where illegal import of exotic birds takes place due to inadequate protection measures. Livestock infection may be chronic and also abortions may occur.

Transmission may occur mainly by inhalation of aerosol containing contaminated dry feces and bird secretions. However, cases of transmission by direct contact have also been reported. The incubation period of *C. psittaci* varies greatly, but usually is 5–20 days.

Psittacosis may present in the form of several syndromes. These may vary from subclinical infection to severe pneumonia or even severe systemic infection with fatal outcome. The most common symptoms are fever with chills and malaise. There may be nonproductive cough, pharyngitis, hepatosplenomegaly, lymphadenopathy and, rarely, pleuritic pain. Apart from the respiratory, other systems may also be implicated, including gastrointestinal and central nervous system. Thus, headache, nausea, photophobia, and drowsiness may also be present. Horder's spots may emerge and resembles the rash of typhoid fever. Psittacosis may be further complicated with *ARDS*, pericarditis, myocarditis, endocarditis, DIC, hepatitis with jaundice, meningitis, encephalitis and seizures.[132-134] Chest radiography may reveal segmental or lobar consolidation in more than 70% of the cases.[135] Hilar enlargement or pleural effusions may also be present. The total and differential white blood cell counts are normal or slightly elevated. Transaminases and bilirubin levels may be elevated, suggesting hepatic complications.

Although *C. psittaci* may be cultured from blood, sputum and pleural fluid, it is not recommended because of the dangers for the laboratory personnel. Serological testing including complement fixation, *ELISA* and molecular techniques, such as *PCR*, are preferred. However, there are shortcomings including delayed appearance of specific antibodies and cross-reactions.

Prevention

There is no vaccine to prevent *C. psittaci* infection. Thus, prevention of the disease can be achieved only by avoiding contact with infected birds. Potential sources of infection should be recognized and infected birds should be treated or eliminated. Human-to-human transmission is rare and patient isolation is not deemed necessary.[136,137] Environmental sanitation should be done because of the pathogen's resistance to usual ambient conditions.

Treatment

C. psittaci is susceptible to tetracycline, chloramphenicol, erythromycin, azithromycin, and moxifloxacin.[138] Doxycycline is the treatment of choice, but in cases of young children and pregnant women macrolides should be used. Although clinical improvement occurs during the first 2–3 days, therapy must continue till 3 weeks have passed to avoid relapse of the disease. It should be noted that quinolones and macrolides are less efficacious and should be used only when there is no alternative.

REFERENCES

1. Spencer RC, Wilcox MH. Agents of biological warfare. *Rev Med Microbiol.* 1993;4:138-43.
2. Borio L, Inglesby T, Peters CJ, et al. Working Group on Civilian Biodefense. Hemorrhagic fever viruses as biological weapons: medical and public health management. *JAMA.* 2002;287:2391-405.
3. Alibek K, Handelman S. Biohazard. The Chilling True Story of the Largest Covert Biological Weapons in the World, Told from the Inside by the Man Who Ran It. New York: Random House; 1999.
4. Wilkening DA. Sverdlovsk revisited: Modeling human inhalation anthrax. *Proc Natl Acad Sci USA.* 2006;103:7589-94.
5. Gubler D. Dengue and dengue haemorrhagic fever. *Clin Microbiol Rev.* 1998;11:480-96.
6. Leroy EM, Kumulungui B, Pourrut X, et al. Fruit bats as reservoirs of Ebola virus. *Nature.* 2005;438:575-6.
7. Towner JS, Pourrut X, Albariño CG, et al. Marburg virus infection detected in a common African bat. *PLoS One.* 2007;2:e764.
8. Franz DR, Jahrling PB, Friedlander AM, et al. Clinical recognition and management of patients exposed to biological warfare agents. *JAMA.* 1997;278:399-411.
9. Bossi P, Tegnell A, Baka A, et al. Task Force on Biological and Chemical Agent Threats, Public Health Directorate, European Commission, Luxembourg. Bichat guidelines for the clinical management of haemorrhagic fever viruses and bioterrorism-related haemorrhagic fever viruses. *Euro Surveill.* 2004;9:E11-E12.
10. Schou S, Hansen AK. Marburg and Ebola virus infections in laboratory non-human primates: a literature review. *Comp Med.* 2000;50:108-23.
11. Centers for Disease Control and Prevention: Outbreak of Ebola haemorrhagic fever-Uganda, August 2000-January 2001. *Wkly Epidemiol Rec.* 2001;76:41-6.
12. Centers for Disease Control and Prevention: Management of patients with suspected viral haemorrhagic fever. *MMWR.* 1988;37:1-16.
13. Feldmann H, Slenczka W, Klenk H. Emerging and reemerging of filoviruses. *Arch Virol.* 1996;11:77-100.
14. Gompf SG, Smith KM. (2012). Arenaviruses. [online] Available from: www.emedicine.com/MED/topic166.htm. April 2012. [Accessed April, 2012].
15. The European Agency for the Evaluation of Medicinal Products. (2002). EMEA/CPMP guidance document on use of medicinal products for treatment and prophylaxis of biological agents that might be used as weapons of bioterrorism. July 2002. [online] Available from www.ema.europa.eu/docs/en_GB/document_library/Regulatory_and_procedural_guideline/2010/01/WC500049399.pdf. [Accessed April, 2012].
16. Bray M, Paragas J. Experimental therapy of filovirus infections. *Antivir Res.* 2002;54:1-17.
17. Feldmann H, Jones SM, Daddario-DiCaprio KM, et al. Effective post-exposure treatment of Ebola infection. *PLoS Pathog.* 2007;3:e2.
18. Martin JE, Sullivan NJ, Enama ME, et al. A DNA vaccine for Ebola virus is safe and immunogenic in a phase I clinical trial. *Clin Vaccine Immunol.* 2006;13:1267-77.
19. The global eradication of smallpox: Final report of the global commission for the certification of smallpox eradication. History of International Public Health, No. 4. Geneva: World Health Organization, 1980. [online] Available from: www.whqlibdoc.who.int/publications/a41438.pdf.
20. Henderson DA. The looming threat of bioterrorism. *Science.* 1999;283:1279-82.
21. Henderson DA, Inglesby TV, Bartlett JG, et al. Smallpox as a biological weapon: medical and public health management. Working Group on Civilian Biodefense. *JAMA.* 1999;281:2127-37.

22. Fenner F, Henderson DA, Arita I, Ježek Z, Ladnyi ID, et al. (1988). Smallpox and its eradication. World Health Organization, Geneva 1988. [online] Available from: www.extranet.who.int/iris/restricted/bitstream/10665/ 39485/1/9241561106.pdf.
23. Moore ZS, Seward JF, Lane JM. Smallpox. *Lancet.* 2006;367: 425-35.
24. Moss B. Poxviridae and their replication. In: Knipe DM, Howley PM (Eds). Field's Virology, 5th Edition. Lippincott Williams & Wilkins: Philadelphia, PA; 2007.
25. Massung RF, Liu LI, Qi J, et al. Analysis of the complete genome of smallpox variola major virus strain Bangladesh-1975. *Virology.* 1994;201:215-40.
26. Shchelkunov SN, Resenchuk SM, Totmenin AV, et al. Comparison of the genetic maps of variola and vaccinia viruses. *FEBS Lett.* 1993;327:321-4.
27. Loveless BM, Mucker EM, Hartmann C, et al. Differentiation of Variola major and Variola minor variants by MGB-Eclipse probe melt curves and genotyping analysis. *Mol Cell Probes.* 2009;23:166-70.
28. Christie AB. Smallpox. In: Christie AB (Ed). Infectious Diseases, Epidemiology and Clinical Practices, 2nd Edition. Edinburgh: Churchill Livingstone; 1974.
29. Koplan JP, Foster SO. Smallpox: clinical types, causes of death, and treatment. *J Infect Dis.* 1979;140:440-1.
30. Albert MR, Ostheimer KG, Liewehr DJ, et al. Smallpox manifestations and survival during the Boston epidemic of 1901 to 1903. *Ann Intern Med.* 2002;137:993-1000.
31. Breman JG, Henderson DA. Diagnosis and management of smallpox. *N Engl J Med.* 2002;346:1300-8.
32. Fauci AS. Smallpox vaccination policy - the need for dialogue. *N Engl J Med.* 2002;346:1319-20.
33. Bicknell WJ. The case for voluntary smallpox vaccination. *N Engl J Med.* 2002;346:1323-5.
34. Supplemental recommendations on adverse events following smallpox vaccine in the pre-event vaccination program: recommendations of the Advisory Committee on Immunization Practices. *MMWR Morb Mortal Wkly Rep.* 2003;52:282-4.
35. Suarez VR, Hankins GD. Smallpox and pregnancy: from eradicated disease to bioterrorist threat. *Obstet Gynecol.* 2002;100:87-93.
36. Capua I, Marangon S. Control of avian influenza in poultry. *Emerg Infect Dis.* 2006;12:1319-24.
37. Yuen KY, Chan PK, Peiris M, et al. Clinical features and rapid viral diagnosis of human disease associated with avian influenza A H5N1 virus. *Lancet.* 1998;351:467-71.
38. Katz JM, Lim W, Bridges CB, et al. Antibody response in individuals infected with avian influenza A (H5N1) viruses and detection of anti-H5 antibody among household and social contacts. *J Infect Dis.* 1999;180:1763-70.
39. Grady D, Broad WJ. (2011). Seeing Terror Risk, U.S. Asks Journals to Cut Flu Study Facts. The New York Times. [online] Available from: <www.nytimes.com/2011/12/21/health/fearing-terrorism-us-asks-journals-to-censor-articles-on-virus.html.[Accessed December, 2011].>
40. Pavia AT. Laboratory Creation of a Highly Transmissible H5N1 Influenza Virus: Balancing Substantial Risks and Real Benefits. *Ann Intern Med.* 2012;156:463-5.
41. Inglesby TV. Engineered H5N1: A Rare Time for Restraint in Science. *Ann Intern Med.* 2012;156:460-2.
42. Fouchier RA, García-Sastre A, Kawaoka Y, et al. Pause on avian flu transmission research. *Science.* 2012;335:400-1.
43. Guan Y, Poon LL, Cheung CY, et al. H5N1 influenza: a protean pandemic threat. *Proc Natl Acad Sci USA.* 2004; 101:8156-61.
44. Kuiken T, Rimmelzwaan G, van Riel D, et al. Avian H5N1 influenza in cats. *Science.* 2004;306:241.
45. Abdel-Ghafar AN, Chotpitayasunondh T, Gao Z, et al. Writing Committee of the Second World Health Organization Consultation on Clinical Aspects of Human Infection with Avian Influenza A (H5N1) Virus, Update on avian influenza A (H5N1) virus infection in humans. *N Engl J Med.* 2008;358:261-73.
46. Tran TH, Nguyen TL, Nguyen TD, et al. Avian influenza A (H5N1) in 10 patients in Vietnam. *N Engl J Med.* 2004; 350:1179-88.
47. Beigel JH, Farrar J, Han AM, et al. Avian influenza A (H5N1) infection in humans. *N Engl J Med.* 2005;353:1374-85.
48. Chotpitayasunondh T, Ungchusak K, Hanshaoworakul W, et al. Human disease from influenza A (H5N1), Thailand, 2004. *Emerg Infect Dis.* 2005;11:201-9.
49. Kawachi S, Luong ST, Shigematsu M, et al. Risk parameters of fulminant acute respiratory distress syndrome and avian influenza (H5N1) infection in Vietnamese children. *J Infect Dis.* 2009;200:510-5.
50. Majury A, Ash J, Toye B, et al. Laboratory diagnosis of human infection with avian influenza. *CMAJ.* 2006;175: 1371.
51. Yob JM, Field H, Rashdi AM, et al. Nipah virus infection in bats (order Chiroptera) in peninsular Malaysia. *Emerg Infect Dis.* 2001;7:439-41.
52. Mohd Nor MN, Gan CH, Ong BL. Nipah virus infection of pigs in peninsular Malaysia. *Rev Sci Tech.* 2000;19:160-5.
53. Goh KJ, Tan CT, Chew NK, et al. Clinical features of Nipah virus encephalitis among pig farmers in Malaysia. *N Engl J Med.* 2000;342:1229-35.
54. Parashar UD, Sunn LM, Ong F, et al. Case-control study of risk factors for human infection with a new zoonotic paramyxovirus, Nipah virus, during a 1998-1999 outbreak of severe encephalitis in Malaysia. *J Infect Dis.* 2000;181: 1755-9.
55. Chew MH, Arguin PM, Shay DK, et al. Risk factors for Nipah virus infection among abattoir workers in Singapore. *J Infect Dis.* 2000;181:1760-3.
56. Tan KS, Tan CT, Goh KJ. Epidemiological aspects of Nipah virus infection. *Neurol J Southeast Asia.* 1999;4:77.
57. Hossain MJ, Gurley ES, Montgomery JM, et al. Clinical presentation of Nipah virus infection in Bangladesh. *Clin Infect Dis.* 2008;46:977-84.
58. Case definitions for the 4 diseases requiring notification to WHO in all circumstances under the IHR (2005). *Wkly Epidemiol Rec.* 2009;84:52-6.
59. Tsang KW, Ho PL, Ooi GC, et al. A cluster of cases of severe acute respiratory syndrome in Hong Kong. *N Engl J Med.* 2003;348:1977-85.
60. Booth TF, Kournikakis B, Bastien N, et al. Detection of airborne severe acute respiratory syndrome (SARS) coronavirus and environmental contamination in SARS outbreak units. *J Infect Dis.* 2005;191:1472-7.
61. Poutanen SM, Low DE, Henry B, et al. Identification of severe acute respiratory syndrome in Canada. *N Engl J Med.* 2003;348:1995-2005.

62. Cheng PK, Wong DA, Tong LK, et al. Viral shedding patterns of coronavirus in patients with probable severe acute respiratory syndrome. *Lancet.* 2004;363:1699-700.
63. Donnelly CA, Ghani AC, Leung GM, et al. Epidemiological determinants of spread of causal agent of severe acute respiratory syndrome in Hong Kong. *Lancet.* 2003; 361:1761-6.
64. Preliminary clinical description of severe acute respiratory syndrome. *MMWR Morb Mortal Wkly Rep.* 2003;52:255-6.
65. Peiris JS, Yuen KY, Osterhaus AD, et al. The severe acute respiratory syndrome. *N Engl J Med.* 2003;349:2431-41.
66. Choi KW, Chau TN, Tsang O, et al. Outcomes and prognostic factors in 267 patients with severe acute respiratory syndrome in Hong Kong. *Ann Intern Med.* 2003;139:715-23.
67. Müller NL, Ooi GC, Khong PL, et al. Severe acute respiratory syndrome: radiographic and CT findings. *AJR Am J Roentgenol.* 2003;181:3-8.
68. Pang X, Zhu Z, Xu F, et al. Evaluation of control measures implemented in the severe acute respiratory syndrome outbreak in Beijing, 2003. *JAMA.* 2003;290:3215-21.
69. Svoboda T, Henry B, Shulman L, et al. Public health measures to control the spread of the severe acute respiratory syndrome during the outbreak in Toronto. *N Engl J Med.* 2004;350:2352-61.
70. Health aspects of chemical and biological weapons: report of WHO Group of Consultants. Geneva, Switzerland. *World Health Organization.* 1970;72:99.
71. Meselson M, Guillemin J, Hugh-Jones M, et al. The Sverdlovsk anthrax outbreak of 1979. *Science.* 1994;266: 1202-8.
72. Abramova FA, Grinberg LM, Yampolskaya OV, et al. Pathology of inhalational anthrax in 42 cases from the Sverdlovsk outbreak of 1979. *Proc Natl Acad Sci USA.* 1993;90:2291-4.
73. Shafazand S, Doyle R, Ruoss S, et al. Inhalational anthrax: epidemiology, diagnosis, and management. *Chest.* 1999;116:1369-76.
74. Pile JC, Malone JD, Eitzen EM, et al. Anthrax as a potential biological warfare agent. *Arch Intern Med.* 1998;158:429-34.
75. Inglesby TV, O'Toole T, Henderson DA, et al. Working Group on Civilian Biodefense. Anthrax as a biological weapon, 2002: updated recommendations for management. *JAMA.* 2002;287:2236-52.
76. Brachman PS. Inhalation anthrax. *Ann NY Acad Sci.* 1980;353:83-93.
77. Hupert N, Bearman GM, Mushlin AI, et al. Accuracy of screening for inhalational anthrax after a bioterrorist attack. *Ann Intern Med.* 2003;139:337-45.
78. Titball R, Turnbull P, Hutson R. The monitoring and detection of Bacillus anthracis in the environment. *Soc Appl Bacteriol Symp Ser.* 1991;20:9S-18S.
79. Braithwaite RS, Fridsma D, Roberts MS. The cost-effectiveness of strategies to reduce mortality from an intentional release of aerosolized anthrax spores. *Med Decis Making.* 2006;26:182-93.
80. Fowler RA, Sanders GD, Bravata DM, et al. Cost-effectiveness of defending against bioterrorism: a comparison of vaccination and antibiotic prophylaxis against anthrax. *Ann Intern Med.* 2005;142:601-10.
81. Doganay M, Aydin N. Antimicrobial susceptibility of Bacillus anthracis. *Scand J Infect Dis.* 1991;23:333-5.
82. Investigation of bioterrorism-related anthrax and interim guidelines for exposure management and antimicrobial therapy, October 2001. MMWR. 2001;50:909-19.
83. www.fda.gov/Drugs/EmergencyPreparedness/BioterrorismandDrugPreparedness/ucm133678.htm. [Accessed April, 2012].
84. Tärnvik A, Berglund L. Tularaemia. *Eur Respir J.* 2003; 21: 361-73.
85. Reintjes R, Dedushaj I, Gjini A, et al. Tularemia outbreak investigation in Kosovo: case control and environmental studies. *Emerg Infect Dis.* 2002;8:69-73.
86. Hubalek Z, Sixl W, Halouzka J, et al. Prevalence of Francisella tularensis in Dermacentor reticulatus ticks collected in adjacent areas of the Czech and Austrian republics. *Cent Eur J Public Health.* 1997;5:199-201.
87. Eliasson H, Lindback J, Nuorti JP, et al. The 2000 tularemia outbreak: A case-control study of risk factors in disease-endemic and emergent areas, Sweden. *Emerg Infect Dis.* 2002;8:956-60.
88. Rodgers BL, Duffield RP, Taylor T, et al. Tularemic meningitis. *Pediatr Infect Dis J.* 1998;17:439-41.
89. Tancik CA, Dillaha JA. Francisella tularensis endocarditis. *Clin Infect Dis.* 2000;30:399-400.
90. Evans ME, Gregory DW, Schaffner W, et al. Tularemia: a 30-year experience with 88 cases. *Medicine (Baltimore).* 1985;64:251-69.
91. Dennis DT, Inglesby TV, Henderson DA, et al. Working Group on Civilian Biodefense. Tularemia as a biological weapon: medical and public health management. *JAMA.* 2001;285:2763-73.
92. Cross JT, Jacobs RF. Tularemia: treatment failures with outpatient use of ceftriaxone. *Clin Infect Dis.* 1993;17:976-80.
93. Aranda EA. Treatment of tularemia with levofloxacin. *Clin Microbiol Infect.* 2001;7:167-8.
94. Slack P. The black death past and present. 2. Some historical problems. *Trans R Soc Trop Med Hyg.* 1989;83:461-3.
95. Perry RD, Fetherston JD. Yersinia pestis - etiologic agent of plague. *Clin Microbiol Rev.* 1997;10:35-66.
96. Inglesby TV, Dennis DT, Henderson DA, et al. Plague as a biological weapon: medical and public health management. Working Group on Civilian Biodefense. *JAMA.* 2000;283:2281-90.
97. Centers for Disease Control and Prevention. Fatal human plague - Arizona and Colorado, 1996. *MMWR.* 1997;46:617-20.
98. Inglesby TV, Henderson DA, Bartlett JG, et al. Anthrax as a biological weapon: medical and public health management. Working Group on Civilian Biodefense. *JAMA.* 1999;281:1735-45.
99. Garner JS. Guideline for isolation precautions in hospitals. The Hospital Infection Control Practices Advisory Committee. *Infect Control Hosp Epidemiol.* 1996;17:53-80.
100. Centers for Disease Control and Prevention. Prevention of plague: recommendations of the Advisory Committee on Immunization Practice (ACIP). *MMWR Recomm Rep.* 1996;45:1-15.
101. Bossi P, Tegnell A, Baka A, et al. Task Force on Biological and Chemical Agent Threats, Public Health Directorate, European Commission, Luxembourg. Bichat guidelines for the clinical management of Q fever and bioterrorism-related Q fever. *Euro Surveill.* 2004;9:E19-20.

102. Norlander L. Q fever epidemiology and pathogenesis. *Microbes Infect.* 2000;2:417-24.
103. Maurin M, Raoult D. Q fever. *Clin Microbiol Rev.* 1999; 12:518-53.
104. Comite Editorial / Editorial Committee. Q fever in Europe. *Euro Surveill.* 1997;2:13-5.
105. Mann JS, Douglas JG, Inglis JM, et al. Q fever: person to person transmission within a family. *Thorax.* 1985;41:974-5.
106. Sawyer L, Fishbein D, McDade JE. Q fever; current concepts. *Rev Infect Dis.* 1987; 9:935-46.
107. Bellamy RJ, Freedman AR. Bioterrorism. *QJM.* 2001;94:227-34.
108. Fenollar F, Fournier PE, Carrieri MP, et al. Risks factors and prevention of Q fever endocarditis. *Clin Infect Dis.* 2001;33:312-6.
109. Antony S, Schaffner W. Q fever pneumonia. *Semin Respir Infect.* 1997;12:2-6.
110. Marrie T. Coxiella burnetii (Q fever) pneumonia. *Clin Infect Dis.* 1995;21:S253-64.
111. Caron F, Meurice JC, Ingrand P, et al. Acute Q fever pneumonia: a review of 80 hospitalized patients. *Chest.* 1998;114:808-13.
112. Zaidi S, Singer C. Gastrointestinal and hepatic manifestations of tick borne diseases in the United States. *Clin Infect Dis.* 2002;34:1206-12.
113. Brouqui P, Dumler JS, Raoult D. Immunohistologic demonstration of C oxiella burnetii in the valves of patients with Q fever endocarditis. *Am J Med.* 1994;97:451-8.
114. Madariaga MG, Rezai K, Trenholme GM, et al. Q fever: a biological weapon in your backyard. *Lancet Infect Dis.* 2003;3:709-21.
115. Whitlock GC, Estes DM, Torres AG. Glanders: off to the races with Burkholderia mallei. *FEMS Microbiol Lett.* 2007;277:115-22.
116. Burtnick MN, Brett PJ, Woods DE. Molecular and physical characterization of Burkholderia mallei O antigens. *J Bacteriol.* 2002;184:849-52.
117. Bossi P, Tegnell A, Baka A, et al. Task Force on Biological and Chemical Agent Threats, Public Health Directorate, European Commission, Luxembourg. Bichat guidelines for the clinical management of glanders and melioidosis and bioterrorism-related glanders and melioidosis. *Euro Surveill.* 2004;9:E17-8.
118. Gilad J, Harary I, Dushnitsky T, et al. Burkholderia mallei and Burkholderia pseudomallei as bioterrorism agents: national aspects of emergency preparedness. *Isr Med Assoc J.* 2007;9:499-503.
119. Peacock SJ, Schweizer HP, Dance DA, et al. Management of accidental laboratory exposure to Burkholderia pseudomallei and B. mallei. *Emerg Infect Dis.* 2008;14:e2.
120. Srinivasan A, Kraus CN, DeShazer D, et al. Glanders in a military research microbiologist. *N Engl J Med.* 2001;345:256-8.
121. United States Medical Research Institute of Infectious Diseases. USAMRIID's Medical Management of Biological Casualties. 5th edition. Fort Detrick: USAMRIID; 2004.
122. Sprague LD, Neubauer H. Melioidosis in animals: a review on epizootiology, diagnosis and clinical presentation. *J Vet Med B Infect Dis Vet Public Health.* 2004;51:305-20.
123. White NJ. Melioidosis. *Lancet.* 2003;361:1715-22.
124. Ip M, Osterberg LG, Chau PY, et al. Pulmonary melioidosis. *Chest.* 1995;108:1420-4.
125. Lim KS, Chong VH. Radiological manifestations of melioidosis. *Clin Radiol.* 2010;65:66-72.
126. Sivalingam SP, Sim SH, Jasper LC, et al. Pre- and post-exposure prophylaxis of experimental Burkholderia pseudomallei infection with doxycycline, amoxicillin/clavulanic acid and co-trimoxazole. *J Antimicrob Chemother.* 2008; 61:674-8.
127. White NJ, Dance DA, Chaowagul W, et al. Halving of mortality of severe melioidosis by ceftazidime. *Lancet.* 1989; 2:697-701.
128. Schlossberg D, Delgado J, Moore MM, et al. An epidemic of avian and human psittacosis. *Arch Intern Med.* 1993;153: 2594-6.
129. Vanrompay D, Andersen AA, Ducatelle R, et al. Serotyping of European isolates of Chlamydia psittaci from poultry and other birds. *J Clin Microbiol.* 1993;31:134-7.
130. Andersen AA. Two new serovars of Chlamydia psittaci from North American birds. *J Vet Diagn Invest.* 1997;9:159-64.
131. Crosse BA. Psittacosis: a clinical review. *J Infect.* 1990;21: 251-9.
132. Yung AP, Grayson ML. Psittacosis-a review of 135 cases. *Med J Aust.* 1988;148:228-33.
133. Schaffner W, Drutz DJ, Duncan GW, et al. The clinical spectrum of endemic psittacosis. *Arch Intern Med.* 1967; 119:433-43.
134. Coutts II, Mackenzie S, White RJ. Clinical and radiographic features of psittacosis infection. *Thorax.* 1985; 40:530-2.
135. Ito I, Ishida T, Mishima M, et al. Familial cases of psittacosis: possible person-to-person transmission. *Intern Med.* 2002;41:580-3.
136. Hughes C, Maharg P, Rosario P, et al. Possible nosocomial transmission of psittacosis. *Infect Control Hosp Epidemiol.* 1997;18:165-8.
137. Gregory DW, Schaffner W. Psittacosis. *Semin Respir Infect.* 1997;12:7-11.

CHAPTER 27

The Role of the Nurse in the Treatment of Respiratory Infections

Sonia O Labeau, Stijn I Blot

ABSTRACT

This chapter discusses nursing care for patients with respiratory tract infections. Preceding the specific aspects of caring for infected patients, the first section elucidates on the importance of nurses' adherence to evidence-based recommendations for preventing these infections. As the assessment of the respiratory tract is an important nurse responsibility, the second section is dedicated to this issue. Third section focuses on the necessity to follow medical orders timely and accurately. Positioning patients with respiratory infections should simultaneously allow maximal expansion of the chest and optimal comfort and are dealt with in the fourth section. The administration of oxygen therapy, care issues for patients on mechanical and non-invasive ventilation are extensively discussed in sections five, six, and seven, respectively. Subsequently, the nurses' role in obtaining laboratory samples is elucidated. The chapter concludes by a section dealing with considerations for supporting patients and their families and providing them with adequate information.

INTRODUCTION

This chapter discusses the role of the nurse in the treatment of respiratory tract infections in adult patients. Respiratory tract infections are multifactorial and patients may present with a variety of symptoms. Optimal nursing care takes into account the diagnosis, condition, and specific needs of each individual patient to contribute to the promotion of his health and well-being. Therefore, the information provided in this chapter merely pertains to major aspects of nursing care for patients with respiratory tract infections and needs to be complemented with interventions tailored to each individual patient's needs.

In adults with respiratory infections, specific nursing goals and desired patient outcomes include but are not limited to the following:

- Improved oxygenation: partial pressure of oxygen in arterial blood (PaO_2) greater than and equal to 60 mmHg, saturation level of oxygen in hemoglobin (SaO_2) greater than and equal to 90%
- Reversal of dyspnea
- Clearance of airway secretions
- Increased activity tolerance
- Decreased breathlessness on exertion.

PREVENTING INFECTION

Hospital-acquired pneumonia (HAP), ventilator-associated pneumonia (VAP), and healthcare-associated pneumonia are healthcare-acquired infections that remain as the important causes of morbidity and mortality, despite the use of a wide range of preventive measures, advances in antimicrobial therapy, and better supportive care modalities.[1-3] Amongst these, VAP, which by definition occurs in critically ill patients is associated with considerable attributable morbidity and mortality, an increased duration of mechanical ventilation and hospitalization, and considerably excessive use of healthcare resources.[2-4]

Nurses must be well aware of the deleterious impact of nosocomial infections. They must also know that the presence of an existing infection does never render further adequate infection prevention superfluous. Importantly, medication administered to combat infections may lower the patients' resistance, making him even more vulnerable. This is especially seen in patients receiving corticosteroids or other types of immunosuppressive drugs, which make them more prone to opportunistic infections.

Various evidence-based recommendations for the prevention of respiratory infections have been issued.[3,5-9] Nurses must adhere to these recommendations and integrate them into individualized patient care. They appear, however, insufficiently aware of their content and importance[10-13] and have often been shown to be non-compliant with the recommended strategies.[14-16]

PERFORMING A NURSING ASSESSMENT OF THE RESPIRATORY TRACT

A nursing assessment of the respiratory tract consists of a thorough and systematical observation of the patient's symptoms. Nurses should be made alert to the possibility of bacterial pneumonia in patients with respiratory symptoms who develop fever, chills, or other potential signs of infection. Also, in patients already diagnosed with respiratory infections, adequate nursing assessment is critical. In patients with pneumonia, the respiratory status is evaluated at least every 2 hours. Moreover, the patient's overall condition must be observed and assessed continuously during patient care.[17]

If the patient's respiratory status deteriorates, nurses must be able to anticipate the need for intubation and mechanical ventilation and take the necessary actions. Abnormalities and alarming symptoms must be reported to the doctor immediately. In order to recognize symptoms and abnormalities and to interpret them correctly, nurses need a thorough knowledge of the anatomy, physiology and pathology of the respiratory tract.[18-22]

The symptoms described below often accompany respiratory tract infections. They should be carefully observed, keeping in mind the diagnosis, treatment and personal history of the individual patient:[20]

- Vital signs: Pulse and blood pressure must be measured regularly, as they provide essential information on the patient's condition
- Fever: It is frequently a symptom of infection and must be monitored throughout the entire course of the treatment. Importantly, antibiotics administration never renders temperature control superfluous. Older patients may lack this typical symptom of infection but may present with atypical symptoms, such as confusion and behavior changes[23,24]
- Coughing: Nurses observe whether a cough is productive or it has changed recently, and if so, in what way. A cough may be dry, such as in mycoplasmal pneumonia or very productive[20]
- Sputum: The nurse observes or asks the patient to estimate the amount of sputum produced as well as its color and consistency. The sputum may be creamy yellow, green, or rust-colored[19]
- Dyspnea: It can be assessed by carefully observing and listening to the patient. It can also be graded by asking the patient to rank his level of dyspnea on a grading scale between 1 (no dyspnea) and 10 (the worst dyspnea the patient has experienced). Evaluation takes place, at least daily
- Orthopnea: A patient with shortness of breath when lying down tends to sleep with upper body elevated. The patient is asked or observed for how many pillows being used, as this reflects the severity of orthopnea
- Breath sounds: Wheezes are high-pitched sounds, first heard on exhalation, occurring when airflow is blocked, and on inhalation, when the severity of the block increases. Ronchi are low-pitched, snoring, rattling sounds that occur primarily on exhalation, although they may also appear on inhalation. They usually change or disappear with coughing and occur when fluid partially blocks the large airways. Crackles are intermittent, brief crackling sounds that are caused by collapsed or fluid-filled alveoli popping open. Heard primarily on inhalation, crackles are classified as either fine or coarse and usually do not clear with coughing. If they do, they are most likely caused by secretions. Stridor is a loud, high-pitched crowing sound that is heard during inspiration, caused by an obstruction in the upper airway. Stridor requires immediate attention[20,25]
- Chest pain: Occurring from a respiratory problem, chest pain is usually the result of pleural inflammation, inflammation of the costochondral junctions, or soreness of chest muscles due to coughing
- Breathing rate and pattern: Adults normally breathe at a rate of 12–20 breaths/min. Rates are always assessed for a full 60 seconds and not taken from the pulse oximeter.[25] The respiratory pattern should be even, coordinated, and regular, with occasional sighs. The inspiration to expiration ratio is about 1:2. A high respiratory rate with shallow breaths may indicate pain preventing normal respiration, whereas a high rate with normal sized breaths may reflect hyperventilation.[18] Both sides of the chest should be

equal at rest and expand equally, as the patient inhales. A chest expanding asymmetrically is a warning sign, as it may indicate that the patient has pleural effusion, atelectasis, pneumonia, or pneumothorax. The use of any accessory muscles must be observed[25]

- Skin color and nail beds: Typically, a patient with a bluish tint to the skin and mucous membranes is considered cyanotic. Cyanosis is a late sign of hypoxemia. The most reliable places to check for cyanosis are the tongue and mucous membranes of the mouth.[19]

Nurses should be aware of the measures that need to be taken in case of emergencies and according to hospital's procedures to secure patient safety until arrival of specialized caregivers. In any case, the attending physician must be contacted if signs of respiratory distress are observed. According to local protocols, nurses can quantify the degree of respiratory distress by adding pulse oximetry monitoring and provide oxygen therapy. Prompt diagnosis by means of pulse oximetry has demonstrated to be beneficial in terms of mortality in patients with severe pneumonia.[26]

FOLLOWING DOCTOR'S ORDERS

To treat an infection, anti-infective agents specific to the causative infectious organism are administered. Oxygen is used to correct hypoxemia. Other treatments vary depending on the patient's diagnosis and symptoms and may include inhaled bronchodilators, cough suppressants, bronchial hygiene therapies, chest physiotherapy, rest, analgesics, and corticosteroids. Some patients may require mechanical ventilation according to their condition.[17]

Nurses must strictly follow doctor's orders. Prescribed medications must be administered to the right patient, at the right time, in the right dosage, and via the right administration route. Adverse effects are to be monitored. Importantly, delay in administration of effective therapy in patients with VAP is associated with increase in mortality rate, length of stay, and cost.[27] As soon as there is a clinical suspicion of HAP, adequate antibiotic treatment is to be implemented.[27,28]

POSITIONING THE PATIENT

Ideally, positioning combines a maximal expansion of the patient's chest with the most comfortable installation for the patient, allowing the patient to rest. Fowler's position usually meets those needs.[19]

Therapeutic beds can deliver patient positioning techniques, such as continuous rotation, proning, semi-recumbent position, and turn-assist options.[29] The evidence for and limitations of therapeutic beds are nevertheless not yet fully known. Several prospective randomized trials have demonstrated that rotational therapy prevents and treats respiratory complications,[30] and this conclusion is supported by a 2007 meta-analysis.[31] A recent randomized clinical trial (RCT) showed that patients in the experimental group, who were continuously, administered rotation therapy in a specialized therapeutic bed, developed less when VAP compared to the control group. Cases also experienced shorter ventilation time and length of stay. Mortality was comparable in both groups.[32] Economic analyses that balance the considerable cost originating from the use of kinetic beds against the gains they bring, need to be conducted.

ADMINISTERING OXYGEN THERAPY

Oxygen therapy aims at preventing or reversing hypoxemia and reducing the work of breathing. A variety of oxygen delivery devices is available. The equipment of choice depends on the patient's age and condition, and on the required fraction of inspired oxygen (FiO_2). High-flow systems, such as Venturi masks and ventilators, deliver a precisely controlled air-oxygen mixture. Low-flow systems, such as nasal prongs, nasal catheter, simple mask, partial rebreather mask, and non-rebreather mask allow variation in the oxygen percentage delivered, based on the patient's respiratory pattern.[17,19,20,22]

Prongs and Catheters

Inexpensive and easy to use, nasal prongs permit talking, eating, and suctioning. They interfere less with the patient's activities than other devices but may cause nasal drying. Nasal prongs deliver oxygen at flow rates from 0.5 to 6 L/min and in concentrations of less than 40% only.[20]

Nasal catheters can deliver low-flow oxygen at somewhat higher concentrations but are not commonly used because of discomfort and drying of the mucous membranes.

Transtracheal oxygen catheters used for patients requiring chronic oxygen therapy, permit highly efficient oxygen delivery and increased mobility with portable oxygen systems and avoid the adverse effects of nasal delivery systems. However, they may become a source of infection and require close monitoring and follow-up after insertion, as well as daily maintenance care.[19-22]

Masks

Simple masks deliver oxygen through an entry port at the bottom of the mask in concentrations of 40–60%. The oxygen exits through large holes on the sides of the mask.[17,20]

With a partial rebreather mask, the patient inspires oxygen from a reservoir bag along with atmospheric air and oxygen from the mask. The first third of exhaled tidal volume enters the bag, the rest exits the mask. Because air entering the reservoir bag comes from the trachea and bronchi where no gas exchange occurs, the patient rebreathes the oxygenated air that was exhaled. Oxygen can be administered in concentrations of 40–60%.[17,20]

With a non-rebreather mask, a 1-way inspiratory valve opens upon inhalation, directing oxygen from a reservoir bag into the mask. On exhalation, gas exits the mask through the 1-way expiratory valves and enters the atmosphere. As the patient breathes air only from the bag, it delivers oxygen at concentrations of 60–90%.[17,20]

A Venturi mask is connected to a Venturi device, which mixes a specific volume of air and oxygen. It delivers highly accurate oxygen concentrations despite the patient's respiratory pattern.[33]

A continuous positive airway pressure (CPAP) mask allows the spontaneously breathing patient to receive CPAP with or without an artificial airway. In mild-to-moderate infectious disorders, CPAP provides an alternative to invasive mechanical ventilation. It increases the functional residual capacity by distending collapsed alveoli, which improves the PaO_2 and decreases intrapulmonary shunting and oxygen consumption. It also reduces the work of breathing.[17,20]

As disadvantages of masks, they may fit poorly, cause discomfort, and must be removed to eat.[17,19,20,34]

Nursing Considerations[19-22,34-37]

- Nurses must ensure that patients receive the prescribed percentage of oxygen
- Oxygen flow exceeding 3 L/min must be humidified to prevent drying of mucous membranes. Humidity is not added with a Venturi mask because water can block the jets
- A cardiopulmonary assessment is performed and it must be checked that baseline arterial blood gas or oximetry values have been obtained. Cardiopulmonary assessments are repeated regularly
- When using a nasal cannula, it is cleaned and the patient's nares ar assessed at least every 8 hours. The nares' patency must be checked; if blocked, a mask might be needed. The attending physician is to be consulted if any change in administration route is required
- All connections are checked regularly. Humidifiers must be checked on bubbling, and oxygen must flow through the mask, catheter, or prongs
- The flow rate is to be set as ordered. Patients with chronically high partial pressure of arterial carbon dioxide ($PaCO_2$), such as those with chronic obstructive pulmonary disease, (COPD) may be stimulated to breathe by a low oxygen level rather than by a slightly high $PaCO_2$ level, as is normal. For such patients, supplemental oxygen therapy should be provided cautiously, because it may depress the stimulus to breathe, thereby, further increasing $PaCO_2$
- If the patient is on bed rest, his position is changed frequently to ensure adequate ventilation and circulation and to prevent pressure sores. Good skin care will prevent irritation and breakdown caused by the tubing, prongs, or mask
- Nurses must assess the patient for signs of hypoxemia, including tachycardia, arrhythmias, diaphoresis, restlessness, altered blood pressure or respiratory rate, clammy skin, and cyanosis. If these occur, the doctor is notified, a pulse oximetry reading is obtained, and the oxygen delivery equipment is checked to see if it is malfunctioning. Especially with changes or discontinuation of the oxygen therapy, special alertness and caution is strongly recommended
- If the patient is on a non-breather mask, the valves are checked periodically to ensure they function properly. If the valves stick closed, the patient is reinhaling CO_2 and not receiving adequate oxygen. The mask is replaced, if necessary
- Patients receiving high oxygen concentrations, i.e., exceeding 50%, for more than 24 hours, should be asked about symptoms of oxygen toxicity, such as burning, substernal chest pain, dyspnea, dry cough, and pulmonary edema. The patient is encouraged to cough and to take deep breathes to help prevent atelectasis. Arterial blood gas levels must be monitored frequently and oxygen concentrations are to be reduced as soon as arterial blood gas values indicate this is feasible
- A low flow rate should be used if the patient has chronic pulmonary disease. However, in this case, use of a simple mask is to be avoided because low flow rates will not flush carbon dioxide from the mask, and the patient will rebreathe it.

CARING FOR THE PATIENT ON INVASIVE MECHANICAL VENTILATION

Invasive mechanical ventilation corrects profoundly impaired ventilation, evidenced by hypercapnia and symptoms of respiratory distress. Invasive mechanical ventilation typically requires an endotracheal tube (ETT) or tracheostomy tube and delivers up to 100% room air under positive pressure or oxygen-enriched air in concentrations up to 100%.

The main types of invasive mechanical ventilation are positive-pressure, negative-pressure, and high-frequency ventilation. Positive-pressure systems can be volume-cycled or pressure-cycled. Negative-pressure systems provide ventilation for patients who cannot generate adequate inspiratory pressures. High frequency ventilation systems provide high ventilation rates with low peak airway pressures, synchronized to the patient's own inspiratory efforts.

Mechanical ventilators can be programmed to assist, control, or assist-control.

Nursing Considerations[17-22,34-37]

- Patients who do not have an ETT or tracheostomy in place, may be started on a noninvasive form of mechanical ventilation to avoid intubation or tracheotomy. If more conservative measures fail or if noninvasive ventilation is contraindicated, the patient may be intubated to establish an artificial airway
- Baseline vital signs and arterial blood gas levels must be obtained and checked as ordered. Overventilation may cause respiratory alkalosis from decreased carbon dioxide levels. Inadequate alveolar ventilation or atelectasis from an inappropriate tidal volume may cause respiratory acidosis
- A bite block may prevent the patient from biting the tube
- Following steps should be performed every 1–2 hours and as needed:
  - All connections between the ventilator and the patient need to be checked and all critical alarms must be turned on. Call bells need to be within the reach of conscious patients
  - Ventilator settings need to be verified as well that the ventilator is operating at those settings
  - Humidifiers are to be refilled if necessary. The corrugated tubing must be checked for condensation and any collected water is to be carefully removed into a container without draining condensation into the patient's airway
  - Oxygen concentration must be checked every 8 hours and arterial blood gas levels whenever ventilator settings are changed. To detect the need for suctioning and to evaluate the response to treatment, the respiratory status needs to be assessed at least every 2 hours in the acute patient and every 4 hours in the stable chronic patient. Suctioning is performed as necessary, noting the amount, color, odor, and consistency of secretions.[38] Nurses may also auscultate for decreased breath sounds on the patient's left side, indicating slipping of the tube into the right mainstem bronchus
- Fluid intake and output are monitored, along with electrolyte balance. The patient is weighed as ordered
- Evidence-based guidelines for the prevention of VAP must continuously be adhered to.[3,39,40] It has recently been demonstrated that intermittent subglottic secretions drainage, continuous lateral rotation therapy, and polyurethane cuffed endotracheal tubes decrease the risk of VAP. Also, ETTs with a taper-shaped cuff appear to better prevent fluid leakage[41]
- All medications are to be administered as ordered
- The patient's bowel sounds and functioning, as well as abdominal distention, which may indicate paralytic ileus, should be monitored
- Adequate oral care must be provided. Mechanisms contributing to a decrease in oral health in ill intubated patients include dental plaque formation, administration of drugs, which cause xerostomia and of antibiotics, which cause colonization of the oral cavity by opportunistic pathogens, change of the oral flora into a predominance of Gram-negative organisms and *Staphylococcus aureus*, and the presence of an endotracheal tube. Moreover, considerable evidence supports the relationship between poor oral health, the oral microflora, and VAP.[42,43] Nurses assess the oral cavity and supply good oral care by means of a thorough mechanical cleaning with use of a toothbrush twice daily and, in addition, chemical decontamination with chlorhexidine or a povidone-iodine oral care solution, at least twice daily[43]
- The patient who is receiving high-pressure ventilation should be assessed for signs of pneumothorax, including absent or diminished breathe sounds on the affected site, acute chest pain, and possibly, tracheal deviation or subcutaneous or mediastinal emphysema. If the patient is receiving a high oxygen concentration, nurses pay attention to signs of toxicity, such as substernal chest pain, increased coughing, tachypnea, decreased lung compliance, and vital capacity, and decreased $PaCO_2$ without a change in oxygen concentration
- Emergency equipment must be readily available in case of ventilator malfunctioning or accidental

extubation. If problems with the ventilator occur, the patient is disconnected from the ventilator and manually ventilated with 100% oxygen, using a handheld resuscitation bag connected to the ETT or tracheostomy tube
- Successful weaning depends on a strong spontaneous respiratory effort, a stable cardiovascular system, and sufficient respiratory muscle strength and level of consciousness to sustain spontaneous breathing
- Nurses must provide emotional support to the patient and his family, who should be reassured that a nurse will always be nearby. A communication system, such as a letter board, is set up with the conscious patient and the call bell is always within his reach. It must be kept in mind that an apprehensive patient may fight the machine.

CARING FOR ENDOTRACHEAL TUBES

By inserting a tube into the patient's lungs through the mouth or nose, a patent airway is established and a route for mechanical ventilation is provided. The tube protects patients from aspiration by sealing off the trachea from the digestive tract and permits removal of tracheobronchial secretions in patients who cannot cough effectively.

Drawbacks of endotracheal intubation include that it bypasses normal respiratory defences against infection, reduces cough effectiveness, may be uncomfortable, and prevents verbal communication.[44,45]

Intubation can be performed nasotracheally or orotracheally. When neither is possible, the alternative of retrograde intubation can be considered in which a wire inserted through the trachea and out of the mouth is used to guide the insertion of an ETT.[20] International VAP prevention guidelines recommend oral intubation above nasal intubation.[3,9,39]

Nursing Considerations[18-22,34-37]

- If possible, the intubation procedure is explained to the patient and his family
- The correct size of ETT must be obtained. The typical size is 7.5 mm for women and 8 mm for men
- ETTs with a taper-shaped cuff appear to better prevent fluid leakage[41,46]
- Medication must be administered as ordered to decrease respiratory secretions, induce amnesia or analgesia, and help calm and relax the conscious patient. Dentures and bridgework are removed
- The ETT must be carefully secured. Before taping an ETT tape in place, the patient's face needs to be clean, dry, and free from beard stubble. If possible, the patient's mouth is suctioned and the tube dried just before taping. Also, the reference mark on the tube is checked to ensure correct placement. Tubes can be secured using adhesive tape or by means of an ETT holder, made of hard plastic or softer material and some of them with bite blocks attached
- After securing the ETT, its placement is reconfirmed by noting bilateral breath sounds and end-tidal carbon dioxide ($ETCO_2$) readings. Breath sounds are auscultated and the patient is watched for chest movement to ensure correct tube placement and full lung ventilation. A chest X-ray may be ordered to confirm tube placement
- Nurses must follow standard precautions and suction through the ETT, as the patient's condition indicates to clear secretions and prevent mucous plugs from obstructing the tube. If available, closed tracheal suction systems are used. Those systems permit the ventilated patient to remain on the ventilator during suctioning and help prevent VAP.[39] Moreover, they can ease removal of secretions and reduce patient complications
- Endotracheal cuff pressure should be maintained at the lowest pressure, i.e., below 20 cmH_2O that prevents cuff leak and should not exceed 30 cmH_2O.[47] Cuff pressure must be high enough to ensure adequate ventilation and prevent aspiration of secretions that accumulate above the ETT cuff. High pressure must nevertheless be avoided in order to prevent tracheal damage from compromised tracheal capillary perfusion pressure.[48] Cuff pressure must be assessed using a calibrated manometer.[49-53] Nowadays, systems that automatically and continuously monitor and adjust cuff pressure in a reliable and safe way are also available.[54-58]

CARING FOR THE PATIENT ON NONINVASIVE VENTILATION

Noninvasive ventilation refers to the provision of ventilatory support through the patient's upper airways using a mask or similar device. Thereby, this technique is distinguished from those bypassing the upper airways with a tracheal tube, laryngeal mask, or tracheostomy and therefore, are considered invasive.[34,59] Modes of noninvasive ventilation include continuous mandatory ventilation, assist control, pressure support, CPAP, bi-level pressure support, and proportional assist ventilation.[34]

Noninvasive ventilation is not suitable for all patients with respiratory failure. In patients with copious respiratory secretions, for example, it is contraindicated.[34] Its use in appropriately selected patients has, however, been shown to improve survival and decrease the need for endotracheal intubation.[34,35,37,60-62]

A large variety of different sizes of interfaces, including nasal masks, total- and full-face masks, and nasal pillows are available for noninvasive ventilation. The interface of choice should match the individual patient's requirements and condition. In the acute setting, a full-face mask can be used initially, changing to a nasal mask after 24 hours, as the patient improves.[34]

Nursing Considerations[18-22,34-37]

- Patients eligible for noninvasive ventilation are, per definition, conscious patients who will not be sedated. Thereby, patients are often anxious and need information and psychological support. Also, the family needs to be informed properly. Patient's cooperation is crucial for the success of noninvasive ventilation. If time permits, the patient is allowed to handle the mask and the equipment
- The permeability of the patient's airways must be checked, secretions aspirated and any objects that could potentially compromise permeability are to be removed
- If a mask is used, the fitting is crucial for the success of the technique. Dentures are kept in, as they may help with producing an adequate seal. If they are nevertheless of poor fitting, they should be removed
- Before starting treatment, the patient is placed in a comfortable position with a call bell within reach. Breaks from noninvasive ventilation can be made, e.g., for drug administration, meals, or general patient comfort
- Pressure sores are prevented by protecting the zones of the patient's body that will be subject to continuous pressure from the interface. Some manufacturers provide padding with the interfaces. If not available, alternatives, such as hydrocolloid strips can be used. These dressings are used at the very onset of ventilation without waiting until the initial signs of pressure sores are observed
- Close observation of the patient and his response to the treatment is paramount. All patients are continuously monitored with oximetry, especially for the first 24 hours of treatment. In critically ill patients, continuous electrocardiogram (ECG) monitoring and insertion of an arterial line may be required. Unless the patient's condition is rapidly deteriorating, arterial blood gas tensions are checked every 30–60 minutes following the establishment of treatment. The frequency of subsequent measures will depend on the patient's progress. Clinical reassessment must routinely take place 1 hour after the patient has been established on noninvasive ventilation
- Improvement in breathlessness is usually seen in 1–2 hours, if the treatment is effective. Mostly, there is an improvement in the neurological status of the patient at the same time
- Nurses should be aware of and anticipate the most common practical problems with the use of noninvasive ventilation, which include mask discomfort, dry nose, air leaks around the mask, eye irritation from air leaks, and gastric distension
- Weaning protocols must be developed with the multidisciplinary team.

AEROSOL THERAPY

Aerosol therapy aids bronchial hygiene by restoring and maintaining mucous blanket continuity, hydrating dried, and retained secretions, promoting expectoration of secretions, humidifying inspired oxygen, and delivering medications.[20-22] The therapy may be administered through nebulizers that have a large or small volume, are ultrasonic, or are placed in-line with the ventilator tubing.

Nursing Considerations[19-22,34-37]

- Nurses should explain the procedure to the patient, whose vital signs are taken and lung fields auscultated to establish a baseline. If possible, the patient is placed in a sitting or high Fowler's position to encourage full lung expansion and to promote aerosol dispersion. The patient is encouraged to take slow, even breaths during the treatment
- During the procedure, the patient is checked frequently to observe for adverse reactions. As ultrasonic nebulizer therapy may hydrate retained secretions and obstruct airways, the patient is observed for labored respiration
- The patient is encouraged to cough and expectorate or suctioned as needed
- The water level in large-volume nebulizers is checked at frequent intervals and replaced as indicated. The nebulizer unit and tubing are to be changed according to the hospital's policy.

CARING FOR PATIENTS WITH TRACHEOTOMY

A tracheotomy provides an airway for an intubated patient who needs prolonged mechanical ventilation. It helps remove lower tracheobronchial secretions in a patient who cannot clear them and is also performed in emergencies and when endotracheal tubing is not possible to prevent an unconscious or paralyzed patient from aspirating food or secretions, and to bypass upper airway obstruction. The doctor creates the surgical opening and inserts a tracheostomy tube to permit access to the airway. He may select from several tube styles, uncuffed, cuffed or fenestrated, depending on the patient's condition.[63,64]

Nursing Considerations

- For an emergency tracheotomy, the procedure is to be explained briefly to the patient as time permits. For a scheduled tracheotomy, the procedure is explained to the patient and his family[63,64]
- If time permits, a communication system with the patient is set up and practiced to ensure that the patient will be able to communicate comfortably while the speech is limited[63,64]
- It must be ensured that samples for arterial blood gas analysis and other diagnostic tests have been collected[20,22]
- After the procedure, breath sounds are checked every 2 hours. Crackles, rhonchi, or diminished breath sounds must be reported[20,22]
- The patient is to be turned every 2 hours to avoid pooling tracheal secretions. As ordered, chest therapy will be provided to help mobilize secretions[20,22]
- For cuff pressure, the same requirements as for ETTs are valid.[63,64]

SPUTUM ANALYSIS

Analysis of a sputum specimen helps determine the causative etiology of respiratory infection. The nature and origin of the specimen, date and time of collection, initial diagnosis, and medication the patient is taking, are included in the request. The specimen is sent to the laboratory immediately after collection. Whatever type of sampling is used, it is pivotal that the specimen is sampled prior to the first antimicrobial dose.[19,20,22]

Collection by Expectoration

The patient is encouraged to increase fluid intake the night before collection to aid expectoration and to obtain a specimen in the morning. Nurses wear gloves and a mask. When the patient is ready to expectorate, the nurse instructs to take 3 deep breaths, to force a deep cough, and to expectorate in the container. If the cough is nonproductive, chest physiotherapy or nebulization, as ordered, can be used to induce sputum. Using an aseptic technique, the container has to be closed securely and placed in a leak-proof bag. The specimen needs to be sputum, not saliva. To prevent contamination with foreign articles, the patient is instructed not to eat, brush teeth or use a mouthwash before expectoration. The patient may rinse the mouth with water.[20,22]

Collection by Tracheal Suctioning

Oxygen must be administered to the patient before and after suctioning and as necessary. Using sterile gloves, a catheter lubricated with normal saline is advanced into the trachea. Suction should not be applied for longer than 15 seconds to obtain the specimen. Catheter and gloves are discarded after the procedure, then the in-line sputum trap from the suction apparatus is detached and the opening is capped.[20,22]

Collection by Bronchoscopy

For bronchoscopy, secretions are collected with a bronchial brush or aspirated through the inner channel of the scope using an irrigating solution, such as normal saline. Following the procedure, the patient is observed for signs of hypoxemia, laryngospasm, bronchospasm, pneumothorax, or trauma to respiratory structures. The nurse checks for breathing or swallowing difficulty. Patients are not to be given any liquids until the gag reflex returns.[20,22,65]

BLOOD ANALYSES

Blood analyses used to diagnose and treat respiratory infections include arterial blood gas analysis, leukocyte count, and differential leukocyte count.[20,65]

Arterial Blood Gas Analysis

Blood for an arterial blood gas analysis is drawn from an arterial line if the patient has one. If a percutaneous puncture must be done, the site must be chosen carefully. The brachial, radial, and femoral arteries can be used.

After Allen's test, which assesses the patient's collateral arterial blood supply before obtaining an arterial blood gas sample, a heparinized blood gas syringe is used. All air is eliminated from the sample, which is transported for analysis immediately. Pressure must be applied to the puncture site for 3–5 minutes, or longer and as necessary if the patient is administered anticoagulants or has a coagulopathy. A gauze pad will be taped firmly over the puncture site. Taping the entire circumference of an arm is avoided as this may restrict the circulation. The site is monitored regularly for bleeding and the arm or leg for signs of circulatory impairment, such as swelling, discoloration, pain, numbness, and tingling. Vital signs are assessed. It is noted on request, whether the patient is breathing room air or oxygen. If oxygen, the number of liters is documented. If the patient is on mechanical ventilation, the fraction of inspired oxygen is mentioned. Nurses wait at least 20 minutes before drawing blood for an arterial blood gas analysis after initiating, changing, or discontinuing oxygen therapy, after initiating or changing settings of mechanical ventilation, after suctioning the patient, or after extubation. The patient is instructed to breathe normally during the test and warned that he may feel brief cramping or throbbing pain at the puncture site.

White Blood Cell Count and Differential White Blood Cell Count

The leukocyte count measures the number of leukocytes in a microliter of whole blood. An elevated count (leukocytosis) commonly signals infection. A differential leukocyte count provides more specific information about a patient's immune system. The laboratory classifies 100 or more WBCs in a stained film of blood according to 5 major types of leukocytes (neutrophils, eosinophils, basophils, lymphocytes, monocytes) and determines the percentage of each type.

To obtain the sample, the nurse performs a venipuncture and collects the sample in a 7 mL tube containing ethylenediaminetetraacetic acid (EDTA). The tube is filled completely and inverted gently several times to adequately mix the sample and anticoagulant.

INFORMING PATIENT AND FAMILY

Nurses play a pivotal role in providing correct and honest information to the patient and his family. As the coordinating members of the multidisciplinary team, they should be alert for information needs and see to the fact that these are fulfilled.

Nurses must know which information they can provide themselves and to whom they are allowed to provide it. They contact the doctor and arrange a meeting for family members who desire to receive specific medical information.

Johnson & Leventhal (1974) promoted combining sensory information with procedural information and coping instructions. Sensory information refers to what the patient will hear, see, smell, taste, during the procedure. Procedural information is information about what will happen before, during, and after the procedure and in the course of the examination. Coping instructions refer to what the patient can do to influence the course of the procedure in a positive way.[66]

SUPPORTING AND EDUCATING PATIENT AND FAMILY

Nurses must be alert for the emotional and social needs of the patient and his family and provide an adequate support. Listening to patients will help nurses know where the nurse needs to be educated.

The patient with pneumonia can be taught how to cough and perform deep-breathing exercises to clear secretions, and is encouraged to do so often. Conscious patients can be educated about taking on the best position to promote full ventilation and drainage of secretions. Encouragement of annual influenza and pneumococcal vaccination for high-risk patients, such as those with COPD and chronic heart disease, may be a nursing educational task. To prevent pneumonia, nurses need to advise their patients to avoid using antibiotics indiscriminately during minor vital infections, because this may result in upper airway colonization with antibiotic-resistant bacteria. All patients are advised to stop smoking and are referred to a local initiative for smoking cessation.

CONCLUSION

As important members of the multidisciplinary team, nurses are responsible for a large variety of care interventions that contribute to the outcome of patients with respiratory tract infections. By completing these interventions adequately, they substantially add to providing high-quality care for this category of patients.

REFERENCES

1. American Thoracic Society; Infectious Diseases Society of America. Guidelines for the management of adults with hospital-acquired, ventilator-associated, and healthcare-associated pneumonia. *Am J Resp Crit Care Med.* 2005;171: 388-416.
2. Depuydt P, Myny D, Blot S. Nosocomial pneumonia: aetiology, diagnosis and treatment. *Curr Opin Pulm Med.* 2006;12:192-7.
3. Coffin SE, Klompas M, Classen D, Arias KM, Podgorny K, Anderson DJ, et al. Strategies to prevent ventilator-associated pneumonia in acute care hospitals. *Infect Control Hosp Epidemiol.* 2008;29:S31-40.
4. Rello J, Ollendorf DA, Oster G, Vera-Llonch M, Bellm L, Redman R, et al. Epidemiology and outcomes of ventilator-associated pneumonia in a large US database. *Chest.* 2002;122:2115-21.
5. Torres A, Ewig S, Lode H, Carlet J; European HAP working group. Defining, treating and preventing hospital acquired pneumonia: European perspective. *Intensive Care Med.* 2009;35:9-29.
6. Niel-Weise BS, Gastmeier P, Kola A, Vonberg RP, Wille JC, van den Broek PJ, et al. An evidence-based

recommendation on bed head elevation for mechanically ventilated patients. *Crit Care.* 2011;15:R111.

7. Muscedere J, Dodek P, Keenan S, Fowler R, Cook D, Heyland D, et al. Comprehensive evidence-based clinical practice guidelines for ventilator-associated pneumonia: Prevention. *J Crit Care.* 2008;23:126-37.
8. Masterton R, Craven D, Rello J, Struelens M, Frimodt-Moller N, Chastre J, et al. Hospital-acquired pneumonia guidelines in Europe: a review of their status and future development. *J Antimicrob Chemother.* 2007;60:206-13.
9. Centers for Disease Control and Prevention. Guidelines for preventing health-care–associated pneumonia, 2003: recommendations of CDC and the Healthcare Infection Control Practices Advisory Committee. *MMWR.* 2004; 53:(RR-3).
10. Pravikoff DS, Tanner AB, Pierce ST. Readiness of U.S. nurses for evidence-based practice: many don't understand or value research and have had little or no training to help them find evidence on which to base their practice. *Am J Nurs.* 2005;105:40-52.
11. Blot SI, Labeau S, Vandijck DM, Van Aken P, Claes B. Evidence-based guidelines for the prevention of ventilator-associated pneumonia. Results of a knowledge test among intensive care nurses. *Intensive Care Med.* 2007;33:1463-7.
12. Labeau S, Vandijck D, Rello J, Adam S, Rosa A, Wenisch C, et al. Evidence-based guidelines for the prevention of ventilator-associated pneumonia: results of a knowledge test among European intensive care nurses. *J Hosp Infect.* 2008;70:180-5.
13. Kaynar AM, Mathew JJ, Hudlin MM, Gingras DJ, Ritz RH, Jackson MR, et al. Attitudes of respiratory therapists and nurses about measures to prevent ventilator-associated pneumonia: a multicenter, cross-sectional survey study. *Respir Care.* 2007;52:1687-94.
14. Sinuff T, Cook D, Giacomini M, Heyland D, Dodek P. Facilitating clinician adherence to guidelines in the intensive care unit: A multicenter, qualitative study. *Crit Care Med.* 2007;35:2083-9.
15. *Ricart M, Lorente C, Diaz E, Kollef MH, Rello J.* Nursing adherence with evidence-based guidelines for preventing ventilator-associated pneumonia. *Crit Care Med.* 2003;31: 2693-6.
16. Kelleher S, Andrews T. An observational study on the open-system endotracheal suctioning practices of critical care nurses. *J Clin Nurs.* 2008;17:360-9.
17. Francis C. Respiratory Care. Oxford: Blackwell Publishing Ltd; 2006.
18. Adam SK, Osborne S. Critical care nursing: Science and practice. 2 ed. Oxford: Oxford University Press; 2006.
19. Brooker C, Nicol M, eds. Nursing adults: the practice of caring. London: Mosby; 2003.
20. Bruck L, Mayer BH, eds. Respiratory care made incredibly easy. Philadelphia, PA: Lipincott Williams & Wilkins; 2005.
21. Bunker Rosdahl C, Kowalski MT. Textbook of basic nursing. 9 ed. Philadelphia, PA: Lippincott Williams & Wilkins; 2008.
22. O'Connell Smeltzer SC, Bare BG, Hinkle JL, Cheever KH. Brunner and Suddarth's Textbook of Medical Surgical Nursing, North American Edition (combined volume). Philadelphia, PA: Lippincott Williams & Wilkins; 2009.
23. Rosenberg G. The significance of pneumonia in the elderly. *Can Fam Physician.* 1987;33:1255-8.
24. Sund-Levander M, Ortqvist A, Grodzinsky E, Klefsgard O, Wahren LK. Morbidity, mortality and clinical presentation of nursing home-acquired pneumonia in a Swedish population. *Scand J Infect Dis.* 2003;35:306-10.
25. Sheppard M, Adam S, Wright M, eds. Principles and practice of high dependency nursing. Philadelphia, PA: Elsevier Health Sciences;2006.
26. Blot SI, Rodriguez A, Sole-Violan J, Blanquer J, Almirall J, Rello J. Effects of delayed oxygenation assessment on time to antibiotic delivery and mortality in patients with severe community-acquired pneumonia. *Crit Care Med.* 2007;35: 2509-14.
27. Blot S. Limiting the attributable mortality of nosocomial infection and multidrug resistance in intensive care units. *Clin Microbiol Infect.* 2008;14:5-13.
28. Rello J, Kollef M, Diaz E, Roderiguez A, eds. Infectious diseases in critical care. Heidelberg:Springer;2007.
29. European Society of Intensive Care Medicine (ESICM), Section on technology assessment & health informatics. Health technology assessment in intensive care medicine: therapeutic beds. Brussels: Imprimerie Cleerebaut 2006.
30. Marklew A. Body positioning and its effect on oxygenation - a literature review. *Nurs Crit Care.* 2006;11:16-22.
31. Goldhill DR, Imhoff M, McLean B, Waldmann C. Rotational bed therapy to prevent and treat respiratory complications: a review and meta-analysis. *Am J Crit Care.* 2007;16:50-62.
32. Staudinger T, Bojic A, Holzinger U, Meyer B, Rohwer M, Mallner F, et al. Continuous lateral rotation therapy to prevent ventilator-associated pneumonia. *Crit Care Med.* 2010;38:486-90.
33. Soto-Ruiz KM, Peacock WF, Varon J. The men and history behind the Venturi mask. *Resuscitation.* 2011;82:244-6.
34. British Thoracic Society Standards of Care Committee. Non-invasive ventilation in acute respiratory failure. *Thorax.* 2002;57:192-211.
35. Ahrens T, Prentice D, Kleinpell RM. Critical care nursing certification: preparation, review, & practice exams. 5th edn. New York: McGraw-Hill; 2007.
36. Burke JP. Infection control-a problem for patient safety. *N Engl J Med.* 2003;348:651-6.
37. Hess DR. The mask for noninvasive ventilation: principles of design and effects on aerosol delivery. *J Aerosol Med.* 2007;20:S85-98.
38. Pedersen CM, Rosendahl-Nielsen M, Hjermind J, Egerod I. Endotracheal suctioning of the adult intubated patient. What is the evidence? *Intensive Crit Care Nurs.* 2009;25:21-30.
39. Dodek P, Keenan S, Cook D, Heyland D, Jacka M, Hand L, et al. Evidence based clinical practice guideline for the prevention of ventilator associated pneumonia. *Ann Intern Med.* 2004;141:305-13.
40. Rello J, Lode H, Cornaglia G, Masterton R; VAP Care Bundle Contributors. A European care bundle for prevention of ventilator-associated pneumonia. *Intensive Care Med.* 2010;36:773-80.

41. Blot S, Rello J, Vogelaers D. What is new in the prevention of ventilator-associated pneumonia? *Curr Opin Pulm Med.* 2011;17:155-9.
42. Blot S, Vandijck D, Labeau S. Oral care of intubated patients. *Clin Pulm Med.* 2008;15:153-60.
43. Labeau SO, Van de Vyver K, Brusselaers N, Vogelaers D, Blot SI. Prevention of ventilator-associated pneumonia with oral antiseptics: a systematic review and meta-analysis. *Lancet Infect Dis.* 2011;11:845-54.
44. Griesdale DE, Henderson WR, Green RS. Airway management in critically ill patients. *Lung.* 2011;189:181-92.
45. Griesdale DE, Bosma TL, Kurth T, Isac G, Chittock DR. Complications of endotracheal intubation in the critically ill. *Intensive Care Med.* 2008;34:1835-42.
46. Dave MH, Frotzler A, Spielmann N, Madjdpour C, Weiss M. Effect of tracheal tube cuff shape on fluid leakage across the cuff: an in vitro study. *Br J Anaesth.* 2010;105:538-43.
47. Rello J, Sonora R, Jubert P, Artigas A, Rue M, Valles J. Pneumonia in intubated patients: Role of respiratory airway care. *Am J Resp Crit Care Med.* 1996;154:111-5.
48. Bernhard WN, Yost L, Joynes D, Cothalis S, Turndorf H. Intracuff pressures in endotracheal and tracheostomy tubes. Related cuff physical characteristics. *Chest.* 1985;87: 720-5.
49. Parwani V, Hoffman RJ, Russell A, Bharel C, Preblick C, Hahn I-H. Practicing paramedics cannot generate or estimate endotracheal tube cuff pressure using standard techniques. *Prehosp Emerg Care.* 2007;11:307-11.
50. O'Donnell J. A comparison of endotracheal tube cuff pressures using estimation techniques and direct intracuff measurement. *AANA J.* 2004;72:250-1.
51. Bhatta K, Greer R. Awareness and monitoring of tracheal tube cuff pressure in a multidisciplinary intensive care unit. *Anaesth Intensive Care.* 2007;35:302-3.
52. Jaber S, El Kamel M, Chanques G, Sebbane M, Cazottes S, Perrigault PF, et al. Endotracheal tube cuff pressure in intensive care unit: The need for pressure monitoring. *Intensive Care Med.* 2007;33:917-8.
53. Fernandez R, Blanch L, Mancebo J, Bonsoms N, Artigas A. Endotracheal tube cuff pressure assessment: pitfalls of finger estimation and need for objective measurement. *Crit Care Med.* 1990;18:1423-6.
54. Valencia M, Ferrer M, Farre R, Navajas D, Badia JR, Nicolas JM, et al. Automatic control of tracheal tube cuff pressure in ventilated patients in semirecumbent position: A randomized trial. *Crit Care Med.* 2007;35:1543-9.
55. Sole ML, Aragon D, Bennett M, Johnson RL. Continuous measurement of endotracheal tube cuff pressure: how difficult can it be? *AACN Adv Crit Care.* 2008;19:235-43.
56. Sole ML, Penoyer DA, Su X, Jimenez E, Kalita SJ, Poalillo E, et al. Assessment of endotracheal cuff pressure by continuous monitoring: A pilot study. *Am J Crit Care.* 2009;18:133-43.
57. Nseir S, Duguet A, Copin MC, De Jonckheere J, Zhang M, Similowski T, et al. Continuous control of endotracheal cuff pressure and tracheal wall damage: a randomized controlled animal study. *Crit Care.* 2007;11:R109.
58. Sole ML, Su X, Talbert S, Penoyer DA, Kalita S, Jimenez E, et al. Evaluation of an Intervention to Maintain Endotracheal Tube Cuff Pressure Within Therapeutic Range. *Am J Crit Care.* 2011;20:109-18.
59. Keenan SP, Sinuff T, Burns KE, Muscedere J, Kutsogiannis J, Mehta S, et al.; Canadian Critical Care Trials Group/Canadian Critical Care Society Noninvasive Ventilation Guidelines Group. Clinical practice guidelines for the use of noninvasive positive-pressure ventilation and noninvasive continuous positive airway pressure in the acute care setting. *CMAJ.* 2011;183:E195-214.
60. Ram FS, Wellington S, Rowe BH, Wedzicha JA. Non-invasive positive pressure ventilation for treatment of respiratory failure due to severe acute exacerbations of asthma. *Cochrane Database Syst Rev.* 2005;(1): CD004360.
61. Confalonieri M, Potena A, Carbone G, Porta RD, Tolley EA, Umberto Meduri G. Acute respiratory failure in patients with severe community-acquired pneumonia. A prospective randomized evaluation of noninvasive ventilation. *Am J Respir Crit Care Med.* 1999; 160:1585-91.
62. Brett A, Sinclair DG. Use of continuous positive airway pressure in the management of community acquired pneumonia. *Thorax.* 1993;48:1280-1.
63. De Leyn P, Bedert L, Delcroix M, Depuydt P, Lauwers G, Sokolov Y, et al. Tracheotomy: clinical review and guidelines. *Eur J Cardiothorac Surg.* 2007;32:412-21.
64. Heffner JE. Management of the chronically ventilated patient with a tracheostomy. *Chron Respir Dis.* 2005;2:151-61.
65. Chatburn RL, Mireles-Cabodevila E. Handbook of Respiratory Care. Sudbury,MA:Jones & Bartlett Learning; 2011.
66. Johnson JE, Leventhal H. Effects of accurate expectations and behavioral instructions on reactions during a noxious medical examination. *J Pers Soc Psychol.* 1974; 29:710-8.

CHAPTER 28

Lung Infections in Cystic Fibrosis

Baroukh M Assael

ABSTRACT

Cystic fibrosis (CF) is a genetic disease caused by mutations in the CF transmembrane conductance regulator gene coding for the protein CFTR which exhibits the properties of a Cl^- epithelial channel. The mutation causes a multiorgan disease with severe pulmonary involvement due to chronic infection, development of bronchiectasis, and eventually, respiratory failure. Typically, infections are caused by *Staphylococcus aureus, Pseudomonas aeruginosa, Stenotrophomonas maltophilia,* and *Burkholderia cepacia,* but new pathogens, including anaerobes, have been identified in the lower airways which can contribute to the progression of the disease. Many of these species are intrinsically resistant to most antibiotics or develop such resistance. Early recognition, intensive treatment, or prevention of these infections is crucial, and can ameliorate quality of life, and prolong life expectancy. Although the role of these bacterial species is clear, there are only hypothesis concerning the pathogenesis of lung damage linking the basic defect of the chloride channel to the increased susceptibility to lung infections by specific microorganisms and an abnormal inflammatory response.

INTRODUCTION

Cystic fibrosis (CF) is a genetic disease transmitted through a Mendelian recessive pathway. It is caused by mutations in the gene, located at chromosome 7q31.2, which encodes for the protein cystic fibrosis transmembrane conductance regulator (CFTR). CFTR exhibits the properties of a chloride channel on the membrane surface of several epithelial cells.

The European CF Registry gathers data from around 29,000 CF patients in Europe,[1] and the CF Foundation Patient Registry reports on data for more than 26,000 patients in the US.[2]

The frequency of CF varies geographically and according to ethnicity. With the Caucasian population, incidence is estimated to be approximately 1 in 3000 births.[3]

Diagnosis of CF is based on an abnormally elevated chloride concentration in sweat, presence of typical symptoms, identification of mutations whose association with the disease has been proven, and/or direct measurement of CFTR function through determination of potential difference in the nasal mucosa. Neonatal screening programs that allow for a definite diagnosis as early as in the first weeks of life have been implemented in many industrialized countries.[4,5]

The term CF refers to the pathological features in the pancreas described in the 1930s,[6] whilst the term "mucoviscidosis" refers to the abnormally dense exocrine pancreas secretions and the abnormally thick sputum observed in sufferers.[7]

In its classical form, CF affects several organs, including the lungs, pancreas, intestine, male reproductive tract, paranasal sinuses, liver, and sweat glands. Around 80% of patients are pancreatic insufficient at birth. Meconium ileus is a complication recognized at birth in approximately 15% of patients and may be diagnosed prenatally;

however, distal intestinal obstruction syndrome can affect patients at any age. Severe liver disease leading to portal hypertension due to the presence of basic defect in the cholangiocyte involves about 3% of patients.[8] Nasal polyps and chronic sinusitis affect a large proportion of patients. Males are usually infertile. Lung disease will be discussed in greater detail further on.

As genetic testing and neonatal screening programs expand, an increasing number of cases are being diagnosed that do not present the complete clinical picture of CF. They may exhibit mild symptoms, are often diagnosed in adulthood or after screening, and sweat test is often borderline. These cases are referred to as atypical or nonclassical CF. Furthermore, evidence of a CFTR dysfunction may be found in some conditions involving a single organ, i.e., in males with isolated congenital bilateral agenesis of vas deferens or in patients with chronic pancreatitis. These conditions may not be defined as CF, either classical or nonclassical (i.e., typical or atypical) and show that the CFTR gene could be involved in a variety of disorders as well as causing what is classically known as CF.[5]

LUNG INFECTION IN CYSTIC FIBROSIS

Until some decades ago, malnutrition due to poor fat absorption in patients with CF was the main cause of shorter life spans. Now, thanks to the introduction of pancreatic enzyme supplementation and aggressive nutritional programs, most infants survive and may grow normally. In the last few decades, lung infection has been the major determinant of morbidity, and mortality and it greatly determines the burden of treatment, both clinically and economically. The age of appearance of respiratory symptoms is extremely variable, although subtle signs can be recognized early in life, often in asymptomatic patients. Signs of lung involvement may be observed before any infection occurs, i.e., increased levels of neutrophils or inflammatory cytokines in bronchial secretions, and this leads us to consider that inflammation might be a primary characteristic of CF. Later, a variety of microorganisms, such as *Pseudomonas aeruginosa, Staphylococcus aureus, Achromobacter* species, *Burkholderia* species, *Stenotrophomonas maltophilia, Haemophilus influenzae,* atypical mycobacteria, and *Aspergillus fumigatus* may chronically colonize the lower respiratory tract, resulting in progressive lung damage, bronchial remodeling, formation of bronchiectasis, eventual development of respiratory insufficiency, and the need for lung transplantation. The particular role of *P. aeruginosa* and *Burkholderia* species is well defined and is clearly associated with worsening of lung functions, but the clinical microbiology of the CF lung is still not entirely understood, and as more bacterial species, including anaerobes, are identified, their role in the progression of lung disease still remains to be clarified.[9]

The early "natural history" of lung infection in CF seems sufficiently clear. Systematic sampling of upper airways shows that most infants are colonized precociously by nontypable *H. influenzae* and *S. aureus*. The latter is often clinically silent and it is debatable as to whether an asymptomatic patient colonized by *S. aureus* should be subjected to antistaphylococcal treatment permanently or not.[10,11] The role of *S. aureus* will be discussed in greater detail further in this chapter.

BASIC DEFECT AND SUSCEPTIBILITY OF THE CYSTIC FIBROSIS AIRWAY TO *PSEUDOMONAS* INFECTIONS

Airway infection and chronic colonization of the lower airways by *P. aeruginosa* are hallmarks of CF. Prevalence increases gradually with age. According to the North American CF Foundation Registry, by the age of 20–24 years, more than 80% of CF patients are chronically colonized by *P. aeruginosa*,[2] although this may no longer be true in centers that implement aggressive anti-pseudomonal strategies.

It is still unclear why CF lungs are particularly susceptible to *P. aeruginosa* infection and what it is that causes the abnormal response of the innate immune system which results in an inability to eliminate the infection. Three main hypotheses should be considered since they are corroborated by a large amount of experimental data; although they are not easily reconcilable in a simple pathogenic model.

- Wild type CFTR is a receptor for *P. aeruginosa* with a role in mediating innate immunity to the pathogen. In CF, this receptor is not functional. The bacteria are not removed, hence, provoking an inflammatory reaction[12]
- The deficiency in solute transport across CF bronchial epithelial cells creates a milieu (airway surface dehydration, reduced oxygen tension) that favors *P. aeruginosa* adaptation mechanisms and induces its capacity to form biofilm[13]
- CFTR plays a role in the maintenance of acidic pH in intracellular vesicles. Mutations in the gene that codes for CFTR cause alkalinization and an imbalance between acid sphingomyelinase and acid ceramidase. The resulting accumulation of ceramide causes pulmonary inflammation, death of respiratory epithelial cells, deposits of DNA in bronchi, and a greatly increased susceptibility to severe *P. aeruginosa* infections.[14]

Interestingly, hypotheses 2 and 3 have opened up new therapeutic perspectives. Hypothesis 2 has led to the consideration of amiloride that inhibits sodium reabsorption in smaller bronchi, as a potential treatment, and also to the use of hypertonic saline aerosols that osmotically increase the water content of CF mucus. Amiloride has been tested clinically and hypertonic saline nebulization is currently recommended in the treatment of CF. In line with these observations, mice overexpressing the β-subunit of the epithelial sodium channels manifest several characteristics of the CF lung, while paradoxically, cftr-/- mice have little pulmonary involvement (however, it is beyond the scope of the present chapter to analyse the lung pathology of mice CF models in detail).[15,16]

Hypothesis 3 has led to experimental pharmacological treatments that demonstrate the potential benefit of drugs, such as amitriptyline or fenretinide which can restore physiological levels of ceramide and prevent *P. aeruginosa* infection in cftr-/- mice. Clinical studies are now going on.[17]

It should be underlined, however, that a number of other abnormal mechanisms have been identified in CF respiratory or inflammatory cells, i.e., abnormal fatty acid metabolism with low levels of eicosapentaenoic acid (EPA) and docosahexaenoic acid (DHA), increased production of reactive oxygen species, defective glutathione metabolism, elevated levels of homocysteine, defective ubiquitination and apoptosis, impaired bicarbonate secretion, and many others.

It seems extremely difficult to reconcile all the available information in a coherent pathogenic model of CF lung disease, its peculiar susceptibility to *Pseudomonas,* and the exaggerated inflammatory response. It is likely that, along with being a chloride channel, CFTR is also involved in the complex regulatory mechanisms of other proteins at different cellular levels.

PSEUDOMONAS INFECTION AND LOWER AIRWAY COLONIZATION IN CYSTIC FIBROSIS: CLINICAL ASPECTS

The first *P. aeruginosa* infection that usually follows a period of colonization by *H. influenzae* and *S. aureus* which can vary in length of time and may be asymptomatic, but it may also occur as early as in the first weeks of life—the result of environmental exposure in CF centers where strict segregation rules for infected patients are not implemented.[18] Schematically, after the first isolation of *P. aeruginosa* in the upper airways or in bronchial secretions, a patient may experience a period of intermittent infection and, eventually, becomes chronically colonized. Intermittency can last for months or years and some patients never become colonized. In the colonization process, *P. aeruginosa* acquires adaptive properties and develops the capacity to grow in the biofilm mode, as opposed to the planktonic mode. Adaptation confers a selectivity advantage and allows *P. aeruginosa* to escape the host immune response. In the biofilm mode, *P. aeruginosa* can survive in a microaerobic environment, such as the thick mucus of the CF airways. It may develop increased resistance to antimicrobials, overproduce alginate, lose properties related to acute virulence, and improve its metabolic fitness. Experimentally, it is possible to show changes in virulence between early and adapted *P. aeruginosa* obtained from CF patients followed longitudinally. This probably accounts for the fact that invasive infections, sepsis, or bacteremia are almost never seen in CF patients despite the fact that they harbor an extremely high number of *P. aeruginosa* colonies in the bronchial tree. Invasive infections almost only occur when patients are immunodepressed after organ transplantation.[19-21]

A clinical definition of chronic colonization is challenging, and currently, none can be considered fully adequate. The assessment of chronicity depends on the frequency and the method of sampling. It is recommended that bacterial culturing is done from the sputum of all CF patients at least 4 times a year, but infants and young children often do not produce sputum, and tests should be performed by oropharyngeal sampling with a swab. Adequacy of culturing procedures in these patients has been discussed. Some centers combine frequent cultures with measurements of anti-*Pseudomonas* immune titers; however, the value of *P. aeruginosa* serology in CF is still debatable. Bronchoalveolar lavage (BAL) may allow better identification of pathogens, which colonize the lower airways, but routine BAL in infants has demonstrated no benefits compared to oropharyngeal cultures in the prevention of *P. aeruginosa* colonization or improvement in lung computed tomography (CT) scores in the early years of life.[22] The possibility of improving early diagnosis by the use of polymerase chain reaction (PCR) analysis is worth evaluation.[22-24]

In general, lung function in patients colonized with *P. aeruginosa* is lower than that of uncolonized patients, although acquisition of *P. aeruginosa* is not necessarily associated with acute lung function deterioration.[25] A case-controlled analysis of longitudinal clinical and microbiological data of F508del homozygous patients included in the CF Foundation registry revealed that patients who developed severe lung disease had acquired permanent *P. aeruginosa* infection in childhood, particularly before 5 years of age. This confirms an earlier observation by Rosenfeld et al.[26] who carried out a prospective study of a cohort of infants wherein BAL was performed annually for bacteriology and quantification of inflammatory markers and patients' lung functions were tested every 6 months. Infants harboring *P. aeruginosa* in the lower airways exhibited more inflammation and poor lung function; however, inflammation was present even in the absence of bacteria. These studies establish an association between early acquisition of *P. aeruginosa* and lung function deterioration, although this does not ascertain a causal relationship.[27]

THE CFTR GENE, MODIFIER-GENE POLYMORPHISMS, LUNG INFECTION, AND PROGRESSION OF LUNG DAMAGE IN CYSTIC FIBROSIS

More than 1800 mutations of the CFTR gene have been found, but relation to disease has been ascertained for only a few of them. The mutations are classified according to their functional effect on the CFTR protein (CF mutations database).[28] Worldwide, the most commonly occurring mutation is F508del that causes an abnormal intracellular processing of the premature CFTR protein preventing its normal localization on the cell membrane. After the recognition of different classes of mutations, the extreme phenotypical variability of CF, including lung disease was initially related to the amount of functional CFTR loss caused by specific mutations. It is now clear that this alone cannot account for the clinical variability, and it is admitted that other genes can influence CF lung disease, most probably by modulating inflammatory mechanisms and susceptibility to *P. aeruginosa* infection. A number of such modifier genes have been described, including interleukin (IL)-1β, transforming growth factor (TGF) β1, mannose-binding lectin (MBL), and long pentraxin 3 (PTX3). PTX3 is a component of the humoral arm which includes molecules that recognize pathogen-associated molecular patterns (PAMPs) and initiates the immune response in coordination with the cellular arm. When administered to mice with experimental *P. aeruginosa* lung infection, PTX3 has been shown to reduce lung damage and inflammation. A specific haplotype of PTX3 exhibits a significantly higher frequency in *P. aeruginosa* uncolonized vs. colonized CF patients, conferring protection. Interestingly, this haplotype also confers protection against tuberculosis. The study of modifier genes, therefore, not only opens up a way to understand the pathogenesis of lung disease in CF but may also lead to new therapeutic perspectives.[29-35]

AIRWAY INFECTION AND INFLAMMATORY RESPONSE IN CYSTIC FIBROSIS

Susceptibility to *P. aeruginosa* infection of CF bronchial epithelial cells is genetically determined by a defect in the CFTR gene. This alone, however, does not account for the development of CF lung disease, i.e., peripheral airway obstructions, inflammatory response, bronchial remodeling, and bronchiectasis. Much interest has been devoted to the inflammatory response of the CF airway and the innate immune system, which seems to play a key role, since a large number of studies have documented that proinflammatory cytokine production is increased in CF. As discussed above, genes encoding for inflammatory cytokines have been systematically investigated for their potential "modifier" role in CF lung disease.[36,37]

Recently, it has also been proposed that genes involved in innate immune response and inflammation can also influence impaired ion conductance in CF epithelia.[38] This suggests that the interaction of inflammatory processes, infection, basic defect, and the progression of lung disease in CF is more complex than thought so far.

Clinical data in infants support the concept that inflammation may even precede infection in CF lung disease. Recently, longitudinal studies of CF infants diagnosed through neonatal screening have been carried out by Pillarisetti et al.[39] Infant lung function tests were performed, and BAL was obtained for microbiological and biochemical measurements. The concentration of neutrophil elastase was elevated in patients with no infection. Lung function declined over time, and this occurred more rapidly in infants infected with *P. aeruginosa*, *S. aureus,* or both. Again, this confirms earlier observations by Rosenfeld et al. that show higher IL-8 concentrations in BALs performed annually during the first 3 years of life, independently of whether CF pathogens were present, although where *P. aeruginosa* was detected, they increased further.[26,40,41]

In conclusion, we can support the hypothesis that loss of CFTR function facilitates *P. aeruginosa* infection, decreases the capacity of the innate immune system to clear *P. aeruginosa,* and leads to increased inflammatory response to the bacterial stimulus. Contemporaneously, the defective CFTR function creates conditions in the air-liquid interface in the lung, favoring changes in *P. aeruginosa* biology and the formation of biofilm. In this mode of growth, *P. aeruginosa* represents a continuous inflammatory stimulus to the airway.

PREVENTION AND EARLY TREATMENT OF *PSEUDOMONAS* LUNG INFECTION IN CYSTIC FIBROSIS PATIENTS

Until a couple of decades ago, the prevalence of *P. aeruginosa* infection in CF increased steadily with age, and most adolescents were inevitably permanently colonized. This picture is changing rapidly, and in many centers, a large proportion of patients can be maintained *P. aeruginosa*-free until adolescence or even into young adulthood. Attempts to develop vaccines to prevent *P. aeruginosa* colonization in CF patients have so far been unsuccessful, despite the fact that 2 vaccines have reached phase III trial levels.[42]

On the contrary, strategies for recognition and eradication of early infection, even if asymptomatic, have achieved important results and should be considered as a major determinant in reported increased patient lung function in many centers over the last 2 decades. Early eradication treatments may help to keep patients *P. aeruginosa*-free for prolonged periods and this can be achieved simply with aerosolized antibiotics, as shown by the Early Pseudomonal Infection Control (EPIC) trial and the Early Inhaled Tobramycing for Eradication (ELITE) study but a number of protocols have been elaborated.[26,43-45]

A recent study conducted over a 3-year period failed to show any advantage of cycled antibiotic prophylaxis in the prevention of *P. aeruginosa* colonization,[46] and thus, the best strategy today seems early recognition of *P. aeruginosa* and aggressive eradication attempts. Despite every effort, a number of patients will eventually be chronically colonized and it is important to identify the genetic mechanisms underlying such susceptibility to *P. aeruginosa* infection. It should also be considered that strict segregation of patients harboring *P. aeruginosa* and epidemic strains of *P. aeruginosa* have also been successful[47] and those rules should be followed. As shall be discussed later these rules should be even more rigorous for pathogens, such as *B. cepacia* or methicillin-resistant *S. aureus* (MRSA). *P. aeruginosa* strains may be transmissible and are associated with epidemics. Segregation rules allow prevention and interruption of transmission.

Burkholderia cepacia Complex

The *B. cepacia* complex is a group of non-fermenting Gram-negative bacilli consisting of several related species, which can infect and colonize patients and are also found in the environment. *B. cenocepacia* (also known as Genomovar III) and *B. multivorans* are a major problem in CF. *B. cepacia* complex infection is associated with a more rapid and sometimes dramatic decline in pulmonary function than in patients with *P. aeruginosa*. Invasive infections may cause the "cepacia syndrome", a highly lethal event. The presence of these pathogens in the airways is considered a contraindication for lung transplantation. *B. cenocepacia* and *multivorans* are transmissible and can cause outbreaks. Strains of *B. cepacia* complex are intrinsically highly resistant to all clinically available antibiotics, including aminoglycosides, quinolones, polymyxins, and β-lactams. Temocillin has been found to have some *in vitro* activity against *B. cepacia* complex, but clinical trials need to be performed.[48,49] The ET-12 strain has caused epidemics in Canada and Europe. It must be said, however, that some patients with *B. cepacia* colonization remain stable over long periods of time. The reasons accounting for such a variable clinical course are not clear. *B. cepacia* strains may differ for the expression of virulence factors, but patients may also vary in their resistance to infection. A large number of molecular studies have been performed on *B. cepacia* complex and have greatly enhanced the knowledge about these bacteria, leading to the identification of several virulence factors. Identification of *B. cepacia* complex and prevention and treatment of infection still remain a challenge for CF centers.[50-55]

Staphylococcus aureus

S. aureus is detected early in the airways of CF patients, and the frequency in CF Centers of methicillin-resistant strains is increasing. Furthermore, the problem of small colony variants of *S. aureus* still needs clarification and the specific impact of *S. aureus* on CF pulmonary disease has not yet been well established. In the author's experience, some patients chronically colonized by *S. aureus* but who are *P. aeruginosa*-free are still severely affected by disease, although this occurs much less frequently than with *P. aeruginosa* infected patients.

Contrary to earlier studies, recent observations reveal that MRSA is associated with more rapid lung function deterioration and worse survival rates. Some patients colonized only by MRSA and not *P. aeruginosa* may develop respiratory insufficiency and need a lung transplant; however, the presence of MRSA may just be a marker of more severe disease, as suggested by an epidemiological North American study which did not detect a change in forced expiratory volume in 1 second (FEV_1) decline after acquisition of MRSA.[56] The controversy is open, since a parallel study conducted on the data of the North American CF Foundation patient registry[57] confirms that patients harboring MRSA exhibit a more rapid decline in lung function.

Early strategies for *S. aureus* and MRSA eradication have been advocated,[58] but there is no consensus on their adoption. Prolonged nebulized vancomycin has been prescribed to patients harboring MRSA with frequent need for intravenous treatments and hospitalization and with rapidly deteriorating lung function. Clinical trials are still needed to support this practice.[10,59-61]

As far as epidemic strains of *P. aeruginosa* are concerned, stringent infection control procedures can keep the prevalence of MSRA low.[62]

While it is clear that *S. aureus* and MRSA in CF are clinically relevant some questions still remain open. Is long-term oral prophylaxis to prevent *S. aureus* colonization in infants justifiable? Is long-term nebulized anti-*S. aureus* and/or anti-MRSA feasible and of any benefit in CF? Since MRSA can be acquired from healthy close contacts whose nostrils are colonized, the role of close contact vs. hospital exposure in CF needs to be clarified in a better way. There is still need for clinical trials for MRSA eradication.

Aspergillus fumigatus and Allergic Aspergillosis

A. fumigatus is found in bronchial secretions of 6–58% of CF patients, although it is debatable whether *Aspergillus* colonization is associated with poorer lung function or not. In a recent study by de Vrankrijker et al.,[63] infected patients did not exhibit a more rapid FEV_1 decline compared to a control group. However, this contradicts another observation that chronic colonization by *A. fumigatus* is associated with poorer pulmonary function, increased incidence of *P. aeruginosa* infection, and increased hospitalization of patients for pulmonary exacerbations.[64]

CT imaging of the lungs of patients infected by *A. fumigatus* shows an increased number of bronchiectasis,[65] and Shoseyov et al.[66] reported cases of patients colonized by *A. fumigatus* who do not fulfill the criteria for allergic bronchopulmonary aspergillosis and who did not respond to antibiotic treatment of an acute exacerbation but improved on antifungal therapy. Therefore, chronic *A. fumigatus* infection, even in the absence of an allergic response to the fungus, may cause harm to CF patients.

Only a subset, approximately 5% of patients colonized by *A. fumigatus* develop allergic bronchopulmonary aspergillosis, a condition characterized by activation of the Th2 response, production of thymus and activation-regulated chemokine (TARC)[67] and a rise in total and specific anti-*Aspergillus* immunoglobulin (Ig) E. Diagnosis is based on immunological markers,[68] such as total IgE, *Aspergillus* IgE, and *Aspergillus* IgG or precipitins. Clinically, this is characterized by the presence of pulmonary infiltrates and pulmonary function deterioration and exacerbations.

Early treatment of allergic bronchopulmonary aspergillosis may prevent deterioration to a severe fibrotic stage as well as permanent lung damage. Systemic steroids are recommended, usually oral prednisone at a dose of 0.5–2 mg/kg/day for 2–4 weeks followed by tapering off slowly. The addition of itraconazole (200–400 mg/day) may allow a reduction in steroid use. Cohen-Cymberknoh et al.[69] have also proposed the use of monthly pulses of high-dose intravenous methylprednisolone to reduce the side effects of oral steroids. Attempts have also been made with inhaled amphotericin B[70] and omalizumab.[71-74]

Other Pathogens

A number of pathogens have been identified in the lower airways of CF patients, either by culturing methods or by DNA analysis. Whilst it is tempting to treat any pathogen identified in a patient whose lung function is deteriorating or during acute exacerbation, the real pathogenic role of many species is still unclear. Some of these pathogens will be considered here.

Stenotrophomonas maltophilia

It is isolated with increasing frequency in CF patients, apparently more so in young adults. Its effects on lung function are still unclear, and the need to treat *S. maltophilia* colonization is still to be proven. In the Copenhagen CF center, 21 chronically colonized patients with no other Gram-negative infections did not show a steeper decline in lung function compared to the pre-colonization period, although patients with *S. maltophilia* had lower FEV_1 and more rapid decline in lung function than a matched control group, which confirms the analysis conducted on data of the CF Foundation Patient Registry.[75] In some studies, patients with *S. maltophilia* were also found to be more frequently coinfected by *A. fumigatus*, which can account for a worse lung function decline. The study of Waters et al. however, suggests that *S. maltophilia* evokes an immune response and is an independent factor in increasing the risk of pulmonary exacerbation; therefore, it is possible that it is a true pathogen in CF and not simply a colonizing agent.[76,77]

Achromobacter (Alcaligenes) xylosoxidans

It is also being isolated with increasing frequency from the airways of CF patients. Colonized patients have been found to exhibit higher serum levels of tumor necrosis factor (TNF)-α compared to CF patients colonized by *P. aeruginosa* or *B. cepacia* complex and similar levels of other proinflammatory cytokines compared to patients colonized by *P. aeruginosa*.[78] This suggests that *A. xylosoxidans* may be a true pathogen in CF and infected patients should be treated, although previous studies have not been able to show any significant decline in lung function once *A. xylosoxidans* infection is established.[79] Rapid increases in specific antibodies have been associated with decline in lung function.[80]

Mycobacteria

A report of Olivier et al.[81] in 2003 showed that non-tuberculous mycobacteria (NTM) was isolated from the sputum of 13% of 986 patients, of which *M. avium* accounted for 72% and *M. abscessus* for 16%. Patients with infection were younger, had poorer respiratory function and exhibited more abnormalities on chest CT scans. An incidence of 6.1% out of a population of 98 children from 6 to 18 years old was found in the Hospital for Sick Children in Toronto. Only 1 patient had a significant lung infection requiring treatment, but the data of Esther et al.[82] led to the conclusion that at least patients who meet the American Thoracic Society (ATS) definition of NTM disease exhibit significant clinical problems and deserve treatment. Olivier et al.[81] followed a cohort of 60 patients from 17 centers from whom NTM had been isolated in more than 1 sputum sample. No significant differences were found in FEV_1, or FEV_1 decline compared to a control group of non-NTM CF patients; however, NTM-positive patients exhibited more frequent progression in lung CT abnormalities.

The isolation of NTM in CF patients before lung transplantation should not be an exclusion criterion for transplantation, although clinicians should be aware that complications may arise, once immunosuppressive therapy is started.[82-85]

Further to these, a number of other pathogens have been isolated in CF patients' bronchial secretions. CF seems to be a risk factor for acquiring *Ralstonia pickettii*,[86] and many patients have been colonized by *Pandoraea* - some of them exhibiting deterioration in lung function.[87] *Inquilinus limosus*[88] can also chronically infect CF patients.

An interesting observation concerns the presence of anaerobic bacteria due to the low oxygen tension present in the mucus of CF patients. Obligatory and facultative anaerobes have been identified in the mucus of CF patients, both in stable conditions and during exacerbations, and their numbers do not decrease when patients are treated by conventional anti-*P. aeruginosa* treatments despite an improvement in lung function. It has been suggested that presence of *P. aeruginosa* increases the likelihood of becoming colonized by anaerobic bacteria. Interestingly, meropenem has been found to have a better *in vitro* activity against anaerobes isolated from CF patients than ampicillin, metronidazole, or piperacillin/tazobactam and this β-lactam has shown superiority in the treatment of acute CF exacerbations. The question of the need to treat anaerobes in CF is still unsolved.[89-91]

ACUTE EXACERBATIONS

Typically, lung disease in CF is characterized by acute episodes of exacerbation. Exacerbations affect quality of life, increase the need for hospitalization, and a large proportion of the healthcare resources for CF are employed in treating them. Although there is no strict definition, exacerbations are distinguished by increased cough, increased sputum production, and changes in sputum appearance (increased density, change in color) usually accompanied by a decrease in lung function, fever, loss of weight, anorexia, fatigue, and exercise intolerance.

Exacerbations may be associated with hemoptysis and be accompanied by upper airway involvement, such as increased sinus discharge and pain. Chest radiography or CT scan may show increased airway trapping, consolidations, mucus plugging, abscesses, atelectasis, and pneumothorax. Acute phase proteins are increased and reflect an activation of the innate immune system as evidenced by increased neutrophils, IL-8, leukotriene B4 (LTB4), and other molecules in blood and sputum. Some studies have documented increased concentrations of inflammatory cytokines in exhaled breath condensate. As the incidence of acute exacerbations and the time to bacterial exacerbations have been adopted as outcome measures to evaluate the effectiveness of therapies, a consensus on criteria for definition seems necessary.

The cause of an abrupt deterioration is usually infection. In patients harboring *P. aeruginosa,* it has been shown that exacerbations are due to clonal expansion and not necessarily to the acquisition of a new strain. Respiratory virus infections can cause acute exacerbations and as shall be discussed later, acute bronchopulmonary aspergillosis can cause episodes, which may be clinically indistinguishable from a bacterial exacerbation.

Acute exacerbations vary in severity but are often a challenging situation. Mild exacerbations may be managed at home by oral antibiotic therapy based on the most recently available sensitivity tests. Home intravenous treatment has been adopted by many centers; however, severe exacerbations need hospitalization and intense treatment. Severely affected patients may experience respiratory insufficiency, increased need for oxygen, limitation of physical activity, anorexia, increased energy consumption, transient glucose intolerance, and a need for insulin. This may progress to respiratory failure, the need for mechanical ventilation, and extracorporeal carbon dioxide removal or oxygenation. Management of exacerbations is complex and based on high dosages of antibiotics, intensification of airway clearance, close monitoring of blood gas analysis, adequate caloric intake, if necessary, by enteral or parenteral routes, and respiratory supportive measures. The duration of treatment is usually 10–14 days, but longer periods, even several weeks, may be necessary in severely affected patients. The goal of treatment is to resolve the acute symptoms and recover the loss in lung function.

A large number of studies have been devoted to the events predicting or associated with exacerbations, as well as to their management and consequences. Excellent recent reviews are available. Dosage recommendation of intravenous antibiotics is higher than those recommended in other conditions. Although very few comparative studies are available, antibiotic combinations that exploit possible synergistic effects (e.g., aminoglycosides and anti-*P. aeruginosa* β-lactams) or have additive effects (e.g., 2 anti-*P. aeruginosa* β-lactams) or for combination with colistin or quinolones are recommended. Repeated exposure to high doses of aminoglycosides, frequently used because of their excellent anti-*P. aeruginosa* activity, is a cause of concern for oto- and nephrotoxicity. Single daily doses of aminoglycosides have been successfully tested in exacerbations and are well tolerated. Colistin has also been associated with toxic effects at high doses, but on the other hand, quinolones are frequently used even in infants, despite the risk of joint toxicity.[92-94]

Many questions remain open: predictiveness of *in vitro* antibiotic tests has been discussed, and testing the synergistic qualities of combinations of antibiotics has been advocated; testing antibiotic activity against biofilm growing bacteria[95-97] might also prove more effective than performing standard testing; management of multiresistant or totally resistant bacteria remains problematic; the benefits of associating steroids with antibiotics is debatable;[98-100] and continuous infusion of β-lactam antibiotic seems to be advantageous in treating resistant *P. aeruginosa*.[101]

Despite efforts, many patients fail to recover to baseline pulmonary function after exacerbation. Frequent episodes are almost universally associated with progression of disease, worsening of structural damage, and deterioration of the clinical condition of the patients. Patients on a waiting list for lung transplantation are more or less constantly maintained on long-term intravenous treatment and may need a permanent intravenous line for drug administration. Management of patients with cultures negative for CF associated pathogens may be problematic.[102] Treatment of mycobacteria, *B. cepacia* and *S. aureus* or MRSA, as well as the management of allergic bronchopulmonary aspergillosis is discussed separately.[103]

ROLE OF VIRAL INFECTIONS

The H1N1 epidemic in 2009–2010 was associated with significant morbidity as demonstrated by a survey of European centers[104] and Italian centers,[105] although adult patients at an UK center were reported to have experienced only mild disease.[106]

A Cochrane review of the use of palivizumab in the prophylaxis of respiratory syncytial virus (RSV) in CF patients did not reach any conclusion in support of this treatment,[107] whilst seasonal vaccination against influenza is recommended. Anti-influenza chemotherapy has been used in CF patients, but there are no specific studies in CF. Airway viral infections can cause acute deterioration of lung function in CF patients. Recent data published by Olesen,[108] obtained in a 12-month prospective study, identified several episodes of viral infections associated with reduction of FEV_1.

MONITORING THE PROGRESSION OF LUNG DISEASE

FEV_1 is the parameter universally used to follow and quantify the progression of lung disease in CF. FEV_1 is related to major outcome measures, such as survival and quality of life. The other important measure is chest X-ray, for which various scoring systems have been developed. Both have major limitations. FEV_1 is not measurable in the uncollaborative, inexperienced patient, and chest X-ray is not sufficiently sensitive to quantify small changes. Furthermore, FEV_1 decline is not linear throughout the whole "natural history" of a patient. In the initial years of life, the curves are rather flat, even in children deteriorating and at low functional levels (<30%), curves are again flat, and the severity of the disease is no longer reflected by changes in FEV_1. Other outcome measures, therefore, need to be evaluated.

The progression of lung disease can be clearly appreciated by longitudinally performed CT scans and subtle structural changes can be quantified even in young, asymptomatic children before classical pulmonary function tests can be reliably performed. Recent observations have been made in severe advanced disease showing that lesions can be quantified even at that stage. Scoring systems have been developed and interobserver agreement is usually high. Changes in high resolution CT scores have proven to be more sensitive than changes in FEV_1; the classical end point in CF pulmonary studies.[109-113] Patients with chronic *Pseudomonas* infections have worse high resolution CT scores and these correlate with markers of inflammation in the exhaled air condensate.[114] A longitudinal epidemiological evaluation was performed in patients enrolled in the Wisconsin newborn screening trial. The presence and severity of bronchiectasis were evaluated by CT scan and were found to be significantly related to mucoid *P. aeruginosa* infection.[115]

Spirometry remains a classical end-point in CF pulmonary studies.[116] Consistent with the precocious localization of *P. aeruginosa* in the small airways,[117] early functional events are loss in forced expiratory flow (FEF) 25–75% followed by a progressive reduction in FEV_1.

Since Spirometry cannot be adequately carried out in children before the age of 5 years, new approaches have been developed, which allow us to determine a loss in respiratory parameters occurring very precociously. How to best evaluate infants and how predictive are tests performed at this age of the progression of lung disease later in life remains to be established.[118-121]

CHRONIC MANAGEMENT OF LUNG INFECTION IN CYSTIC FIBROSIS PATIENTS

Managing lung infections and the progression of lung disease in CF patients are the main problems encountered in clinical practice. In addition to prevention, which has been discussed earlier, management is complex, and is based on a multiplicity of interventions aimed at facilitating expectoration, mucus fluidification, early identification and treatment of pathogens, recognition and treatment of exacerbations, and long-term treatment of the vicious circle of infection or inflammation. Such a wide spectrum of problems has been faced for decades, and it is surprising how few formally acceptable clinical trials exist that validate treatments. Most randomized, interventional clinical studies have been performed only in the last decade.

Limitations in performing clinical studies are related to the lack of adequate clinical end points, the extreme genetic and phenotypical variability of the disease, the small number of patients in single centers, and the need for long-term studies in order to establish clinically relevant outcomes.

In the last few decades survival rates for CF patients have greatly improved. Once considered a pediatric disease, median survival age now approaches and in some centers, surpasses 40 years. In parallel, lung function has greatly improved and most patients reach adulthood exhibiting only mild pulmonary involvement. This is the result of complex management methods, carried out mostly in specialized centers equipped to deal with the complex nature of the disease. It is impossible to manage pulmonary disease without effective nutritional support and adequate diabetes treatment, and it is necessary to recognize and provide action mechanisms to deal with the potential barriers patients face in adhering to the medical prescription.

Chest Physiotherapy

Once diagnosis has been made almost all CF patients undergo chest physiotherapy to remove thick mucus from the airways. Different techniques for this have been elaborated, i.e., autogenous drainage, postural drainage, positive airway pressure, etc. Whilst there is unanimous consensus about the necessity to treat symptomatic patients, there is still a debate about the management of asymptomatic infants.[122] Unfortunately, there are few comparative trials that establish the superiority of one technique over the others, and the same is the case regarding the superiority of chest physiotherapy vs. exercise in certain conditions.[123] This is mostly due to the numerous difficulties encountered in the design of such studies in the small number of patients, which can be recruited by single centers, and by the fact that long periods of time are necessary to assess their efficacy. Physiotherapy is time consuming for the patient and for the parents of sick children, and adherence is a major problem; nonetheless, it represents a typical aspect of CF Centre activities.

Changing Mucus Composition

Hypertonic saline

The inhalation of hypertonic saline may osmotically increase the water content of mucus. A double-blind prospective trial showed that inhaled hypertonic saline may decrease the frequency of pulmonary exacerbations and, subsequently, the incidence of hospitalization of CF patients. Further studies have documented its safety for infants and preschool children and also, a potential anti-inflammatory effect. The positive effects of hypertonic saline are also seen in patients undergoing treatment with DNAse.[124-126]

DNAse

DNAse is one of the best studied drugs in the management of pulmonary disease in CF. Its use is supported by the results of a number of randomized comparative trials lasting as long as for 3 years. DNA is present in high concentrations in the mucus of CF patients and contributes greatly to its viscosity. DNAse breaks down the DNA in the CF sputum through enzymatic hydrolysis, thereby, increasing its fluidity and leading to a reduction in the rate of FEV_1 decline in patients of 5 years of age or older. The development and introduction of human recombinant DNAse in treatment has solved the safety problems related to the bovine compound. Recent data have also shown that DNAse may improve ventilation inhomogeneity (lung clearance index) in patients 8–18 years old with FEV_1 more than 80% and by targeting and directing the aerosol to small airways, DNAse may also promote improvement of FEF25. No serious side effects for DNAse treatment have been reported.[127-131]

Amiloride

Sodium hyper-reabsorption is considered to be important in the pathogenesis of lung disease, and amiloride inhibits the epithelial sodium channel involved in sodium reabsorption. Clinical trials have demonstrated no significant benefits for inhaled amiloride, but this could be due to the relatively short action of the drug on the bronchial epithelium. Recent experimental data have shown that, if given preventively and before bronchiectasis or mucus plugs have formed, amiloride may still have a therapeutic potential in CF. Molecules with longer duration of action are now under development.[132]

Mannitol

Mannitol is a potent osmotic agent and it can hydrate mucus after inhalation. Preliminary clinical data have shown that it is a potentially therapeutic molecule in CF. Phase III clinical trials are ongoing to further document its efficacy.[133]

Inhaled Antibiotics

Long-term suppression of chronic infection by *P. aeruginosa* is an important goal in the management of lung disease in CF patients. Elevated concentrations of antibiotic in the sputum can be achieved when the antibiotics are inhaled whereas systemic concentrations are lower. It is still unclear about the relative importance of reaching the bronchial tree through the vascular side or from the air-liquid interface. Data exist to support the theory that during acute exacerbations, it is better to have high systemic levels of antibiotics, with the antibiotics having arrived at the respiratory epithelia through the vascular system. Aerosol antibiotic delivery, however, being used as a chronic suppressive treatment in CF, has gained popularity among clinicians through several decades of empirical use. Early observations concerned carbenicillin and gentamicin. Nebulized antibiotic treatment is supported by the results of controlled trials.

In parallel with its popularity among clinicians, there is a desire to improve and optimize the devices used in the aerosol administration of the drugs.

This field of research is extremely active and a number of compounds have now reached the level of phases II–III clinical trial. It is expected that an increasing number of inhaled antibiotics will be available over the coming years and will become a major arm of lung disease management in CF. Administration of dry powder antibiotics is also expected to be of great interest in the near future, and some are already in the market.

The effects of tobramycin nebulized solution, colesthimate sodium, and aztreonam lysinate have been examined in prospective randomized, placebo-controlled studies, and results of comparative studies between them are now available.

Aerosol treatments have been shown to improve spirometry results, reduce the need for intravenous treatment, lower the incidence of hospitalization for acute exacerbations, and improve patients' reported outcomes. In general, antibiotics are poorly absorbed systemically but concentrations in sputum reach levels that are much higher than minimum inhibitory concentrations (MICs). In particular, aminoglycosides have not been shown to reach oto- or nephrotoxic levels potentially. Side effects are usually limited to airway irritation and cough. In some cases, they can cause transient decrease in spirometry results. Administration of a bronchodilator 15–30 min before administration of the nebulized antibiotic is normally recommended. After the first tobramycin nebulized solution (TNS) trial, the recommendation was to administer antibiotics following a pattern of 28 days on and 28 days off. It was thought that this would decrease the probability of developing resistant flora while assuring clinical efficacy. It is not clear if this is still logical with newer antibiotics. A common practice has been to use 2 aerosol antibiotics in alternating months (i.e., TNS and cholestimate) in more severe patients. Nebulized quinolones, amikacin, and new antibiotic associations are under development.

A logical assumption is that these treatments will lead to a decrease in the global costs of care of CF patients, since they have proven to decrease the number of exacerbations and need for hospitalization. Similarly, their use is associated with a better quality of life.

Although most studies concern the treatment of *P. aeruginosa* infections, there is also an interest in the use of aerosol drug delivery in the treatment of *S. aureus*, *A. fumigatus*, and *B. cepacia*. In these cases, however, controlled trials are still lacking, although results from empirical use in limited cases with vancomycin or amphotericin are encouraging.[134]

Anti-inflammatory Treatment

Since inflammation is intrinsically activated in CF airways, anti-inflammatory strategies are a major area of research. The systemic administration of prednisone has proven its efficacy in CF patients, but it is limited by the severity of its side effects.[135,136] As an alternative, nonsteroidal anti-inflammatory molecules have been studied. Ibuprofen has also been shown to have some efficacy in ameliorating lung disease progression in CF.[137,138] In recent years, the potential anti-inflammatory effect of macrolide antibiotics has gained much interest. Several studies show that drugs like azithromycin or clarithromycin can modulate the innate immune response and inflammation in the airway epithelium, improve lung function in patients, not only in CF but also in chronic obstructive pulmonary disease (COPD) and diffuse panbronchiolitis (DPB) and bronchiolitis obliterans patients. Probably, the most impressive effects of macrolides have been seen in Japan with the prolongation in survival of DPB patients. Despite the fact that macrolides have no anti-*P. aeruginosa* activity, neither bactericidal nor bacteriostatic, it has been hypothesized that they can modulate the production of the toxic products of *P. aeruginosa* and the formation of biofilm. These drugs are therefore, now used extensively in CF and in some centers patients have now been treated continuously for more than a decade. Macrolides are given orally, usually 3 times a week. In the long-term, they have proven to be surprisingly safe, although some patients exhibit gastric intolerance and some bacterial resistance has been reported.[138] However, recent data suggest that prolonged use of azithromycin may be associated with increased infections from NTM.[139]

Managing the Severe Patient and Lung Transplant Programs

Despite aggressive treatment, a large proportion of patients deteriorate. FEV_1 levels decrease, and high resolution CT scores increase. When hypercapnia develops and patients need frequent antibiotic courses, the only alternative left is being listed for lung transplantation. Noninvasive ventilation has been proposed as a bridge to transplantation and some specific experience is available in CF. Studies have shown that gas exchange improves, as well as oxygenation during physiotherapy. It is not known whether noninvasive ventilation prolongs survival.

Lung transplantation is the ultimate choice for the severely deteriorating patient. CF is one of the leading reasons for lung transplantation in children and young adults. A number of publications have shown that lung transplantation is at least as successful in CF as in other diseases and that it can prolong survival. Median survival time after surgery is now more than 6 years, but several centers have reported continuous improvement as experience increases.

It is still problematic to establish the time for listing a patient. FEV_1 of less than 30, a need for elevated oxygen support, hypercapnia, a need for continuous antibiotics, and poor quality of life are considered as indicators. *B. cenocepacia* infection and colonization by pan-resistant *P. aeruginosa* are considered specific contraindications in CF. A small number of CF patients develop portal hypertension and liver failure. Some of them have been lung and liver transplanted or have been lung transplanted after portal shunts had been positioned. These procedures have so far been performed in a limited number of patients but with reasonably good success rates.[140-143]

CONCLUSION

Although much is known on bacterial species typically associated with the progression of lung disease in CF, much less is known on the pathogenesis of the infection and the inflammatory response to bacteria in the airways. Recent research has identified new microbial species, i.e., anaerobes, in the lower airways of patients with CF, but their specific role in the progression of lung disease still needs to be clarified. Due to the development of bacterial resistance and the necessity of prolonged treatment, new antibiotics and new devices to deliver aerosolized drugs into the lungs are needed. The role of chronic anti-inflammatory drugs in modulating host response to infection also requires further research.

REFERENCES

1. McCormick J, Mehta G, Olesen HV, Viviani L, Macek M Jr, Mehta A; European Registry Working Group. Comparative demographics of the European cystic fibrosis population: a cross-sectional database analysis. *Lancet*. 2010;375:1007-13.
2. Available from: www.cffoundation.org/patients registry report
3. Walters S, Mehta A. Epidemiology of cystic fibrosis. In: Hodson M, Geddes DM, Bush A, editors. Cystic fibrosis, 3rd edition. London:Edward Arnold Ltd;2007. p. 21-45.

4. Farrell PM, Rosenstein BJ, White TB, Accurso FJ, Castellani C, Cutting GR, et al.; Cystic Fibrosis Foundation. Guidelines for diagnosis of cystic fibrosis in newborns through older adults: Cystic Fibrosis Foundation consensus report. *J Pediatr.* 2008;153:S4-14.
5. De Boeck K, Wilschanski M, Castellani C, Taylor C, Cuppens H, Dodge J, et al.; Diagnostic Working Group. Cystic fibrosis: terminology and diagnostic algorithms. *Thorax.* 2006;61:627-35.
6. Andersen, DH. Cystic fibrosis of the pancreas and its relation.to celiac disease. *Am J Dis Child.* 19385;6:344-99.
7. Farber S. Some organic digestive disturbances in early life. *J Mich State Med Soc.* 1945;44:587-94. cit in Quinton P.M. Physiological Basis of Cystic Fibrosis: A Historical Perspective. *Physiol Rev.* 1999;79:S3-S22.
8. Wilschanski M, Durie PR. Pathology of pancreatic and intestinal disorders in cystic fibrosis. *J R Soc Med.* 1998;91: 40-9.
9. Lipuma JJ. The changing microbial epidemiology in cystic fibrosis. *Clin Microbiol Rev.* 2010;23:299-323.
10. Kahl BC. Impact of Staphylococcus aureus on the pathogenesis of chronic cystic fibrosis lung disease. *Int J Med Microbiol.* 2010;300:514-9.
11. Goerke C, Wolz C. Adaptation of Staphylococcus aureus to the cystic fibrosis lung. *Int J Med Microbiol.* 2010;300:520-5.
12. Campodónico Victoria L, Gadjeva Mihaela, Paradis-Bleau Catherine, Uluer Ahmet, Pier Gerald B. Airway epithelial control of Pseudomonas aeruginosa infection in cystic fibrosis. *Trends Mol Med.* 2008;14:120-33.
13. Boucher RC. Cystic fibrosis: a disease of vulnerability to airway surface dehydration. *Trends Mol Med.* 2007;13:231-40.
14. Teichgräber V, Ulrich M, Endlich N, Riethmüller J, Wilker B, De Oliveira-Munding C C, et al. Ceramide accumulation mediates inflammation, cell death and infection susceptibility in cystic fibrosis. *Nat Med.* 2008;14:382-91.
15. Livraghi A, Grubb BR, Hudson EJ, Wilkinson KJ, Sheehan JK, Mall MA, et al. Airway and lung pathology due to mucosal surface dehydration in {beta}-epithelial Na+ channel-overexpressing mice: role of TNF-{alpha} and IL-4R{alpha} signaling, influence of neonatal development, and limited efficacy of glucocorticoid treatment. *J Immunol.* 2009;182:4357-67.
16. Bragonzi A. Murine models of acute and chronic lung infection with cystic fibrosis pathogens. *Int J Med Microbiol.* 2010;300:584-93.
17. Guilbault C, De Sanctis JB, Wojewodka G, Saeed Z, Lachance C, Skinner TA, et al. Fenretinide corrects newly found ceramide deficiency in cystic fibrosis. *Am J Respir Cell Mol Biol.* 2008;38:47-56.
18. Li Z, Kosorok MR, Farrell PM, Laxova A, West SE, Green CG, et al. Longitudinal development of mucoid Pseudomonas aeruginosa infection and lung disease progression in children with cystic fibrosis. *JAMA.* 2005;293:581-8.
19. Lei Y, Lars J, Søren M. Microbial ecology and adaptation in cystic fibrosis airways. *Environ Microbiol.* 2011;13:1682-9.
20. Bragonzi A, Paroni M, Nonis A, Cramer N, Montanari S, Rejman J, et al. Pseudomonas aeruginosa microevolution during cystic fibrosis lung infection establishes clones with adapted virulence. *Am J Respir Crit Care Med.* 2009; 180:138-45.
21. Hogardt M, Heesemann J. Adaptation of Pseudomonas aeruginosa during persistence in the cystic fibrosis lung. *Int J Med Microbiol.* 2010;300:557-62.
22. Wainwright CE, Vidmar S, Armstrong DS, Byrnes CA, Carlin JB, Cheney J, et al.; ACFBAL Study Investigators. Effect of bronchoalveolar lavage-directed therapy on Pseudomonas aeruginosa infection and structural lung injury in children with cystic fibrosis: a randomized trial. *JAMA.* 2011;306:163-71.
23. Pressler T, Bohmova C, Conway S, Dumcius S, Hjelte L, Hoiby N, et al. Chronic *Pseudomonas aeruginosa* infection definition: EuroCareCF Working Group report. *J Cyst Fibros.* 2011;10:S75-8.
24. Farrell PM, Govan JRW. Pseudomonas serology: confusion, controversy, and challenges. *Thorax.* 2006;61:645-7.
25. Kerem E, Corey M, Gold R, Levison H. Pulmonary function and clinical course in patients with cystic fibrosis after pulmonary colonisation with Pseudomonas-aeruginosa. *J Pediatr.* 1990;116:714-9.
26. Rosenfeld M, Gibson RL, McNamara S, Emerson J, Burns JL, Castile R, et al. Early pulmonary infection, inflammation, and clinical outcomes in infants with cystic fibrosis. *Pediatr Pulmonol.* 2001;32:356-66.
27. Pittman JE, Calloway EH, Kiser M, Yeatts J, Davis SD, Drumm ML, et al. Age of Pseudomonas aeruginosa acquisition and subsequent severity of cystic fibrosis lung disease. *Pediatr Pulmonol.* 2011;46:497-504.
28. Zielenski J. Genotype and Phenotype in Cystic Fibrosis. *Respiration.* 2000; 67:117-33.
29. Levy H, Murphy A, Zou F, Gerard C, Klanderman B, Schuemann B, et al. IL1β polymorphisms modulate cystic fibrosis lung disease. *Pediatr Pulmonol.* 2009;44:580-93.
30. Corvol Harriet, Boelle Pierre-Yves, Brouard Jacques, Knauer Nicola, Chadelat Katarina, Henrion-Caude Alexandra, et al. Genetic variations in inflammatory mediators influence lung disease progression in cystic fibrosis. *Pediatr Pulmonol.* 2008;43:1224-32.
31. Levy H, Murphy A, Zou F, Gerard C, Klanderman BJ, Schuemann B, et al. Polymorphisms in the IL-1 Gene Family and Lung Disease Severity in Patients with Cystic Fibrosis. *Proc Am Thorac Soc.* 2008;5:373-4.
32. Chiarini M, Sabelli C, Melotti P, Garlanda C, Savoldi G, Mazza C, et al. PTX3 genetic variations affect the risk of Pseudomonas aeruginosa airway colonisation in cystic fibrosis patients. *Genes Immun.* 2010;11:665-70.
33. Moalli F, Paroni M, Véliz Rodriguez T, Riva F, Polentarutti N, Bottazzi B, et al. The therapeutic potential of the humoral pattern recognition molecule ptx3 in chronic lung infection caused by Pseudomonas aeruginosa. *J Immunol.* 2011;186:5425-34.
34. Knowles MR. Gene modifiers of lung disease. *Curr Opin Pulm Med.* 2006;12:416-21.
35. Schluchter MD, Konstan MW, Drumm ML, Yankaskas JR, Knowles MR. Classifying severity of cystic fibrosis lung disease using longitudinal pulmonary function data. *Am J Respir Crit Care Med.* 2006;174:780-6.
36. Elizur A, Cannon CL, Ferkol TW. Airway inflammation in cystic fibrosis. *Chest.* 2008;133:489-95.
37. Nichols DP, Konstan MW, Chmiel JF. Anti-inflammatory therapies for cystic fibrosis-related lung disease. *Clin Rev Allergy Immunol.* 2008;35:135-53.

38. Stanke F, Becker T, Kumar V, Hedtfeld S, Becker C, Cuppens H, et al. Genes that determine immunology and inflammation modify the basic defect of impaired ion conductance in cystic fibrosis epithelia. *J Med Genet.* 2011; 48:24-31.
39. Pillarisetti N, Williamson E, Linnane B, Skoric B, Robertson CF, Robinson P, et al.; Australian Respiratory Early Surveillance Team for Cystic Fibrosis (AREST CF). Infection, inflammation and lung function decline in infants with cystic fibrosis. *Am J Respir Crit Care Med.* 2011;184:75-81.
40. Accurso FJ, Khan TZ, Wagener JS. Does Inflammation Precede Infection in Early Airways Disease? *Pediatr Pulmonol.* 1995;12:71-2.
41. Khan TZ, Wagener JS, Bost T, Martinez J, Accurso FJ. Early pulmonary inflammation in infants with cystic fibrosis. *Am J Respir Crit Care Med.* 1995;151:1075-82.
42. Döring G. Prevention of Pseudomonas aeruginosa infection in cystic fibrosis patients. *Int J Med Microbiol.* 2010; 300:573-7.
43. Ratjen F, Munck A, Kho P, Angyalosi G, Angyalosi G. Treatment of early Pseudomonas aeruginosa infection in patients with cystic fibrosis: the ELITE trial. *Thorax.* 2010; 65:286-91.
44. Lebecque P, Leal T, Zylberberg K, Reychler G, Bossuyt X, Godding V. Towards zero prevalence of chronic Pseudomonas aeruginosa infection in children with cystic fibrosis. *J Cyst Fibros.* 2006;5:237-44.
45. Stuart B, Lin JH, Mogayzel PJ. Early eradication of Pseudomonas aeruginosa in patients with cystic fibrosis. *Paediatr Respir Rev.* 2010;11:177-84.
46. Tramper-Stranders GA, Wolfs TF, van Haren Noman S, van Aalderen WM, Nagelkerke AF, Nuijsink M, et al. Controlled trial of cycled antibiotic prophylaxis to prevent initial Pseudomonas aeruginosa infection in children with cystic fibrosis. *Thorax.* 2010;65:915-20.
47. Griffiths AL, Jamsen K, Carlin JB, Grimwood K, Carzino R, Robinson PJ, et al. Effects of segregation on an epidemic Pseudomonas aeruginosa strain in a cystic fibrosis clinic. *Am J Respir Crit Care Med.* 2005;171:1020-5.
48. Van Acker H, Van Snick E, Nelis HJ, Coenye T. In vitro activity of temocillin against planktonic and sessile Burkholderia cepacia complex bacteria. *J Cyst Fibros.* 2010;9:450-4.
49. Avgeri SG, Matthaiou DK, Dimopoulos G, Grammatikos AP, Falagas ME. Therapeutic options for Burkholderia cepacia infections beyond co-trimoxazole: a systematic review of the clinical evidence. *Int J Antimicrob Agents.* 2009;33:394-404.
50. Sousa SA, Ramos CG, Leitão JH. Burkholderia cepacia complex: emerging multihost pathogens equipped with a wide range of virulence factors and determinants. *Int J Microbiol.* 2011;2011.
51. St Denis M, Ramotar K, Vandemheen K, Tullis E, Ferris W, Chan F, et al. Infection with Burkholderia cepacia complex bacteria and pulmonary exacerbations of cystic fibrosis. *Chest.* 2007;131:1188-96.
52. De Boeck K, Malfroot A, Van Schil L, Lebecque P, Knoop C, Govan JR, et al. Epidemiology of Burkholderia cepacia complex colonisation in cystic fibrosis patients. *Eur Respir J.* 2004;23:851-6.
53. Jones AM, Dodd ME, Govan JR, Barcus V, Doherty CJ, Morris J, et al. Burkholderia cenocepacia and Burkholderia multivorans: influence on survival in cystic fibrosis. *Thorax.* 2004,59:948-51.
54. Vandamme P, Dawyndt P. Classification and identification of the Burkholderia cepacia complex: Past, present and future. *Syst Appl Microbiol.* 2011,34:87-95.
55. Courtney JM, Dunbar KE, McDowell A ,Moore JE ,Warke TJ, Stevenson M, et al. Clinical outcome of Burkholderia cepacia complex infection in cystic fibrosis adults. *J Cyst Fibros.* 2004,3:93-8.
56. Sawicki GS, Rasouliyan L, Pasta DJ, Regelmann WE, Wagener JS, Waltz DA, et al.; Investigators and Coordinators of the Epidemiologic Study of Cystic Fibrosis. The impact of incident methicillin resistant Staphylococcus aureus detection on pulmonary function in cystic fibrosis. *Pediatr Pulmonol.* 2008;43:1117-23.
57. Dasenbrook EC, Merlo CA, Diener-West M, Lechtzin N, Boyle MP. Persistent methicillin-resistant Staphylococcus aureus and rate of FEV1 decline in cystic fibrosis. *Am J Respir Crit Care Med.* 2008;178:814-21.
58. Solis A, Brown D, Hughes J, Van Saene HK, Heaf DP. Methicillin-resistant Staphylococcus aureus in children with cystic fibrosis: An eradication protocol. *Pediatr Pulmonol.* 2003;36:189-95.
59. Miall LS, McGinley NT, Brownlee KG, Conway SP. Methicillin Resistant Staphylococcus Aureus (MRSA) Infection in Cystic Fibrosis. *Arch Disease Child.* 2001;184:160-2.
60. Dasenbrook EC, Checkley W, Merlo CA, Konstan MW, Lechtzin N, Boyle MP. Association between respiratory tract methicillin-resistant Staphylococcus aureus and survival in cystic fibrosis. *JAMA.* 2010;303:2386-92.
61. Stone A, Saiman L. Update on the epidemiology and management of Staphylococcus aureus, including methicillin-resistant Staphylococcus aureus, in patients with cystic fibrosis. *Curr Opin Pulm Med.* 2007;13:515-21.
62. Doe SJ, McSorley A, Isalska B, Kearns AM, Bright-Thomas R, Brennan AL, et al. Patient segregation and aggressive antibiotic eradication therapy can control methicillin-resistant Staphylococcus aureus at large cystic fibrosis centres. *J Cyst Fibros.* 2010;9:104-9.
63. de Vrankrijker AM, van der Ent CK, van Berkhout FT, Stellato RK, Willems RJ, Bonten MJ, et al. Aspergillus fumigatus colonisation in cystic fibrosis: implications for lung function? *Clin Microbiol Infect.* 2011;17:1381-6.
64. Amin R, Dupuis A, Aaron SD, Ratjen F. The effect of chronic infection with Aspergillus fumigatus on lung function and hospitalisation in patients with cystic fibrosis. *Chest.* 2010;137:171-6.
65. McMahon MA, Chotirmall SH, McCullagh B, Branagan P, McElvaney NG, Logan PM. Radiological abnormalities associated with Aspergillus colonisation in a cystic fibrosis population. *Eur J Radiol.* 2012;81:e197-202.
66. Shoseyov D, Brownlee KG, Conway SP, Kerem E. Aspergillus bronchitis in cystic fibrosis. *Chest.* 2006;130:222-6.
67. Latzin P, Hartl D, Regamey N, Frey U, Schoeni MH, Casaulta C. Comparison of serum markers for allergic bronchopulmonary aspergillosis in cystic fibrosis. *Eur Respir J.* 2008;31:36-42.

68. Barton RC, Hobson RP, Denton M, Peckham D, Brownlee K, Conway St, et al. Serologic diagnosis of allergic bronchopulmonary aspergillosis in patients with cystic fibrosis through the detection of immunoglobulin G to Aspergillus fumigatus. *Diagn Microbiol Infect Dis.* 2008;62:287-91.
69. Cohen-Cymberknoh M, Blau H, Shoseyov D, Mei-Zahav M, Efrati O, Armoni S, et al. Intravenous monthly pulse methylprednisolone treatment for ABPA in patients with cystic fibrosis. *J Cyst Fibros.* 2009;8:253-7.
70. Proesmans M, Vermeulen F, Vreys M, De Boeck K. Use of nebulised amphotericin B in the treatment of allergic bronchopulmonary aspergillosis in cystic fibrosis. *Int J Pediatr.* 2010;2010:376287.
71. Zirbes Jacquelyn M, Milla Carlos E. Steroid-sparing effect of omalizumab for allergic bronchopulmonary aspergillosis and cystic fibrosis. *Pediatr Pulmonol.* 2008;43:607-10.
72. Kanu A, Patel K. Treatment of allergic bronchopulmonary aspergillosis (ABPA) in CF with anti-IgE antibody (omalizumab). *Pediatr Pulmonol.* 2008;43:1249-51.
73. Randhawa I, Chin T, Nussbaum E. Resolution of corticosteroid-induced diabetes in allergic bronchopulmonary aspergillosis with omalizumab therapy: a novel approach. *J Asthma.* 2009;46:445-7.
74. Moss RB. Allergic bronchopulmonary aspergillosis and Aspergillus infection in cystic fibrosis. *Curr Opin Pulm Med.* 2010;16:598-603.
75. Goss CH, Mayer-Hamblett N, Aitken ML, Rubenfeld GD, Ramsey BW. Association between Stenotrophomonas maltophilia and lung function in cystic fibrosis. *Thorax.* 2004;59:955-9.
76. Dalbøge CS, Hansen CR, Pressler T, Høiby N, Johansen HK. Chronic pulmonary infection with Stenotrophomonas maltophilia and lung function in patients with cystic fibrosis. *J Cyst Fibros.* 2011;10:318-25.
77. Waters V, Yau Y, Prasad S, Lu A, Atenafu E, Crandall I, et al. Stenotrophomonas maltophilia in Cystic Fibrosis: Serologic response and effect on lung disease. *Am J Respir Crit Care Med.* 2011;183:635-40.
78. Hansen CR, Pressler T, Nielsen KG, JensenPØ, Bjarnsholt T, Høiby N. Inflammation in Achromobacter xylosoxidans infected cystic fibrosis patients. *J Cyst Fibros.* 2010;9:51-8.
79. De Baets F, Schelstraete P, Van Daele S, Haerynck F, Vaneechoutte M. Achromobacter xylosoxidans in cystic fibrosis: prevalence and clinical relevance. *J Cyst Fibros.* 2007;6:75-8.
80. Rønne Hansen C, Pressler T, Høiby N, Gormsen M. Chronic infection with Achromobacter xylosoxidans in cystic fibrosis patients, a retrospective case control study. *J Cyst Fibros.* 2006;5:245-51.
81. Olivier KN, Weber DJ, Lee JH, Handler A, Tudor G, Molina PL, et al. Nontuberculous mycobacteria. II: nested-cohort study of impact on cystic fibrosis lung disease. *Am J Respir Crit Care Med.* 2003;167:835-40.
82. Chalermskulrat W, Sood N, Neuringer IP, Hecker TM, Chang L, Rivera MP, et al. Non-tuberculous mycobacteria in end stage cystic fibrosis: implications for lung transplantation. *Thorax.* 2006;61:507-13.
83. Radhakrishnan DK, Yau Y, Corey M, Richardson S, Chedore P, Jamieson F, et al. Non-tuberculous mycobacteria in children with cystic fibrosis: isolation, prevalence, and predictors. *Pediatr Pulmonol.* 2009;44:1100-6.
84. Pierre-Audigier C, Ferroni A, Sermet-Gaudelus I, Le Bourgeois M, Offredo C, Vu-Thien H, et al. Age-related prevalence and distribution of nontuberculous mycobacterial species among patients with cystic fibrosis. *J Clin Microbiol.* 2005;43:3467-70.
85. Mussaffi H, Rivlin J, Shalit I, Ephros M, Blau H. Nontuberculous mycobacteria in cystic fibrosis associated with allergic bronchopulmonary aspergillosis and steroid therapy. *Eur Respir J.* 2005;25:324-8.
86. Stelzmueller I, Biebl M, Wiesmayr S, Eller M, Hoeller E, Fille M, et al. Ralstonia pickettii-innocent bystander or a potential threat? *Clin Microbiol Infect.* 2006;12:99-101.
87. Jorgensen IM, Johansen HK, Frederiksen B, Pressler T, Hansen A, Vandamme P, et al. Epidemic spread of Pandoraea apista, a new pathogen causing severe lung disease in cystic fibrosis patients. *Pediatr Pulmonol.* 2003; 36:439-46.
88. Bittar F, Leydier A, Bosdure E, Toro A, Reynaud-Gaubert M, Boniface S, et al. Inquilinus limosus and cystic fibrosis. *Emerg Infect Dis.* 2008;14:993-5.
89. Blumer JL, Saiman L, Konstan MW, Melnick D. The efficacy and safety of meropenem and tobramycin vs ceftazidime and tobramycin in the treatment of acute pulmonary exacerbations in patients with cystic fibrosis. *Chest.* 2005;128:2336-46.
90. Worlitzsch D, Rintelen C, Böhm K, Wollschläger B, Merkel N, Borneff-Lipp M, et al. Antibiotic-resistant obligate anaerobes during exacerbations of cystic fibrosis patients.. *Clin Microbiol Infect.* 2009;15:454-60.
91. Tunney MM, Field TR, Moriarty TF, Patrick S, Doering G, Muhlebach MS, et al. Detection of anaerobic bacteria in high numbers in sputum from patients with cystic fibrosis. *Am J Respir Crit Care Med.* 2008;177:995-1001.
92. Goss CH, Burns Jane L. Exacerbations in cystic fibrosis. 1: Epidemiology and pathogenesis. *Thorax.* 2007;62:360-7.
93. Bell Scott C, Robinson Philip J. Exacerbations in cystic fibrosis: 2. prevention. *Thorax.* 2007;62:723-32.
94. Smyth A, Elborn JS. Exacerbations in cystic fibrosis: 3-Management.*Thorax.* 2008;63:180-4.
95. Dales L, Ferris W, Vandemheen K, Aaron SD. Combination antibiotic susceptibility of biofilm-grown Burkholderia cepacia and Pseudomonas aeruginosa isolated from patients with pulmonary exacerbations of cystic fibrosis. *Eur J Clin Microbiol Infect Dis.* 2009;28:1275-9.
96. Keays T, Ferris W, Vandemheen KL, Chan F, Yeung S-W, Mah T-F, et al. A retrospective analysis of biofilm antibiotic susceptibility testing: a better predictor of clinical response in cystic fibrosis exacerbations. *J Cyst Fibros.* 2009;8:122-7.
97. Moskowitz SM, Emerson JC, McNamara S, Shell RD, Orenstein DM, Rosenbluth D, et al. Randomized trial of biofilm testing to select antibiotics for cystic fibrosis airway infection. *Pediatr Pulmonol.* 2011;46:184-92.
98. Ghdifan S, Couderc L, Michelet I, Leguillon C, Masseline B, Marguet C. Bolus methylprednisolone efficacy for uncontrolled exacerbation of cystic fibrosis in children. *Pediatrics.* 2010;125:e1259-64.

99. Dovey M, Aitken ML, Emerson J, McNamara S, Waltz DA, Gibson RL. Oral corticosteroid therapy in cystic fibrosis patients hospitalized for pulmonary exacerbation: a pilot study. *Chest.* 2007;132:1212-8.
100. Hester KLM, Powell T, Downey DG, Elborn JS, Jarad NA. Glucocorticoids as an adjuvant treatment to intravenous antibiotics for cystic fibrosis pulmonary exacerbations: a UK Survey. *J Cyst Fibros.* 2007;6:311-3.
101. Hubert D, Le Roux E, Lavrut T, Wallaert B, Scheid P, Manach D, et al. Continuous versus intermittent infusions of ceftazidime for treating exacerbation of cystic fibrosis. *Antimicrob Agents Chemother.* 2009;53:3650-6.
102. Zemanick ET, Wagner BD, Harris JK, Wagener JS, Accurso FJ, Sagel SD. Pulmonary exacerbations in cystic fibrosis with negative bacterial cultures. *Pediatr Pulmonol.* 2010; 45:569-77.
103. Rosenfeld M, Emerson J, Williams-Warren J, Pepe M, Smith A, Montgomery AB, et al. Defining a pulmonary exacerbation in cystic fibrosis. *J Pediatr.* 2001,139:359-65.
104. Viviani L, Assael B, Kerem E. Impact of the H1N1 pandemic influenza (season 2009-2010) on patients with cystic fibrosis. *J Cyst Fibros.* 2011;10:370-6.
105. Colombo C, Battezzati PM, Lucidi V, Magazzù G, Motta V, Alicandro G, et al. Influenza A/H1N1 in patients with cystic fibrosis in Italy: a multicentre cohort study. *Thorax.* 2011;66:260-1.
106. Nash EF, Whitmill R, Barker B, Rashid R, Whitehouse JL, Honeybourne D. Clinical outcomes of pandemic (H1N1) 2009 influenza (swine flu) in adults with cystic fibrosis. *Thorax.* 2011;66:259.
107. Robinson KA, Odelola OA, Saldanha I, McKoy N. Palivizumab for prophylaxis against respiratory syncytial virus infection in children with cystic fibrosis. *Cochrane Database Syst Rev.* 2010;2:CD007743.
108. Olesen HV, Nielsen LP, Schiotz PO. Viral and atypical bacterial infections in the outpatient pediatric cystic fibrosis clinic. *Pediatr Pulmonol.* 2006;41:1197-204.
109. Brody AS. Early morphologic changes in the lungs of asymptomatic infants and young children with cystic fibrosis. *J Pediatr.* 2004;144:145-6.
110. de Jong PA, Tiddens HA. Cystic fibrosis specific computed tomography scoring. *Proc Am Thorac Soc.* 2007;4:338-42.
111. Tiddens HA, de Jong PA. Update on the application of chest computed tomography scanning to cystic fibrosis. *Curr Opin Pulm Med.* 2006;12:433-9.
112. Tiddens HA, Brody Alan S. Monitoring cystic fibrosis lung disease in clinical trials: is it time for a change? *Proc Am Thorac Soc.* 2007;4:297-8.
113. Ramsey BW. Use of lung imaging studies as outcome measures for development of new therapies in cystic fibrosis. *Proc Am Thorac Soc.* 2007;4:359-63.
114. Robroeks CM, Roozeboom MH, de Jong PA, Tiddens HA, Jöbsis Q, Hendriks HJ, et al. Structural lung changes, lung function, and non-invasive inflammatory markers in cystic fibrosis. *Pediatr Allergy Immunol.* 2010;21:493-500.
115. Farrell PM, Collins J, Broderick LS, Rock MJ, Li Z, Kosorok MR, et al. Association between mucoid Pseudomonas infection and bronchiectasis in children with cystic fibrosis. *Radiology.* 2009;252:534-43.
116. Tiddens HA, Donaldson SH, Rosenfeld M, Paré PD. Cystic fibrosis lung disease starts in the small airways: can we treat it more effectively? *Pediatr Pulmonol.* 2010;45:107-17.
117. Baltimore RS, Christie C, Smith W. Immunohistopathologic localisation of Pseudomonas aeruginosa in lungs from patients with cystic fibrosis. *Am Rev Respir Dis.* 1989;140: 1650-61.
118. Davis SD, Rosenfeld M, Kerby GS, Brumback L, Kloster MH, Acton JD, et al. Multicentre evaluation of infant lung function tests as cystic fibrosis clinical trial endpoints. *Am J Respir Crit Care Med.* 2010;182:1387-97.
119. Linnane BM, Hall GL, Nolan G, Brennan S, Stick SM, Sly PD, et al.; AREST-CF. Lung function in infants with cystic fibrosis diagnosed by newborn screening. *Am J Respir Crit Care Med.* 2008;178:1238-44.
120. Davies JC, Cunningham S, Alton EW, Innes JA. Lung clearance index in CF: a sensitive marker of lung disease severity. *Thorax.* 2008;63:96-7.
121. Lum S, Gustafsson P, Ljungberg H, Hülskamp G, Bush A, Carr SB, et al.; London Cystic Fibrosis Collaboration. Early detection of cystic fibrosis lung disease: multiple-breath washout versus raised volume tests. *Thorax.* 2007;62:341-7.
122. Prasad SA, Main E, Dodd ME; Association of Chartered Physiotherapists. Finding consensus on the physiotherapy management of asymptomatic infants with cystic fibrosis. *Pediatr Pulmonol.* 2008;43:236-44.
123. Main E, Prasad A, Schans C. Conventional chest physiotherapy compared to other airway clearance techniques for cystic fibrosis. *Cochrane Database Syst Rev.* 2005;(1): CD002011.
124. Elkins MR, Robinson M, Rose BR, Harbour C, Moriarty CP, Marks GB, et al.; National Hypertonic Saline in Cystic Fibrosis (NHSCF) Study Group . A controlled trial of long-term inhaled hypertonic saline in patients with cystic fibrosis. *N Engl J Med.* 2006;354:229-40.
125. Subbarao P, Balkovec S, Solomon M, Ratjen F. Pilot study of safety and tolerability of inhaled hypertonic saline in infants with cystic fibrosis. *Pediatr Pulmonol.* 2007;42:471-6.
126. Dellon EP, Donaldson SH, Johnson R, Davis SD. Safety and tolerability of inhaled hypertonic saline in young children with cystic fibrosis. *Pediatr Pulmonol.* 2008;43:1100-6.
127. Quan JM, Tiddens HA., Sy JP, McKenzie SG, Montgomery MD, Robinson PJ, et al. A two-year randomised, placebo-controlled trial of dornase alfa in young patients with cystic fibrosis with mild lung function abnormalities. *J Pediatr.* 2001;139:813-20.
128. Amin R, Subbarao P, Lou W, Jabar A, Balkovec S, Jensen R, et al. The effect of dornase alfa on ventilation inhomogeneity in patients with cystic fibrosis. *Eur Respir J.* 2011; 37:806-12.
129. Konstan MW, Wagener JS, Pasta DJ, Millar SJ, Jacobs JR, Yegin A, et al. Clinical use of dornase alfa is associated with a slower rate of FEV(1) decline in cystic fibrosis. *Pediatr Pulmonol.* 2011;46:545-53.
130. Jones AP, Wallis C. Dornase alfa for cystic fibrosis. *Cochrane Database Syst Rev.* 2010;3:CD001127.
131. Fuchs HJ, Borowitz S, Christiansen DH, Morris EM, Nash ML, Ramsey RW, et al. Effect of aerosolized recombinant human DNase on exacerbations of respiratory symptoms

and on pulmonary function in patients with cystic fibrosis. *N Engl J Med.* 1994;331:637-42.

132. Ratjen F, Bush A. Amiloride: still a viable treatment option in cystic fibrosis? *Am J Respir Crit Care Med.* 2008; 178:1191-2.
133. Bilton D, Robinson P, Cooper P, Gallagher CG, Kolbe J, Fox H, et al. Inhaled dry powder mannitol in cystic fibrosis: an efficacy and safety study. *Eur Respir J.* 2011;38:1071-80.
134. Ryan G, Mukhopadhyay S, Singh M. Nebulised anti-pseudomonal antibiotics for cystic fibrosis. *Cochrane Database Syst Rev.* 2011;(3):CD001021.
135. Auerbach HS, Williams M, Kirkpatrick JA, Colten HR. Alternate-day prednisone reduces morbidity and improves pulmonary function in cystic fibrosis. *Lancet.* 1985;2:686-8.
136. Eigen H, Rosenstein BJ, Fitzsimmons S, Schidlow DV. A multicentre study of alternate-day prednisone therapy in patients with cystic fibrosis. *J Pediatr.* 1995;126:515-23.
137. Konstan MW. Ibuprofen therapy for cystic fibrosis lung disease: revisited. *Curr Opin Pulm Med.* 2008;14:567-73.
138. Crosbie PA, Woodhead MA. Long-term macrolide therapy in chronic inflammatory airway diseases. *Eur Respir J.* 2009;33:171-81.
139. Renna M, Schaffner C, Brown K, Shang S, Tamayo MH, Hegyi K, et al. Azithromycin blocks autophagy and may predispose cystic fibrosis patients to mycobacterial infection. *J Clin Invest.* 2011;121:3554-63.
140. Nash EF, Volling C, Gutierrez, CA, Tullis E, Coonar A, McRae K, et al. Outcomes of patients with cystic fibrosis undergoing lung transplantation with and without cystic fibrosis-associated liver cirrhosis. *Clin Transplant.* 2012; 26:34-41.
141. Weiss ES, Allen JG, Merlo CA, Conte JV, Shah AS. Factors Indicative of Long-term Survival After Lung Transplantation: A Review of 836 10-Year Survivors. *J Heart Lung Transplant.* 2010;29:240-6.
142. Rosenblatt RL. Lung transplantation in cystic fibrosis. *Respir Care.* 2009;54:777-86.
143. Mason DP, Thuita L, Nowicki ER, Murthy SC, Pettersson GB, Blackstone EH. Should lung transplantation be performed for patients on mechanical respiratory support? The US experience. *J Thorac Cardiovasc Surg.* 2010;139: 765-73.

Index

Page numbers followed by *f* refer to figure, *t* refer to table and *b* refer to box.

D

E

J

K

L

M

N

O

P

Q

R

S

T

U

V

W

Y

Z